KAPLAN

MCAT®

Behavioral Sciences Review 2027–2028

Edited by Alexander Stone Macnow, MD

ACKNOWLEDGMENTS

Editor-in-Chief, 2027–2028 Edition
M. Dominic Eggert

Contributing Editors, 2027–2028 Edition
Ae-Ri Kim, PhD; Elizabeth Minten, MD PhD; Gregory J. Riviello, MA; Christopher Vestuto

Prior Edition Editorial Staff: Elisabeth Fassas, MD MSc

Published by Kaplan North America, LLC
1515 West Cypress Creek Road
Fort Lauderdale, Florida 33309

Printed in India.

ISBN: 979-8-3497-0103-0

10 9 8 7 6 5 4 3 2 1

TABLE OF CONTENTS

THE *KAPLAN MCAT REVIEW* TEAM

Alexander Stone Macnow, MD
Editor-in-Chief

Áine Lorié, PhD
Editor

Derek Rusnak, MA
Editor

Mikhail Alexeeff
Kaplan MCAT Faculty

Laura L. Ambler
Kaplan MCAT Faculty

Krista L. Buckley, MD
Kaplan MCAT Faculty

Kristen L. Russell, ME
Editor

Pamela Willingham, MSW
Editor

Melinda Contreras, MS
Kaplan MCAT Faculty

Samantha Fallon
Kaplan MCAT Faculty

Jason R. Selzer
Kaplan MCAT Faculty

M. Dominic Eggert
Editor

Faculty Reviewers and Editors: Elmar R. Aliyev; James Burns; Jonathan Cornfield; Alisha Maureen Crowley; Nikolai Dorofeev, MD; Benjamin Downer, MS; Colin Doyle; Christopher Durland; Marilyn Engle; Eleni M. Eren; Raef Ali Fadel; Elizabeth Flagge; Adam Grey; Rohit Gupta, Jonathan Habermacher; Tyra Hall-Pogar, PhD; Justine Harkness, PhD; Scott Huff; Samer T. Ismail; Ae-Ri Kim, PhD; Elizabeth A. Kudlaty; Kelly Kyker-Snowman, MS; Ningfei Li; John P. Mahon; Brandon McKenzie; Matthew A. Meier; Nainika Nanda; Caroline Nkemdilim Opene; Kaitlyn E. Prenger; Uneeb Qureshi; Jason Selzer; Allison St. Clair; Bela G. Starkman, PhD; Chris Sun; Michael Paul Tomani, MS; Bonnie Wang; Ethan Weber; Lauren K. White; Nicholas M. White; Allison Ann Wilkes, MS; Kerranna Williamson, MBA; and Tony Yu.

Thanks to Kevin Anderson; Rebecca Anderson; Jeff Batzli; Jurre Blom; Hari Priya Chandran; Eric Chiu; James Coleman; Deepika Devan; Tim Eich; Samantha Fallon; Tyler Fara; Owen Farcy; Dan Frey; Robin Garmise; Rita Garthaffner; Joanna Graham; Allison Gudenau; Allison Harm; Beth Hoffberg; Aaron Lemon-Strauss; Keith Lubeley; Diane McGarvey; Leonard Mendoza; Petros Minasi; Elizabeth Minten, MD, PhD; Beena P V; John Polstein; Deeangelee Pooran-Kublall, MD, MPH; Andrea Repole; Rochelle Rothstein, MD; Larry Rudman; Tor Sanden; Srividhya Sankar; Sylvia Tidwell Scheuring; Carly Schnur; Aiswarya Sivanand; Todd Tedesco; Karin Tucker; Lee Weiss; Christina Wheeler; Kristen Workman; Amy Zarkos; and the countless others who made this project possible.

GETTING STARTED CHECKLIST

Getting Started Checklist

- [ ] Register for your free online assets: if you bought this book new as part of a set, scan the QR code on the front of the book set's slipcase and enter the unique code there; if you bought this book separately, instead go to **www.kaptest.com/moreonline**.
- [ ] Create a study calendar that ensures you complete content review and sufficient practice by Test Day!
- [ ] As you finish a chapter and the online practice for that chapter, check it off on the table of contents.
- [ ] Register to take the MCAT at **www.aamc.org/mcat.**
- [ ] Set aside time during your prep to make sure the rest of your application—personal statement, recommendations, and other materials—is ready to go!
- [ ] Take a moment to admire your completed checklist, then get back to the business of prepping for this exam!

PREFACE

And now it starts: your long, yet fruitful journey toward wearing a white coat. Proudly wearing that white coat, though, is hopefully only part of your motivation. You are reading this book because you want to be a healer.

If you're serious about going to medical school, then you are likely already familiar with the importance of the MCAT in medical school admissions. While the holistic review process puts additional weight on your experiences, extracurricular activities, and personal attributes, the fact remains: along with your GPA, your MCAT score remains one of the two most important components of your application portfolio—at least early in the admissions process. Each additional point you score on the MCAT pushes you in front of thousands of other students and makes you an even more attractive applicant. But the MCAT is not simply an obstacle to overcome; it is an opportunity to show schools that you will be a strong student and a future leader in medicine.

We at Kaplan take our jobs very seriously and aim to help students see success not only on the MCAT, but as future physicians. We work with our learning science experts to ensure that we're using the most up-to-date teaching techniques in our resources. Multiple members of our team hold advanced degrees in medicine or associated biomedical sciences, and are committed to the highest level of medical education. Kaplan has been working with the MCAT for over 50 years and our commitment to premed students is unflagging; in fact, Stanley Kaplan created this company when he had difficulty being accepted to medical school due to unfair quota systems that existed at the time.

We stand now at the beginning of a new era in medical education. As citizens of this 21st-century world of healthcare, we are charged with creating a patient-oriented, culturally competent, cost-conscious, universally available, technically advanced, and research-focused healthcare system, run by compassionate providers. Suffice it to say, this is no easy task. Problem-based learning, integrated curricula, and classes in interpersonal skills are some of the responses to this demand for an excellent workforce—a workforce of which you'll soon be a part.

We're thrilled that you've chosen us to help you on this journey. Please reach out to us to share your challenges, concerns, and successes. Together, we will shape the future of medicine in the United States and abroad; we look forward to helping you become the doctor you deserve to be.

Good luck!

Alexander Stone Macnow, MD
Editor-in-Chief
Department of Pathology and Laboratory Medicine
Hospital of the University of Pennsylvania

BA, Musicology—Boston University, 2008
MD—Perelman School of Medicine at the University of Pennsylvania, 2013

ABOUT THE MCAT

Anatomy of the MCAT

Here is a general overview of the structure of Test Day:

Section	Number of Questions	Time Allotted
Test-Day Certification		4 minutes
Tutorial (optional)		10 minutes
Chemical and Physical Foundations of Biological Systems	59	95 minutes
Break (optional)		10 minutes
Critical Analysis and Reasoning Skills (CARS)	53	90 minutes
Lunch Break (optional)		30 minutes
Biological and Biochemical Foundations of Living Systems	59	95 minutes
Break (optional)		10 minutes
Psychological, Social, and Biological Foundations of Behavior	59	95 minutes
Void Question		3 minutes
Satisfaction Survey (optional)		5 minutes

The structure of the four sections of the MCAT is shown below.

Chemical and Physical Foundations of Biological Systems	
Time	95 minutes
Format	• 59 questions • 10 passages • 44 questions are passage-based, and 15 are discrete (stand-alone) questions. • Score between 118 and 132
What It Tests	• Biochemistry: 25% • Biology: 5% • General Chemistry: 30% • Organic Chemistry: 15% • Physics: 25%

Critical Analysis and Reasoning Skills (CARS)	
Time	90 minutes
Format	• 53 questions • 9 passages • All questions are passage-based. There are no discrete (stand-alone) questions. • Score between 118 and 132
What It Tests	Disciplines: • Humanities: 50% • Social Sciences: 50% Skills: • *Foundations of Comprehension*: 30% • *Reasoning Within the Text*: 30% • *Reasoning Beyond the Text*: 40%
Biological and Biochemical Foundations of Living Systems	
Time	95 minutes
Format	• 59 questions • 10 passages • 44 questions are passage-based, and 15 are discrete (stand-alone) questions. • Score between 118 and 132
What It Tests	• Biochemistry: 25% • Biology: 65% • General Chemistry: 5% • Organic Chemistry: 5%
Psychological, Social, and Biological Foundations of Behavior	
Time	95 minutes
Format	• 59 questions • 10 passages • 44 questions are passage-based, and 15 are discrete (stand-alone) questions. • Score between 118 and 132
What It Tests	• Biology: 5% • Psychology: 65% • Sociology: 30%
Total	
Testing Time	375 minutes (6 hours, 15 minutes)
Total Seat Time	447 minutes (7 hours, 27 minutes)
Questions	230
Score	472 to 528

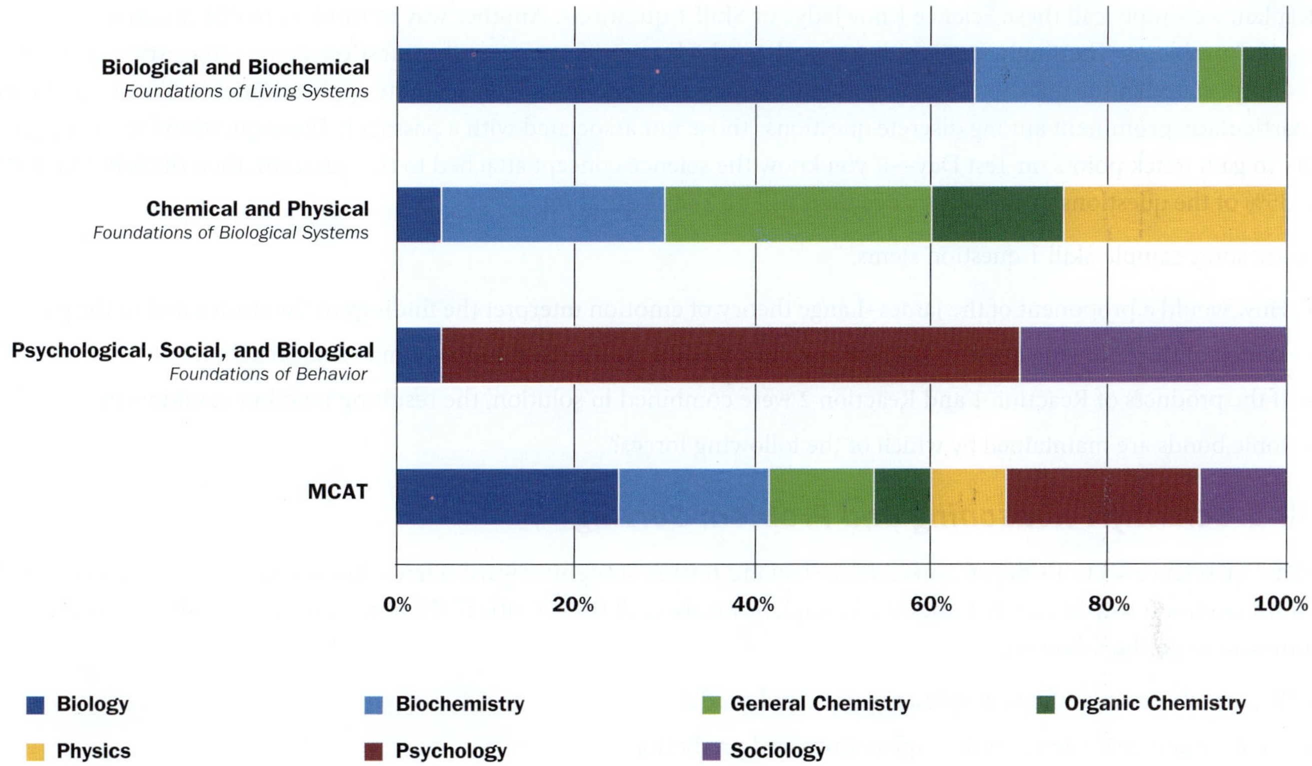

Scientific Inquiry and Reasoning Skills (SIRS)

The AAMC has defined four *Scientific Inquiry and Reasoning Skills* (SIRS) that will be tested in the three science sections of the MCAT:

1. *Knowledge of Scientific Concepts and Principles* (35% of questions)
2. *Scientific Reasoning and Problem-Solving* (45% of questions)
3. *Reasoning About the Design and Execution of Research* (10% of questions)
4. *Data-Based and Statistical Reasoning* (10% of questions)

Let's see how each one breaks down into more specific Test Day behaviors. Note that the bullet points of specific objectives for each of the SIRS are taken directly from the *Official Guide to the MCAT Exam*; the descriptions of what these behaviors mean and sample question stems, however, are written by Kaplan.

Skill 1*: Knowledge of Scientific Concepts and Principles*

This is probably the least surprising of the four SIRS; the testing of science knowledge is, after all, one of the signature qualities of the MCAT. Skill 1 questions will require you to do the following:

- Recognize correct scientific principles
- Identify the relationships among closely related concepts
- Identify the relationships between different representations of concepts (verbal, symbolic, graphic)
- Identify examples of observations that illustrate scientific principles
- Use mathematical equations to solve problems

At Kaplan, we simply call these Science Knowledge or Skill 1 questions. Another way to think of Skill 1 questions is as "one-step" problems. The single step is either to realize which scientific concept the question stem is suggesting or to take the concept stated in the question stem and identify which answer choice is an accurate application of it. Skill 1 questions are particularly prominent among discrete questions (those not associated with a passage). These questions are an opportunity to gain quick points on Test Day—if you know the science concept attached to the question, then that's it! On Test Day, 35% of the questions in each science section will be Skill 1 questions.

Here are some sample Skill 1 question stems:

- How would a proponent of the James–Lange theory of emotion interpret the findings of the study cited in the passage?
- Which of the following most accurately describes the function of FSH in the human menstrual cycle?
- If the products of Reaction 1 and Reaction 2 were combined in solution, the resulting reaction would form:
- Ionic bonds are maintained by which of the following forces?

Skill 2: *Scientific Reasoning and Problem-Solving*

The MCAT science sections do, of course, move beyond testing straightforward science knowledge; Skill 2 questions are the most common way in which it does so. At Kaplan, we also call these Critical Thinking questions. Skill 2 questions will require you to do the following:

- Reason about scientific principles, theories, and models
- Analyze and evaluate scientific explanations and predictions
- Evaluate arguments about causes and consequences
- Bring together theory, observations, and evidence to draw conclusions
- Recognize scientific findings that challenge or invalidate a scientific theory or model
- Determine and use scientific formulas to solve problems

Just as Skill 1 questions can be thought of as "one-step" problems, many Skill 2 questions are "two-step" problems, and more difficult Skill 2 questions may require three or more steps. These questions can require a wide spectrum of reasoning skills, including integration of multiple facts from a passage, combination of multiple science content areas, and prediction of an experiment's results. Skill 2 questions also tend to ask about science content without actually mentioning it by name. For example, a question might describe the results of one experiment and ask you to predict the results of a second experiment without actually telling you what underlying scientific principles are at work—part of the question's difficulty will be figuring out which principles to apply in order to get the correct answer. On Test Day, 45% of the questions in each science section will be Skill 2 questions.

Here are some sample Skill 2 question stems:

- Which of the following experimental conditions would most likely yield results similar to those in Figure 2?
- All of the following conclusions are supported by the information in the passage EXCEPT:
- The most likely cause of the anomalous results found by the experimenter is:
- An impact to a person's chest quickly reduces the volume of one of the lungs to 70% of its initial value while not allowing any air to escape from the mouth. By what percentage is the force of outward air pressure increased on a 2 cm^2 portion of the inner surface of the compressed lung?

Skill 3: *Reasoning About the Design and Execution of Research*

The MCAT is interested in your ability to critically appraise and analyze research, as this is an important day-to-day task of a physician. We call these questions Skill 3 or Experimental and Research Design questions for short. Skill 3 questions will require you to do the following:

- Identify the role of theory, past findings, and observations in scientific questioning
- Identify testable research questions and hypotheses
- Distinguish between samples and populations and distinguish results that support generalizations about populations
- Identify independent and dependent variables
- Reason about the features of research studies that suggest associations between variables or causal relationships between them (such as temporality and random assignment)
- Identify conclusions that are supported by research results
- Determine the implications of results for real-world situations
- Reason about ethical issues in scientific research

Over the years, the AAMC has received input from medical schools to require more practical research skills of MCAT test takers, and Skill 3 questions are the response to these demands. This skill is unique in that the outside knowledge you need to answer Skill 3 questions is not taught in any one undergraduate course; instead, the research design principles needed to answer these questions are learned gradually throughout your science classes and especially through any laboratory work you have completed. It should be noted that Skill 3 comprises 10% of the questions in each science section on Test Day.

Here are some sample Skill 3 question stems:

- What is the dependent variable in the study described in the passage?
- The major flaw in the method used to measure disease susceptibility in Experiment 1 is:
- Which of the following procedures is most important for the experimenters to follow in order for their study to maintain a proper, randomized sample of research subjects?
- A researcher would like to test the hypothesis that individuals who move to an urban area during adulthood are more likely to own a car than are those who have lived in an urban area since birth. Which of the following studies would best test this hypothesis?

Skill 4: *Data-Based and Statistical Reasoning*

Lastly, the science sections of the MCAT test your ability to analyze the visual and numerical results of experiments and studies. We call these Data and Statistical Analysis questions. Skill 4 questions will require you to do the following:

- Use, analyze, and interpret data in figures, graphs, and tables
- Evaluate whether representations make sense for particular scientific observations and data
- Use measures of central tendency (mean, median, and mode) and measures of dispersion (range, interquartile range, and standard deviation) to describe data
- Reason about random and systematic error

- Reason about statistical significance and uncertainty (interpreting statistical significance levels and interpreting a confidence interval)
- Use data to explain relationships between variables or make predictions
- Use data to answer research questions and draw conclusions

Skill 4 is included in the MCAT because physicians and researchers spend much of their time examining the results of their own studies and the studies of others, and it's very important for them to make legitimate conclusions and sound judgments based on that data. The MCAT tests Skill 4 on all three science sections with graphical representations of data (charts and bar graphs), as well as numerical ones (tables, lists, and results summarized in sentence or paragraph form). On Test Day, 10% of the questions in each science section will be Skill 4 questions.

Here are some sample Skill 4 question stems:

- According to the information in the passage, there is an inverse correlation between:
- What conclusion is best supported by the findings displayed in Figure 2?
- A medical test for a rare type of heavy metal poisoning returns a positive result for 98% of affected individuals and 13% of unaffected individuals. Which of the following types of error is most prevalent in this test?
- If a fourth trial of Experiment 1 was run and yielded a result of 54% compliance, which of the following would be true?

SIRS Summary

Discussing the SIRS tested on the MCAT is a daunting prospect given that the very nature of the skills tends to make the conversation rather abstract. Nevertheless, with enough practice, you'll be able to identify each of the four skills quickly, and you'll also be able to apply the proper strategies to solve those problems on Test Day. If you need a quick reference to remind you of the four SIRS, these guidelines may help:

Skill 1 (**Science Knowledge**) questions ask:

- Do you remember this science content?

Skill 2 (**Critical Thinking**) questions ask:

- Do you remember this science content? And if you do, could you please apply it to this novel situation?
- Could you answer this question that cleverly combines multiple content areas at the same time?

Skill 3 (**Experimental and Research Design**) questions ask:

- Let's forget about the science content for a while. Could you give some insight into the experimental or research methods involved in this situation?

Skill 4 (**Data and Statistical Analysis**) questions ask:

- Let's forget about the science content for a while. Could you accurately read some graphs and tables for a moment? Could you make some conclusions or extrapolations based on the information presented?

Critical Analysis and Reasoning Skills (CARS)

The *Critical Analysis and Reasoning Skills* (CARS) section of the MCAT tests three discrete families of textual reasoning skills; each of these families requires a higher level of reasoning than the last. Those three skills are as follows:

1. *Foundations of Comprehension* (30% of questions)
2. *Reasoning Within the Text* (30% of questions)
3. *Reasoning Beyond the Text* (40% of questions)

These three categories of skills are tested through nine humanities- and social sciences-themed passages, with approximately 5 to 7 questions per passage. Let's take a more in-depth look into these three types. Again, the bullet points of specific objectives for each of the CARS are taken directly from the *Official Guide to the MCAT Exam*; the descriptions of what these behaviors mean and sample question stems, however, are written by Kaplan.

Foundations of Comprehension

Questions in this category will ask for basic facts and simple inferences about the passage; the questions themselves will be similar to those seen on reading comprehension sections of other standardized exams like the SAT® and ACT®. *Foundations of Comprehension* questions will require you to do the following:

- Understand the basic components of the text
- Infer meaning from rhetorical devices, word choice, and text structure

This covers a wide range of question skills (Summarize Text, Recognize Opinion, Paraphrase Detail, and Interpret Meaning), but finding the correct answer to all *Foundations of Comprehension* questions will follow from a basic understanding of the passage and the point of view of its author (and occasionally that of other voices in the passage). Because these questions tend to avoid digging too deeply into the passage, Kaplan calls these *surface* questions.

Here are some sample *Foundations of Comprehension* question stems:

- **Summarize Text**—The author's primary thesis in this passage is:
- **Recognize Opinion**—Based on the information in the second paragraph, which of the following is the most accurate summary of the opinion held by Schubert's critics?
- **Paraphrase Detail**—According to the passage, which of the following is FALSE about literary reviews in the 1920s?
- **Interpret Meaning**—The word "obscure" (paragraph 3), when used in reference to the historian's actions, most nearly means:

Reasoning Within the Text

While *Foundations of Comprehension* questions will usually depend on interpreting a single piece of information in the passage or understanding the passage as a whole, *Reasoning Within the Text* questions require more thought because they will ask you to identify the purpose of a particular piece of information in the context of the passage, or ask how one piece of information relates to another. *Reasoning Within the Text* questions will require you to:

- Integrate different components of the text to draw relevant conclusions

In other words, questions in this type often ask either *How do these two details relate to one another?* or *What else must be true that the author didn't say?* The CARS section will also ask you to judge certain parts of the passage or even judge the author. These questions, which fall under the *Reasoning Within the Text* skill, can ask you to identify authorial bias, evaluate the credibility of cited sources, determine the logical soundness of an argument, identify the importance of a particular fact or statement in the context of the passage, or search for relevant evidence in the passage to support a given conclusion. This category, which Kaplan refers to as *deep* questions because of their tendency to venture into the deep reasoning of the passage, encompasses the following skills: Describe Purpose, Evaluate Reasoning, and Make Deduction.

Here are some sample *Reasoning Within the Text* question stems:

- **Describe Purpose**—The author's discussion of the effect of socioeconomic status on social mobility primarily serves which of the following functions?
- **Evaluate Reasoning**—Which of the following facts is used in the passage as the most prominent piece of evidence in favor of the author's conclusions?
- **Make Deduction**—In putting together the argument in the passage, the author most likely assumes:

Reasoning Beyond the Text

The distinguishing factor of *Reasoning Beyond the Text* questions is in the title of the category: the word *Beyond*. Questions of this type, which make up a larger share of the CARS section than questions from either of the other two types, will always introduce a completely new situation that was not present in the passage itself; these questions will ask you to determine how one influences the other. *Reasoning Beyond the Text* questions will require you to:

- Apply or extrapolate ideas from the passage to new contexts
- Assess the impact of introducing new factors, information, or conditions to ideas from the passage

Because they always introduce ideas not discussed in the passage, Kaplan refers to these as *new info* questions. They test the following skills: Anticipate Response, Predict Outcome/Explanation, Imagine Example/Analogy, and Strengthen/Weaken Argument.

Here are some sample *Reasoning Beyond the Text* question stems:

- **Anticipate Response**—If a document were located that demonstrated Berlioz intended to include a chorus of at least 700 in his *Grande Messe des Morts*, how would the author likely respond?
- **Imagine Example/Analogy**—Which of the following is the best example of a "virtuous rebellion," as it is defined in the passage?
- **Predict Outcome/Explanation**—Extending the author's discussion of ancient Greek history, a conflict between a democracy and an oligarchy would most likely result in:
- **Strengthen/Weaken Argument**—Which of the following sentences, if added to the end of the passage, would most WEAKEN the author's conclusions in the last paragraph?

CARS Summary

Through the *Foundations of Comprehension* category of skills, the CARS section tests many of the reading skills you have been building on since grade school, albeit in the context of very challenging doctorate-level passages. But through the two other categories (*Reasoning Within the Text* and *Reasoning Beyond the Text*), the MCAT demands that you understand the deep structure of passages and the arguments within them at an advanced level. And, of course, all of this is tested under very tight timing restrictions: only 102 seconds per question—and that doesn't even include the time spent reading the passages.

Here's a quick reference guide to the three categories and 11 skills tested in CARS:

Foundations of Comprehension skills:

- Interpret Meaning: Use context to determine what a word/phrase from the passage is intended to communicate.
- Recognize Opinion: Identify what the author or someone else feels about a passage idea based on word choice or other context clues.
- Paraphrase Detail: Recognize a specific piece of information that is stated or strongly implied at one location in the passage.
- Summarize Text: Articulate the main idea of the passage or of a part of it.

Reasoning Within the Text skills:

- Describe Purpose: Identify why the author wrote the passage or a part of it.
- Evaluate Reasoning: Characterize logical connections between ideas in the passage.
- Make Deduction: Infer a claim that follows from multiple parts of the passage, such as an assumption in an argument.

Reasoning Beyond the Text skills:

- Anticipate Response: Identify what the author or someone else would feel/say/do about a new situation based on its similarities to passage ideas.
- Predict Outcome/Explanation: Apply causal reasoning or another connection from the passage to a new situation.
- Strengthen/Weaken Argument: Characterize the logical relationship between a new claim and arguments from the passage.
- Imagine Example/Analogy: Identify new examples of categories defined in the passage or analogies of passage concepts.

Scoring

Each of the four sections of the MCAT is scored between 118 and 132, with the median at approximately 125. This means the total score ranges from 472 to 528, with the median at about 500. Why such peculiar numbers? The AAMC stresses that this scale emphasizes the importance of the central portion of the score distribution, where most students score (around 125 per section, or 500 total), rather than putting undue focus on the high end of the scale.

Note that there is no wrong answer penalty on the MCAT, so you should select an answer for every question—even if it is only a guess.

The AAMC has released the 2022–2024 correlation between scaled score and percentile, as shown on the following page. It should be noted that the percentile scale is adjusted and renormalized over time and thus can shift slightly from year to year. Percentile rank updates are released by the AAMC around May 1 of each year.

Total Score	Percentile	Total Score	Percentile
528	100	499	46
527	100	498	42
526	100	497	39
525	100	496	36
524	100	495	34
523	99	494	31
522	99	493	28
521	98	492	25
520	97	491	23
519	96	490	21
518	95	489	18
517	94	488	16
516	92	487	14
515	91	486	12
514	89	485	11
513	87	484	9
512	84	483	8
511	82	482	6
510	79	481	5
509	77	480	4
508	74	479	3
507	71	478	2
506	68	477	2
505	65	476	1
504	62	475	1
503	58	474	<1
502	55	473	<1
501	52	472	<1
500	49		

Source: AAMC. 2025. Summary of MCAT Total and Section Scores. Accessed October 2025.
https://students-residents.aamc.org/mcat-research-and-data/percentile-ranks-mcat-exam

Further information on score reporting is included at the end of the next section (see *After Your Test*).

MCAT Policies and Procedures

We strongly encourage you to download the latest copy of *MCAT® Essentials*, available on the AAMC's website, to ensure that you have the latest information about registration and Test Day policies and procedures; this document is updated annually. A brief summary of some of the most important rules is provided here.

MCAT Registration

The only way to register for the MCAT is online. You can access AAMC's registration system at **www.aamc.org/mcat**.

The AAMC posts the schedule of testing, registration, and score release dates in the fall before the MCAT testing year, which runs from January into September. See the AAMC's website for the exact dates that registration opens each year. There is one standard registration fee, but the fee for changing your test date or test center increases the closer you get to your MCAT.

Fees and the Fee Assistance Program (FAP)

Payment for test registration must be made by American Express, Discover, MasterCard, or VISA. As described earlier, the fee for rescheduling your exam or changing your testing center increases as one approaches Test Day. In addition, it is not uncommon for test centers to fill up well in advance of the registration deadline. For these reasons, we recommend identifying your preferred Test Day as soon as possible and registering. There are ancillary benefits to having a set Test Day, as well: when you know the date you're working toward, you'll study harder and are less likely to keep pushing back the exam. The AAMC offers a Fee Assistance Program (FAP) for students with financial hardship to help reduce the cost of taking the MCAT, as well as for the American Medical College Application Service (AMCAS®) application. Further information on the FAP can be found at **www.aamc.org/students/applying/fap**.

Testing Security

On Test Day, you will be required to present a qualifying form of ID. Generally, a current driver's license or United States passport will be sufficient (consult the AAMC website for the full list of qualifying criteria). When registering, take care to spell your first and last names (middle names, suffixes, and prefixes are not required and will not be verified on Test Day) precisely the same as they appear on this ID; failure to provide this ID at the test center or differences in spelling between your registration and ID will be considered a "no-show," and you will not receive a refund for the exam.

During Test Day registration, other identity data collected may include: a digital palm vein scan, a Test Day photo, a digitization of your valid ID, and signatures. Some testing centers may use a metal detection wand to ensure that no prohibited items are brought into the testing room. Prohibited items include all electronic devices, including watches and timers, calculators, cell phones, and any and all forms of recording equipment; food, drinks (including water), and cigarettes or other smoking paraphernalia; hats and scarves (except for religious purposes); and books, notes, or other study materials. If you require a medical device, such as an insulin pump or pacemaker, you must apply for accommodated testing. During breaks, you are allowed access to food and drink, but not to electronic devices, including cell phones.

Testing centers are under video surveillance and the AAMC does not take potential violations of testing security lightly. The bottom line: *know the rules and don't break them.*

Accommodations

Students with disabilities or medical conditions can apply for accommodated testing. Documentation of the disability or condition is required, and requests may take two months—or more—to be approved. For this reason, it is recommended that you begin the process of applying for accommodated testing as early as possible. More information on applying for accommodated testing can be found at **www.aamc.org/students/applying/mcat/accommodations**.

After Your Test

When your MCAT is all over, no matter how you feel you did, be good to yourself when you leave the test center. Celebrate! Take a nap. Watch a movie. Get some exercise. Plan a trip or outing. Call up all of your neglected friends or message them on social media. Go out for snacks or drinks with people you like. Whatever you do, make sure that it has absolutely nothing to do with thinking too hard—you deserve some rest and relaxation.

Perhaps most importantly, do not discuss specific details about the test with anyone. For one, it is important to let go of the stress of Test Day, and reliving your exam only inhibits you from being able to do so. But more significantly, the Examinee Agreement you sign at the beginning of your exam specifically prohibits you from discussing or disclosing exam content. The AAMC is known to seek out individuals who violate this agreement and retains the right to prosecute these individuals at their discretion. This means that you should not, under any circumstances, discuss the exam in person or over the phone with other individuals—including us at Kaplan—or post information or questions about exam content to Facebook, Student Doctor Network, or other online social media. You are permitted to comment on your "general exam experience," including how you felt about the exam overall or an individual section, but this is a fine line. In summary: *if you're not certain whether you can discuss an aspect of the test or not, just don't do it!* Do not let a silly Facebook post stop you from becoming the doctor you deserve to be.

Scores are typically released approximately one month after Test Day. The release is staggered during the afternoon and evening, ending at 5 p.m. Eastern Standard Time. This means that not all examinees receive their scores at exactly the same time. Your score report will include a scaled score for each section between 118 and 132, as well as your total combined score between 472 and 528. These scores are given as confidence intervals. For each section, the confidence interval is approximately the given score ± 1; for the total score, it is approximately the given score ± 2. You will also be given the corresponding percentile rank for each of these section scores and the total score.

AAMC Contact Information

For further questions, contact the MCAT team at the Association of American Medical Colleges:

MCAT Resource Center
Association of American Medical Colleges
www.aamc.org/mcat
(202) 828-0600
www.aamc.org/contactmcat

HOW THIS BOOK WAS CREATED

The *Kaplan MCAT Review* project began shortly after the release of the *Preview Guide for the MCAT 2015 Exam*, 2nd edition. Through thorough analysis by our staff psychometricians, we were able to analyze the relative yield of the different topics on the MCAT, and we began constructing tables of contents for the books of the *Kaplan MCAT Review* series. A dedicated staff of 30 writers, 7 editors, and 32 proofreaders worked over 5,000 combined hours to produce these books. The format of the books was heavily influenced by weekly meetings with Kaplan's learning science team.

In the years since this book was created, a number of opportunities for expansion and improvement have occurred. This edition is the product of our largest revision since the series' creation more than a decade ago.

To better accommodate students who prefer learning visually, our six science titles have added more than 500 new images and updated more than a hundred existing figures. All of these new images were chosen by an expert team of MCAT faculty members, led by veteran teachers and tutors with advanced science or medical degrees. Our objective with these new images was not to add visual flair but to enhance student learning outcomes. Toward that end, our team of medical illustrators partnered with our MCAT experts to ensure scientific accuracy and relevance for the exam.

On top of this extensive science image expansion, we completely rewrote *Critical Analysis and Reasoning Skills Review* based on what we've learned from more than ten years of helping students improve on the CARS section in our classrooms. In addition to this collective experience, internal data suggests that our new approach is more effective at helping students get higher CARS scores. Our streamlined and simplified CARS strategies accompany an extended focus on the critical thinking skills tested on the exam, best embodied by our new Skillbuilder activities that enable targeted skill practice in a lower pressure setting.

These books were submitted for publication in January 2026. For any updates after this date, please visit www.kaptest.com/retail-book-corrections-and-updates.

If you have any questions about the content presented here, email KaplanMCATfeedback@kaplan.com. For other questions not related to content, email booksupport@kaplan.com.

Each book has been vetted through at least ten rounds of review. To that end, the information presented in these books is true and accurate to the best of our knowledge. Still, your feedback helps us improve our prep materials. Please notify us of any inaccuracies or errors in the books by sending an email to KaplanMCATfeedback@kaplan.com.

USING THIS BOOK

Kaplan MCAT Behavioral Sciences Review, and the other six books in the *Kaplan MCAT Review* series, bring the Kaplan classroom experience to you—right in your home, at your convenience. This book offers the same Kaplan content review, strategies, and practice that make Kaplan the #1 choice for MCAT prep.

This book is designed to help you review the behavioral sciences topics covered on the MCAT. Please understand that content review—no matter how thorough—is not sufficient preparation for the MCAT! The MCAT tests not only your science knowledge but also your critical reading, reasoning, and problem-solving skills. Do not assume that simply memorizing the contents of this book will earn you high scores on Test Day; to maximize your scores, you must also improve your reading and test-taking skills through MCAT-style questions and practice tests.

Learning Objectives

At the beginning of each section, you'll find a short list of objectives describing the skills covered within that section. Learning objectives for these texts were developed in conjunction with Kaplan's learning science team, and have been designed specifically to focus your attention on tasks and concepts that are likely to show up on your MCAT. These learning objectives will function as a means to guide your study, and indicate what information and relationships you should be focused on within each section. Before starting each section, read these learning objectives carefully. They will not only allow you to assess your existing familiarity with the content, but also provide a goal-oriented focus for your studying experience of the section.

MCAT Concept Checks

At the end of each section, you'll find a few open-ended questions that you can use to assess your mastery of the material. These MCAT Concept Checks were introduced after numerous conversations with Kaplan's learning science team. Research has demonstrated repeatedly that introspection and self-analysis improve mastery, retention, and recall of material. Complete these MCAT Concept Checks to ensure that you've got the key points from each section before moving on!

Science Mastery Assessments

At the beginning of each chapter, you'll find 15 concept-focused multiple-choice questions. These are designed to help you assess your understanding of the chapter before you begin reading the chapter. Using the guidance provided with the assessment, you can determine the best way to review each chapter based on your personal strengths and weaknesses. Most of the questions in the Science Mastery Assessments focus on the first of the *Scientific Inquiry and Reasoning Skills* (*Knowledge of Scientific Concepts and Principles*), although there are occasional questions that fall into the second or fourth SIRS (*Scientific Reasoning and Problem-Solving* and *Data-Based and Statistical Reasoning*, respectively). You can complete each chapter's assessment in a testing interface in your online resources, where you'll also find a test-like passage set covering the same content you just studied to ensure you can also apply your knowledge the way the MCAT will expect you to!

Guided Examples with Expert Thinking

Embedded in each chapter of this book is a Guided Example with Expert Thinking. Each of these guided examples will be located in the same section as the content used in that example. Each example will feature an MCAT-level scientific article, that simulates an MCAT experiment passage. Read through the passage as you would on the real MCAT, referring to the Expert Thinking material to the right of the passage to clarify the key information you should be gathering from each paragraph. Read and attempt to answer the associated question once you have worked through the passage. There is a full explanation, including the correct answer, following the given question. These passages and questions are designed to help build your critical thinking, experimental reasoning, and data interpretation skills as preparation for the challenges you will face on the MCAT.

Sidebars

The following is a guide to the five types of sidebars you'll find in *Kaplan MCAT Behavioral Sciences Review:*

- **Bridge:** These sidebars create connections between science topics that appear in multiple chapters throughout the *Kaplan MCAT Review* series.
- **Key Concept:** These sidebars draw attention to the most important takeaways in a given topic, and they sometimes offer synopses or overviews of complex information. If you understand nothing else, make sure you grasp the Key Concepts for any given subject.
- **MCAT Expertise:** These sidebars point out how information may be tested on the MCAT or offer key strategy points and test-taking tips that you should apply on Test Day.
- **Mnemonic:** These sidebars present memory devices to help recall certain facts.
- **Real World:** These sidebars illustrate how a concept in the text relates to the practice of medicine or the world at large. While this is not information you need to know for Test Day, many of the topics in Real World sidebars are excellent examples of how a concept may appear in a passage or discrete (stand-alone) question on the MCAT.

What This Book Covers

The information presented in the *Kaplan MCAT Review* series covers everything listed on the official MCAT content lists. Every topic in these lists is covered in the same level of detail as is common to the undergraduate and postbaccalaureate classes that are considered prerequisites for the MCAT. Note that your premedical classes may include topics not discussed in these books, or they may go into more depth than these books do. Additional exposure to science content is never a bad thing, but all of the content knowledge you are expected to have walking in on Test Day is covered in these books.

Chapter profiles, on the first page of each chapter, represent a holistic look at the content within the chapter, and will include a pie chart as well as text information. The pie chart analysis is based directly on data released by the AAMC, and will give a rough estimate of the importance of the chapter in relation to the book as a whole. Further, the text portion of the Chapter Profiles includes which AAMC content categories are covered within the chapter. These are referenced directly from the AAMC MCAT exam content listing, available on the testmaker's website.

You'll also see High-Yield badges scattered throughout the sections of this book:

In This Chapter

1.1 Amino Acids Found in Proteins High Yield

LEARNING OBJECTIVES

After Chapter 1.1, you will be able to:

These badges represent the top 100 topics most tested by the AAMC. In other words, according to the testmaker and all our experience with their resources, a High-Yield badge means more questions on Test Day.

This book also contains a thorough glossary and index for easy navigation of the text.

In the end, this is your book, so write in the margins, draw diagrams, highlight the key points—do whatever is necessary to help you get that higher score. We look forward to working with you as you achieve your dreams and become the doctor you deserve to be!

Studying with This Book

In addition to providing you with the best practice questions and test strategies, Kaplan's team of learning scientists are dedicated to researching and testing the best methods for getting the most out of your study time. Here are their top four tips for improving retention:

Review multiple topics in one study session. This may seem counterintuitive—we're used to practicing one skill at a time in order to improve each skill. But research shows that weaving topics together leads to increased learning. Beyond that consideration, the MCAT often includes more than one topic in a single question. Studying in an integrated manner is the most effective way to prepare for this test.

Customize the content. Drawing attention to difficult or critical content can ensure you don't overlook it as you read and re-read sections. The best way to do this is to make it more visual—highlight, make tabs, use stickies, whatever works. We recommend highlighting only the most important or difficult sections of text. Selective highlighting of up to about 10 percent of text in a given chapter is great for emphasizing parts of the text, but over-highlighting can have the opposite effect.

Repeat topics over time. Many people try to memorize concepts by repeating them over and over again in succession. Our research shows that retention is improved by spacing out the repeats over time and mixing up the order in which you study content. For example, try reading chapters in a different order the second (or third!) time around. Revisit practice questions that you answered incorrectly in a new sequence. Perhaps information you reviewed more recently will help you better understand those questions and solutions you struggled with in the past.

Take a moment to reflect. When you finish reading a section for the first time, stop and think about what you just read. Jot down a few thoughts in the margins or in your notes about why the content is important or what topics came to mind when you read it. Associating learning with a memory is a fantastic way to retain information! This also works when answering questions. After answering a question, take a moment to think through each step you took to arrive at a solution. What led you to the answer you chose? Understanding the steps you took will help you make good decisions when answering future questions.

Online Resources

In addition to the resources located within this text, you also have online resources awaiting you. If you purchased this book as part of a 7-book set, scan the QR code that appears on your slipcase (the illustrated box that originally contained the books) and enter your unique access code, which appears on a sticker on the front of that slipcase. If you purchased this book separately, book-specific resources are available at **www.kaptest.com/booksonline**. Make sure to log on and take advantage of free practice and additional resources!

Please note that access to the online resources is limited to the original owner of this book.

STUDYING FOR THE MCAT

The first year of medical school is a frenzied experience for most students. To meet the requirements of a rigorous work schedule, students either learn to prioritize their time or else fall hopelessly behind. It's no surprise, then, that the MCAT, the test specifically designed to predict success in medical school, is a high-speed, time-intensive test. The MCAT demands excellent time-management skills, endurance, and grace under pressure both during the test as well as while preparing for it. Having a solid plan of attack and sticking with it are key to giving you the confidence and structure you need to succeed.

Creating a Study Plan

The best time to create a study plan is at the beginning of your MCAT preparation. If you don't already use a calendar, you will want to start. You can purchase a planner, print out a free calendar from the Internet, use a built-in calendar or app on one of your smart devices, or keep track using an interactive online calendar. Pick the option that is most practical for you and that you are most likely to use consistently. If you purchased this book new as part of a set, your online resources come with a study plan to space out your readings, chapter quizzes, full-length practice tests, and other study materials (see the previous page for how to log on).

Once you have a calendar, you'll be able to start planning your study schedule with the following steps:

1. **Fill in your obligations and choose a day off.**

   Write in all your school, extracurricular, and work obligations first: class sessions, work shifts, and meetings that you must attend. Then add in your personal obligations: appointments, lunch dates, family and social time, etc. Making an appointment in your calendar for hanging out with friends or going to the movies may seem strange at first, but planning social activities in advance will help you achieve a balance between personal and professional obligations even as life gets busy. Having a happy balance allows you to be more focused and productive when it comes time to study, so stay well-rounded and don't neglect anything that is important to you.

   In addition to scheduling your personal and professional obligations, you should also plan your time off. Taking some time off is just as important as studying. Kaplan recommends taking at least one full day off per week, ideally from all your study obligations but at minimum from studying for the MCAT.

2. **Add in study blocks around your obligations.**

   Once you have established your calendar's framework, add in study blocks around your obligations, keeping your study schedule as consistent as possible across days and across weeks. Studying at the same time of day as your official test is ideal for promoting recall, but if that's not possible, then fit in study blocks wherever you can.

   To make your studying as efficient as possible, block out short, frequent periods of study time throughout the week. From a learning perspective, studying one hour per day for six days per week is much more valuable than studying for six hours all at once one day per week. Specifically, Kaplan recommends studying for no longer than three hours in one sitting. Within those three-hour blocks, also plan to take ten-minute breaks every hour. Use these breaks to get up from your seat, do some quick stretches, get a snack and drink, and clear your mind. Although ten minutes of break for every

50 minutes of studying may sound like a lot, these breaks will allow you to deal with distractions and rest your brain so that, during the 50-minute study blocks, you can remain fully engaged and completely focused.

3. **Add in your full-length practice tests.**

   Next, you'll want to add in full-length practice tests. You'll want to take one test very early in your prep and then spread your remaining full-length practice tests evenly between now and your test date. Staggering tests in this way allows you to form a baseline for comparison and to determine which areas to focus on right away, while also providing realistic feedback throughout your prep as to how you will perform on Test Day.

When planning your calendar, aim to finish your full-length practice tests and the majority of your studying by one week before Test Day, which will allow you to spend that final week completing a final review of what you already know. In your online resources, you'll find a sample study calendar to use as a starting point. This sample calendar may include more focus than you need in some areas, and less in others, and it may not fit your timeline to Test Day. You will need to customize your study calendar to your needs using the steps above.

The total amount of time you spend studying each week will depend on your schedule, your personal prep needs, and your time to Test Day, but it is recommended that you spend somewhere in the range of 300–350 hours preparing before taking the official MCAT. One way you could break this down is to study for three hours per day, six days per week, for four months, but this is just one approach. You might study six days per week for more than three hours per day. You might study over a longer period of time if you don't have much time to study each week. No matter what your plan is, ensure you complete enough practice to feel completely comfortable with the MCAT and its content. A good sign you're ready for Test Day is when you begin to earn your goal score consistently in practice.

How to Study

The MCAT covers a large amount of material, so studying for Test Day can initially seem daunting. To combat this, we have some tips for how to take control of your studying and make the most of your time.

Goal Setting

To take control of the amount of content and practice required to do well on the MCAT, break the content down into specific goals for each week instead of attempting to approach the test as a whole. A goal of "I want to increase my overall score by 5 points" is too big, abstract, and difficult to measure on the small scale. More reasonable goals are "I will read two chapters each day this week." Goals like this are much less overwhelming and help break studying into manageable pieces.

Active Reading

As you go through this book, much of the information will be familiar to you. After all, you have probably seen most of the content before. However, be very careful: Familiarity with a subject does not necessarily translate to knowledge or mastery of that subject. Do not assume that if you recognize a concept you actually know it and can apply it quickly at an appropriate level. Don't just passively read this book. Instead, read actively. Highlighting can be an excellent tool, but use it sparingly: highlighting every sentence isn't active reading, it's coloring. Frequently stop and ask yourself questions while you read (e.g., *What is the main point? How does this fit into the overall scheme of things? Could I thoroughly explain this to someone else?*). By making connections and focusing on the grander scheme, not only will you ensure you know the essential content, but you also prepare yourself for the level of critical thinking required by the MCAT.

Focus on Areas of Greatest Opportunity

If you are limited by only having a minimal amount of time to prepare before Test Day, focus on your biggest areas of opportunity first. Areas of opportunity are topic areas that are highly tested and that you have not yet mastered. You likely won't have time to take detailed notes for every page of these books; instead, use your results from practice materials to determine which areas are your biggest opportunities and seek those out. After you've taken a full-length test, make sure you are using your performance report to best identify areas of opportunity. Skim over content matter for which you are already demonstrating proficiency, pausing to read more thoroughly when something looks unfamiliar or particularly difficult. Begin with the Science Mastery Assessment at the beginning of each chapter. If you can get all of those questions correct within a reasonable amount of time, you may be able to quickly skim through that chapter, but if the questions prove to be more difficult, then you may need to spend time reading the chapter or certain subsections of the chapter more thoroughly.

Practice, Review, and Tracking

Leave time to review your practice questions and full-length tests. You may be tempted, after practicing, to push ahead and cover new material as quickly as possible, but failing to schedule ample time for review will actually throw away your greatest opportunity to improve your performance. The brain rarely remembers anything it sees or does only once. When you carefully review the questions you've solved (and the explanations for them), the process of retrieving that information reopens and reinforces the connections you've built in your brain. This builds long-term retention and repeatable skill sets—exactly what you need to beat the MCAT!

One useful tool for making the most of your review is the How I'll Fix It (HIFI) sheet. You can create a HIFI sheet, such as the sample below, to track questions throughout your prep that you miss or have to guess on. For each such question, figure out why you missed it and supply at least one action step for how you can avoid similar mistakes in the future. As you move through your MCAT prep, adjust your study plan based on your available study time and the results of your review. Your strengths and weaknesses are likely to change over the course of your prep. Keep addressing the areas that are most important to your score, shifting your focus as those areas change.

Section	Q #	Topic or skill	Why I missed it	How I'll fix it
Chem/Phys	*42*	*Nuclear chem.*	*Confused electron absorption and emission*	*Reread Physics Chapter 9.2*
Chem/Phys	*47*	K_{eq}	*Didn't know right equation*	*Memorize equation for* K_{eq}
CARS	*2*	*Paraphrase Detail*	*Didn't read "not" in answer choice*	*Slow down when finding match*
CARS	*4*	*Make Deduction*	*Forgot to research answer*	*Reread passage and predict first*

Where to Study

One often-overlooked aspect of studying is the environment where the learning actually occurs. Although studying at home is many students' first choice, several problems can arise in this environment, chief of which are distractions. Studying can be a mentally draining process, so as time passes, these distractions become ever more tempting as escape routes. Although you may have considerable willpower, there's no reason to make staying focused harder than it needs to be. Instead of studying at home, head to a library, quiet coffee shop, or another new location whenever possible. This will eliminate many of the usual distractions and also promote efficient studying; instead of studying off and on at home over the course of an entire day, you can stay at the library for three hours of effective studying and enjoy the rest of the day off from the MCAT.

No matter where you study, make your practice as much like Test Day as possible. Just as is required during the official test, don't have snacks or chew gum during your study blocks. Turn off your music, television, and phone. Practice on the computer with your online resources to simulate the computer-based test environment. When completing practice questions, do your work on scratch paper or noteboard sheets rather than writing directly on any printed materials since you won't have that option on Test Day. Because memory is tied to all of your senses, the more test-like you can make your studying environment, the easier it will be on Test Day to recall the information you're putting in so much work to learn.

CHAPTER 1

BIOLOGY AND BEHAVIOR

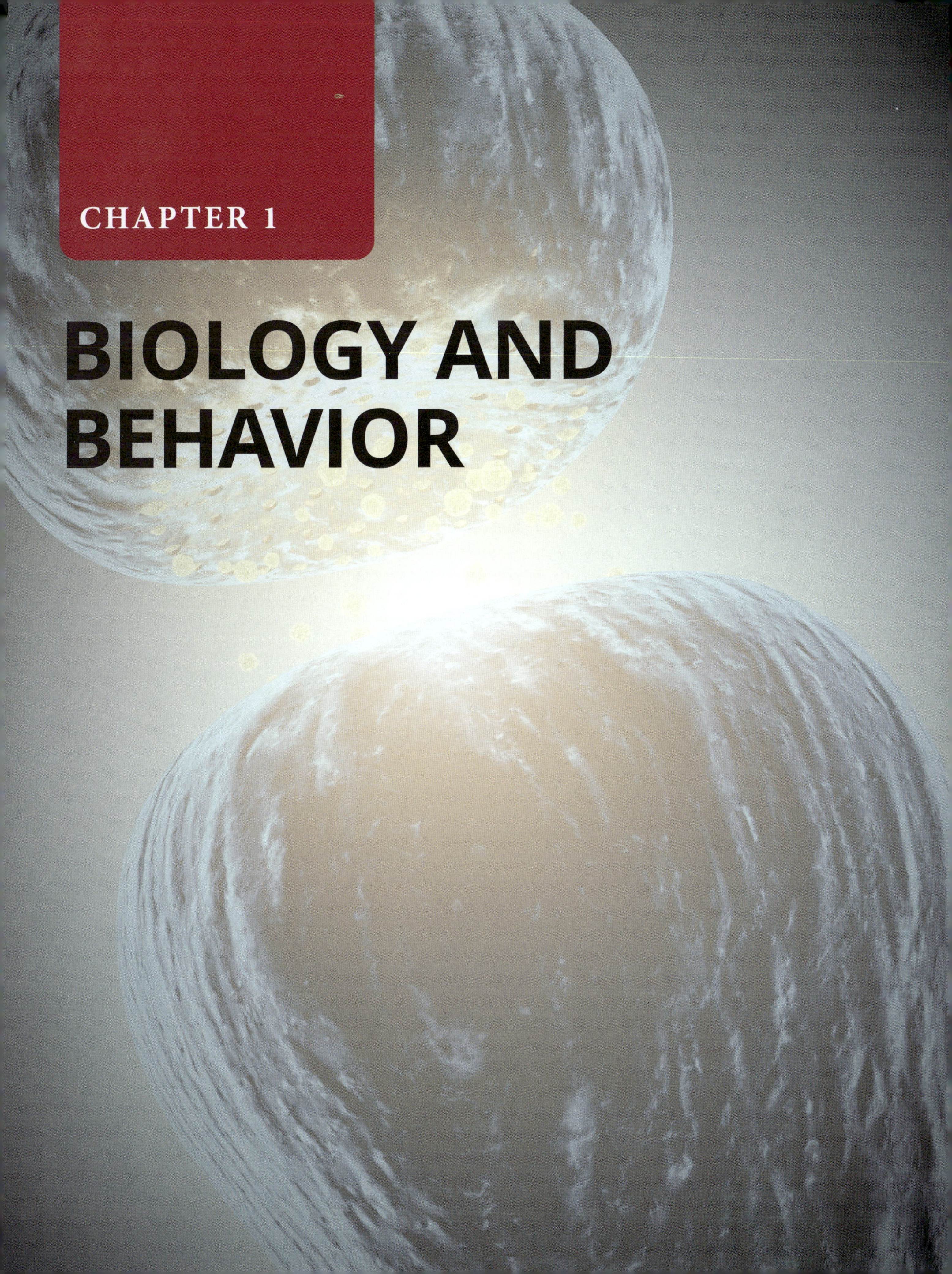

SCIENCE MASTERY ASSESSMENT

Every pre-med knows this feeling: there is so much content I have to know for the MCAT! How do I know what to do first or what's important?

While the high-yield badges throughout this book will help you identify the most important topics, this Science Mastery Assessment is another tool in your MCAT prep arsenal. This quiz (which can also be taken in your online resources) and the guidance below will help ensure that you are spending the appropriate amount of time on this chapter based on your personal strengths and weaknesses. Don't worry though—skipping something now does not mean you'll never study it. Later on in your prep, as you complete full-length tests, you'll uncover specific pieces of content that you need to review and can come back to these chapters as appropriate.

How to Use This Assessment

If you answer 0–7 questions correctly:

Spend about 1 hour to read this chapter in full and take limited notes throughout. Follow up by reviewing **all** quiz questions to ensure that you now understand how to solve each one.

If you answer 8–11 questions correctly:

Spend 20–40 minutes reviewing the quiz questions. Beginning with the questions you missed, read and take notes on the corresponding subchapters. For questions you answered correctly, ensure your thinking matches that of the explanation and you understand why each choice was correct or incorrect.

If you answer 12–15 questions correctly:

Spend less than 20 minutes reviewing all questions from the quiz. If you missed any, then include a quick read-through of the corresponding subchapters, or even just the relevant content within a subchapter, as part of your question review. For questions you answered correctly, ensure your thinking matches that of the explanation and review the Concept Summary at the end of the chapter.

1. A researcher deletes a gene from an organism to determine the gene's function. This approach is most analogous to the work of which of the following scientists?
   - **A.** Paul Broca
   - **B.** Pierre Flourens
   - **C.** Franz Gall
   - **D.** Sir Charles Sherrington

2. Which component of the nervous system is NOT involved in the initial reflexive response to pain?
   - **A.** Spinal cord
   - **B.** Cerebral cortex
   - **C.** Interneuron
   - **D.** Motor neuron

3. A child has experienced nervous system damage and can no longer coordinate the movements to dribble a basketball, although the child can still walk in an uncoordinated fashion. Which region of the central nervous system was most likely affected?
   - **A.** Forebrain
   - **B.** Midbrain
   - **C.** Hindbrain
   - **D.** Spinal cord

4. The temporal lobe deals with all of the following EXCEPT:
   - **A.** language comprehension.
   - **B.** memory.
   - **C.** emotion.
   - **D.** motor skills.

5. Which part of the brain deals with both homeostasis and emotions?
   - **A.** Cerebellum
   - **B.** Pons
   - **C.** Hypothalamus
   - **D.** Thalamus

6. Which of the following activities would most likely be completed by the right hemisphere of a left-handed person?
   - **A.** Finding a car in a parking lot
   - **B.** Learning a new language
   - **C.** Reading a book for pleasure
   - **D.** Jumping rope with friends

7. Which of the following is/are true with regard to neurulation?
   - **I.** The neural tube differentiates from endoderm.
   - **II.** The neural tube becomes the peripheral nervous system.
   - **III.** Neural crest cells migrate from their original site.
   - **A.** I only
   - **B.** III only
   - **C.** II and III only
   - **D.** I, II, and III

8. Which of the following neurotransmitters is NOT classified as a catecholamine?
   - **A.** Epinephrine
   - **B.** Norepinephrine
   - **C.** Dopamine
   - **D.** Acetylcholine

9. If the amount of acetylcholinesterase, an enzyme that breaks down acetylcholine, is increased, which of the following would likely be the result?
   - **A.** Weakness of muscle movements
   - **B.** Excessive pain or discomfort
   - **C.** Mood swings and mood instability
   - **D.** Auditory and visual hallucinations

10. The adrenal glands do all of the following EXCEPT:
    - **A.** promote the fight-or-flight response via estrogen.
    - **B.** produce stress responses via cortisol.
    - **C.** produce both hormones and neurotransmitters.
    - **D.** release estrogen in males and testosterone in females.

11. A disorder of the pineal gland would most likely result in which of the following disorders?
    - **A.** High blood pressure
    - **B.** Diabetes
    - **C.** Insomnia
    - **D.** Hyperthyroidism

12. Which of the following conclusions would William James most likely support?
    - **A.** Mental processes help individuals adapt to their environments.
    - **B.** Psychological attributes could be measured by feeling the skull.
    - **C.** Specific functional impairments can be linked to specific lesions in the brain.
    - **D.** Synaptic transmission is an electrical process.

13. A scientist designs a study to determine if different regions of the brain are activated when a person speaks their native language vs. a second language. Which of the following methods would the scientist most likely choose?
    - **A.** MRI
    - **B.** CT scan
    - **C.** fMRI
    - **D.** EEG

14. During a physical examination, a physician brushes the bottom of the foot of a patient who is fifty years old with multiple sclerosis. The patient's toes are observed to curl toward the bottom of the foot, with no fanning of the toes. This response is:
    - **A.** abnormal, and evidence that the patient is exhibiting a primitive reflex.
    - **B.** normal, and evidence that the patient is exhibiting a primitive reflex.
    - **C.** abnormal, and evidence that the patient is not exhibiting a primitive reflex.
    - **D.** normal, and evidence that the patient is not exhibiting a primitive reflex.

15. Which of the following fine motor tasks would one expect to see first in an infant?
    - **A.** Grasping for objects with two fingers
    - **B.** Following objects with the eyes
    - **C.** Scribbling with a crayon
    - **D.** Moving a toy from one hand to the other

Answer Key

1. **B** (See section 1.1)
2. **B** (See section 1.2)
3. **C** (See section 1.2)
4. **D** (See section 1.4)
5. **C** (See section 1.4)
6. **A** (See section 1.4)
7. **B** (See section 1.6)
8. **D** (See section 1.5)
9. **A** (See section 1.5)
10. **A** (See section 1.5)
11. **C** (See section 1.4)
12. **A** (See section 1.1)
13. **C** (See section 1.2)
14. **D** (See section 1.6)
15. **B** (See section 1.6)

The relevant section of the chapter to review for each question is given in parentheses after the correct answer. Detailed explanations can be found at the end of the chapter.

CHAPTER 1

BIOLOGY AND BEHAVIOR

In This Chapter

CHAPTER PROFILE

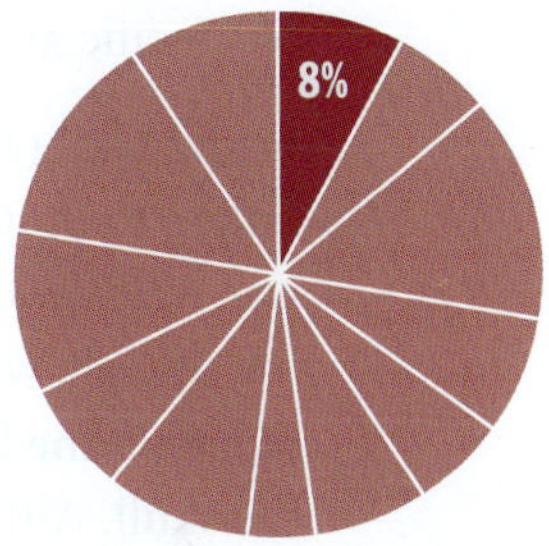

The content in this chapter should be relevant to about 8% of all questions about the behavioral sciences on the MCAT.

This chapter covers material from the following AAMC content categories:

3A: Structure and functions of the nervous and endocrine systems and ways in which these systems coordinate the organ systems

7A: Individual influences on behavior

Introduction

When you woke up this morning and got ready to start reading *MCAT Behavioral Sciences Review*, you almost certainly had specific feelings about it—perhaps you were excited to crack open the book and start learning some of the material that will get you that top score on the MCAT; perhaps you dreaded the size and rich detail of the information in the book. Either way, your body began to respond to these impulses from your mind: increasing heart rate, increasing breathing rate, dilating the eyes, and slowing down digestion. This link between the mind and the body is still a hot topic in medicine, although we've been exploring the effects of psychology on well-being for almost two centuries now.

In this chapter, we'll begin our exploration of psychology and sociology by looking at the biological side of psychology. After a quick survey of the history of neuropsychology, we'll look at the structure and organization of the human nervous system, communication between the nervous and endocrine systems, the effects of genes and environment on behavior, and some aspects of psychological development.

1.1 A Brief History of Neuropsychology

LEARNING OBJECTIVES

After Chapter 1.1, you will be able to:

- Recall the major contributions to early neuropsychology
- Connect the major contributors of early neuropsychology to their contributions

Researchers in the 19th century began to think about behavior from a physiological perspective. Many of these early thinkers formed the foundation of current knowledge about neuroanatomy, linking the functions of specific areas of the brain with thought and behavior.

Franz Gall (1758–1828) had one of the earliest theories that behavior, intellect, and even personality might be linked to brain anatomy. He developed the doctrine of phrenology. The basic idea was that if a particular trait was well-developed, then the part of the brain responsible for that trait would expand. This expansion, according to Gall, would push the area of the skull that covered that part of the brain outward and therefore cause a bulge on the head. Gall believed that one could thus measure psychological attributes by feeling or measuring the skull. Although phrenology was shown to be false, it did generate serious research on brain functions and was the impetus for the work of other psychologists through the remainder of the 19th century.

Pierre Flourens (1794–1867) was the first person to study the functions of the major sections of the brain. He did this by **extirpation**, also known as **ablation**, on rabbits and pigeons. In extirpation, various parts of the brain are surgically removed and the behavioral consequences are observed. Flourens's work led to his assertion that specific parts of the brain had specific functions, and that the removal of one part weakens the whole brain.

William James (1842–1910), known as the founder of American psychology, studied how the mind adapts to the environment. His views formed the foundation for the system of thought in psychology known as **functionalism**, which studies how mental processes help individuals adapt to their environments.

John Dewey (1859–1952) is another important name in functionalism because his 1896 article is seen as its inception. This article criticized the concept of the reflex arc, which breaks the process of reacting to a stimulus into discrete parts. Dewey believed that psychology should focus on the study of the organism as a whole as it functioned to adapt to the environment.

Around 1860, **Paul Broca** (1824–1880) added to the knowledge of physiology by examining the behavioral deficits of people with brain damage. He was the first person to demonstrate that specific functional impairments could be linked with specific brain lesions. Broca studied a person who was unable to speak and discovered that the person's disability was due to a lesion in a specific area on the left side of the person's brain. This area of the brain is now referred to as Broca's area (Figure 1.1).

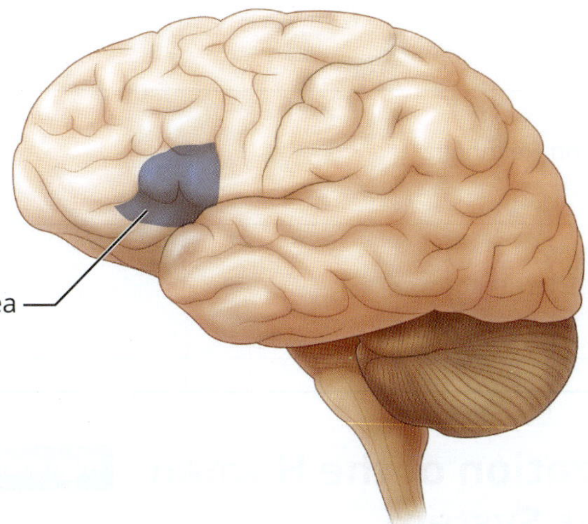

Figure 1.1 Broca's Area

Hermann von Helmholtz (1821–1894) was the first to measure the speed of a nerve impulse. He also related the measured speed of such impulses to reaction time, providing an important early link between behavior and underlying nervous system activity. Because Helmholtz provided one of the earliest measurable links between psychology and physiology, he is often credited with the transition of psychology out of the realm of philosophy and into the realm of quantifiable natural science.

Around the turn of the century, **Sir Charles Sherrington** (1857–1952) first inferred the existence of synapses. Many of his conclusions have held over time—except for one. He thought that synaptic transmission was an electrical process, but we now know that it is primarily a chemical process.

MCAT CONCEPT CHECK 1.1

Before you move on, assess your understanding of the material with this question.

1. Briefly list the main contributions of each of the following scientists to neuropsychology.
   - Franz Gall:

   ____

   - Pierre Flourens:

   ____

   - William James:

   ____

   - John Dewey:

   ____

BRIDGE

Solutions to concept checks for a given chapter in *MCAT Behavioral Sciences Review* can be found near the end of the chapter in which the concept check is located, following the Concept Summary for that chapter.

- Paul Broca:

- Hermann von Helmholtz:

- Sir Charles Sherrington:

1.2 Organization of the Human Nervous System High Yield

MCAT EXPERTISE

The "High-Yield" badge on this section indicates that the content is frequently tested on the MCAT.

LEARNING OBJECTIVES

After Chapter 1.2, you will be able to:

- Correctly associate regions of the nervous system with the CNS or PNS
- Distinguish between afferent and efferent neurons
- Describe the functions of the somatic and autonomic nervous systems, as well as the sympathetic and parasympathetic nervous systems:

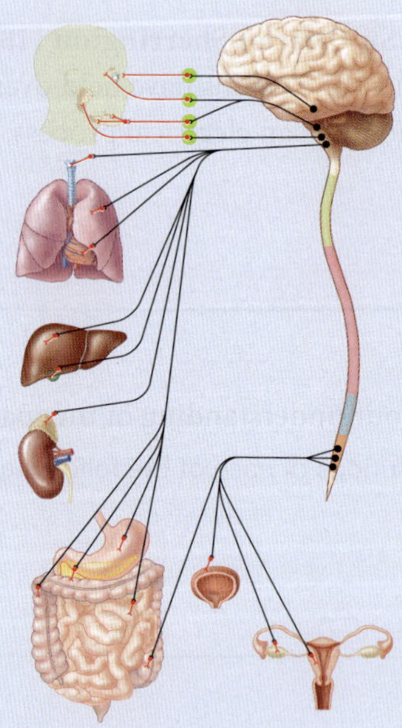

The human nervous system is a complex web of over 100 billion cells that communicate, coordinate, and regulate signals for the rest of the body. Mental and physical action occurs when the body can react to external stimuli using the nervous system. In this section, we will look at the nervous system and its basic organization.

Note: Much of the information contained in this section is also discussed in Chapter 4 of MCAT Biology Review.

Central and Peripheral Nervous Systems

There are three kinds of nerve cells in the nervous system: sensory neurons, motor neurons, and interneurons. **Sensory neurons** (also known as **afferent neurons**) transmit sensory information from receptors to the spinal cord and brain. **Motor neurons** (also known as **efferent neurons**) transmit motor information from the brain and spinal cord to muscles and glands. **Interneurons** are found between other neurons and are the most numerous of the three types of neurons. Interneurons are located predominantly in the brain and spinal cord and are often linked to reflexive behavior. Neural circuits called **reflex arcs** control this type of reflexive behavior. For example, look at Figure 1.2 and consider what occurs when someone steps on a nail. Receptors in the foot detect pain and the pain signal is transmitted by sensory neurons up to the spinal cord. At that point, the sensory neurons connect with interneurons, which then relay pain impulses up to the brain. However, rather than waiting for the brain to send out a signal, interneurons in the spinal cord send signals to the muscles of both legs directly, causing the individual to reflexively withdraw the foot in pain while simultaneously reflexively transferring weight to the other foot. The original sensory information still makes its way up to the brain; however, by that time, the muscles have already responded to the pain, thanks to the cooperation of these several reflex arcs.

MNEMONIC

Afferent neurons **a**scend in the cord toward the brain; **e**fferent neurons **e**xit the cord on their way to the rest of the body.

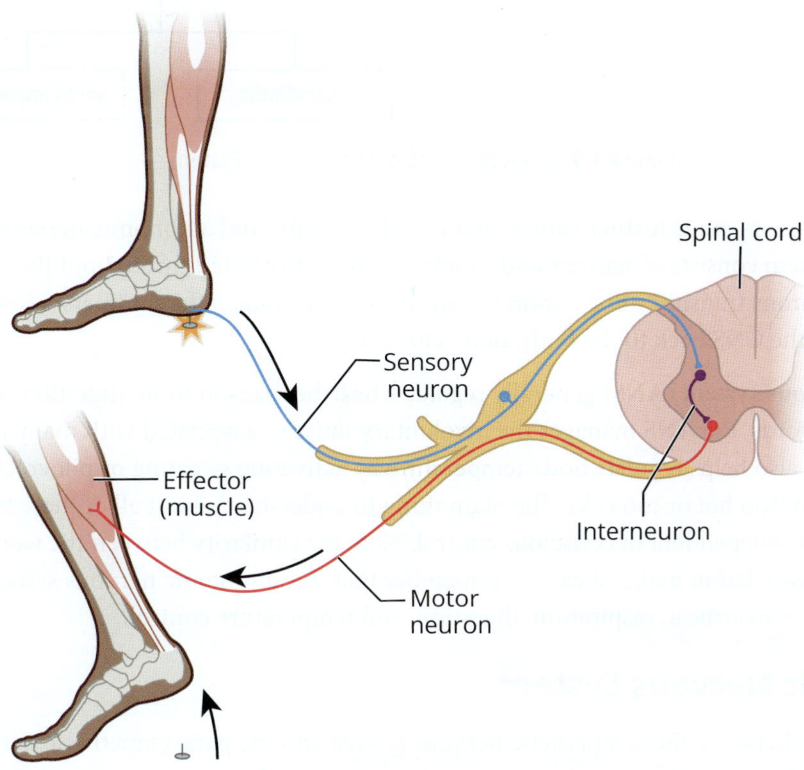

Figure 1.2 Reflex Arc

Let's turn to the overall structure of the human nervous system, which is diagrammed in Figure 1.3. The nervous system can be broadly divided into two primary components: the central and peripheral nervous systems. The **central nervous system** (**CNS**) is composed of the brain and spinal cord. The **peripheral nervous system** (**PNS**), in contrast, is made up of nerve tissue and fibers outside the brain and spinal cord. Note that the peripheral nervous system includes all 31 pairs of nerves emanating from the spinal cord, which are called **spinal nerves**, and 12 pairs of nerves emanating directly from the brain, called **cranial nerves**. The olfactory and optic nerves (cranial nerves I and II) are structurally outgrowths of the central nervous system, but are still considered components of the peripheral nervous system. The PNS thus connects the CNS to the rest of the body.

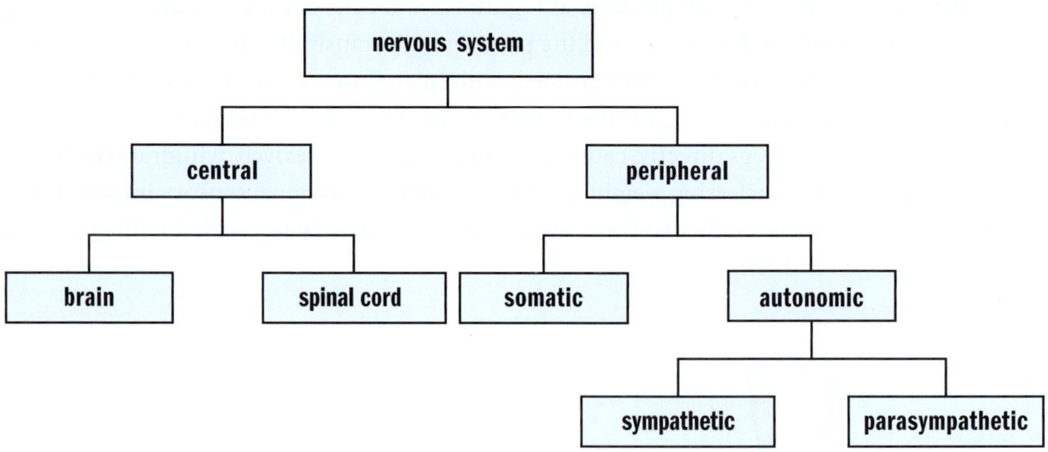

Figure 1.3 Major Divisions of the Nervous System

The peripheral nervous system is further subdivided into the somatic and autonomic nervous systems. The **somatic nervous system** consists of sensory and motor neurons distributed throughout the skin, joints, and muscles. Sensory neurons transmit information toward the CNS through afferent fibers. Motor impulses, in contrast, travel from the CNS back to the body along efferent fibers.

The **autonomic nervous system** (**ANS**) generally regulates heartbeat, respiration, digestion, and glandular secretions. In other words, the ANS manages the involuntary muscles associated with many internal organs and glands. The ANS also helps regulate body temperature by activating sweating or piloerection, depending on whether the body is too hot or too cold. The main thing to understand about all of these functions is that they are automatic, or independent of conscious control. Note the similarity between the words autonomic and automatic. This association makes it easy to remember that the autonomic nervous system manages automatic functions such as heartbeat, respiration, digestion, and temperature control.

The Autonomic Nervous System

The ANS has two subdivisions: the sympathetic nervous system and the parasympathetic nervous system. These two branches often act in opposition to one another, meaning they are antagonistic. For example, the sympathetic nervous system acts to accelerate heart rate and inhibit digestion, while the parasympathetic nervous system decelerates heart rate and increases digestion.

The main role of the **parasympathetic nervous system** is to conserve energy. It is associated with resting and sleeping states, and acts to reduce heart rate and constrict the bronchi. The parasympathetic nervous system is also responsible for managing digestion by increasing peristalsis and exocrine secretions. Acetylcholine is the neurotransmitter responsible for parasympathetic responses in the body. The functions of the parasympathetic nervous system are summarized in Figure 1.4.

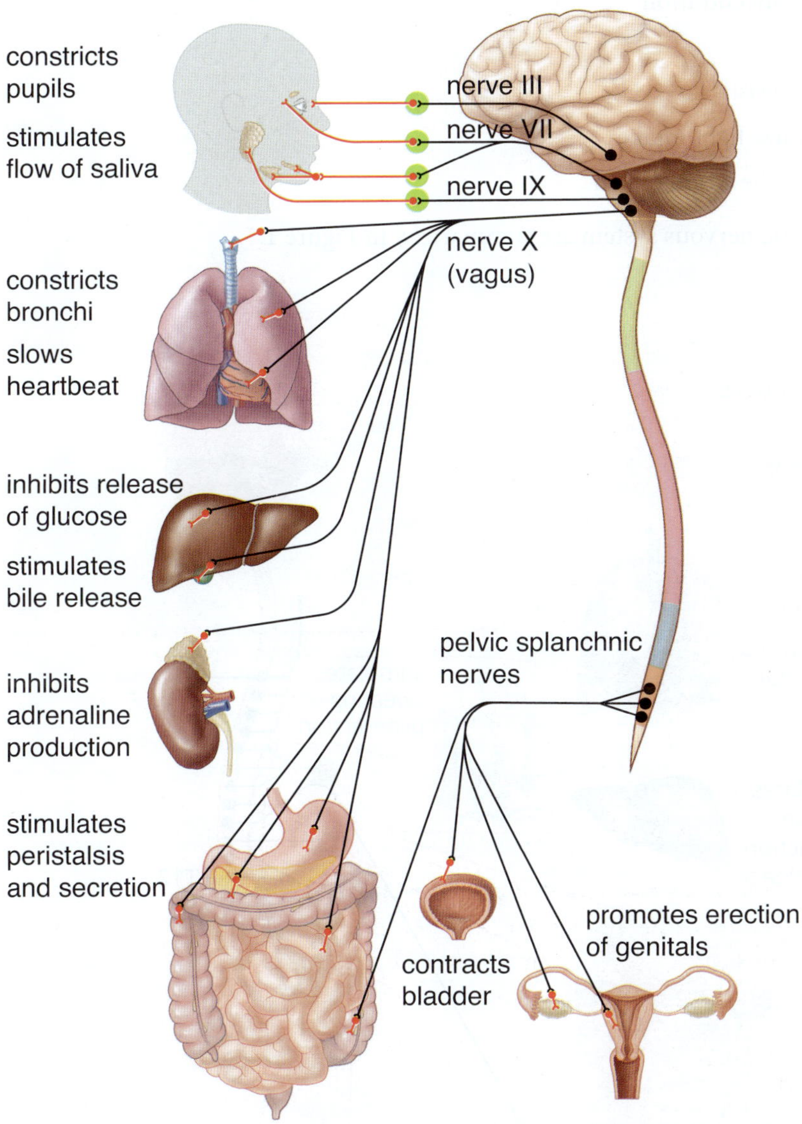

Figure 1.4 Functions of the Parasympathetic Nervous System

In contrast, the **sympathetic nervous system** is activated by stress. This can include everything from a mild stressor, such as keeping up with schoolwork, to emergencies that mean the difference between life and death. The sympathetic nervous system is closely associated with rage and fear reactions, also known as "fight-or-flight" reactions.

MNEMONIC

Sympathetic and parasympathetic nervous systems:

- Sympathetic: "**fight**-or-**flight**"
- Parasympathetic: "**rest**-and-**digest**"

When activated, the sympathetic nervous system:

- Increases heart rate
- Redistributes blood to muscles of locomotion
- Increases blood glucose concentration
- Relaxes the bronchi
- Decreases digestion and peristalsis
- Dilates the eyes to maximize light intake
- Releases epinephrine into the bloodstream

The functions of the sympathetic nervous system are summarized in Figure 1.5.

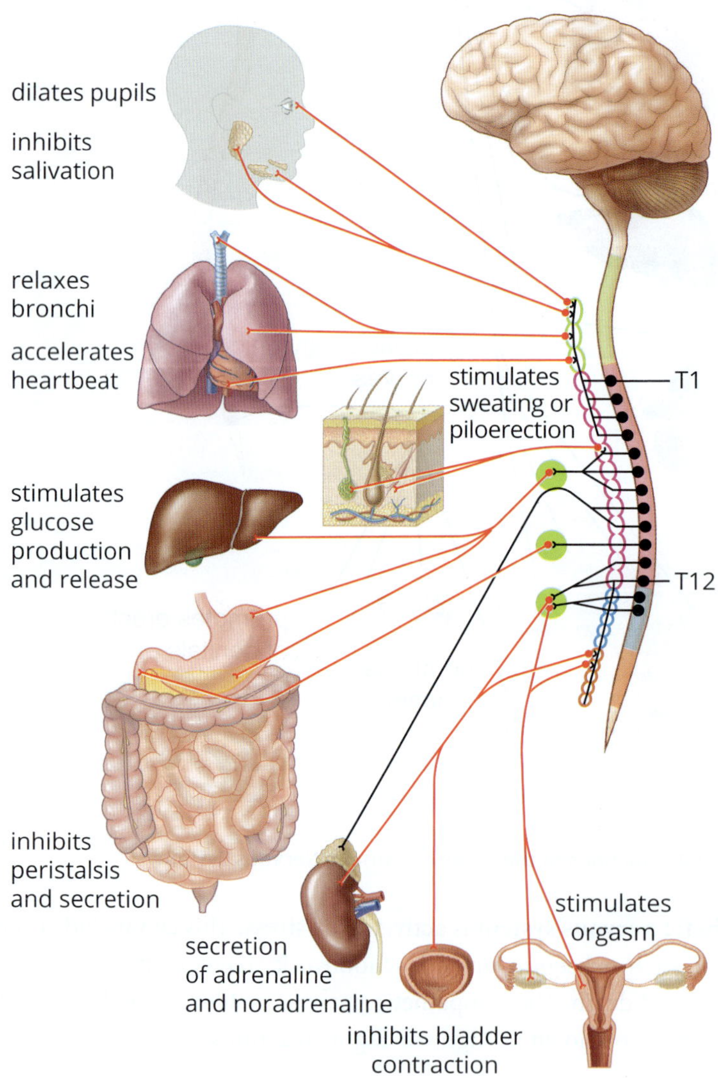

Figure 1.5 Functions of the Sympathetic Nervous System

MCAT CONCEPT CHECK 1.2

Before you move on, assess your understanding of the material with these questions.

1. What parts of the nervous system are in the central nervous system (CNS)? Peripheral nervous system (PNS)?
   - CNS:
   - PNS:
2. What do afferent neurons do? Efferent neurons?
   - Afferent:
   - Efferent:
3. What functions are accomplished by the somatic nervous system? The autonomic nervous system?
   - Somatic:
   - Autonomic:
4. What are the effects of the sympathetic nervous system? The parasympathetic nervous system?
   - Sympathetic:
   - Parasympathetic:

1.3 Organization of the Brain **High Yield**

LEARNING OBJECTIVES

After Chapter 1.3, you will be able to:

- Describe the major functions of the hindbrain, midbrain, and forebrain
- Recognize the most commonly used methods for mapping the brain
- Identify the structures protecting and surrounding the brain

Throughout this section, refer to Figure 1.6, which identifies various anatomical structures inside the human brain. As we discuss different parts of the brain, it's important to remember the functions of these brain structures. Different parts of the brain perform remarkably different functions. For instance, one part of the brain processes sensory information while an entirely different part of the brain maintains activities of the internal organs. For complex functions such as playing a musical instrument, several brain regions work together. For the MCAT, you will need to know some of the basics about how the brain integrates input from different regions.

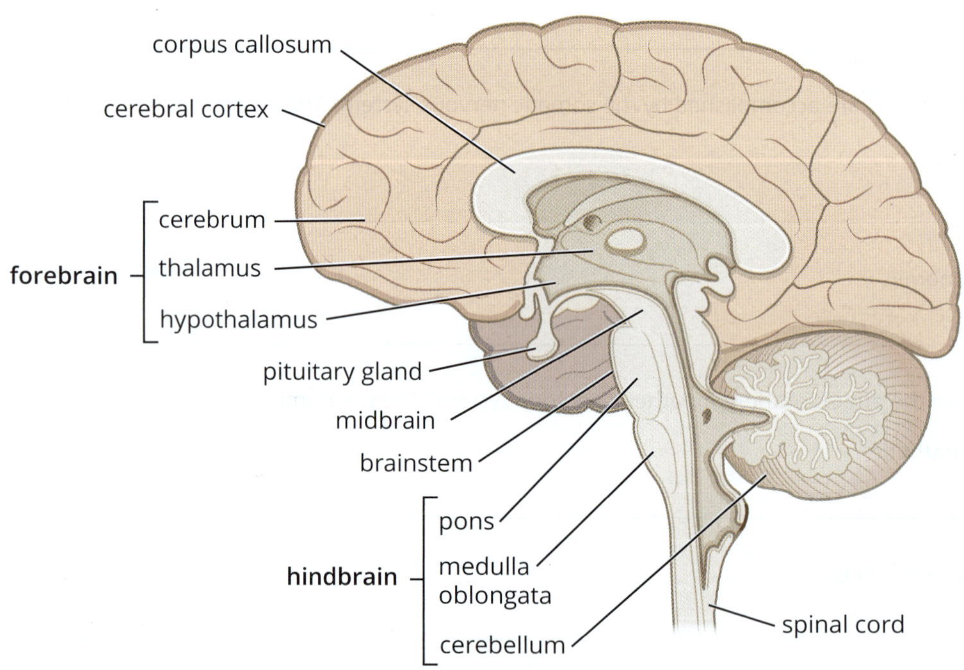

Figure 1.6 Anatomical Structures Inside the Human Brain

The brain is covered with a thick, three-layered sheath of connective tissue collectively called the **meninges**. The outer layer of connective tissue is the **dura mater**, and is connected directly to the skull. The middle layer is a fibrous, weblike structure called **arachnoid mater**. And the inner layer, connected directly to the brain, is known as the **pia mater**. These three layers of connective tissue are shown in Figure 1.7. The meninges help protect the brain by keeping it anchored within the skull, and the meninges also resorb **cerebrospinal fluid**, which is the aqueous solution that nourishes the brain and spinal cord and provides a protective cushion. Cerebrospinal fluid is produced by specialized cells that line the **ventricles** (internal cavities) of the brain.

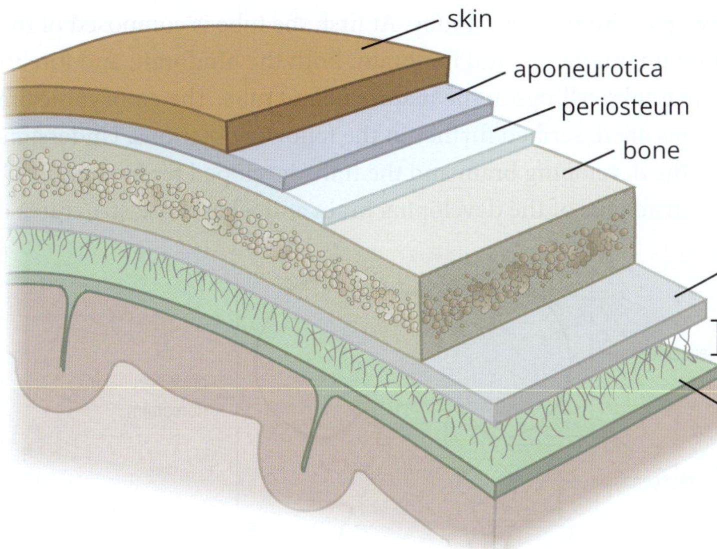

Figure 1.7 Layers of the Meninges

The human brain can be divided into three basic parts: the hindbrain, the midbrain, and the forebrain. Notice that brain structures associated with basic survival are located at the base of the brain and brain structures with more complex functions are located higher up. The meaningful connection between brain location and functional complexity is no accident. In evolutionary terms, the hindbrain and midbrain were brain structures that developed earlier. Together they form the **brainstem**, which is the most primitive region of the brain. The forebrain developed later, including the **limbic system**, a group of neural structures primarily associated with emotion and memory. Aggression, fear, pleasure, and pain are all related to the limbic system. The most recent evolutionary development of the human brain is the **cerebral cortex**, which is the outer covering of the cerebral hemispheres. In humans, the cerebral cortex is associated with everything from language processing to problem solving, and from impulse control to long-term planning. Most of the key brain regions described in the following sections are summarized in Table 1.1.

Major Divisions and Principal Structures	Functions
Forebrain	
Cerebral cortex	Complex perceptual, cognitive, and behavioral processes
Basal ganglia	Movement
Limbic system	Emotion and memory
Thalamus	Sensory relay station
Hypothalamus	Hunger and thirst; emotion
Midbrain	Sensorimotor reflexes
Inferior and superior colliculi	
Hindbrain	
Cerebellum	Refined motor movements
Medulla oblongata	Heart, vital reflexes (vomiting, coughing)
Reticular formation	Arousal and alertness
Pons	Communication within the brain, breathing

Table 1.1 Anatomical Subdivisions of the Brain

In prenatal life, the brain develops from the neural tube. At first, the tube is composed of three swellings, which correspond to the hindbrain, midbrain, and forebrain. Both the hindbrain and forebrain later divide into two swellings, creating five total swellings in the mature neural tube. The embryonic brain is diagrammed in Figure 1.8, and its subdivisions are described further in the following sections. Understanding the relationship between the structures of the developing brain and the fully developed brain is important. So the following sections describe both the structures of the developing brain and what those structures develop into.

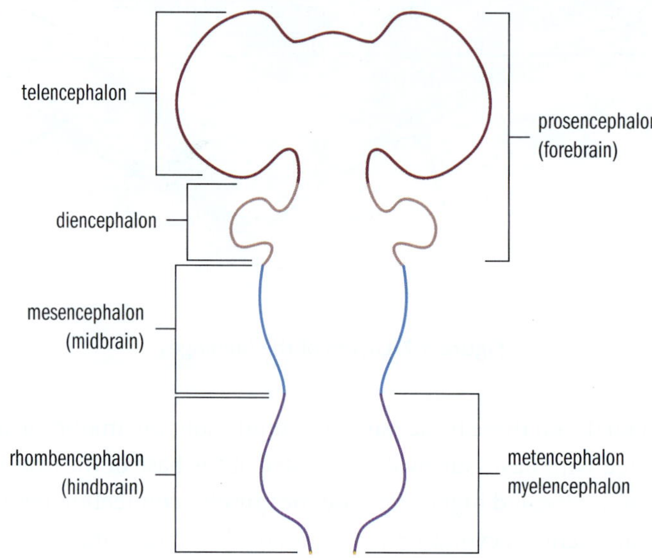

Figure 1.8 Subdivisions of the Embryonic Brain

Hindbrain

Located where the brain meets the spinal cord, the **hindbrain** (**rhombencephalon**) controls balance, motor coordination, breathing, digestion, and general arousal processes such as sleeping and waking. In short, the hindbrain manages vital functioning necessary for survival. During embryonic development, the rhombencephalon divides to form the **myelencephalon** (which becomes the medulla oblongata) and the **metencephalon** (which becomes the pons and cerebellum). In the developed brain, the **medulla oblongata** is a lower brain structure that is responsible for regulating vital functions such as breathing, heart rate, and digestion. The **pons** lies above the medulla and contains sensory and motor pathways between the cortex and the medulla. At the top of the hindbrain, mushrooming out of the back of the pons, is the **cerebellum**, a structure that helps maintain posture and balance and coordinates body movements. Damage to the cerebellum causes clumsiness, slurred speech, and loss of balance. Notably, alcohol impairs the functioning of the cerebellum, and consequently affects speech and balance.

Midbrain

Just above the hindbrain is the **midbrain** (**mesencephalon**), which receives sensory and motor information from the rest of the body. The midbrain is associated with involuntary reflex responses triggered by visual or auditory stimuli. There are several prominent nuclei in the midbrain, two of which are collectively called **colliculi**. The **superior colliculus** receives visual sensory input, and the **inferior colliculus** receives sensory information from the auditory system. The inferior colliculus has a role in reflexive reactions to sudden loud noises.

Forebrain

Above the midbrain is the **forebrain** (**prosencephalon**), which is associated with complex perceptual, cognitive, and behavioral processes. Among its other functions, the forebrain is associated with emotion and memory; it is the forebrain that has the greatest influence on human behavior. Its functions are not absolutely necessary for survival, but are associated instead with the intellectual and emotional capacities most characteristic of humans. During prenatal development, the prosencephalon divides to form the **telencephalon** (which forms the cerebral cortex, basal ganglia, and limbic system) and the **diencephalon** (which forms the thalamus, hypothalamus, posterior pituitary gland, and pineal gland).

Methods of Mapping the Brain

Neuropsychology refers to the study of functions and behaviors associated with specific regions of the brain. It is most often applied in research settings, where researchers attempt to associate very specific areas in the brain to behavior. Neuropsychology is also applied in clinical settings with evaluations of patient cognitive and behavioral functioning, as well as the diagnosis and treatment of brain disorders. Neuropsychology has its own experimental methodology and technology.

Studying human patients with brain lesions is one way that researchers have determined the functions of the brain. In order to conclude that a specific structure of the brain is responsible for a specific function, researchers look for patients that exhibit damage to that structure coupled with a loss of the function. One problem in studying human brain lesions, however, is that such lesions are rarely isolated to specific brain structures. When several brain structures are damaged, the impairment could be attributed to any of the damaged structures, and pinpointing a specific link between brain structure and function becomes difficult.

One method for studying the relationship of brain regions and behaviors is to study brain lesions in lab animals. The advantage of this approach is that precisely defined brain lesions can be created in animals by extirpation. Researchers can also produce lesions by inserting tiny electrodes inside the brain and then selectively applying intense heat, cold, or electricity to specific brain regions. Such electrodes can be placed with great precision by using stereotactic instruments, which provide high-resolution, three-coordinate images of the brain. Ethical or cruelty concerns notwithstanding, such studies have greatly increased our understanding of comparable neural structures in humans.

Another neuropsychology method involves electrically stimulating the brain and recording consequent brain activity. While operating on the brain, a surgeon can stimulate a patient's cortex with a small electrode. This stimulation causes groups of neurons to fire, thereby activating the behavioral or perceptual processes associated with those neurons. For instance, if the electrode stimulates neurons in the motor cortex, the stimulation can lead to specific muscle movements. If the electrode stimulates the visual cortex, the patient may "see" flashes of light that are not really there. By using electrical stimulation, neurosurgeons can thus create **cortical maps**. This method relies on the assistance of the patient, who is awake and alert. Because there are no pain receptors in the brain, only local anesthesia is required. Electrodes have also been used in lab animals to study deeper regions of the brain. Depending on where these electrodes are implanted, they can elicit sleep, sexual arousal, rage, or terror. Once the electrode is turned off, these behaviors cease.

Electrodes can also be used to record electrical activity produced by the brain itself. In some studies, individual neurons are recorded by inserting ultrasensitive microelectrodes into individual brain cells and recording their electrical activity. Electrical activity generated by larger groups of neurons can be studied using an **electroencephalogram** (**EEG**), which involves placing several electrodes on the scalp. Broad patterns of electrical activity can thus be detected and recorded. Because this procedure is noninvasive (it does not cause any damage), electroencephalograms are commonly used with human subjects. In fact, research on sleep, seizures, and brain lesions relies heavily on EEGs, like the one shown in Figure 1.9.

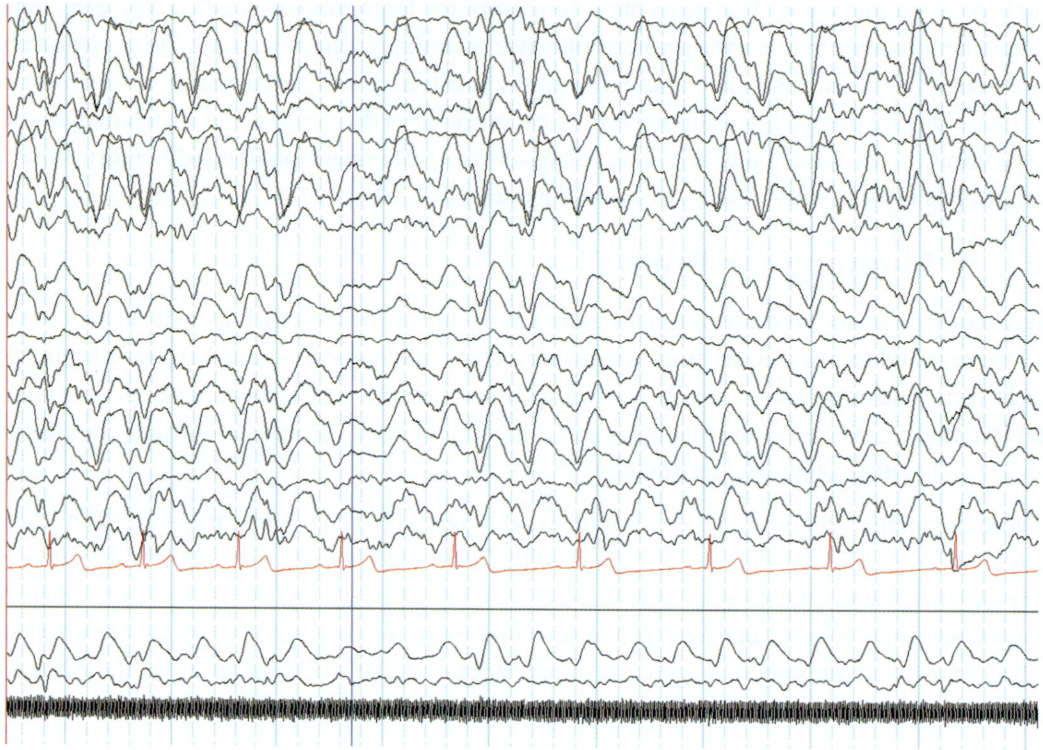

Figure 1.9 Electroencephalogram (EEG) during REM Sleep

Another noninvasive mapping procedure is **regional cerebral blood flow (rCBF)**, which detects broad patterns of neural activity based on increased blood flow to different parts of the brain. rCBF relies on the assumption that blood flow increases to regions of the brain that are engaged in cognitive function. For example, listening to music may increase blood flow to the right auditory cortex because music is processed in that region in most individuals' brains. To measure blood flow, the patient inhales a harmless radioactive gas; a special device that can detect radioactivity in the bloodstream can then correlate radioactivity levels with regional cerebral blood flow. This research method uses noninvasive computerized scanning devices.

Some of the other common scanning devices and methods of visualization used for brain imaging include:

- **CT (computed tomography)**, also known as **CAT (computed axial tomography) scan**, in which multiple X-rays are taken at different angles and processed by a computer to produce cross-sectional images of the tissue.
- **PET (positron emission tomography) scan**, in which a radioactive sugar is injected and absorbed into the body, and its dispersion and uptake throughout the target tissue is imaged.
- **MRI (magnetic resonance imaging)**, in which a magnetic field that interacts with hydrogen atoms is used to map out hydrogen dense regions of the body.

BRIDGE

MRI techniques are dependent on the reaction of hydrogen to a magnetic field, and the scientific principles behind MRI scans are also applied in NMR techniques, which can be found in Chapter 11 of *MCAT Organic Chemistry Review.*

- **fMRI (functional magnetic resonance imaging)**, which uses the same base technique as MRI, but specifically measures changes associated with blood flow. fMRI is especially useful for monitoring neural activity, since increased blood flow to a region of the brain is typically coupled with its neuronal activation.

Visual examples of each imaging type can be seen in Figure 1.10.

fMRI (functional MRI) | MRI (magnetic resonance imaging) | CT (computed tomography) | PET (positron emission tomography)

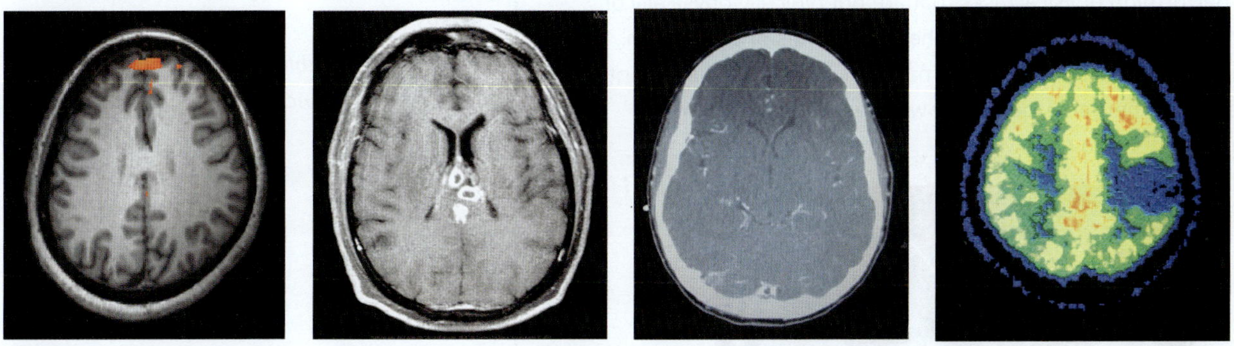

Matthews K. / CC BY 2.5 | Krishna Rao / Uniformed Services University | CCO | Public domain

- fMRI: Reveals brain function in real-time by tracking changes in blood flow
- MRI: Generates high-resolution images of soft tissue using magnetic fields
- CT: Combines a series of X-ray slices to create a detailed image of the tissue
- PET: Measures brain activity by monitoring the uptake of radiolabeled glucose

Figure 1.10 Brain Imaging Methods

MCAT CONCEPT CHECK 1.3

Before you move on, assess your understanding of the material with these questions.

1. What are the main functions of the hindbrain? Midbrain? Forebrain?

Subdivision	Functions
Hindbrain	
Midbrain	
Forebrain	

2. What are some of the methods used for mapping the brain?

____

3. What structures surround and protect the brain?

____

BEHAVIORAL SCIENCES GUIDED EXAMPLE WITH EXPERT THINKING

Multiple sclerosis is a demyelinating disease that results in a host of neurological and physiological symptoms including muscle weakness, numbness, spasms, visual problems, pain, unstable mood, and fatigue. This last symptom is interesting because it is effort-independent; patients express a subjective feeling of fatigue as a result of performing physical tasks that are not typically physically or mentally taxing. To investigate a mechanism for this phenomenon, researchers used the following fMRI mask to highlight regions of interest in measuring neural resource use with respect to subjective fatigue in patients who have MS:

MS symptoms. The author finds fatigue interesting because it is subjective. Used fMRI to investigate.

Independent Variable (IV): MS (probably versus control)

Dependent Variable (DV): fMRI activity detection differences

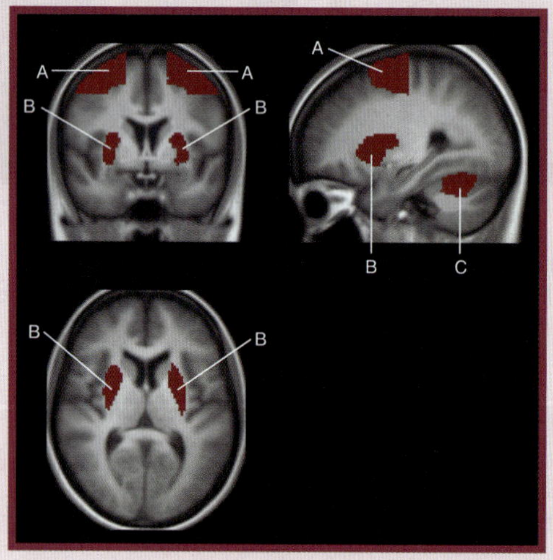

Figure 1 fMRI mask

Mask shows regions of interest for the study

Region B is a structure called the putamen, a part of the basal ganglia. It is connected to and provides pathways of communication for many structures in the brain, and generally influences and regulates motor behaviors such as planning, learning, preparation, and execution of motor sequences.

Region B = putamen: communication and motor behaviors

Researchers found no difference in activity in region B between patients with relapsing-remitting MS and controls. However, it was found that region C showed increased activation over the course of a non-fatiguing tonic grip task in patients who have MS. This increased activation correlated positively with subjective fatigue, and was not present in healthy control subjects. Furthermore, control subjects showed increased activation in region A over the course of the task, and no such activation occurred in patients who have MS.

Results: region B not implicated in MS-related fatigue, but C shows more activity and A shows less.

Adapted from: Svolgaard O, Andersen KW, Bauer C, Madsen KH, Blinkenberg M, Selleberg F, et al. (2018) Cerebellar and premotor activity during a non-fatiguing grip task reflects motor fatigue in relapsing-remitting multiple sclerosis. *PLoS ONE* 13(10): e0201162. https://doi.org/10.1371/journal.pone.0201162

Based on the functions of the regions studied, what do these results suggest about the nature of subjective fatigue in patients who have MS compared to healthy participants?

Our first step in answering this question is to identify the regions presented in the study that are referenced in the question stem. For this particular question, we don't have to worry too much about the structure of the experiment, as most of the information we need is in the results and the description of the regions. The authors give us the name and function of region B: the putamen, described in paragraph 2. This information is helpful because the actual brain isn't color coded and labeled, and due to the low structural resolution of the image, it's tough to tell exactly what region B is from the shape of the mask. On Test Day, using the image alone, we might be able to infer that region B is part of the midbrain and therefore, like other structures of the midbrain, it is probably involved in some kind of relay system. But the additional information in the passage text gives us insight that the picture alone just cannot provide. The passage also says that activity in region B is the same in patients who have MS and controls, allowing us to infer that difficulties in relaying motor signals are probably not the cause of subjective fatigue.

Based on our outside content knowledge, region C is the cerebellum, which we know is responsible for coordinating movement and for maintaining posture and balance. A differential increase in activity here implies that patients with MS may need more resources to perform motor tasks the longer these tasks are maintained.

Region A is in the forebrain. If we've studied the regions of the cerebrum, we might recognize this region as the premotor cortex, which is responsible for higher-level motor control and motivation. However, even without the specifics, we can guess that this region of the forebrain has something to do with executive motor control because of its general location. From the noted activity pattern in the final paragraph, we can guess that increased activity in region A helps to prevent subjective fatigue; thus, for patients who have MS, a lack of activation in this region may contribute to their experience of increased subjective fatigue.

We now have enough information to form a general picture of events here. In patients who have MS, the cerebellum is more active, presumably consuming more resources during maintained motor movements than the cerebellum of their healthy counterparts. This increase in resource consumption could be the patient's brain attempting to accommodate for functions from other regions that have been lost as a result of disease, or could indicate a greater overall demand on cognitive processes involving movement. This overtaxing of cerebellar resources is most likely related to the increase in subjective fatigue experienced by patients who have MS.

1.4 Parts of the Forebrain

LEARNING OBJECTIVES

After Chapter 1.4, you will be able to:

- Link the regions of the forebrain to their functions
- Describe the laterality of brain–body communication and the role of hemispheric dominance
- Describe the functions of the four lobes of the cerebral cortex:

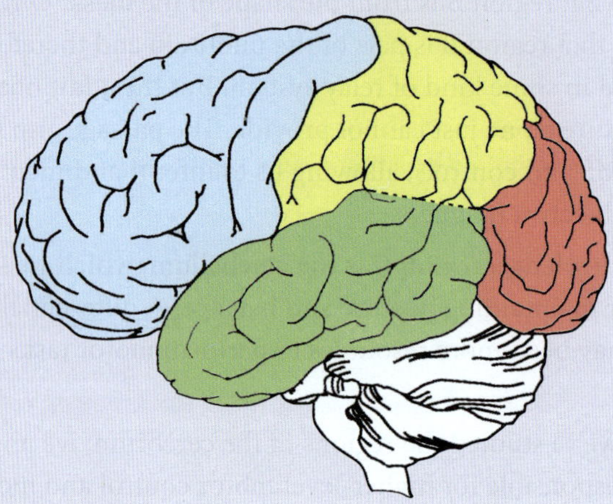

The forebrain is the most "modern" portion of the brain, and—in humans—forms the largest portion of the brain by weight and volume. The forebrain contains regions derived from the diencephalon, such as the thalamus, hypothalamus, posterior pituitary, and pineal gland; it also includes derivatives of the telencephalon, such as the cerebral cortex, basal ganglia, and limbic system.

Thalamus

The **thalamus** is a structure within the forebrain that serves as an important relay station for incoming sensory information, including all senses except for smell. After receiving incoming sensory impulses, the thalamus sorts and transmits them to the appropriate areas of the cerebral cortex. The thalamus can be viewed as the "mail deliverer" for the brain's sensory information, as depicted in Figure 1.11.

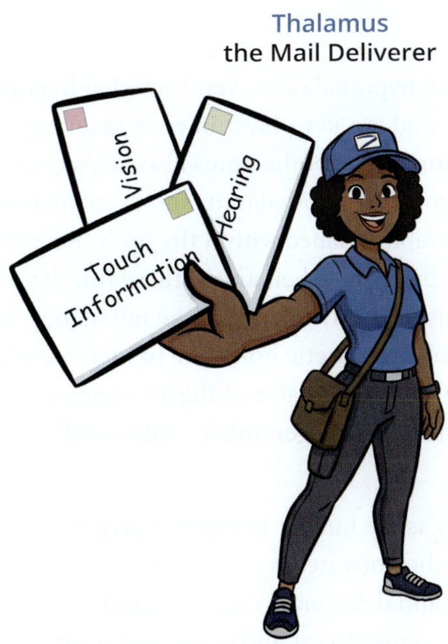

Figure 1.11 The Thalamus as Mail Deliverer

MNEMONIC

The Four **F**s of the Hypothalamus (see Figure 1.12):

- **F**eeding
- **F**ighting
- **F**lighting
- (Sexual) **F**unctioning

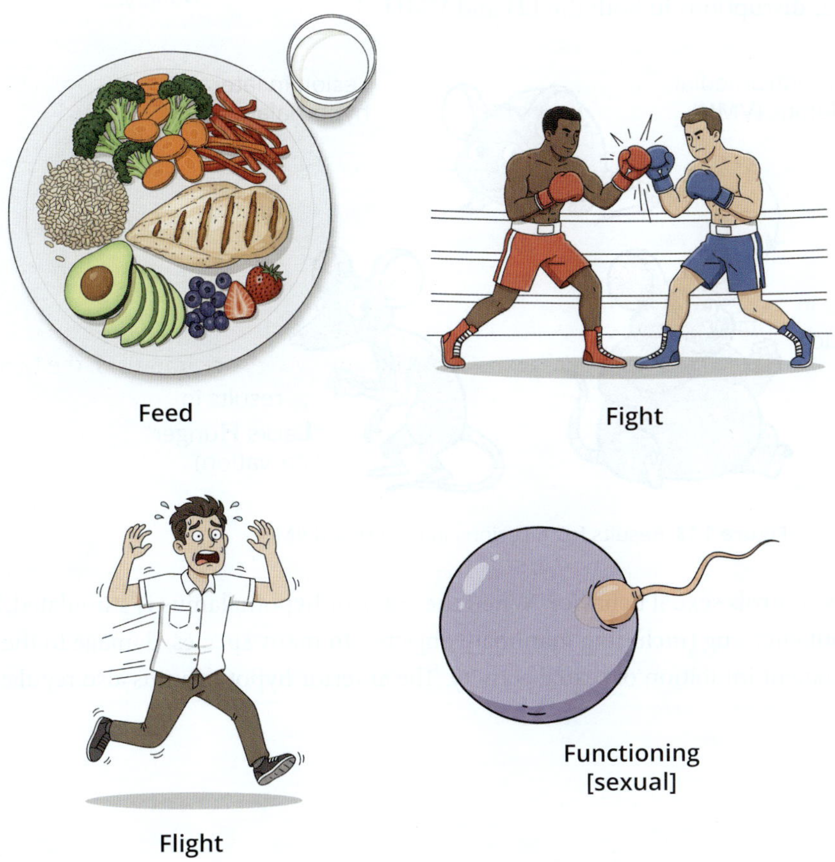

Figure 1.12 The Four Fs of the Hypothalamus

Hypothalamus

The **hypothalamus**, subdivided into the lateral hypothalamus, ventromedial hypothalamus, and anterior hypothalamus, serves homeostatic functions, and is a key player in emotional experiences during high arousal states, aggressive behavior, and sexual behavior. The hypothalamus also helps control some endocrine functions, as well as the autonomic nervous system. The hypothalamus serves many homeostatic functions, which are self-regulatory processes that maintain a stable balance within the body. Receptors in the hypothalamus regulate metabolism, temperature, and water balance. When any of these functions are out of balance, the hypothalamus detects the problem and signals the body to correct the imbalance; for example, osmoreceptors in the hypothalamus may trigger the release of antidiuretic hormone to increase water reabsorption as part of fluid balance. The hypothalamus is also the primary regulator of the autonomic nervous system and is important in drive behaviors: hunger, thirst, and sexual behavior.

The **lateral hypothalamus** (**LH**) is referred to as the hunger center because it has special receptors thought to detect when the body needs more food or fluids. In other words, the LH triggers eating and drinking. When this part of the hypothalamus is removed in lab rats, they refuse to eat and drink and must be force-fed with tubes to survive.

The **ventromedial hypothalamus** (**VMH**) is identified as the "satiety center," and provides signals to stop eating. Brain lesions to this area usually lead to obesity. Figure 1.13 visualizes disruptions in both the LH and VMH.

MNEMONIC

When the **L**ateral **H**ypothalamus (**LH**) is removed, one **L**acks **H**unger.

MNEMONIC

When the **V**entro**M**edial **H**ypothalamus (**VMH**) is destroyed, one is **V**ery **M**uch **H**ungry.

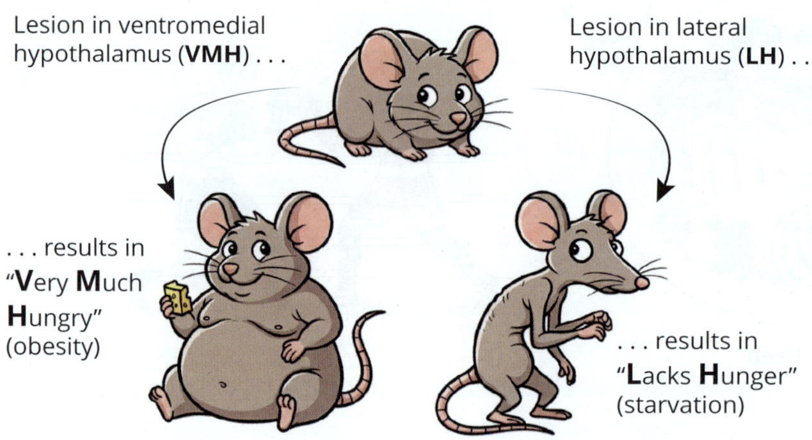

Figure 1.13 Results from Lesions in the LH and VMH

The **anterior hypothalamus** controls sexual behavior. When the anterior hypothalamus is stimulated, lab animals will mount just about anything (including inanimate objects). In many species, damage to the anterior hypothalamus leads to permanent inhibition of sexual activity. The anterior hypothalamus also regulates sleep and body temperature.

Other Parts of the Diencephalon

The diencephalon also differentiates to form the posterior pituitary gland, pineal gland, and connecting pathways to other brain regions. The **posterior pituitary** is comprised of axonal projections from the hypothalamus and is the site of release for the hypothalamic hormones **antidiuretic hormone** (**ADH**, also called **vasopressin**) and **oxytocin**. The functions of these hormones are described in Chapter 5 of *MCAT Biology Review*. The **pineal gland** is the key player in several biological rhythms. Most notably, the pineal gland secretes a hormone called **melatonin**, which regulates circadian rhythms. The pineal gland receives direct signals from the retina for coordination with sunlight.

Basal Ganglia

In the middle of the brain are a group of structures known as the basal ganglia. The **basal ganglia** coordinate muscle movement as they receive information from the cortex and relay this information (via the extrapyramidal motor system) to the brain and the spinal cord. The **extrapyramidal system** gathers information about body position and carries this information to the central nervous system, but does not function directly through motor neurons. Essentially, the basal ganglia help make our movements smooth and our posture steady. **Parkinson's disease** is one chronic illness associated with destruction of portions of the basal ganglia. This disease is characterized by jerky movements and uncontrolled resting tremors. The basal ganglia may also play a role in schizophrenia and obsessive–compulsive disorder.

Limbic System

The **limbic system**, diagrammed in Figure 1.14, comprises a group of interconnected structures looping around the central portion of the brain and is primarily associated with emotion and memory. Its primary components include the septal nuclei, amygdala, hippocampus, and anterior cingulate cortex. In Chapter 5 of *MCAT Behavioral Sciences Review*, we will also explore the roles of the thalamus, hypothalamus, and cortex in the limbic system.

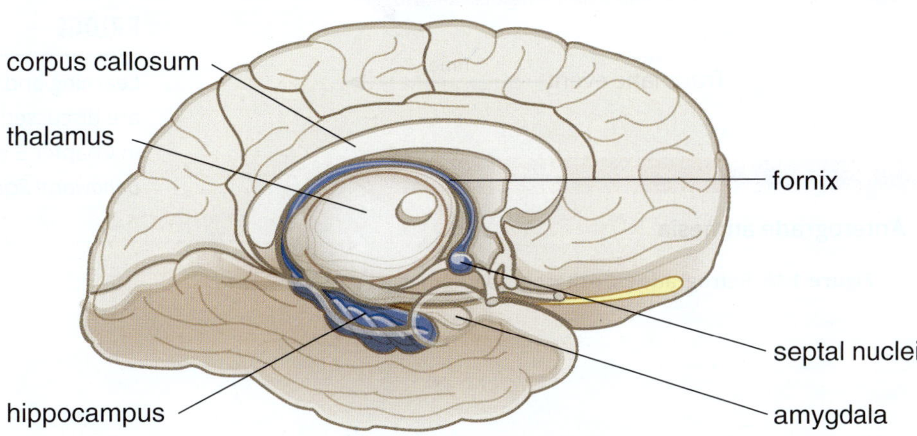

Figure 1.14 The Limbic System

REAL WORLD

In the early 1920s, researchers first discovered the hypothalamus's role in rage and fighting through classic experiments conducted with cats. When researchers removed the cat's cerebral cortex but left the hypothalamus in place, the cat displayed a pattern of pseudoaggressive behavior that was called "sham rage"—lashing of the tail, arching of the back, clawing, and biting—except that rage was spontaneous or triggered by the mildest touch. The researchers concluded that the cortex typically inhibits this type of response. When the researchers removed the cat's cortex and hypothalamus together, the outcome was very different. The cat no longer showed any signs of sham rage, and much rougher stimulation was required before the cats showed any defensive behavior at all.

Septal Nuclei

The **septal nuclei** contain one of the primary pleasure centers in the brain. Mild stimulation of the septal nuclei is reported to be intensely pleasurable; there is an association between these nuclei and addictive behavior.

Amygdala

The **amygdala** is a structure that plays an important role in defensive and aggressive behaviors, including fear and rage. Researchers base this observation on studies of animals and humans with brain lesions. When the amygdala is damaged, aggression and fear reactions are markedly reduced. Lesions to the amygdala result in docility and hypersexual states.

Hippocampus

The **hippocampus** plays a vital role in learning and memory processes; specifically, the hippocampus helps consolidate information to form long-term memories, and can redistribute remote memories to the cerebral cortex. The hippocampus communicates with other portions of the limbic system through a long projection called the **fornix**. Researchers originally discovered the connection between memory and the hippocampus through a famous patient named Henry Molaison (known as H.M. in the scientific literature until his death in 2008). Parts of H.M.'s temporal lobes—including the amygdala and hippocampus—were removed in an effort to control epileptic seizures. After surgery, H.M.'s intelligence was largely intact but he suffered a drastic and irreversible loss of memory for any new information. This kind of memory loss is called **anterograde amnesia** and is characterized by not being able to establish new long-term memories, whereas memory for events that occurred before brain injury is usually intact. The opposite kind of memory loss, **retrograde amnesia**, refers to memory loss of events that transpired before brain injury. A helpful visual for these two amnesias can be seen in Figure 1.15.

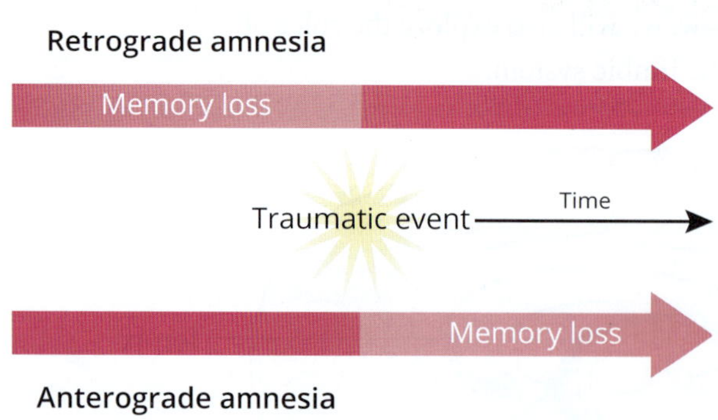

Figure 1.15 Retrograde vs. Anterograde Amnesia

REAL WORLD

James Olds and Peter Milner discovered the association between the septal nuclei and addictive behavior in the 1950s. They demonstrated that when rats could stimulate their septal regions at will by pushing a lever, they found it so pleasurable that they preferred it to eating or any other activities, even after going 24 hours without food or sleep.

REAL WORLD

Heinrich Klüver and Paul Bucy performed studies that linked the amygdala with defensive and aggressive behavior in monkeys. When the amygdala of the Rhesus monkey was removed, they noted increased sexual behavior, decreased fear responses, and hyperorality, or the examination of inanimate or animate objects by mouth. These symptoms are now referred to as Klüver–Bucy syndrome.

BRIDGE

Learning and memory are discussed thoroughly in Chapter 3 of *MCAT Behavioral Sciences Review*.

Anterior Cingulate Cortex

Due to the connection with the frontal and parietal lobes, the **anterior cingulate cortex** functions in higher order cognitive processes, including regulation of impulse control and decision-making. It also maintains connections to other parts of the limbic system, and thus plays a role in emotion and motivation.

Cerebral Cortex

The outer surface of the brain is called the **cerebral cortex**. The cortex is sometimes called the **neocortex**, a reminder that the cortex is the most recent brain region to evolve. Rather than having a smooth surface, the cortex has numerous bumps and folds called **gyri** and **sulci**, respectively. The convoluted structure of the brain provides increased surface area. The cerebrum is divided into two halves, called **cerebral hemispheres**. The surface of the cortex is divided into four lobes—the frontal lobe, parietal lobe, occipital lobe, and temporal lobe. These lobes are identified in Figure 1.16, which shows a side view of the left cerebral hemisphere.

MNEMONIC

Lobes of the brain: **F-POT**

- **F**rontal
- **P**arietal
- **O**ccipital
- **T**emporal

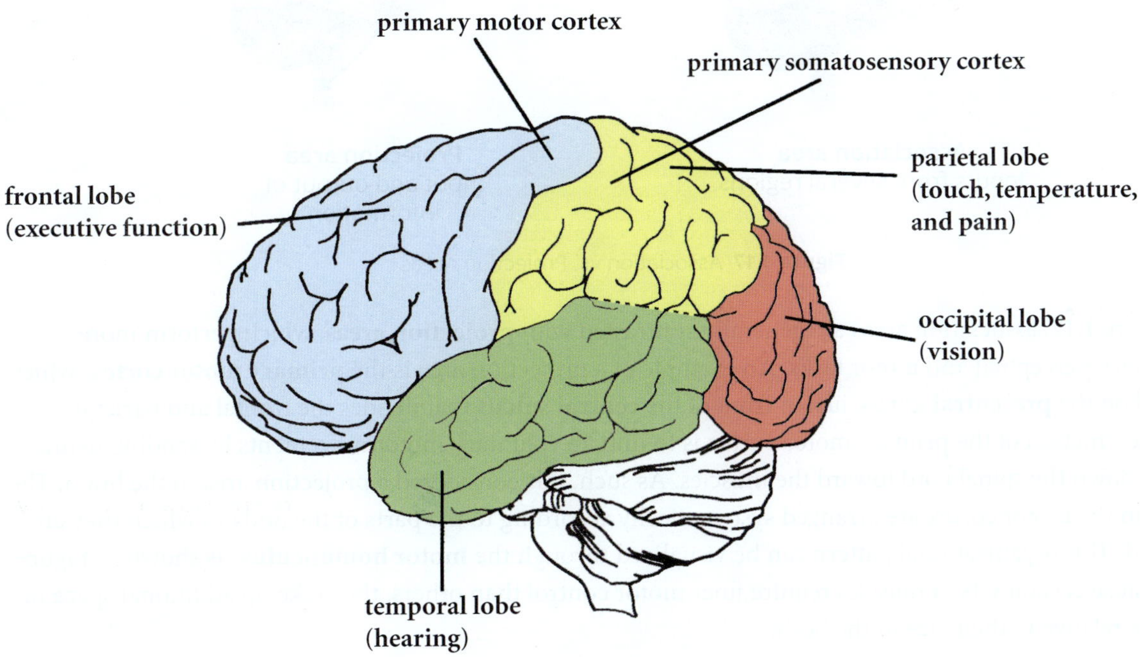

Figure 1.16 Lobes of the Brain

Frontal Lobe

The **frontal lobe** is comprised of two basic regions: the prefrontal cortex and the motor cortex. The **prefrontal cortex** manages executive function by supervising and directing the operations of other brain regions. To regulate attention and alertness, the prefrontal cortext communicates with the reticular formation in the brainstem, telling an individual either to wake up or to relax, depending on the situation. This region also supervises processes associated with perception, memory, emotion, impulse control, and long-term planning. In memory, for instance, the role of the prefrontal cortex is not to store any memory traces, but rather to remind individuals that they have something to remember at all.

Damage to the prefrontal cortex impairs its overall supervisory functions. People with prefrontal lesions may be more impulsive and generally less in control of their behavior. As a result, these individuals can have an increased tendency towards angry outbursts, as well as a higher predisposition to crying. Additionally, it is not unusual for someone with a prefrontal lesion to make vulgar and inappropriate sexual remarks, or to be apathetic to the emotional responses of others.

Because the prefrontal cortex integrates information from different cortical regions, the prefrontal cortex is a good example of an **association area**, which is an area that integrates input from diverse regions of the brain. For example, multiple inputs may be necessary to solve a complex puzzle, to plan ahead for the future, or to reach a difficult decision.

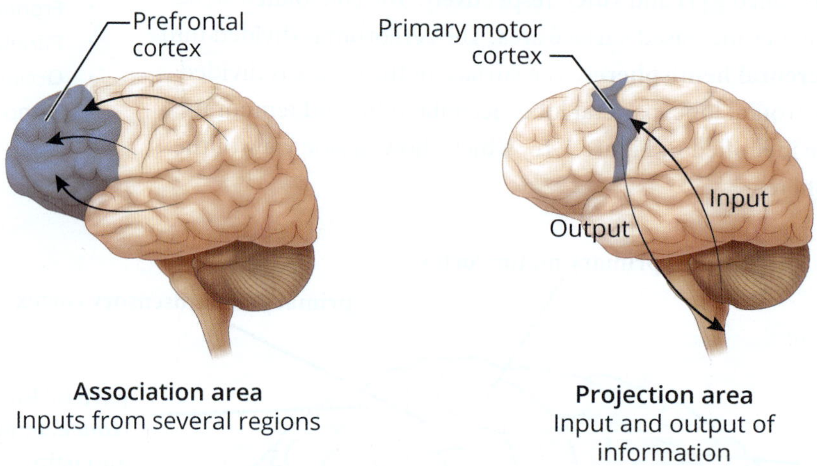

Figure 1.17 Association vs. Projection Areas

As in Figure 1.17, association areas are generally contrasted with **projection areas**, which perform more rudimentary perceptual and motor tasks. An example of a projection area is the **primary motor cortex**, which is located on the **precentral gyrus**, just in front of the **central sulcus** that divides the frontal and parietal lobes. The function of the primary motor cortex is to initiate voluntary motor movements by sending neural impulses down the spinal cord toward the muscles. As such, it is considered a projection area in the brain. The neurons in the motor cortex are arranged systematically according to the parts of the body to which they are connected. This organizational pattern can be visualized through the **motor homunculus**, as shown in Figure 1.18. Because certain sets of muscles require finer motor control than others, they take up additional space in the cortex relative to their size in the body.

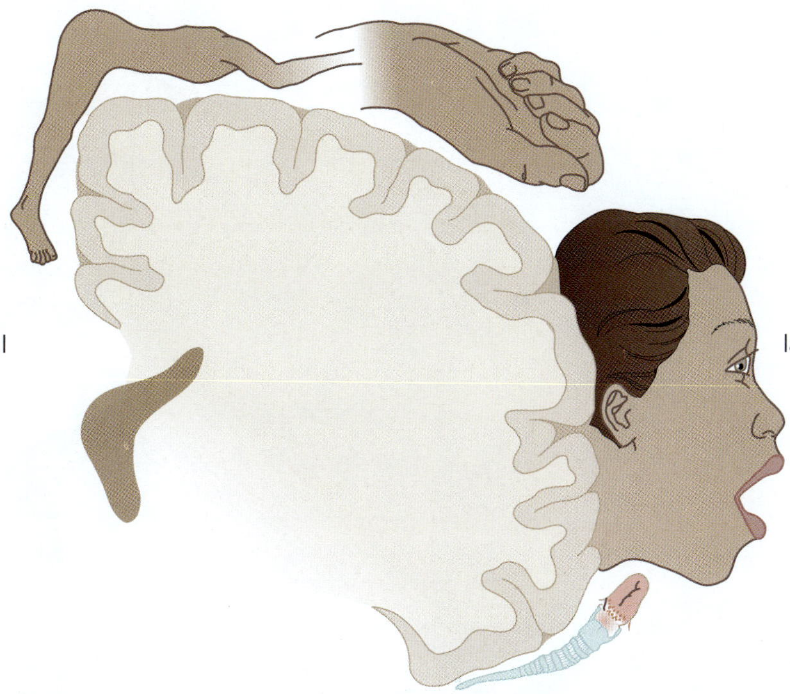

Figure 1.18 Motor Homunculus on the Precentral Gyrus of the Frontal Lobe

A third important part of the frontal lobe is **Broca's area**, which is vitally important for speech production. Broca's area is usually found in only one hemisphere, the so-called "dominant" hemisphere; for most people—both right- and left-handed—this is the left hemisphere.

Parietal Lobe

The **parietal lobe** is located to the rear of the frontal lobe. The **somatosensory cortex** is located on the **post-central gyrus** (just behind the central sulcus) and is involved in somatosensory information processing. This projection area is the destination for all incoming sensory signals for touch, pressure, temperature, and pain. Despite certain differences, the somatosensory cortex and motor cortex are very closely related. In fact, they are so interrelated they sometimes are described as a single unit: the sensorimotor cortex. The somatosensory homunculus is shown in Figure 1.19. The central region of the parietal lobe is associated with spatial processing and manipulation. This region makes it possible to orient oneself and other objects in three-dimensional space, to do spatial manipulation of objects, and to apply spatial orientation skills such as those required for map reading.

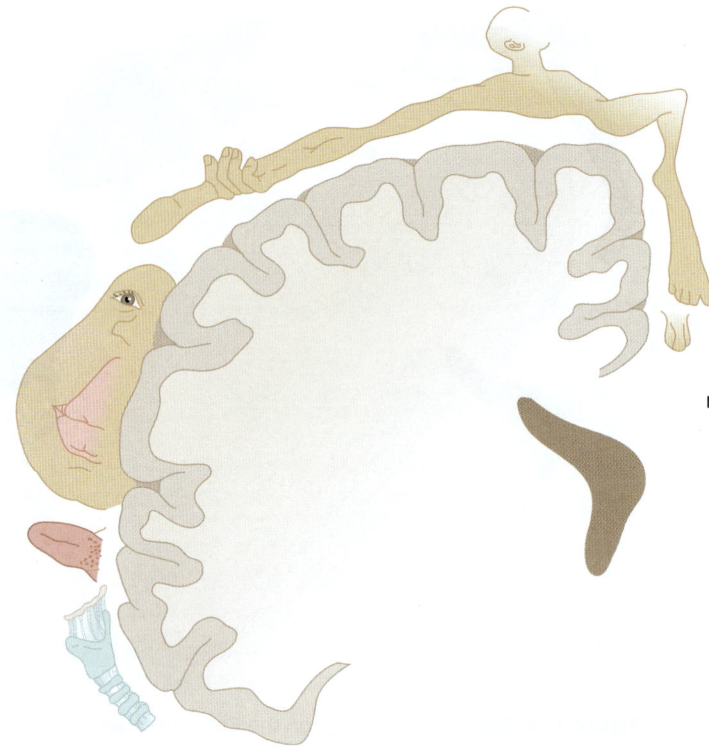

Figure 1.19 Somatosensory Homunculus on the Postcentral Gyrus of the Parietal Lobe

REAL WORLD

Several techniques have been developed to assess the function of brain regions, especially those associated with language and auditory processing. One such technique is called **speech shadowing**, which is a technique used to research both stuttering and speech perception. Speech shadowing involves participants reciting along with auditory inputs, which can be presented to one or both ears. If different messages are presented to each ear, as in a dichotic listening test, speech shadowing can ensure that the participant is paying attention to the auditory input to the correct ear. This seemingly simple experimental task requires successful functioning of the temporal lobe, parietal lobe, and frontal cortex!

Occipital Lobe

The **occipital lobes**, at the very rear of the brain, contain the **visual cortex**, which is sometimes called the **striate cortex**. *Striate* means furrowed or striped, which is how the visual cortex appears when examined under a microscope. The visual cortex is one of the best-understood brain regions, owing to the large amount of research that has been done on visual processing. Research has revealed curious phenomena such as **blindsight**. Blindsight occurs when the primary visual cortex, or pathways to it, have been damaged, leaving a person unable to see normally. On the other hand, the occipito-parietal pathway remains intact. This allows the person to perform certain visual tasks without being consciously aware of the visual stimulus. Sensation and perception of visual information are discussed thoroughly in Chapter 2 of *MCAT Behavioral Sciences Review*. Areas in the occipital lobe have also been implicated in learning and motor control.

Temporal Lobe

The **temporal lobes** are associated with a number of functions. The auditory cortex and Wernicke's area are located in the temporal lobe. The **auditory cortex** is the primary site of most sound processing, including speech, music, and other sound information. **Wernicke's area** is associated with language reception and comprehension. The temporal lobe also functions in memory processing, emotion, and language. Studies have shown that electrical stimulation of the temporal lobe can evoke memories for past events. This makes sense because the hippocampus is located deep inside the temporal lobe. It is important to note that the lobes, although having seemingly independent functions, are not truly independent of one another. Often, a sensory modality may be represented in more than one area.

Cerebral Hemispheres and Laterality

In most cases, one side of the brain communicates with the opposite side of the body. In such cases, we say a cerebral hemisphere communicates **contralaterally**. For example, the motor neurons on the left side of the brain activate movements on the right side of the body. In other cases (for instance, hearing), cerebral hemispheres communicate with the same side of the body. In such cases, the hemispheres communicate **ipsilaterally**.

We distinguish between dominant and nondominant hemispheres. The dominant hemisphere is typically defined as the one that is more heavily stimulated during language reception and production. In the past, hand dominance was used as a proxy for hemispheric dominance; that is, right-handed individuals were assumed to have left-dominant brains and left-handed individuals were assumed to have right-dominant brains (because the brain communicates contralaterally with the hand). However, this correlation has not held up under scrutiny; 95 percent of right-handed individuals are indeed left brain dominant, but only 18 percent of left-handed individuals are right brain dominant.

REAL WORLD

The **corpus callosum** connects and shares information between the two cerebral hemispheres; its function was discovered in patients who have epilepsy whose corpora callosa were severed in a last-ditch effort to limit their convulsive seizures. In these "split-brain" patients (see Figure 1.20), in whom the corpus callosum has been severed, each hemisphere has its own function and specialization that is no longer accessible by the other. As an example of the result: an object felt only by the left hand (which projects to the right hemisphere) could not be named (because language function is usually in the left hemisphere).

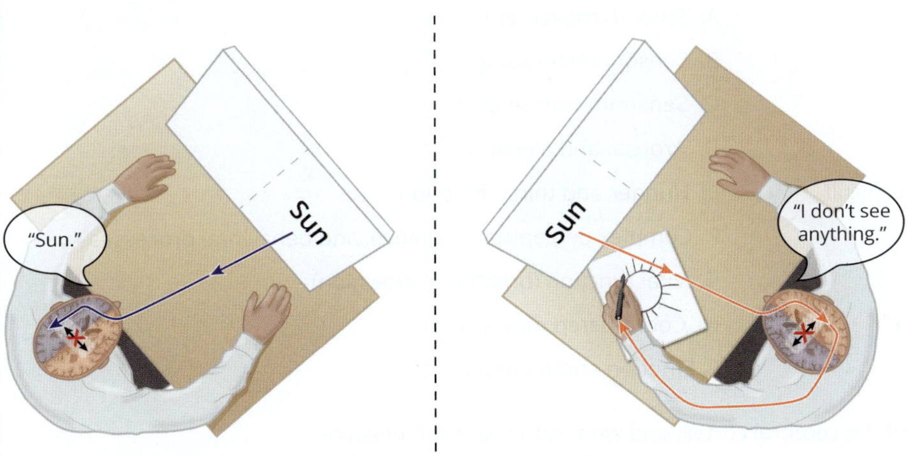

Figure 1.20 Split-Brain Syndrome

The **dominant hemisphere** (usually the left) is primarily analytic in function, making it well-suited for managing details. For instance, language, logic, and math skills are all located in the dominant hemisphere. Again, language production (Broca's area) and language comprehension (Wernicke's area) are primarily driven by the dominant hemisphere.

The **nondominant hemisphere** (usually the right) is associated with intuition, creativity, music cognition, and spatial processing. The nondominant hemisphere simultaneously processes the pieces of a stimulus and assembles them into a holistic image. The nondominant hemisphere serves a less prominent role in language. It is more sensitive to the emotional tone of spoken language, and permits us to recognize others' moods based on visual and auditory cues, which adds to communication. The dominant hemisphere thus screens incoming language to analyze its content, and the nondominant hemisphere interprets it according to its emotional tone. The roles of the dominant and nondominant hemispheres are summarized in Table 1.2; remember that the left hemisphere is the dominant hemisphere in most individuals, regardless of handedness.

Function	Dominant Hemisphere	Nondominant Hemisphere
Visual system	Letters, words	Faces
Auditory system	Language-related sounds	Music
Language	Speech, reading, writing, arithmetic	Emotions
Movement	Complex voluntary movement	–
Spatial processes	–	Geometry, sense of direction

Table 1.2 Comparison of Dominant and Nondominant Hemispheres' Functions

MCAT CONCEPT CHECK 1.4

Before you move on, assess your understanding of the material with these questions.

1. Match the parts of the brain below to their functions:

1. Basal ganglia	A. Smooth movement
2. Cerebellum	B. Sensory relay station
3. Cerebral cortex	C. Sensorimotor reflexes
4. Hypothalamus	D. Arousal and alertness
5. Inferior and superior colliculi	E. Hunger and thirst; emotion
6. Limbic system	F. Complex perceptual, cognitive, and behavioral processes
7. Medulla oblongata	G. Vital function (breathing, digestion)
8. Reticular formation	H. Coordinated movement
9. Thalamus	I. Emotion and memory

2. What are the four lobes of the cerebral cortex, and what is the function of each?

Lobe	Function

3. What is the difference between ipsilateral and contralateral communication between the brain and the body?

____

4. How is the dominant hemisphere typically defined?

____

1.5 Influences on Behavior High Yield

LEARNING OBJECTIVES

After Chapter 1.5, you will be able to:

- Associate major neurotransmitters with their common functions
- Detail the links between the endocrine system and the brain
- Explain the nature vs. nurture debate and the different study types used to explore this question

Merely describing the functions of brain regions does not fully explain the wide variety of human behaviors that are possible. Other influences on behavior include chemical controls (neurotransmitters, hormones in the endocrine system), heredity, and the environment.

Neurotransmitters

A **neurotransmitter** is a chemical used by neurons to send signals to other neurons; more than 100 neurotransmitters have been identified. Several of the most important are described in this section and are summarized in Table 1.3. Some drugs mimic the action of neurotransmitters by binding to the same receptor to produce the same biological response. A drug that mimics the action of some neurotransmitter is called an **agonist**. Drugs can also act by blocking the action of neurotransmitters, and such drugs are called **antagonists**. Agonistic and antagonistic effects are shown in Figure 1.21.

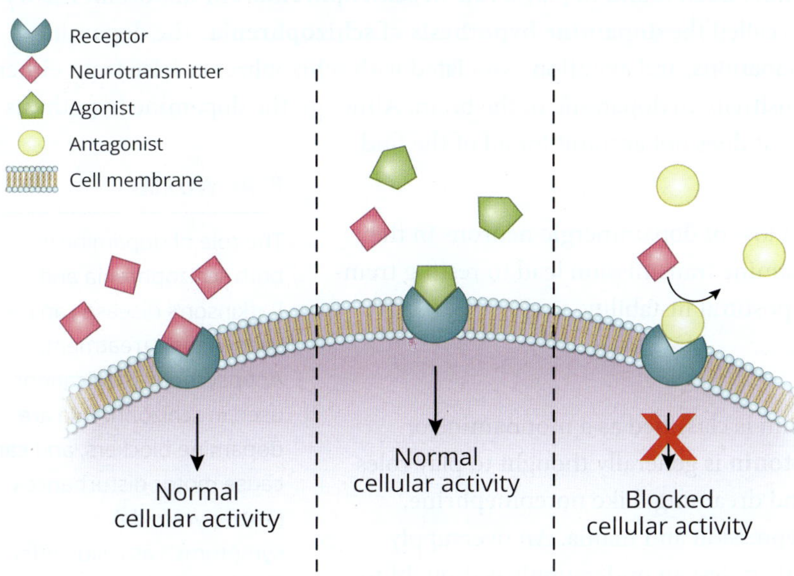

Figure 1.21 Agonist vs. Antagonist

KEY CONCEPT

Acetylcholine is the neurotransmitter used by the efferent limb of the somatic nervous system and the parasympathetic nervous system. Acetylcholine can act as an excitatory or inhibitory neurotransmitter in muscle cells, dependent on the type of receptor found on the cell. For example, acetylcholine will transmit an inhibitory response in cardiac muscle cells, but it can also transmit an excitatory response if acting on skeletal muscle cells. Acetylcholine within the central nervous system largely functions as an excitatory neurotransmitter.

Acetylcholine

Acetylcholine is a neurotransmitter found in both the central and peripheral nervous systems. In the peripheral nervous system, acetylcholine is used to transmit nerve impulses to the muscles. It is the neurotransmitter used by the parasympathetic nervous system and a small portion of the sympathetic nervous system (in ganglia and for innervating sweat glands). In the central nervous system, acetylcholine has been linked to attention and arousal. In fact, loss of cholinergic neurons connecting with the hippocampus is associated with Alzheimer's disease, an illness resulting in progressive and incurable memory loss.

Epinephrine and Norepinephrine

Epinephrine, norepinephrine, and dopamine are three closely related neurotransmitters known as **catecholamines**. Due to similarities in their molecular composition, these three transmitters are also classified as **monoamines** or **biogenic amines**. The most important thing to know about the catecholamines is that they all play important roles in the experience of emotions.

Epinephrine (**adrenaline**) and **norepinephrine** (**noradrenaline**) are involved in controlling alertness and wakefulness. As the primary neurotransmitter of the sympathetic nervous system, they promote the fight-or-flight response. Whereas norepinephrine more commonly acts at a local level as a neurotransmitter, epinephrine is more often secreted from the adrenal medulla to act systemically as a hormone. Low levels of norepinephrine are associated with depression; high levels are associated with anxiety and mania.

Dopamine

Dopamine is another catecholamine, created by the enzyme dopamine decarboxylase from L-dihydroxyphenylalanine (L-DOPA), that plays an important role in movement and posture. High concentrations of dopamine are normally found in the basal ganglia, which help smooth movements and maintain postural stability.

Imbalances in dopamine transmission have been found to play a role in **schizophrenia**. An important theory about the origin of this mental illness is called the **dopamine hypothesis of schizophrenia**. The dopamine hypothesis argues that delusions, hallucinations, and agitation associated with schizophrenia arise from either too much dopamine or from an oversensitivity to dopamine in the brain. Although the dopamine hypothesis of schizophrenia is an important theory, it does not account for all of the findings of the disease.

Parkinson's disease is associated with a loss of dopaminergic neurons in the basal ganglia. These disruptions of dopamine transmission lead to resting tremors and jerky movements, as well as to postural instability.

REAL WORLD

The role of dopamine in both schizophrenia and Parkinson's disease can be seen in their treatment. Antipsychotic medications used in schizophrenia are dopamine blockers, and can cause motor disturbances ("extrapyramidal symptoms") as a side effect. Parkinson's disease can be treated with L-DOPA, which increases dopamine levels in the brain; an overdose of L-DOPA can lead to psychotic symptoms similar to schizophrenia.

Serotonin

Along with the catecholamines, serotonin is classified as a monoamine or biogenic amine neurotransmitter. **Serotonin** is generally thought to play roles in regulating mood, eating, sleeping, and dreaming. Like norepinephrine, serotonin is thought to play a role in depression and mania. An oversupply of serotonin is thought to produce manic states; an undersupply is thought to produce depression.

GABA, Glycine, and Glutamate

The neurotransmitter **γ-aminobutyric acid** (**GABA**) produces inhibitory postsynaptic potentials and is thought to play an important role in stabilizing neural activity in the brain. GABA exerts its effects by causing hyperpolarization of the postsynaptic membrane.

Glycine may be better known as one of the twenty proteinogenic amino acids, but it also serves as an inhibitory neurotransmitter in the central nervous system by increasing chloride influx into the neuron. This hyperpolarizes the postsynaptic membrane, similar to the function of GABA.

Finally, **glutamate**, another of the twenty proteinogenic amino acids, also acts as a neurotransmitter in the central nervous system. In contrast to glycine, however, it is an excitatory neurotransmitter.

Peptide Neurotransmitters

Studies suggest that peptides are also involved in neurotransmission. The synaptic action of these **neuromodulators** (also called **neuropeptides**) involves a more complicated chain of events in the postsynaptic cell than that of regular neurotransmitters. Neuromodulators are therefore relatively slow and have longer effects on the postsynaptic cell than neurotransmitters. The **endorphins**, which are natural painkillers produced in the brain, are the most important peptides to know. Endorphins (and their relatives, **enkephalins**) have actions similar to morphine or other opioids in the body.

Neurotransmitter	Behavior
Acetylcholine	Voluntary muscle control, parasympathetic nervous system, attention, alertness
Epinephrine and Norepinephrine	Fight-or-flight responses, wakefulness, alertness
Dopamine	Smooth movements, postural stability
Serotonin	Mood, sleep, eating, dreaming
GABA and Glycine	Brain "stabilization"
Glutamate	Brain excitation
Endorphins	Natural painkillers

Table 1.3 Neurotransmitters and Their Functions

The Endocrine System

We've already discussed the relatively fast communication network—the nervous system—that uses chemical messages called neurotransmitters. The **endocrine system** is the other internal communication network in the body, and it uses chemical messengers called **hormones**. The endocrine system is somewhat slower than the nervous system because hormones travel to their target destinations through the bloodstream. The endocrine system is covered extensively in Chapter 5 of *MCAT Biology Review*, so our focus here will be on the role of certain endocrine organs on behavior.

BRIDGE

The entire endocrine system is covered in Chapter 5 of *MCAT Biology Review*.

The hypothalamus links the endocrine and nervous systems and, in addition to the roles described earlier, regulates the hormonal function of the pituitary gland. The hypothalamus and pituitary gland are spatially close to each other, and control is maintained through endocrine release of hormones into the **hypophyseal portal system** that directly connects the two organs, as shown in Figure 1.22.

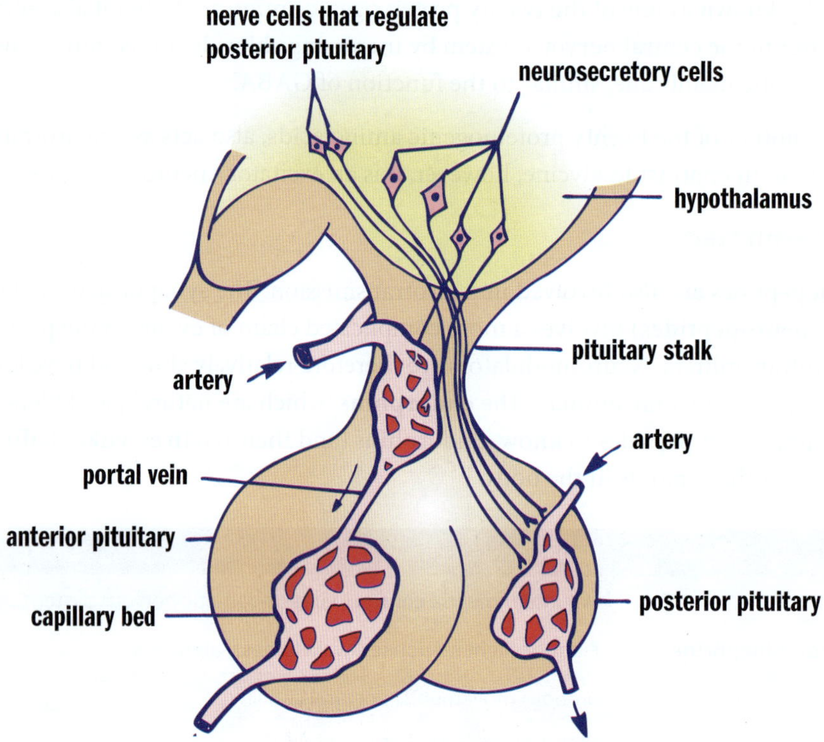

Figure 1.22 The Hypophyseal Portal System

The **pituitary gland**, sometimes referred to as the "master" gland, is located at the base of the brain and is divided into two parts: anterior and posterior. It is the **anterior pituitary** that is the "master" because it releases hormones that regulate activities of endocrine glands elsewhere in the body. However, the anterior pituitary itself is controlled by the hypothalamus. The pituitary secretes various hormones into the bloodstream that travel to other endocrine glands located elsewhere in the body to activate them. Once activated by the pituitary, a given endocrine gland manufactures and secretes its own characteristic hormone into the bloodstream.

The **adrenal glands** are located on top of the kidneys and are divided into two parts: the adrenal medulla and adrenal cortex. The **adrenal medulla** releases epinephrine and norepinephrine as part of the sympathetic nervous system. The **adrenal cortex** produces many hormones called **corticosteroids**, including the stress hormone **cortisol**. The adrenal cortex also contributes to sexual functioning by producing sex hormones, such as **testosterone** and **estrogen**.

The **gonads** are the sex glands of the body—ovaries in females and testes in males. These glands produce sex hormones in higher concentrations, leading to increased levels of testosterone in males and increased levels of estrogen in females. These sex hormones increase **libido** and contribute to mating behavior and sexual function. Higher levels of testosterone also increase aggressive behavior.

Genetics and Behavior

Just as physical traits are inherited from parents, behavioral traits can be inherited as well. Evidence for the inherited nature of behavior comes from the fact that many behaviors are species specific. For example, many animals exhibit mating behaviors only seen within their species. Behaviors can also be bred into a species; many breeds of dog have been bred for certain traits and behaviors. Behaviors are also seen to run in families. Often times, violence and aggression are observed passing along a family line, as are mental illnesses.

Innate behavior is genetically programmed as a result of evolution and is seen in all individuals regardless of environment or experience. In contrast, other behaviors are considered learned. **Learned behaviors** are not based on heredity but instead are based on experience and environment. **Adaptive value** is the extent to which a trait or behavior positively benefits a species by influencing the evolutionary fitness of the species, thus leading to **adaptation** through **natural selection**.

REAL WORLD

Bipolar disorder is considered one of the most heritable disorders, including medical illnesses. In one study, having a monozygotic (identical) twin with bipolar disorder was associated with a 43% risk of being diagnosed with the same disorder.

BRIDGE

Natural selection is discussed in greater detail in Chapter 12 of *MCAT Biology Review*.

How much of an individual's behavior is based on genetic makeup and how much is based on environment and experiences? This controversial question is often referred to as the **nature vs. nurture** question. Here, **nature** is the influence of inherited characteristics on behavior. **Nurture** refers to the influence of environment and physical surroundings on behavior. There is no easy answer to this long-debated question. An individual's behavior is not only influenced by both genetics and environment, but also by how these two factors may influence each other. For example, hereditary traits may make a certain person more likely to have an addictive personality. But, the individual would still have to be exposed to drugs, alcohol, or gambling to develop an addiction.

To determine the degree of genetic influence on behavior, researchers often use one of three methods: family studies, twin studies, and adoption studies. **Family studies** rely on the fact that genetically related individuals are more similar genotypically than unrelated individuals. Researchers may compare rates of a given trait among family members to rates of that trait among unrelated individuals. For example, family studies have determined that the risk of developing schizophrenia for children of a patient who has schizophrenia is 13 times higher than in the general population. For siblings of a patient who has schizophrenia, the rate is 9 times higher. Observations such as these have led psychologists to conclude that schizophrenia has a hereditary component. Family studies are limited, however, because families share both genetics and environment. Family studies cannot distinguish shared environmental factors from shared genetic factors. For example, what if the increased rates of schizophrenia in families are a result of experiencing the same emotional climate in the home rather than genetically shared characteristics?

Twin studies, comparing concordance rates for a trait between **monozygotic** (**MZ**; identical) and **dizygotic** (**DZ**; fraternal) twins, are better able to distinguish the relative effects of shared environment and genetics. **Concordance rates** refer to the likelihood that both twins exhibit the same trait. MZ twins are genetically identical, sharing 100 percent of their genes, whereas DZ twins share approximately 50 percent of their genes. The assumption made by twin studies is that the two individuals in each MZ or DZ twin pair share the same environment; thus, differences between MZ and DZ twins are thought to reflect hereditary factors. Twin studies can also be used to measure genetic effects relative to environmental effects. In this version of the twin study, researchers compare traits in twins raised together versus twins raised apart. For example, one study of personality characteristics showed that MZ (identical) twins raised in separate families were still more similar than DZ (fraternal) twins raised together. Such a result offers convincing evidence for a strong genetic component to personality.

Finally, **adoption studies** also help us understand environmental and genetic influences on behavior. These studies compare the similarities between biological relatives and the child who was adopted to similarities between adoptive relatives and the child. For example, researchers have found that the IQ of children who were adopted is more similar to their biological parents' IQ than to their adoptive parents' IQ (see Figure 1.23). This research suggests that IQ is heritable. Criminal behavior among teenagers shows a similar pattern of heritability.

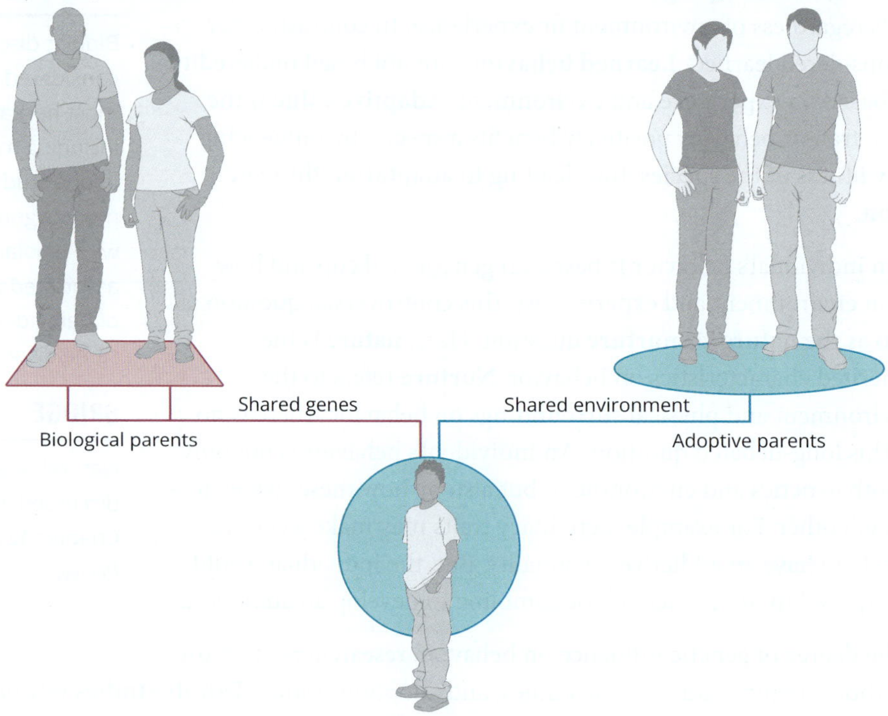

Figure 1.23 Adoption Studies

MCAT CONCEPT CHECK 1.5

Before you move on, assess your understanding of the material with these questions.

1. Match the neurotransmitters below to their functions:

1. Acetylcholine	A. Wakefulness and alertness, fight-or-flight responses
2. Dopamine	B. Brain "stabilizer"
3. Endorphins	C. Mood, sleep, eating, dreaming
4. Epinephrine/norepinephrine	D. Natural painkiller
5. GABA/glycine	E. Smooth movements and steady posture
6. Glutamate	F. Voluntary muscle control
7. Serotonin	G. Brain excitation

2. Which endocrine organs influence behavior? What hormones do they use, and what do they accomplish?

____

3. Briefly discuss the influence of nature vs. nurture on behavior.

____

4. In each of the study types below, what is the sample group? The control group?

Study	Sample Group	Control Group
Family study		
Twin study		
Adoption study		

1.6 Development

LEARNING OBJECTIVES

After Chapter 1.6, you will be able to:

- Describe the process of neurulation
- Link the primitive reflexes with the behaviors to which they correspond
- Identify the main themes that dictate stages of motor development in children

The developmental process begins at the moment of conception. Physiological changes are rapid from embryonic to fetal stages, and well into infancy. Children exhibit surprisingly consistent patterns of motor abilities, as well as physiological changes based on age. Understanding these changes and when they occur is important in the discussion of developmental psychology. There are specific periods in development where children are particularly susceptible to environmental factors, called **critical periods**. Absence of the appropriate environmental factors may result in failure to learn a given skill or trait during the critical period, which may also mean learning that skill later on is difficult or even impossible.

Prenatal

The development of the nervous system starts with neurulation, at three to four weeks' gestational age. **Neurulation** occurs when the ectoderm overlying the notochord begins to furrow, forming a **neural groove** surrounded by two **neural folds**, as shown in Figure 1.24. Cells at the leading edge of the neural fold are called the **neural crest**, and will migrate throughout the body to form disparate tissues, including dorsal root ganglia, melanocytes (pigment-producing cells), and calcitonin-producing cells of the thyroid. The remainder of the furrow closes to form the **neural tube**, which will ultimately form the central nervous system (CNS). The neural tube has an **alar plate**, which differentiates into sensory neurons, and a **basal plate**, which differentiates into motor neurons. Over time, the neural tube invaginates and folds on itself many times; the embryonic brain begins as three swellings (prosencephalon, mesencephalon, rhombencephalon) that become five swellings (telencephalon, diencephalon, mesencephalon, metencephalon, myelencephalon) as it becomes the mature brain, as demonstrated in Figure 1.8 earlier in this chapter.

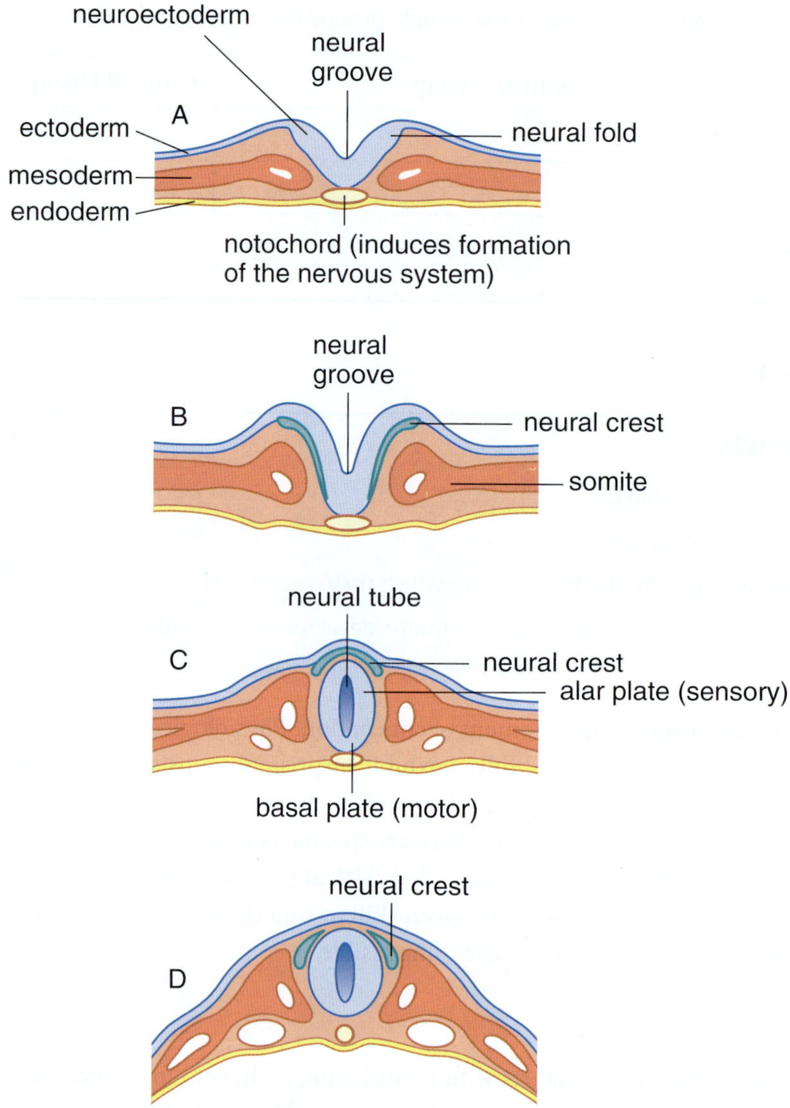

Figure 1.24 Development of the Nervous System

Prenatal development does not occur in a vacuum, of course, but in the mother's uterus. Within this environment, temperature, chemical balance, orientation of the fetus with respect to gravity, and atmospheric pressure are all carefully controlled and remain relatively constant. The fetus is attached to the uterine wall and placenta by the **umbilical cord**. The **placenta** transmits food, oxygen, and water to the fetus while returning water and waste to the mother. Maternal blood supplies many of the proteins and amino acids needed for growth, although the embryo begins to produce its own proteins and amino acids as well.

A variety of external influences can have deleterious effects on the development of the fetus. A number of viruses or bacteria can cross the placenta and cause damage to the developing fetus, including rubella (German measles), which may cause cataracts, deafness, heart defects, and intellectual disability. Other viral infections—such as measles, mumps, hepatitis, influenza, varicella (chickenpox), and herpes—have been linked to various birth defects.

An unfortunate side effect of the revolution in pharmaceutical development is that many drugs that help the mother can have damaging effects on the fetus she carries. The most notorious of these drugs is *thalidomide*, which was prescribed in the late 1950s and early 1960s to reduce morning sickness. Mothers who took this drug while pregnant often gave birth to babies with missing and malformed limbs and defects of the heart, eyes, ears, digestive tract, and kidneys. Antiepileptic medications are associated with neural tube defects, in which the neural tube fails to close completely, leading to malformations such as *spina bifida* or *anencephaly*.

A host of environmental factors and exposures may also affect maturation. Maternal malnutrition is considered to be a leading cause of abnormal development. Protein deficiency can slow growth, lead to intellectual disability, and reduce immunity to disease. Maternal narcotic addiction produces chemically dependent infants who must undergo severe withdrawal after birth. Regular cigarette smoking can lead to slowed growth, increased fetal heart rate, and a greater chance of premature birth. Daily use of alcohol also leads to slowed growth, both physically and psychologically. Finally, prenatal exposure to X-rays has been strongly linked to intellectual disabilities; defects of the skull, spinal cord, and eyes; cleft palate; and limb deformities.

Motor

Although they may seem helpless, infants are equipped with well-developed somatic structures and a broad array of reflexes that help ensure survival. A **reflex** is a behavior that occurs in response to a given stimulus without higher cognitive input. While motor and startle reflexes exist in adults, infants have a number of **primitive reflexes** that disappear with age. For example, the **rooting reflex** is the automatic turning of the head in the direction of a stimulus that touches the cheek—such as a nipple during feeding. Sucking and swallowing when an object is placed in the mouth are also examples of reflexes related to feeding.

Other primitive reflexes may have served an adaptive purpose in earlier stages of human evolution, but are currently used mainly in assessing infant neurological development. By comparing the point in time at which each of these reflexes disappears relative to the established norms, it is possible to tell whether neurological development is taking place in a normal fashion. One such reflex is the **Moro reflex**, illustrated in Figure 1.25. Infants react to abrupt movements of their heads by flinging out their arms, then slowly retracting their arms and crying. It has been speculated that this reflex may have developed during a time when our prehuman ancestors lived in trees and falling could have been prevented by instinctive clutching. The Moro reflex usually disappears after four months and its continuation at one year is a strong suggestion of developmental difficulties. Asymmetry of the Moro reflex may hint at underlying neuromuscular problems.

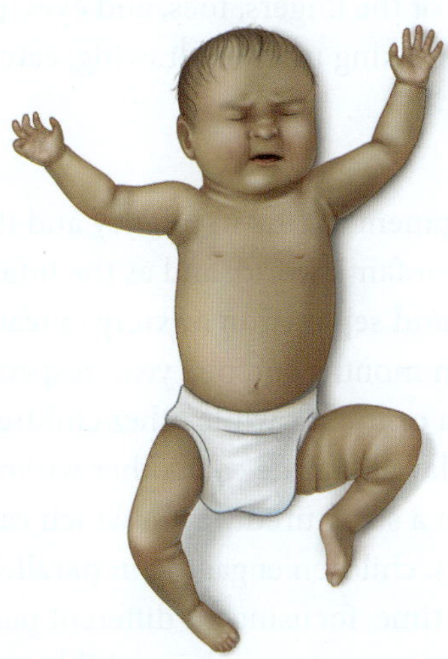

Figure 1.25 The Moro Reflex
The infant extends the arms, then slowly withdraws them and cries.

The **Babinski reflex** causes the toes to spread apart automatically when the sole of the foot is stimulated, as seen in Figure 1.26. The **grasping reflex** occurs when infants close their fingers around an object placed in the hand. Adults with neurological diseases may exhibit these primitive reflexes, especially in illnesses that cause demyelination (loss of the myelin sheath).

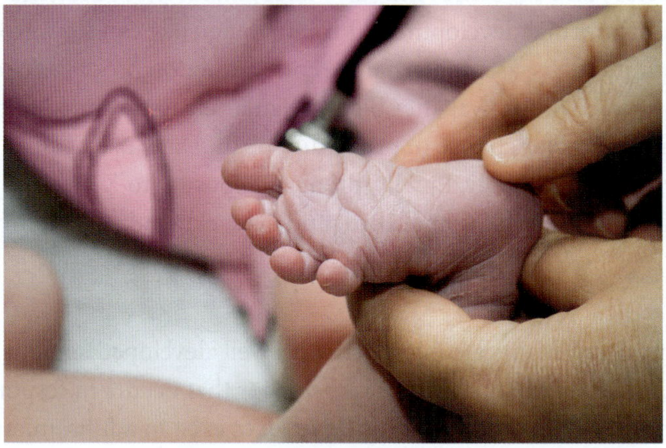

Figure 1.26 The Babinski Reflex
The big toe extends while the other toes fan outward.

Although reflexive behavior dominates the repertoire of the neonate, other behaviors occur as well. Newborn infants also kick, turn, and wave their arms. These uncoordinated, unconnected behaviors form the basis for later, more coordinated movements.

Infants typically develop motor skills at about the same age, in the same order. Due to this pattern, most psychologists and doctors agree that these are innately programmed abilities for human infants. However, the educational richness of the environment has been observed to affect the rate of learning, with more enriched environments promoting quicker development.

Motor skills are broken down into two classes: gross and fine motor skills. **Gross motor skills** incorporate movement from large muscle groups and whole body motion, such as sitting, crawling, and walking. **Fine motor skills** involve the smaller muscles of the fingers, toes, and eyes, providing more specific and delicate movement. Fine motor abilities include tracking motion, drawing, catching, and waving.

Social

In addition to motor skills, social development occurs in infancy and through adolescence. At birth, the parental figure becomes the center of the infant's world, and as the infant ages, **stranger anxiety** (a fear and apprehension of unfamiliar individuals) and **separation anxiety** (a fear of being separated from the parental figure) develop at approximately seven months and one year, respectively. During this time, the child progresses from **solitary play** to being an **onlooker** while other children play, and at two years they begin to **parallel play**, in which children will play alongside each other without influencing each other's behavior. For example, instead of playing a game in a structured way in which each child takes their turn and then sits patiently while others take their turns, children engaging in parallel play with a game may act on game materials (board, cards, etc.) at the same time, focusing on different parts of it without directly interacting. Figure 1.27 depicts this transition in play stages. At age three, children have an awareness of their assigned gender at birth, engage in gender-stereotyped play, and know their full name.

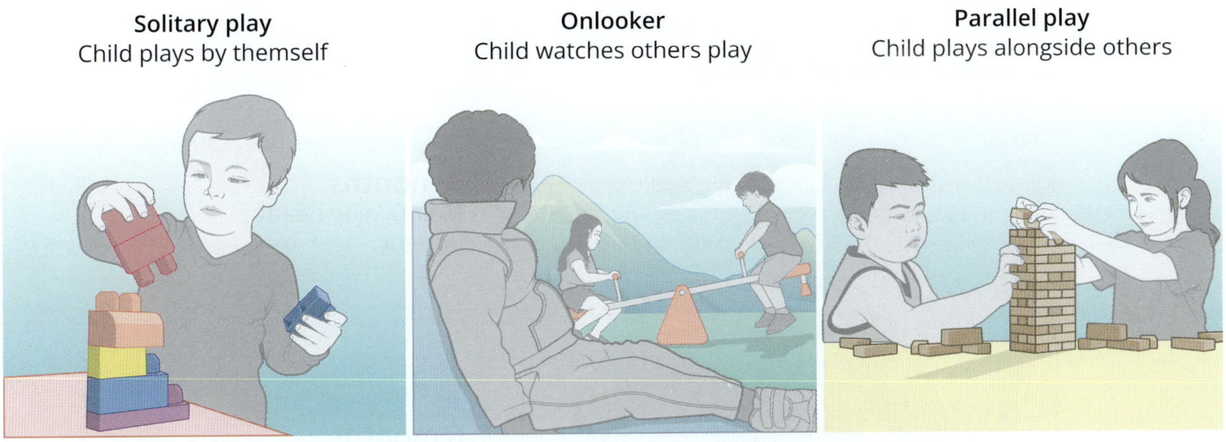
Solitary play
Child plays by themself
Onlooker
Child watches others play
Parallel play
Child plays alongside others

Figure 1.27 Developmental Play Stages

By age five, conformity to peers and romantic feelings for others begin to develop. From ages six through twelve, friend circles tend to be of the same gender without expression of romantic feelings. In the teenage years, children become more self-sufficient, and often express their desire for independence by rebelling against their parents. Inter-gender friendships become more common. Individuals also become more aware of their gender identity and sexual orientation and may begin sexual relationships.

In this chapter we have described several abilities and behaviors that are expected to emerge at particular times in a person's development. These skills are known as **developmental milestones**. The developmental milestones of the first three years of life are listed in Table 1.4. While this is a general timetable based on averages, most children fall within plus or minus two months of the chart. The goal is not to memorize this chart, but to recognize some themes. As shown in Figure 1.28, gross motor skills progress in a head-to-toe order: children first develop the ability to lift the head, then to stabilize the trunk, and finally to walk. There is also a correlation between the development of motor skills and proximity to the center of the body, with skills being developed at the core prior to extremities. Social skills move from being parent-oriented to self-oriented to other-oriented. Language skills, discussed in Chapter 4 of *MCAT Behavioral Sciences Review*, become more complex and structured.

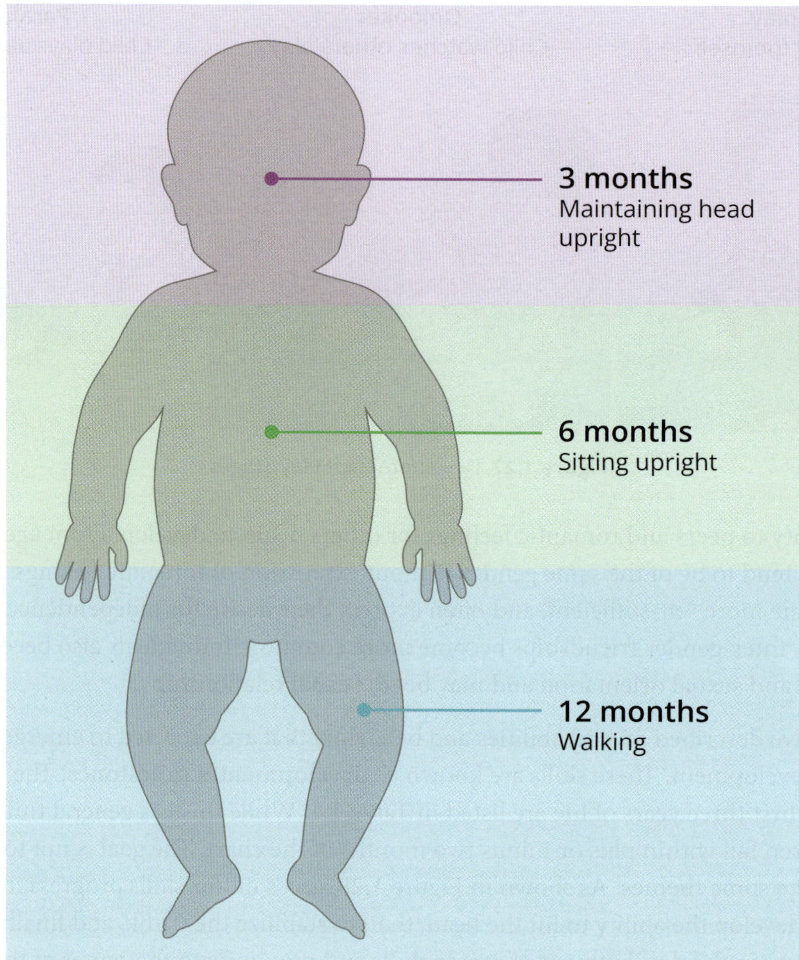

Figure 1.28 Head-to-Toe Development of Gross Motor Skills

Age	Physical and Motor Developments	Social Developments	Language Developments
1st year of life	• Puts everything in mouth • Sits with support (4 mo) • Stands with help (8 mo) • Crawls, fear of falling (9 mo) • Pincer grasp (10 mo) • Follows objects to midline (4 wk) • One-handed approach/grasp of toy • Feet in mouth (5 mo) • Bang and rattle stage • Changes hands with toy (6 mo)	• Parental figure central • Issues of trust are key • Stranger anxiety (7 mo) • Play is solitary and exploratory • Pat-a-cake, peek-a-boo (10 mo)	• Laughs aloud (4 mo) • Repetitive responding (8 mo) • "mama, dada" (10 mo)
Age 1	• Walks alone (13 mo) • Climbs stairs alone (18 mo) • Emergence of hand preference (18 mo) • Kicks ball, throws ball • Pats pictures in book • Stacks three cubes (18 mo)	• Separation anxiety (12 mo) • Dependency on parental figure • Onlooker play	• Great variation in timing of language development • Uses 10 words
Age 2	• High activity level • Walks backward • Can turn doorknob, unscrew jar lid • Scribbles with crayon • Stacks six cubes (24 mo) • Stands on tiptoes (30 mo) • Able to aim thrown ball	• Selfish and self-centered • Imitates mannerisms and activities • May be aggressive • Recognizes self in mirror • "No" is favorite word • Parallel play	• Use of pronouns • Parents understand most • Two-word sentences • Uses 250 words • Identifies body parts by pointing
Age 3	• Rides tricycle • Stacks nine cubes (36 mo) • Alternates feet going up stairs • Bowel and bladder control (toilet training) • Draws recognizable figures • Catches ball with arms • Cuts paper with scissors • Unbuttons buttons	• Awareness of assigned gender • Gender-stereotyped play • Understands "taking turns" • Knows full name	• Complete sentences • Uses 900 words • Understands 3600 words • Strangers can understand • Recognizes common objects in pictures • Can answer, "Tell me what we wear on our feet?" "Which block is bigger?"

Table 1.4 Child Development Milestones

MCAT CONCEPT CHECK 1.6

Before you move on, assess your understanding of the material with these questions.

1. Describe the process of neurulation.

   ___

2. For each of the primitive reflexes below, briefly describe the observed behavior.

Primitive Reflex	Behavior
Rooting	
Moro	
Babinski	
Grasping	

3. What are the two main themes that dictate the stages of motor development in early childhood?

   1. ___
   2. ___

Conclusion

Behavioral psychology is the study of all physical and mental actions based on the response of the body to external stimuli, specifically the activity of the nervous and endocrine systems. The nervous system is a complex organization of structures and neurons that communicate and coordinate information. The endocrine system, in conjunction with the nervous system, controls human behavior. Aside from neurotransmitter and hormonal control of behavior, certain behaviors are genetically passed from generation to generation, as are many other physical traits. The genetic aspects of behavior are thought to interact with the learned components of behavior. Human behavior is also studied as it correlates to the development from embryo to fetus to infant and well into adolescence and adulthood. The development of motor skills and social behavior is seen to progress at a consistent rate across the species.

In the next chapter, our focus will be on the neurological systems used to interact with the world—most notably, those systems that exist for sensation and perception of the environment. These include vision, hearing, smell and taste, somatosensation, and others.

GO ONLINE

You've reviewed the content, now test your knowledge and critical thinking skills by completing a test-like passage set in your online resources!

CONCEPT SUMMARY

A Brief History of Neuropsychology

- **Neuropsychology** is the study of the connection between the nervous system and behavior. It most often focuses on the functions of various brain regions.

Organization of the Human Nervous System

- There are three types of neurons in the nervous system: **sensory** (**afferent**) neurons, **motor** (**efferent**) neurons, and **interneurons**.
- **Reflex arcs** use the ability of interneurons in the spinal cord to relay information to the source of stimuli while simultaneously routing it to the brain.
- The nervous system is made up of the **central nervous system** (**CNS**; brain and spinal cord) and **peripheral nervous system** (**PNS**; most cranial and spinal nerves).
  - The PNS is divided into the **somatic** (voluntary) and **autonomic** (automatic) divisions.
  - The autonomic system is further divided into the **parasympathetic** (rest-and-digest) and **sympathetic** (fight-or-flight) branches.

Organization of the Brain

- The brain has three subdivisions: hindbrain, midbrain, and forebrain.
  - The **hindbrain** contains the cerebellum, medulla oblongata, and reticular formation.
  - The **midbrain** contains the inferior and superior colliculi.
  - The **forebrain** contains the thalamus, hypothalamus, basal ganglia, limbic system, and cerebral cortex.
- Methods of studying the brain include studying humans and animals with lesions, electrical stimulation and activity recording (including **electroencephalography** [**EEG**]), and **regional cerebral blood flow**.

Parts of the Forebrain

- The **thalamus** is a relay station for sensory information.
- The **hypothalamus** maintains homeostasis and integrates with the endocrine system through the **hypophyseal portal system** that connects it to the **anterior pituitary**.
- The **basal ganglia** smoothen movements and help maintain postural stability.
- The **limbic system**, which contains the septal nuclei, amygdala, and hippocampus, controls emotion and memory.
  - The **septal nuclei** are involved with feelings of pleasure, pleasure-seeking behavior, and addiction.
  - The **amygdala** controls fear and aggression.
  - The **hippocampus** consolidates memories and communicates with other parts of the limbic system through an extension called the **fornix**.
- The **cerebral cortex** is divided into four lobes: frontal, parietal, occipital, and temporal.
  - The **frontal lobe** controls executive function, impulse control, long-term planning, motor function, and speech production.

- The **parietal lobe** controls sensations of touch, pressure, temperature, and pain; spatial processing; orientation; and manipulation.
- The **occipital lobe** controls visual processing.
- The **temporal lobe** controls sound processing, speech perception, memory, and emotion.

- The brain is divided into two **cerebral hemispheres**, left and right. In most individuals, the left hemisphere is the dominant hemisphere for language.

Influences on Behavior

- **Neurotransmitters** are released by neurons and carry a signal to another neuron or effector (a muscle fiber or a gland).
  - **Acetylcholine** is used by the somatic nervous system (to move muscles), the parasympathetic nervous system, and the central nervous system (for alertness).
  - **Dopamine** maintains smooth movements and steady posture.
  - **Endorphins** and **enkephalins** act as natural painkillers.
  - **Epinephrine** and **norepinephrine** maintain wakefulness and alertness and mediate fight-or-flight responses. Epinephrine tends to act as a hormone, and norepinephrine tends to act more classically as a neurotransmitter.
  - γ-**Aminobutyric acid** (**GABA**) and **glycine** act as brain "stabilizers."
  - **Glutamate** acts as an excitatory neurotransmitter in the brain.
  - **Serotonin** modulates mood, sleep patterns, eating patterns, and dreaming.
- The endocrine system is tied to the nervous system through the hypothalamus and the anterior pituitary, as well as a few other hormones.
  - **Cortisol** is a stress hormone released by the adrenal cortex.
  - **Testosterone** and **estrogen** mediate libido; testosterone also increases aggressive behavior. Both are released by the adrenal cortex. In males, the testes also produce testosterone. In females, the ovaries also produce estrogen.
  - **Epinephrine** and **norepinephrine** are released by the adrenal medulla and cause physiological changes associated with the sympathetic nervous system.
- **Nature vs. nurture** is a classic debate regarding the relative contributions of genetics (nature) and environment (nurture) to an individual's traits. For most traits, both nature and nurture play a role. The relative effects of each can be studied.
  - **Family studies** look at the relative frequency of a trait within a family compared to the general population.
  - **Twin studies** compare concordance rates between monozygotic (identical) and dizygotic (fraternal) twins.
  - **Adoption studies** compare similarities between children who were adopted and their adoptive parents, relative to similarities with their biological parents.

Development

- The nervous system develops through neurulation, in which the notochord stimulates overlying ectoderm to fold over, creating a **neural tube** topped with **neural crest** cells.
  - The **neural tube** becomes the central nervous system (CNS).
  - The **neural crest** cells spread out throughout the body, differentiating into many different tissues.
- **Primitive reflexes** exist in infants and should disappear with age. Most primitive reflexes serve (or served, in earlier times) a protective role. They can reappear in certain nervous system disorders.
  - In the **rooting reflex**, infants turn their heads toward anything that brushes the cheek.
  - In the **Moro reflex**, the infant extends the arms, then slowly retracts them and cries in response to a sensation of falling.
  - In the **Babinski reflex**, the big toe is extended and the other toes fan in response to the brushing of the sole of the foot.
  - In the **grasping reflex**, infants grab anything put into their hands.
- Developmental milestones give an indication of what skills and abilities a child should have at a given age. Most children adhere closely to these milestones, deviating by only one or two months.
  - Gross and fine motor abilities progress head to toe and core to periphery.
  - Social skills shift from parent-oriented to self-oriented to other-oriented.
  - Language skills become increasingly complex.

ANSWERS TO CONCEPT CHECKS

1.1

1. - Franz Gall: phrenology; associated development of a trait with growth of its relevant part of the brain.
   - Pierre Flourens: extirpation/ablation; concluded that different brain regions have specific functions.
   - William James: "founder of American psychology"; pushed for importance of studying adaptations of the individual to the environment.
   - John Dewey: credited with the landmark article on functionalism; argued for studying the entire organism as a whole.
   - Paul Broca: correlated pathology with specific brain regions, such as speech production from Broca's area.
   - Hermann von Helmholtz: measured speed of a nerve impulse.
   - Sir Charles Sherrington: inferred the existence of synapses.

1.2

1. The central nervous system includes the brain and spinal cord. The peripheral nervous system includes most of the cranial and spinal nerves and sensors.
2. Afferent (sensory) neurons bring signals from a sensor to the central nervous system. Efferent (motor) neurons bring signals from the central nervous system to an effector.
3. The somatic nervous system is responsible for voluntary actions; most notably, moving muscles. The autonomic nervous system is responsible for involuntary actions, like heart rate, bronchial dilation, dilation of the eyes, exocrine gland function, and peristalsis.
4. The sympathetic nervous system promotes a fight-or-flight response, with increased heart rate and bronchial dilation, redistribution of blood to locomotor muscles, dilation of the eyes, and slowing of digestive and urinary functions. The parasympathetic nervous system promotes rest-and-digest functions, slowing heart rate and constricting the bronchi, redistributing blood to the gut, promoting exocrine secretions, constricting the pupils, and promoting peristalsis and urinary function.

1.3

1.

Subdivision	Functions
Hindbrain	Balance, motor coordination, breathing, digestion, general arousal processes (sleeping and waking); "vital functioning"
Midbrain	Receives sensory and motor information from the rest of the body; reflexes to auditory and visual stimuli
Forebrain	Complex perceptual, cognitive, and behavioral processes; emotion and memory

2. Methods used for mapping the brain include studying humans with brain lesions, extirpation, stimulation or recording with electrodes (cortical mapping, single-cell electrode recordings, electroencephalogram [EEG]), and regional cerebral blood flow (rCBF).
3. From most deep to most superficial, the structures surrounding the brain are the meninges, bone, periosteum, and skin.

1.4

1. 1–A, 2–H, 3–F, 4–E, 5–C, 6–I, 7–G, 8–D, 9–B
2.

Lobe	Function
Frontal	Executive function, impulse control, long-term planning (prefrontal cortex), motor function (primary motor cortex), speech production (Broca's area)
Parietal	Sensation of touch, pressure, temperature, and pain (somatosensory cortex); spatial processing, orientation, and manipulation
Occipital	Visual processing
Temporal	Sound processing (auditory cortex), speech perception (Wernicke's area), memory, and emotion (limbic system)

3. Ipsilateral communication occurs when cerebral hemispheres communicate with the same side of the body. Contralateral communication occurs when cerebral hemispheres communicate with the opposite side of the body.
4. The dominant hemisphere is typically defined as the one that is more heavily stimulated during language reception and production.

1.5

1. 1–F, 2–E, 3–D, 4–A, 5–B, 6–G, 7–C
2. The hypothalamus controls release of pituitary hormones; the pituitary is the "master gland" that triggers hormone secretion in many other endocrine glands. The adrenal medulla produces adrenaline (epinephrine), which causes sympathetic nervous system effects throughout the body. The adrenal cortex produces cortisol, a stress hormone. The adrenal cortex and testes produce testosterone, which is associated with libido.
3. Nature is defined as heredity, or the influence of inherited characteristics on behavior. Nurture refers to the influence of environment and physical surroundings on behavior. It has long been debated whether nature or nurture has the larger influence; it is a complicated situation, but for most traits, both exert some influence.
4.

Study	Sample Group	Control Group
Family study	Family of genetically related individuals	Unrelated individuals (general population)
Twin study	Monozygotic (MZ, identical) twins	Dizygotic (DZ, fraternal) twins
Adoption study	Adoptive family (relative to child who was adopted)	Biological family (relative to child who was adopted)

1.6

1. Neurulation occurs when a furrow is produced from ectoderm overlying the notochord and consists of the neural groove and two neural folds. As the neural folds grow, the cells at their leading edge are called neural crest cells. When the neural folds fuse, this creates the neural tube, which will form the CNS.

2.

Primitive Reflex	Behavior
Rooting	Turns head toward direction of any object touching the cheek
Moro	In response to sudden head movement, arms extend and slowly retract; baby usually cries
Babinski	Extension of big toe and fanning of other toes in response to brushing the sole of the foot
Grasping	Holding onto any object placed in the hand

3. Gross motor development proceeds from head to toe, and from the core to the periphery.

SCIENCE MASTERY ASSESSMENT EXPLANATIONS

1. **B**

Creating knockouts to study gene function is similar to ablation, or extirpation, in which specific parts of an organism's anatomy are removed. This approach was used by Pierre Flourens to show that specific parts of the brain served particular functions, supporting **(B)** as the correct answer. Unlike Pierre, Paul Broca, choice **(A)**, did not ablate regions of the brain; rather he studied the functional impairments in individuals with different brain lesions.

2. **B**

The cerebral cortex is not involved in the initial reflexive response to pain. Instead, the sensory receptors send information to the interneurons in the spinal cord, which stimulate a motor neuron to allow quick withdrawal. While the brain does ultimately get the signal, the reflexive withdrawal has already occurred by that time.

3. **C**

The hindbrain is responsible for balance and motor coordination, which would be necessary for dribbling a basketball. The midbrain, **(B)**, manages sensorimotor reflexes that also promote survival. The forebrain, **(A)**, is associated with emotion, memory, and higher-order cognition. The spinal cord, **(D)**, is likely not damaged as the child can still walk.

4. **D**

The temporal lobes have many functions, but motor skills are not associated with this area. The temporal lobes contain Wernicke's area, which is responsible for language comprehension, **(A)**. The temporal lobes also function in memory and emotion, **(B)** and **(C)**, because they contain the hippocampus and amygdala. Motor skills are associated with the frontal lobe (primary motor cortex), basal ganglia (smooth movements), and cerebellum (coordination).

5. **C**

The hypothalamus is responsible for homeostatic and emotional functions. The cerebellum, **(A)**, is responsible for maintaining posture and balance while the pons, **(B)**, is above the medulla and contains sensory and motor tracts between the cortex and the medulla. The thalamus, **(D)**, acts as a relay station for sensory information.

6. **A**

The right hemisphere is usually the nondominant hemisphere, even in left-handed individuals. Sense of direction is an ability of the nondominant hemisphere. The other answer choices are all abilities attributed to the dominant hemisphere.

7. **B**

Neurulation occurs when the notochord causes differentiation of overlying ectoderm into the neural tube and neural crest cells. The neural tube ultimately becomes the central nervous system (brain and spinal cord), and neural crest cells migrate to other sites in the body to differentiate into a number of different tissues. Thus, only statement III is true.

8. **D**

Catecholamines are the hormones produced by the adrenal glands during the fight-or-flight response, and include epinephrine, norepinephrine, and dopamine. Acetylcholine is produced by cholinergic neurons and is, thus, not a catecholamine.

9. **A**

If there were increased amounts of acetylcholinesterase, more acetylcholine would be degraded, lowering acetylcholine levels in the body. Low levels of acetylcholine would result in weakness or paralysis of muscles. Pain, **(B)**, could result if one were injured and endorphins were found in low levels. Mood swings, **(C)**, could be a result of varying levels of serotonin. Hallucinations, **(D)**, have been seen to result from high levels of dopamine.

10. **A**

The adrenal glands do promote the fight-or-flight response, but through epinephrine and norepinephrine, not estrogen. The adrenal cortex produces both estrogen and testosterone in both sexes, as mentioned in **(D)**, thus serving as a source of estrogen in males and testosterone in females.

11. **C**

The pineal gland is responsible for producing melatonin, which controls the body's circadian rhythm. Insomnia would be a disturbance of this circadian rhythm, and may be attributable to a pineal gland disorder in some cases. Hypertension, diabetes, and hyperthyroidism would be unrelated to issues with the pineal gland.

12. **A**

William James studied how the mind adapts to the environment and formed the foundation of functionalism. Thus, **(A)** is correct. The remaining wrong answer choices can be ascribed to other scientists. Answer **(B)** describes phrenology, the theory of Franz Gall. Answer **(C)** describes the conclusions of Paul Broca. Answer **(D)** describes one of the conclusions of Sir Charles Sherrington (although we now know that his conclusion was false).

13. **C**

Activity in different regions of the brain is assumed to positively correlate with blood flow. Thus, regions that are more active should have increased blood flow. Changes in blood flow can be measured via fMRI, supporting **(C)** as the preferred methodology. On the other hand, MRI and CT scans are used to image tissues, ruling out **(A)** and **(B)**, and EEGs are useful in measuring broad brain activity and not specific brain regions, eliminating **(D)**.

14. **D**

The Babinski reflex is a primitive reflex that refers to an extension of the big toe accompanied by fanning of the other toes. It is normal in infants, but should disappear with time—certainly by the time a child begins to walk. In a person who is fifty years old, the Babinski reflex would be abnormal. However, despite having a neurological illness, this patient is exhibiting a normal response to the brushing of the foot; that is, the patient is not showing the Babinski reflex.

15. **B**

Motor skills tend to develop from the core toward the periphery. Following objects with the eyes occurs around four weeks of age. The other actions all require movements of the hand, which do not occur in an organized fashion until later.

GO ONLINE

Consult your online resources for additional practice.

SHARED CONCEPTS

Behavioral Sciences Chapter 2
Sensation and Perception

Behavioral Sciences Chapter 3
Learning and Memory

Behavioral Sciences Chapter 4
Cognition, Consciousness, and Language

Biology Review Chapter 3
Embryogenesis and Development

Biology Review Chapter 4
The Nervous System

Biology Review Chapter 5
The Endocrine System

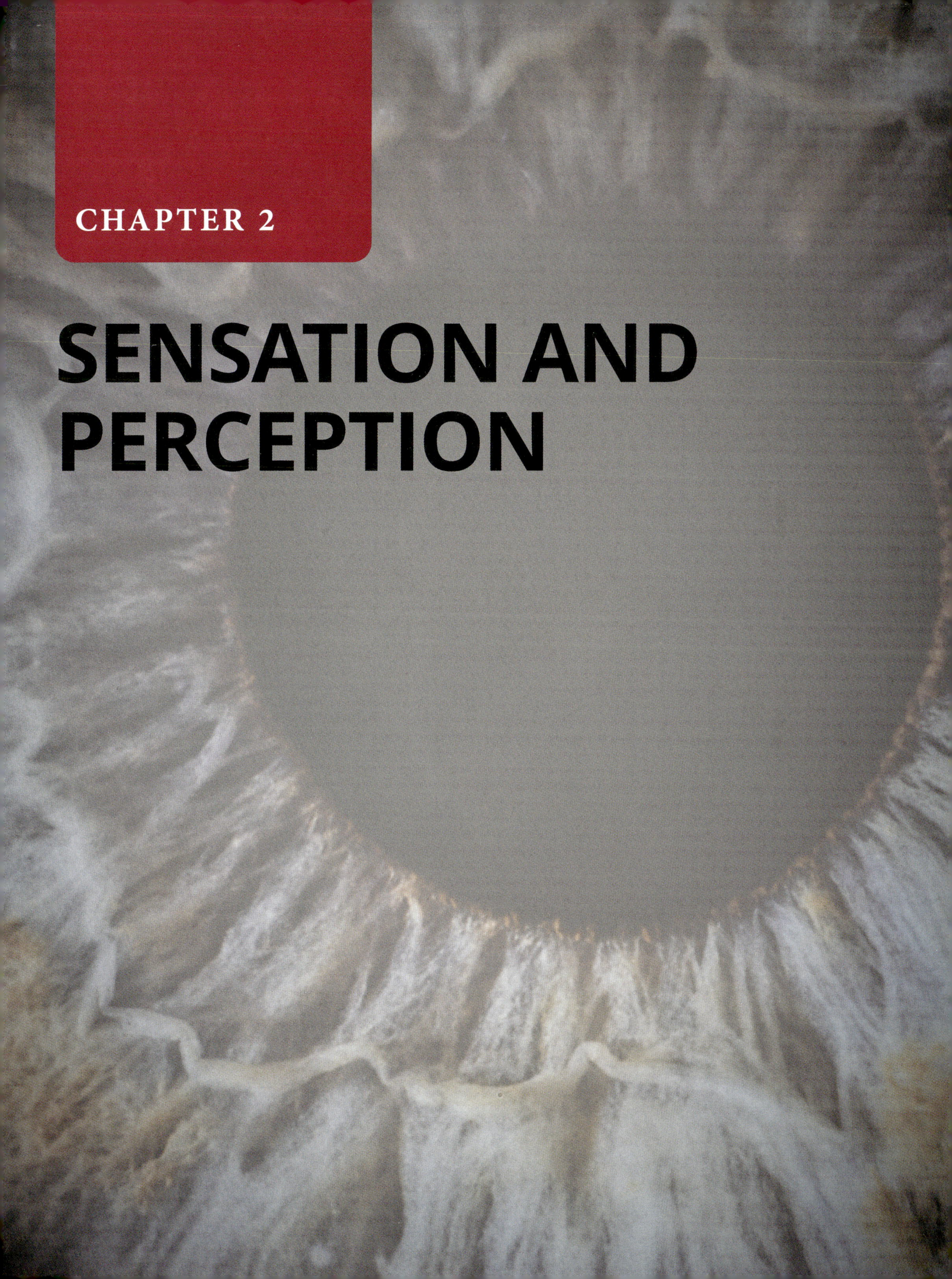

CHAPTER 2

SENSATION AND PERCEPTION

SCIENCE MASTERY ASSESSMENT

Every pre-med knows this feeling: there is so much content I have to know for the MCAT! How do I know what to do first or what's important?

While the high-yield badges throughout this book will help you identify the most important topics, this Science Mastery Assessment is another tool in your MCAT prep arsenal. This quiz (which can also be taken in your online resources) and the guidance below will help ensure that you are spending the appropriate amount of time on this chapter based on your personal strengths and weaknesses. Don't worry though—skipping something now does not mean you'll never study it. Later on in your prep, as you complete full-length tests, you'll uncover specific pieces of content that you need to review and can come back to these chapters as appropriate.

How to Use This Assessment

If you answer 0–7 questions correctly:

Spend about 1 hour to read this chapter in full and take limited notes throughout. Follow up by reviewing **all** quiz questions to ensure that you now understand how to solve each one.

If you answer 8–11 questions correctly:

Spend 20–40 minutes reviewing the quiz questions. Beginning with the questions you missed, read and take notes on the corresponding subchapters. For questions you answered correctly, ensure your thinking matches that of the explanation and you understand why each choice was correct or incorrect.

If you answer 12–15 questions correctly:

Spend less than 20 minutes reviewing all questions from the quiz. If you missed any, then include a quick read-through of the corresponding subchapters, or even just the relevant content within a subchapter, as part of your question review. For questions you answered correctly, ensure your thinking matches that of the explanation and review the Concept Summary at the end of the chapter.

1. A weight lifter is just able to tell the difference between 100 and 125 pounds. According to Weber's law, the lifter would notice a difference between:
   - **A.** 125 and 150 pounds.
   - **B.** 5 and 6 pounds.
   - **C.** 25 and 35 pounds.
   - **D.** 225 and 275 pounds.

2. A person is at a party with a friend. There is loud music in the background and the location is crowded. While listening to the music, the person hears what seems like the friend's laughter and turns around to investigate. The person is exhibiting:
   - **A.** feature detection.
   - **B.** bottom-up processing.
   - **C.** vestibular sense.
   - **D.** signal detection.

3. A person is at a restaurant and orders a spicy entrée. After the first bite, the person experiences burning in the mouth and becomes concerned that the food is too hot. The next few bites are similarly uncomfortable, but after a while the spiciness seems to subside somewhat, and by the end of the meal, the person doesn't notice the spice level. The end of the meal experience is best described as:
   - **A.** adaptation.
   - **B.** signal detection.
   - **C.** a difference threshold.
   - **D.** pain perception.

4. Which sensory receptors send signals in response to tissue damage?
   - **A.** Chemoreceptors
   - **B.** Nociceptors
   - **C.** Osmoreceptors
   - **D.** Photoreceptors

5. Which part of the eye is responsible for gathering and focusing light?
   - **A.** Cornea
   - **B.** Pupil
   - **C.** Iris
   - **D.** Retina

6. A person is looking for change to do laundry and decides to look under the seats of the household car. Even using a flashlight allows no more than an obscured look at the space below. There are various items such as wrappers and papers, but the person sees the glint of silver from an object laying flat and determines it to be a coin. To make this determination, this person used:
   - **A.** signal detection.
   - **B.** sensory adaptation.
   - **C.** feature detection.
   - **D.** kinesthetic sense.

7. Upon which part of the eye are images projected and transduced into electrical signals?
   - **A.** Cornea
   - **B.** Pupil
   - **C.** Retina
   - **D.** Lens

8. The ability to sense stimuli against one's own skin is known as:
   - **A.** somatosensation.
   - **B.** kinesthetic sense.
   - **C.** vestibular sense.
   - **D.** chemoreception.

9. Which of the following is NOT a taste modality?
   - **A.** Sweet
   - **B.** Floral
   - **C.** Savory
   - **D.** Bitter

10. Which of the following best describes the difference between endolymph and perilymph?
    - **A.** Endolymph is found in the vestibule, while perilymph is found in the cochlea.
    - **B.** Endolymph is found in the cochlea, while perilymph is found in the vestibule.
    - **C.** Endolymph is found in the membranous labyrinth, while perilymph is found in the bony labyrinth.
    - **D.** Endolymph is found in the bony labyrinth, while perilymph is found in the membranous labyrinth.

11. Chemicals that compel behavior after binding with chemoreceptors are known as:
    - **A.** pheromones.
    - **B.** olfactory receptors.
    - **C.** somatostimuli.
    - **D.** papillae.

12. Prolonged vitamin B_{12} deficiency can be associated with subacute combined degeneration of the spinal cord. Patients with this disease have difficulty walking because they lose the ability to feel where their feet are in space. This represents a loss of:
    - **A.** vestibular sense.
    - **B.** kinesthetic sense.
    - **C.** parallel processing.
    - **D.** feature detection.

13. A person proofreading a paper reads over a long, misspelled word in which an "e" is replaced with an "o." The person does not recognize the error and reads the word as correct. Which of the following could explain why the proofreader read the word as correct?
    - **A.** Parallel processing
    - **B.** Feature detection
    - **C.** Top-down processing
    - **D.** Bottom-up processing

14. A corporate logo uses five unconnected angles equally spaced in a circular fashion. When viewed, it appears to be a star. Which of the following is the logo artist using to create a complete pattern to viewers?
    - **A.** Bottom-up processing
    - **B.** Top-down processing
    - **C.** Gate theory
    - **D.** Gestalt principles

15. A patient comes in with a tumor of the pituitary gland which has grown upward into the optic chiasm and caused a visual field defect. The most likely defect from compression of the optic chiasm is:
    - **A.** complete blindness in one eye.
    - **B.** loss of the upper visual fields in both eyes.
    - **C.** loss of the nasal visual fields in both eyes.
    - **D.** loss of the temporal visual fields in both eyes.

Answer Key

1. **C** (See section 2.1)
2. **D** (See section 2.1)
3. **A** (See section 2.4)
4. **B** (See section 2.4)
5. **A** (See section 2.2)
6. **C** (See section 2.5)
7. **C** (See section 2.2)
8. **A** (See section 2.4)
9. **B** (See section 2.4)
10. **C** (See section 2.3)
11. **A** (See section 2.4)
12. **B** (See section 2.3)
13. **C** (See section 2.5)
14. **D** (See section 2.5)
15. **D** (See section 2.2)

The relevant section of the chapter to review for each question is given in parentheses after the correct answer. Detailed explanations can be found at the end of the chapter.

CHAPTER 2

SENSATION AND PERCEPTION

In This Chapter

CHAPTER PROFILE

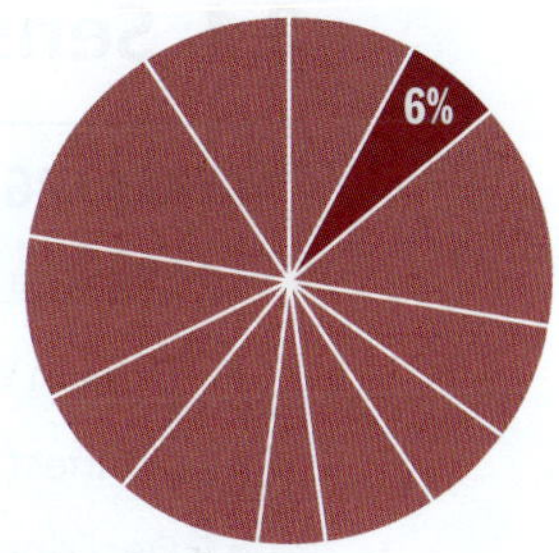

The content in this chapter should be relevant to about 6% of all questions about the behavioral sciences on the MCAT.

This chapter covers material from the following AAMC content category:

6A: Sensing the environment

Introduction

It's your first time visiting a new city. You can't wait to explore the area, try out a new café or restaurant, and see famous landmarks there. You want to take in the sights and sounds of this new place—you want to have a sensory experience. To truly experience any location, your sensory receptors—for vision, hearing, taste, smell, and somatosensation—gather all of the information from the world around you, and your brain filters and processes that information to focus on the most salient details. This activity involves a complex interplay between sensory processes, neural tracts, and the brain itself.

You finally arrive in the new city and begin to explore. You turn the corner on one street and are suddenly overwhelmed with an odd feeling of familiarity. *But . . . I've never been here before!* you think as the strange sensation of *déjà vu* sets in. Everything just seems "right": the signs are in the proper place, the cars look familiar, and everything is bizarrely where you expect it to be. *Déjà vu* (French for "already seen") comes from many sources, including processing information faster than expected. When you process an image (or other sensory input) for the first time, it actually takes longer than the next time you are exposed to that same stimulus. Thus, an exposure to the same scenery at an earlier time through a movie or television show may have primed you for *déjà vu*.

But we don't feel *déjà vu* every time we see an image again; that's where memory comes in—a topic we'll discuss in Chapter 3 of *MCAT Behavioral Sciences Review*. Indeed, this phenomenon of *déjà vu* comes from the brain's sensory receptors saying, *Yes, you have seen this before!* in tandem with the memory system saying, *But I don't know when or where!*

In this chapter, we will focus on the concept of sensation and its associated receptors, including the eyes and hair cells in the ear, as well as perception and the complex brain functions associated with processing sensory information. We'll briefly touch on the other sensory modalities, including vestibular sense, taste, smell, somatosensation, and kinesthetic sense, and consider the roles these senses play in helping us interact with the world.

2.1 Sensation vs. Perception

LEARNING OBJECTIVES

After Chapter 2.1, you will be able to:

- Explain the pathway for a stimulus to reach conscious perception
- Connect the common sensory receptors to their functions
- Describe absolute threshold, threshold of conscious perception, and difference threshold
- Explain Weber's law and signal detection theory
- Describe how sensory adaptation affects a difference threshold

In common parlance, we often use the terms "sensation" and "perception" interchangeably, as synonyms. However, in the field of psychology, these two terms have very specific definitions and are commonly contrasted. **Sensation** more appropriately aligns with **transduction**, which means taking the physical, electromagnetic, auditory, and other information from our internal and external environment and converting this information into electrical signals in the nervous system. Sensation is performed by receptors in the peripheral nervous system, which forward the stimuli to the central nervous system in the form of action potentials and neurotransmitters. Sensation can therefore be thought of as a raw signal, which is unfiltered and unprocessed until it enters the central nervous system.

Perception, on the other hand, refers to processing this information within the central nervous system in order to make sense of the information's significance. The complex manipulations involved in perception include both the external sensory experience and the internal activities of the brain and spinal cord (see Figure 2.1). Regions of the brain like the thalamus help organize and process incoming signals. Perception thus helps us make sense of the world. The difference between sensation and perception is key to the challenge of creating autonomous robots that can navigate and interact with the real world: we can easily create sensors for robots to pick up information from their environment, but teaching them how to comprehend and respond to that information is far more challenging.

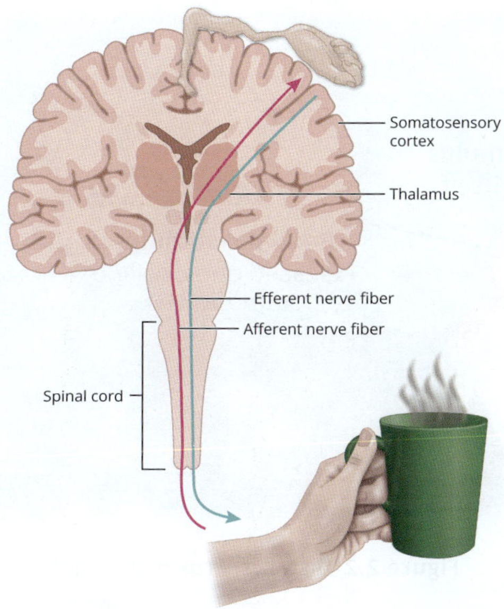

Figure 2.1 The Pathway of Conscious Stimuli

Sensory processing is a common topic on the MCAT; you should not only understand the definitions of these terms, but also be able to apply the concepts herein to your own day-to-day sensory experiences.

Sensory Receptors

Sensory receptors are neurons that respond to stimuli by triggering electrical signals that carry information to the central nervous system. Physical objects outside of the body are referred to as **distal stimuli**. These objects often produce photons, sound waves, heat, pressure, or other stimuli that directly interact with sensory receptors; these sensory-stimulating byproducts are called **proximal stimuli**. For example, a campfire is a distal stimulus (Figure 2.2). The photons that are emitted by the fire, the sounds of crackling and popping, and the energetic gas particles that transfer heat energy are all proximal stimuli. So, proximal stimuli directly interact with and affect the sensory receptors, and thereby inform the observer about the presence of distal stimuli. Sensory receptors may encode multiple aspects of a stimulus. For example, photoreceptors respond to light and can encode not only the brightness of the light, but also its color and shape. The relationship between the physical nature of stimuli and the sensations and perceptions these stimuli evoke is studied in the field of **psychophysics**.

MNEMONIC

Distal = in the **distan**ce

Proximal = in close **proxim**ity

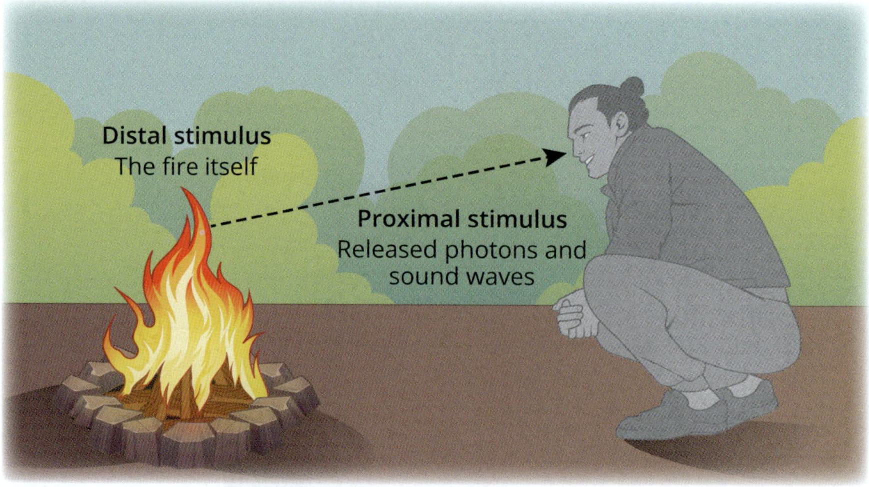

Figure 2.2 Distal vs. Proximal Stimuli

In order to inform the central nervous system, the signals from these stimuli must pass through specific sensory pathways. In each case, different types of receptors—generally nerve endings or specific sensory cells—receive the stimulus, transduce the stimulus into electrical signals, and transmit the data to the central nervous system through sensory ganglia. **Ganglia** are collections of neuron cell bodies found outside the central nervous system. Once transduction from these sensory ganglia occurs, the electrochemical energy is sent along neural pathways to various **projection areas** in the brain, which further analyze the sensory input.

Sensory receptors differ from one sense to another. There are over a dozen recognized sensory receptors, but the MCAT is unlikely to test even half of those. The most heavily tested receptors include:

- Photoreceptors: respond to electromagnetic waves in the visible spectrum (sight)
- Mechanoreceptors: respond to pressure or movement. Hair cells, for example, respond to movement of fluid in the inner ear structures (movement, vibration, hearing, rotational and linear acceleration)
- Nociceptors: respond to painful or noxious stimuli (somatosensation)
- Thermoreceptors: respond to changes in temperature (thermosensation)
- Osmoreceptors: respond to the osmolarity of the blood (water homeostasis)
- Olfactory receptors: respond to volatile compounds (smell)
- Taste receptors: respond to dissolved compounds (taste)

Thresholds

Perception, like sensation, is closely tied to the biology and physiology of interpreting the world around us. However, unlike sensation, perception is inextricably linked to experience as well as to internal and external biases. Sensations are relayed to the brain, which perceives the significance of the stimulus. To illustrate the significance of perception, keep in mind that all sensory information is sent to the central nervous system in the form of action potentials, which the central nervous system must then interpret and act upon. For example, the central nervous system must determine whether incoming action potentials from thermoreceptors are indicating whether an object is hot or is cold, and whether that temperature difference is enough to cause us harm. Moreover, the same sensation can produce radically different perceptions in different people, and because these variations must be explained by central nervous system activity, perception is considered a part of psychology.

A good example of the psychological element of perception is a **threshold**—the minimum amount of a stimulus that renders a difference in perception. For example, the temperature may noticeably change from warm to cool when the sun sets, but subtle fluctuations in temperature throughout the day are generally unnoticeable because they are below the difference threshold. If sound volume increases 10 dB (ten times the sound intensity), the change is usually very obvious; but, if volume increases only 0.1 dB, the change might be too small to detect. There are three main types of thresholds: the absolute threshold, the threshold of conscious perception, and the difference threshold.

Absolute Threshold

The **absolute threshold** is the minimum of stimulus energy that is needed to activate a sensory system. This threshold is therefore a threshold in sensation, not in perception. While most human sensory systems are extremely sensitive, all systems also have an absolute threshold below which the stimulus will not be transduced into action potentials, and the information will therefore never be sent to the central nervous system. For example, sounds of extremely low intensity may still cause slight vibrations in the sensory receptors of the inner ear, but these vibrations might not be significant enough to open ion channels linked to these sensory receptors. The absolute threshold for sweet taste is a teaspoon of sucrose dissolved in two gallons of water. On a clear, dark night with no other lights shining, the eye can just detect the light of one candle burning thirty miles away. When we are talking about an absolute threshold, we're talking about how bright, loud, or intense a stimulus must be before it is sensed.

Threshold of Conscious Perception

It is possible for sensory systems to send signals to the central nervous system without a person perceiving these signals. This lack of conscious perception may be because the stimulus is too subtle to demand our attention, or may last for too brief a duration for the brain to fully process the information. The level of intensity that a stimulus must pass in order to be consciously perceived by the brain is the **threshold of conscious perception**. By way of contrast, information that is received by the central nervous system but that does not cross this threshold is called **subliminal perception**. Figure 2.3 utilizes a graph to explain these perception thresholds. Note the difference between the absolute threshold and the threshold for conscious perception: a stimulus below the absolute threshold will not be transduced, and thus never reaches the central nervous system. A stimulus below the threshold of conscious perception arrives at the central nervous system, but does not reach the higher-order brain regions that control attention and consciousness. Contrary to common thinking, there is actually little practical value to using subliminal perception to sell products.

MCAT EXPERTISE

On the MCAT, thresholds will frequently be used in conjunction with subjects in studies. Be on the lookout for experimental design questions when thresholds appear in a passage.

KEY CONCEPT

The absolute threshold is the minimum intensity at which a stimulus will be transduced (converted into action potentials).

BRIDGE

You may already know one of the absolute thresholds from the discussion of sound in Chapter 7 of *MCAT Physics and Math Review*. Remember that I_0 $(10^{-12}\frac{W}{m^2})$ in the equation for sound level is the absolute threshold of normal human hearing.

REAL WORLD

The Latin word for "thresholds" is *limina*. Hence, something that is "subliminal" is literally "below threshold." The threshold referred to in the term "subliminal perception" is the threshold of conscious perception. So, signals that are "subliminal" are strong enough to pass the absolute threshold, but not strong enough to pass the threshold of conscious perception.

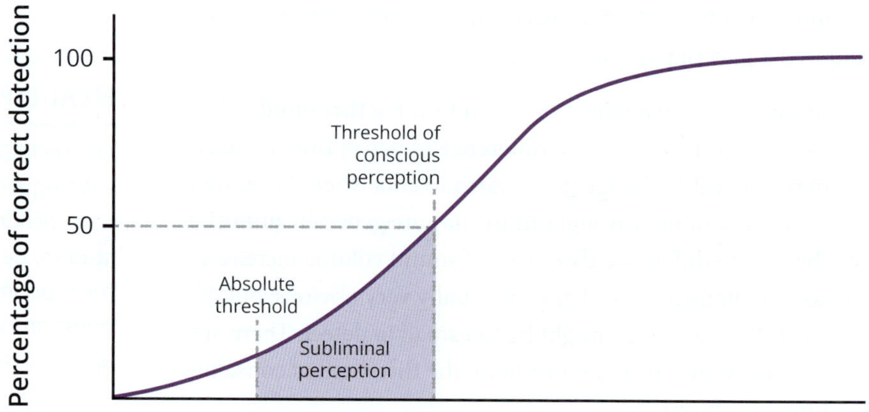

Figure 2.3 Perception Threshold Curve

Difference Threshold

A third commonly studied threshold is the **difference threshold**, sometimes called the **just-noticeable difference (jnd)** between two stimuli. The difference threshold refers to the minimum change in magnitude required for an observer to perceive that two different stimuli are, in fact, different. If the difference between stimuli is below the difference threshold, the two stimuli will seem to the observer to be the same. For example, imagine two sound waves are played one after the other, the first having frequency 440 Hz and then the second having frequency 441 Hz. These sounds are different. But without formal ear training, most individuals cannot hear the difference. In this range of sound frequencies, the just-noticeable difference for most listeners is about 3 Hz. So, for the average person to hear a difference in pitch, the sound waves need to be 440 Hz and 443 Hz. Below this difference threshold, the two pitches will sound the same.

The previous example illustrates one common experimental technique researchers use to explore the difference threshold. The technique is called psychophysical discrimination testing, or sometimes just **discrimination testing**. In a common discrimination testing experiment, a participant is presented with a stimulus. The stimulus is then varied slightly and researchers ask the participant to report whether they perceive a change. Often, the difference continues to be increased until the participant reports they notice the change, and this interval is recorded as the just noticeable difference.

Returning to the example of two sounds: The difference between a 440 Hz sound and a 443 Hz sound is just noticeable for most people. But, by using discrimination testing, researchers have discovered that the absolute difference (3 Hz, in this case) is far less important than the percent difference. For this reason, the just noticeable difference is usually reported as a fraction or a percent. To compute this percent, divide the change in stimulus by the magnitude of the original stimulus. In our example, we would compute 3 Hz / 440 Hz = 0.0068 = 0.68%. To illustrate why percentages are used, consider a 1000 Hz sound. An increase of 0.68% results in a sound of frequency 1007 Hz. So, to the average person, the difference in pitch from 1000 Hz to 1007 Hz would be just noticeable. By contrast, the difference from 1000 Hz to 1003 Hz would not be noticeable. While a 3 Hz difference was noticeable in the lower frequency range, that same 3 Hz difference is not noticeable in the higher frequency range. This auditory example is illustrated in Figure 2.4.

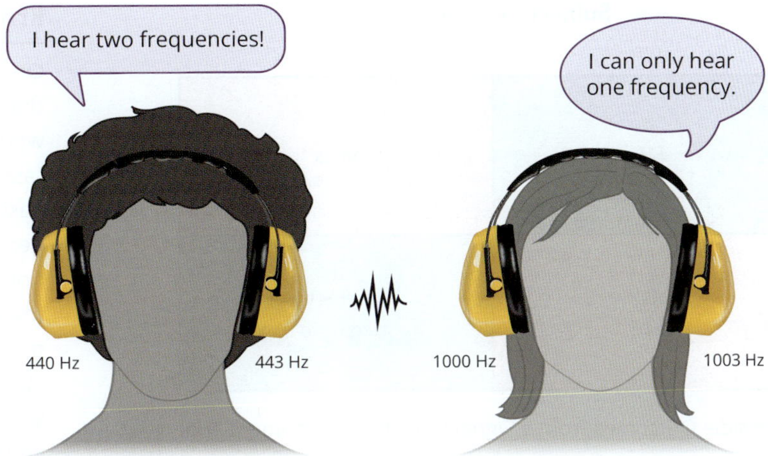

Figure 2.4 An Auditory Example of Weber's Law

Ernst Heinrich Weber (1795–1878) is often credited with the observation that difference thresholds are proportional and must be computed as percentages. This idea is therefore often called **Weber's law**. Weber's law applies to the perception of a number of senses, including the perception of loudness and pitch of sounds, the perception of brightness of light, and the perception of weight of objects.

MCAT EXPERTISE

When the MCAT brings up Weber's law, questions will usually give a numerical relationship and then ask for it to be applied; typically, the solution simply amounts to applying a ratio.

Signal Detection Theory

Perception of stimuli can also be affected by nonsensory factors, such as experiences (memory), motives, and expectations. **Signal detection theory** studies how internal (psychological) and external (environmental) factors influence thresholds of sensation and perception. For example, how loud would someone need to yell your name in a crowd to get your attention? The answer depends on environmental factors, like the size of the crowd; social factors, like the makeup of the crowd and your comfort with the individuals around you; psychological factors, like whether or not you are expecting to have your name called; and personality factors, like your level of introversion or extroversion. In signal detection theory, these factors are treated like independent variables. For example, researchers can measure how likely a person is to hear their name called when the person is informed that at some point their name will be called, versus when the person is left uninformed.

A basic signal detection experiment consists of many trials; during each trial, a stimulus (signal) may or may not be presented. Trials in which the signal is presented are called **noise trials**, whereas those in which the signal is not presented are called **catch trials**. After each trial, the subject is asked to indicate whether or not a signal was presented. There are therefore four possible outcomes for each trial, as illustrated in Figure 2.5. A **hit** is a trial in which the signal is presented and the subject correctly perceives the signal; a **miss** is a trial in which the subject fails to perceive the presented signal. A **false alarm** is a trial in which the subject indicates perceiving the signal, even though the signal was not presented; a **correct negative** is a trial in which the subject correctly identifies that no signal was presented. By tracking the rates of these various outcomes, researchers are able to identify factors that influence perception.

	Subject's Response: "Yes"	Subject's Response: "No"
Signal Present	Hit	Miss
Signal Absent	False alarm	Correct negative

Figure 2.5 Possible Outcomes from a Signal Detection Experiment Trial

Adaptation

Our ability to detect a stimulus can change over time through **adaptation**. Adaptation can have both a physiological (sensory) component and a psychological (perceptual) component. For example, the pupils of the eyes will dilate in the dark and constrict in the light (Figure 2.6), which illustrates physiological adaptation. Similarly, in loud environments, small muscles in the middle ear will reflexively contract in order to dampen the vibration of the ossicles, reducing sound intensity. We also adapt to somatosensory stimuli; cold water no longer seems so cold once our bodies "get used to it." Once we're dressed, we stop feeling the clothes on our bodies until we have a reason to think about them. Adaptation is one way the mind and body try to focus attention on only the most relevant stimuli, which are usually changes in the environment around us.

REAL WORLD

On the surface, signal detection experiments would appear to be easy tasks—shouldn't individuals easily be able to tell if they perceived something or not? However, consider the thought processes that occur when you're quietly studying in the library with your phone on silent and you suddenly think you may have heard a buzz. *Is my phone ringing?* you wonder. You freeze in place and wait for another buzz; even if it doesn't come, you may still be so convinced you heard a signal that you still check your phone. Perception is not a passive matter!

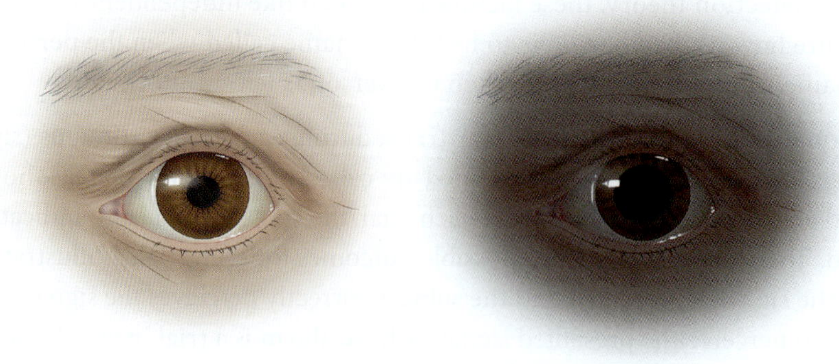

Figure 2.6 Sensory Adaptation of the Pupil

MCAT CONCEPT CHECK 2.1

Before you move on, assess your understanding of the material with these questions.

1. What is the pathway for a stimulus to reach conscious perception?

____

2. Match each sensory receptor to its function:

1. Hair cell	A. Sense painful or bothersome physical stimuli
2. Nociceptor	B. Sense changes in temperature
3. Olfactory receptor	C. Sense electromagnetic radiation in the visible range
4. Osmoreceptor	D. Sense changes in blood concentration
5. Photoreceptor	E. Sense volatile chemicals
6. Taste receptor	F. Sense motion of fluid in the inner ear
7. Thermoreceptor	G. Sense dissolved chemicals

3. For each of the thresholds below, provide a brief description:

 - Absolute threshold:

____

 - Threshold of conscious perception:

____

 - Difference threshold:

____

4. What aspect of thresholds do Weber's law and signal detection theory focus on?

 - Weber's law:

____

 - Signal detection theory:

____

5. How does sensory adaptation affect a difference threshold?

____

2.2 Vision High Yield

LEARNING OBJECTIVES

After Chapter 2.2, you will be able to:

- List the functions of the parts of the eye, including the cornea, pupil, iris, ciliary body, canal of Schlemm, lens, retina, and sclera
- Describe parallel processing
- Identify the cell types responsible for color, shape, and motion detection
- Recall the structures in the visual pathway:

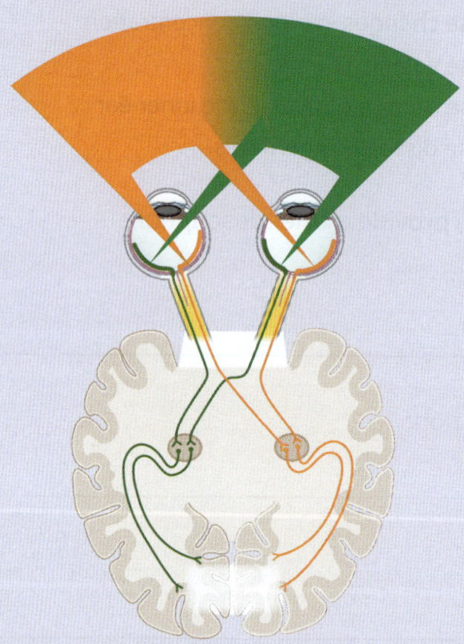

Vision is a highly adapted sense in human beings. With the ability to sense brightness, color, shape, and movement, and then to integrate this information to create a cohesive three-dimensional model of the world, the visual pathways are extremely important to everyday life. In fact, vision is the only sense to which an entire lobe of the brain is devoted: the occipital lobe. While some individuals experience vision differently, such as those who are color deficient or partially sighted, the MCAT focuses primarily on the details of unimpaired vision.

Structure and Function of the Eye

The anatomy of the eye is shown in Figure 2.7.

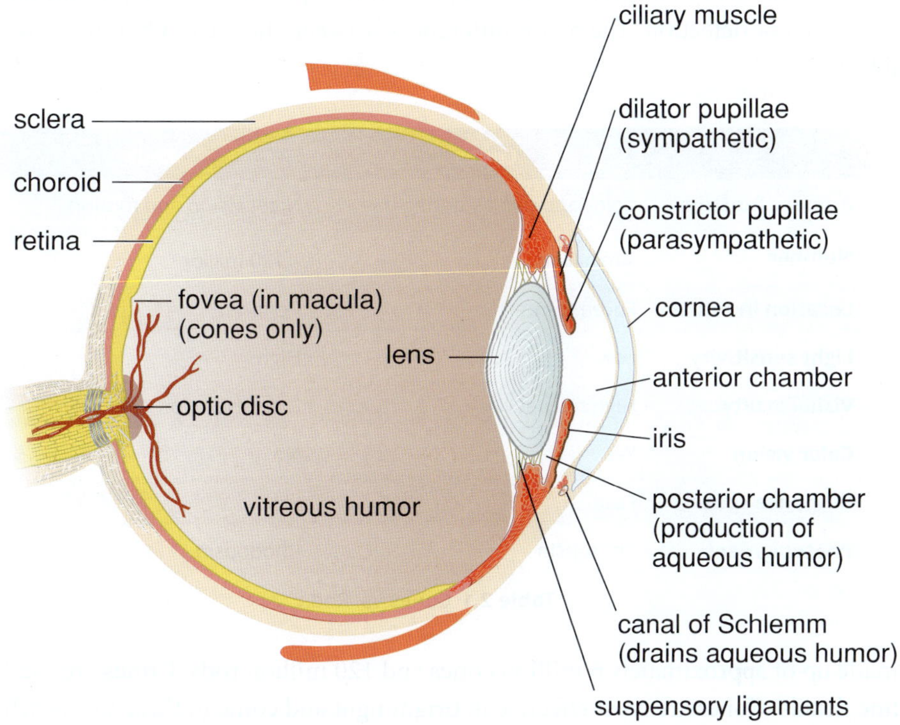

Figure 2.7 Anatomy of the Eye

The eye is a specialized organ used to detect light in the form of photons. Most of the exposed portion of the eye is covered by a thick structural layer known as the **sclera**, or the white of the eye. The sclera does not cover the frontmost portion of the eye, the cornea. The eye is supplied with nutrients by two sets of blood vessels: the **choroidal vessels**, a complex intermingling of blood vessels between the sclera and the retina, and the **retinal vessels**. The innermost layer of the eye is the **retina**, which contains the actual photoreceptors that transduce light into electrical information the brain can process.

When entering the eye, light passes first through the **cornea**, a clear, domelike window in the front of the eye, which gathers and focuses the incoming light. The front of the eye is divided into the **anterior chamber**, which lies in front of the iris, and the **posterior chamber** between the iris and the lens. The **iris**, which is the colored part of the eye, is composed of two muscles: the **dilator pupillae**, which opens the pupil under sympathetic stimulation; and the **constrictor pupillae**, which constricts the pupil under parasympathetic stimulation. The iris is continuous with the **choroid**, which is a vascular layer of connective tissue that surrounds and provides nourishment to the retina. The iris is also continuous with the the **ciliary body**, which produces the **aqueous humor** that bathes the front part of the eye before draining into the **canal of Schlemm**. The **lens** lies right behind the iris and helps control the refraction of the incoming light. Contraction of the **ciliary muscle**, a component of the ciliary body, is under parasympathetic control. As the muscle contracts, it pulls on the **suspensory ligaments** and changes the shape of the lens to focus on an image as the distance varies, a phenomenon known as **accommodation**. Behind the lens lies the **vitreous humor**, a transparent gel that supports the retina.

The **retina** is in the back of the eye and is like a screen consisting of neural elements and blood vessels. Its function is to convert incoming photons of light to electrical signals. It is actually considered part of the central nervous system and develops as an outgrowth of brain tissue. The **duplexity** or **duplicity theory of vision** states that the retina contains two kinds of photoreceptors: those specialized for light-and-dark detection and those specialized for color detection. The major differences between these two photoreceptor types are summarized in Table 2.1.

	Cones	Rods
Primary function	Color and details during day	Night vision and motion
Number	~6 million	~120 million
Location in retina	Fovea (center)	Periphery
Light sensitivity	Low	High
Visual acuity	High resolution	Low resolution
Color vision	Yes	No
Response speed	Fast	Slow
Photopigment	Photopsin	Rhodopsin

Table 2.1 Cones vs. Rods

The retina is made up of approximately 6 million cones and 120 million rods. **Cones** are used for color vision and to sense fine details. Cones are most effective in bright light and come in three forms, which are named for the wavelengths of light they best absorb, as shown in Figure 2.8. Additionally, there is an **opponent-process theory** of vision for cones. It states that there are three opposing channels: red versus green, blue versus yellow, and black versus white. These opposing pairs work via a process in which the activation of one color in a pair inhibits the perception of the other.

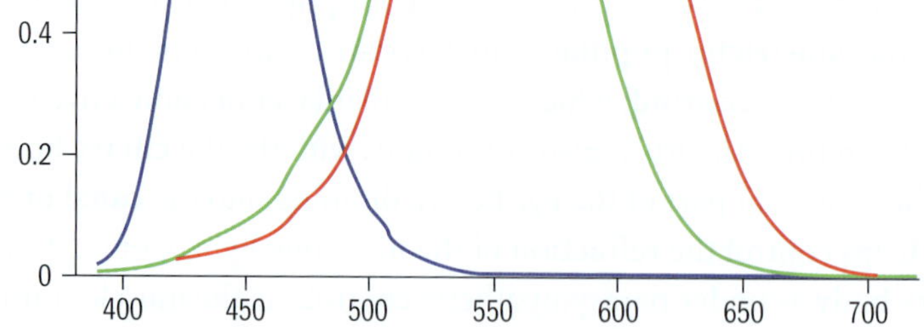

Figure 2.8 Relative Absorption of the Three Types of Cones at Different Wavelengths
The cones are named for the wavelengths at which they have highest light absorption: short (S, also called blue), medium (M, green), and long (L, red).

MNEMONIC

Cones are for **c**olor vision. **Rods** function best in "**rod**uced" light.

In reduced illumination, **rods** are more functional than cones because each rod cell is highly sensitive to photons and is somewhat easier to stimulate than a cone cell. In part, the sensitivity of rods has to do with the fact that all rods contain only a single pigment type called **rhodopsin**. In general, color vision requires far more light because each cone responds only to certain wavelengths of light. By contrast, a rod can be stimulated by light of any color. However, while rods permit vision in reduced light, the tradeoff is that rods only allow sensation of light and dark. Also, even though individual rods are highly sensitive to light, as a whole they are less useful for detecting fine details because rods are spread over a much larger area of the retina.

While there are many more rods than cones in the human eye, the central section of the retina, called the **macula**, has a high concentration of cones; in fact, the centermost region of the macula, called the **fovea**, contains only cones. As one moves further away from the fovea towards the **peripheral retina**, the concentration of rods increases while the concentration of cones decreases. Therefore, visual acuity is best at the fovea, and the fovea is most sensitive in normal daylight vision. Some distance away from the center of the retina, the optic nerve leaves the eye. This region of the retina, which is devoid of photoreceptors, is called the optic disk, and gives rise to a **blind spot**, as shown in Figure 2.9.

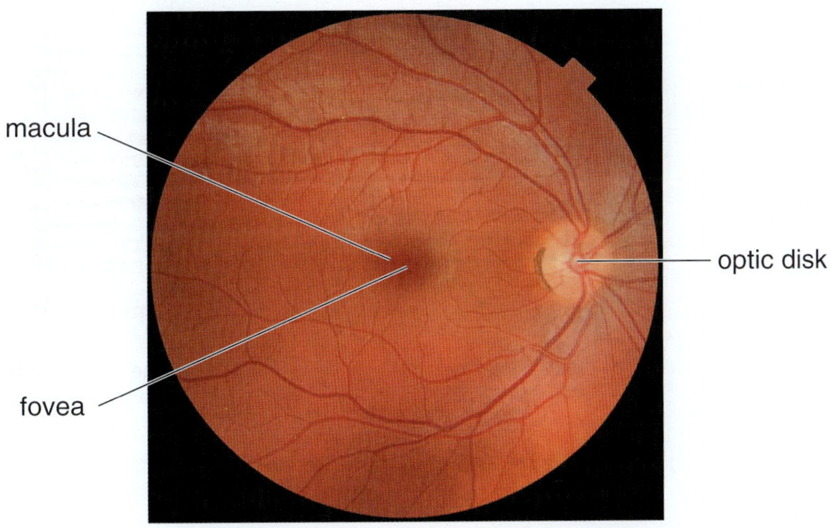

Figure 2.9 Specialized Regions of the Retina

Rods and cones are specialized neurons and, like most neurons, connect with other neurons through synapses. However, rods and cones do not connect directly to the optic nerve. Rather, there are several layers of neurons in between, as shown in Figure 2.10. Rods and cones synapse directly with **bipolar cells**, which highlight gradients between adjacent rods or cones. Bipolar cells then synapse with **ganglion cells**, the axons of which group together to form the **optic nerve**. These bipolar and ganglion cells not only fall "in between" the rods and cones and the optic nerve, but also the bipolar and ganglion cells are actually located in front of the rods and cones, closer to the front of the eye. This arrangement means that a photon must actually navigate past several layers of cells to reach the rods and cones at the "back" of the retina; the information is then transmitted "forward" (in the form of action potentials) from the rod and cone cells until the signal reaches the ganglion cells. Observe in Figure 2.10 that there are significantly more photoreceptor cells than ganglion cells, so the output from each ganglion cell represents the combined activity of many rods and cones. The result is a pruning of details as information from the photoreceptors is combined.

As the number of receptors that converge through the bipolar neurons onto one ganglion cell increases, the resolution decreases. On average, the number of cones converging onto an individual ganglion cell is smaller than for rods. This arrangement helps explain why color vision has a greater sensitivity to fine detail than black-and-white vision does.

Also shown in Figure 2.10 are **amacrine** and **horizontal cells**, which receive input from multiple retinal cells in the same area before the information is passed on to ganglion cells. Amacrine and horizontal cells can thereby accentuate slight differences between the visual information in each bipolar cell. For example, these cells are important for edge detection, as they increase our perception of contrasts.

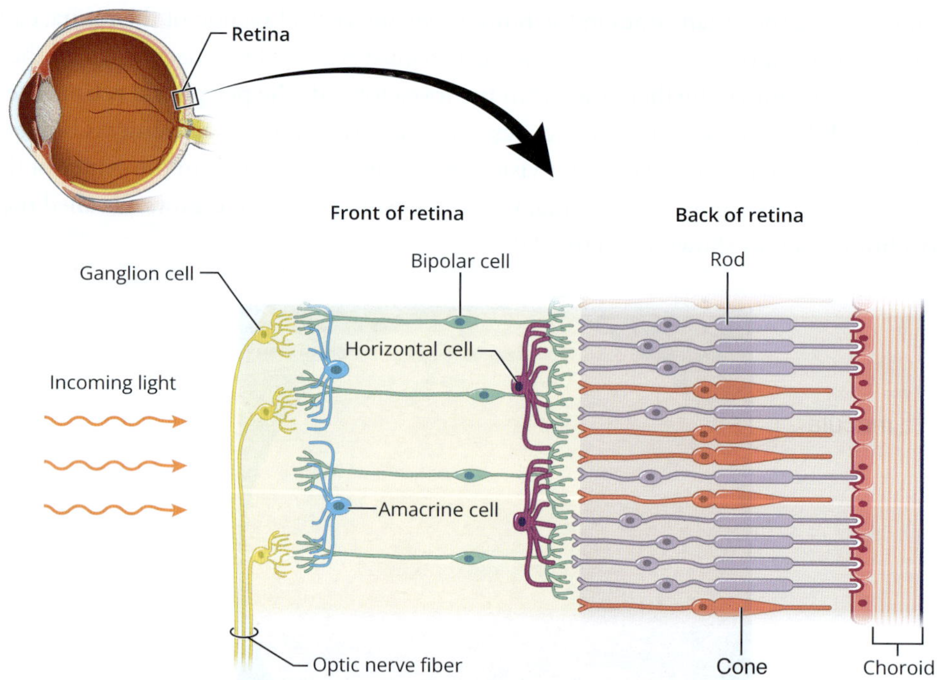

Figure 2.10 Cells of the Retina

Visual Pathways

Visual pathways refer to both the anatomical connections between the eyes and brain and to the flow of visual information along these connections. These pathways are illustrated in Figure 2.11. The terminology for these pathways can seem confusing. So here is a simple rule of thumb to start: If an object is to your left, then photons from that object stimulate the right side of the retina in each eye. To help visualize this result, look at Figure 2.11. In this figure, an object to your left is in the orange field. Photons from that object enter each eye and stimulate the retinal fibers that are illustrated using the color orange. This result is due to simple geometry! If an object is to your left, then photons from that object must travel to the right to reach your eyes, and in so doing, these photons enter your eyes and continue travelling to the right, thereby stimulating the right side of each of your eyes' retinas. From there, retinal fibers from each eye project to the right side of your brain. All of this leads to a famous result: Visual information from objects to your left is processed by the right side of your brain. Similarly, if an object is to your right (the blue patches in the figure), then photons from this object stimulate the left side of each retina (the green nerves), and this visual data is sent to the left side of your brain.

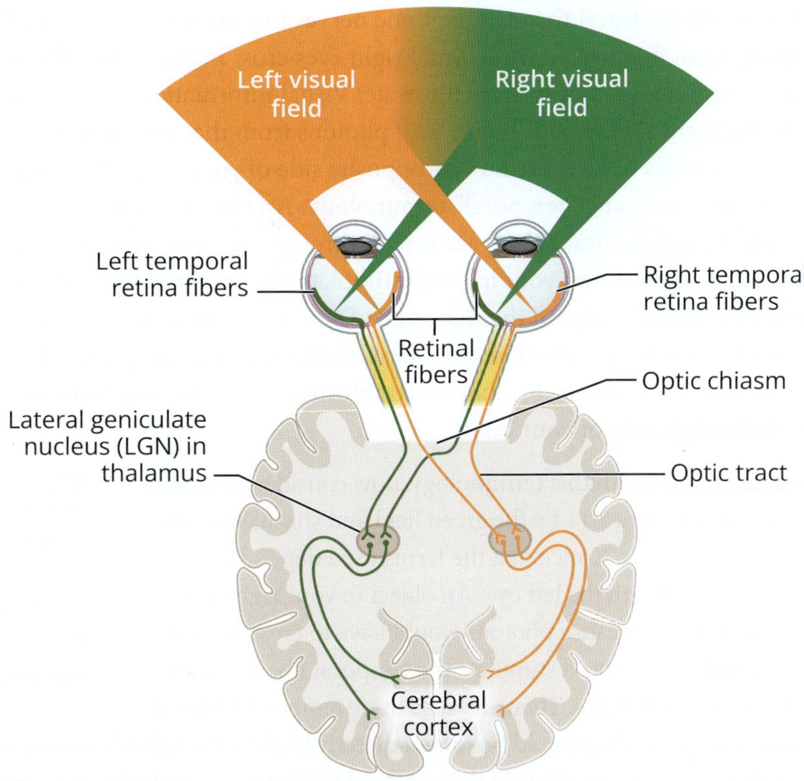

Figure 2.11 Visual Pathways

To help describe these phenomena with more specificity, scientists use the terms **temporal** and **nasal retinal fibers**. Here's an example. Consider an object to your left, depicted in the orange field in Figure 2.11. In each eye, photons from this object strike the retinal fibers that are illustrated in Figure 2.11 using the color orange. But notice: In the right eye, those orange fibers are on the lateral side of the retina, closer to your temple, and so these fibers are called the temporal fibers of the right eye. In the left eye, the orange fibers are medial, closer to your nose, and so are called the nasal fibers of the left eye.

Scientists also describe the placement of the object in space, relative to your eyes, using the terms "temporal" and "nasal," but now referring to the **temporal** and **nasal visual fields**. Again, this terminology is best explained by example. Imagine an object is a little to your left. Then photons from that object must cross in front of your nose in order to reach your right eye. So, this object is described as being in the nasal field of your right eye. Think carefully about what happens to these photons next. They enter your right eye, continue heading to the right, and ultimately strike the temporal fibers on the right side of your right eye. Pay close attention to the terminology: We're saying that an object in the *nasal field* of the right eye stimulates the *temporal fibers* of that eye! This mixing of terminology—nasal field stimulates temporal fibers—illustrates the crossing over of visual information. By contrast, for that same object, which, remember, is spatially to your left, photons can enter your left eye directly. Therefore, this object is described as being in the temporal field of your left eye. Then, these photons strike the nasal fibers of the left eye. So again, there is mixing of the terminology—the object is in the *temporal field* of the left eye, and photons strike the *nasal fibers* of the left eye.

MNEMONIC

If photons from an object would need to cross your nose to reach your eye (or if the object is right in front of your nose) then the object is said to be in the nasal visual field for that eye.

As the retinal fibers from each eye travel through the optic nerves toward the brain, a significant event occurs at the **optic chiasm**. Here, nasal fibers from the left and right eyes cross paths. Notice that only the nasal fibers cross at the optic chiasm. Again, an example helps illustrate: Visual information from an object to your left is ultimately processed by the right side of your brain. So if photons from that object are captured by the left eye, then this visual information needs to be routed to the opposite side of your brain. That routing is done using the optic chiasm. To use the "nasal" and "temporal" terminology: An object to your left will stimulate the nasal fibers of your left eye, and then these nasal fibers are routed through the optic chiasm to the right side of your brain. By contrast, that same object, off to your left, will stimulate the temporal fibers of your right eye. Because these temporal fibers are already on the right side of your body, there is no need to cross them. Therefore, only nasal fibers cross at the optic chiasm. These reorganized pathways are called **optic tracts** after leaving the optic chiasm. And the end result is that visual information emanating from an object to your left is ultimately processed on the right side of your brain.

To summarize, and to gain practice with this terminology, now consider an object off to your right, represented in Figure 2.11 by the green field and stimulating the fibers illustrated using the color green. Notice that the terms used depend on which eye is considered. Let's start with the left eye. An object to your right would be in the nasal field of your left eye, because photons would have to cross your nose to reach your left eye. These photons would stimulate the temporal fibers of the left eye—nasal field stimulates temporal fibers. Then, because these temporal fibers are already on the left side of your body, they would be routed directly back to the left side of your brain. Now consider the right eye. An object spatially to your right is in the temporal field of your right eye, and stimulates the nasal fibers of that eye. Then, in order to bring this visual information to the left side of your brain, these nasal fibers are routed through the optic chiasm. Through all of this, keep these two trends in mind: First, the temporal field of each eye stimulates the nasal fibers of each eye, and vice versa. Second, the nasal fibers cross at the optic chiasm.

MNEMONIC

For each eye, the temporal visual field stimulates the nasal retinal fibers. The nasal visual field stimulates the temporal retinal fibers.

From the optic chiasm, the information goes to several different places in the brain: some nerve fibers pass to the **lateral geniculate nucleus (LGN)** of the **thalamus** where they synapse with nerves that then pass through radiations in the temporal and parietal lobes to the **visual cortex** in the **occipital lobe**. This connectivity makes sense because the thalamus is a well-known connecting and routing center of the forebrain. Other nerve fibers branch off from the optic tracts, skip the thalamus, and head directly to the **superior colliculi** in the midbrain, which control some reflexive responses to visual stimuli and reflexive eye movements.

REAL WORLD

When there is a sudden, bright flash of light, the superior colliculus aligns the eyes with the likely stimulus. In other words, it's the superior colliculus (as well as the sympathetic nervous system) that gives us the "deer in the headlights" appearance during the startle response.

Processing

The ability to sense light information in the environment around us is useful in its own right. But, to effectively interact with the environment, we must also be able to make sense of visual stimuli. The connections between optic tract, LGN, and visual cortex help create a cohesive image of the world through a phenomenon known as parallel processing. Visual **parallel processing** is the brain's ability to analyze information regarding color, form, motion, and depth simultaneously, i.e. "in parallel," using independent pathways in the brain. For example, most people can quickly and easily recognize a moving car from a distance. The speed of recognition is facilitated, in part, by the fact that the form of the car (i.e. its shape) and the motion of the car are processed simultaneously in separate, parallel pathways in the brain. In contrast, **serial processing** occurs when cognitive processes are executed in a sequential, step-by-step manner. While slower than parallel processing, serial processing allows for the processing of tasks that require a high level of focus and attention, leading to greater accuracy.

Now let's explore where each of these four aspects of vision is processed and the specialized cells that contribute to their detection. As described previously, cones are responsible for our perception of color. **Form** refers not only to the shape of an object, but also our ability to discriminate an object of interest from the background by detecting its boundaries. The neurons responsible for processing form, color, and motion have distinct specializations, as summarized in Table 2.2. Neurons carrying information from the fovea and surrounding central portion of the retina synapse with **parvocellular cells** in the lateral geniculate nucleus. These cells have very high color **spatial resolution**; that is, these cells permit us to detect very fine detail when thoroughly examining an object. However, parvocellular cells can only work with stationary or slow-moving objects because these cells have very low **temporal resolution**.

	Parvocellular Cells	Magnocellular Cells
Function	Form and color	Motion
Spatial resolution	High, provides fine detai	Low, provides a blurry image
Temporal resolution	Low, suitable for slow-moving objects	High, suitable for detecting motion

Table 2.2 Parvocellular vs. Magnocellular Cells

Conversely, **magnocellular cells** are well-suited for detecting motion because these cells have very high temporal resolution. Reflecting the fact that form and motion are processed in parallel, magnocellular cells and parvocellular cells are located in distinct layers of the lateral geniculate nucleus. Also, magnocellular cells predominantly receive inputs from the periphery of our vision, allowing more rapid detection of objects approaching us from the sides. However, magnocellular cells have low spatial resolution, so much of the rich detail of an object can no longer be seen once the object is in motion. Magnocellular cells therefore provide a blurry but moving image of an object.

MNEMONIC

Magnocellular cells specialize in **m**otion detection.

Depth perception, our ability to discriminate the three-dimensional shape of our environment and judge the distance of objects within it, is largely based on discrepancies between the inputs the brain receives from our two eyes (more on this to follow in *MCAT Behavioral Sciences Review*, Section 2.5, Object Recognition). Specialized cells in the visual cortex known as **binocular neurons** are responsible for comparing the inputs to each hemisphere and detecting these differences.

Finally, our brains wouldn't be very good at processing visual information if they didn't learn to associate certain patterns of stimuli with expected behaviors or outcomes. **Perceptual learning** is the ability to distinguish between two perceptually similar objects and keep those differences in memory. To assist in this, a whole slew of even more specialized cells called **feature detectors** exist in the visual cortex. Each feature detector cell type detects a very particular, individual feature of an object in the visual field. For example, if we were to look at a stop sign we would activate: a feature detector for the color red, while another feature detector would respond to the white border and letters. Yet another type of feature detector would recognize the horizontal lines, while still others would be activated by the angled lines of the octagon. Rather than needing to individually process each of these features every time, the overall combination of feature detectors become activated in parallel. Finally, our response to the stop sign, i.e. to STOP, also is stored for future retrieval.

MCAT CONCEPT CHECK 2.2

Before you move on, assess your understanding of the material with these questions.

1. List the functions of the various parts of the eye:
   - Cornea:
   - Pupil:
   - Iris:
   - Ciliary body:
   - Canal of Schlemm:
   - Lens:
   - Retina:
   - Sclera:
2. List the structures in the visual pathway, from where light enters the cornea to the visual projection areas in the brain.
3. What is parallel processing?

4. In feature detection, what type of cells are responsible for color? Form? Motion? Depth?
    - Color:

    - Form:

    - Motion:

    - Depth:

2.3 Hearing and Vestibular Sense

LEARNING OBJECTIVES

After Chapter 2.3, you will be able to:

- Identify the structures used to detect linear acceleration and rotational acceleration
- Explain how the structural features of the cochlea and the hair cells are able to transmit information about pitch of an incoming sound to the brain
- List the structures in the auditory pathway

The ear is a complex organ responsible not only for our sense of hearing, but also for our **vestibular sense**, which is our ability to both detect rotational and linear acceleration and to use this information to inform our sense of balance and spatial orientation. These senses are critically important to our ability to get around in the world, and their associated structures are encased in some of the densest bone of the body to protect these structures from damage. While recognizing that individuals can differ in their hearing and vestibular senses, as with vision, the MCAT primarily focuses on the standard healthy operations of these senses.

Structure and Function of the Ear

The ear is divided into three parts, as shown in Figure 2.12: the outer, middle, and inner ear. A sound wave first reaches the cartilaginous outside part of the ear, called the **pinna** or **auricle**. The main function of the pinna is to channel sound waves into the **external auditory canal**, which directs the sound waves to the **tympanic membrane (eardrum)**. The membrane vibrates in phase with the incoming sound waves. The frequency of the sound wave determines the rate at which the tympanic membrane vibrates: it moves back and forth at a high rate for high-frequency sounds and more slowly for low-frequency sounds. Louder sounds have greater **intensity**, which corresponds to an increased amplitude of vibration.

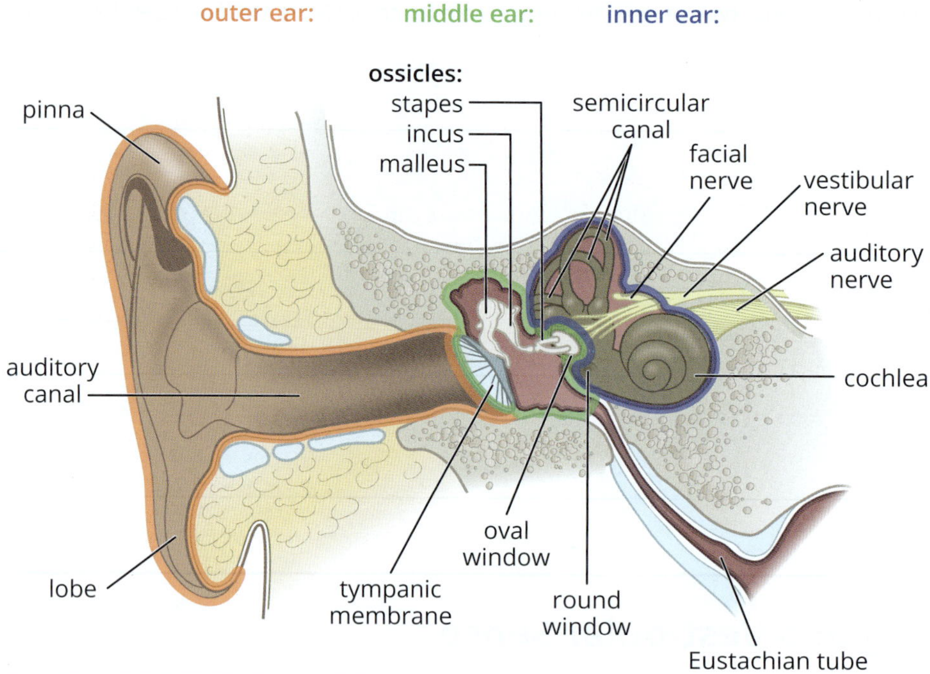

Figure 2.12 Anatomy of the Ear

The tympanic membrane divides the outer ear from the middle ear. The middle ear houses the three smallest bones in the body, called **ossicles**. The ossicles help transmit and amplify the vibrations from the tympanic membrane to the inner ear. The **malleus** (**hammer**) is affixed to the tympanic membrane; it acts on the **incus** (**anvil**), which acts on the **stapes** (**stirrup**). The baseplate of the stapes rests on the oval window of the cochlea, which is the entrance to the inner ear. The middle ear is connected to the nasal cavity via the **Eustachian tube**, which helps equalize pressure between the middle ear and the environment.

The inner ear sits within a **bony labyrinth**, which is a hollow region of the temporal bone containing the cochlea, vestibule, and semicircular canals, as shown in Figure 2.13. Inside the bony labyrinth rests a continuous collection of tubes and chambers called the **membranous labyrinth**. This collection of structures contains receptors for the sense of equilibrium and hearing. The membranous labyrinth is filled by a potassium-rich fluid called **endolymph**, and is suspended within the bony labyrinth by a thin layer of another fluid called perilymph. **Perilymph** simultaneously transmits vibrations from the outside world and cushions the inner ear structures.

BRIDGE

Remember that sound is a longitudinal wave carried through air (or another medium), which causes displacement of particles parallel to the axis of sound propagation. In other words, when a sound wave hits your eardrum, it literally causes it to oscillate back and forth because of moving air particles. Sound is discussed in Chapter 7 of *MCAT Physics and Math Review*.

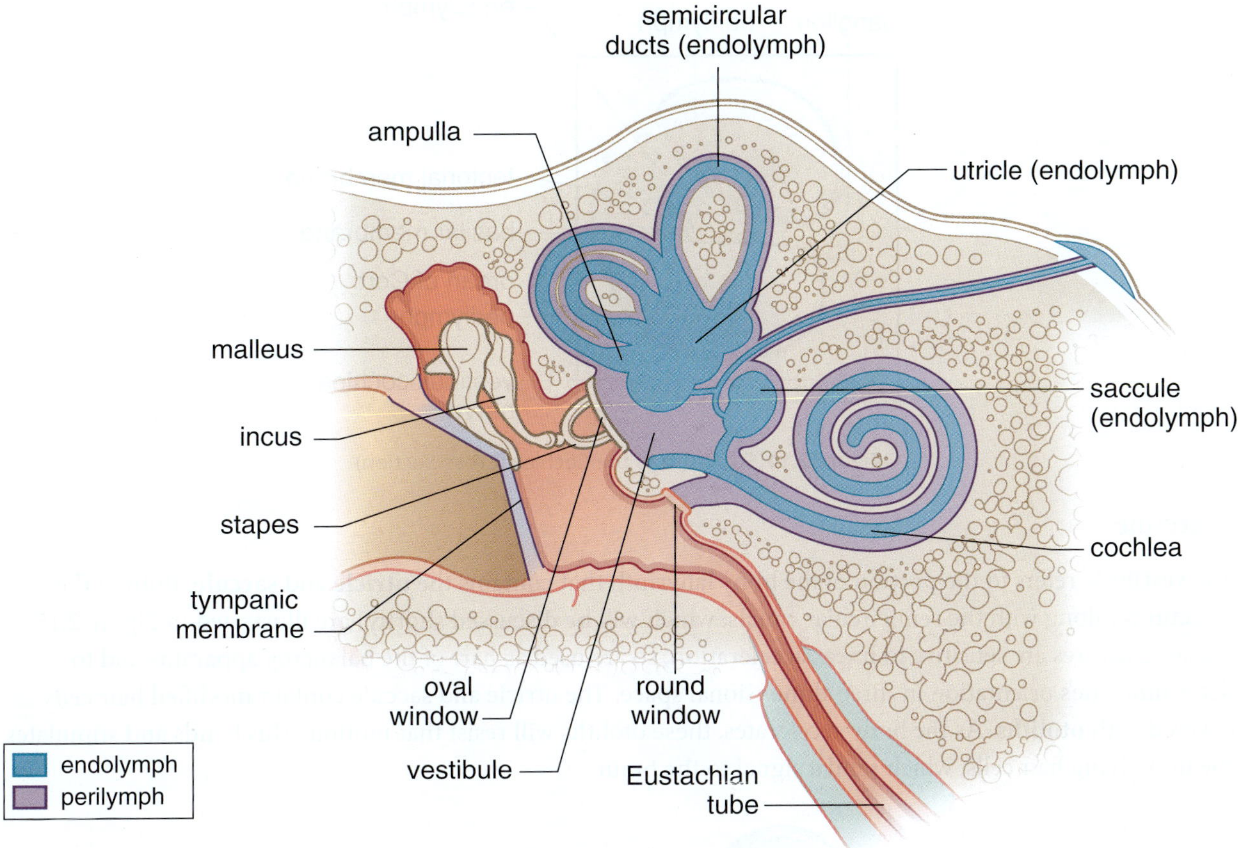

Figure 2.13 The Membranous and Bony Labyrinth
The membranous labyrinth is filled with endolymph (blue); it is suspended within the bony labyrinth, which is filled with perilymph (purple).

Cochlea

The **cochlea** is a spiral-shaped organ that contains the receptors for hearing; it is divided into three parts called **scalae**, as shown in Figure 2.14. All three scalae run the entire length of the cochlea. The middle scala houses the actual hearing apparatus, called the **organ of Corti**, which rests on a thin, flexible membrane called the **basilar membrane**. The organ of Corti is composed of thousands of hair cells, which are bathed in endolymph. On top of the organ of Corti is a relatively immobile membrane called the **tectorial membrane**. The other two scalae, filled with perilymph, surround the hearing apparatus and are continuous with the oval and round windows of the cochlea. Thus, sound entering the cochlea through the oval window causes vibrations in perilymph, which are transmitted to the basilar membrane. Because fluids are essentially incompressible, the **round window**, a membrane-covered hole in the cochlea, permits the perilymph to actually move within the cochlea. Like the rods and cones of the eye, the hair cells in the organ of Corti transduce the physical stimulus into an electrical signal, which is carried to the central nervous system by the **auditory (vestibulocochlear) nerve**.

BRIDGE

The junction between the stapes and the oval window is extremely similar to a thermodynamic gas–piston system, as described in Chapter 3 of *MCAT Physics and Math Review*. However, fluids are not as compressible as gases; therefore, the round window must be present to allow the perilymph in the cochlea to actually move back and forth with the stapedial footplate.

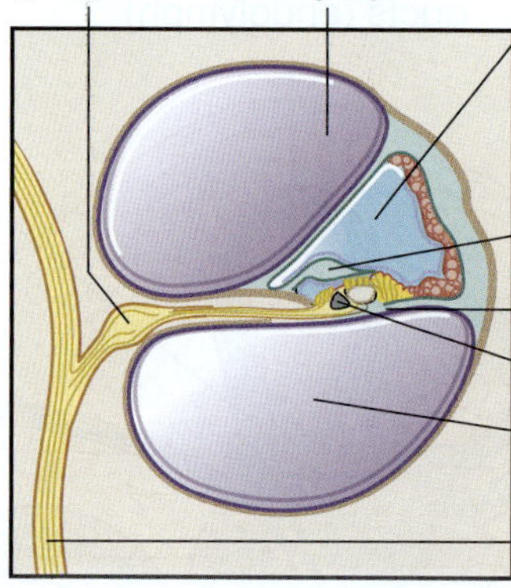

Figure 2.14 Structure of the Cochlea (Cross-Section)

Vestibule

The **vestibule** refers to the portion of the bony labyrinth that contains the **utricle** and **saccule**. Both of these structures (along with the semicircular canals, which will be discussed shortly) are illustrated in Figure 2.15. These structures are sensitive to linear acceleration, so are used as part of the balancing apparatus and to determine one's orientation in three-dimensional space. The utricle and saccule contain modified hair cells covered with **otoliths**. As the body accelerates, these otoliths will resist that motion. This bends and stimulates the underlying hair cells, which send a signal to the brain.

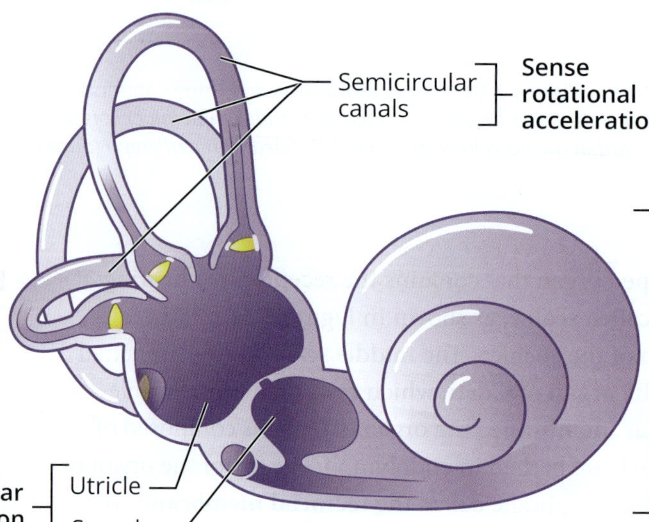

Figure 2.15 The Utricle, Saccule, and Semicircular Canals

Semicircular Canals

While the utricle and saccule are sensitive to linear acceleration, the three **semicircular canals** are sensitive to rotational acceleration. The semicircular canals are arranged perpendicularly to each other, and each ends in a swelling called an **ampulla**, where hair cells are located. When the head rotates, endolymph in the semicircular canal resists this motion, bending the underlying hair cells, which send a signal to the brain.

Auditory Pathways

The **auditory pathways** in the brain are a bit more complex than the visual pathways. Most sound information passes through the vestibulocochlear nerve to the brainstem, where it ascends to the **medial geniculate nucleus** (MGN) of the thalamus. From there, nerve fibers project to the **auditory cortex** in the temporal lobe for sound processing. Some information is also sent to the **superior olive**, which localizes the sound, and the **inferior colliculus**, which is involved in the startle reflex and helps keep the eyes fixed on a point while the head is turned (vestibulo–ocular reflex).

MNEMONIC

The **l**ateral geniculate nucleus (**L**GN) is for **l**ight; the **m**edial geniculate nucleus (**M**GN) is for **m**usic.

Hair Cells

Hair cells are named for the long tufts of **stereocilia** on their top surface, shown in Figure 2.16. As vibrations reach the basilar membrane underlying the organ of Corti, the stereocilia adorning the hair cells begin to sway back and forth within the endolymph. The swaying causes the opening of ion channels, which cause a receptor potential. Certain hair cells are also directly connected to the immobile tectorial membrane; these hair cells are involved in amplifying the incoming sound.

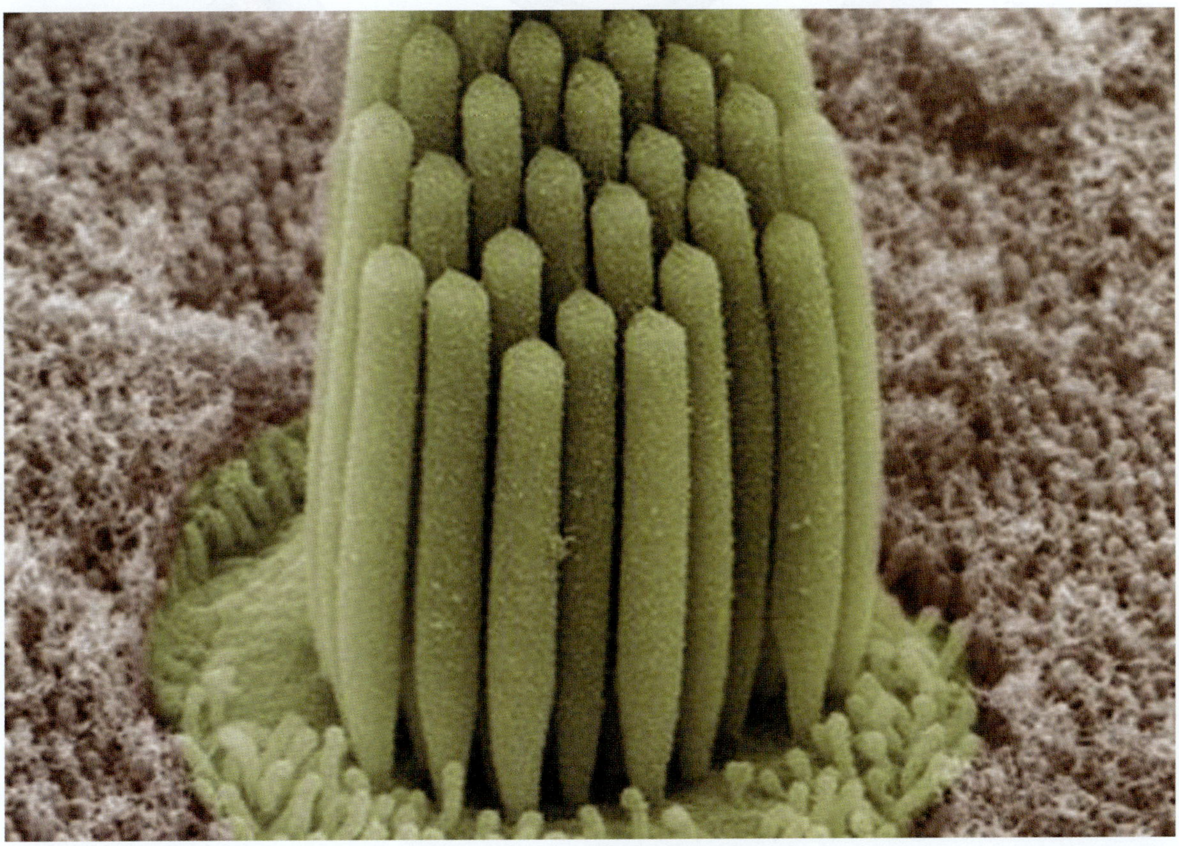

Figure 2.16 Stereocilia of a Hair Cell
Movement of fluid inside the cochlea leads to depolarization of the neuron associated with the hair cell.

The basilar membrane changes thickness depending on its location in the cochlea. The accepted theory on sound perception is **place theory**, which states that the location of a hair cell on the basilar membrane determines the perception of pitch when that hair cell is vibrated. The mapping of the cochlea in place theory can be seen in Figure 2.17. The highest-frequency pitches cause vibrations of the basilar membrane very close to the oval window, whereas low-frequency pitches cause vibrations at the apex, away from the oval window. Thus, the cochlea is **tonotopically** organized: which hair cells are vibrating gives the brain an indication of the pitch of the sound.

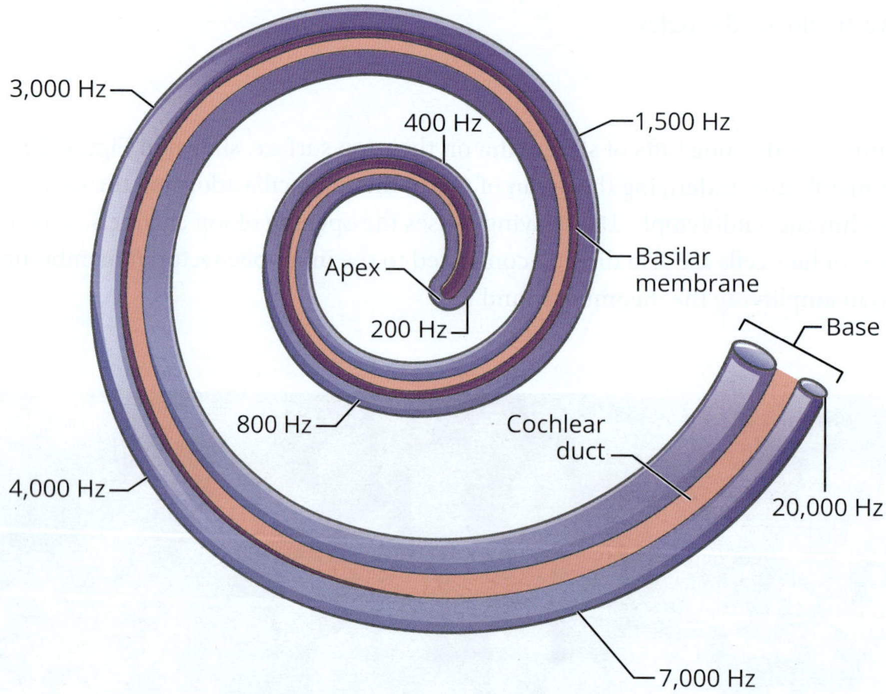

Figure 2.17 Place Theory

BEHAVIORAL SCIENCES GUIDED EXAMPLE WITH EXPERT THINKING

Researchers sought to explain a puzzling phenomenon: that differences in frequency of auditory stimuli sometimes correspond with greater than proportional increases in perceived pitch, even when taking Weber's law into account.

Translated: even if a noise "should" sound high (high frequency), it isn't necessarily perceived as high (high pitch). This is a reference to my outside knowledge: I'll need to recall what Weber's law is!

The researchers hypothesized that differences in pitch specifically for sounds that are familiar, such as human speech, would be amplified perceptually when compared to those of unfamiliar sounds. Participants listened to recordings of both human vocalizations and synthesized tones at 165 Hz and 175 Hz.

There are a couple of independent variables here: type of sound and frequency. The dependent variable must be what the participants report hearing.

Adapted from: Monson BB, Han S, Purves D (2013) Are Auditory Percepts Determined by Experience? *PLoS ONE* 8(5): e63728. https://doi.org/10.1371/journal.pone.0063728

What results would help to support the researchers' hypothesis? What effect would these results have on the place theory of sound perception?

When we encounter experimental passages on the MCAT, there are a few things we should always be on the lookout for: what is the hypothesis, and what are the independent and dependent variables? What results are presented, and what effect do they have on the hypothesis? What conclusion did the researchers come to, and is this conclusion reasonable given the results? If any of these pieces are missing, we should anticipate questions asking us to identify possibilities that would fit with the passage and our outside content knowledge. Here, we are given a hypothesis without results, and the question asks us for results that would support the hypothesis. We'll need to dive into the scenario to identify what is being tested and why, and then use that information in conjunction with our content knowledge to answer this question.

The researchers hypothesized that differences in perceived pitch are amplified for more commonly encountered sounds. Take a moment to consider what the researchers should expect if this hypothesis is correct. It would stand to reason that the difference between perceived pitch for the 165 Hz and 175 Hz samples would be larger for voices (which we hear all the time) than for synthesized tones (which we don't hear too often). In other words, a result that would help support the researchers' hypothesis would be experimental evidence that human vocalizations sounded more different in pitch than the synthesized tones, despite the absolute difference in frequency remaining the same.

For the second part of the question, we need to recall that place theory predicts that perceived pitch results directly from the location of the hair cells that are vibrated when exposed to that frequency; higher frequencies vibrate hair cells closer to the oval window, and lower frequencies vibrate hair cells that are farther away. What is important here is that, according to place theory, the type of sound is irrelevant; sounds of the same frequency should be perceived in the same way. However, the hypothesis of this study (and the hypothetical results we've just imagined in support of that hypothesis), call place theory into question as, according to the passage, similar changes in vibrations are not perceived as the same change in pitch. According to this study, the perceived pitch instead depends at least in part on the nature of the sound perceived by the listener. Note that this new finding wouldn't affect a place theory of sound sensation/detection, which could still be accurate: this experiment is specifically about how sounds are *perceived*, not about how they are *sensed*.

In sum, to support the researchers, the results must find a greater perceived difference in pitch between the vocal samples as compared to the synthesized audio samples. This finding would contradict the place theory of sound perception.

MCAT CONCEPT CHECK 2.3

Before you move on, assess your understanding of the material with these questions.

1. What structures are used to detect linear acceleration? Rotational acceleration?
   - Linear acceleration:

   ____

   - Rotational acceleration:

   ____

2. List the structures in the auditory pathway, from where sound enters the pinna to the auditory projection areas in the brain.

   ____

3. How does the organization of the cochlea indicate the pitch of an incoming sound?

   ____

2.4 Other Senses High Yield

LEARNING OBJECTIVES

After Chapter 2.4, you will be able to:

- List the structures in the olfactory pathway
- Distinguish between the chemicals detected by the nose and mouth
- Recall the four main modalities of somatosensation

While vision and hearing are, by far, the most heavily tested senses on the MCAT, the other senses are still considered fair game on Test Day. These include the chemical senses of smell and taste; somatosensation, which includes all of the modalities of "touch"; and kinesthetic sense.

Smell

Smell is considered one of the chemical senses, which means that it responds to incoming chemicals from the outside world. Specifically, the sense of smell responds to volatile or aerosolized compounds through the use of **chemoreceptors**, or receptors that detect sensory information by binding to chemical stimuli. These **olfactory chemoreceptors** (**olfactory nerves**) are located in the olfactory epithelium in the upper part of the nasal cavity. There are a tremendous number of specific chemoreceptors, which allows us to recognize subtle differences in similar scents, such as lavender and jasmine.

REAL WORLD

Smell is an impressive motivator for behavior. Food aromas may make a person hungry, a familiar fragrance may remind a person of a significant other from years ago, and an unpleasant smell may signify that an unknown bottle contains a dangerous chemical rather than water. Smell is the only sense that does not pass through the thalamus, but rather travels—unfiltered—into higher-order brain centers.

Smell can also carry interpersonal information through the medium of **pheromones**, which are chemicals secreted by one animal, and which, once bonded with chemoreceptors, compel or urge another animal to behave in a specific way. Pheromones have debatable effects on humans, but play an enormous role in many animals' social, foraging, and sexual behaviors.

As is true with all senses, there is a defined **olfactory pathway** to the brain. Odor molecules are inhaled into the nasal passages and then contact the olfactory nerves in the olfactory epithelium. These receptor cells are activated, sending signals to the **olfactory bulb**. These signals are then relayed via the **olfactory tract** to higher regions of the brain, including the limbic system.

Taste

As a sense, taste is often simpler than we imagine. There are five basic tastes: sweet, sour, salty, bitter, and umami (savory). Flavor is not synonymous with taste, but rather refers to the complex interplay between smell and taste, which can be affected by nonchemical stimuli like texture and the individual's mood.

Similar to smell, tastes are detected using chemoreceptors. These chemoreceptors are sensitive to dissolved compounds. Saltiness, for example, is a reaction to alkali metals, and is generally triggered by the sodium found in table salt. Sourness, on the other hand, is a reaction to acid, such as lemon juice or vinegar. Sweet, bitter, and savory flavors are also triggered by specific molecules binding to receptors. The receptors for taste are groups of cells called **taste buds**, which are found in little bumps on the tongue called **papillae**. Taste information travels from taste buds to the brainstem, and then ascends to the **taste center** in the thalamus before traveling to higher-order brain regions.

Somatosensation

Somatosensation is often reduced to "touch" when listed as a sense, but is actually quite complex. Somatosensation is usually described as having four modalities: pressure, vibration, pain, and temperature. At least five different types of receptor receive tactile information, including:

- **Pacinian corpuscles:** respond to deep pressure and vibration
- **Meissner corpuscles:** respond to light touch
- **Merkel cells (discs):** respond to deep pressure and texture
- **Ruffini endings:** respond to stretch
- **Free nerve endings:** respond to pain and temperature

Transduction occurs in the receptors, which send the signal to the central nervous system where it eventually travels to the **somatosensory cortex** in the parietal lobe.

REAL WORLD

Pain and temperature actually use a different pathway than pressure and vibration through the spinal cord. This can be seen in Brown-Séquard syndrome, in which half of the spinal cord is severed. Patients lose pressure and vibration sense on the same side as the lesion, but lose pain and temperature sensation on the opposite side.

There are three additional concepts related to touch perception that are important to know: two-point thresholds, physiological zero, and gate theory of pain. A **two-point threshold** refers to the minimum distance necessary between two points of stimulation on the skin such that the points will be felt as two distinct stimuli. Below the two-point threshold, the two stimuli will be felt as one. The size of the two-point threshold depends on the density of nerves in the particular area of skin being tested.

Temperature is judged relative to **physiological zero**, or the normal temperature of the skin (between 86° and 97°F). Thus, an object feels "cold" because it is under physiological zero; an object feels "warm" because it is above physiological zero.

Pain perception is part of the somatosensory system and can result from signals sent from a variety of sensory receptors, most commonly **nociceptors**. Pain also relies on thresholds, which may vary greatly from person to person. For example, the temperature of water that is perceived to be "so hot it hurts" may vary by several degrees between individuals. The **gate theory of pain** proposes that a special "gating" mechanism can turn pain signals on or off, affecting whether or not we perceive pain. In this theory, the spinal cord is able to preferentially forward the signals from other touch modalities (pressure, temperature) to the brain, thus reducing the sensation of pain. Gate theory has been superseded by other theories, but is still a useful model for understanding how touch is processed at the spinal cord.

REAL WORLD

The gate theory of pain explains why rubbing an injury (like bumping your knee on a table) seems to reduce the pain of the injury.

Kinesthetic Sense

Kinesthetic sense is also called **proprioception** and refers to the ability to tell where one's body is in space. For example, even with your eyes closed, you could still describe the location and position of your hand. The receptors for proprioception, called **proprioceptors**, are found mostly in muscle and joints, and play critical roles in hand–eye coordination, balance, and mobility.

Synesthesia

Synesthesia is a phenomena in which the activation of one sense triggers the perception of another sense. For example, a person with synesthesia who is listening to music may also perceive certain colors, or they may see shapes when they smell certain odors. Synesthesia highlights how interconnected and complex the senses and their associated perceptions can be.

MCAT CONCEPT CHECK 2.4

Before you move on, assess your understanding of the material with these questions.

1. List the structures in the olfactory pathway, from where odor molecules enter the nose to where olfactory signals project in the brain.

____

____

2. Both smell and taste are sensitive to chemicals. What is different about the types of chemicals each one can sense?

____

____

3. What are the four main modalities of somatosensation?

   1. _______________
   2. _______________
   3. _______________
   4. _______________

2.5 Object Recognition High Yield

LEARNING OBJECTIVES

After Chapter 2.5, you will be able to:

- Compare and contrast bottom-up processing and top-down processing
- Describe each of the Gestalt principles: proximity, similarity, good continuation, subjective contours, closure, and prägnanz

Modern theories of object recognition assume at least two major types of psychological processing: bottom-up processing and top-down processing. Examples of both types of processing are contained in Figure 2.18. **Bottom-up (data-driven) processing** refers to object recognition by parallel processing and feature detection, as described earlier. Essentially, the brain takes the individual sensory stimuli and combines them together to create a cohesive image before determining what the object is. **Top-down (conceptually driven) processing** is driven by memories and expectations that allow the brain to recognize the whole object and then recognize the components based on these expectations. In other words, top-down processing allows us to quickly recognize objects without needing to analyze their specific parts. Neither system is sufficient by itself: if we only performed bottom-up processing, we would be extremely inefficient at recognizing objects; every time we looked at an object, it would be like looking at the object for the first time. On the other hand, if we only performed top-down processing, we would have difficulty discriminating slight differences between similar objects. This distinction is also partially responsible for the feeling of *déjà vu* described in the introduction to this chapter: when we believe we are experiencing something for the first time, we expect to rely on bottom-up processing; however, when the mind is able to recognize an experience more quickly than expected (through top-down processing), the mind searches for a reason for this recognition. In other words, *déjà vu* is often evoked when we have recognition without an obvious reason: *I know that person from somewhere . . . but where?* The distinction between top-down and bottom-up processing is relevant for all senses, but is most commonly applied in the context of vision.

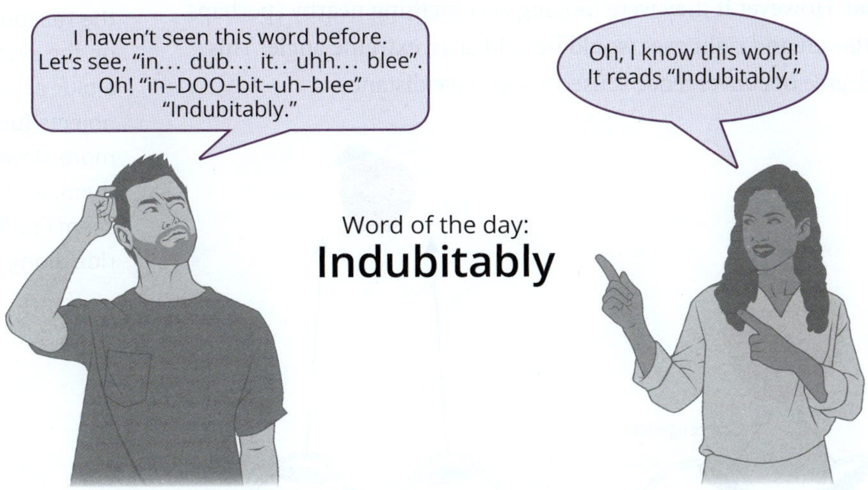
I haven't seen this word before. Let's see, "in... dub... it.. uhh... blee". Oh! "in–DOO–bit–uh–blee" "Indubitably."
Oh, I know this word! It reads "Indubitably."
Word of the day:
Indubitably

Figure 2.18 Top-Down vs. Bottom-Up Processing

Perceptual organization refers to the ability to create a complete picture or idea by combining top-down and bottom-up processing with all of the other sensory clues gathered from an object. Most of the images we see in everyday life are incomplete; often, we may only be able to see a part of an object and we must infer what the rest of the object looks like. By using what information is available in terms of depth, form, motion, constancy, and other clues, we can often "fill in the gaps" using Gestalt principles (described below).

Depth perception relies on a number of visual cues that are interpreted by the brain to deduce an object's distance. These visual cues are separated into monocular and binocular cues. **Monocular cues** only require one eye and include relative size, interposition, linear perspective, motion parallax, and other minor cues. Some of these monocular cues are shown in Figure 2.19. **Relative size** refers to the idea that objects appear larger the closer they are. **Interposition** means that when two objects overlap, the one in front is closer. **Linear perspective** refers to the convergence of parallel lines at a distance: the greater the convergence, the further the distance. **Motion parallax** is the perception that objects closer to us seem to move faster when we change our field of vision (look at something else).

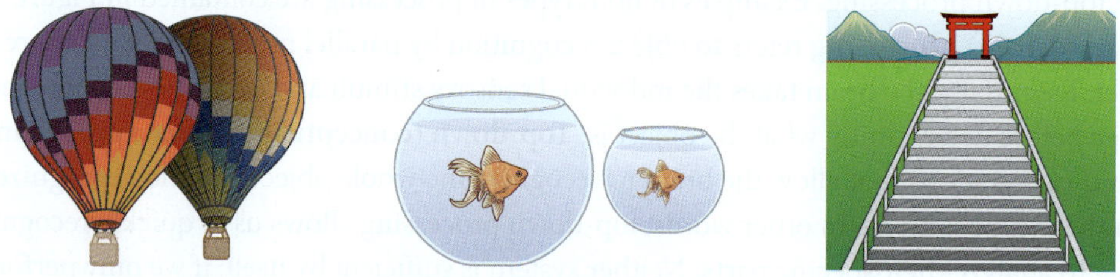

Figure 2.19 Monocular Cues for Distance

Binocular cues primarily involve **retinal disparity** which refers to the slight difference in images projected on the two retinas. This feature of depth perception is exploited in virtual reality (VR) devices: the images supplied to each eye are slightly different, giving the perception of depth even though the VR device displays 2D images. A secondary binocular cue is **convergence**, in which the brain detects the angle between the two eyes required to bring an object into focus (see Figure 2.20). If a person was looking at a distant object, both of their eyes would stare straight ahead. However if they were looking at something nearby (perhaps their own nose!) the left and right eyes would be held at an extreme angle. This difference in the degree of convergence is used to perceive distance.

REAL WORLD

If you've ever looked out the side window of a car, bus, or train on a clear night, you've experienced motion parallax. Parallax is the reason why the objects on the side of the road are a blur as you go past, why objects further away move more slowly as you pass them, and why the moon seems to follow you as you ride along.

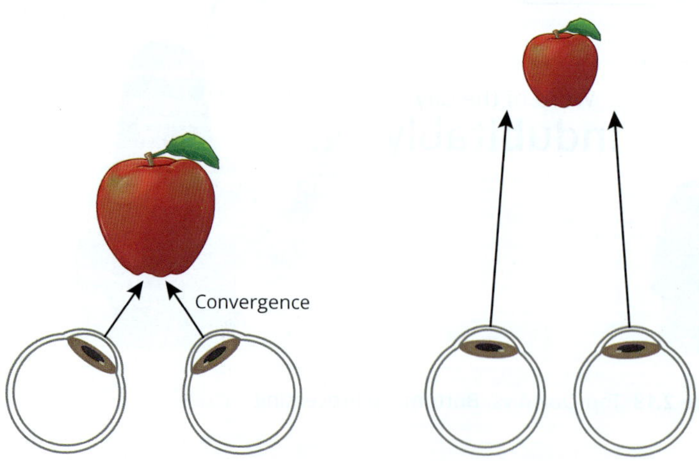

Figure 2.20 The Binocular Cue of Convergence

The form of an object is usually determined through parvocellular cells and feature detection, and the motion of an object is perceived through magnocellular cells, as described earlier. **Constancy** refers to our ability to perceive that certain characteristics of objects remain the same, despite changes in the environment. For example, we perceive a white piece of paper as essentially the same color whether the paper is illuminated by fluorescent lights, incandescent bulbs, or sunlight—this type of constancy is called color constancy. We also have constancy for brightness, size, and shape, depending on context.

Gestalt Principles

The brain constantly uses incomplete information to try to create a complete picture of the environment. **Gestalt principles** are a set of general rules that account for the fact that the brain tends to view incomplete stimuli in organized, patterned ways. There are dozens of Gestalt principles, but the highest-yield are summarized below and can be visualized in Figure 2.21.

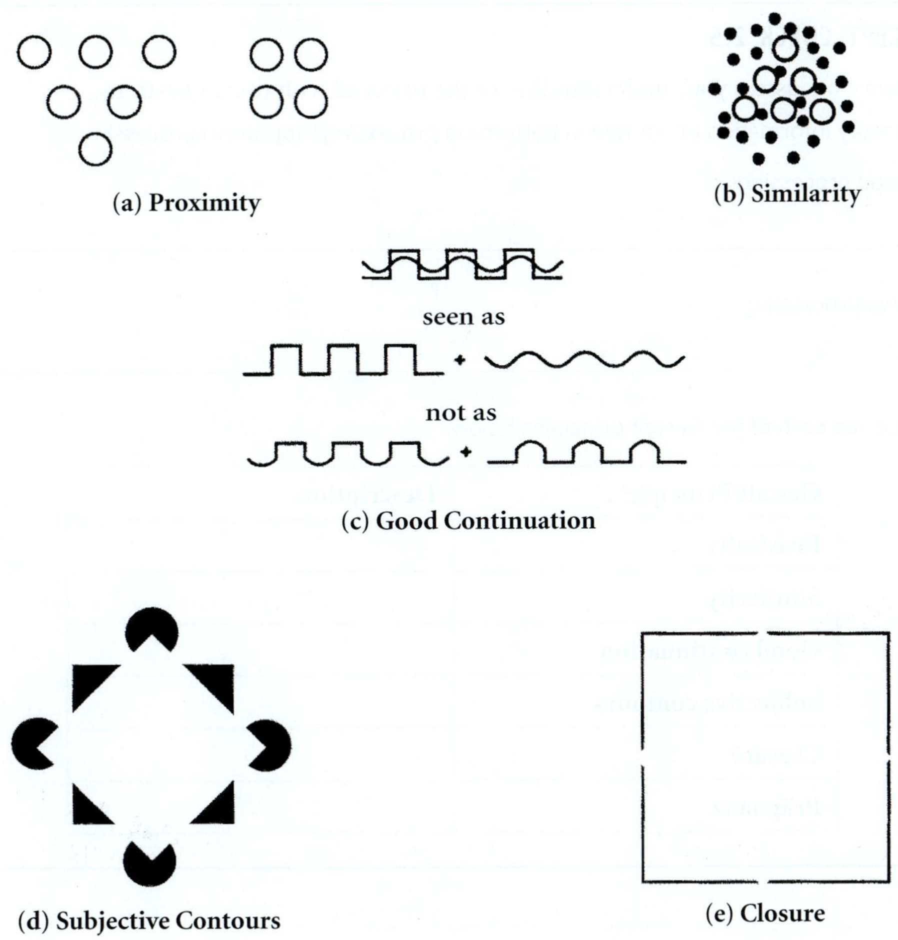

Figure 2.21 Gestalt Principles

The **law of proximity** says that elements close to one another tend to be perceived as a unit. In Figure 2.21(a), we do not see ten unrelated dots; rather, we see a triangle and a square, each composed of a certain number of dots. The **law of similarity** says that objects that are similar tend to be grouped together. In Figure 2.21(b), we see the big hollow dots as being distinct from the others, forming a triangle against a background of small filled-in dots. The **law of good continuation** says that elements that appear to follow in the same pathway tend to be grouped together. That is, there is a tendency to perceive continuous patterns in stimuli rather than abrupt changes. As seen in Figure 2.21(c), our mind tends to break down this complex figure into a sawtooth line and a wavy line, rather than two lines that contain both sawtooth and wavy elements. Some researchers have argued that the phenomena of subjective contours may arise from this law. **Subjective contours** have to do with perceiving contours and, therefore, shapes that are not actually present in the stimulus. In Figure 2.21(d), subjective contours lead to the perception of a white diamond on a black square with its corners lying on the four circles. Finally, the **law of closure** says that when a space is enclosed by a contour, the space tends to be perceived as a complete figure. Closure also refers to the fact that certain figures tend to be perceived as more complete (or closed) than they really are. In Figure 2.21(e), we don't see four right angles; instead, we see a square, even though the four sides aren't complete. All these laws operate to create the most stable, consistent, and simplest figures possible within a given visual field. Taken altogether, the Gestalt principles are governed by the **law of prägnanz**, which says that perceptual organization will always be as regular, simple, and symmetric as possible.

MCAT CONCEPT CHECK 2.5

Before you move on, assess your understanding of the material with these questions.

1. How is sensory information integrated in bottom-up processing? Top-down processing?
   - Bottom-up processing:

   ____

   - Top-down processing:

   ____

2. Briefly describe each of the Gestalt principles below:

Gestalt Principle	Description
Proximity	
Similarity	
Good continuation	
Subjective contours	
Closure	
Prägnanz	

Conclusion

The sensory systems described in this chapter are key to your success on Test Day. Not only are the eye, ear, and other senses high-yield in their own right, but connections to topics in physics, biology, research design, and other concepts in the behavioral sciences make these key topics for passages. But sensation is only one part of the system; we must then take this raw information and process it in the brain to truly perceive the world around us. We use complex neurological pathways to integrate and sort sensory information. We then process sensory information through multiple systems, analyzing individual features and components of the environment while building expectations based on our memories and past experiences. We fill in gaps in our sensorium using Gestalt principles. And what reaches our conscious awareness is the final product: a cohesive concept of the world around us.

You've completed your visit to the new city. You used your rods and cones to see the sites, your chemoreceptors to taste and smell the local food, your hair cells to listen to the local sounds, and your kinesthetic and vestibular senses to help navigate through physical space. As you get ready to head home, all you're left with are your memories—a topic we'll turn to in the next chapter.

GO ONLINE

You've reviewed the content, now test your knowledge and critical thinking skills by completing a test-like passage set in your online resources!

CONCEPT SUMMARY

Sensation vs. Perception

- **Sensation** is the conversion, or transduction, of physical, electromagnetic, auditory, and other information from the internal and external environment into electrical signals in the nervous system.
- **Perception** is the processing of sensory information to make sense of its significance.
- **Sensory receptors** are nerves that respond to stimuli and trigger electrical signals.
  - Sensory neurons are associated with **sensory ganglia**: collections of cell bodies outside the central nervous system.
  - Sensory stimuli are transmitted to **projection areas** in the brain, which further analyze the sensory input.
  - Common sensory receptors include photoreceptors, hair cells, nociceptors, thermoreceptors, osmoreceptors, olfactory receptors, and taste receptors.
- A **threshold** is the minimum stimulus that causes a change in signal transduction.
  - The **absolute threshold** is the minimum of stimulus energy that is needed to activate a sensory system.
  - The **threshold of conscious perception** is the minimum of stimulus energy that will create a signal large enough in size and long enough in duration to be brought into awareness.
  - The **difference threshold** or **just-noticeable difference** (**jnd**) is the minimum difference in magnitude between two stimuli before one can perceive this difference.
  - **Weber's law** states that the jnd for a stimulus is proportional to the magnitude of the stimulus, and that this proportion is constant over most of the range of possible stimuli.
  - **Signal detection theory** refers to the effects of nonsensory factors, such as experiences, motives, and expectations, on perception of stimuli.
  - Signal detection experiments allow us to look at **response bias**. In a signal detection experiment, a stimulus may or may not be given, and the subject is asked to state whether or not the stimulus was given. There are four possible outcomes: hits, misses, false alarms, or correct negatives.
- **Adaptation** refers to a decrease in response to a stimulus over time.

Vision

- The eye is an organ specialized to detect light in the form of photons.
  - The **cornea** gathers and filters incoming light.
  - The **iris** divides the front of the eye into the **anterior** and **posterior chambers**. It contains two muscles, the **dilator** and **constrictor pupillae**, which open and close the **pupil**.
  - The **lens** refracts incoming light to focus it on the retina and is held in place by **suspensory ligaments** connected to the **ciliary muscle**.
  - The ciliary body produces **aqueous humor**, which drains through the **canal of Schlemm**.
  - The retina contains rods and cones. **Rods** detect light and dark; **cones** come in three forms (short-, medium-, and long-wavelength) to detect colors.

- The retina contains mostly cones in the **macula**, which corresponds to the central visual field. The center of the macula is the **fovea**, which contains only cones.
- Rods and cones synapse on **bipolar cells**, which synapse on **ganglion cells**. Integration of the signals from ganglion cells and edge-sharpening is performed by **horizontal** and **amacrine cells**.
- The bulk of the eye is supported by the **vitreous** on the inside and the **sclera** and **choroid** on the outside.

- The visual pathway starts from the eye, and travels through the **optic nerves**, **optic chiasm**, **optic tracts**, **lateral geniculate nucleus** (**LGN**) of the thalamus, and **visual radiations** to get to the **visual cortex**.
  - The optic chiasm contains fibers crossing from the nasal side of the retina (temporal visual fields) of both eyes.
  - The visual radiations run through the temporal and parietal lobes.
  - The visual cortex is in the occipital lobe.
- Vision, like all senses, is processed through **parallel processing**: the ability to simultaneously analyze and combine information regarding color, form, motion, and depth.
  - Color is detected by **cones**.
  - Form is detected by **parvocellular cells**, with high spatial resolution and low temporal resolution.
  - Motion is detected by **magnocellular cells**, with low spatial resolution and high temporal resolution.
  - Depth is detected by **binocular neurons**.

Hearing and Vestibular Sense

- The ear is divided into the outer, middle, and inner ear.
  - The **outer ear** consists of the **pinna** (**auricle**), **external auditory canal**, and **tympanic membrane**.
  - The **middle ear** consists of the **ossicles**: **malleus** (hammer), **incus** (anvil), and **stapes** (stirrup). The footplate of the stapes rests on the **oval window** of the cochlea. The middle ear is connected to the nasal cavity by the **Eustachian tube**.
  - The **inner ear** contains the **bony labyrinth**, within which is the **membranous labyrinth**. The bony labyrinth is filled with **perilymph**; the membranous labyrinth is filled with **endolymph**. The membranous labyrinth consists of the **cochlea**, which detects sound; **utricle** and **saccule**, which detect linear acceleration; and **semicircular canals**, which detect rotational acceleration.
- The auditory pathway starts from the cochlea and travels through the **vestibulocochlear nerve** and **medial geniculate nucleus** (**MGN**) of the thalamus to get to the **auditory cortex** in the temporal lobe.
- Sound information also projects to the **superior olive**, which localizes the sound, and the **inferior colliculus**, which is involved in the startle reflex.

Other Senses

- Smell is the detection of volatile or aerosolized chemicals by the **olfactory chemoreceptors** (**olfactory nerves**) in the olfactory epithelium.
  - The olfactory pathway starts from the olfactory nerves and travels through the **olfactory bulb** and **olfactory tract** to get to higher-order brain areas, such as the limbic system.
  - Pheromones are chemicals given off by animals that have an effect on social, foraging, and sexual behavior in other members of that species.
- Taste is the detection of dissolved compounds by **taste buds** in **papillae**. It comes in five modalities: sweet, sour, salty, bitter, and umami (savory).
- **Somatosensation** refers to the four touch modalities: pressure, vibration, pain, and temperature.
  - A **two-point threshold** is the minimum distance necessary between two points of stimulation on the skin such that the points will be felt as two distinct stimuli.
  - **Physiological zero** is the normal temperature of the skin to which objects are compared to determine if they feel "warm" or "cold."
  - **Nociceptors** are responsible for pain perception. The **gate theory of pain** states that pain sensation is reduced when other somatosensory signals are present.
- **Kinesthetic sense** (**proprioception**) refers to the ability to tell where one's body is in three-dimensional space.

Object Recognition

- **Bottom-up** (**data-driven**) **processing** refers to recognition of objects by parallel processing and feature detection. It is slower, but less prone to mistakes.
- **Top-down** (**conceptually driven**) **processing** refers to recognition of an object by memories and expectations, with little attention to detail. It is faster, but more prone to mistakes.
- Perceptual organization refers to our synthesis of stimuli to make sense of the world, including integration of depth, form, motion, and constancy.
- **Gestalt principles** are ways that the brain can infer missing parts of a picture when a picture is incomplete.
  - The **law of proximity** says that elements close to one another tend to be perceived as a unit.
  - The **law of similarity** says that objects that are similar appear to be grouped together.
  - The **law of good continuation** says that elements that appear to follow the same pathway tend to be grouped together.
  - **Subjective contours** refer to the perception of nonexistent edges in figures, based on surrounding visual cues.
  - The **law of closure** says that when a space is enclosed by a group of lines, it is perceived as a complete or closed line.
  - The **law of prägnanz** says that **perceptual organization** will always be as regular, simple, and symmetric as possible.

ANSWERS TO CONCEPT CHECKS

2.1

1. Sensory receptor → afferent neuron → sensory ganglion → spinal cord → brain (projection areas)
2. 1–F, 2–A, 3–E, 4–D, 5–C, 6–G, 7–B
3. Absolute threshold is the minimum stimulus that can evoke an action potential in a sensory receptor. Threshold of conscious perception is the minimum stimulus that can evoke enough action potentials for a long enough time that the brain perceives the stimulus. The difference threshold (just-noticeable difference) is the minimum difference between two stimuli that can be detected by the brain.
4. Weber's law explains that just-noticeable differences are best expressed as a ratio, which is constant over most of the range of sensory stimuli. Signal detection theory concerns the threshold to sense a stimulus, given obscuring internal and external stimuli.
5. Adaptation generally raises the difference threshold for a sensory response; as one becomes used to small fluctuations in the stimulus, the difference in stimulus required to evoke a response must be larger.

2.2

1. Cornea: gathers and focuses the incoming light
   Pupil: allows passage of light from the anterior to posterior chamber
   Iris: controls the size of the pupil
   Ciliary body: produces aqueous humor; accommodation of the lens
   Canal of Schlemm: drains aqueous humor
   Lens: refracts the incoming light to focus it on the retina
   Retina: detects images
   Sclera: provides structural support
2. Cornea → pupil → lens → vitreous → retina (rods and cones → bipolar cells → ganglion cells) → optic nerve → optic chiasm → optic tract → lateral geniculate nucleus (LGN) of thalamus → radiations through parietal and temporal lobes → visual cortex (occipital lobe)
3. Parallel processing is the ability to simultaneously analyze color, shape, and motion of an object and to integrate this information to create a cohesive image of the world. Parallel processing also calls on memory systems to compare a visual stimulus to past experiences to help determine the object's identity.
4. Cones are responsible for color. Parvocellular cells are responsible for form. Magnocellular cells are responsible for motion. Binocular neurons are responsible for depth.

2.3

1. Linear acceleration is detected by the utricle and saccule. Rotational acceleration is detected by the semicircular canals.
2. Pinna → external auditory canal → tympanic membrane → malleus → incus → stapes → oval window → perilymph in cochlea → basilar membrane → hair cells → vestibulocochlear nerve → brainstem → medial geniculate nucleus (MGN) of thalamus → auditory cortex (temporal lobe)
3. The basilar membrane is tonotopically organized: high-pitched sounds cause vibrations at the base of the cochlea, whereas low-pitched sounds cause vibrations at the apex of the cochlea.

2.4

1. Nostril → nasal cavity → olfactory chemoreceptors (olfactory nerves) on olfactory epithelium → olfactory bulb → olfactory tract → higher-order brain regions, including limbic system
2. Smell is sensitive to volatile or aerosolized compounds; taste is sensitive to dissolved compounds.
3. The four main modalities of somatosensation are pressure, vibration, pain, and temperature.

2.5

1. Bottom-up processing requires each component of an object to be interpreted through parallel processing and then integrated into one cohesive whole. Top-down processing starts with the whole object and, through memory, creates expectations for the components of the object.
2.

Gestalt Principle	Description
Proximity	Components close to one another tend to be perceived as a unit.
Similarity	Components that are similar (in color, shape, size) tend to be grouped together.
Good continuation	Components that appear to follow in the same pathway tend to be grouped together; abrupt changes in form are less likely than continuation of the same pattern.
Subjective contours	Edges or shapes that are not actually present can be implied by the surrounding objects (especially if good continuation is present).
Closure	A space enclosed by a contour tends to be perceived as a complete figure; such figures tend to be perceived as more complete (or closed) than they really are.
Prägnanz	Perceptual organization will always be as regular, simple, and symmetric as possible.

SCIENCE MASTERY ASSESSMENT EXPLANATIONS

1. **C**

Weber's law posits that thresholds are proportional. Going from 100 to 125 pounds is a 25 percent increase. **(C)** is a 40 percent increase while all the rest are all under 25 percent.

2. **D**

The person is discerning a specific noise within a field of many noises. This is the definition of signal detection. In an experimental setup, the person's response would be considered a hit if the friend was indeed laughing; it would be considered a false alarm if the friend was not laughing.

3. **A**

The spicy food can be considered an extreme stimulus because it eclipses what the person believes can be handled in terms of heat. However, after experiencing the stimulus over and over, the experience of spice drops to barely perceptible. This is sensory adaptation: a reduction in response to a stimulus over time.

4. **B**

Nociceptors are important for pain sensation, which would be expected during tissue damage. Chemoreceptors, **(A)**, respond to chemicals, whether volatile or aerosolized (olfaction) or dissolved (taste). Osmoreceptors, **(C)**, respond to changes in blood osmolarity, and photoreceptors, **(D)**, respond to light.

5. **A**

The cornea is responsible for gathering and focusing light. The pupil and iris, **(B)** and **(C)**, are both involved in regulating the amount of light coming into the eye but not in focusing it. The retina, **(D)**, transduces the light into electrical signals that are sent to the brain. The lens serves a similar function to the cornea and would also be a valid answer to this question.

6. **C**

This person was able to distinguish the coin from other items by recognizing specific features of the coin; in this case, it was the glint of the metal surface and its position in the car. This phenomenon is called feature detection.

7. **C**

The retina is the part of the eye upon which images are projected. Rods and cones in the retina then convert the electromagnetic radiation into electrical signals.

8. **A**

Somatosensation refers to the various modalities of touch: pressure, vibration, temperature, and pain. Kinesthetic sense, **(B)**, refers to the ability to tell where one's body is in space. Vestibular sense, **(C)**, refers to the detection of linear and rotational acceleration in the middle ear. Finally, chemoreception, **(D)**, refers to sensing chemicals in the environment.

9. **B**

The five tastes are sweet, sour, salty, bitter, and umami. Floral would be related to smell rather than taste.

10. **C**

Endolymph is the potassium-rich fluid that bathes the hair cells of the inner ear, all of which are found within the membranous labyrinth. Perilymph is found in the space between the membranous labyrinth and the bony labyrinth. Both the membranous labyrinth and bony labyrinth contribute to the cochlea and the vestibule, eliminating **(A)** and **(B)**.

11. **A**

Pheromones are the volatile chemicals given off by organisms that bind with olfactory chemoreceptors and influence behavior. It is debatable if pheromones serve a role in humans, but they are known to affect foraging and sexual behavior in some animals.

12. **B**

Kinesthetic sense, or proprioception, refers to the ability to tell where body parts are in three-dimensional space. The sensors for proprioception are found predominantly in the muscles and joints. Loss of vestibular sense, **(A)**, would also cause difficulty walking, but this would be due to a sense of dizziness or vertigo, not an inability to feel one's feet.

13. **C**

The proofreader used a larger pattern to identify the word and expected to see an "e," thus missing the error. This is related to top-down processing; the proofreader used recognition and expectations, which led to missing a detail. Bottom-up processing, **(D)**, would be the analysis of each detail individually before creating a cohesive image.

14. **D**

Gestalt principles are the basis for many optical illusions and include the tendency of people to see continuity even when lines are unconnected. Specifically, this logo appears to rely on the law of closure to create one complete star from five nontouching angles.

15. **D**

The optic chiasm houses the crossing fibers from each optic nerve. Specifically, the fibers coming from the nasal half of the retina in each eye cross in the chiasm to join the optic tract on the opposite side. Remember that the lens of the eye causes inversion, so images on the nasal half of the retina actually originate in the temporal visual field. This condition is called bitemporal hemianopsia.

GO ONLINE

Consult your online resources for additional practice.

SHARED CONCEPTS

Behavioral Sciences Chapter 1
Biology and Behavior

Biology Chapter 4
The Nervous System

Biology Chapter 10
Homeostasis

Physics and Math Chapter 3
Thermodynamics

Physics and Math Chapter 7
Waves and Sound

Physics and Math Chapter 8
Light and Optics

CHAPTER 3

LEARNING AND MEMORY

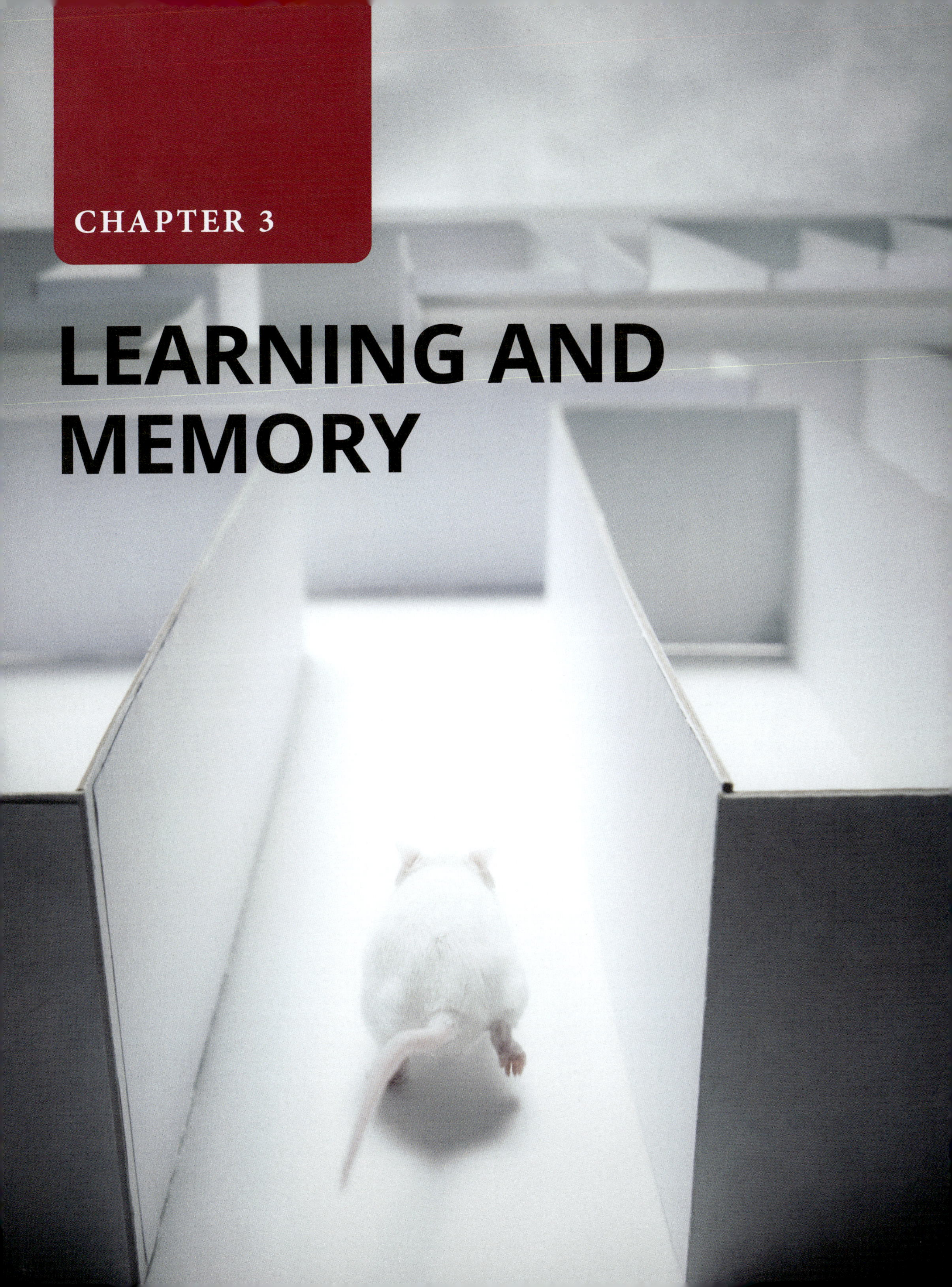

SCIENCE MASTERY ASSESSMENT

Every pre-med knows this feeling: there is so much content I have to know for the MCAT! How do I know what to do first or what's important?

While the high-yield badges throughout this book will help you identify the most important topics, this Science Mastery Assessment is another tool in your MCAT prep arsenal. This quiz (which can also be taken in your online resources) and the guidance below will help ensure that you are spending the appropriate amount of time on this chapter based on your personal strengths and weaknesses. Don't worry though—skipping something now does not mean you'll never study it. Later on in your prep, as you complete full-length tests, you'll uncover specific pieces of content that you need to review and can come back to these chapters as appropriate.

How to Use This Assessment

If you answer 0–7 questions correctly:

Spend about 1 hour to read this chapter in full and take limited notes throughout. Follow up by reviewing **all** quiz questions to ensure that you now understand how to solve each one.

If you answer 8–11 questions correctly:

Spend 20–40 minutes reviewing the quiz questions. Beginning with the questions you missed, read and take notes on the corresponding subchapters. For questions you answered correctly, ensure your thinking matches that of the explanation and you understand why each choice was correct or incorrect.

If you answer 12–15 questions correctly:

Spend less than 20 minutes reviewing all questions from the quiz. If you missed any, then include a quick read-through of the corresponding subchapters, or even just the relevant content within a subchapter, as part of your question review. For questions you answered correctly, ensure your thinking matches that of the explanation and review the Concept Summary at the end of the chapter.

1. Researchers repeatedly startle a participant with a loud buzzer. After some time, the participant stops being startled by the buzzer. If the researchers interrupt the study with the sound of pans banging together, which of the following would likely be observed?
   - **A.** Increased startle response to the buzzer
   - **B.** Decreased startle response to the buzzer
   - **C.** No change in the response to the buzzer
   - **D.** Generalization to previously nonaversive stimuli

2. Many pets will run toward the kitchen when they hear the sound of a can opener opening a can of pet food. The sound of the can opener is a(n):
   - **A.** conditioned response.
   - **B.** unconditioned response.
   - **C.** conditioned stimulus.
   - **D.** unconditioned stimulus.

3. A person suffers from food poisoning after eating a spoiled orange and later finds that the smell of lemon and other citrus fruits causes a feeling of nausea. This is an example of:
   - **A.** acquisition.
   - **B.** generalization.
   - **C.** discrimination.
   - **D.** negative reinforcement.

4. Which of the following processes would increase the likelihood of a behavior?
   - **A.** Extinction
   - **B.** Negative punishment
   - **C.** Positive punishment
   - **D.** Avoidance learning

5. The presynaptic neuron becomes more efficient at releasing neurotransmitters while receptor density increases on the postsynaptic neuron. These changes are consistent with:
   - **A.** long term potentiation.
   - **B.** synaptic pruning.
   - **C.** an increase in neuroplasticity.
   - **D.** amnesia.

6. A rat is trained to press a lever to obtain food under a fixed-interval schedule. Which of the following behaviors would the rat most likely exhibit?
   - **A.** Pressing the lever continuously whenever it is hungry.
   - **B.** Pressing the lever exactly once and waiting for the food pellet before pressing it again.
   - **C.** Pressing the lever slowly at first, but with increasing frequency as the end of the interval approaches.
   - **D.** None of the above; the association formed by fixed-interval schedules is too weak to increase behavior.

7. Which of the following is true of teaching an animal a complicated, multistage behavior?
   - **I.** The individual parts of the behavior should not run counter to the animal's natural instincts.
   - **II.** The behaviors must be tied to a food reward of some kind.
   - **III.** Rewarding individual parts of the behavior on their own interferes with reinforcement of the entire behavior.
   - **A.** I only
   - **B.** I and III only
   - **C.** II and III only
   - **D.** I, II, and III

8. Which of the following is true of controlled processing?
   - **A.** It is the means through which information enters short-term memory.
   - **B.** Information that requires controlled processing cannot become automatic.
   - **C.** It always requires active attention to the information being encoded.
   - **D.** Most information we can later recall is encoded using controlled processing.

9. Which of the following methods of encoding is most conducive to later recall?
   A. Semantic
   B. Visual
   C. Iconic
   D. Acoustic

10. A hemisphere of the brain can be removed to prevent the recurrence of severe seizures. How would the ability of the other hemisphere to adopt functionalities of the removed section differ between a two year old and a twenty year old?
    A. The brain of the twenty year old would be more adaptable due to higher neuroplasticity.
    B. The brain of the twenty year old would be more adaptable due to lower neuroplasticity.
    C. The brain of the two year old would be more adaptable due to higher neuroplasticity.
    D. The brain of the two year old would be more adaptable due to lower neuroplasticity.

11. An individual memorizes a shopping list by associating each item with an image that corresponds with a number. This individual is using which of the following mnemonics?
    A. Clustering
    B. Method of loci
    C. Elaborative rehearsal
    D. Peg-words

12. A researcher uses a partial-report procedure after presenting participants with an array of nine numbers for a fraction of a second. Which of the following is the most likely result of this procedure?
    A. The participants will be able to recall any of the rows or columns in great detail but only immediately after presentation.
    B. The participants will only be able to recall the first few numbers in the array due to the serial position effect.
    C. The participants will be able to recall approximately seven of the numbers for a few seconds following presentation of the stimulus.
    D. The participants will not be able to recall any of the numbers verbally, but will be able to draw the full array under hypnosis.

13. Which of the following is an example of a semantic memory?
    A. Having the ability to drive a car
    B. Knowing the parts of a car engine
    C. Remembering the experience of learning to drive
    D. Associating a car with other vehicles in a semantic network

14. Which of the following is an example of a circumstance that could cause a state-dependent recall effect?
    I. The individual is outside on a rainy day.
    II. The individual is intoxicated on cannabis.
    III. The individual is experiencing a manic episode.
    A. I only
    B. III only
    C. II and III only
    D. I, II, and III

15. Which of the following would an older adult be most likely to have trouble recalling?
    A. The circumstances of meeting a significant other in college
    B. A doctor's appointment scheduled for 1:00 p.m.
    C. The names of the characters in a favorite television show
    D. That a library book needs to be returned when passing by the library on a morning walk

Answer Key

1. **A** (See section 3.1)
2. **C** (See section 3.1)
3. **B** (See section 3.1)
4. **D** (See section 3.1)
5. **A** (See section 3.3)
6. **C** (See section 3.1)
7. **A** (See section 3.1)
8. **C** (See section 3.2)
9. **A** (See section 3.2)
10. **C** (See section 3.3)
11. **D** (See section 3.2)
12. **A** (See section 3.2)
13. **B** (See section 3.2)
14. **C** (See section 3.2)
15. **B** (See section 3.2)

The relevant section of the chapter to review for each question is given in parentheses after the correct answer. Detailed explanations can be found at the end of the chapter.

CHAPTER 3

LEARNING AND MEMORY

In This Chapter

CHAPTER PROFILE

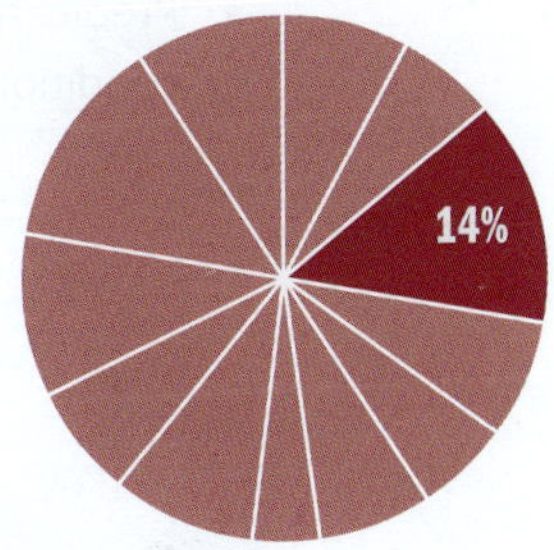

The content in this chapter should be relevant to about 14% of all questions about the behavioral sciences on the MCAT.

This chapter covers material from the following AAMC content categories:

6B: Making sense of the environment

7C: Attitude and behavior change

Introduction

A college student sits hunched over a desk in a quiet library, poring over a small stack of textbooks. It's 11 p.m. the night before the organic chemistry midterm, and there seems to be a near endless list of reactions to commit to memory before tomorrow. The situation seems bleak, but the student has been here before and has taken every precaution to make sure that this study session will be successful: drinking coffee will increase alertness, while the quiet of the library will reduce distractions to aid concentration. It's stressful, to be sure, but the student has been able to study this way before and do quite well, reinforcing this current set of behaviors. The student works through a set of flashcards—reactants on one side, products on the other—and is able to identify most of them but misses a few. Those cards are placed in a separate pile to be reviewed later. Sure, this rehearsal will most likely help for the exam tomorrow, but will the student be able to recall this information again for the final in two months? The student takes another sip of coffee and tries to put everything else out of mind, focusing intently on the book sitting open on the desk.

Sound familiar? If you're like most students, you've found yourself in a similar scenario at least once. This chapter will discuss the ways in which you both memorize new information and learn new behaviors. This will not only help you to directly prepare to answer MCAT questions about this content, but also to learn a few new tricks about how to effectively commit all of the MCAT content to memory. This is a skill that will be helpful both now and later in your career as a doctor.

3.1 Learning High Yield

LEARNING OBJECTIVES

After Chapter 3.1, you will be able to:

- Apply principles of habituation, dishabituation, and sensitization to real-life scenarios
- Identify the conditioned stimulus, unconditioned stimulus, conditioned response, and unconditioned response in a Pavlovian learning paradigm
- Distinguish between negative reinforcement, positive reinforcement, negative punishment, and positive punishment
- Predict how reinforcement schedule will affect relative frequency of behavioral response in an operant conditioning scenario:

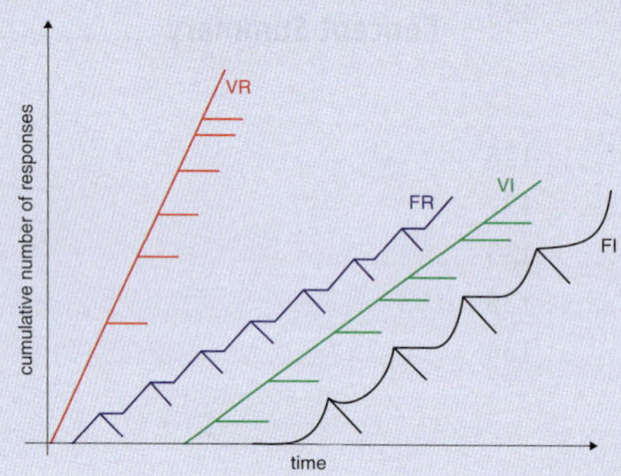

To a psychologist, **learning** refers specifically to the way in which we acquire new behaviors. To understand learning, we must start with the concept of a stimulus. A **stimulus** can be defined as anything to which an organism can respond, including all of the sensory inputs we discussed in Chapter 2 of *MCAT Behavioral Sciences Review*. The combination of stimuli and responses serves as the basis for all behavioral learning.

Responses to stimuli can change over time depending on the frequency and intensity of the stimulus. For instance, repeated exposure to the same stimulus can cause a decrease in response called **habituation**. This is seen in many first-year medical students: students often have an intense physical reaction the first time they see a cadaver or treat a severe laceration, but as they get used to these stimuli, the reaction lessens until they are unbothered by these sights. Note that a stimulus too weak to elicit a response is called **subthreshold** stimulus.

The opposite process can also occur. **Dishabituation** is defined as the recovery of a response to a stimulus after habituation has occurred. Dishabituation is often noted when, late in the habituation of a stimulus, a second stimulus is presented. As can be seen in Figure 3.1, the second stimulus interrupts the habituation process and thereby causes an increase in response to the original stimulus. Imagine, for example, that you're taking a long car trip and driving for many miles on a highway. After a while, your brain will get used to the sights, sounds, and sensations of highway driving: the dashed lines dividing the lanes, the sound of the engine and the tires on the road, and so on. Habituation has occurred. At some point you use an exit ramp, and these sensations change. As you merge onto the new highway, you pay more attention to the sensory stimuli coming in. Even if the stimuli are more or less the same as on the previous highway, the presentation of a different stimulus (using the

KEY CONCEPT

Dishabituation is the recovery of a response to a stimulus, usually after a different stimulus has been presented. Note that the term refers to changes in response to the original stimulus, not the new one.

exit ramp) causes dishabituation and a new awareness of—and response to—these stimuli. Dishabituation is temporary and always refers to changes in response to the original stimulus, not the new one.

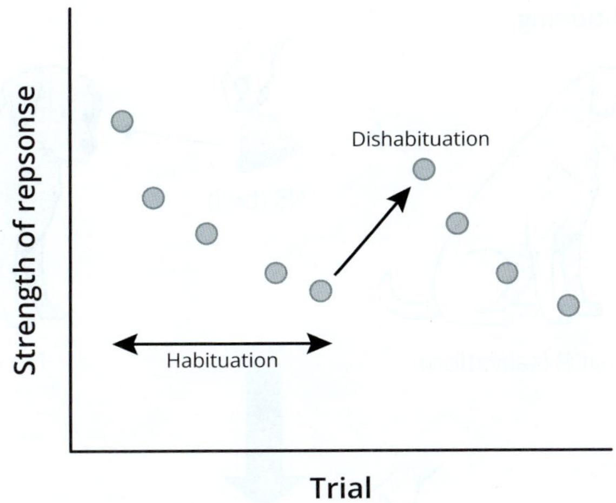

Figure 3.1 Habituation and Dishabituation

Learning, then, is a change in behavior that occurs in response to a stimulus. While there are many types of learning, the MCAT focuses on two types: associative learning and observational learning.

Associative Learning

Associative learning is the creation of a pairing, or association, either between two stimuli or between a behavior and a response. On the MCAT, you'll be tested on two kinds of associative learning: classical and operant conditioning.

Classical Conditioning

Classical conditioning is a type of associative learning that takes advantage of biological, instinctual responses to create associations between two unrelated stimuli. For many people, the first name that comes to mind for research in classical conditioning is Ivan Pavlov. His experiments on dogs were not only revolutionary, but also provide a template for the way the MCAT will test classical conditioning.

Classical conditioning works, first and foremost, because some stimuli cause an innate or reflexive physiological response. For example, we reflexively salivate when we smell bread baking in an oven, or we may jump or recoil when we hear a loud noise. Any stimulus that brings about such a reflexive response is called an **unconditioned stimulus**, and the innate or reflexive response is called an **unconditioned response**. Many stimuli do not produce a reflexive response and are known as **neutral stimuli**.

In Pavlov's experiment, the unconditioned stimulus was meat, which would cause the dogs to salivate reflexively, and the neutral stimulus was a ringing bell. Through the course of the experiment, Pavlov repeatedly rang the bell before placing meat in the dogs' mouths. Initially, the dogs did not react much when they only heard the bell ring without receiving meat. However, after this procedure was repeated several times, the dogs began to salivate when they heard the bell ring. In fact, the dogs would salivate even if Pavlov only rang the bell and did not deliver any meat. Pavlov thereby turned a neutral stimulus into a **conditioned stimulus**: a normally neutral stimulus that, through association, now causes a reflexive response called a **conditioned response**. The process of using a reflexive, unconditioned stimulus to turn a neutral stimulus into a conditioned stimulus is termed **acquisition**, as shown in Figure 3.2. The experiment used **appetitive conditioning**, a type of classical conditioning in which the unconditioned stimulus is pleasant or desirable; this type of stimulus, referred to as an **appetitive stimulus**, functions to increase the frequency of a response.

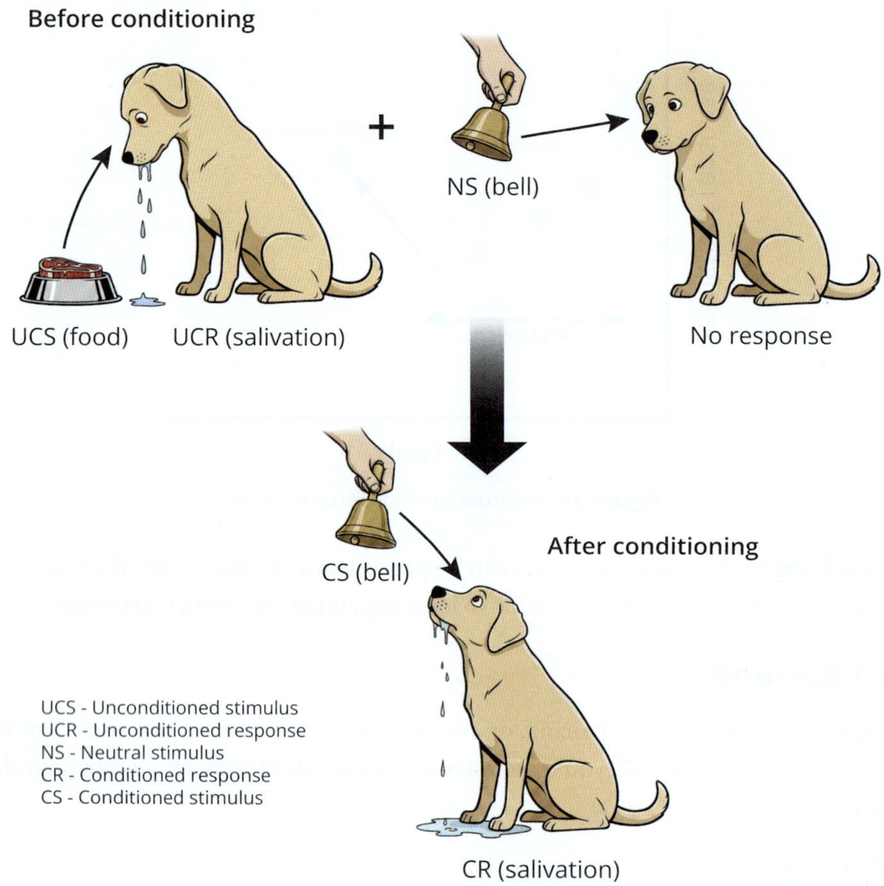

Figure 3.2 Acquisition in Classical Conditioning

Notice that the stimuli change in this experiment, but the response is the same throughout. Because salivation in response to food is natural and requires no conditioning, it is an unconditioned response in this context. On the other hand, when paired with the conditioned stimulus of the bell, salivation is considered a conditioned response.

However, it is important to recognize that just because a conditioned response has been acquired, that does not mean that the conditioned response is permanent. **Extinction** refers to the loss of a conditioned response, and can occur if the conditioned stimulus is repeatedly presented without the unconditioned stimulus. Applying this concept to the Pavlov example, if the bell rings often enough without the dog getting meat, the dog may stop salivating when the bell sounds. Interestingly, this extinction of a response is not always permanent; after some time, presenting subjects again with an extinct conditioned stimulus will sometimes produce a weak conditioned response, a phenomenon called **spontaneous recovery**. Figure 3.3 contains a graphical depiction of the acquisition, extinction, and spontaneous recovery phases in behavioral learning.

MCAT EXPERTISE

On the MCAT, the key to telling conditioned and unconditioned responses apart will be to look at which stimulus is causing them: unconditioned stimuli cause an unconditioned response, while conditioned stimuli cause a conditioned response.

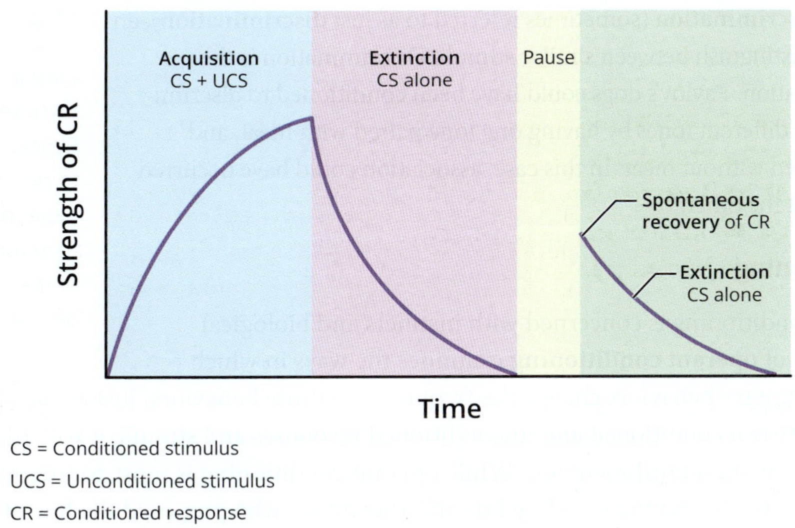

Figure 3.3 Acquisition, Extinction, and Spontaneous Recovery

There are a few processes that can modify the response to a conditioned stimulus after acquisition has occurred. **Generalization** is a broadening effect by which a stimulus similar enough to the conditioned stimulus can also produce the conditioned response. In one famous and ethically controversial experiment, researchers conditioned a child called Little Albert to be afraid of a white rat by pairing the presentation of the rat with a loud noise. Subsequent tests showed that Little Albert's conditioning had generalized such that he also exhibited a fear response to a white stuffed rabbit, a white sealskin coat, and even a man with a white beard. See a depiction of this experiment in Figure 3.4.

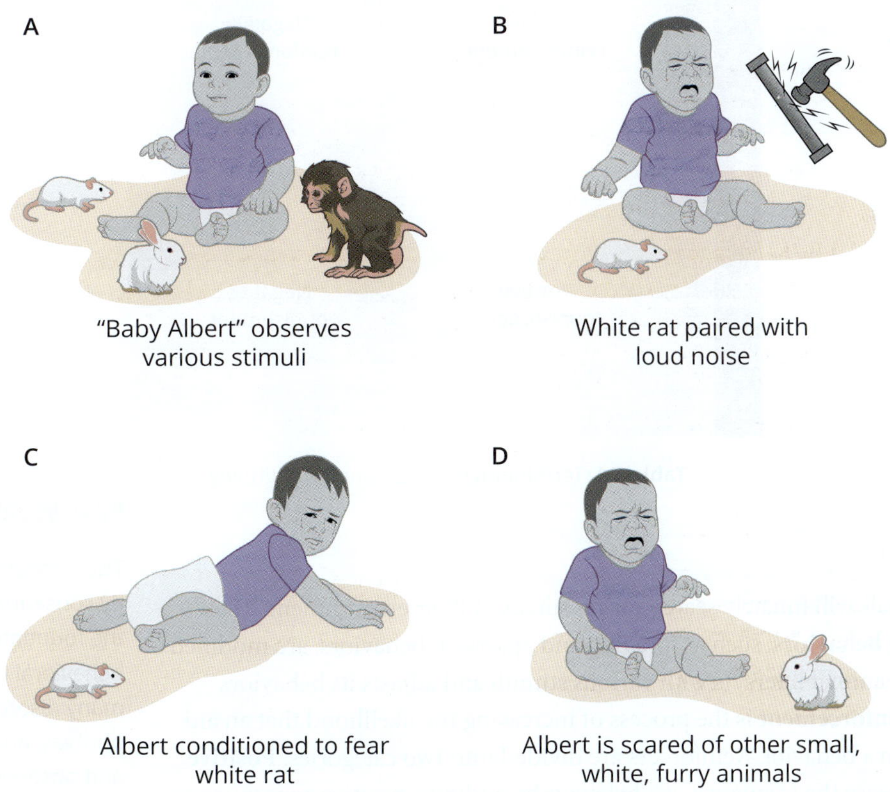

Figure 3.4 The Little Albert Experiment

Finally, in **stimuli discrimination** (sometimes referred to as just **discrimination**), an organism learns to distinguish between similar stimuli. Discrimination is the opposite of generalization. Pavlov's dogs could have been conditioned to discriminate between bells of different tones by having one tone paired with meat, and another tone presented without meat. In this case, association could have occurred with one tone but not the other.

MCAT EXPERTISE

Classical conditioning is a favorite topic on the MCAT. Expect at least one question to describe a Pavlovian experiment and ask you to identify the role of one of the stimuli or responses described.

Operant Conditioning

Whereas classical conditioning is concerned with instincts and biological responses, the study of **operant conditioning** examines the ways in which consequences of voluntary behaviors change the frequency of those behaviors. Just as the MCAT will test you on the difference between conditioned and unconditioned responses and stimuli, it will ask you to distinguish between reinforcement and punishment too. While operant conditioning is most commonly associated with B. F. Skinner, it was actually first theorized by Edward Thorndike, who proposed the **law of effect** based on experiments with cages and cats. The law of effect states that behaviors that produce desirable outcomes (like pressing a button to open the cage) will be repeated. Skinner continued Thorndike's work, and is considered one of the founders of **behaviorism**, the theory that all behaviors are conditioned. The four possible relationships between stimulus and behavior are summarized in Table 3.1.

		Stimulus	
		Added	Removed
Behavior	Continues	Positive reinforcement	Negative reinforcement
	Stops	Positive punishment	Negative punishment

Table 3.1 Terminology of Operant Conditioning

Reinforcement

Almost all animals will innately search for resources in their environment. These **reward-seeking behaviors**, such as foraging and approach behaviors, are modified over time as the animal interacts with various stimuli and adjusts its behaviors accordingly. **Reinforcement** is the process of increasing the likelihood that an animal will perform a behavior. Reinforcers are divided into two categories. **Positive reinforcers** increase the frequency of a behavior by adding a positive consequence

REAL WORLD

This concept of learning by consequence forms the foundation for behavioral therapies for many disorders including phobias, anxiety disorders, and obsessive–compulsive disorder.

or incentive following the desired behavior. Money is an example of a common and strong positive reinforcer: employees will continue to work if they are paid. **Negative reinforcers** act similarly in that they increase the frequency of a behavior, but they do so by removing something unpleasant. For example, taking an aspirin reduces a headache, so the next time you have a headache, you are more likely to take one. Negative reinforcement is often confused with punishment, which will be discussed in the next section, but remember that the frequency of the behavior is the distinguishing factor: any reinforcement—positive or negative—increases the likelihood that a behavior will be performed.

Negative reinforcement can be subdivided into escape learning and avoidance learning, which differ in whether the unpleasant stimulus occurs or not. **Escape learning** describes a situation where the animal experiences the unpleasant stimulus and, in response, displays the desired behavior in order to trigger the removal of the stimulus. So, in this type of learning, the desired behavior is used to escape the stimulus. In contrast, **avoidance learning** occurs when the animal displays the desired behavior in anticipation of the unpleasant stimulus, thereby avoiding the unpleasant stimulus.

Avoidance learning often develops from multiple experiences of escape learning. An example of this progression from escape learning to avoidance learning is the seat belt warning in a car (Figure 3.5). If a driver begins driving without buckling the seat belt, then the car will produce an annoying beeping noise, which only ends when the seat belt is buckled. In this example, the desired behavior is to buckle the seat belt. This behavior is reinforced by the removal of an unpleasant stimulus (the audible beeping), so this type of learning is negative reinforcement. More specifically, this example illustrates escape learning, since the driver first experiences the unpleasant stimulus, then exhibits the desired behavior in order to escape the unpleasant stimulus. However, after forgetting to buckle the seat belt several times, the driver will eventually learn to preemptively buckle up before driving the car in order to avoid the beeping sound. At that point, the escape learning has progressed to avoidance learning. Finally, this example illustrates an important misconception about the term *negative reinforcement:* Buckling one's seat belt is generally considered a "positive" behavior, in that it protects one's health. Nevertheless, the terms "positive" and "negative" in operant conditioning only refer to the addition or removal of a stimulus. So even though buckling up is a "good" thing, this example illustrates several types of negative reinforcement!

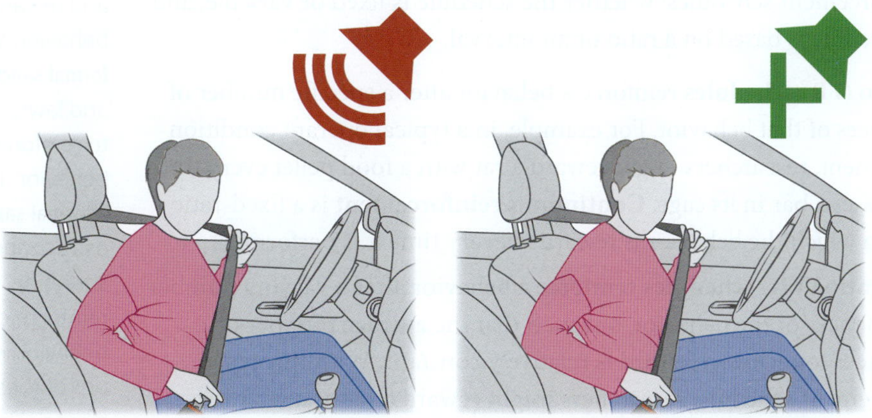

Figure 3.5 Escape vs. Avoidance Learning

Classical and operant conditioning can be used hand-in-hand. For example, some dog trainers take advantage of reinforcers when training dogs to perform tricks. Sometimes, the trainers will feed the dog a bit of meat after it performs a trick. The meat can be said to be a **primary reinforcer** because the meat is a treat that the dog responds to naturally. Dog trainers also use tiny handheld devices that emit a clicking sound. This clicker would not normally be a reinforcer on its own, but the trainers use classical conditioning to pair the clicker with meat to elicit the same response. The clicker is thus a **conditioned reinforcer**, which is sometimes called a **secondary reinforcer**. Eventually, the dog may even associate the presence of the trainer with the possibility of reward, making the presence of the trainer a **discriminative stimulus**. A discriminative stimulus indicates that reward is potentially available in an operant conditioning paradigm. If the dog had to wait an extended period of time between performing the trick and getting the treat, then the treat would be considered a **delayed reinforcement**, which tends to be less effective than immediate reinforcement.

Punishment

In contrast to reinforcement, **punishment** uses conditioning to reduce the occurrence of a behavior. **Positive punishment** adds an unpleasant consequence in response to a behavior to reduce that behavior; for example, receiving a ticket and having to pay a fine for parking illegally. Because positive punishment involves using something unpleasant to discourage a behavior, it is sometimes referred to as **aversive conditioning**. By contrast, **negative punishment** is removing a stimulus in order to cause reduction of a behavior. For example, a parent or guardian may forbid a child from watching television as a consequence for bad behavior, with the goal of preventing the behavior from happening again.

KEY CONCEPT

Negative reinforcement is often confused with positive punishment. Negative reinforcement is the *removal* of a bothersome stimulus to *encourage* a behavior; positive punishment is the *addition* of a bothersome stimulus to *reduce* a behavior.

Reinforcement Schedules

The presence or absence of reinforcing or punishing stimuli is just a part of the story. The rate at which desired behaviors are acquired is also affected by the **reinforcement schedule** being used to deliver the stimuli. There are two key factors to reinforcement schedules: whether the schedule is fixed or variable, and whether the schedule is based on a ratio or an interval.

- **Fixed-ratio (FR) schedules** reinforce a behavior after a specific number of performances of that behavior. For example, in a typical operant conditioning experiment, researchers might reward a rat with a food pellet every third time it presses a bar in its cage. **Continuous reinforcement** is a fixed-ratio schedule in which the behavior is rewarded every time it is performed.
- **Variable-ratio (VR) schedules** reinforce a behavior after a varying number of performances of the behavior, but such that the average number of performances to receive a reward is relatively constant. With this type of reinforcement schedule, researchers might reward a rat first after two button presses, then eight, then four, then finally six.
- **Fixed-interval (FI) schedules** reinforce the first instance of a behavior after a specified time period has elapsed. For example, once our rat gets a pellet, it has to wait 60 seconds before it can get another pellet. The first lever press after 60 seconds gets a pellet, but subsequent presses during those 60 seconds accomplish nothing.

BRIDGE

Sociological institutions often rely on punishments and rewards to adjust behavior. Within a society, **formal sanctions**, or rules and laws, can be used to reinforce or punish behavior. Likewise, **informal sanctions**, such as ostracization, praise, and shunning, can be used to reinforce or punish social behavior without depending on rules established by social institutions. Socialization and social institutions are discussed in Chapters 8 and 11 of *MCAT Behavioral Sciences Review*, respectively.

- **Variable-interval (VI) schedules** reinforce a behavior the first time that behavior is performed after a varying interval of time. Instead of waiting exactly 60 seconds, for example, our rat might have to wait 90 seconds, then 30 seconds, then three minutes. In each case, once the interval elapses, the next press gets the rat a pellet.

Of these schedules, variable-ratio works the fastest for learning a new behavior, and is also the most resistant to extinction. The effectiveness of the various reinforcement schedules is demonstrated in Figure 3.6.

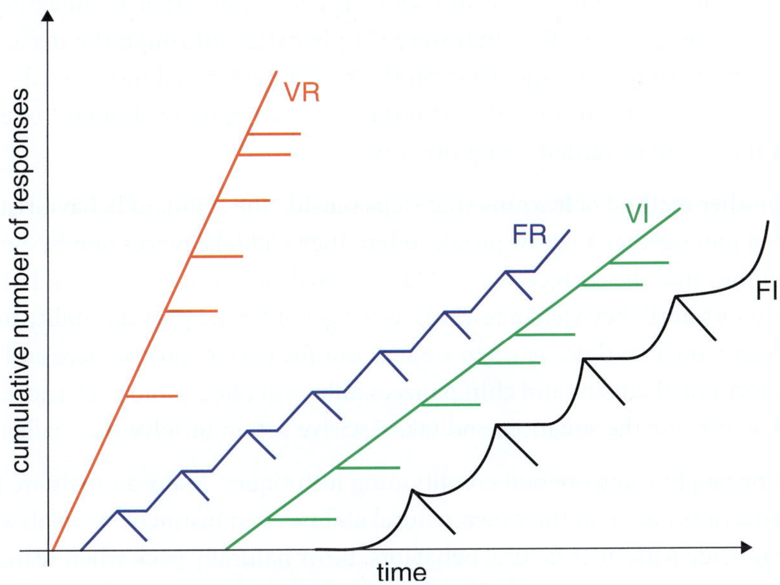

Figure 3.6 Reinforcement Schedules
Hatches correspond to instances of reinforcement. The start of each line corresponds to time zero for that schedule.

There are a few things to note in this graph. First, variable-ratio schedules have the fastest response rate: the rat will continue pressing the bar quickly with the hope that the next press will be the "right one." Also note that fixed schedules (fixed-ratio and fixed-interval) often have a brief moment of no responses after the behavior is reinforced: the rat will stop hitting the lever until it wants another pellet, once it has figured out what behavior is necessary to receive the pellet.

One final idea associated with operant conditioning is the concept of **shaping**, which is the process of rewarding increasingly specific behaviors that become closer to a desired response. For example, if you wanted to train a bird to spin around in place and then peck a key on a keyboard, you might first give the bird a treat for turning slightly to the left, then only for turning a full 90 degrees, then 180, and so on, until the bird has learned to spin around completely. Then you might only reward this behavior if done near the keyboard until eventually the bird is only rewarded once the full set of behaviors is performed. While it may take some time, the use of shaping in operant conditioning can allow for the training of extremely complicated behaviors.

MNEMONIC

VR stands for **V**ariable-**R**atio, but it can also stand for **V**ery **R**apid and **V**ery **R**esistant to extinction.

REAL WORLD

Gambling (and gambling addiction) is so difficult to extinguish because most gambling games are based on variable-ratio schedules. While the probability of winning the jackpot on any individual pull of a slot machine is the same, we get caught in the idea that the next pull will be the "right one."

Cognitive and Biological Factors in Associative Learning

It would be incorrect to say that classical and operant conditioning are the only factors that affect behavior, nor would it be correct to say that we are all mindless and robotic, unable to resist the rewards and punishments that occur in our lives. Since Skinner's initial perspectives, it has been found that many cognitive and biological factors are at work that can change the effects of associative learning or allow us to resist them altogether.

Many organisms undergo **latent learning**, which is learning that occurs without a reward but that is spontaneously demonstrated once a reward is introduced. The classic experiment associated with latent learning involves rats running a maze. Rats that were simply carried through the maze and then incentivized with a food reward for completing the maze on their own performed just as well—and in some cases better—than those rats that had been trained to run the maze using more standard operant conditioning techniques by which they were rewarded along the way.

Problem solving is another method of learning that steps outside the standard behaviorist approach. Think of the way young children put together a jigsaw puzzle: often, they will take pieces one-by-one and try to make them fit together until they find the correct match. Many animals will also use this kind of trial-and-error approach, testing behaviors until they yield a reward. As we get older, we gain the ability to analyze the situation and respond correctly the first time, as when we seek out the correct puzzle piece and orientation based on the picture we are forming. Humans and chimpanzees alike will often avoid trial-and-error learning and instead take a step back, observe the situation, and take decisive action to solve the challenges they face.

Not all behaviors can be taught using operant conditioning techniques. Many animals are predisposed to learn (or not learn) behaviors based on their own natural abilities and instincts. Animals are most able to learn behaviors that coincide with their natural behaviors: birds naturally peck when searching for food, so rewarding them with food in response to a pecking-based behavior works well. This predisposition is known as **preparedness**. Similarly, it can be very difficult to teach animals behaviors that work against their natural instincts. When animals revert to an instinctive behavior after learning a new behavior that is similar, the animal has undergone **instinctive** (or **instinctual**) **drift**. For example, researchers used behavioral techniques to train raccoons to place coins in a piggy bank (see Figure 3.7). Their efforts were ultimately unsuccessful as the learned behaviors were only temporary. Eventually, rather than placing the coins in the bank, the raccoons would pick up the coins, rub them together, and dip them into the bank before pulling them back out. The researchers concluded that the task they were trying to train the raccoons to perform was conflicting with their natural food-gathering instinct, which was to rub seeds together and wash them in a stream to clean them before eating. The researchers had far better luck training the raccoons to place a ball in a basketball net, as the ball was too large to trigger the food-washing instinct.

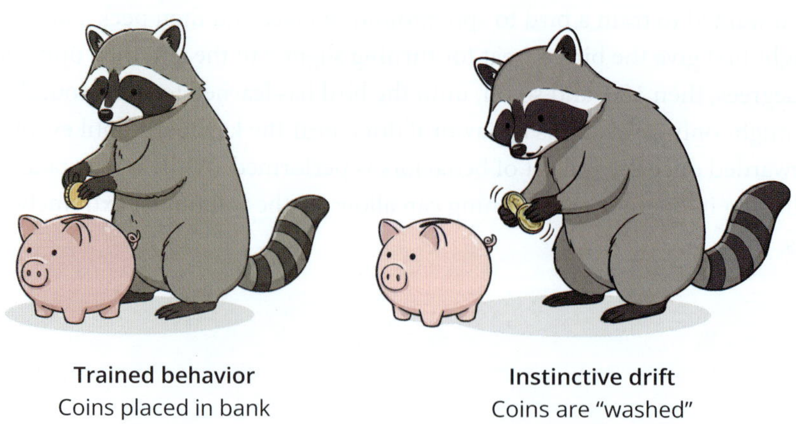

Figure 3.7 Instinctual Drift Experiment: Raccoons and Coins

Observational Learning

Observational learning is the process of learning a new behavior or gaining information by watching others. The most famous and perhaps most controversial study into observational learning is Albert Bandura's Bobo doll experiment, in which children watched an adult in a room full of toys punching and kicking an inflatable clown toy. When the children were later allowed to play in the room, many of them ignored the other toys in the room and inflicted similar violence on the Bobo doll just as they had seen the adult do. It's important to note that observational learning is not simply imitation because observational learning can be used to teach individuals to avoid behavior as well. In later iterations of the Bobo doll experiment, children who watched the adult get scolded after attacking the Bobo doll were less likely to be aggressive toward the Bobo doll themselves.

Like associative learning, there are a few neurological factors that affect observational learning. The most important of these are **mirror neurons**. These neurons are located in the frontal and parietal lobes of the cerebral cortex and fire both when an individual performs an action and when that individual observes someone else performing that action. Mirror neurons are largely involved in motor processes, but additionally are thought to be related to empathy and vicarious emotions; some mirror neurons fire both when we experience an emotion and also when we observe another experiencing the same emotion. Mirror neurons also play a role in imitative learning by a number of primates, as shown in Figure 3.8.

REAL WORLD

The connection between violent video games and aggressive behavior is still under active debate. While there are many interest groups on both sides of the controversy, the American Academy of Pediatrics (a major medical society) published one report in which they attributed a 13 to 22% increase in aggressive behavior to observational learning from video games.

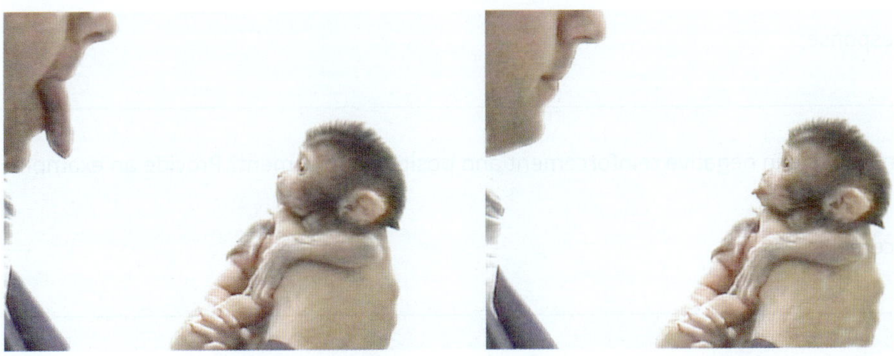

Figure 3.8 Use of Mirror Neurons in a Macaque
Many neonatal primates imitate facial expressions using mirror neurons.

Research suggests that observational learning through **modeling** is an important factor in determining people's behavior throughout their lifetime. People learn what behaviors are acceptable by watching others perform them. Much attention is focused on violent media as a model for antisocial behavior, but prosocial modeling can be just as powerful. Of course, observational learning is strongest when a model's words are consistent with actions. Many parents and guardians adopt a *Do as I say, not as I do* approach when teaching their children, but research suggests that children will disproportionately imitate what the model *did*, rather than what the model *said*.

MCAT CONCEPT CHECK 3.1

Before you move on, assess your understanding of the material with these questions.

1. Which of the following might cause a person to eat more food during a meal: eating each course separately and moving to the next only when finished with the current course, or interrupting the main course several times by eating side dishes?

 ____

2. A college student plays a prank on a roommate by popping a balloon behind the roommate's head after every time making popcorn. Before long, the smell of popcorn makes the roommate nervous. Which part of the story corresponds to each of the classical conditioning concepts below?
   - Conditioned stimulus:

 ____

   - Unconditioned stimulus:

 ____

   - Conditioned response:

 ____

   - Unconditioned response:

 ____

3. What is the difference between negative reinforcement and positive punishment? Provide an example of each.
   - Negative reinforcement:

 ____

 ____

   - Positive punishment:

 ____

 ____

3.2 Memory **High Yield**

LEARNING OBJECTIVES

After Chapter 3.2, you will be able to:

- Order the three modes of encoding from strongest to weakest
- Distinguish between maintenance rehearsal and elaborative rehearsal
- Predict how learning environments may impact recall
- Describe factors and phenomena that can lead to flaws in memory
- Define each type of human memory:

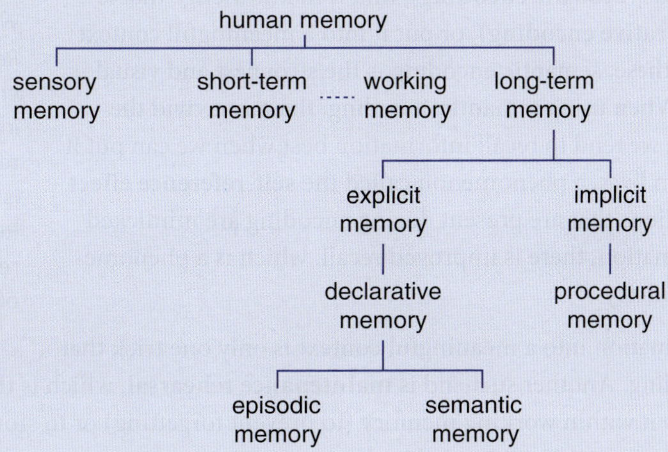

While learning is mostly concerned with behavior, the study of memory focuses on how we gain the knowledge that we accumulate over our lifetimes. The formation of memories can be divided into three major processes: encoding, storage, and retrieval.

Encoding

Encoding refers to the process of putting new information into memory. Information gained without any effort is the result of **automatic processing**. This type of cognitive processing is unintentional, and information is passively absorbed from the environment. As you walk down the street, you are constantly bombarded with information that seeps into your brain: you notice the temperature; you keep track of the route that you're taking; you might stop for coffee and realize that the same cashier has been working each day this week.

There are, however, times when we must actively work to gain information. In studying for the MCAT, for example, you may create flashcards to memorize the enzymes of digestion or the functions of endocrine hormones. This active memorization is known as **controlled (effortful) processing**.

MCAT EXPERTISE

Do not allow yourself to study for the MCAT using automatic processing! Just reading the text "to get through it" won't cut it for the MCAT. Engage with the text: fill out the MCAT Concept Checks, write notes in the margins, ask yourself questions. Scientific studies of learning have demonstrated, time and time again, that controlled processing improves comprehension, retention, and speed and accuracy on Test Day.

With practice, controlled processing can become automatic. Think back to a time when you were learning a foreign language. At first, each word required a great deal of processing to decipher: you had to hear the word and consciously translate it into your native language in order to understand what was being said. This process took an amount of time and effort that was probably difficult to maintain for prolonged periods. However, as you gained more experience with the language, this process became easier until you may have been able to understand those same words intuitively, without having to think very hard about them at all. At that point, this skill that once required controlled processing became automatic.

There are a few different ways that we encode the meaning of information when controlled processing is required. We can visualize information (**visual encoding**), store the way it sounds (**acoustic encoding**), link it to knowledge that is already in memory (**elaborative encoding**), or put it into a meaningful context (**semantic encoding**). Of these, semantic encoding is the strongest and visual encoding is the weakest. When using semantic encoding, the more vivid the context, the better. In fact, we tend to recall information best when we can put it into the context of our own lives, a phenomenon called the **self-reference effect**. Similarly, when the conditions that are present during encoding are mimicked when retrieving the information, there is improved recall, which is a phenomenon called **encoding specificity**.

REAL WORLD

The purpose of the Real World sidebars in your *MCAT Review* books is semantic encoding: by putting content into a meaningful context, retention of the information is improved. Most of our Real World sidebars are related to medicine because of the self-reference effect.

Of course, grouping information into a meaningful context is only one trick that we can use to aid in encoding. Another such aid is **maintenance rehearsal**, which is the repetition of a piece of information to either keep it within working memory (to prevent forgetting) or to store it in short-term and eventually long-term memory—topics discussed in the next section.

Mnemonics are another common way to memorize information, particularly lists. As you've seen in your Kaplan study materials, mnemonics are often acronyms or rhyming phrases that provide a vivid organization of the information we are trying to remember. Two other mnemonic techniques are commonly employed by memory experts. The **method of loci** (Figure 3.9) involves associating each item in a list with a location along a route through a building that has already been memorized. For example, in memorizing a grocery list, someone might picture a carton of eggs sitting on their doorstep, a person spilling milk in the front hallway, a giant stick of butter in the living room, and so on. Later, when the person wishes to recall the list, they simply take a mental walk through the locations and recall the images they formed earlier. Similarly, the **peg-word system** associates numbers with items that rhyme with or resemble the numbers. For example, one might be associated with the sun, two with a shoe, three with a tree, and so on. As groundwork, the individual memorizes their personal peg-list. When another list needs to be memorized, the individual can simply pair each item in the list with their peg-list. In this example, the individual may visualize eggs being fried by the sun (1), a pair of shoes (2) filled with milk, and a tree (3) with leaves made of butter. Because of the serial nature of both the method-of-loci and peg-word systems, they are very useful for memorizing large lists of objects in order.

REAL WORLD

Many feats of memory are accomplished via mnemonic techniques. In fact, the method of loci is a favorite among participants in the World Memory Championships.

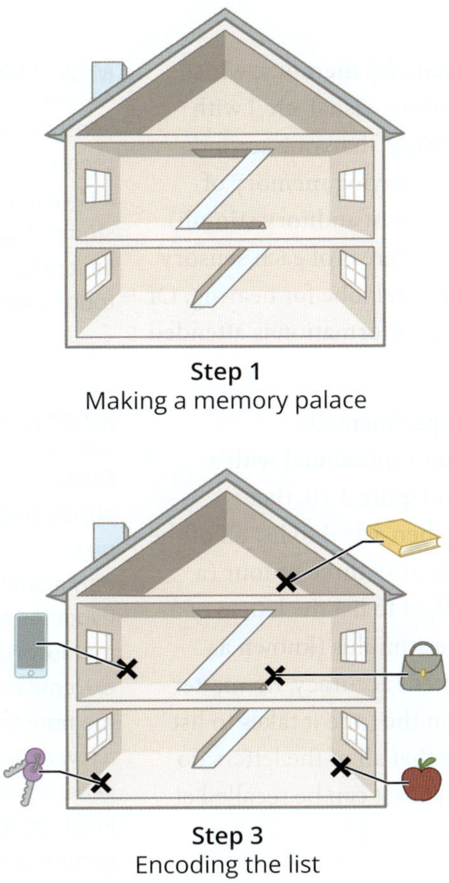

Figure 3.9 The Method of Loci

Finally, **chunking** (sometimes referred to as **clustering**) is a memory trick that involves taking individual elements of a large list and grouping them together into groups of elements with related meaning. For example, consider the following list of 16 letters: E-N-A-L-P-K-C-U-R-T-R-A-C-S-U-B. Memorizing the list in order by rote might prove difficult until we realize that we can reverse the items and group them into meaningful chunks: BUS, CAR, TRUCK, PLANE.

Storage

Following encoding, information must be stored if it is to be remembered. There are several types of memory storage.

Sensory Memory

The first and most fleeting kind of memory storage is **sensory memory**, which preserves information in its original sensory form (auditory, visual, etc.) with high accuracy and lasts only a very short time, generally less than one second. Sensory memory consists of both **iconic memory** (fast-decaying memory of visual stimuli) and **echoic memory** (fast-decaying memory of auditory stimuli). Sensory memories are maintained by the major projection areas of each sensory system, such as the occipital lobe for vision and the temporal lobe for hearing. Of course, sensory memory fades very quickly, so unless the information is attended to, it will be lost.

The nature of sensory memory can be demonstrated experimentally. Consider the following procedure: a research participant is presented with a three-by-three array of letters, such as that presented in Figure 3.10, that is flashed onto a screen for a mere fraction of a second. When asked to list all of the letters in the array, the participant is able to correctly identify three or four (a procedure known as **whole-report**). However, when asked to list the letters of a particular row immediately after the presentation of the stimulus (known as **partial-report**), the participant can do so with 100 percent accuracy, no matter which row is chosen. This is iconic memory in action: in the time it takes to list out a few of the items, the entire list fades; yet it is clear that all of the letters do make their way into iconic memory because any small subset can be recalled at will.

MCAT EXPERTISE

Sensory memory theoretically encompasses all five major senses, but studies have been mostly limited to sight, hearing, and touch (haptic memory).

MCAT EXPERTISE

Eidetic memory refers to the ability to recall, with high precision, an image after only a brief exposure. It is hypothesized that eidetic memory represents an extreme example of iconic memory that endures for a few minutes. Although generally not observed in adults, it is reported to occur in a small percentage of children.

B	X	O
R	T	P
W	Q	L

Figure 3.10 A Sample 3-by-3 Array for Studying Sensory Memory

Short-Term Memory

Of course, we do pay attention to some of the information that we are exposed to, and that information enters our **short-term memory**. Similar to sensory memory, short-term memory fades quickly, over the course of approximately 30 seconds without rehearsal. In addition to having a limited duration, the number of items we can hold in our short-term memory at any given time, our **memory capacity**, is limited to approximately seven items, usually stated as the 7 ± 2 rule. As discussed in the previous section, the capacity of short-term memory can be increased by clustering information, and the duration can be extended using maintenance rehearsal. Short-term memory is housed primarily in the **hippocampus**, which is also responsible for the consolidation of short-term memory into long-term memory.

Working Memory

Working memory is closely related to short-term memory and is similarly supported by the hippocampus. It enables us to keep a few pieces of information in our consciousness simultaneously and to manipulate that information. To do this, one must integrate short-term memory, attention, and executive function; accordingly, the frontal and parietal lobes are also involved. This is the form of memory that allows us to do simple math in our heads.

Long-Term Memory

With enough rehearsal, information moves from short-term to **long-term memory**, an essentially limitless warehouse for knowledge that we are then able to recall on demand, sometimes for the rest of our lives. One of the ways that information is consolidated into long-term memory is **elaborative rehearsal**. Unlike maintenance rehearsal, which is simply a way of keeping the information at the forefront of consciousness, elaborative rehearsal is the association of the information to knowledge already stored in long-term memory. Elaborative rehearsal is closely tied to the self-reference effect noted earlier; those ideas that we are able to relate to our own lives are more likely to find their way into our long-term memory. While long-term memory is primarily controlled by the hippocampus, it should be noted that memories are moved, over time, back to the cerebral cortex. Thus, very long-term memories—our names and birthdates, the faces of our parents—are generally not affected by damage to the hippocampus.

REAL WORLD

Have you ever looked at a picture of a simple unfinished puzzle, and been able to fit the pieces together mentally? This skill is explained by one of the major theories that underlies working memory, which includes the concept of a visuospatial sketchpad. The visuospatial sketchpad was proposed by Baddeley and Hitch as part of their three-part working memory model along with the other two components they proposed: the central executive and the phonological loop. The visuospatial sketchpad explains our ability to not only store visual and spatial information, but to manipulate it as well.

BEHAVIORAL SCIENCES GUIDED EXAMPLE WITH EXPERT THINKING

A musical melody is a series of tones played in succession that form a coherent musical idea. Melodies can be played in many different keys: absolute pitch of each of the notes changes as one changes keys, but as long as the relative pitches remain the same, the melody should still be recognizable. For example, the familiar melody of the song "Happy Birthday" should sound the same regardless of whether the first note is a C, an F, or a B-flat. While most people cannot name the key of a piece of music just by listening to it, they might still implicitly remember the way it "is supposed to sound" such that they could distinguish between the same melody played in different keys.

The passage provides the definition of melody, and the difference between absolute and relative pitch. Helpful if I'm not a musician, but really just setting the stage for the experiment.

Researchers interested in musical memory conducted an experiment with three groups of participants: 7- to 8-year-olds, 9- to 11-year-olds, and adults. Twenty-four British and Irish folk melodies were selected to be used as stimuli. The researchers expected that because these melodies share the sorts of patterns that are common in much North American and European music, they should thereby be recognizable as melodies rather than simply a series of tones. It was also expected that these melodies were uncommon enough to be unfamiliar to the participants prior to the beginning of the study.

Setup: Three groups, two children, one adult, presented with melodies. The melodies were intended to be unfamiliar.

IV: age

In the exposure phase, participants were presented with twelve of the twenty-four melodies to listen to. In the recognition phase, all twenty-four melodies were presented. Of the melodies that were presented in the exposure phase, six were then presented in the recognition phase transposed to a higher or lower key. Participants were asked to rate whether each melody they heard in the recognition phase had been presented in the exposure phase, and rated this recognition on a scale from 1 ("definitely new") to 6 ("definitely heard before").

Finally, the description of the procedure. I'll want to parse this carefully. In the second phase, some melodies were heard earlier and some weren't. Some of those that have been heard before were presented in a different key.

Second IV: transposition

DV: recognition

To eliminate bias, researchers used an Area Under the Curve (AUC) score, which measures the relative difference in recognition rather than the absolute difference. If all of the recognition scores for old melodies are higher than the recognition scores for new melodies for a given participant, the AUC score is 1.0, which represents perfect discrimination. A score of 0.5 represents chance performance, such that the old and new melodies are indistinguishable.

I've never heard of an AUC score before, but the passage explains it. I'll probably need this to interpret the results.

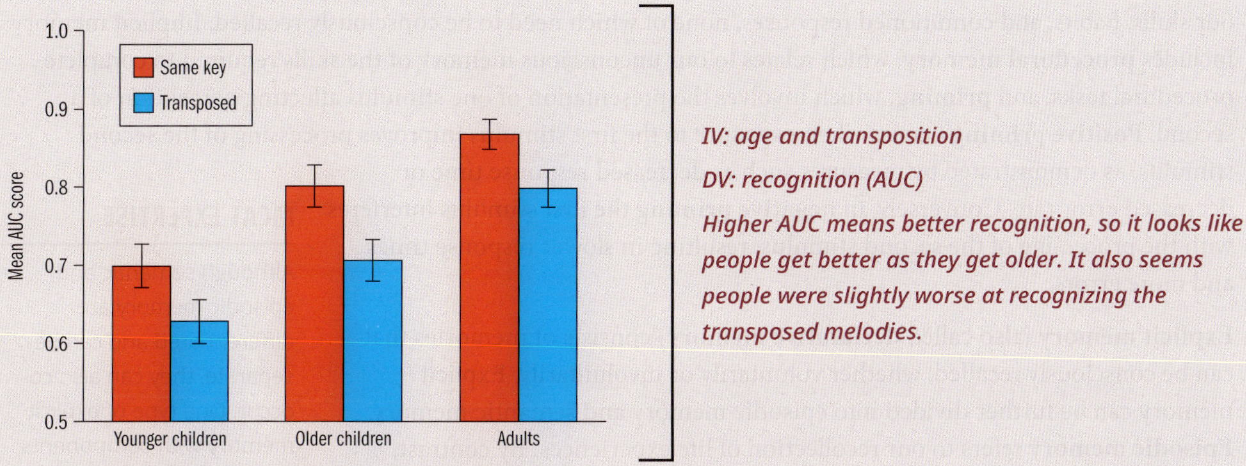

Figure 1 Mean AUC score for each group

Adapted from: Schellenberg EG, Poon J, Weiss MW (2017) Memory for melody and key in childhood. *PLoS ONE* 12(10): e0187115. https://doi.org/10.1371/journal.pone.0187115

What do these results suggest about between-group and within-group trends with respect to explicit and implicit memory for music?

To answer this question, we're going to have to make use of the results of this study, but we'll also have to recall and apply content knowledge from outside this passage. The prompt asks about differences in explicit and implicit memory, so we'll want to start by figuring out how these terms apply in this general context, then apply these ideas specifically to the experiment. For the MCAT, we should know that explicit and implicit memory are both subdivisions of long-term memory. Explicit memory is the encoding of facts, and particularly relevant to the present study is episodic memory, the kind of explicit memory that involves experiences. The question "have I heard this melody before?" is answered by accessing an explicit memory. The relevance of implicit memory is more difficult here, since we typically think of implicit memories as procedural, involving skills and conditioned responses. Whenever we're not sure of how a concept in a question is related to the passage, we should go back to the passage and search for clues. The passage does provide a clue: in the first paragraph, the author describes the memory of the key of a melody as implicit rather than explicit. Now that we know what we're looking for, we can examine the results of the study with these concepts, and the way in which they relate to the passage, already in mind.

The AUC score system used by the researchers might be unfamiliar, but the concept isn't that much different from what we might normally see in a study like this one. A score of 0.5 represents random chance, and a score higher than that means that the participants were able to distinguish the melodies they'd heard from the ones they hadn't. The higher the score, the better the recognition. From the figure, we can see two trends: as participants get older, recognition gets better, but when the melody is transposed, recognition gets worse for all participants by approximately the same amount.

We must apply the memory vocabulary words to these trends. We can conclude from these results that explicit memory for music improved by age across groups. Further, within each group, implicit memory did play a significant role in recognition, because melodies that matched those heard earlier explicitly but not implicitly (i.e., they were the same melody but transposed to a different key) were less readily recognized. The role of implicit memory on recognition seems to be consistent between groups.

There are two types of long-term memory. **Implicit memory** (also called **nondeclarative memory**) consists of our skills, habits, and conditioned responses, none of which need to be consciously recalled. Implicit memory includes **procedural memory**, which relates to our unconscious memory of the skills required to complete procedural tasks, and **priming**, which involves the presentation of one stimulus affecting perception of a second. **Positive priming** occurs when exposure to the first stimulus improves processing of the second stimulus, as demonstrated by measures such as decreased response time or decreased error rate. Conversely, in **negative priming** the first stimulus interferes with the processing of the second stimulus, resulting in slower response times and more errors.

Explicit memory (also called **declarative memory**) consists of memories that can be consciously recalled, whether voluntarily or involuntarily. Explicit memory can be further divided into episodic memory and semantic memory. **Episodic memory** refers to our recollection of life experiences. By contrast, **semantic memory** refers to ideas, concepts, or facts that we know, but are not tied to specific life experiences. **Autobiographical memory** is the name given to our explicit memories about our lives and ourselves, and includes all of our episodic memories of our own life experiences, but also includes semantic memories that relate to our personal traits and characteristics. Interestingly, memory disorders can affect one type of memory but leave others alone. For example, a patient who has amnesia might not remember learning to ride a bicycle (episodic memory) or the names of the parts of a bicycle (semantic memory), but may, surprisingly, retain the skill of riding a bicycle when given one (procedural memory). The various major categories of memory are summarized in Figure 3.11.

MCAT EXPERTISE

Although semantic and episodic memory are differentiated and can be separate, they can also co-occur. One type of explicit memory with components of both episodic and semantic memory is **flashbulb memory**, which is the detailed recollection of stimuli immediately surrounding an important (or emotionally arousing) event. Flashbulb memory helps you answer the question "Do you remember where you were when...?"

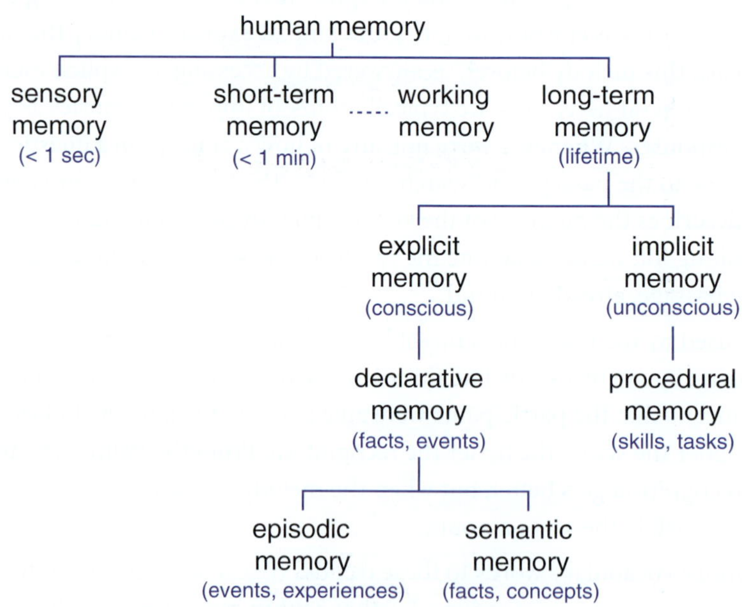

Figure 3.11 Types of Memory

Retrieval

Of course, memories that are stored are of no use unless we can pull them back out to use them. **Retrieval** is the name given to the process of demonstrating that something that has been learned has been retained. Most people think about retrieval in terms of **recall**, or the retrieval and statement of previously learned information, but learning can be additionally demonstrated by recognizing or quickly relearning information.

Recognition, the process of merely identifying a piece of information that was previously learned, is far easier than recall. This difference is something you can take advantage of because the MCAT, as a multiple-choice test, is largely based on recognizing information. If the MCAT were a fill-in-the-blank style exam, your approach to studying would have to be vastly different and far more in-depth.

REAL WORLD

Think back to elementary school. How many of your classmates do you think you could list? Chances are, not many. On the other hand, glancing through your class photo, you would probably recognize the vast majority of your former classmates. This gap is the difference between recall and recognition.

Relearning is another way of demonstrating that information has been stored in long-term memory. In studying the memorization of lists, Hermann Ebbinghaus found that his recall of a list of short words he had learned the previous day was often quite poor. However, he was able to rememorize the list much more quickly the second time through. Ebbinghaus interpreted this to mean that the information had been stored, even though it wasn't readily available for recall. Through additional research, he discovered that the longer the amount of time between sessions of relearning, the greater the retention of the information later on. Ebbinghaus dubbed this phenomenon the **spacing effect** (Figure 3.12), and it helps to explain why cramming is not nearly as effective as spacing out studying over an extended period of time.

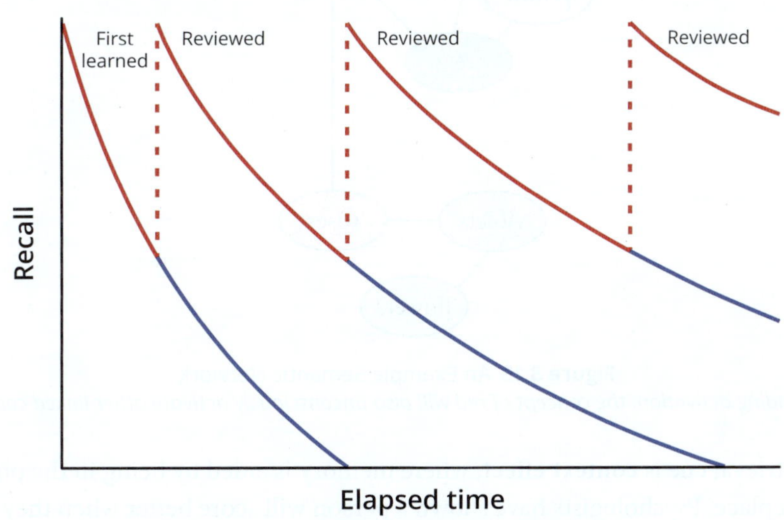

Figure 3.12 Recall Ability with Spacing Effect

Recalling a fact at a moment's notice can be difficult. Fortunately, the brain has ways of organizing information so that it can take advantage of environmental cues to tell it where to find a given memory. Psychologists think of memory not as simply a stockpile of unrelated facts, but rather as a network of interconnected ideas. The brain organizes ideas into a **semantic network**, as shown in Figure 3.13, in which concepts are linked together based on similar meaning, not unlike an Internet encyclopedia wherein each page includes links for similar topics. For example, the concept of *red* might be closely linked to other colors, like *orange* and *green*, as well as objects, like *fire engine* and *roses*. When one node of our semantic network is activated, such as seeing the word *red* on a sign, the other linked concepts around it are also unconsciously activated, a process known as **spreading activation**. Spreading activation is at the heart of the previously mentioned positive priming, as recall is aided by first being presented with a word or phrase, a **recall cue**, that is close to the desired semantic memory.

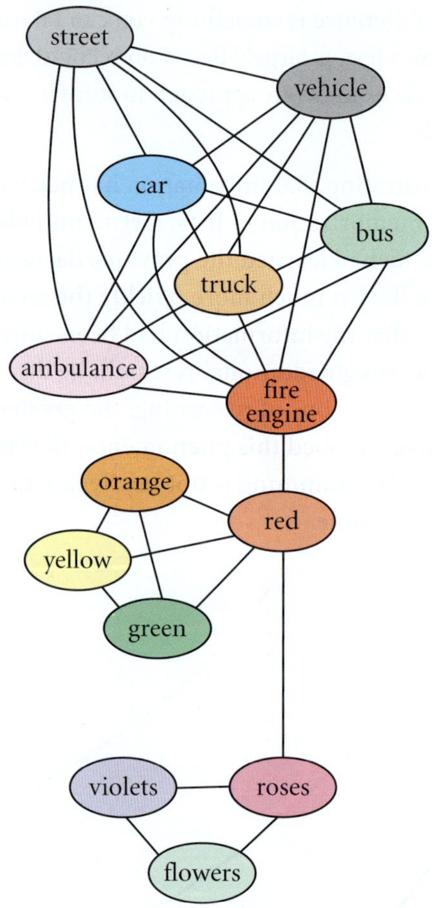

Figure 3.13 An Example Semantic Network
In spreading activation, the concept of red will also unconsciously activate other linked concepts.

Another common retrieval cue is **context effect**, where memory is aided by being in the physical location where encoding took place. Psychologists have shown a person will score better when they take an exam in the same room in which they learned the information. Context effects can go even further than this; facts learned underwater are better recalled when underwater than when on land. Similarly, **source monitoring** is a part of the retrieval process that involves determining the origin of memories, and whether they are factual (real and accurate) or fictional (from a dream, novel, or movie).

A person's mental state can also affect their ability to recall. **State-dependent memory,** alternately referred to as a **state-dependent effect**, is a retrieval cue based on performing better when in the same mental state as when the information was learned. People who learn facts or skills while intoxicated, for example, will show better recall or proficiency when performing those same tasks while intoxicated as compared to performing them while sober. Emotions work in a similar way: being in a foul mood primes negative memories, which in turn work to sustain the foul mood. So not only will memory be better for information learned when in a similar mood, but recall of negative or positive memories will lead to the persistence of the mood.

Finally, studies on list memorization have indicated that an item's position in the list affects participants' ability to recall, which Ebbinghaus termed the **serial-position effect**. A classic graph demonstrating this effect appears in Figure 3.14. When researchers give participants a list of items to memorize, the participants have much higher recall for both the first few and last few items on the list. The tendency to remember early items is called the **primacy effect**, while the similar tendency for late items is the **recency effect**. However, when asked to remember the list later, people show strong recall for the first few items while recall of the last few items fades. Psychologists interpret this to mean that the recency effect is a result of the last items still being in short-term memory on initial recall.

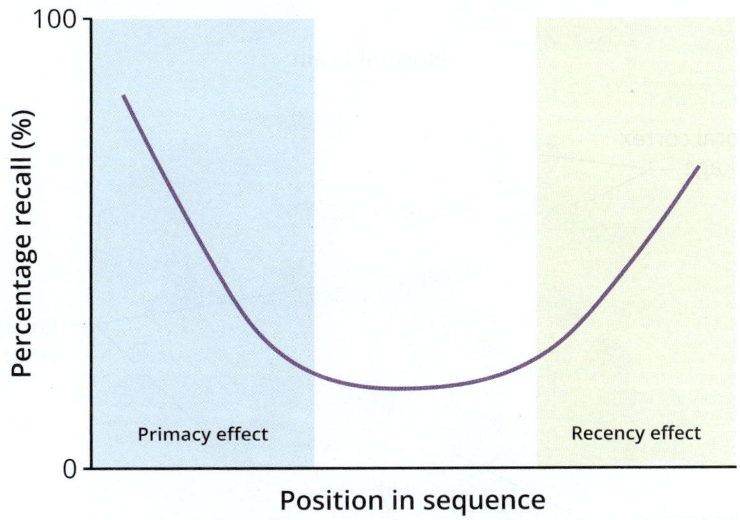

Figure 3.14 The Serial-Position Effect

Forgetting

Unfortunately, even long-term memory is not always permanent. Several phenomena can result in **amnesia**, a significant loss of memorized information. The inability to remember where, when, or how one has obtained knowledge is called **source amnesia**.

Brain Disorders

There are several disorders that can lead to decline in memory. The most common is **Alzheimer's disease**, which is a degenerative brain disorder thought to be linked to a loss of acetylcholine in neurons that link to the hippocampus, although its exact causes are not well understood. Alzheimer's is marked by progressive **dementia** (a loss of cognitive function) and memory loss, with atrophy of the brain, as shown in Figure 3.15. While not perfectly linear, memory loss in Alzheimer's disease tends to proceed in a retrograde fashion, with loss of recent memories before distant memories. Microscopic findings of Alzheimer's include **neurofibrillary tangles** and **β-amyloid plaques**. One common phenomenon that occurs in individuals with middle- to late-stage Alzheimer's is **sundowning**, an increase in dysfunction in the late afternoon and evening.

BRIDGE

The β-amyloid plaques of Alzheimer's disease are incorrectly folded copies of the amyloid precursor protein, in which insoluble β-pleated sheets form and then deposit in the brain. Protein folding is discussed in detail in Chapter 1 of *MCAT Biochemistry Review*.

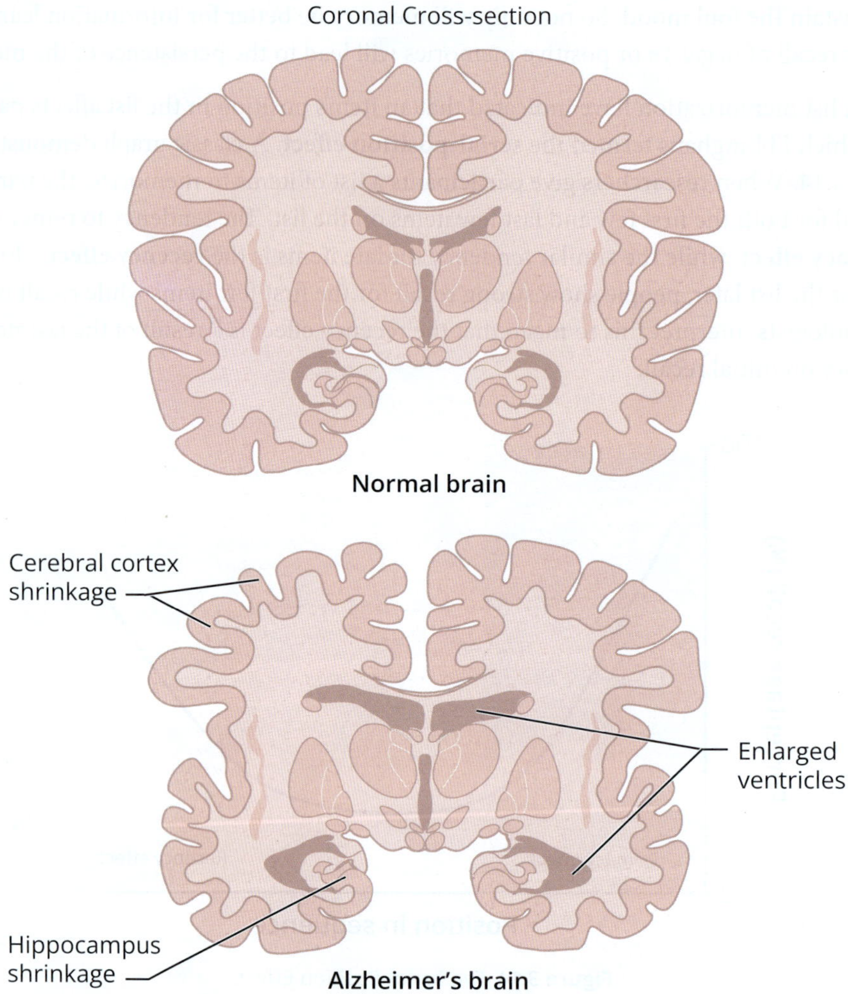

Figure 3.15 The Brain with Alzheimer's Disease

Korsakoff's syndrome is another form of memory loss caused by thiamine deficiency in the brain. The disorder is marked by both **retrograde amnesia** (the loss of previously formed memories) and **anterograde amnesia** (the inability to form new memories). Another common symptom is **confabulation**, or the process of creating vivid but fabricated memories, typically thought to be an attempt made by the brain to fill in the gaps of missing memories.

Agnosia is the loss of the ability to recognize objects, people, or sounds, though usually only one of the three. Agnosia is usually caused by physical damage to the brain, such as that caused by a stroke or a neurological disorder such as multiple sclerosis.

Decay

Of course, not all memory loss is due to a disorder. Through a process known as **decay**, memories are simply lost naturally over time as the neurochemical trace of a short-term memory fades. In his word memorization experiment, Ebbinghaus noted what he called a "curve of forgetting," formally called the **retention function**, as shown in Figure 3.16. For a day or two after learning the list, recall fell sharply but then leveled off.

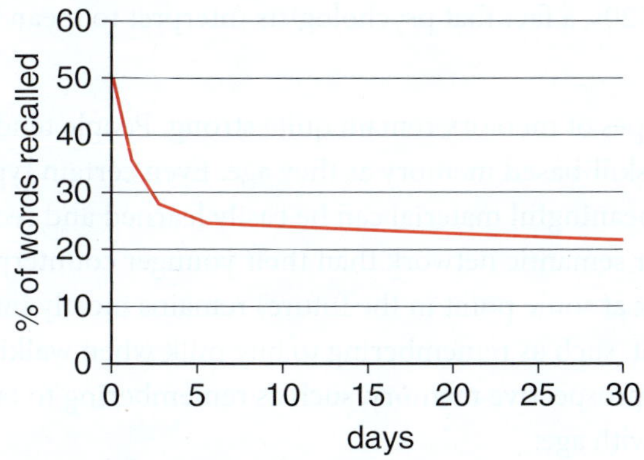

Figure 3.16 Ebbinghaus's Curve of Forgetting

Interference

Another common reason for memory loss is **interference** (also referred to as an **interference effect**), a retrieval error caused by the existence of other, usually similar, information. Interference can be classified by its "forward" or "backward" direction (see Figure 3.17). When we experience **proactive interference**, old information is interfering with new learning. For example, think back to a time when you moved to a new address. For a short time, you may have had trouble recalling individual pieces of the new address because you were so used to the old one. Similarly, Ebbinghaus found that with each successive list he learned, his recall for new lists decreased over time, an effect he attributed to interference caused by older lists.

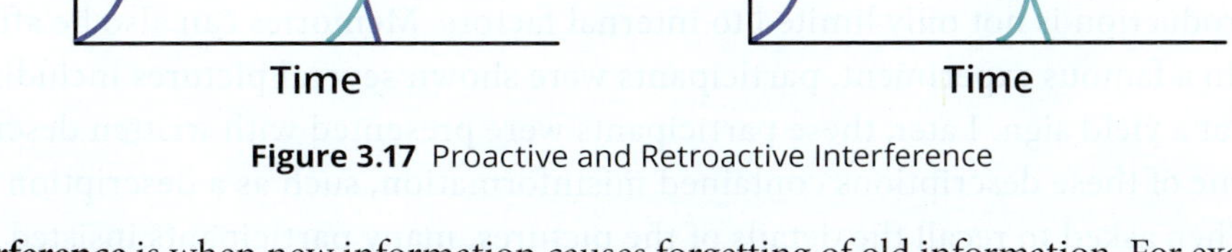

Figure 3.17 Proactive and Retroactive Interference

Retroactive interference is when new information causes forgetting of old information. For example, at the beginning of a school year, teachers learning a new set of students' names often find that they can no longer remember the names of the previous year's students. One way of preventing retroactive interference is to reduce the number of interfering events, which is why it is often best to study in the evening about an hour before falling asleep (although this also depends on your personal style!).

Aging and Memory

Contrary to popular belief, aging does not necessarily lead to significant memory loss; while there are many individuals whose memory fades in old age, this is not always the case. In fact, studies show that there is a larger range of memory ability for 70-year-olds than there is for 20-year-olds. There are, however, some trends that can be demonstrated when evaluating the memories of older individuals. When asked about the most pivotal events in their lives, people in their 70s and 80s tend to say that their most vivid memories are of events that occurred in their teens and 20s, a fact that psychologists interpret to mean that this time is a peak period for encoding in a person's life.

Even for older adults, certain types of memory remain quite strong. People tend not to demonstrate much degeneration in recognition or skill-based memory as they age. Even certain types of recall will remain strong for most people; semantically meaningful material can be easily learned and recalled, most likely due to older individuals having a larger semantic network than their younger counterparts. **Prospective memory** (remembering to perform a task at some point in the future) remains mostly intact when it is event-based—that is, primed by a trigger event, such as remembering to buy milk when walking past the grocery store. On the other hand, time-based prospective memory, such as remembering to take a medication every day at 7:00 a.m., does tend to decline with age.

Memory Reconstruction

We often think of memory as a record of our experiences or a kind of video recording that is stored to be accessed later; this accurate recall of past events is defined as **reproductive memory**. Nothing could be further from the truth. **Reconstructive memory** is a theory of memory recall in which cognitive processes such as imagination, semantic memory, and perception affect the act of remembering. This theory explains how two people can recall the same event as occurring in completely different ways. A memory that incorrectly recalls actual events or recalls events that never occurred is known as a **false memory**. Despite their unsettling nature, false memories are common and are to be expected when we consider the many factors that can affect memory. Most memories are encoded with little detail, only focusing on the details deemed important in the moment. Also, as previously discussed, if a person repeatedly rehearses the memory in their mind, then that person may fill in missing details with unreliable information. Repressed memories, memories stored in the unconscious mind and blocked from recall, have also been a topic of controversy. Some psychologists believe repressed memories can be brought back into our conscious mind either spontaneously or through psychotherapy. Such memories are called **recovered memories**. However, it is not possible to distinguish between false memories and recovered memories without evidence and some research psychologists believe psychotherapy is more likely to lead to the creation of false memories. So, the act of recalling a memory can result in the production of a false memory.

False memory production is not only limited to internal factors. Memories can also be affected by outside sources as well. In a famous experiment, participants were shown several pictures including one picture of a car stopped at a yield sign. Later, these participants were presented with written descriptions of the pictures, and some of these descriptions contained misinformation, such as a description of a car stopped at a stop sign. When asked to recall the details of the pictures, many participants insisted they had seen a stop sign in the picture. This example illustrates the **misinformation effect**, where a person's recall of an event becomes less accurate due to the injection of outside information into the memory.

The misinformation effect can also be seen at the point of recall. In another experiment, participants were shown a video of an automobile accident. Some participants were then asked, *How fast were the cars moving when they collided?*, while others were asked about the accident using more descriptive language such as

How fast were the cars moving when they crashed? Those participants who were asked the question with leading language were much more likely to overstate the severity of the accident than those who had been asked the question with less descriptive language.

Intrusion errors refers to false memories that have included a false detail into a particular memory. This is similar to the misinformation effect but distinct in that the intrusion error is not from an outside source. Instead, the intruding memory is injected into original memory due to both memories being related or sharing a theme. Upon memory recall, the brain incorrectly associates the intruding memory with the source memory, leading to a false memory. For example, if over the years you've attended multiple New Year's Eve celebrations in two different cities, then your memories of the two cities are linked. A possible intrusion error could be recalling that a particular restaurant is located in Vancouver, because you recall eating at the restaurant on New Year's Eve and celebrating New Year's Eve in Vancouver. However, the restaurant is really in Toronto, where you have also celebrated on New Year's.

Source-monitoring error involves confusion between semantic and episodic memory: a person remembers the details of an event, but confuses the context under which those details were gained. Source-monitoring error often manifests when a person hears a story of something that happened to someone else, and later recalls the story as a personal memory.

REAL WORLD

During a Congressional Medal of Honor ceremony in 1983, Ronald Reagan relayed a vivid story about a heroic World War II pilot who received a posthumous medal. Skeptical reporters, unaware of any incident matching the details of Reagan's story, checked into the story and found that the pilot had existed—in the 1944 movie *A Wing and a Prayer*. Reagan had remembered the details of the pilot's heroic actions but had forgotten their source.

MCAT CONCEPT CHECK 3.2

Before you move on, assess your understanding of the material with these questions.

1. List the three modes in which information can be encoded, from strongest to weakest.
   1. ______________________________
   2. ______________________________
   3. ______________________________
2. In what ways is maintenance rehearsal different from elaborative rehearsal?

   ____
3. In terms of recall, why might it be a bad idea to study for the MCAT while listening to music?

   ____
4. What are some factors that might cause eyewitness courtroom testimony to be unreliable?

   ____

3.3 Neurobiology of Learning and Memory

LEARNING OBJECTIVES

After Chapter 3.3, you will be able to:

- Describe neuroplasticity and changes that occur throughout the human life span
- Recall the terms involved with removing and strengthening memory connections

Even as you read this text, your brain is changing. Memory, and therefore learning, involves changes in brain physiology, such that with each new concept you learn your brain is altering its synaptic connections in response. You may have heard that it is far easier for children to learn a new language than it is for adults. Indeed, the saying *you can't teach an old dog new tricks*, while not strictly true, does have its roots in neurobiology.

As infants, we are born with many more neurons than we actually need. As our brains develop, neural connections form rapidly in response to stimuli via a phenomenon called **neuroplasticity** (also known as **neural plasticity**). In fact, the brains of young children are so plastic that they can reorganize drastically in response to injury, as evidenced by studies of children who have had entire hemispheres of their brains removed to prevent severe seizures. The remaining hemisphere will change to take over functions of the missing parts of the brain, allowing these children to grow up to lead unimpaired lives. While our brains do maintain a degree of plasticity throughout our lives, adult brains display nowhere near the degree of plasticity as those of a child. Another way our brains change is through a process called **synaptic pruning**. As we grow older, weak neural connections are broken while strong ones are bolstered, increasing the efficiency of our brains' ability to process information.

This concept of plasticity is important because it is closely linked to learning and memory. As you learned in Chapter 4 of *MCAT Biology Review*, stimuli cause activation of neurons, which release their neurotransmitters into the **synaptic cleft**, the gap between a neuron and a target cell. These neurotransmitters continue to stimulate activity until degradation, reuptake, or diffusion out of the synaptic cleft. In the interim, this neural activity forms a memory trace that is thought to be the cause of short-term memory. As discussed earlier, if the stimulus isn't repeated or rehearsed, the memory trace disappears, and the consequence is the loss of the short-term memory. However, as the stimulus is repeated, the stimulated neurons become more efficient at releasing their neurotransmitters and at the same time receptor sites on the other side of the synapse increase, increasing receptor density. The strengthening of neural connections through repeated use is known as **long-term potentiation**, and is believed to be the neurophysiological basis of long-term memory. Figure 3.18 is an illustration of the increase in receptor concentration as a result of the potentiation process.

MCAT EXPERTISE

Recent research has begun to elucidate the mechanism of long-term potentiation. It has been observed that a specific type of glutamate receptor, the **NMDA receptor**, is required for the strengthening of synaptic connections.

MNEMONIC

The word *potentiate* means to increase the potency or strength of something. Long-term potentiation can be thought of as the strengthening of a "long-term" synaptic connection.

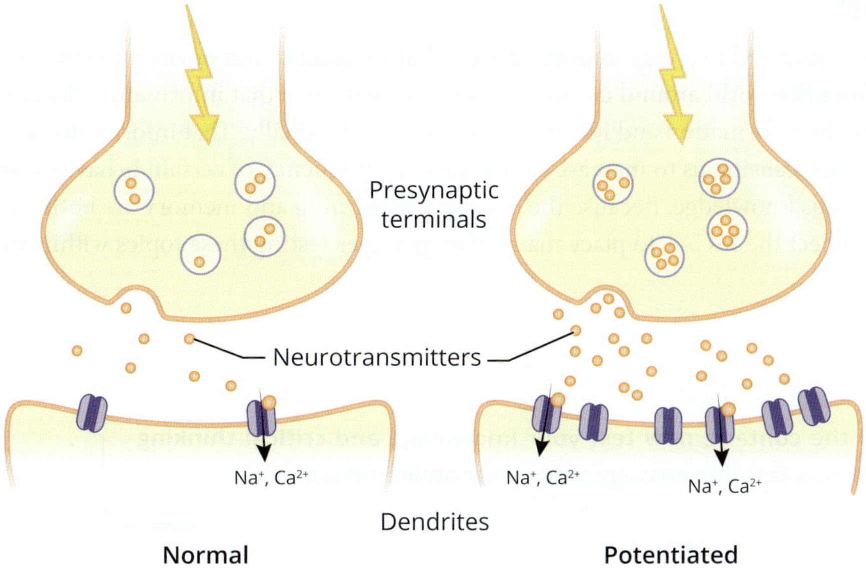

Figure 3.18 Long-Term Potentiation

As described in the previous section, a memory begins its life as a sensory memory in the projection area of a given sensory modality. This sensory memory is brief, unless maintained in consciousness and moved, as a short-term memory, into the hippocampus in the temporal lobe. The memory can then be manipulated through working memory while in the hippocampus (in tandem with the frontal and parietal lobes), and even stored for later recall. Over very long periods of time, memories are gradually moved from the hippocampus back to the cerebral cortex. Note that this general pathway is a drastic oversimplification of the complex interplay of brain regions involved in memory, but is a useful paradigm for Test Day.

MCAT CONCEPT CHECK 3.3

Before you move on, assess your understanding of the material with these questions.

1. What is neuroplasticity? How does neuroplasticity change during life?

___

___

2. What is the term for removing weak neural connections? What is the term for strengthening memory connections through increased neurotransmitter release and receptor density?
   - Removing weak connections:

   ___

   - Strengthening connections:

   ___

Conclusion

In this chapter, we discussed two very important ways that we react to our environments. We are constantly receiving input from the world around us, and the way we memorize that information depends greatly on both the nature of the information and its importance to us individually. That information can also have a profound effect on us, causing us to increase or decrease the frequency of certain behaviors, sometimes without our conscious knowledge. Because the concepts of learning and memory are both used heavily in research, we can expect the MCAT to place many of its passages testing these topics within an experimental context.

GO ONLINE

You've reviewed the content, now test your knowledge and critical thinking skills by completing a test-like passage set in your online resources!

CONCEPT SUMMARY

Learning

- **Habituation** is the process of becoming used to a stimulus. **Dishabituation** can occur when a second stimulus intervenes, causing a resensitization to the original stimulus.
- **Associative learning** is a way of pairing together stimuli and responses, or behaviors and consequences.
- In **classical conditioning**, an unconditioned stimulus that produces an instinctive, unconditioned response is paired with a neutral stimulus. With repetition, the neutral stimulus becomes a conditioned stimulus that produces a conditioned response.
- In **operant conditioning**, behavior is changed through the use of consequences.
  - **Reinforcement** increases the likelihood of a behavior.
  - **Punishment** decreases the likelihood of a behavior.
  - The schedule of reinforcement affects the rate at which the behavior is performed. Schedules can be based either on a ratio of behavior to reward or on an amount of time, and can be either fixed or variable. Behaviors learned through variable-ratio schedules are the hardest to extinguish.
- **Observational learning**, or **modeling**, is the acquisition of behavior by watching others.

Memory

- **Encoding** is the process of putting new information into memory. It can be **automatic** or **effortful**. Semantic encoding is stronger than both acoustic and visual encoding.
- **Sensory** and **short-term memory** are transient and are based on neurotransmitter activity. **Working memory** requires short-term memory, attention, and executive function to manipulate information.
- **Long-term memory** requires elaborative rehearsal and is the result of increased neuronal connectivity.
  - **Explicit (declarative) memory** stores facts and stories.
  - **Implicit (nondeclarative) memory** stores skills and conditioning effects.
- Facts are stored via **semantic networks**.
- **Recognition** of information is stronger than **recall**.
- **Retrieval** of information is often based on **priming** interconnected nodes of the semantic network.
- Memories can be lost through disorders such as Alzheimer's disease, Korsakoff's syndrome, or agnosia; decay; or interference.
- Memories are highly subject to influence by outside information and mood both at the time of encoding and at recall.

Neurobiology of Learning and Memory

- Both learning and memory rely on changes in brain chemistry and physiology, the extent of which depends on **neuroplasticity**, which decreases as we age.
- **Long-term potentiation**, responsible for the conversion of short-term to long-term memory, is the strengthening of neuronal connections resulting from increased neurotransmitter release and adding of receptor sites.

ANSWERS TO CONCEPT CHECKS

3.1

1. Eating each course of a meal before moving on to the next causes habituation; each bite causes less pleasurable stimulation, so people feel less desire to keep eating. On the other hand, mixing up the courses of a meal causes dishabituation for taste, which would cause people to eat more overall.
2. The conditioned stimulus is the smell of popcorn. The unconditioned stimulus is the popping of the balloon. The conditioned response is nervousness (fear) in response to the presence of popcorn. The unconditioned response is fear in response to the popping of the balloon.
3. Negative reinforcement causes an increase of a given behavior by removing something unpleasant, while positive punishment reduces behavior by adding something unpleasant. Examples will vary, but common negative reinforcers include medicines that reduce pain or avoiding uncomfortable situations to reduce anxiety. Common examples of positive punishments include having to pay a fine for speeding while driving or getting detention in school for bad behavior.

3.2

1. Of the three modes in which information can be encoded, semantic is the strongest, followed by acoustic. Visual is the weakest.
2. Maintenance rehearsal is the repetition of information to keep it within short-term memory for near-immediate use. Elaborative rehearsal is the association of information to other stored knowledge and is a more effective way to move information from short-term to long-term memory.
3. Because you will be taking the MCAT in a quiet room, studying under similar circumstances will aid recall due to context effects. Music may also compete for attention, reducing your ability to focus on the relevant study material.
4. Several factors can affect the accuracy of eyewitness testimony, including the manner in which questions are asked; the nature of information shared with the witness by police, lawyers, and other witnesses following the event; the misinformation effect; source-monitoring error; and the amount of time elapsed between the event and the trial. Even watching crime dramas, watching the news, or witnessing similar events can cause source-monitoring error.

3.3

1. Neuroplasticity is the ability of the brain to form new connections rapidly. The brain is most plastic in young children, and plasticity quickly drops off after childhood.
2. Pruning is the term for removing weak neural connections. Long-term potentiation is the strengthening of memory connections through increased neurotransmitter release and receptor density.

SCIENCE MASTERY ASSESSMENT EXPLANATIONS

1. **A**

After a while, the participant became habituated to the sound of the buzzer. Introducing a new stimulus, such as the banging pans, should dishabituate (resensitize) the original stimulus, causing a temporary increase in response to the sound of the buzzer.

2. **C**

The sound of a can opener would not normally produce a response on its own, making it a stimulus that must have been conditioned by association with food.

3. **B**

Generalization is the process by which similar stimuli can produce the same conditioned response. Here, the response to the taste and smell of oranges has generalized to that of all citrus.

4. **D**

Avoidance learning is a type of negative reinforcement in which a behavior is increased to prevent an unpleasant future consequence. Extinction, **(A)**, is a decreased response to a conditioned stimulus when it is no longer paired with an unconditioned stimulus. Punishment, **(B)** and **(C)**, leads to decreased behaviors in operant conditioning.

5. **A**

Long term potentiation is believed to be the neurophysiological basis of long-term memory, making **(A)** the correct answer. As synapses are reinforced, the neuroplasticity of the brain decreases, eliminating **(C)**. Also, synaptic pruning, **(B)**, refers to the removal of infrequently used synapses, which is not consistent with the description in the question stem.

6. **C**

In a fixed-interval schedule, the desired behavior is rewarded the first time it is exhibited after the fixed interval has elapsed. Both fixed-interval and fixed-ratio schedules tend to show this phenomenon: almost no response immediately after the reward is given, but the behavior increases as the rat gets close to receiving the reward.

7. **A**

Complicated, multistage behaviors are typically taught through shaping, so statement III must not be part of the correct answer. Reinforcers do not necessarily need to be food-based, and instinctive drift can interfere with learning of complicated behaviors; therefore, only statement I is accurate.

8. **C**

This is the definition of controlled processing and is the only answer choice that is necessarily true of controlled processing. Effortful processing is used to create long-term memories, and—with practice—can become automatic, invalidating **(A)** and **(B)**. Most of our day-to-day activities are processed automatically, making **(D)** incorrect.

9. **A**

Semantic encoding, or encoding based on the meaning of the information, is the strongest of the methods of encoding. Visual encoding, **(B)**, is the weakest, and acoustic encoding, **(D)**, is intermediate between the two. Iconic memory, **(C)**, is a type of sensory memory.

10. **C**

We are born with an overabundance of neurons and quickly form many new synapses in the first few years of life. As we age, the plasticity of our brains decreases, although we do retain some plasticity throughout adulthood. Thus, the brain of a two year old, due to its higher neuroplasticity, would better adapt, supporting **(C)** as the correct answer.

11. D

The association of words on a list to a preconstructed set of ideas is common to both the method-of-loci and peg-word mnemonics. Method-of-loci systems, **(B)**, associate items with locations, while peg-word systems use images associated with numbers.

12. A

Partial-report procedures, in which the individual is asked to recall a specific portion of the stimulus, are incredibly accurate, but only for a very brief time. This is a method of studying sensory (specifically, iconic) memory. Both the serial position effect, **(B)**, and the 7 ± 2 rule, **(C)**, are characteristics of short-term memory.

13. B

Semantic memory is the category of long-term memory that refers to recall of facts, rather than experiences or skills. Be careful not to confuse semantic memory with semantic networks, **(D)**, which are the associations of similar concepts in the mind to aid in their retrieval.

14. C

State-dependent recall is concerned with the internal rather than external states of the individual. As such, both statements II and III are examples of state-dependent circumstances, while statement I might cause a context effect instead.

15. B

Older adults may have trouble with time-based prospective memory, which is remembering to do an activity at a particular time. Other forms of memory are generally preserved, or may decline slightly but less significantly than time-based prospective memory.

GO ONLINE

Consult your online resources for additional practice.

SHARED CONCEPTS

Behavioral Sciences Chapter 1
Biology and Behavior

Behavioral Sciences Chapter 2
Sensation and Perception

Behavioral Sciences Chapter 4
Cognition, Consciousness, and Language

Behavioral Sciences Chapter 5
Motivation, Emotion, and Stress

Behavioral Sciences Chapter 7
Psychological Disorders

Biology Chapter 4
The Nervous System

CHAPTER 4

COGNITION, CONSCIOUSNESS, AND LANGUAGE

SCIENCE MASTERY ASSESSMENT

Every pre-med knows this feeling: there is so much content I have to know for the MCAT! How do I know what to do first or what's important?

While the high-yield badges throughout this book will help you identify the most important topics, this Science Mastery Assessment is another tool in your MCAT prep arsenal. This quiz (which can also be taken in your online resources) and the guidance below will help ensure that you are spending the appropriate amount of time on this chapter based on your personal strengths and weaknesses. Don't worry though—skipping something now does not mean you'll never study it. Later on in your prep, as you complete full-length tests, you'll uncover specific pieces of content that you need to review and can come back to these chapters as appropriate.

How to Use This Assessment

If you answer 0–7 questions correctly:

Spend about 1 hour to read this chapter in full and take limited notes throughout. Follow up by reviewing **all** quiz questions to ensure that you now understand how to solve each one.

If you answer 8–11 questions correctly:

Spend 20–40 minutes reviewing the quiz questions. Beginning with the questions you missed, read and take notes on the corresponding subchapters. For questions you answered correctly, ensure your thinking matches that of the explanation and you understand why each choice was correct or incorrect.

If you answer 12–15 questions correctly:

Spend less than 20 minutes reviewing all questions from the quiz. If you missed any, then include a quick read-through of the corresponding subchapters, or even just the relevant content within a subchapter, as part of your question review. For questions you answered correctly, ensure your thinking matches that of the explanation and review the Concept Summary at the end of the chapter.

1. Which of the following terms describes how existing schemata are modified to incorporate new information?
   A. Assimilation
   B. Adaptation
   C. Affirmation
   D. Accommodation

2. After completing final exams, a student reports to student health complaining of paranoia, lack of appetite, and elevated heart rate. After some questioning, the student admits to having been awake for over 48 hours after having bought pills from another student in the library. Which of the following drugs has this student likely taken?
   A. Phenobarbitol
   B. Dextroamphetamine
   C. Oxycodone
   D. Lysergic acid diethylamide

3. A student is volunteering in a hospital with a stroke center. When asked what the prevalence of stroke is among those greater than 65 years old, the student states that it is probably about 40% even though data analysis indicates that it is significantly lower. What accounts for this error?
   A. Deductive reasoning
   B. Representativeness heuristic
   C. Base rate fallacy
   D. Confirmation bias

4. Which of the following types of intelligence is NOT described by Gardner's theory of multiple intelligences?
   A. Fluid intelligence
   B. Bodily–kinesthetic intelligence
   C. Visual–spatial intelligence
   D. Linguistic intelligence

5. EEG waveforms during REM sleep most resemble which of the following states of consciousness?
   A. Alertness
   B. Slow-wave sleep
   C. Stage 1 sleep
   D. Meditation

6. Which of the following indicates the pattern of sleep stages during a complete sleep cycle early in the night?
   A. 1–2–3–4–1–2–REM
   B. 1–2–3–4–3–2–REM
   C. 4–3–2–1–2–3–REM
   D. 4–3–2–4–3–1–REM

7. Which of the following best explains a student's ability to sit on the couch and watch reruns of a favorite TV show while studying for a chemistry exam?
   A. Selective attention
   B. Divided attention
   C. Shadowing
   D. Parallel processing

8. Which theory of dreaming states that dreams and thoughts during wakeful periods use the same stream-of-consciousness system?
   A. Activation–synthesis theory
   B. Problem solving theory
   C. Cognitive process theory
   D. Neurocognitive theory

9. A 19-year-old college student with bloodshot eyes is picked up by campus police after shoplifting a large bag of corn chips and a dozen ice cream sandwiches. During questioning, the student cannot stop giggling and repeatedly asks for water, complaining of dryness in the mouth. What is the psychoactive substance in the drug this student has most likely recently taken?

- **A.** Alprazolam
- **B.** 3,4-Methylenedioxy-*N*-methylamphetamine
- **C.** Diacetylmorphine
- **D.** Tetrahydrocannabinol

10. Language consists of multiple components. Which of the following involves the order in which words are put together?

- **A.** Phonology
- **B.** Semantics
- **C.** Syntax
- **D.** Pragmatics

11. A child speaks in sentences of at least 3 words, but makes grammatical errors including misuse of the past tense. How old is this child likely to be?

- **A.** 14 months
- **B.** 22 months
- **C.** 30 months
- **D.** 5 years

12. Which language theory states that language development occurs due to preferential reinforcement of certain phonemes by parents and caregivers?

- **A.** Nativist theory
- **B.** Learning theory
- **C.** Social interactionist theory
- **D.** Neurocognitive theory

13. A stroke patient comprehends speech but cannot properly move the mouth to form words. Which of the following brain areas is likely affected?

- **A.** Broca's area
- **B.** Wernicke's area
- **C.** Arcuate fasciculus
- **D.** Superior temporal gyrus

14. A person sits at a terminal of the airport and works on a challenging sudoku puzzle. The individual ignores most of the intercom announcements but, after an announcement indicates that boarding for the flight has begun, quickly gets in line. Which of the following best explains the person's rapid response for boarding?

- **A.** Cocktail party phenomenon
- **B.** Divided attention
- **C.** Automatic processing
- **D.** Effortful processing

15. During which of the following stages does dreaming occur?

- **I.** Stage 3
- **II.** Stage 4
- **III.** REM

- **A.** I only
- **B.** II only
- **C.** III only
- **D.** I, II, and III

Answer Key

1. **D** (See section 4.1)
2. **B** (See section 4.4)
3. **C** (See section 4.2)
4. **A** (See section 4.2)
5. **A** (See section 4.3)
6. **B** (See section 4.3)
7. **B** (See section 4.5)
8. **C** (See section 4.3)
9. **D** (See section 4.4)
10. **C** (See section 4.6)
11. **C** (See section 4.6)
12. **B** (See section 4.6)
13. **A** (See section 4.6)
14. **A** (See section 4.5)
15. **D** (See section 4.3)

The relevant section of the chapter to review for each question is given in parentheses after the correct answer. Detailed explanations can be found at the end of the chapter.

CHAPTER 4

COGNITION, CONSCIOUSNESS, AND LANGUAGE

In This Chapter

CHAPTER PROFILE

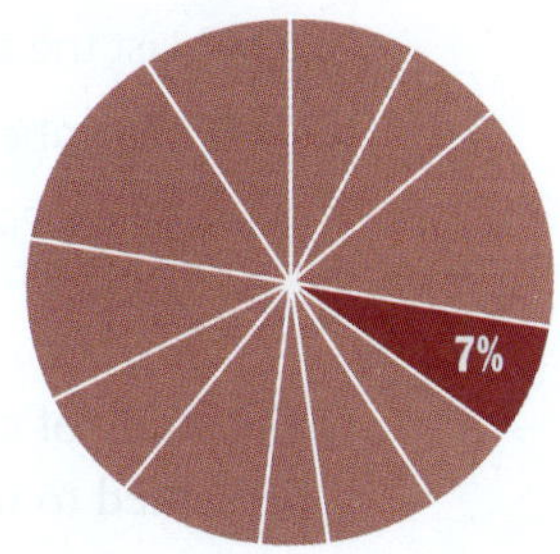

The content in this chapter should be relevant to about 7% of all questions about the behavioral sciences on the MCAT.

This chapter covers material from the following AAMC content category:

6B: Making sense of the environment

Introduction

As you think and move through the world, you often take your brain for granted. As you read, speak, ponder, make decisions, and perform complex motor functions, your brain is rapidly using electrical and chemical impulses to encode, store, and retrieve information. Most of these processes occur without your awareness or conscious thought. Imagine going to the grocery store. You fill your cart while comparing prices, assessing the produce, and planning what meals to make in the near future. After the cashier totals your purchases, you pull out a debit card, punch in a PIN, and leave with your groceries. While you were shopping in that grocery store, your brain was busy taking in all of the information around it and deciding which stimuli required attention. At the same time, you were making conscious decisions about your purchases, likely daydreaming, and maybe even singing along to music playing in the background. But, to your awareness, this was still just a simple trip to the store because most of the time, you don't even notice the tremendous processing power of your brain as you navigate the world.

But in some ways, this capacity for simultaneous conscious thinking, daydreaming, and decision making is what makes us human. Many of these functions are under the province of the frontal lobe, which—in comparison to other species on this planet—is disproportionately large in *H. sapiens*. Your frontal lobe enables you to eschew instantaneous reward and to seek out delayed gratification, like studying for the MCAT to get that high score you deserve. The frontal lobe also controls your production of language, which permits you to transmit ideas between individuals, cultures, and time. Finally, the frontal lobe helps you coordinate your thinking by deciding which stimuli deserve your attention. These are functions that are indispensable to your daily functioning and will be the focus of this chapter.

4.1 Cognition High Yield

LEARNING OBJECTIVES

After Chapter 4.1, you will be able to:

- List the steps in the information processing model of cognition
- Describe the effects of aging, heredity, and environment on cognitive function
- Recall Piaget's four stages of cognitive development and their key features

The study of **cognition** looks at how our brains process and react to the incredible information overload presented to us by the world. Cognition, overall, is not a uniquely human trait, but we are certainly the most advanced species on the planet in terms of complex thought. As described in the introduction, the frontal lobe is disproportionately large in our subspecies; a comparison to our recent anthropological ancestors demonstrates that our skull is shaped to accommodate this enlarged lobe, as shown in Figure 4.1.

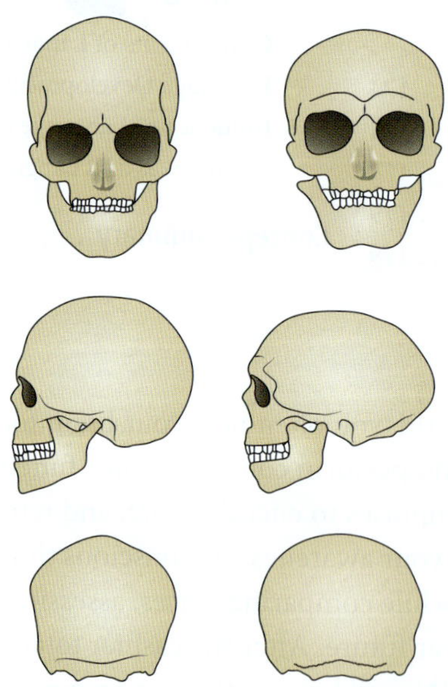

Figure 4.1 Skulls of *H. sapiens* (left) and *H. neanderthalensis* (right)

Information Processing Model

In the 1950s, much of science and engineering turned toward the production of computers and artificial intelligence. It was noted that certain steps were required in order to use a computer to store and process information. First, the information must be encoded in a language that the computer understands. Then, the information must be stored in such a way that it can be found later. Finally, the computer must be able to retrieve that information when required.

Psychologists took this model of information processing and applied it to the human brain. They theorized that the brain is somewhat like a computer. It must encode information into a series of chemical and electrical signals. Then, the brain must be able to store this information such that it can be retrieved when needed. Then, there must be a process by which the brain is able to retrieve information.

The manner in which information is encoded, stored, and retrieved has been a consistent source of debate. One prominent theory, Paivio's **dual-coding theory**, states that both verbal association and visual images are used to process and store information. For example, the word "tree" can recall some information, and a picture of a tree can recall that same information. The fact that we can code this information in two different ways builds redundancy and increases the chance that the information can be retrieved and used effectively when cued, much like search engine optimization within a computer program.

However, the human brain is not a computer. While the computer analogy creates a simple paradigm by which information is processed by the brain, it does not tell the whole story. The human brain doesn't just handle information in the form of facts: it also handles emotions, sensations such as smell and taste, as well as memories. As discussed in Chapter 3 of *MCAT Behavioral Sciences Review*, encoding, storage, and retrieval are often flavored by context and emotion.

BRIDGE

The key memory processes of encoding, storage, and retrieval are covered in Chapter 3 of *MCAT Behavioral Sciences Review.*

The **information processing model** has four key components, depicted in Figure 4.2 and summarized as follows:

- Thinking requires sensation, encoding, and storage of stimuli.
- Stimuli must be analyzed by the brain (rather than responded to automatically) to be useful in decision making.
- Decisions made in one situation can be extrapolated and adjusted to help solve new problems (also called situational modification).
- Problem solving is dependent not only on the person's cognitive level, but also on the context and complexity of the problem.

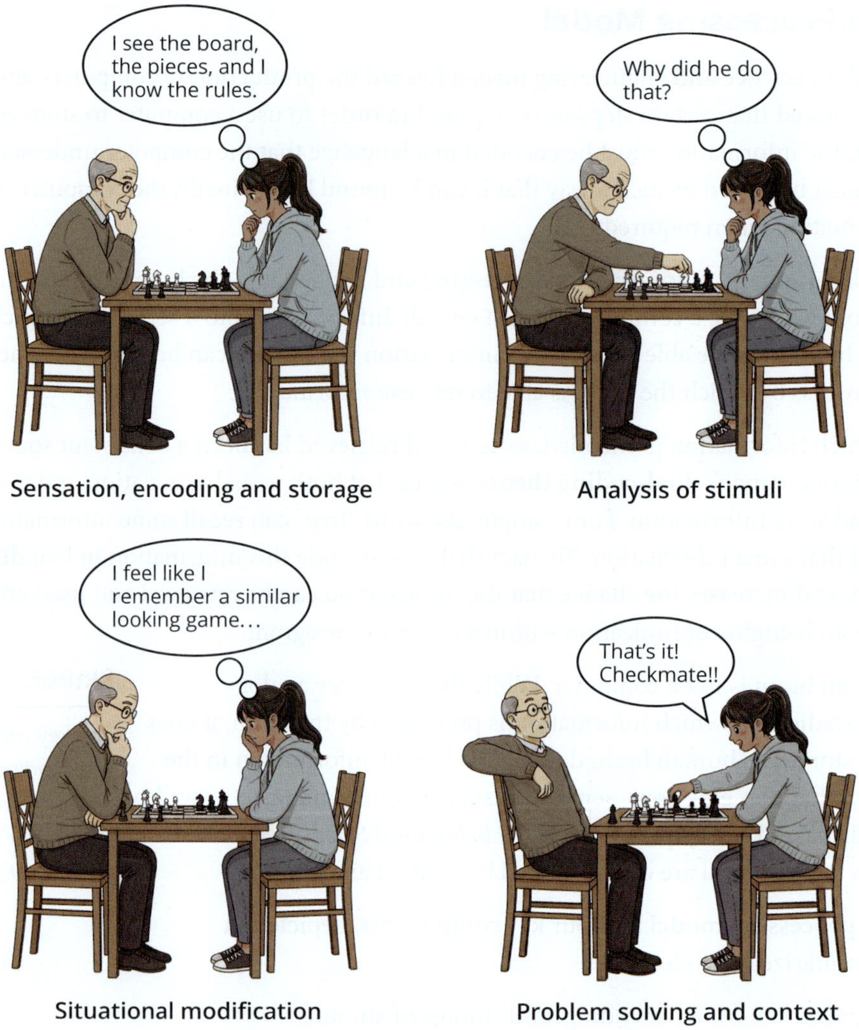
I see the board, the pieces, and I know the rules.
Why did he do that?
I feel like I remember a similar looking game...
That's it! Checkmate!!
Sensation, encoding and storage
Analysis of stimuli
Situational modification
Problem solving and context

Figure 4.2 The Information Processing Model

Cognitive Development

Cognitive development is the development of one's ability to think and solve problems across the life span. Interestingly, during childhood, cognitive development is limited by the pace of brain maturation. Early cognitive development includes learning control of one's own body as well as learning how to interact with and manipulate the environment. Early cognitive development is characterized by mastering the physical environment. As physical tasks are mastered, a new challenge looms for a developing child: abstract thinking. As discussed in Chapter 1 of *MCAT Behavioral Sciences Review*, social skills also develop during the lifetime.

As you will see during our review of Piaget's stages of cognitive development, the development of the ability to think abstractly is developed throughout childhood. The development of abstract thinking is also dependent upon increases in working memory and mental capacities. As the brain develops, the ability to process information in an abstract manner also develops.

REAL WORLD

Abstract thought, the ability to think about things that are not physically present, can be lost in some mental disorders. For example, a common cognitive test with patients who have schizophrenia is to ask them to interpret a cliché, such as *Don't count your chickens before they hatch*. These patients have concrete thinking and will give an answer focused on the chickens themselves—not the underlying concept.

Piaget's Stages of Cognitive Development

Jean Piaget was one of the most influential figures in developmental psychology. Piaget's model of cognitive development proposes that there are qualitative differences between the way that children and adults think, and that these differences can be explained by dividing the life span into four stages of cognitive development: sensorimotor, preoperational, concrete operational, and formal operational. Piaget believed that passage through each of these stages was a continuous and sequential process in which completion of each stage prepares the individual for the stage that follows.

KEY CONCEPT

Piaget's stages of cognitive development:

- Sensorimotor
- Preoperational
- Concrete operational
- Formal operational

Before delving into the actual stages, we have to look at how Piaget explained learning. According to Piaget, infants learn mainly through instinctual interaction with the environment. For example, infants possess a grasping reflex. Through experience with this reflex, the infant learns that it is possible to grasp objects. Piaget referred to these organized patterns of behavior and thought as schemata. A **schema** can include a concept (What is a *dog*?), a behavior (What do you do when someone asks you your name?), or a sequence of events (What do you normally do in a sit-down restaurant?). As a child proceeds through the stages, new information has to be placed into the different schemata. Piaget theorized that new information is processed via **adaptation**. According to Piaget, adaptation to information comes about by two complementary processes: assimilation and accommodation. **Assimilation** is the process of classifying new information into existing schemata. If the new information does not fit neatly into existing schemata, then accommodation occurs. **Accommodation** is the process by which existing schemata are modified to encompass this new information. As shown in Figure 4.3, a classic example of assimilation and accommodation is when a young child calls a cute, furry animal a dog when, in reality, it is a cat.

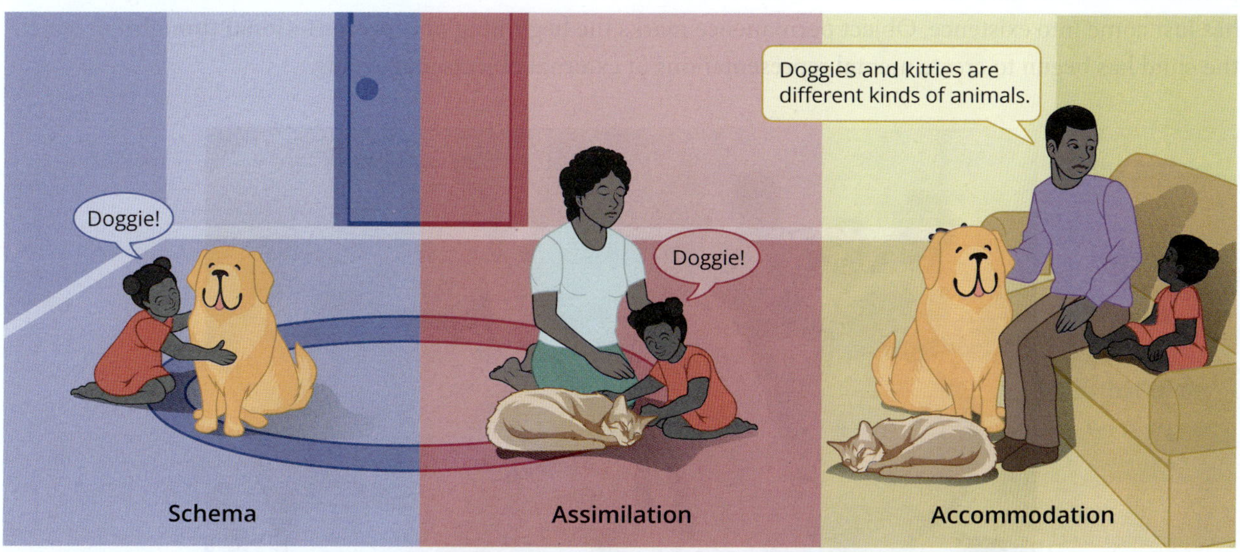

Figure 4.3 Assimilation and Accommodation

The first stage in Piaget's model is the **sensorimotor stage**, starting at birth and lasting until about two years of age. In this stage, a child learns to manipulate the environment in order to meet physical needs and learns to coordinate sensory input with motor actions (hence the name *sensorimotor*). To explore their surroundings, infants in the sensorimotor stage begin to exhibit three types of behavior patterns known for their repetitive natures called **circular reactions** (see Figure 4.4). **Primary circular reactions** are repetitions of body movements that originally occurred by chance, such as sucking the thumb. Usually such behaviors are repeated because the child finds these behaviors soothing. **Secondary circular reactions** occur when manipulation is focused on something outside the body, such as repeatedly throwing toys from a high chair. These behaviors are often repeated because the child gets a response from the environment, such as a parent picking up the dropped toy. **Tertiary circular reactions**, which emerge around the first year of life, involve the child experimenting with actions to observe different outcomes, such as hitting a toy against various surfaces to see the different sounds it makes.

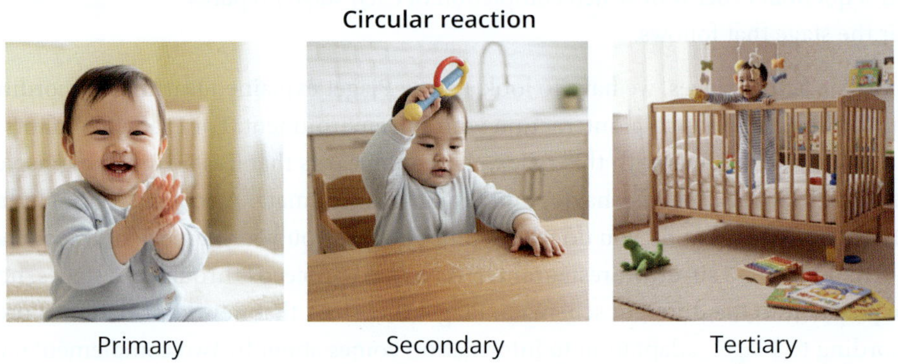

Figure 4.4 Circular Reactions

The key milestone that ends the sensorimotor stage is the development of **object permanence**, which is the understanding that objects continue to exist even when out of view. Object permanence is the idea behind "peek-a-boo," shown in Figure 4.5. This game is so entertaining to young infants because they lack object permanence. Each time an adult reveals the face from behind hands, the child interprets it as though the adult has just come into existence. Object permanence marks the beginning of **representational thought**, in which the child has begun to create mental representations of external objects and events.

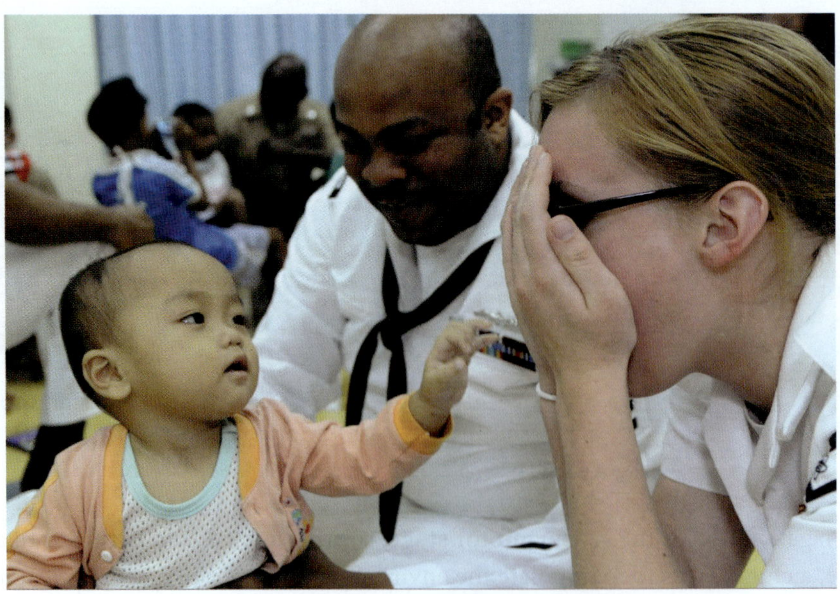

Figure 4.5 Peek-a-Boo
This game depends on the child being in the sensorimotor stage, prior to the development of object permanence.

The **preoperational stage** lasts from about two to seven years of age and is characterized by symbolic thinking and egocentrism. **Symbolic thinking** refers to the ability to pretend, play make-believe, and have an imagination. **Egocentrism** refers to the inability to imagine what another person may think or feel. The preoperational stage also includes the inability to grasp the concept of **conservation**, which is the understanding that a physical amount remains the same, even if there is a change in shape or appearance. For example, imagine a child presented with two equal quantities of pizza. On one plate is a single large slice, while the other plate has the exact same quantity in two slices. A child in the preoperational stage will be unable to tell that the quantities are equal and will focus mainly on the number of slices on the plate rather than the actual quantity. (Another classic example of conservation that uses water is shown in Figure 4.6.) Piaget believed that this flaw in cognition was due to **centration**, which is the tendency to focus on only one aspect of a phenomenon, for example the number of slices, while ignoring other important elements.

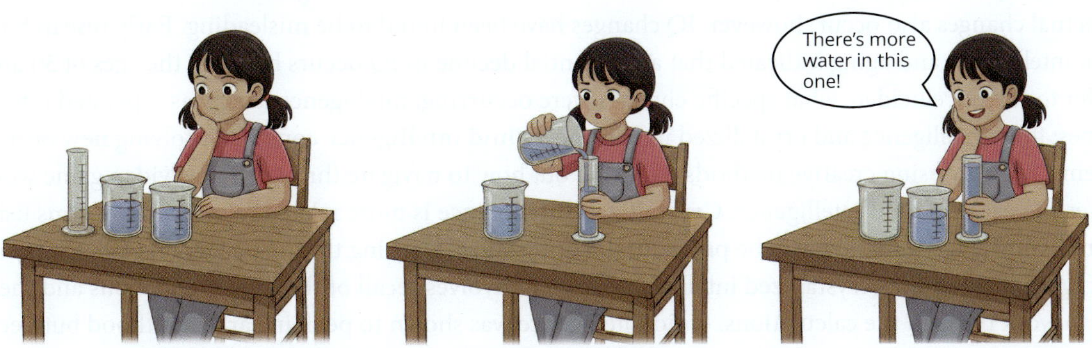

Figure 4.6 A Child Lacking the Concept of Conservation

The **concrete operational stage** lasts from about 7 to 11 years of age. In this stage, children can understand conservation and consider the perspectives of others. This consideration results in the loss of egocentrism. Additionally, they are able to engage in logical thought as long as they are working with concrete objects or information that is directly available. These children have not yet developed the ability to think abstractly.

The **formal operational stage** starts around 11 years of age, and is marked by the ability to think logically about abstract ideas. Generally coinciding with adolescence, this stage is marked by the ability to reason about abstract concepts and problem solve. The difference between this type of thought and concrete operations is illustrated by Piaget's pendulum experiment. Children were given a pendulum in which they could vary the length of the string, the weight of the pendulum, the force of the push, and the initial angle of the swing. They were asked to find out what determined the frequency of the swing. Children in the concrete operational stage manipulated the variables at random and even distorted the data to fit preconceived hypotheses. Adolescents, on the other hand, were able to hold all variables but one constant at a given time, proceeding methodically to discover that only the length of the string affects the frequency. The ability to mentally manipulate variables in a number of ways, generally within the scope of scientific experiments, is an important component of the formal operational stage, and is termed **hypothetical reasoning**.

Role of Culture in Cognitive Development

Cognitive development is very much related to culture, as one's culture will determine what one is expected to learn. Some cultures will place a higher value on social learning, including cultural traditions and roles, while other cultures will value knowledge. In addition, one's culture will also influence the rate of cognitive development as children can be treated very differently from culture to culture.

BRIDGE

Culture has profound effects on cognitive development, as well as social structure, rules, and mores. Culture is discussed in detail in Chapter 11 of *MCAT Behavioral Sciences Review.*

Lev Vygotsky, a prominent educational psychologist, proposed that the engine driving cognitive development is children's internalization of their culture, including interpersonal and societal rules, symbols, and language. As children develop, their skills and abilities are still in formative stages. With help from adults or other children, those skills can develop further. That help may come in the form of instruction from a teacher or even watching another child perform the skill.

BRIDGE

Lev Vygotsky is also a key figure in the psychology of identity. Along with Kohlberg, Freud, and Erikson, he proposed a staged system of identity formation. These theorists are discussed in Chapter 6 of *MCAT Behavioral Sciences Review.*

Cognitive Changes in Late Adulthood

Aging brings about many changes in cognition. Reaction time increases steadily in early adulthood, while time-based prospective memory—the ability to remember to perform a task at a specific time in the future—declines with age. Intellectual changes also occur; however, IQ changes have been found to be misleading. Early research into the field of intelligence and aging indicated that a substantial decline in IQ occurs between the ages of 30 and 40. In order to further elucidate what specific changes were occurring, intelligence itself was separated into two subtypes: fluid intelligence and crystallized intelligence. **Fluid intelligence** consists of solving new or novel problems, possibly using creative methods. Figuring out how to navigate through a new video game world involves the usage of fluid intelligence. **Crystallized intelligence** is more related to solving problems using acquired knowledge, and often can be procedural. For instance, working through a General Chemistry stoichiometry problem requires crystallized intelligence since it involves recall of the proper equations and the steps taken to work through the calculations. Fluid intelligence was shown to peak in early adulthood but decline with age, while crystallized intelligence peaked in middle adulthood and remains stable with age (Figure 4.7).

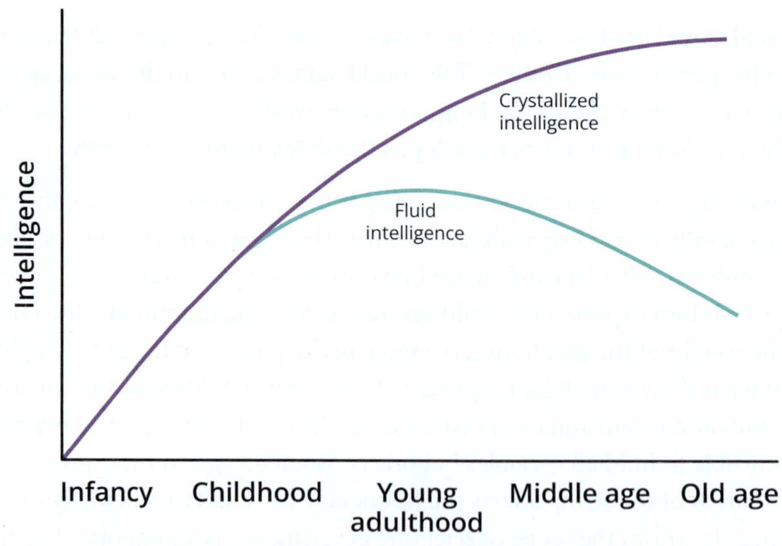

Figure 4.7 Fluid and Crystallized Intelligence throughout Life

Decline in intellectual abilities in adulthood has been linked with how long an older adult retains the ability to function in what are known as **activities of daily living** (eating, bathing, toileting, dressing, and ambulation). It appears, however, that this decline is not uniform. Certain characteristics, such as higher level of education, more frequent performance of intellectual activities, socializing, and a stimulating environment have been found to be protective against intellectual decline.

Intellectual decline is not always benign. Some types of intellectual decline are very common and indicate a progressive loss of function beyond that of old age. Disorders and conditions that are characterized by a general loss of cognitive function are collectively known as **dementia**. Dementia often begins with impaired memory, but later progresses to impaired judgment and confusion. Personality changes are also very common as dementia progresses. The most common cause of dementia is Alzheimer's disease. Vascular (multi-infarct) dementia, caused by high blood pressure and repeated microscopic clots in the brain, is also a very common cause. It is also important to note that people with dementia often require full-time supportive care in order to carry out activities of daily living. This causes tremendous stress on families, including children and spouses of those with dementia, as the care for the person with dementia often falls on family members.

REAL WORLD

Alzheimer's disease accounts for approximately 60 to 80% of all dementia cases.

Heredity, Environment, and Biologic Factors

Cognition can be affected by a wide variety of conditions. These may include actual problems with the brain itself (organic brain disorders), genetic and chromosomal conditions, metabolic derangements, and long-term drug use. The environment can also affect both cognitive development and day-to-day cognition.

Parenting styles may influence cognitive development by reward, punishment, or indifference for an emerging skill. In addition, genetics can predispose to a state that may make cognitive development difficult. For example, many genetic and chromosomal diseases such as Down syndrome and Fragile X syndrome are associated with delayed cognitive development. Antisocial personality disorder has also been shown to have a strong genetic component. The presence of genes for this disorder may make it difficult for a child to appreciate the rights of others.

Intellectual disabilities in children can also be caused by chemical exposures, illness, injury, or trauma during birth. Alcohol use during pregnancy can cause fetal alcohol syndrome, which results in slowed cognitive development and distinct craniofacial features, shown in Figure 4.8. Infections in the brain may result in electrical abnormalities and slowed development. Complications during birth—especially those causing reduced oxygen delivery to the brain—may also affect cognition. Finally, reduced cognition can also occur following trauma to the brain, as occurs with shaken baby syndrome.

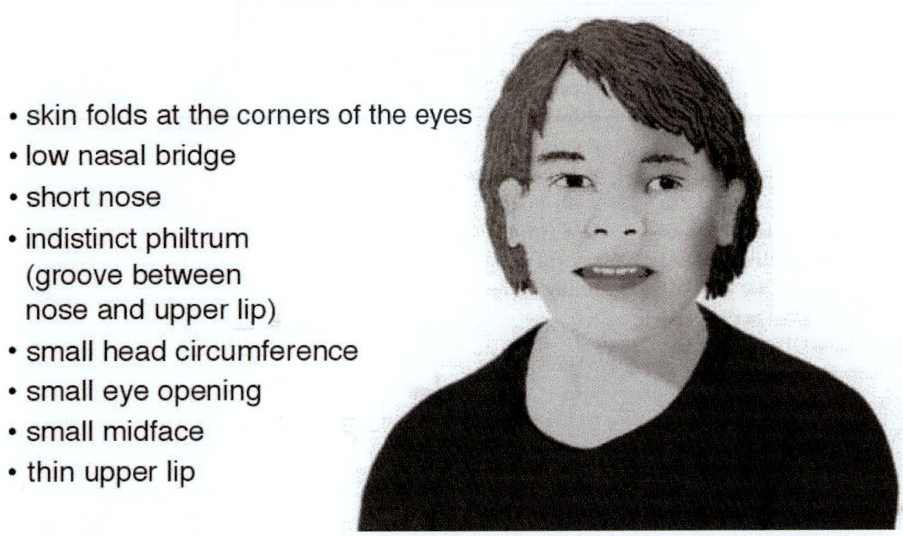

Figure 4.8 Craniofacial Features of Fetal Alcohol Syndrome

However, not all cognitive decline in adulthood is slow. If there has been a rapid decline in cognition, this may be the result of delirium. **Delirium** is rapid fluctuation in cognitive function that is reversible and caused by medical (nonpsychological) causes. It can be caused by a variety of issues, including electrolyte and pH disturbances, malnutrition, low blood sugar, infection, a drug reaction, alcohol withdrawal, and pain.

REAL WORLD

The delirium associated with alcohol withdrawal, called *delirium tremens*, can be life threatening. As a depressant, alcohol is the only major drug of abuse in which both overdose and withdrawal can be lethal.

MCAT CONCEPT CHECK 4.1

Before you move on, assess your understanding of the material with these questions.

1. The three steps in the information processing model are:
   1. ______________________
   2. ______________________
   3. ______________________
2. A person brings a parent, who is an older adult, to the doctor. During the past two days, the parent has been overheard speaking to a spouse who has been deceased for four years. Prior to that, the parent was completely normal. The parent most likely has:

   ____
3. List Piaget's four stages of cognitive development and the key features of each.

Stage	Key Features

4.2 Problem Solving and Decision Making

High Yield

LEARNING OBJECTIVES

After Chapter 4.2, you will be able to:

- Identify examples of functional fixedness, mental sets, trial-and-error problem solving, algorithms, and deductive reasoning
- Recall key fallacies and biases, including base rate fallacy, disconfirmation principle, confirmation bias, overconfidence, and belief perseverance
- Describe models of intellectual functioning and tests of intellectual ability
- Explain the availability and representativeness heuristics

Every day you are faced with problems. Many of these problems you solve without any real conscious thought about what is happening. However, much like the scientific method, problem solving itself has a process. First, we must frame the problem; that is, we create a mental image or schematic of the issue. Then, we generate potential solutions and begin to test them. These potential solutions may be derived from a **mental set**, which is the tendency to approach similar problems in the same way. Once solutions have been tested, we evaluate the results, considering other potential solutions that may have been easier or more effective in some way.

KEY CONCEPT

The first step in problem solving (framing the problem) may seem obvious; however, when we get "stuck" on a problem, it is most often because the manner in which we have framed the problem is inefficient or not useful.

Problem solving can be impeded by an inappropriate mental set, as well as by functional fixedness, which is demonstrated by Duncker's candle problem. Consider the following scenario: You walk into a room and see a box of matches, some tacks, and a candle. Your task is to mount the candle on the wall so that it can be used without the wax dropping on the floor. Before reading on, try to solve the problem.

Most people find the task challenging. You might have thought of tacking the candle to the wall, but that solution doesn't work because the wax would still drop to the floor. The key is to realize that the matchbox can serve not just as a container for the matches, but as a holder for the candle. The solution, therefore, is to tack the box to the wall and put the candle in the box. **Functional fixedness** can thus be defined as the inability to consider how to use an object in a nontraditional manner.

Types of Problem Solving

In psychology, different approaches to problem solving include trial-and-error, algorithms, deductive reasoning, and inductive reasoning.

Trial-and-Error

Trial-and-error is a less sophisticated type of problem solving in which various solutions are tried until one is found that seems to work. While an educated approach may be used, this type of problem solving is usually only effective when there are relatively few possible solutions.

Algorithms

An **algorithm** is a formula or procedure for solving a certain type of problem. Algorithms can be mathematical or a set of instructions, designed to automatically produce the desired solution.

Deductive Reasoning

Deductive (top-down) reasoning starts from a set of general rules and draws conclusions from the information given. An example of deductive reasoning is a logic puzzle, as shown in Figure 4.9. In these puzzles, one has to synthesize a list of logical rules to come up with the single possible solution to the problem.

	Black	Turnip	Spade	Yuka	Patch	Liam	1	2	3
Jim	●	X	X	●	X	X	X	●	X
Tylor	X	●	X	X			X	X	●
Meera	X	X	●	X			●	X	X
1				X	X	●			
2						X			
3	X		X			X			
Yuka			X						
Patch									
Liam									

Figure 4.9 A Logic Puzzle Grid
Logic puzzles are applications of deductive reasoning in which only one possible solution can be deduced based on the information given.

MCAT EXPERTISE

Remember that a deduction is a solution that *must* be true based on the information given. This is why answers on the MCAT that merely *might* be true (but don't *have* to be) are never the correct answer.

Inductive Reasoning

Inductive (bottom-up) reasoning seeks to create a theory via generalizations. This type of reasoning starts with specific instances, and then draws a conclusion from them. Both inductive and deductive reasoning have their beneficial roles in the medical field, as demonstrated in Figure 4.10.

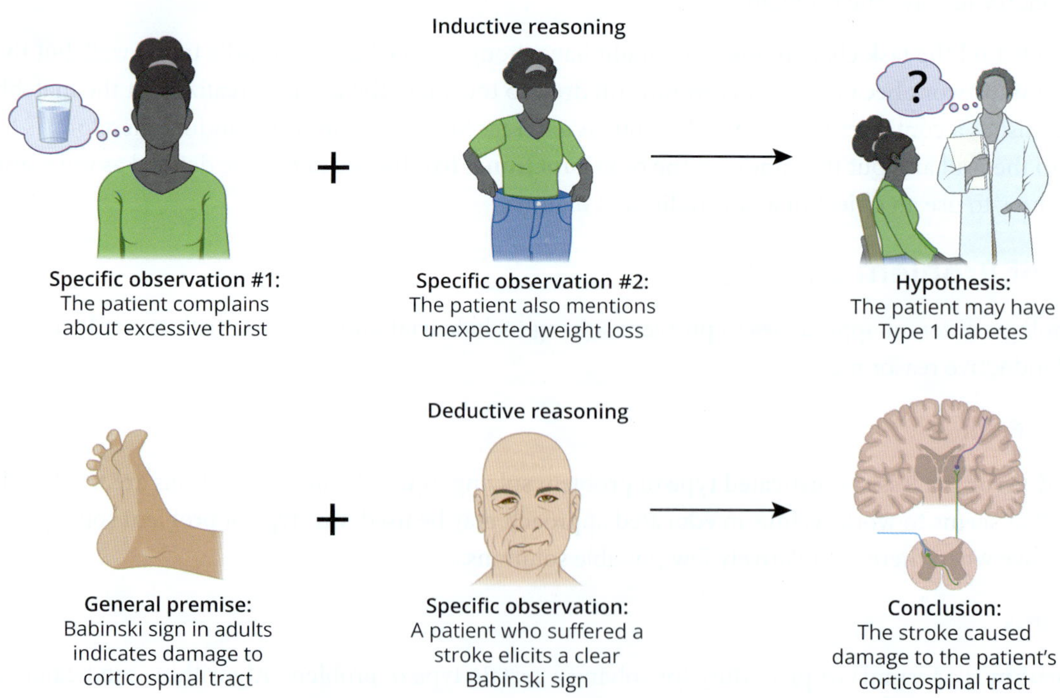

Figure 4.10 Deductive vs. Inductive Reasoning

Heuristics, Biases, Intuition, and Emotion

We make decisions every day. Some are related to our daily routines: *What should I wear today?* Others concern our broader life goals: *Where am I going to apply to medical school?* Decision making is a complicated process, but we use a number of tools, such as heuristics, biases, intuition, and emotions, to speed up or simplify the process. While useful from a time and complexity standpoint, these tools can also lead us to shortsighted or problematic solutions.

Heuristics

Heuristics are simplified principles used to make decisions; they are colloquially called "rules of thumb." The **availability heuristic** is a heuristic used when we base the likelihood of an event on how easily examples of that event come to mind. Often, the use of this heuristic leads us to a correct decision, but not always. As an example, answer the following question: *Are there more words in the English language that start with the letter "K" or that have "K" as their third letter?*

Most people respond that there are more words that begin with the letter "K" than have "K" as their third letter. In fact, there are actually at least twice as many words in English that have "K" as the third letter than begin with "K." Most people approach this question by trying to think of words that fit into each category. Because we so often classify words by their first letter, most people can easily think of words beginning with "K." However, most people have a harder time thinking of words with "K" as their third letter. Thus, in this case, the availability heuristic tends to lead to an incorrect answer.

The **representativeness heuristic** involves categorizing items on the basis of whether they fit the prototypical, stereotypical, or representative image of the category. For example, consider a standard coin that is flipped ten times in a row and lands on heads every time. What is the probability of the coin landing on heads the next time? Mathematically, the probability must still be 50 percent, but most individuals will either overestimate the probability based on the pattern that has been established, or underestimate the probability with the logic that the number of heads and tails must "even out." Hence, like the availability heuristic, the use of the representativeness heuristic can sometimes lead us astray. Using prototypical or stereotypical factors while ignoring actual numerical information is called the **base rate fallacy**.

While heuristics can lead us astray, they are essential to speedy and effective decision making. Heuristics are often used by experts in a given field. For instance, to win at chess, one must be able to think several moves ahead. On any particular turn, there may be 15 or 20 possible moves, each one of which may have multiple consequences; analyzing every possibility would take far too long. There are heuristics, however, that can quickly rule out some of the possible moves: the king must be protected, it is generally good to control the center squares, and pieces should not be put in danger when possible. In this way, heuristics provide a more efficient—although sometimes inaccurate—method for problem solving.

Bias and Overconfidence

When a potential solution to a problem fails during testing, this solution should be discarded. This is known as the **disconfirmation principle**: the evidence obtained from testing demonstrated that the solution does not work. However, the presence of a confirmation bias may prevent an individual from eliminating this solution. **Confirmation bias** is the tendency to focus on information that fits an individual's beliefs, while rejecting information that goes against them. Confirmation bias also contributes to **overconfidence**, or a tendency to erroneously interpret one's decisions, knowledge, and beliefs as infallible. An additional type of bias is **hindsight bias**, which is the tendency for people to overestimate their ability to predict the outcome of events that already happened. The similar phenomenon of **belief perseverance** refers to the inability to reject a particular belief despite clear evidence to the contrary. Together, confirmation bias, overconfidence, hindsight bias, and belief perseverance can seriously impede a person's analysis of available evidence.

Intuition

Intuition can be defined as the ability to act on perceptions that may not be supported by available evidence. Often, people may have beliefs that are not necessarily supported by evidence, but that a person "feels" to be correct. Intuition is often developed by experience. For example, an emergency room physician, over the course of seeing thousands of patients with chest pain, may develop a keen sense of which patients are actually having a heart attack without even looking at an electrocardiogram (EKG) or a patient's vital signs. This intuition can be more accurately described by the **recognition-primed decision model**: the doctor's brain is actually sorting through a wide variety of information to match a pattern. Over time, the doctor has gained an extensive level of experience that can be accessed without awareness.

Emotion

Emotion is the subjective experience of a person in a certain situation. How a person feels often influences how a person thinks and makes decisions. For example, a person who is angry is often more likely to engage in more risky decision making. In addition, emotions in decision making are not limited to the emotion experienced while the decision is being made; emotions that a person *expects* to feel from a particular decision are also involved. For example, if people believe a car will make them feel more powerful, they may be more likely to purchase that car.

Intellectual Functioning

Intellectual functioning is a highly studied area of psychology. How is intelligence defined? What makes someone more intelligent than someone else? These are multifaceted questions that are difficult to answer; however, theorists have proposed models for some aspects of intelligence.

Theories of Intelligence

There has been much debate concerning the definition of intelligence. Howard Gardner's theory of **multiple intelligences** is one of the most all-encompassing definitions, with at least eight defined types of intelligence: linguistic, logical–mathematical, musical, visual–spatial, bodily–kinesthetic, interpersonal, intrapersonal, and naturalist. Gardner argues that some cultures value the first two abilities over the others. After all, linguistic ability and logical–mathematical ability are the two abilities tested on traditional intelligence quotient (IQ) tests. Despite not being the central focus of the cultures Gardner discusses, people's interpersonal and intrapersonal intelligence can heavily impact their quality of life. **Interpersonal intelligence** is the ability to detect and navigate the moods and motivations of others. Gardner believed that people with high interpersonal intelligence would make great sales representatives and therapists. While intrapersonal intelligence centers around being mindful of one's own emotions, strengths, and weaknesses, which can provide clear guidance what role one should take in a group or society.

KEY CONCEPT

Gardner's multiple intelligences include linguistic, logical–mathematical, musical, visual–spatial, bodily–kinesthetic, interpersonal, intrapersonal, and naturalist.

Robert Sternberg pioneered a cognitive perspective that focused on how people use their intelligence, rather than taking the traditional approach of trying to measure an individual's level of intelligence. More specifically, Sternberg's triarchic theory of human intelligence defines three subtypes: **analytical intelligence**, which involves the ability to evaluate and reason; **creative intelligence**, which is the ability to solve problems using novel methods; and **practical intelligence**, which involves dealing with everyday problems at home or at work.

Successful navigation of our social world also requires us to have a good understanding of both our own emotions and the emotions of those around us. The theory of **emotional intelligence** addresses our emotional awareness in four components: the ability to express and perceive emotions in ourself and others, the ability to comprehend and analyze our emotions, the ability to regulate our emotions, and awareness of how emotions shape our thoughts and decisions. Empathy is often given as an example of emotional intelligence because empathy requires individuals to understand their own emotions well enough to recognize those emotions in other people.

Variations in Intellectual Ability

There are a number of tests and studies that have historically attempted to quantify intelligence. A founding concept behind these tests is Charles Spearman's "g factor," or general intelligence factor. The theory behind the existence of a g factor is based on the observation that performance on different cognitive tasks is in many cases positively correlated, indicating an underlying factor or variable is playing a role. This underlying variable of intelligence is often measured with standardized tests that generate an **intelligence quotient** (IQ) for the test taker. IQ tests were largely pioneered by Alfred Binet in the early twentieth century. A professor at Stanford University took Binet's work and created what is known as the **Stanford–Binet IQ test**.

BEHAVIORAL SCIENCES GUIDED EXAMPLE WITH EXPERT THINKING

Many decisions we make use the affect heuristic; that is, we make quick judgments that depend on our emotional state as well as the emotional content of the decision. Specifically, options that provoke positive emotions are more likely to be chosen than those that evoke negative emotions when the choices are quantitatively identical, and even in cases in which the choice associated with negative feelings is quantitatively better. The following three studies were conducted:

Definition of new term: affect heuristic

Study 1: Researchers provided participants with quantitative information about one of two issues: violent crime (steadily declining) and deer overpopulation (steadily increasing). The participants were asked to rate the severity of each problem on a scale from "very bad" to "very good."

Two problems which differ in severity and emotional content.

IV: issue

DV: rating

Study 2: Participants were asked to set a price for a listing of retail electronics. One listing included ten unused items and another included 18 items, 14 of which were unused and 4 of which were described as being used and in "poor working order."

Comparison between two sets of items, varying in content.

IV: list contents (broken items)

DV: price

Study 3: Participants were asked to determine punishments for a number of hypothetical college students who had committed some form of academic dishonesty. The participants were provided a photograph and description for each student. The same student was used, but one group of participants was provided a picture of the student smiling, and the other group was provided a picture of the student with a neutral expression.

Meting out punishment for people, some of whom are smiling in pictures.

IV: photograph

DV: punishment

Adapted from: Wilson, Robyn S.; Arvai, Joseph L. (March 2006). "When Less Is More: How Affect Influences Preferences When Comparing Low and High-risk Options". *Journal of Risk Research.* **9** (2): 165–178.

LaFrance, M.; Hecht, M.A. (March 1995). "Why Smiles Generate Leniency". *Personality and Social Psychology Bulletin.* **21** (3): 207–214.

If the affect heuristic is shown to be a factor in each of the studies described, what can be predicted about the results of each?

When the MCAT asks us to predict the outcome of an experiment, we want to first consider any content, either from the passage or from our outside knowledge, that might be relevant. Fortunately, this passage provides us with what we need: a definition of the affect heuristic in paragraph one. For each study, then, you'll want to select the result that prioritizes emotional content. For Study 1, the notion of "violent crime" likely provokes a strong negative feeling, while for most people, the idea of "deer overpopulation" would not be expected to be associated with the same emotional response. It is likely, then, that participants would rate violent crime as a worse problem than deer overpopulation regardless of the actual outcome of analyzing the quantitative impact of each issue. The same heuristic explains why people are more afraid of being attacked by a shark at the beach than of other, more likely causes of death, even though statistically injury or death by shark attack is extremely unlikely.

In Study 2, we would predict that the broken items would cause the second listing to be valued the same as or lower than the first listing, even though the second listing actually contains more items that are unused. This is because the additional broken items would be expected to provoke a negative feeling about the second listing. In fact, further research supports the idea that participants do not add up the value of each item separately, but rather evaluate heuristically what they perceive as an average value of the set of items as a whole.

Finally, in Study 3, we should expect that the smiling students were judged less harshly than those presented with a neutral expression. This is based on the same decision-making heuristic we've been using all along: the smiling student is more likely to be associated with positive emotions, and the decision is likely to be altered based on this emotional input.

To summarize: we should predict based on the affect heuristic that in Study 1 the violent crime will be rated as the more problematic of the two issues, that in Study 2 the batch of items containing broken goods will be rated as less valuable, and that in Study 3 the smiling student will be judged less harshly than the neutral student.

While later iterations of the test use different methodologies to arrive at a score, it is useful to know the original formula for calculating IQ:

$$\text{IQ} = \frac{\text{mental age}}{\text{chronological age}} \times 100$$

Equation 4.1

Using this equation, a four-year-old with intelligence abilities at the level of the average six-year-old would have an IQ of 150. The distribution of IQ scores from the original study of the Stanford–Binet IQ test is shown in Figure 4.11.

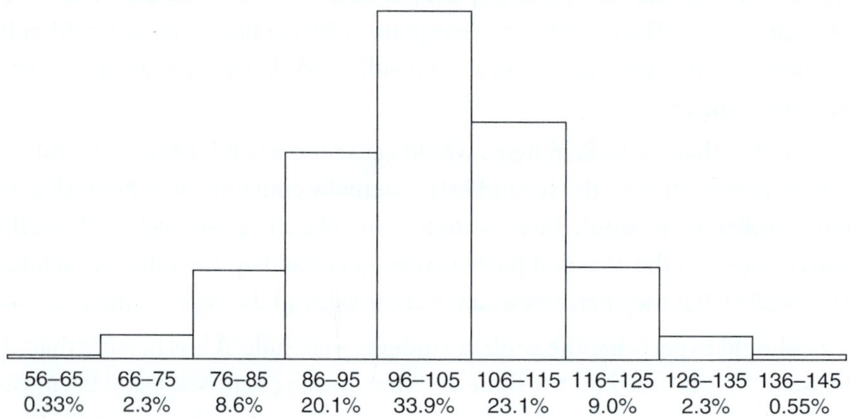

Figure 4.11 Distribution of IQ Scores for Children 5 to 14 Years of Age
Mean = 100; SD = 15

Some theorists have argued heavily for intelligence as a hereditary trait, most notably Galton in his novel *Hereditary Genius.* In reality, variations in intellectual ability can be attributed to many determinants, including genes, environment, and educational experiences. Intellectual ability does appear to run in families, which may be due to both genetics and the environment; some environments are simply more enriching than others. Parental expectations, socioeconomic status, and nutrition have all been shown to correlate with intelligence.

The educational system plays a significant role in the development of intelligence. Children who attend school tend to have greater increases in IQ, and IQ actually decreases slightly during summer vacations. Early intervention in childhood also improves IQ, especially for children in low-enrichment environments. Finally, both children with high IQs and those with cognitive disabilities benefit from specialized educational environments. For students with cognitive disabilities, this is often defined as the least restrictive environment, in which they are encouraged to participate as much as possible in the regular mainstream classroom, with individualized help as needed.

REAL WORLD

The Stanford-Binet IQ test, while still popular, has been found to have variable levels of success in assessing intelligence with different ages and cultural groups. In practice, a variety of intelligence assessments can be found in use around the world. Some of these tests still use measures similar to IQ but are specialized for a subpopulation, such as the Wechsler Intelligence Scale for Children (WISC) exam. Other assessments eschew the concept of IQ entirely and instead follow alternative theories, including Gardner's theory of multiple intelligences.

MCAT CONCEPT CHECK 4.2

Before you move on, assess your understanding of the material with these questions.

1. A child plays with a tool set, noting that a nail can only be hit with a hammer. When a friend suggests that the handle of a screwdriver can be used to hit a nail, the child passionately objects. This is an example of:

 ____

2. A doctor uses a flowchart to treat a patient with sepsis. Given its use in problem solving, a flowchart is an example of a(n):

 ____

3. A patient in a mental health facility believes that the sky is pink. Despite several trips outside, the patient still declares the sky is pink. Which psychological principle does this represent?

 ____

4. Provide a brief definition of the availability and representativeness heuristics.
 - Availability heuristic:

 ____

 - Representativeness heuristic:

 ____

4.3 Consciousness High Yield

LEARNING OBJECTIVES

After Chapter 4.3, you will be able to:

- Identify the two hormones most associated with circadian rhythms
- Distinguish between dyssomnia and parasomnia
- Associate the stages of sleep with their EEG waveforms and other main features:

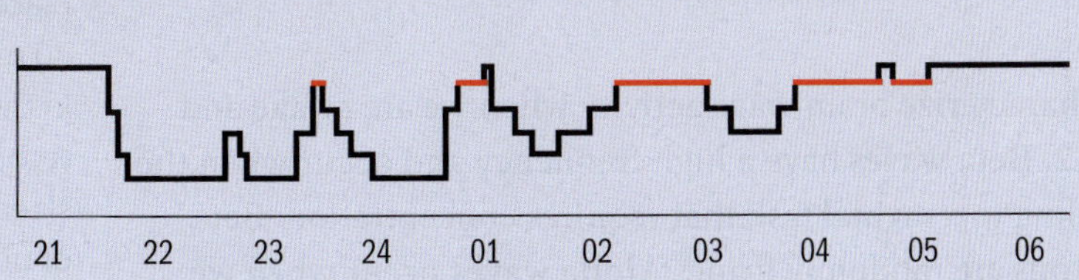

Consciousness is one's level of awareness of both the world and one's own existence within that world.

States of Consciousness

The accepted states of consciousness are alertness, sleep, dreaming, and altered states of consciousness. Technically, sleep and dreaming are also considered altered states, but we will consider these states separately from hypnosis, meditation, and drug-induced altered states of consciousness. Altered states of consciousness may also result from sickness, dementia, delirium, and coma.

Alertness

Alertness is a state of consciousness in which we are awake and able to think. In this state, we are able to perceive, process, access, and verbalize information. In the alert state, we also experience a certain level of **physiological arousal**, which is characterized by physiological reactions such as increased heart rate, breathing rate, blood pressure, and so on. Cortisol levels tend to be higher, and electroencephalogram (EEG) waves indicate a brain in the waking state.

Alertness is maintained by neurological circuits in the prefrontal cortex at the very front of the brain. Fibers from the prefrontal cortex communicate with the **reticular formation** (reticular activation system), a neural structure located in the brainstem, to keep the cortex awake and alert. A brain injury that results in disruption of these connections results in coma.

Sleep

Sleep is important to consider while studying for the MCAT or any other major exam. While it may be tempting to pull all-nighters in an attempt to maximize your test score, this may not be the best strategy for success. In fact, long-term sleep deprivation has been linked with diminished cognitive performance as well as the development of chronic diseases such as diabetes and obesity.

Stages of Sleep

Sleep is studied by recording brain wave activity occurring during the course of a night's sleep. This is done with **electroencephalography**, or **EEG**, which records an average of the electrical patterns within different portions of the brain. There are four characteristic EEG patterns correlated with different stages of waking and sleeping: beta, alpha, theta, and delta waves. There is a fifth wave that corresponds to REM sleep, which is the time during the night when we have most of our dreams. These sleep stages form a complete cycle lasting about 90 minutes.

Beta and alpha waves characterize brain wave activity when we are awake and are shown in Figure 4.12. **Beta waves** have a high frequency and occur when the person is alert or attending to a mental task that requires concentration. Beta waves occur when neurons are randomly firing. **Alpha waves** occur when we are awake but relaxing with our eyes closed, and are somewhat slower than beta waves. Alpha waves are also more synchronized than beta waves.

MCAT EXPERTISE

One of the best ways to enhance your recall and test performance is to maintain a regular schedule of sleep. Regular sleep, exercise, and a healthy diet help to make Test Day successful.

REAL WORLD

An electroencephalogram (EEG) is a test used to monitor electrical activity in the brain. It consists of 19 recording electrodes placed on the scalp for 20 to 40 minutes, or continuously in the inpatient setting. This technique is used to study sleep and to identify areas of unusual brain activity, as seen during seizures.

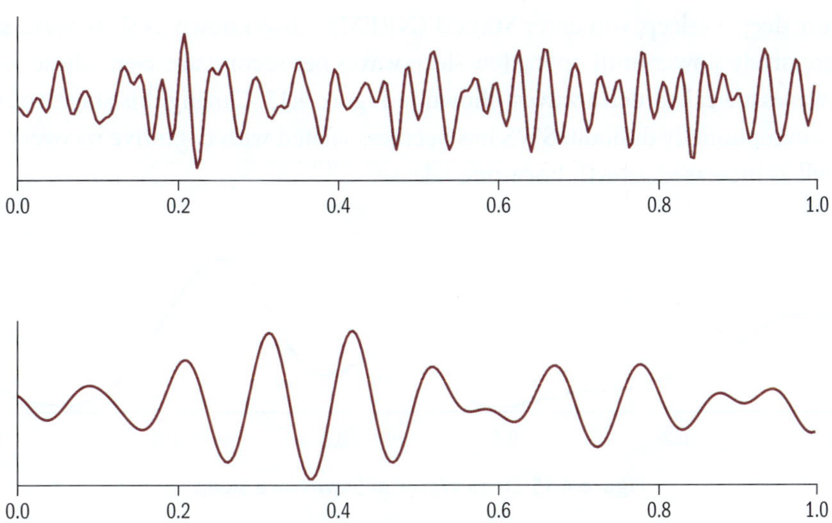

Figure 4.12 Beta (top) and Alpha (bottom) Waves on EEG
Beta and alpha waves are seen during alertness.

As soon as you doze off, you enter **Stage 1** (also known as NREM1), which is detected on the EEG by the appearance of **theta waves**, shown in Figure 4.13. At this point, EEG activity is characterized by irregular waveforms with slower frequencies and higher voltages.

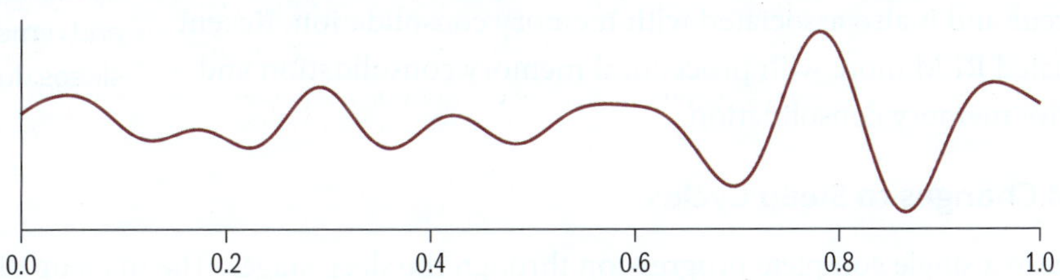

Figure 4.13 Theta Waves
Theta waves are seen during Stage 1 and 2 sleep.

As you fall more deeply asleep, you enter **Stage 2** (NREM2). The EEG shows theta waves along with **sleep spindles**, which are bursts of high-frequency waves, and **K complexes**, which are singular high-amplitude waves, shown in Figure 4.14.

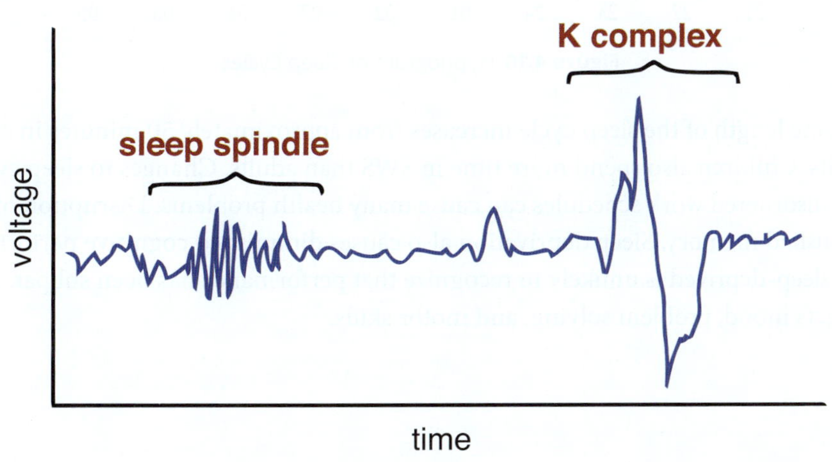

Figure 4.14 Sleep Spindle and K Complex in Stage 2 Sleep

As you fall even more deeply asleep, you enter **Stage 3** (NREM3), also known as **slow-wave sleep** (**SWS**). EEG activity grows progressively slower until only a few sleep waves per second are seen. These low-frequency, high-voltage sleep waves are called **delta waves**, shown in Figure 4.15. During this stage, rousing someone from sleep becomes exceptionally difficult. SWS has been associated with cognitive recovery and memory consolidation, as well as increased growth hormone release.

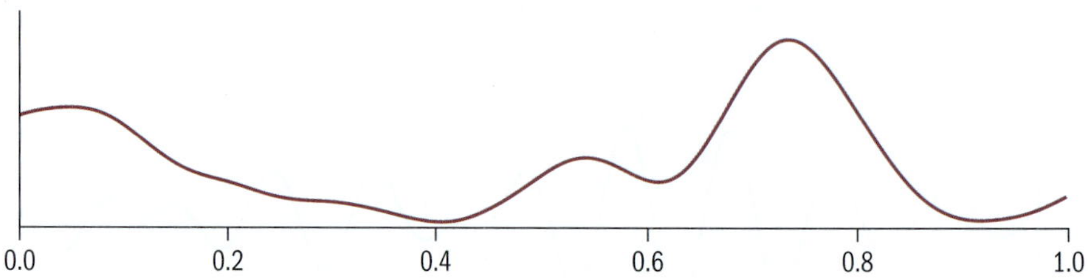

Figure 4.15 Delta Waves of Slow-Wave Sleep

The stages above are collectively called **non-rapid eye movement sleep**, which is where the acronym *NREM* comes from. Interspersed between cycles of the NREM stages is **rapid eye movement** (**REM**) **sleep**. In REM sleep, arousal levels reach that of wakefulness, but the muscles are paralyzed. REM sleep is also called **paradoxical sleep** because one's heart rate, breathing patterns, and EEG mimic wakefulness, but the individual is still asleep. This is the stage in which dreaming is most likely to occur and is also associated with memory consolidation. Recent studies have associated REM more with procedural memory consolidation and SWS with declarative memory consolidation.

MNEMONIC

Remember the sequential order of these brain waves—**b**eta, **a**lpha, **t**heta, **d**elta—by combining their first letters to form **BAT-D** and remember that a **bat** sleeps during the **d**ay.

Sleep Cycles and Changes to Sleep Cycles

A **sleep cycle** refers to a single complete progression through the sleep stages. The makeup of a sleep cycle changes during the course of the night, as shown in Figure 4.16. Early in the night, SWS predominates as the brain falls into deep sleep and then into more wakeful states. Later in the night, REM sleep predominates.

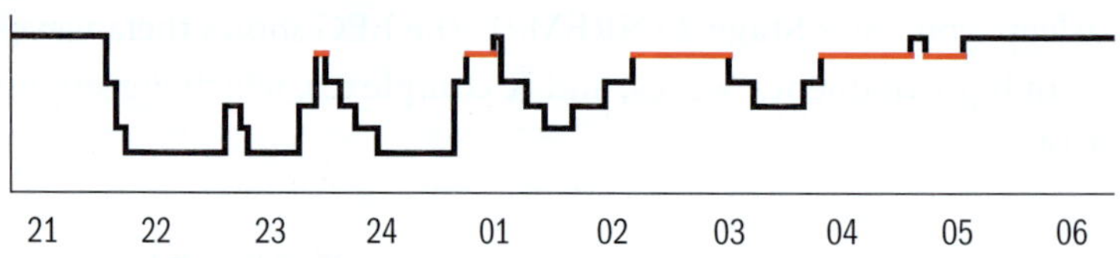

Figure 4.16 Hypnogram of Sleep Cycles

Over the life span, the length of the sleep cycle increases from approximately 50 minutes in children to 90 minutes in adults. Children also spend more time in SWS than adults. Changes to sleep cycles from disrupted sleep or disordered work schedules can cause many health problems. Disruption of SWS and REM can result in diminished memory. Sleep deprivation also causes diminished cognitive performance, although the person who is sleep-deprived is unlikely to recognize that performance has been subpar. Sleep deprivation also negatively affects mood, problem solving, and motor skills.

Sleep and Circadian Rhythms

Our daily cycle of waking and sleeping, as seen in Figure 4.17, is regulated by internally generated rhythms or **circadian rhythms**. In humans and other animals, the circadian rhythm approximates a 24-hour cycle that is somewhat affected by external cues such as light. Biochemical signals underlie circadian rhythms. Sleepiness can partially be attributed to blood levels of **melatonin**, a serotonin-derived hormone from the **pineal gland**. The retina has direct connections to the hypothalamus, which controls the pineal gland; thus, decreasing light can cause the release of melatonin.

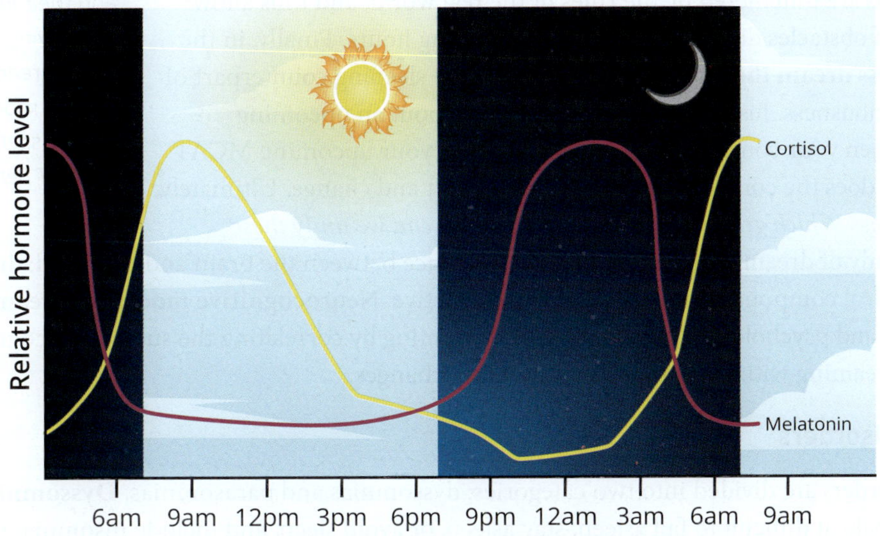

Figure 4.17 The Circadian Rhythm

Cortisol, a steroid hormone produced in the **adrenal cortex**, is also related to the sleep–wake cycle. Its levels slowly increase during early morning because increasing light causes the release of **corticotropin-releasing factor** (**CRF**) from the hypothalamus. CRF causes release of **adrenocorticotropic hormone** (**ACTH**) from the anterior pituitary, which stimulates cortisol release. Cortisol contributes to wakefulness.

MNEMONIC

Melatonin **mel**lows you out. Corti**sol** helps you get up with the sun (*sol* is Latin for sun).

Dreaming

Philosophers and those interested in the human experience have hypothesized about the purpose, meaning, and function of dreaming since antiquity. The ancient Egyptians believed that dreams were messages sent from the supernatural world to tell of future events. In ancient Greece, people believed dreams to carry messages from the gods, but the dream required the help of a priest to interpret. Dreams have long been a subject of wonder.

Most dreaming occurs during REM; however, soon after we enter Stage 2 sleep, our mental experience starts to shift to a dreamlike state. Throughout the night, approximately 75% of dreaming occurs during REM. REM dreams tend to be longer and more vivid than those experienced during NREM sleep.

BRIDGE

The hypothalamic–pituitary–adrenal axis is an example of how the endocrine system can regulate behavior. The endocrine system is discussed in Chapter 5 of *MCAT Biology Review.*

While the purpose and meaning of dreams is not fully understood, a few theories have been proposed. In the **activation–synthesis theory**, dreams are caused by widespread, random activation of neural circuitry. This activation can mimic incoming sensory information, and may also consist of pieces of stored memories, current and previous desires, met and unmet needs, and other experiences. The cortex then tries to stitch this unrelated information together, resulting in a dream that is both bizarre and somewhat familiar. In the **problem solving dream theory**, dreams are a way to solve problems while you are sleeping. Dreams are untethered by the rules of the real world, and thus allow interpretation of obstacles differently than during waking hours. Finally, in the **cognitive process dream theory**, dreams are merely the sleeping counterpart of stream-of-consciousness. Just as you may be thinking about an upcoming weekend trip when your consciousness quickly shifts to your upcoming MCAT Test Day, so too does the content of a dream rapidly shift and change. Ultimately, the question is less *Which group is right?* and more *How can we unify these theories?* The study of dreaming is limited by the difference between the brain and the mind: dreaming must have a neurological component, but is still highly subjective. **Neurocognitive models of dreaming** seek to unify biological and psychological perspectives on dreaming by correlating the subjective, cognitive experience of dreaming with measurable physiological changes.

BRIDGE

Other psychologists have proposed explanations for dreams. One of the most notable is Freud, who separated dreams into their *manifest content* (what one actually sees and hears) and their *latent content* (the underlying significance of these dream elements). Freud's model of personality is discussed in Chapter 6 of *MCAT Behavioral Sciences Review*.

Sleep-Wake Disorders

Sleep-wake disorders are divided into two categories: dyssomnias and parasomnias. **Dyssomnias** refer to disorders that make it difficult to fall asleep, stay asleep, or avoid sleep, and include insomnia, narcolepsy, and sleep apnea. **Parasomnias** are abnormal movements or behaviors during sleep, and include night terrors and sleepwalking. Most sleep-wake disorders occur during NREM sleep.

Insomnia is difficulty falling asleep or staying asleep. It is the most common sleep-wake disorder and may be related to anxiety, depression, medications, or disruption of sleep cycles and circadian rhythms. **Narcolepsy**, in contrast, is a condition characterized by lack of voluntary control over the onset of sleep. The symptoms of narcolepsy are unique and include **cataplexy**, a loss of muscle control and sudden intrusion of REM sleep during waking hours, usually caused by an emotional trigger; **sleep paralysis**, a sensation of being unable to move despite being awake; and **hypnagogic** and **hypnopompic hallucinations**, which are hallucinations when going to sleep or awakening. Another dyssomnia is **sleep apnea**, which is an inability to breathe during sleep. People with this disorder awaken often during the night in order to breathe. Sleep apnea can be either obstructive or central. Obstructive sleep apnea occurs when a physical blockage in the pharynx or trachea prevents airflow; central sleep apnea occurs when the brain fails to send signals to the diaphragm to breathe.

MNEMONIC

Hypna**go**gic hallucinations occur when one is **go**ing to bed. Hypno**p**o**mp**ic hallucinations occur when one is **pop**ping up out of bed.

Night terrors, which are most common in children, are periods of intense anxiety that occur during slow-wave sleep. Children will often thrash and scream during these terrors, and will show signs of sympathetic overdrive, with a high heart rate and rapid breathing. Because these usually occur during SWS, the child experiencing the episode is very difficult to wake, and usually does not remember the dream the next morning. **Sleepwalking**, or **somnambulism**, also usually occurs during SWS. Some people who sleepwalk may eat, talk, have sexual intercourse, or even drive great distances while sleeping with absolutely no recollection of the event. Most return to their beds and awake in the morning, with no knowledge of their nighttime activities.

Contrary to popular belief, awakening a person who is sleepwalking will not harm the person; however, it is generally suggested to quietly guide the individual back to bed to avoid disturbing SWS.

Sleep deprivation can result from as little as one night without sleep, or from multiple nights with poor-quality, short-duration sleep. Sleep deprivation results in irritability, mood disturbances, decreased performance, and slowed reaction time. Extreme deprivation can cause psychosis. While one cannot make up for lost sleep, people who are permitted to sleep normally after sleep deprivation often exhibit **REM rebound**, an earlier onset and greater duration of REM sleep compared to normal.

Hypnosis

Hypnosis, named after the ancient Greek god of sleep, *Hypnos*, was first documented in the eighteenth century. **Hypnosis** can be defined as a state in which a person appears to be in control of normal functions, but is in a highly suggestible state. In other words, a hypnotized person easily succumbs to the suggestions of others. Hypnosis starts with **hypnotic induction**, in which the hypnotist seeks to relax the subject and increase the subject's level of concentration. Then, the hypnotist can suggest perceptions or actions to the hypnotized person. In practice, hypnosis is not the same as its sensationalized version in the media, in which a hypnotist will snap his fingers and cause an individual to exhibit bizarre behavior. Rather, hypnosis has been used successfully for pain control, psychological therapy, memory enhancement, weight loss, and smoking cessation. Brain imaging has indicated that hypnotic states are indeed real; however, effective hypnosis requires a willing personality and lack of skepticism on the part of the patient.

BRIDGE

Hypnosis has been used to recover repressed memories of trauma; however, these memories are not admissible in a court of law. This is because the suggestible state of hypnotism makes an individual vulnerable to creating false memories, which can be perceived as completely real. False memories are discussed in Chapter 3 of *MCAT Behavioral Sciences Review*.

Meditation

Defining **meditation** can be tricky and is highly dependent on the practitioners of meditation and their beliefs. Meditation has been a central practice in many religions. Meditation usually involves quieting of the mind for some purpose, whether spiritual, religious, or related to stress reduction. In the secular Western tradition, meditation is often used for counseling and psychotherapy because it produces a sense of relaxation and relief from anxiety and worrying. To that end, meditation causes physiological changes such as decreased heart rate and blood pressure. On EEG, meditation resembles Stage 1 sleep with theta and slow alpha waves.

MCAT EXPERTISE

Recent studies have demonstrated that mindful meditation not only improves psychological well-being, but may even help improve test scores and student performance. Take time for yourself while studying for the MCAT; keep your mind calm to keep it sharp.

MCAT CONCEPT CHECK 4.3

Before you move on, assess your understanding of the material with these questions.

1. For each of the sleep stages below, list its EEG waveforms and main features.

Stage	EEG Waves	Features
Awake		
Stage 1		
Stage 2		
Stage 3		
Stage 4		
REM		

2. Which two hormones are most associated with maintaining circadian rhythms?
   -
   -

3. What is the difference between a dyssomnia and a parasomnia? Provide an example of each.
   - Dyssomnia:
   - Parasomnia:

4.4 Consciousness-Altering Drugs

LEARNING OBJECTIVES

After Chapter 4.4, you will be able to:

- List the drugs (or drug classes) known to increase GABA activity in the brain
- Recall the drugs (or drug classes) known to upregulate dopamine, norepinephrine, or serotonin activity
- Identify the three main structures in the mesolimbic reward pathway and the primary neurotransmitter of the pathway:

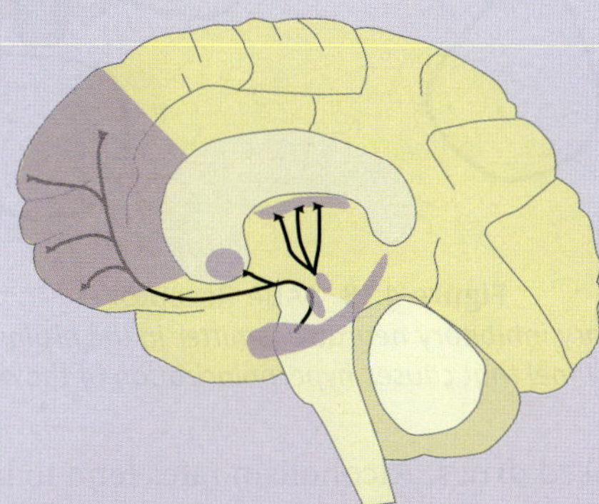

Consciousness-altering drugs, also known as psychoactive drugs, are generally described in four different groups: depressants, stimulants, opiates, and hallucinogens. Biologically speaking, marijuana has depressant, stimulant, and hallucinogenic effects, and will be considered separately.

Depressants

Depressants reduce nervous system activity, resulting in a sense of relaxation and reduced anxiety. Of the depressants, alcohol is certainly the most common. Another is sedatives, or "downers," which calm and induce sleep.

Alcohol

Alcohol has several different effects on the brain. It increases activity of the GABA receptor, a chloride channel that causes hyperpolarization of the membrane, as shown in Figure 4.18. This hyperpolarization causes generalized brain inhibition at the physiological level, resulting in diminished arousal at moderate doses. The changes in brain activity also cause changes in outward behavior. For example, excessive consumption of alcohol may be associated with a notable a lack of self-control known as **disinhibition**, which occurs because the centers of the brain that prevent inappropriate behavior are also depressed. Alcohol also increases dopamine levels, causing a sense of mild euphoria. At higher doses, brain activity becomes more disrupted. Logical reasoning and motor skills are affected, and fatigue may result. One of the main effects on logical reasoning is the inability to recognize consequences of actions, creating a short-sighted view of the world called **alcohol myopia**. Alcohol use is implicated in many automobile accidents, homicides (for both perpetrator and victim), and hospital admissions. Intoxication with alcohol is often measured using blood alcohol level.

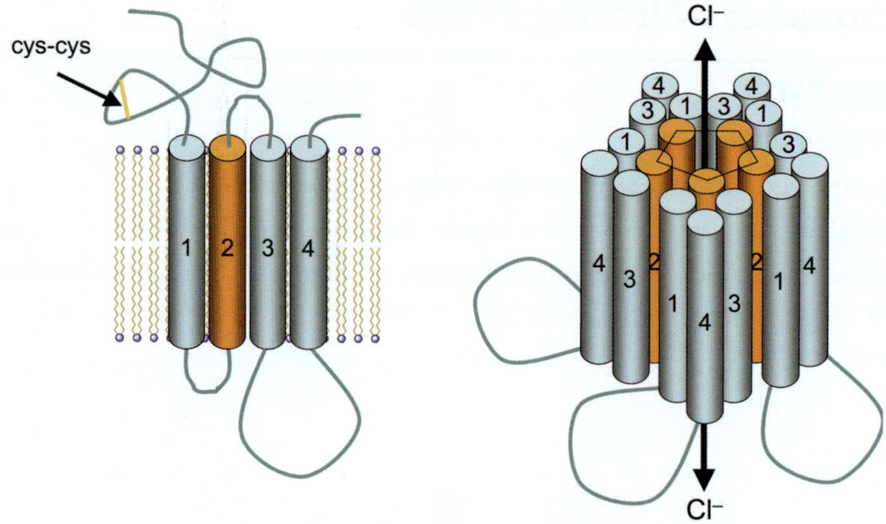

Figure 4.18 GABA Receptor
GABA is the primary inhibitory neurotransmitter in the brain; its receptor is a chloride channel that causes hyperpolarization of the membrane.

Alcohol is one of the most widely abused drugs. Alcoholism rates tend to be higher for those of lower socioeconomic status (SES), but people with a lower SES who have alcoholism tend to enter recovery sooner and at higher rates. Alcoholism tends to run in families, and children of people with alcoholism are also likely to suffer from major depressive disorder. Long-term consequences of alcoholism include cirrhosis and liver failure, pancreatic damage, gastric or duodenal ulcers, gastrointestinal cancer, and brain disorders including **Wernicke–Korsakoff syndrome**, caused by a deficiency of thiamine (vitamin B_1) and characterized by severe memory impairment with changes in mental status and loss of motor skills.

Sedatives

Sedatives tend to depress central nervous system activity, resulting in feelings of calm, relaxation, and drowsiness. Two types of sedatives are barbiturates and benzodiazepines. **Barbiturates** were historically used as anxiety-reducing (anxiolytic) and sleep medications, but have mostly been replaced by **benzodiazepines**, which are less prone to overdose. Barbiturates include *amobarbital* and *phenobarbital*; benzodiazepines include *alprazolam*, *lorazepam*, *diazepam*, and *clonazepam*. These drugs also increase GABA activity, causing a sense of relaxation. However, both of these drug types can be highly addictive. If taken with alcohol, overdoses of barbiturates or benzodiazepines may result in coma or death.

Stimulants

Stimulants cause an increase in arousal in the nervous system. Each drug increases the frequency of action potentials, but does so by different mechanisms.

Amphetamines

Amphetamines cause increased arousal by increasing release of dopamine, norepinephrine, and serotonin at the synapse and decreasing their reuptake. This increases arousal and causes a reduction in appetite and decreased need for sleep. Physiological effects include an increase in heart rate and blood pressure. Psychological effects include euphoria, hypervigilance (being "on edge"), anxiety, delusions of grandeur, and paranoia. Prolonged use of high doses of amphetamines can result in stroke or brain damage. People who take amphetamines often suffer from withdrawal after discontinuation, leading to depression, fatigue, and irritability.

Cocaine

Cocaine originates from the coca plant, grown in the high-altitude regions of South America. Cocaine can be purified from these leaves or created synthetically. Similar to amphetamines, cocaine also acts on dopamine, norepinephrine, and serotonin synapses, but cocaine decreases reuptake of the neurotransmitters instead. Hence, the effects of cocaine intoxication and withdrawal are therefore similar to amphetamines, as listed above. Cocaine also has anesthetic and vasoconstrictive properties, and is therefore sometimes used in surgeries in highly vascularized areas, such as the nose and throat. These vasoconstrictive properties can also lead to heart attacks and strokes when used recreationally. **Crack** is a form of cocaine that can be smoked. With quick and potent effects, this drug is highly addictive.

Ecstasy (3,4-methylenedioxy-*N*-methylamphetamine, MDMA)

Ecstasy, commonly called "E," acts as a hallucinogen combined with an amphetamine. As a designer amphetamine, its mechanism and effects are similar to other amphetamines. Physiologically, ecstasy causes increased heart rate, increased blood pressure, blurry vision, sweating, nausea, and hyperthermia. Psychologically, ecstasy causes feelings of euphoria, increased alertness, and an overwhelming sense of well-being and connectedness. Ecstasy is an example of a club or rave drug, and is often packaged in colorful pills, as shown in Figure 4.19.

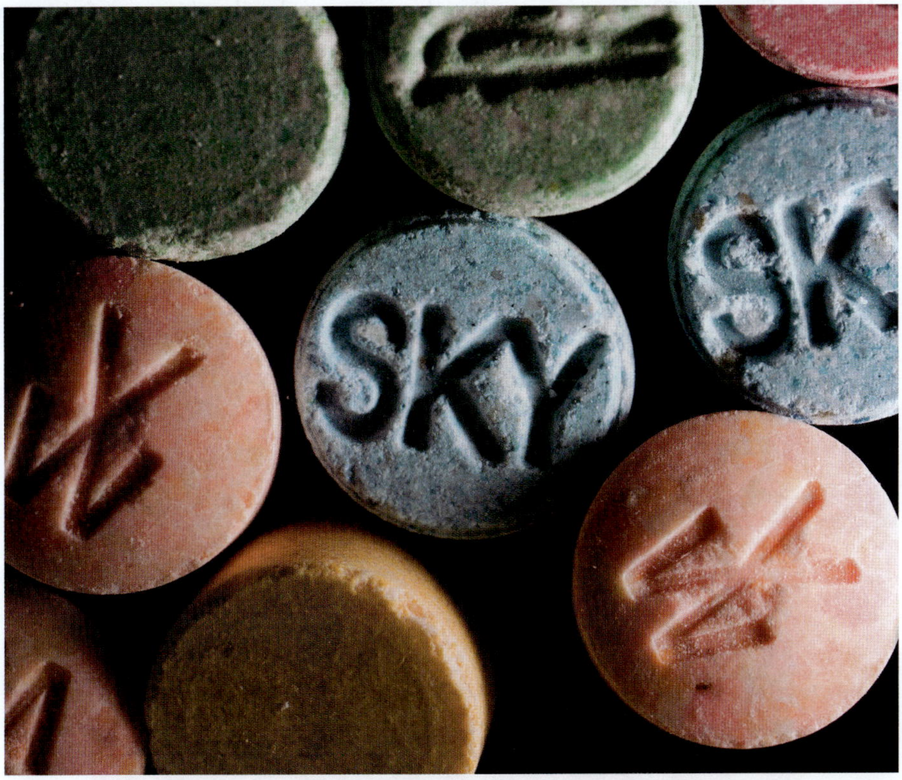

Figure 4.19 Pills of Ecstasy (MDMA)

Opiates and Opioids

Opiates and opioids are types of narcotics, also known as painkillers. Derived from the poppy plant, **opium** has been used and abused for centuries. Today, we have numerous drugs, used both recreationally and therapeutically, derived from opium. Naturally occurring forms, called **opiates**, include *morphine* and *codeine*. Semisynthetic derivatives, called **opioids**, include *oxycodone, hydrocodone*, and *heroin*. These compounds bind to opioid receptors in the peripheral and central nervous system. They act as endorphin agonists and cause a decreased reaction to pain and a sense of euphoria. Overdose, however, can cause death by respiratory suppression, in which the brain stops sending signals to breathe.

Heroin, or *diacetylmorphine*, was originally created as a substitute for morphine. Once injected, the body rapidly metabolizes heroin to morphine. Usually smoked or injected, heroin was once the most widely abused opioid; however, this designation has shifted to prescription opioids like oxycodone and hydrocodone. Treatment for opioid addiction may include use of *methadone*, a long-acting opioid with lower risk of overdose.

Hallucinogens

Hallucinogens are drugs which typically cause introspection, distortions of reality and fantasy, and enhancement of sensory experiences. Physiologic effects include increased heart rate and blood pressure, dilation of pupils, sweating, and increased body temperature. Examples of hallucinogens include **lysergic acid diethylamide (LSD)**, shown in Figure 4.20, *peyote, mescaline, ketamine*, and *psilocybin*-containing mushrooms. The exact mechanism of most hallucinogens is unknown, but is thought to be a complex interaction between various neurotransmitters, especially serotonin.

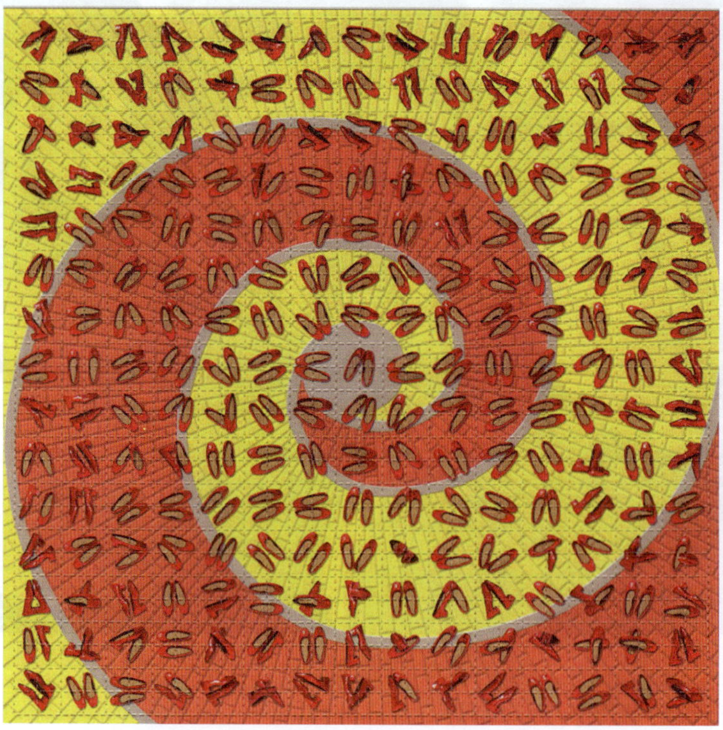

Figure 4.20 Sheet of LSD Blotter Paper
LSD is often sold on colorful paper, reflecting the fact that, like ecstasy, LSD is considered a club drug.

Marijuana

Marijuana, shown in Figure 4.21, primarily refers to the leaves and flowers of two plant species: *Cannabis sativa* and *Cannabis indica*. It has been the subject of many news reports in the last few years as many states move toward the legalization of marijuana for medical or recreational use. While talks about the legal status of marijuana in the United States are fairly recent, marijuana has been used for centuries, with the earliest known accounts originating from approximately 3 B.C.E.

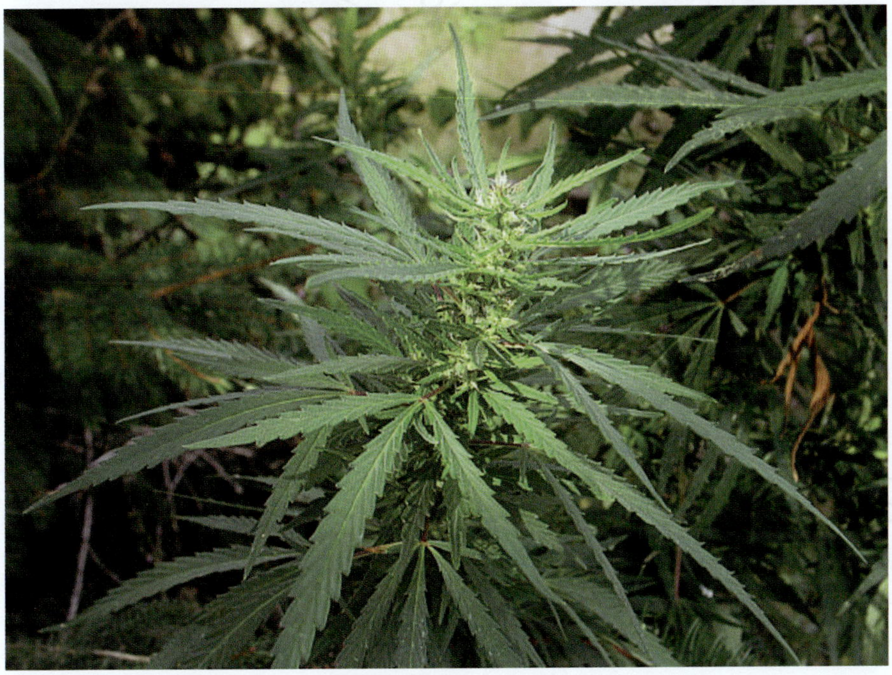

Figure 4.21 Cannabis

The active chemical in marijuana is known as **tetrahydrocannabinol** (**THC**). THC exerts its effects by acting at cannabinoid receptors, glycine receptors, and opioid receptors. How these receptors interact to create the "high" achieved from marijuana use is unknown. It is known, however, that THC inhibits GABA activity and indirectly increases dopamine activity (causing pleasure). Physiological effects are mixed, including eye redness, dry mouth, fatigue, impairment of short-term memory, increased heart rate, increased appetite, and lowered blood pressure. Psychologically, effects seem to fall into the categories of stimulant, depressant, and hallucinogen.

Drug Addiction

Drug addiction is highly related to the **mesolimbic reward pathway**, one of four dopaminergic pathways in the brain, as shown in Figure 4.22. This pathway includes the **nucleus accumbens** (**NAc**), the **ventral tegmental area** (**VTA**), and the connection between them called the **medial forebrain bundle** (**MFB**). This pathway is normally involved in motivation and emotional response, and its activation accounts for the positive reinforcement of substance use. This addiction pathway is activated by all substances that produce psychological dependence. Gambling and falling in love also activate this pathway.

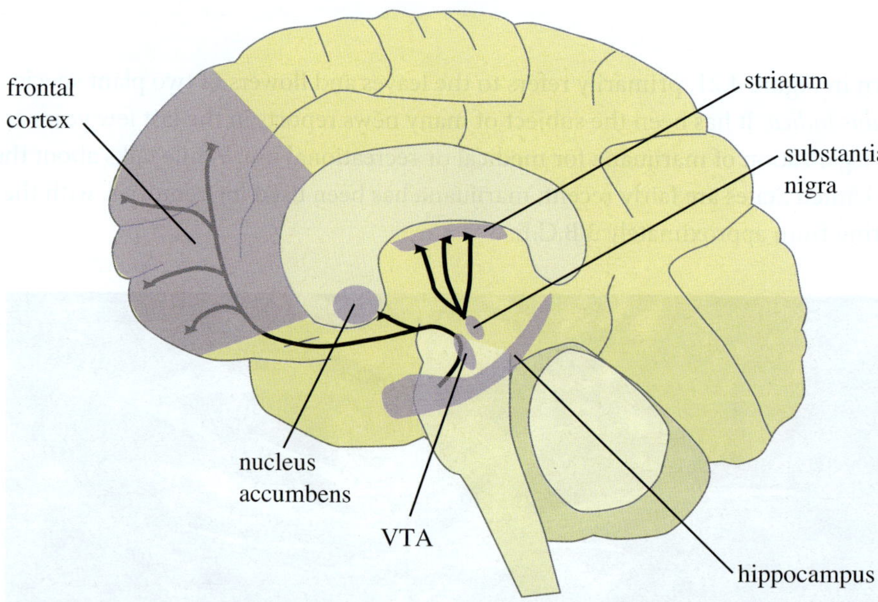

Figure 4.22 Dopaminergic Pathways in the Brain
The reward pathway is composed of the nucleus accumbens, ventral tegmental area (VTA), and the medial forebrain bundle between them (not labeled).

MCAT CONCEPT CHECK 4.4

Before you move on, assess your understanding of the material with these questions.

1. Which three drugs (or drug classes) are known to increase GABA activity in the brain?
    - ____
    - ____
    - ____

2. Which three drugs (or drug classes) are known to increase dopamine, norepinephrine, and serotonin activity in the brain?
    - ____
    - ____
    - ____

3. What are the three main structures in the mesolimbic reward pathway? What is this pathway's primary neurotransmitter?
   - Structure:

   ___

   - Structure:

   ___

   - Structure:

   ___

   - Neurotransmitter:

   ___

4.5 Attention

LEARNING OBJECTIVES

After Chapter 4.5, you will be able to:

- Compare and contrast controlled processing and automatic processing
- Describe the role of the "filter" used in selective attention

Attention refers to concentrating on one aspect of the sensory environment, or **sensorium**. While this definition is straightforward, an understanding of how attention works and the mechanism by which we can shift our attention from one set of stimuli to another is still somewhat unclear.

Selective Attention

Selective attention is focusing on one part of the sensorium while ignoring other stimuli. It therefore acts as a filter between sensory stimuli and our processing systems. If a stimulus is attended to, it is passed through a filter and analyzed further. If the stimulus is not attended to, it is lost. In its original conceptualization, selective attention was viewed as an all-or-nothing process: if we choose a particular stimulus to give our attention to, the other stimuli are lost. However, recent evidence indicates that this is not the case.

Imagine this: You are at a party, talking with a friend. However, your ears perk up when you hear your name spoken halfway across the room. Even though you were engaged in conversation and presumably paying attention, you were able to perceive your name being mentioned. This is sometimes called the **cocktail party phenomenon** and is evidence of a different interpretation of selective attention. Selective attention is probably more of a filter that allows us to focus on one thing while allowing other stimuli to be processed in the background. Only if the other stimuli are particularly important—one's name being mentioned, a sudden flash of light, pain—do we shift our attention to them.

Dichotic listening tests (one of which is shown in Figure 4.23) are designed to test selective attention. Participants are given headphones that have distinct auditory stimuli going to each ear. Participants are then asked to pay attention to either or both stimuli, then asked to repeat out loud what they heard in the attended ear, which is termed **shadowing**. This task tests selective attention because participants are asked to filter out information from the unattended ear. Alternatively, the task can test whether participants can subconsciously gain information from the unattended ear.

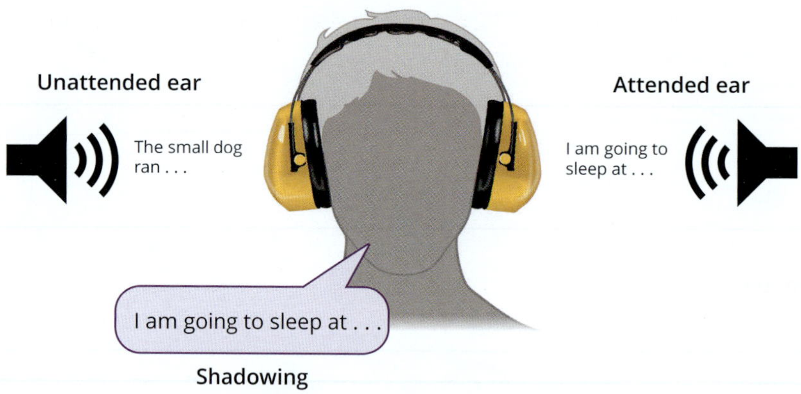

Figure 4.23 Dichotic Listening Test

Divided Attention

Divided attention is the ability to perform multiple tasks at the same time. Most new or complex tasks require undivided attention and utilize **controlled (effortful) processing**, discussed in Chapter 3 of *MCAT Behavioral Sciences Review*. In contrast, familiar or routine actions can be performed with **automatic processing**, which permits the brain to focus on other tasks with divided attention. Consider learning to drive: at first, drivers intensely grip the steering wheel and pay undivided attention to the road ahead. But as you become more accustomed to driving, you can relegate some aspects of driving—like knowing how hard to push on the pedal—to automatic processing. This lets a driver perform secondary tasks such as changing the radio station. That being said, automatic processing is far from perfect. It does not allow for innovation or rapid response to change, which may contribute to the high incidence of car accidents that result from distracted driving.

MCAT CONCEPT CHECK 4.5

Before you move on, assess your understanding of the material with these questions.

1. Compare and contrast controlled (effortful) processing and automatic processing:
   - Controlled (effortful) processing:

     ____

   - Automatic processing:

     ____

2. Briefly describe the function of the “filter” used in selective attention:

   ____

   ____

4.6 Language High Yield

LEARNING OBJECTIVES

After Chapter 4.6, you will be able to:

- Recall the expected milestones of language development and the ages at which they should occur
- Identify the primary characteristics of the nativist, behaviorist, and social interactionist theories of language development
- Describe the symptoms and brain regions associated with Broca's, Wernicke's, and conduction aphasia:

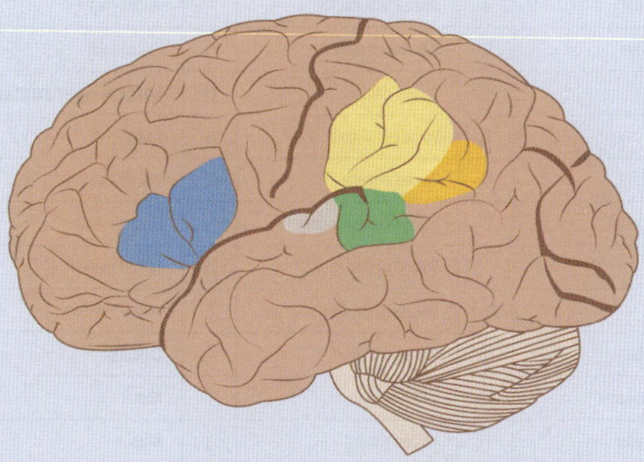

Whether it is written, spoken, or signed, **language** is fundamental to the creation of communities. As humans began to live in groups, the ability to communicate became essential. Division of labor and a sense of shared history require that the meaning of the language be the same for all speakers of the language.

Components of Language

There are five basic components of language: phonology, morphology, semantics, syntax, and pragmatics.

Phonology

Phonology refers to the actual sound of language. There are about 40 speech sounds or **phonemes** in English, although many more exist in other languages, as shown in Figure 4.24. Children must learn to produce and recognize the sounds of language, separating them from environmental noises and other human-created sounds, like coughing. Additionally, when a language has subtle differences in speech sounds that represent a change in meaning, children learn to distinguish those phonemes; this ability is called **categorical perception**. The ability to recognize a word as being the same, even if the pronunciation of the word varies between people is an auditory example of **constancy**, which is described in Chapter 2 of *MCAT Behavioral Sciences Review*.

International Phonetic Alphabet

Plosive

Name	Text
Voiceless bilabial	p
Voiced bilabial	b
Voiceless alveolar	t
Voiced alveolar	d
Voiceless retroflex	ʈ
Voiced retroflex	ɖ
Voiceless palatal	c
Voiced palatal	ɟ
Voiceless velar	k
Voiced velar	ɡ
Voiceless uvular	q
Voiced uvular	ɢ
Voiceless glottal	ʔ

Nasal

Name	Text
Voiced bilabial	m
Voiced labiodental	ɱ
Voiced alveolar	n
Voiced retroflex	ɳ
Voiced palatal	ɲ
Voiced velar	ŋ
Voiced uvular	ɴ

Trill

Name	Text
Voiced bilabial	ʙ
Voiced alveolar	r
Voiced uvular	ʀ

Tap or Flap

Name	Text
Voiced alveolar	ɾ
Voiced retroflex	ɽ

Fricative

Name	Text
Voiceless bilabial	ɸ
Voiced bilabial	β
Voiceless labiodental	f
Voiced labiodental	v
Voiceless dental	θ
Voiced dental	ð
Voiceless alveolar	s
Voiced alveolar	z
Voiceless postalveolar	ʃ
Voiced postalveolar	ʒ
Voiceless retroflex	ʂ
Voiced retroflex	ʐ
Voiceless palatal	ç
Voiced palatal	ʝ
Voiceless velar	x
Voiced velar	ɣ
Voiceless uvular	χ
Voiced uvular	ʁ
Voiceless pharyngeal	ħ
Voiced pharyngeal	ʕ
Voiceless glottal	h
Voiced glottal	ɦ
Voiceless dorso-palatal	ɧ

Lateral Fricative

Name	Text
Voiceless alveolar	ɬ
Voiced alveolar	ɮ

Approximant

Name	Text
Voiced labiodental	ʋ
Voiced alveolar	ɹ
Voiced retroflex	ɻ
Voiced palatal	j
Voiced velar	ɰ

Lateral Approximant

Name	Text
Voiced alveolar	l
Voiced retroflex	ɭ
Voiced palatal	ʎ
Voiced velar	ʟ

Clicks

Name	Text
Bilabial	ʘ
Dental	ǀ
(Post)alveolar	!
Palatoalveolar	ǂ
Alveolar lateral	ǁ

Figure 4.24 A Section of the International Phonetic Alphabet
The IPA is an unambiguous system of writing all of the known phonemes of all human languages.

Morphology

Morphology refers to the structure of words. Many words are composed of multiple building blocks called **morphemes**, each of which connotes a particular meaning. Consider the word *redesigned*, which can be broken into three morphemes: *re–*, indicating *to do again*; *–design–*, the verb root; and *–ed*, indicating an action in the past.

Semantics

Semantics refers to the association of meaning with a word. A child must learn that certain combinations of phonemes represent certain physical objects or events, and that words may refer to entire categories, such as *animal*, while others refer to specific members of categories, such as *doggy*. One can see this skill developing in young children as they may refer to all animals as *doggy*.

Syntax

Syntax refers to how words are put together to form sentences. A child must notice the effects of word order on meaning: *Nathan has only three pieces of candy* has a very different meaning than *Only Nathan has three pieces of candy*.

Pragmatics

Finally, **pragmatics** refers to the dependence of language on context and preexisting knowledge. In other words, the manner in which we speak may differ depending on the audience and our relationship to that audience. Imagine asking to share a seat on a bus. Depending on whom we ask, we may word this request in wildly different ways. To a stranger, we may be more formal: *Pardon me, do you mind if I share this seat?* To a close friend, we may be less so: *Hey, move over!* Pragmatics are also affected by **prosody**—the rhythm, cadence, and inflection of our voices.

Language Development

To effectively interact with society, a child must learn to communicate through language, whether oral or signed. An important precursor to language is **babbling**. Almost without exception, children—including children who are hearing impaired—spontaneously begin to babble during their first year. For children who can hear, babbling reaches its highest frequency between nine and twelve months. For children who are hearing impaired or deaf, verbal babbling often ceases soon after it begins.

The timeline of language acquisition is fairly consistent among children. From 12 to 18 months, children add about one word per month. Starting around 18 months, an explosion of language begins. During this **naming explosion**, the child quickly learns dozens of words, and uses each word with varying inflection and gestures to convey a desired meaning. For example, a child may ask, *Apple?* while pointing at an apple in a bowl of fruit, in an effort to request the apple. During this naming explosion, children may also frequently fall into **overextension**, in which they inappropriately apply a term to an object that bears cursory similarities to the term. For example, in an attempt to request a kiwi from a fruit bowl, a child might point at the kiwi and ask, *Apple?* For children at this age, gestures, inflection, and context are essential for the parent or caregiver to identify the meaning.

KEY CONCEPT

Timeline of language acquisition:

- 9 to 12 months: babbling
- 12 to 18 months: about one word per month
- 18 to 20 months: "explosion of language" and combining words
- 2 to 3 years: longer sentences (3 words or more)
- 5 years: language rules largely mastered

Between 18 and 20 months of age, children begin to combine words. For example, children may say, *Eat apple* to indicate that they would like to eat an apple. In the grocery store, the same children may ask, *That apple?* to distinguish between fruit. In this way, context and gesture becomes less important as the ability to assemble sentences develops.

By the age of two or three years, children can speak in longer sentences. Vocabulary grows exponentially. As a child creates longer sentences, grammatical errors increase as the child internalizes the complex rules of grammar. These include **errors of growth** in which a child applies a grammatical rule (often a morpheme) in a situation where it does not apply: *runned* instead of *ran*, or *funner* instead of *more fun*. Interestingly, caregivers are less likely to correct errors of grammar than errors of word choice.

REAL WORLD

Pediatricians often monitor language development to determine if there is a developmental delay. For example, a two-year-old child who uses fewer than 10 words has a significant developmental delay and should be referred for speech therapy. This would also prompt a search for other developmental issues.

For the most part, language is substantially mastered by the age of five. The acquisition of language appears easy for most children, which has led to significant speculation on exactly how this occurs.

Nativist (Biological) Theory

The **nativist (biological) theory**, largely credited to linguist Noam Chomsky, advocates for the existence of some innate capacity for language. Chomsky is known for his study of **transformational grammar**. He focused on syntactic transformations, or changes in word order that retain the same meaning; for example, *I took the MCAT* vs. *The MCAT was taken by me*. Chomsky noted that children learn to make such transformations effortlessly at an early age. He therefore concluded that this ability must be innate. In this theory, this innate ability is called the **language acquisition device (LAD)**, a theoretical pathway in the brain that allows infants to process and absorb language rules.

Nativists believe in a **critical period** for language acquisition between two years and puberty. If no language exposure occurs during this time, later training is largely ineffective. This idea came to light through an unfortunate test case: a victim of child abuse. This child had been isolated from all human contact from age two to thirteen, when she was discovered by authorities. Even with later language exposure, she was unable to master many rules of language, although she was able to learn some aspects of syntax. The fact that this child was able to learn some rules may indicate that there is a sensitive period for language development, rather than a critical period. A **sensitive period** is a time when environmental input has maximal effect on the development of an ability. Most psychologists consider the sensitive period for language development to be before the onset of puberty.

Learning (Behaviorist) Theory

The **learning (behaviorist) theory**, proposed by B. F. Skinner, explained language acquisition by operant conditioning. Very young babies are capable of distinguishing between phonemes of all human languages, but by six months of age show a strong preference for phonemes in the language spoken by their parents. Skinner explained language acquisition by **reinforcement**. That is, caregivers repeat and reinforce sounds that sound most like the language they speak. Thus, over time, the infant perceives that certain sounds have little value and are not reinforced, while other sounds have value and are reliably reinforced by caregivers. While this may account for the development of words and speech, many psycholinguists point out that this theory cannot fully explain the explosion in vocabulary that occurs during early childhood.

Social Interactionist Theory

The **social interactionist theory** of language development focuses on the interplay between biological and social processes. That is, language acquisition is driven by the child's desire to communicate and behave in a social manner, such as interacting with caretakers and other children. Interactionist theory allows for the role of brain development in the acquisition of language. As the biological foundation for language develops and children are exposed to language, the brain groups sounds and meanings together. Then, as the child interacts with others, certain brain circuits are reinforced, while others are de-emphasized, resulting in atrophy of those circuits.

Influence of Language on Cognition

Psycholinguistics has long focused on the relationship between language and thinking. Linguist Benjamin Whorf proposed the **Whorfian hypothesis**, also called the **linguistic relativity hypothesis**, which suggests that our perception of reality—the way we think about the world—is determined by the content of language. In essence, language affects the way we think rather than the other way around. For instance, some Inuit dialects have a wide variety of names for different types of snow, whereas the English language has very few. Therefore, according to the Whorfian hypothesis, people who speak one of those Inuit dialects are better at discriminating subtleties between different types of snow than English speakers are. This is a somewhat controversial notion that depends on the definition of "a word" but most linguists agree that language can influence how we think to some degree. Word choice, inflection, context, and speaker all play a role in our perception of a message. In addition, language often provides an original framework for understanding information. A more expansive framework with more specific vocabulary allows for more sophisticated processing of that information and enhanced communication of that information to others.

Brain Areas and Language

Two different areas of the brain are responsible for speech production and language comprehension, as shown in Figure 4.25. Both, however, are located in the dominant hemisphere, which is usually the left hemisphere. **Broca's area**, located in the inferior frontal gyrus of the frontal lobe, controls the motor function of speech via connections with the motor cortex. **Wernicke's area**, located in the superior temporal gyrus of the temporal lobe, is responsible for language comprehension. Broca's area and Wernicke's area are connected by the **arcuate fasciculus**, a bundle of axons that allows appropriate association between language comprehension and speech production.

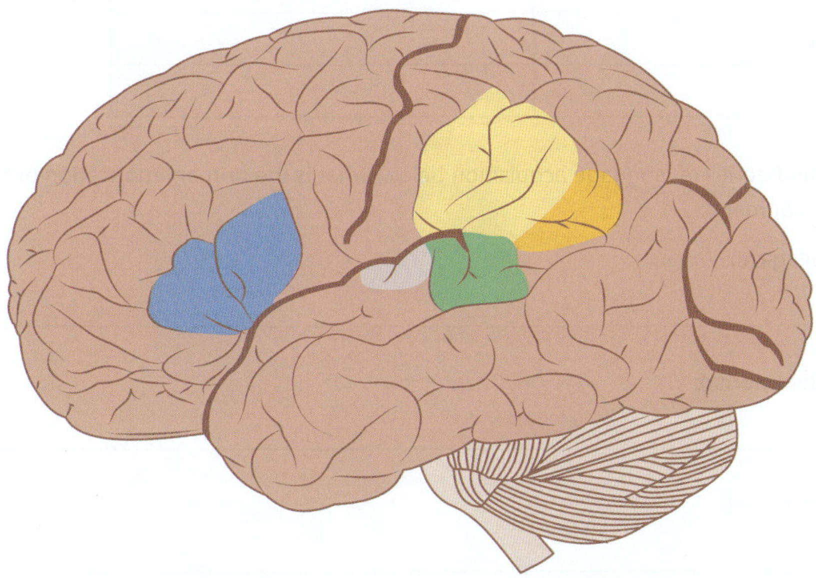

Figure 4.25 Brain Areas Associated with Language
Blue = Broca's area; Green = Wernicke's area. Other colored regions are associated with other aspects of language beyond the scope of the MCAT (yellow = supramarginal gyrus; orange = angular gyrus; light pink = primary auditory cortex).

Aphasia is a deficit of language production or comprehension. Much of what we know regarding language and aphasia is through observations of people with damage to speech-related areas. When damage occurs to Broca's area, speech comprehension is intact but the patient will have a reduced or absent ability to produce spoken language. This is known as **Broca's (expressive) aphasia**. These patients are often very frustrated because they are stuck with the sensation of having every word on the tip of their tongue.

On the other hand, when Wernicke's area is damaged, motor production and fluency of speech is retained but comprehension of speech is lost. This is known as **Wernicke's (receptive) aphasia**. Because speech comprehension is lost, these patients speak nonsensical sounds and inappropriate word combinations devoid of meaning. Patients with Wernicke's aphasia often believe that they are speaking and understanding perfectly well, even though the people around them have no comprehension of what is being said. This can also be very frustrating to patients.

Finally, if the arcuate fasciculus is affected, the resulting aphasia is known as **conduction aphasia**. Because Broca's and Wernicke's areas are unaffected, speech production and comprehension are intact. However, the patient is unable to repeat something that has been said because the connection between these two regions has been lost. This is a very rare form of aphasia.

MCAT CONCEPT CHECK 4.6

Before you move on, assess your understanding of the material with these questions.

1. For each of the ages below, list the expected milestone(s) of language development:

Age	Milestone(s)
9 to 12 months	
12 to 18 months	
18 to 20 months	
2 to 3 years	
5 years	

2. For each of the theories of language acquisition below, what is the primary motivation or trigger for language development?

    - Nativist (Biological):

    ____

    - Learning (Behaviorist):

    ____

    - Social interactionist:

    ____

3. Briefly describe the clinical features of each type of aphasia listed below:

    - Broca's aphasia:

    ____

    - Wernicke's aphasia

    ____

    - Conduction aphasia:

    ____

Conclusion

One of the biggest questions that psychology and biology seek to answer is how the brain, an organ consisting of lipids, water, and neurotransmitters, becomes the mind. Cognition and consciousness allow us to think about who we are, where we are, and what we are doing at a given moment, and this all occurs due to a complex interaction between individual neurons within the brain. Not only do we experience consciousness, but our behaviors are also intricately intertwined with physiological brain function. Language is one of the most complex cognitive processes, requiring intact comprehension and production mechanisms and an understanding of the rules of our native language.

As much as we research what the mind is and how it works, there is as much interest in *why* we do what we do and how we *feel* about it. This is the function of motivation (both internal and external) and emotion, which we will explore in detail in the next chapter.

GO ONLINE

You've reviewed the content, now test your knowledge and critical thinking skills by completing a test-like passage set in your online resources!

CONCEPT SUMMARY

Cognition

- Thought is more than just that of which we are conscious. The brain processes and makes decisions about the importance of various stimuli below the level of conscious awareness.
- The **information processing model** states that the brain encodes, stores, and retrieves information much like a computer.
- The ability to think abstractly develops over the life span. Early cognitive development is limited by brain maturation. Culture, genes, and environment also influence cognitive development.
- **Piaget's stages of cognitive development** are sensorimotor, preoperational, concrete operational, and formal operational.
  - The **sensorimotor stage** focuses on manipulating the environment to meet physical needs through **circular reactions**. **Object permanence** ends this stage.
  - The **preoperational stage** focuses on **symbolic thinking**, **egocentrism**, and **centration**.
  - The **concrete operational stage** focuses on understanding the feelings of others and manipulating physical (concrete) objects.
  - The **formal operational stage** focuses on abstract thought and problem solving.
- A mild level of cognitive decline while aging is normal; significant changes in cognition may signify an underlying disorder.
- Biological factors that affect cognition include organic brain disorders, genetic and chromosomal conditions, metabolic derangements, and drug use.

Problem Solving and Decision Making

- **Problem solving** requires identification and understanding of the problem, generation of potential solutions, testing of potential solutions, and evaluation of results.
  - A **mental set** is a pattern of approach for a given problem. An inappropriate mental set may negatively impact problem solving.
  - **Functional fixedness** is the tendency to use objects only in the way they are normally utilized, which may create barriers to problem solving.
- Types of problem solving include **trial-and-error**, **algorithms**, **deductive reasoning** (deriving conclusions from general rules), and **inductive reasoning** (deriving generalizations from evidence).
- Heuristics, biases, intuition, and emotions may assist decision making but may also lead to erroneous or problematic decisions.
  - **Heuristics** are shortcuts or rules of thumb used to make decisions.
  - **Biases** exist when an experimenter or decision maker is unable to objectively evaluate information.
  - **Intuition** is a "gut feeling" regarding a particular decision. However, intuition can often be attributed to experience with similar situations.
  - Emotional state often plays a role in decision making.

- Gardner's theory of **multiple intelligences** proposes at least eight areas of intelligence including: linguistic, logical–mathematical, musical, visual–spatial, bodily–kinesthetic, interpersonal, intrapersonal, and naturalist.
- Variations in intellectual ability can be attributed to combinations of environment, education, and genetics.

Consciousness

- States of consciousness include alertness, sleep, dreaming, and altered states of consciousness.
- **Alertness** is the state of being awake and able to think, perceive, process, and express information. **Beta** and **alpha waves** predominate on **electroencephalography** (**EEG**).
- **Sleep** is important for health of the brain and body.
  - **Stage 1** is light sleep and is dominated by **theta waves** on EEG. **Stage 2** is slightly deeper and includes theta waves, **sleep spindles**, and **K complexes**.
  - **Stages 3** and **4** are deep (**slow-wave**) sleep (**SWS**). **Delta waves** predominate on EEG. Most sleep-wake disorders occur during Stage 3 and 4 **non-rapid eye movement** (**NREM**) **sleep**. Dreaming in SWS focuses on consolidating declarative memories.
  - **Rapid eye movement** (**REM**) **sleep** is sometimes called **paradoxical sleep**: the mind appears close to awake on EEG, but the person is asleep. Eye movements and body paralysis occur in this stage. Dreaming in REM focuses on consolidating procedural memories.
  - The **sleep cycle** is approximately 90 minutes for adults; the normal cycle is Stage 1–2–3–4–3–2–REM or just 1–2–3–4–REM, although REM becomes more frequent toward the morning.
  - Changes in light in the evening trigger release of **melatonin** by the **pineal gland**, resulting in sleepiness. **Cortisol** levels increase in the early morning and help promote wakefulness. **Circadian rhythms** normally trend around a 24-hour day.
  - Most **dreaming** occurs during REM, but some dreaming occurs during other sleep stages. There are many different models that attempt to account for the content and purpose of dreaming.
  - Sleep-wake disorders include **dyssomnias**, such as insomnia, narcolepsy, sleep apnea, and sleep deprivation; and **parasomnias**, such as night terrors and sleepwalking (somnambulism).
- **Hypnosis** is a state of consciousness in which individuals appear to be in control of their normal faculties but are in a highly suggestible state. Hypnosis is often used for pain control, psychological therapy, memory enhancement, weight loss, and smoking cessation.
- **Meditation** involves a quieting of the mind and is often used for relief of anxiety. It has also played a role in many of the world's religions.

Consciousness-Altering Drugs

- Consciousness-altering drugs are grouped by effect into depressants, stimulants, opiates, and hallucinogens.
  - **Depressants** include alcohol, barbiturates, and benzodiazepines. They promote or mimic GABA activity in the brain.
  - **Stimulants** include amphetamines, cocaine, and ecstasy. They increase dopamine, norepinephrine, and serotonin concentration at the synaptic cleft.

- **Opiates** and **opioids** include heroin, morphine, opium, and prescription pain medications such as oxycodone and hydrocodone. They can cause death by respiratory depression.
- **Hallucinogens** include lysergic acid diethylamide (LSD), peyote, mescaline, ketamine, and psilocybin-containing mushrooms.
- **Marijuana** has depressant, stimulant, and hallucinogenic effects. Its active ingredient is **tetrahydrocannabinol**.

- Drug addiction is mediated by the **mesolimbic pathway**, which includes the **nucleus accumbens**, **medial forebrain bundle**, and **ventral tegmental area**. Dopamine is the main neurotransmitter in this pathway.

Attention

- **Selective attention** allows one to pay attention to a particular stimulus while determining if additional stimuli in the background require attention.
- **Divided attention** uses **automatic processing** to pay attention to multiple activities at one time.

Language

- Language consists of phonology, morphology, semantics, syntax, and pragmatics.
  - **Phonology** refers to the actual sound of speech.
  - **Morphology** refers to the building blocks of words, such as rules for pluralization (–*s* in English), past tense (–*ed*), and so forth.
  - **Semantics** refers to the meaning of words.
  - **Syntax** refers to the rules dictating word order.
  - **Pragmatics** refers to the changes in language delivery depending on context.
- Theories of language development focus on different reasons or motivations for language acquisition.
  - The **nativist (biological) theory** explains language acquisition as being innate and controlled by the **language acquisition device (LAD)**.
  - The **learning (behaviorist) theory** explains language acquisition as being controlled by operant conditioning and reinforcement by caregivers.
  - The **social interactionist theory** explains language acquisition as being caused by a motivation to communicate and interact with others.
- The **Whorfian (linguistic relativity) hypothesis** states that the lens through which we view and interpret the world is created by language.
- Speech areas in the brain are found in the dominant hemisphere, which is usually the left.
  - The motor function of speech is controlled by **Broca's area**. Damage results in **Broca's aphasia**, a nonfluent aphasia in which generating each word requires great effort.
  - Language comprehension is controlled by **Wernicke's area**. Damage results in **Wernicke's aphasia**, a fluent, nonsensical aphasia with lack of comprehension.
  - The **arcuate fasciculus** connects Wernicke's area and Broca's area. Damage results in **conduction aphasia**, marked by the inability to repeat words heard despite intact speech generation and comprehension.

ANSWERS TO CONCEPT CHECKS

4.1

1. The three steps in the information processing model are encoding, storage, and retrieval.
2. The older adult most likely has delirium. The time course is incompatible with the slow decline of dementia.
3.

Stage	Key Features
Sensorimotor	Focuses on manipulating environment for physical needs; circular reactions; ends with object permanence
Preoperational	Symbolic thinking, egocentrism, and centration
Concrete operational	Understands conservation and the feelings of others; can manipulate concrete objects logically
Formal operational	Can think abstractly and problem solve

4.2

1. Functional fixedness
2. Algorithm
3. Belief perseverance
4. The availability heuristic is used for making decisions based on how easily similar instances can be imagined. The representativeness heuristic is used for making decisions based on how much a particular item or situation fits a given prototype or stereotype.

4.3

1.

Stage	EEG Waves	Features
Awake	Beta and alpha	Able to perceive, process, access information, and express that information verbally
Stage 1	Theta	Light sleep and dozing
Stage 2	Theta	Sleep spindles and K complexes
Stage 3	Delta	Slow-wave sleep; dreams; declarative memory consolidation; sleep-wake disorders occur in this stage
Stage 4	Delta	Slow-wave sleep; dreams; declarative memory consolidation; sleep-wake disorders occur in this stage
REM	Mostly beta	Appears awake physiologically; dreams; procedural memory consolidation; body is paralyzed

2. The two hormones most associated with maintaining circadian rhythms are melatonin and cortisol.
3. Dyssomnias are disorders in which the duration or timing of sleep is disturbed. Examples include insomnia, narcolepsy, and sleep apnea. Parasomnias are disorders in which abnormal behaviors occur during sleep. Examples include night terrors and sleepwalking (somnambulism).

4.4

1. Drugs known to increase GABA activity in the brain include alcohol, barbiturates, and benzodiazepines. Note that marijuana inhibits GABA activity.
2. Drugs known to increase dopamine, norepinephrine, and serotonin activity in the brain include amphetamines, cocaine, and ecstasy (MDMA). Ecstasy is a designer amphetamine; it is mentioned separately here because of its hallucinogenic properties.
3. The three main structures in the mesolimbic reward pathway are the nucleus accumbens, medial forebrain bundle, and ventral tegmental area. The neurotransmitter of this pathway is dopamine.

4.5

1. Controlled (effortful) processing is used when maintaining undivided attention on a task, and is usually used for new or complex actions. Automatic processing is used for less critical stimuli in divided attention, and is usually used for familiar or repetitive actions.
2. The filter in selective attention permits us to focus on one set of stimuli while scanning other stimuli in the background for important information (such as our name or a significant change in the environment).

4.6

1.

Age	Milestone(s)
9 to 12 months	Babbling
12 to 18 months	Increase of about one word per month
18 to 20 months	"Explosion of language" and combining words (two-word sentences)
2 to 3 years	Longer sentences of three or more words
5 years	Language rules largely mastered

2. The primary trigger in the nativist theory is an innate ability to pick up language via the language acquisition device. In the learning theory, it is operant conditioning with reinforcement by caregivers. In the social interactionist theory, it is a desire to communicate and act socially.
3. Broca's aphasia is marked by difficulty producing language, with hesitancy and great difficulty coming up with words. Wernicke's aphasia is fluent, but includes nonsensical sounds and words devoid of meaning; language comprehension is lost. Conduction aphasia is marked by difficulty repeating speech, with intact speech production and comprehension.

SCIENCE MASTERY ASSESSMENT EXPLANATIONS

1. **D**

Jean Piaget hypothesized that new information is processed by adaptation, **(B)**. Adaptation is too broad of an answer because it includes both assimilation, **(A)**, and accommodation, **(D)**. Assimilation is incorporation of new information into existing schemata. If the new information doesn't fit, then accommodation occurs. Accommodation is the modification of existing schemata to account for new information and is thus the correct answer.

2. **B**

While many drugs can cause paranoia, the elevation in heart rate combined with prolonged alertness and a decrease in appetite suggests amphetamines, matching choice **(B)**.

3. **C**

The base rate fallacy occurs when prototypical or stereotypical factors are used for analysis rather than actual data. Because the student is volunteering in a hospital with a stroke center, the student sees more patients who have experienced a stroke than would be expected in a hospital without a stroke center. Thus, this experience changes the student's perception and results in base rate fallacy. Deductive reasoning, **(A)**, refers to drawing conclusions by integrating different pieces of evidence. The representativeness heuristic, **(B)**, involves categorization and classification based on how well an individual example fits its category. Confirmation bias, **(D)**, occurs when people only seek information that reinforces their opinions.

4. **A**

Fluid intelligence consists of problem-solving skills and is not one of Gardner's eight multiple intelligences. Gardner's theory lists linguistic, logical–mathematical, musical, visual–spatial, bodily–kinesthetic, interpersonal, intrapersonal, and naturalist intelligences.

5. **A**

EEG during REM is composed mainly of beta waves, which are present during alertness. SWS, **(B)**, consists mainly of delta waves, which are not typically present during REM sleep. Stage 1 sleep, **(C)**, consists mainly of theta waves. Meditation, **(D)**, is quieting of the mind, and consists mainly of slow alpha and theta waves.

6. **B**

Early in the evening, sleep cycles include deepening of sleep (Stages 1–2–3–4), followed either by lightening of sleep (Stages 4–3–2) and then REM, or just directly moving from Stage 4 into REM. Later in the evening, the cycle may be shortened as slow-wave sleep becomes less common.

7. **B**

Divided attention is the ability to perform several tasks simultaneously. Routine actions, such as rewatching familiar episodes of a favorite TV show, are completed via automatic processing which allows the brain to focus on other tasks. Working on two tasks simultaneously means the student is using divided attention, supporting **(B)** as the correct answer. By contrast, parallel processing, **(D)**, refers to the brain's ability to analyze imagery by processing several aspects of the image (shape, color, motion, etc.) independently and simultaneously.

8. **C**

Cognitive theorists proposed in the cognitive process dream theory that wakeful and dreaming states use the same mental systems within the brain, particularly stream-of-consciousness. The activation–synthesis theory, **(A)**, states that dreams are caused by widespread, random activation of neural circuitry. The problem solving dream model, **(B)**, indicates that dreams are used to solve problems while sleeping due to untethering of dreams from obstacles perceived while awake. The neurocognitive theorists, **(D)**, seek to unify cognitive and biological perspectives by correlating the subjective dream experience with the physiological experience of dreaming.

9. **D**

The description of the student matches the clinical features of marijuana (cannabis) use: hunger (presumably, based on what was shoplifted), redness of the eyes, dry mouth, and euphoria. Marijuana may also cause an increased heart rate, short-term memory loss, paranoia, and—in high doses—hallucinations. Tetrahydrocannabinol is the primary active substance in marijuana.

10. **C**

Syntax refers to how words are put together to form sentences and create meaning. Phonology, **(A)**, refers to the actual sounds of a language. Semantics, **(B)**, refers to the association of meaning with a word. Pragmatics, **(D)**, refers to changes in usage, wording, and inflection based on context.

11. **C**

A child who speaks in three-word sentences but has not yet mastered most of the fundamental rules of language, including past tense, is likely to be between two and three years old.

12. **B**

Learning theory, largely based on the work of B. F. Skinner, states that parents reinforce phonemes that sound most like their language, resulting in preferential preservation of these phonemes. Nativist theory, **(A)**, posits a critical period during which language acquisition occurs. Social interactionist theory, **(C)**, indicates that language develops via interaction with parents and caregivers as well as a desire of the child to communicate. Neurocognitive theory, **(D)**, is concerned with the subjective experience of dreaming and the physiology of dreaming.

13. **A**

Broca's area governs the motor function of language. A stroke that affects Broca's area will leave receptive language intact, but word formation will be affected. A stroke affecting Wernicke's area, **(B)**, will make it so the individual is unable to comprehend speech. A stroke affecting the arcuate fasciculus, **(C)**, will result in an inability to repeat words heard but spontaneous language production is intact. The superior temporal gyrus, **(D)**, is where Wernicke's area is located.

14. **A**

With selective attention, a person focuses on a specific task while filtering out background stimuli. In this way, the individual in the airport ignored most of the background noise while working on a puzzle. However, the brain can shift attention quickly when a stimulus is particularly important, such as the specific call for boarding the flight. This shift is known as the cocktail party phenomenon, named for a person's ability to quickly reorient their focus when they hear their name at a party. Thus, **(A)** is the correct answer. By contrast, while effortful processing, **(D)**, describes this person's intense focus on the puzzle, it does not explain the ability to respond quickly to the boarding announcement. Similarly, divided attention, **(B)**, works best on simple tasks and the question stem uses the word "challenging" to describe the puzzle.

15. **D**

About 75% of dreaming occurs during REM, but dreams occur in all other stages of sleep as well. More bizarre dreams are likely to occur during REM.

GO ONLINE

Consult your online resources for additional practice.

EQUATION TO REMEMBER

(4.1) **Stanford–Binet intelligence quotient:** $IQ = \frac{\text{mental age}}{\text{chronological age}} \times 100$

SHARED CONCEPTS

Behavioral Sciences Chapter 1
Biology and Behavior

Behavioral Sciences Chapter 3
Learning and Memory

Behavioral Sciences Chapter 6
Identity and Personality

Behavioral Sciences Chapter 11
Social Structure and Demographics

Biology Chapter 4
The Nervous System

CHAPTER 5

MOTIVATION, EMOTION, AND STRESS

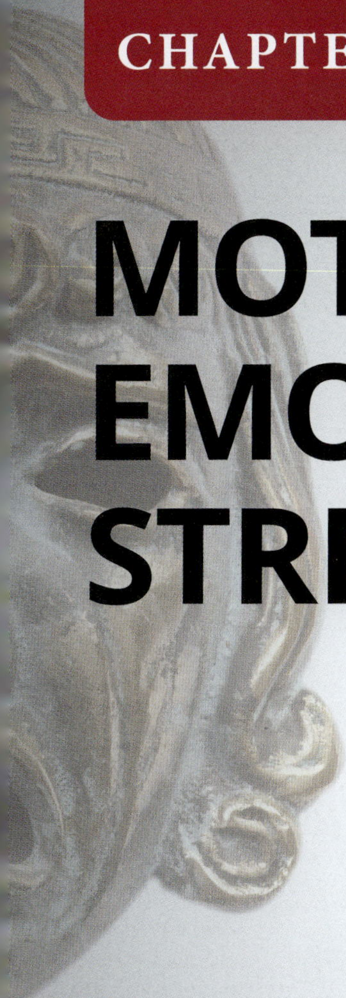

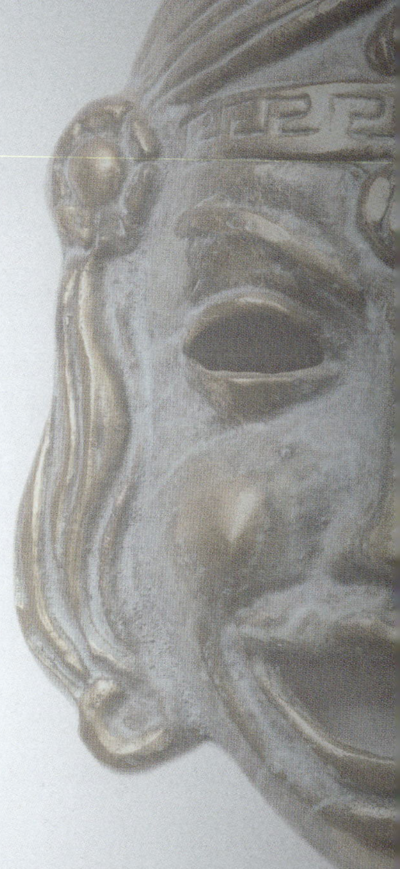

SCIENCE MASTERY ASSESSMENT

Every pre-med knows this feeling: there is so much content I have to know for the MCAT! How do I know what to do first or what's important?

While the high-yield badges throughout this book will help you identify the most important topics, this Science Mastery Assessment is another tool in your MCAT prep arsenal. This quiz (which can also be taken in your online resources) and the guidance below will help ensure that you are spending the appropriate amount of time on this chapter based on your personal strengths and weaknesses. Don't worry though—skipping something now does not mean you'll never study it. Later on in your prep, as you complete full-length tests, you'll uncover specific pieces of content that you need to review and can come back to these chapters as appropriate.

How to Use This Assessment

If you answer 0–7 questions correctly:

Spend about 1 hour to read this chapter in full and take limited notes throughout. Follow up by reviewing **all** quiz questions to ensure that you now understand how to solve each one.

If you answer 8–11 questions correctly:

Spend 20–40 minutes reviewing the quiz questions. Beginning with the questions you missed, read and take notes on the corresponding subchapters. For questions you answered correctly, ensure your thinking matches that of the explanation and you understand why each choice was correct or incorrect.

If you answer 12–15 questions correctly:

Spend less than 20 minutes reviewing all questions from the quiz. If you missed any, then include a quick read-through of the corresponding subchapters, or even just the relevant content within a subchapter, as part of your question review. For questions you answered correctly, ensure your thinking matches that of the explanation and review the Concept Summary at the end of the chapter.

1. A college student strives for excellent grades and hopes to graduate with a better GPA than an older sibling. This type of motivation is considered:
   - **A.** extrinsic motivation.
   - **B.** intrinsic motivation.
   - **C.** a primary drive.
   - **D.** a secondary drive.

2. When practicing a recital song at home, a student sounds perfectly in pitch to family and friends. However, when performing at the recital in front of a large audience of peers, strangers, and coaches, the student's pitch and tone are off, resulting in a poor performance. This second performance is best explained by:
   - **A.** drive reduction theory.
   - **B.** instinct approach theory.
   - **C.** Maslow's hierarchy of needs.
   - **D.** the Yerkes–Dodson law.

3. Seeking homeostasis to reduce an uncomfortable internal state is associated with which motivational theory?
   - **A.** Drive reduction theory
   - **B.** Instinct theory
   - **C.** Arousal theory
   - **D.** Incentive theory

4. People from cultures around the world can identify which of the following emotions?
   - **A.** Happiness, sadness, and surprise
   - **B.** Happiness, anger, and apathy
   - **C.** Sadness, anticipation, and happiness
   - **D.** Excitement, anger, and disgust

5. Experiencing emotion involves three components, which are:
   - **A.** behavioral, reactionary, and cognitive.
   - **B.** emotional, physical, and mental.
   - **C.** physiological, cognitive, and behavioral.
   - **D.** emotional, cognitive, and behavioral.

6. The statement "I noticed my heart racing and breathing rate increasing when I saw a bear, so I am afraid" corresponds most closely with which theory of emotion?
   - **A.** Schachter–Singer theory
   - **B.** Yerkes–Dodson theory
   - **C.** Cannon–Bard theory
   - **D.** James–Lange theory

7. Which theory of motivation is most significantly informed by Darwin's theory of evolution?
   - **A.** Arousal theory
   - **B.** Drive reduction theory
   - **C.** Instinct theory
   - **D.** Incentive theory

8. Simultaneous processing of conscious emotions and physiological activation is the defining feature of which theory of emotion?
   - **A.** Schachter–Singer theory
   - **B.** James–Lange theory
   - **C.** Incentive theory
   - **D.** Cannon–Bard theory

9. All of the following brain regions are primarily responsible for the experience of emotions EXCEPT the:
   A. amygdala.
   B. prefrontal cortex.
   C. basal ganglia.
   D. thalamus.

10. A person with high left frontal lobe activity is most likely experiencing which emotion?
   A. Happiness
   B. Sadness
   C. Surprise
   D. Disgust

11. Determination of the intensity and risk of a stressor occurs during which stage(s) of stress appraisal?
   A. Primary appraisal only
   B. Secondary appraisal only
   C. Both primary and secondary appraisal
   D. Neither primary nor secondary appraisal

12. A medical student is feeling a high level of stress due to upcoming exams and pressure from family to engage in activities at home. The student chooses to go to the gym for a workout to help relax. This workout is which type of stress?
   A. Hassle
   B. Frustration
   C. Distress
   D. Eustress

13. Which type of conflict is associated with the LEAST amount of stress?
   A. Approach–approach conflict
   B. Avoidance–avoidance conflict
   C. Approach–avoidance conflict
   D. Avoidance–escape conflict

14. While cleaning your house, you notice a large spider on the wall by your head and feel your heart rate jump up and your skin temperature grow warm. Which stage of stress response are you experiencing?
   A. Alarm
   B. Resistance
   C. Exhaustion
   D. Homeostasis

15. Each of the following responses to stress is considered maladaptive EXCEPT:
   A. drug use.
   B. social withdrawal.
   C. progressive muscle relaxation.
   D. avoiding the stressor.

Answer Key

1. **A** (See section 5.1)
2. **D** (See section 5.1)
3. **A** (See section 5.1)
4. **A** (See section 5.2)
5. **C** (See section 5.2)
6. **D** (See section 5.2)
7. **C** (See section 5.1)
8. **D** (See section 5.2)
9. **C** (See section 5.2)
10. **A** (See section 5.2)
11. **B** (See section 5.3)
12. **D** (See section 5.3)
13. **A** (See section 5.3)
14. **A** (See section 5.3)
15. **C** (See section 5.3)

The relevant section of the chapter to review for each question is given in parentheses after the correct answer. Detailed explanations can be found at the end of the chapter.

CHAPTER 5

MOTIVATION, EMOTION, AND STRESS

In This Chapter

CHAPTER PROFILE

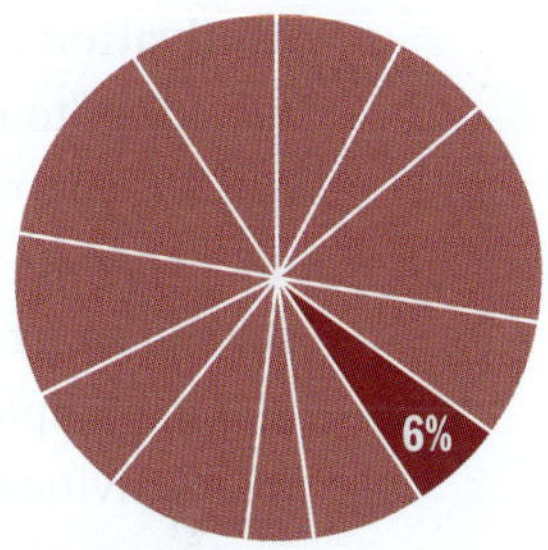

The content in this chapter should be relevant to about 6% of all questions about the behavioral sciences on the MCAT.

This chapter covers material from the following AAMC content categories:

6C: Responding to the world

7A: Individual influences on behavior

Introduction

A heart condition, substantial bone density decreases, esophageal and stomach ulcers, a loss of 25 percent of body mass—these are some of the possible consequences of anorexia nervosa. Sometimes those who develop this condition have been put under extreme pressure in their work or personal lives to look a certain way. Over time, this pressure can motivate weight loss in an unhealthy manner. Patients are sometimes motivated by feelings of disgust and guilt that go directly against the body's basic needs. A combination of stress from job and peers, intrinsic and extrinsic motivation, and negative emotions can result in what could be a life-threatening condition.

In this chapter, we'll discuss motivation, emotion, and stress. We will look at factors that influence motivation, the components of emotion, and the stressors that lead to the stress response. We will also look at theories used to explain these processes and associated behaviors. The physiological, cognitive, and behavioral elements will be examined in order to understand the role that these topics play in everyday life. Exploring these ideas will enable us to tackle any question related to these concepts on Test Day.

5.1 Motivation High Yield

LEARNING OBJECTIVES

After Chapter 5.1, you will be able to:

- Describe the sources of motivation posited by instinct theory, arousal theory, drive reduction theory, and the need-based theories
- Order Maslow's proposed hierarchy of needs from most to least essential
- Apply opponent-process theory to drug use and withdrawal

Motivation is the purpose, or driving force, behind our actions. The word derives from the Latin *movere*, meaning "to move." There are many examples of motivation in our everyday lives. As you sit, studying for the MCAT, you realize you are thirsty, so you reach for your water bottle. When you realize it is empty, the need to quench your thirst drives you to get up, walk to the kitchen, and fill the bottle with water. Thus, the physical state of thirst motivated an action. The desire to go to medical school and become a physician has motivated you to complete required undergraduate coursework, strive for a competitive GPA, participate in extracurricular activities, and dedicate your time to study for a standardized test. The goal of staying fit and healthy motivates many to spend hours in the gym, while the initial discomfort of physical activity might motivate others to stay sedentary. Motivation can be directed toward minimizing pain, maximizing pleasure, or it can be rooted in the desire, or **appetite**, to fullfil a physical need. Though the term appetite is commonly used to refer to a need for food, this term can more generally be applied to any need such as eating, drinking, sleeping, or social acceptance.

Motivation can manifest from external forces, such as rewards and punishments, or internal forces, where the behavior is personally gratifying. External forces, coming from outside oneself, create extrinsic motivation. **Extrinsic motivation** can include rewards for showing a desired behavior or avoiding punishment if the desired behavior is not achieved. Examples of such motivation include working hard at your job for praise from your boss, practicing regularly for a sport so that you will perform strongly in an upcoming game, or studying for months on end to achieve a high score on the MCAT. Each of these acts results in external, tangible rewards. Extrinsic motivation can also include doing chores to avoid punishment and working to avoid being fired. Competition is a strong form of external motivation because people are incentivized to beat others and not only to win, perform, or achieve for themselves. Motivation that comes from within oneself is referred to as **intrinsic motivation**. This can be driven by interest in a task or pure enjoyment. A student who takes interest in the subject matter at hand and has the goal of mastering the content is driven by intrinsic motivation, while the goal of achieving high grades is considered extrinsic. The distinction between extrinsic and intrinsic motivation is playfuly shown in Figure 5.1, where two players are striving to win for two different reasons.

REAL WORLD

Intrinsic motivation can be reduced by introducing external reward into a scenario. In one study, children were given art supplies and told to draw. Some children were told they would receive a gold ribbon for their drawing, while others were not. Those who knew of the potential reward were driven by extrinsic motivation and spent less time drawing, acting only to receive the reward. Children who did not know about the reward drew for the sake of drawing—by intrinsic motivation—and spent more time drawing.

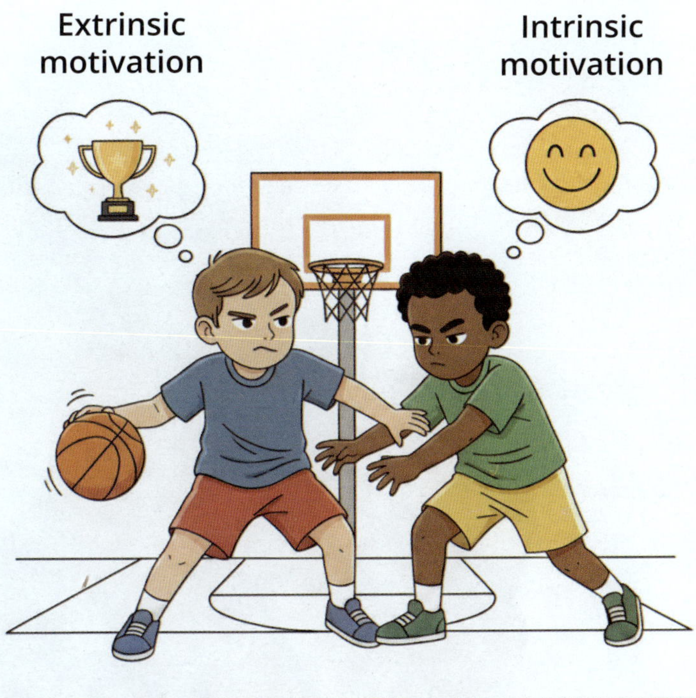

Figure 5.1 Extrinsic vs. Intrinsic Motivation

The primary views of motivation focus on instincts that elicit natural behavior, the desire to maintain optimal levels of arousal, the drive to reduce uncomfortable states, and the goal of satisfying physiological and psychological needs.

Instinct Theory

Early attempts to understand the basis of motivation focused on **instincts**, which are innate, fixed patterns of behavior. For example, wolves are instinctively pack creatures that naturally follow the alpha male of their group. Additionally, they are highly territorial creatures, protecting areas that are much larger than needed to hunt and dwell. This protection includes scent-marking, howling, and direct aggressive attacks on intruders. Humans also have instinctive behavior; for example, thumb sucking is an instinctual response to stress in babies that is aimed at self-soothing. As discussed in Chapter 1 of *MCAT Behavioral Sciences Review*, primitive reflexes like the grasp reflex, shown in Figure 5.2, are also instinctual. Note that some instincts last for the entire lifetime, while others may appear or disappear with age.

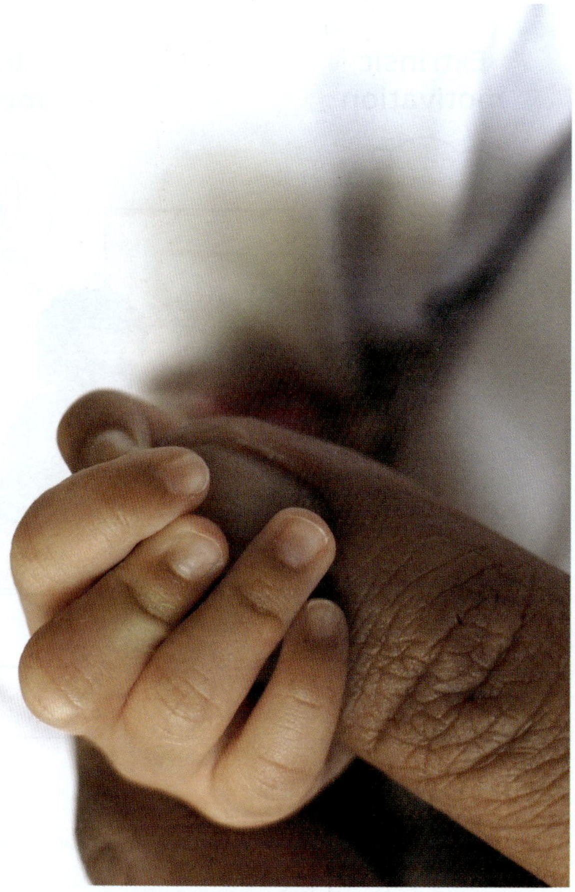

Figure 5.2 The Grasp Reflex
Primitive reflexes are examples of instincts seen in infants that extinguish with age.

According to the **instinct theory** of motivation, certain behaviors are based on evolutionarily programmed instincts. This theory was one of the first to describe motivation and was derived from Darwin's theory of evolution. William James, the father of modern psychology, was one of the first to write about human instincts in his 1890 publication of *Principles of Psychology*. He stated that humans were motivated by many instincts, possibly more than any other animal studied. James suggested that human actions are derived from 20 physical instincts, including suckling and locomotion, and 17 mental instincts, including curiosity and fearfulness. However, he said that many of these instincts were in direct conflict with each other and could be overridden by experience. Arguably the greatest proponent of instinct theory was William McDougall, who proposed that humans were led to all thoughts and behaviors by 18 distinctive instincts, including flight and acquisition. James and McDougall postulated that the instincts of suckling and carrying food to the mouth result in naturally motivating one to eat.

KEY CONCEPT

An instinct is an innate, fixed pattern of behavior. It may be consistent throughout life, or it may appear or disappear with time.

Arousal Theory

Another factor that influences motivation is **arousal**, the psychological and physiological state of being awake and reactive to stimuli. Arousal involves the brainstem, autonomic nervous system, and endocrine system and plays a vital role in behavior and cognition.

Arousal theory states that people perform actions in order to maintain an optimal level of arousal: seeking to increase arousal when it falls below their optimal level, and to decrease arousal when it rises above their optimum level. Additionally, the **Yerkes–Dodson law** postulates a U-shaped function between the level of arousal and performance. This law states that performance is worst at extremely high and low levels of arousal and optimal at some intermediate level, as depicted in Figure 5.3. The optimal level of arousal varies between different types of tasks: lower levels are optimal for highly cognitive tasks, while higher levels are optimal for activities that require physical endurance and stamina. Further, simple tasks generally require slightly higher arousal than complex tasks.

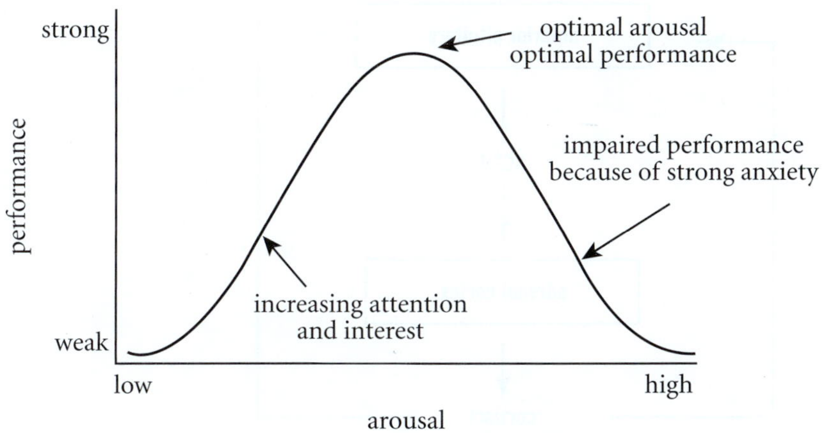

Figure 5.3 Yerkes–Dodson Law

REAL WORLD

While a moderate level of arousal is optimal for performance, certain individuals seek out higher levels of arousal. Such people may seek out dangerous activities, such as skydiving or bungee jumping. These individuals are sometimes found to have lower levels of monoamine oxidase (MAO), which breaks down catecholamines. Low levels of MAO result in higher neurotransmitter levels, which may lead to motivation to experience high levels of arousal.

Drive Reduction Theory

Drives are defined as internal states of tension that activate particular behaviors focused on goals. Drives are thought to originate within an individual without requiring any external factors to motivate behavior. In other words, drives help humans survive by creating an uncomfortable state, ensuring motivation to eliminate this state or to relieve the internal tension created by unmet needs. **Primary drives**, including the need for food, water, and warmth, motivate us to sustain bodily processes in homeostasis. **Homeostasis** is the regulation of the internal environment to maintain an optimal, stable set of conditions. In homeostatic regulation, external factors are encountered, and the system will react to push the system back to its optimal state.

Homeostasis is usually controlled by **negative feedback** loops. A common real-life example of a negative feedback loop is a thermostat. A thermostat is set to a desired temperature, and then sensors monitor the air temperature in relation to this desired temperature. If the air temperature gets too cold, the heater will turn on; if the temperature gets too warm, the heater will turn off. Negative feedback loops in the body operate the same way. Likewise when our bodies are lacking nutrients and energy, feedback systems release hormones like ghrelin that create hunger and motivate eating. After we consume food, feedback is sent to the brain to turn off the hunger drive through hormones like leptin. Hunger is a complex feedback system involving these hormones, receptors in the walls of the stomach, levels of glucose (maintained by the liver), and insulin and glucagon levels (released by the pancreas).

REAL WORLD

One well-characterized drive is the hunger (food) drive, which has been studied for more than 60 years. The hunger drive is a primary drive, in that food is necessary for life. Given the necessity of food to life, many species possess multiple processes that drive the individual to consume food. These biological processes include tie-ins to the sense of smell and taste, which were demonstrated by many studies, notably those of Janowitz and Grossman.

The concentrations of many hormones of the endocrine system are regulated by three-organ "axes," such as the hypothalamic–pituitary–adrenal axis shown in Figure 5.4.

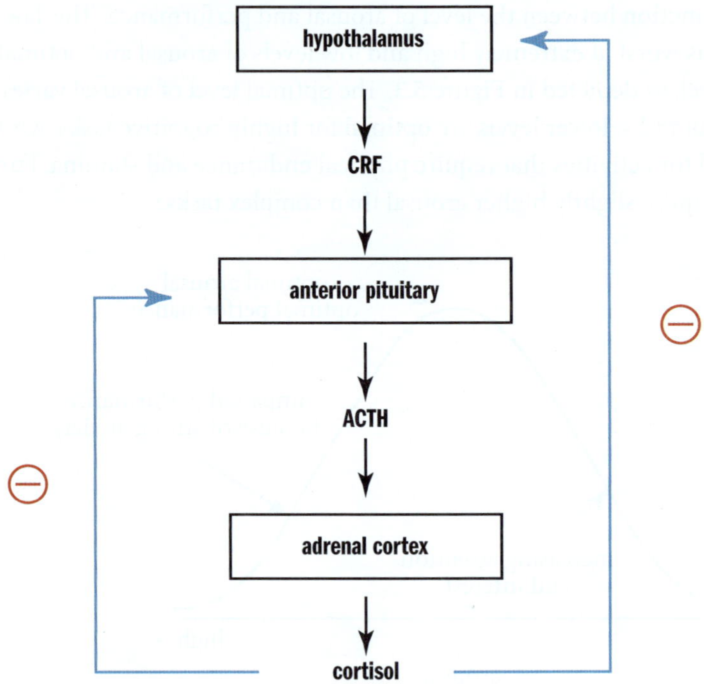

Figure 5.4 Negative Feedback in the Endocrine System

Additional drives that are not directly related to biological processes are called **secondary drives**. These drives are thought to stem from learning. The drive to matriculate into medical school and become a physician is an example of a secondary drive. Secondary drives also include certain emotions, such as the desire for nurturing, love, achievement, and aggression.

Drive reduction theory explains that motivation is based on the goal of eliminating uncomfortable states. Theorists hypothesize that certain physiological conditions result in a negative internal environment. This internal environment then drives motivation and seeks homeostasis in order to reduce the uncomfortable internal state.

Need-Based Theories

In need-based theories of motivation, energy and resources are allocated to best satisfy human needs. These needs may be **primary needs**, which are generally physiological needs such as the need for food, water, sleep, and shelter. Or these needs might be **secondary needs**, which are generally mental states, like a desire for power, achievement, or social belonging.

KEY CONCEPT

Primary drives are those that motivate us to sustain necessary biological processes. Secondary drives are those that motivate us to fulfill nonbiological, emotional, or "learned" desires.

BRIDGE

Drive reduction theory can be applied to motivation in terms of learning, and is commonly used to define motivational states within behavioral conditioning. Conditioning and learning are discussed in Chapter 3 of *MCAT Behavioral Sciences Review*.

Abraham Maslow defined **needs** as relatively long-lasting feelings that require relief or satisfaction and tend to influence action. He observed that certain needs will yield a greater influence on our motivation and he established what is referred to as **Maslow's hierarchy of needs**. Maslow classified needs into five groups, and assigned different levels of priority to each group. The hierarchy is typically displayed as a pyramid, as shown in Figure 5.5, where the most primitive, essential, and important needs are at the base. The first four levels of the pyramid correspond to physiological needs, safety and security, love and belonging, and self-esteem. The highest level of the pyramid corresponds to **self-actualization**, or the need to realize one's fullest potential. Maslow theorized that if the lowest level of need is not met, motivation to meet that need will be the highest priority. Once the lowest level of needs is met, if additional needs exist, they will be satisfied based on priority. For example, a person's most basic motivation will be to satisfy physiological needs, followed by the need to establish a safe and secure environment.

MCAT EXPERTISE

Knowing the four primary factors that influence motivation is key for Test Day: instincts, arousal, drives, and needs. The MCAT will expect you to know the common theories for explaining motivation.

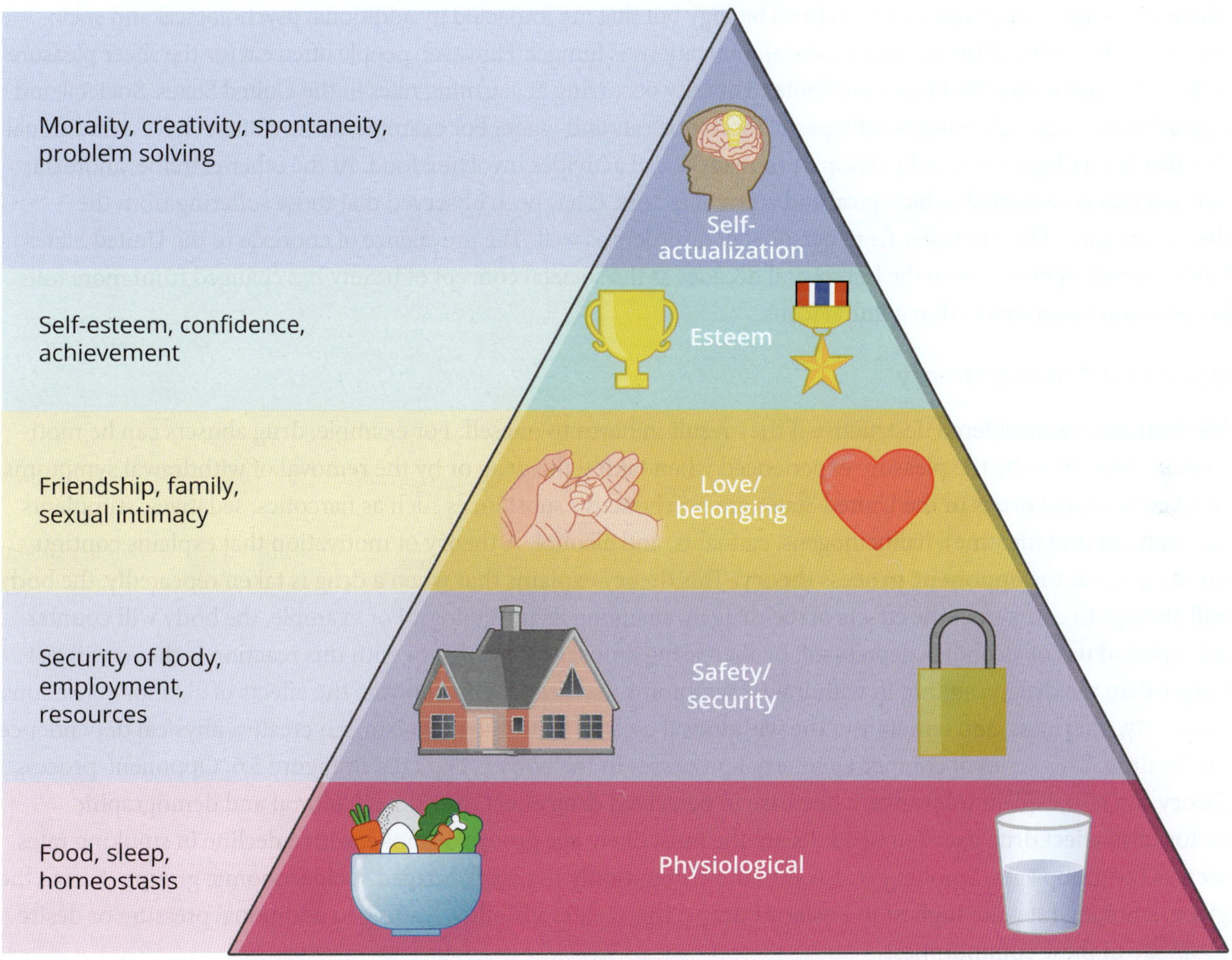

Figure 5.5 Maslow's Hierarchy of Needs

Another need-based motivational theory is the **self-determination theory** (**SDT**), which emphasizes the role of three universal needs: autonomy, the need to be in control of one's actions and ideas; competence, the need to complete and excel at difficult tasks; and relatedness, the need to feel accepted and wanted in relationships. Theorists explain that these three needs must be met in order to develop healthy relationships with oneself and others.

Additional Theories and Applications

There are a few other theories of motivation that you should know for the MCAT: opponent-process theory, sexual motivation, incentive theory, and expectancy-value theory. Opponent-process theory and sexual motivation will be discussed in more detail below. **Incentive theory** explains that behavior is motivated not by need or arousal, but by the desire to pursue rewards and to avoid punishments. **Expectancy–value theory** states that the amount of motivation needed to reach a goal is the result of both the individual's expectation of success in reaching the goal and the degree to which the individual values succeeding at the goal.

There are many motivations that stem from biology but that are impacted by additional psychological and sociocultural factors. One of the strongest natural motivations is hunger. However, people often eat for the sheer pleasure of the act, a motivation that may contribute to obesity occurring at alarming rates in the United States. Societal and cultural norms can determine what types of foods one eats and when. For example, some cultures have a traditional diet that is very high in fat and participate in many social activities involving food. At the other extreme, anorexia nervosa is also correlated to biological and cultural factors. It has been observed that those suffering from the disease are more likely to suffer from personality disorders as well. The prevalence of anorexia in the United States has increased significantly in the last several decades as the societal concept of beauty has changed from more full-bodied idols to extremely thin cultural icons.

Opponent-Process Theory

Motivations are considered destructive if they result in harm to oneself. For example, drug abusers can be motivated to take drugs by the pleasure experienced when taking the drug or by the removal of withdrawal symptoms. Most recreational drugs in the United States are psychoactive substances such as narcotics, sedatives, stimulants (e.g. caffeine and nicotine), hallucinogens, cannabis, and alcohol. A theory of motivation that explains continuous drug use is the **opponent-process theory**. This theory explains that when a drug is taken repeatedly, the body will attempt to counteract the effects of the drug by changing its physiology. For example, the body will counteract repeated use of alcohol, a depressant, by increasing arousal. The problem with this reaction is that it will last longer than the drug, resulting in withdrawal symptoms that are exactly opposite the effects of alcohol: sensations of anxiety, jitteriness, and irritability. The withdrawal created by this mechanism can create a physical dependence on the drug. This series of competing internal processes in the body is depicted in Figure 5.6. Opponent-process theory can also explain **tolerance**, a decrease in perceived drug effect over time. Cultural and demographic factors also affect drug use. Young adults are the most likely age group to smoke, with a decline in smoking rates seen as the group ages. Smoking is also seen more commonly in disadvantaged socioeconomic groups. Across the globe, smoking rates are highest in Eastern Europe; this creates visibility, leading to additional pressure or desire to smoke in these communities.

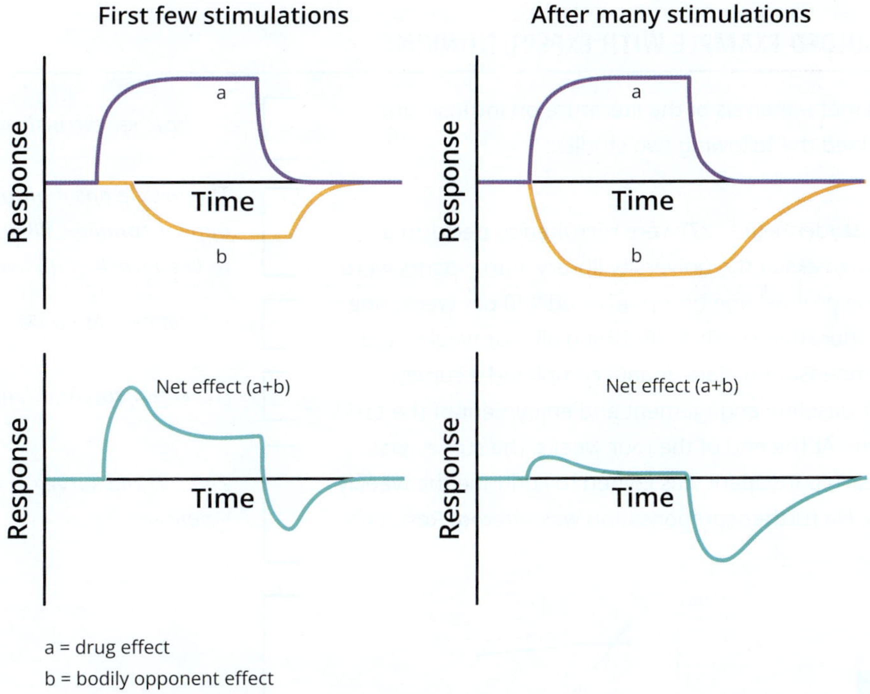

Figure 5.6 The Opponent-Process Theory of Motivation

It is worth mentioning that there is also an opponent-process theory of emotion. This theory proposes that there are two emotional responses that occur to a given situation. One emotion is expressed immediately due to a stimulus, and then another emotion follows in order to bring back a "homeostasis" of emotion. For example, someone on a roller coaster might feel intense fear during the ride, but then feels a strong sense of relief or happiness afterwards. This strong relief, according to the opponent-process theory, is returning the mind back to an emotional equilibrium.

BEHAVIORAL SCIENCES GUIDED EXAMPLE WITH EXPERT THINKING

Researchers conducting a meta-analysis of the literature on intrinsic and extrinsic motivation examined the following two studies:

Intrinsic vs. extrinsic motivation

Study 1:

Undergraduate university students ($n = 27$) were recruited to perform a weekly filing task over four weeks at the university library. Participants were randomly divided into three groups: one group received $20 per week, one group received a general education credit for finishing all four weeks, and one group received no compensation. Participants completed a survey designed to measure their baseline engagement and enjoyment of the tasks they were asked to perform. At the end of the four weeks, the survey was administered again, and each participant was invited to continue the weekly tasks on a volunteer basis. No further compensation was offered. Results are shown in Figure 1.

This article has multiple studies that appear complex. I'll need to make sure to keep track of all variables.

IV: compensation ($)

DV: engagement in/enjoyment of task

2nd DV: 2nd survey + willingness to volunteer

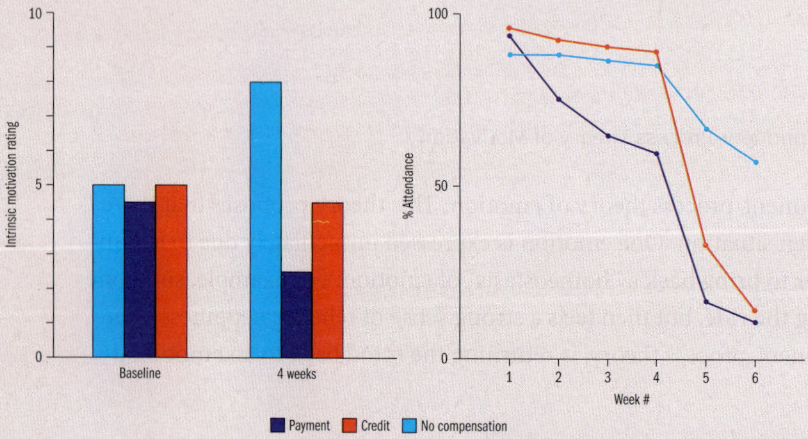

The no-compensation group seemed to enjoy the task much more than the other two groups compared to baseline, and more of them continued to volunteer after the study was over.

Figure 1 Enjoyment survey results and participation

Study 2:

A sample of men identified as being at high risk of heart disease ($n = 128$) were recruited for a multifaceted intervention program which required attending a clinic once per week for medication, physical exercise, and counseling. Participants came from both medium and low socioeconomic status (SES) households. All individuals in the low SES group experienced food insecurity. Participants in each SES group were divided into three conditions: monetary compensation for attendance, grocery credit for attendance, and no compensation for attendance. Compensation was offered for a six-month period. Participants completed an inventory designed to measure baseline intrinsic motivation to improve their health, with items such as "The reason I am participating in this course of treatment as prescribed is because participation in this treatment is consistent with my life goals." The inventory was administered again at six months and at twelve months. Results are shown in Figure 2.

IVs: SES and compensation for attendance

DV: intrinsic motivation, measured by survey

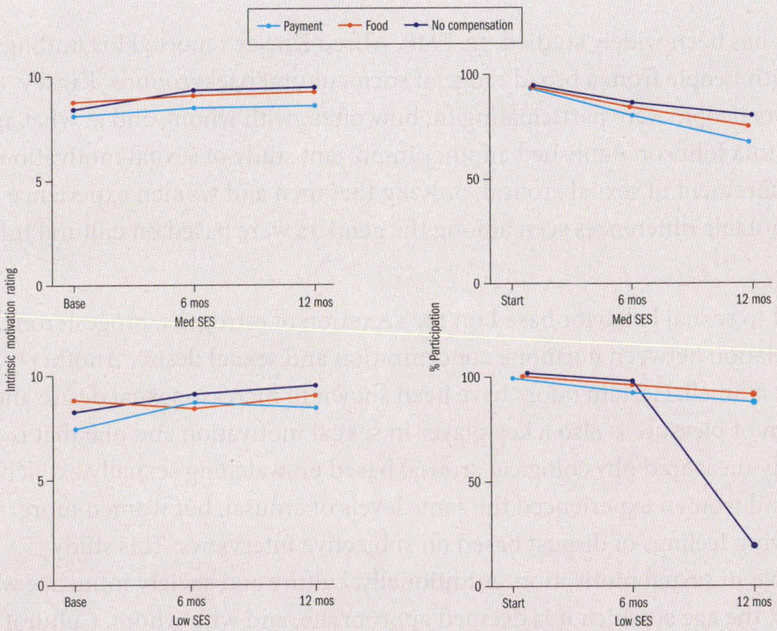

Motivation is high for all groups, as is participation, with the exception of the no-compensation low SES group once compensation ends.

Figure 2 Motivation and participation over 12 months

Adapted from: Czaicki NL, Dow WH, Njau PF, McCoy SI (2018) Do incentives undermine intrinsic motivation? Increases in intrinsic motivation within an incentive-based intervention for people living with HIV in Tanzania. *PLoS ONE* 13(6): e0196616. https://doi.org/10.1371/journal.pone.0196616

What do the results of these two studies suggest about the role of intrinsic and extrinsic factors in motivation?

This question is asking for a fairly high-level analysis of the three different conditions across the two studies. To answer, first we will need to consider what was being tested and the results from each study. Identifying the variables as we read the studies will make this task much more manageable and, as we have seen in guided examples from other chapters, is a generally good approach to reading any study. In Study 1, the only difference between groups is the offer of compensation, which is an extrinsic motivator. The results are consistent with conventional wisdom (and our outside content knowledge) that when an extrinsic motivator is introduced, intrinsic motivation decreases. Therefore, when the compensation is removed, participation declines. We can specifically see this within the data: groups receiving compensation see a substantial decline in intrinsic motivation and attendance as compared to the no-compensation group. Additionally, the lack of an extrinsic motivator increases intrinsic motivation, as demonstrated by the volunteerism rate in the no-compensation group.

Given the results of Study 1, Study 2 may seem surprising. Based on the results in the figure for Study 2, for the medium SES and low SES groups receiving compensation, intrinsic motivation remained consistent throughout the study. For the low SES group, however, participation declined sharply for the non-compensated group.

Fortunately, on Test Day we will never be asked to write an essay explaining these results, so we are not responsible for coming up with an explanation on our own. Among the answer choices will be an explanation that is consistent with both the scientific content we studied and the analysis of the results we conducted.

If a question like this shows up on the real MCAT, take a moment to consider what we know and what we've learned from the passage, and make a general prediction that targets the *kind* of information a correct answer could provide. In this case we are looking for a difference between the low and medium SES groups that might explain the observed difference in the no-compensation group. We might consider the implications of SES generally, but the passage provided a potential clue when it mentioned that the low SES group had food insecurity. Given what we know about Maslow's hierarchy of needs we might anticipate an answer that implies motivation to obtain food is more important than reducing the risk of heart disease.

Sexual Motivation

Sexual motivation is another area that has been widely studied. In 1948, Alfred Kinsey reported his findings on sexual behavior from interviews with people from a broad range of sociocultural backgrounds. Kinsey hoped to identify what sexual behaviors people were participating in, how often, with whom, and at what age they began. William Masters and Virginia Johnson published another important study of sexual motivation. The study involved physiological measurement of sexual arousal, proving that men and women experience similar physical responses. The most notable differences seen among the genders were based on cultural influences and learned behavior.

Physiologically, humans are motivated to sexual behavior based on the secretion of estrogens, progesterone, and androgens. There is a strong correlation between hormone concentration and sexual desire. Another biological factor for sexual motivation is smell. Certain odors have been shown to increase sexual desire and activity. Pleasure and the interpretation of pleasure is also a key player in sexual motivation and one that is highly influenced by culture. One study measured physiological arousal based on watching sexually explicit videos. The results showed that men and women experienced the same levels of arousal, but women more often reported being unaroused or having feelings of disgust based on subjective interviews. This study demonstrated that cognition plays a role in sexual motivation. Additionally, culture and society influence what is deemed appropriate sexual behavior, the age at which it is deemed appropriate, and with whom. Cultural norms and conditioning influence the desire for sexual interaction, or lack thereof.

MCAT CONCEPT CHECK 5.1

Before you move on, assess your understanding of the material with these questions.

1. For each of the theories listed below, what creates motivation?

Theory	Factor for Motivation
Instinct theory	
Arousal theory	
Drive reduction theory	
Need-based theories	

2. List Maslow's hierarchy of needs in decreasing priority:

- ______________________________
- ______________________________
- ______________________________

-

-

3. Based on opponent-process theory, what clinical features would be expected with withdrawal from cocaine use?

5.2 Emotion

High Yield

LEARNING OBJECTIVES

After Chapter 5.2, you will be able to:

- Describe the three elements of emotion: psychological response, behavioral response, and cognitive response
- Recall the seven universal facially expressed emotions
- Compare and contrast the James–Lange, Cannon–Bard, and Schachter–Singer theories of emotion
- Identify the names and functions of the parts of the limbic system

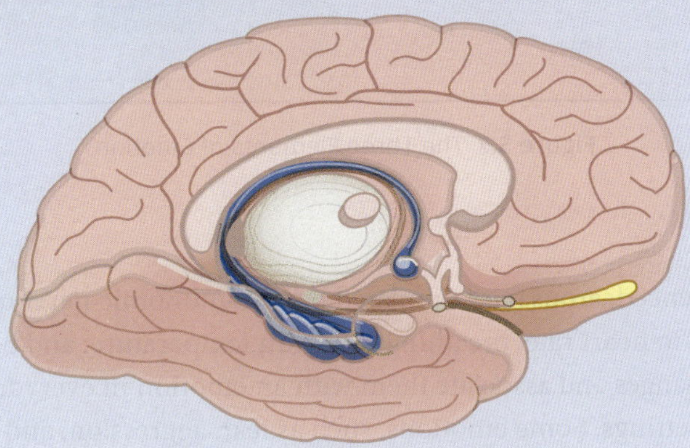

Emotion is a natural instinctive state of mind derived from one's circumstances, mood, or relationships with others. The word emotion is derived from the same Latin word as motivation.

Three Elements of Emotion

There are three elements of an emotion: the physiological response, the behavioral response, and the cognitive response. These elements are depicted in Figure 5.7.

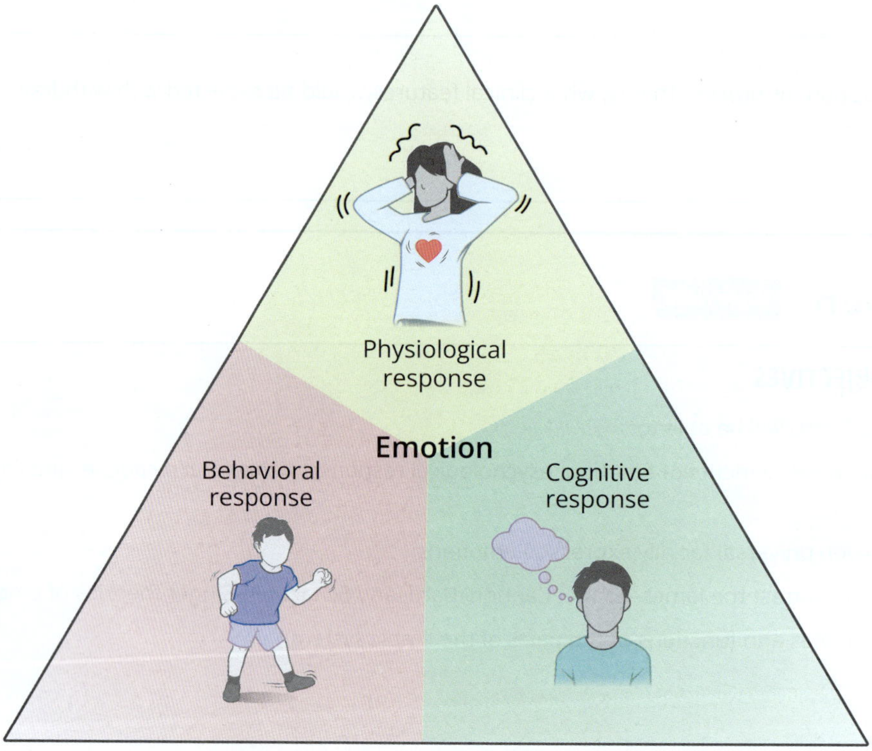

Figure 5.7 The Three Elements of Emotion

Physiological Response

When a feeling is first experienced, arousal is stimulated by the autonomic nervous system. The physiological component includes changes in heart rate, breathing rate, skin temperature, and blood pressure. While it may be hard to recognize these changes and associate them with an emotion in everyday life, these changes have been detected in laboratory settings. Some emotions, such as fear, aggression, and embarrassment, are associated with more pronounced physiological changes than others.

Behavioral Response

The behavioral component of an emotion includes facial expressions and body language. For example, a smile, a friendly hand gesture, or even a subtle head tilt toward someone are commonly recognized as warm and happy signals. On the other hand, a frown, slumping of the shoulders, and looking downward are recognized as sad or downtrodden signals.

Cognitive Response

Finally, the cognitive component of emotion is the subjective interpretation of the feeling being experienced. Determination of one's emotion is an evaluative process largely based on memories of past experiences and perception of the cause of the emotion.

Universal Emotions

Darwin made the argument that emotions are a result of evolution; thus, emotions and their corresponding expressions are universal. He explained that all humans evolved the same set of facial muscles to show the same expressions when communicating emotion, regardless of their society or culture. This sparked an ongoing discussion of the relationship between emotion and culture among psychologists and sociologists. Paul Ekman described a set of basic emotions that are recognized by societies around the world and further identified that six emotions are associated with consistent facial expressions across cultures. Ekman and other psychologists have revised this list; one of the more well-recognized sets consists of seven universal facially expressed emotions and includes: happiness, sadness, contempt, surprise, fear, disgust, and anger. These emotions correspond to the distinctive facial expressions explained in Table 5.1 and depicted in Figure 5.8.

MCAT EXPERTISE

The AAMC lists fear, anger, happiness, surprise, contempt, disgust, and sadness as universal emotions. Given the lack of consensus in the scientific community, the MCAT is more likely to test the topic conceptually than specifically.

Emotion	Facial Expression Cues
Happiness	Smile, wrinkling around eyes, raised cheeks
Sadness	Frown, inner eyebrows pulled up and together
Contempt	One corner of the mouth pulled upwards
Surprise	Eyes widen, eyebrows pulled up and curved, jaw opens
Fear	Eyes widen, eyebrows pulled up and together, lips pulled toward ears
Disgust	Nose wrinkling and/or raising of upper lip
Anger	Glaring, eyebrows pulled down and together, lips pressed together

Table 5.1 Seven Universal Emotions

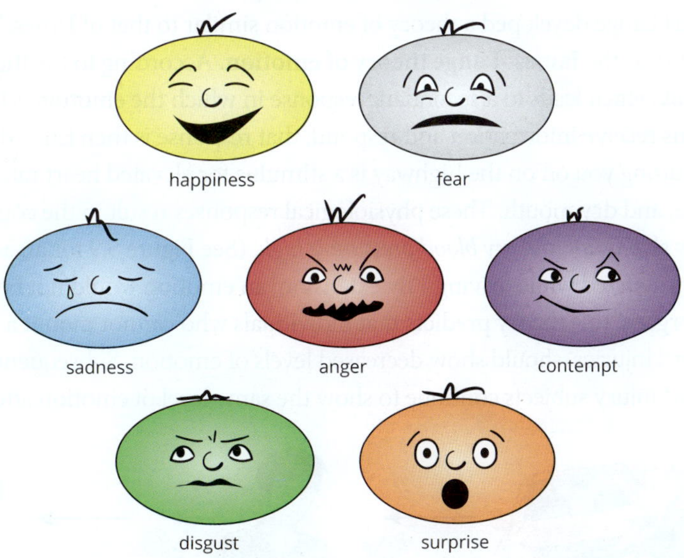

Figure 5.8 Seven Universal Emotions

While emotions are experienced universally, it is argued that they can be affected greatly by culture. Cultural dissimilarities in emotion include varying reactions to similar events, differences in the emotional experience itself, the behavior exhibited in response to an emotion, and the perception of that emotion by others within the society.

Facial-Feedback Effect

Charles Darwin was also one of the first people to suggest that not only did emotion affect one's expression, but that physiological changes also can affect emotion. The **facial-feedback effect**, also known as the **facial-feedback hypothesis**, is a theory that certain facial expressions can influence emotions. There are two versions of this theory that are commonly referenced: the weak version, which hypothesizes that facial expressions have a minor ability to affect emotions, and the strong version, which states that facial feedback is the primary cause of an emotional state.

Adaptive Role of Emotion

In accordance with Darwin's thoughts on universal emotion, the **evolutionary perspective** states that everything we do, think, and feel is based on specialized functional programs designed for any problem we encounter. These programs are functionally coordinated in order to produce a cohesive response. Emotions are thought to be evolutionary adaptations due to situations encountered over the evolutionary history of the human species that guide sensory processing, physiological response, and behavior. Further, different emotions are thought to have evolved during different periods in history. Among the earliest to develop were primal emotions, such as fear; other, more evolutionarily progressive emotions include social emotions, such as guilt and pride.

Theories of Emotion

Early psychologists believed that the cognitive component of emotion led to the physiological component, which then produced the behavioral component. In other words, the feeling of anger started with perception of a negative stimulus, which caused physiological changes, such as increased skin temperature, which then resulted in behavior, such as yelling. This explanation assumes that feeling precedes arousal, which precedes action.

James–Lange Theory

William James, the founder of functionalist theory, viewed the progression of these emotional elements differently. Around the same time, Carl Lange developed a theory of emotion similar to that of James. The explanation developed by the two is referred to as the **James–Lange theory of emotion**. According to the theory, a stimulus results first in physiological arousal, which leads to a secondary response in which the emotion is labeled. James believed that when peripheral organs receive information and respond, that response is then labeled as an emotion by the brain. For example, a car cutting you off on the highway is a stimulus for elevated heart rate and blood pressure, increased skin temperature, and dry mouth. These physiological responses result in the cognitive labeling of anger: *I must be angry because my skin is hot and my blood pressure is high.* (See Figure 5.9 for an additional example in which a driver starts feeling agitated while driving.) By extension, an emotion would not be processed without feedback from the peripheral organs; this theory predicts that individuals who cannot mount a sympathetic response, like patients with spinal cord injuries, should show decreased levels of emotion. Subsequent studies have proven this claim to be false; spinal cord injury subjects continue to show the same level of emotion after their injuries as before.

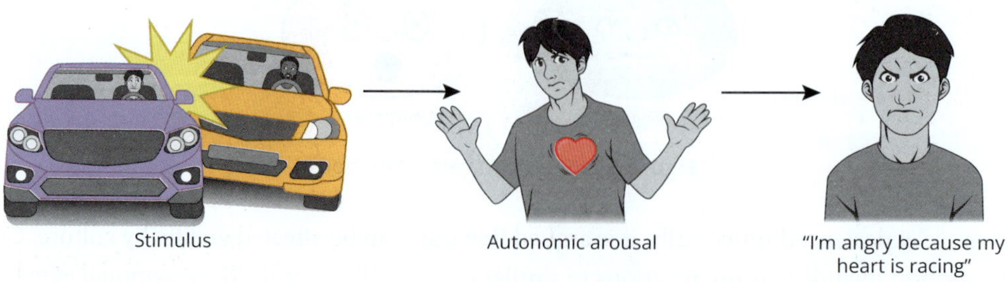

Figure 5.9 James-Lange Theory of Emotion

Cannon–Bard Theory

Walter Cannon and Philip Bard developed another scheme for explaining emotional components, referred to as the Cannon–Bard theory of emotion. In an attempt to test the James–Lange theory, Cannon studied the expression of emotion and its relationship to feedback from the sympathetic nervous system using cats whose afferent nerves had been severed. He hypothesized that physiological arousal and feeling an emotion occur at the same time, not in sequence. Thus, severing the feedback should not alter the emotion experienced. In this theory, a person will respond with action after experiencing the emotion both mentally and physically. Bard, a student of Cannon's, further explained that when exposed to a stimulus, sensory information is received and sent to both the cortex and the sympathetic nervous system simultaneously by the thalamus. Thus, the **Cannon–Bard theory of emotion**, depicted in Figure 5.10, states that the conscious experience of emotion and physiological arousal occur simultaneously, and then the behavioral component of emotion (i.e., action) follows: *I see a snake, so I feel afraid and my heart is racing . . . Let me out of here!*

While critics of the James–Lange theory cite the severed afferent nerve study as support for the Cannon–Bard theory, there are also weaknesses in this theory. The Cannon–Bard theory fails to explain the vagus nerve, a cranial nerve that functions as a feedback system, conveying information from the peripheral organs back to the central nervous system.

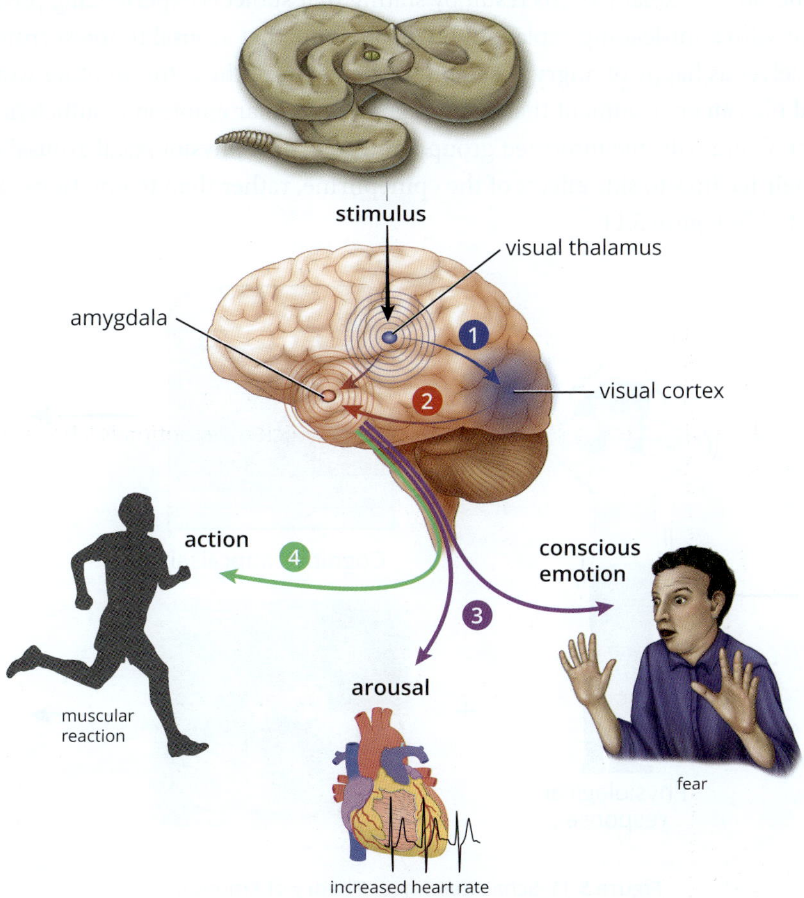

Figure 5.10 Cannon–Bard Theory of Emotion
Visual stimuli pass through the thalamus, and rough information is sent to the amygdala (fear) and the sympathetic nervous system (arousal). Action (muscle contraction) quickly follows. The visual cortex can either strengthen or quell this fear response once it has identified the stimulus.

Schachter–Singer Theory

A third theory is the **Schachter–Singer theory of emotion**, also termed the **cognitive arousal theory** or the **two-factor theory**, which states that two factors (physiological arousal and a cognitive label) are needed to experience emotion. According to this theory, physiological arousal alone is insufficient to elicit an emotional response. To feel an emotion, the mind must also identify the environmental stimulus causing that physiological arousal: *I am excited because my heart is racing and everyone else is happy*.

MCAT EXPERTISE

The MCAT will expect that you have a solid understanding of the differences in emotional processing described by each of the three theories of emotion. It is best to mentally sort these theories by "first response" and "second response" to the stimulus.

What is unique to the Schachter–Singer theory is this aspect of cognitive appraisal: to feel an emotion, one must consciously analyze the environment in relation to nervous system arousal. To study this phenomenon, Stanley Schachter and Jerome Singer gave injections of epinephrine or placebo to groups of subjects that were either informed, ignorant, or misinformed. They also manipulated external cues in the study by having an actor act either happy or angry. They observed that epinephrine did result in increased physiological arousal; however, they also discovered that the environment and cognitive processing affected the emotion experienced by the subjects. The groups who were misinformed or ignorant experienced the highest levels of emotion. Schachter and Singer explained this result by stating that subjects experiencing physiological arousal with no explanation or with a misleading explanation will attribute that arousal to the surrounding environment, and label themselves as happy or angry based on the behavior of the actor. In other words, the presence of unexpected arousal plus an environment that encourages a particular emotion is sufficient to create that emotion in the subject. Contrarily, the informed group knew to expect physiological arousal from the drug, and thus attributed their feelings to side effects of the epinephrine, rather than to emotions. The Schachter-Singer theory is depicted in Figure 5.11.

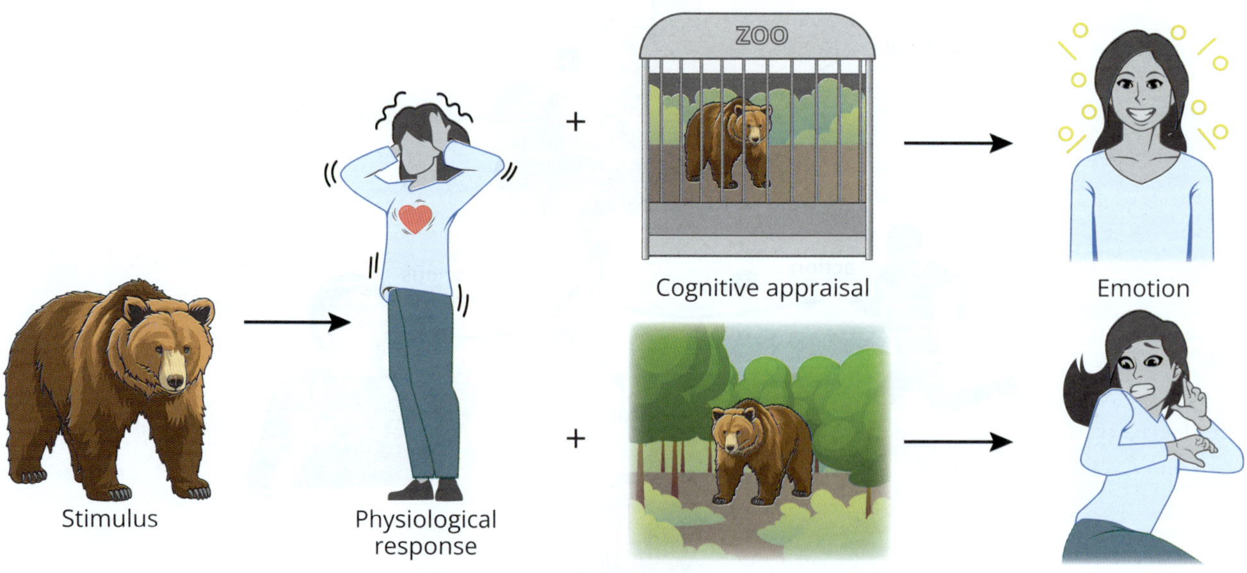

Figure 5.11 Schachter-Singer Theory of Emotion

The three theories of emotion discussed in this section are summarized in Table 5.2.

Theory		First Response	Second Response
James–Lange	**Stimulus**	Nervous system arousal	Conscious emotion
Cannon–Bard	**Stimulus**	Nervous system arousal and conscious emotion	Action
Schachter–Singer	**Stimulus**	Nervous system arousal and cognitive appraisal	Conscious emotion

Table 5.2 Theories of Emotion

The Limbic System

Experiencing emotion is a complex process involving many parts of the brain. The most notable of these circuits is the **limbic system**, a complex set of structures that reside below the cerebrum on either side of the thalamus, as shown in Figure 5.12. The system is made up of the amygdala, thalamus, hypothalamus, hippocampus and fornix, septal nuclei, and parts of the cerebral cortex; it plays a large role in both motivation and emotion.

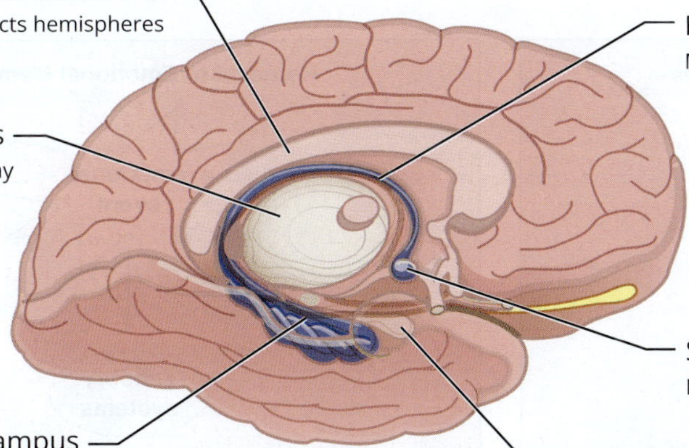

Figure 5.12 The Limbic System

REAL WORLD

When specific areas of the limbic system are stimulated during brain surgery, patients have described sensations such as happiness, contentment, and pleasure; in other areas, they report fear and anxiety.

REAL WORLD

Research on rats has shown that when the amygdalae are damaged, the rats can no longer be classically conditioned to establish new fears. Similar effects have also been seen in humans wherein damage to this region prevents fear conditioning. This has been measured by autonomic nervous system responses as well as functional imaging.

The **amygdala** is a small round structure that signals the cortex about stimuli related to attention and emotions. The amygdala processes the environment, detects external cues, and learns from the person's surroundings in order to produce emotion. This region is associated with fear and also plays a role in human emotion through interpretation of facial expressions.

The **thalamus** functions as a preliminary sensory processing station and routes information to the cortex and other appropriate areas of the brain. The **hypothalamus**, located below the thalamus, synthesizes and releases a variety of neurotransmitters. It serves many homeostatic functions, and is involved in modulating emotion. Indeed, by controlling the neurotransmitters that affect mood and arousal, the hypothalamus largely dictates emotional states.

The **hippocampus**, within the temporal lobe, is primarily involved in creating long-term memories. Along with the functions of the amygdala and hypothalamus, the storage and retrieval of emotional memories is key in producing an emotional response. The hippocampus also aids in creating context for stimuli to lead to an emotional experience. As described in Chapter 3 of *MCAT Behavioral Sciences Review*, memory systems can be divided into two categories: explicit and implicit. When an emotion is experienced, sensory systems transmit this information into both the explicit memory system, primarily controlled by the hippocampus in the medial temporal lobe, and the implicit memory system, controlled by the amygdala. Both memory systems are used for both the formation and retrieval of emotional memories, as shown in Figure 5.13. The conscious (explicit) memory is the memory of experiencing the actual emotion: remembering that you were happy at your high school graduation or that you were sad when you lost a loved one is explicit memory. Note that these are episodic memories: they are more properly considered memories *about* emotions than stored emotions. The unconscious (implicit) memory is referred to as **emotional memory**; this is the storage of the actual feelings of emotion associated with an event. When experiencing a similar event later on, these emotions may be retrieved. Thus, explicit memory of the emotion produces a conscious memory of the experience, and implicit memory determines the expression of past emotions. This distinction can be further identified when looking at individuals with posttraumatic stress disorder (PTSD). The explicit memory is the "story" of the event: what happened, where it occurred, who was involved, the fact that the scenario was traumatic, and so forth. The implicit memory corresponds to the sensations of unease and anxiety when put back into a similar environment.

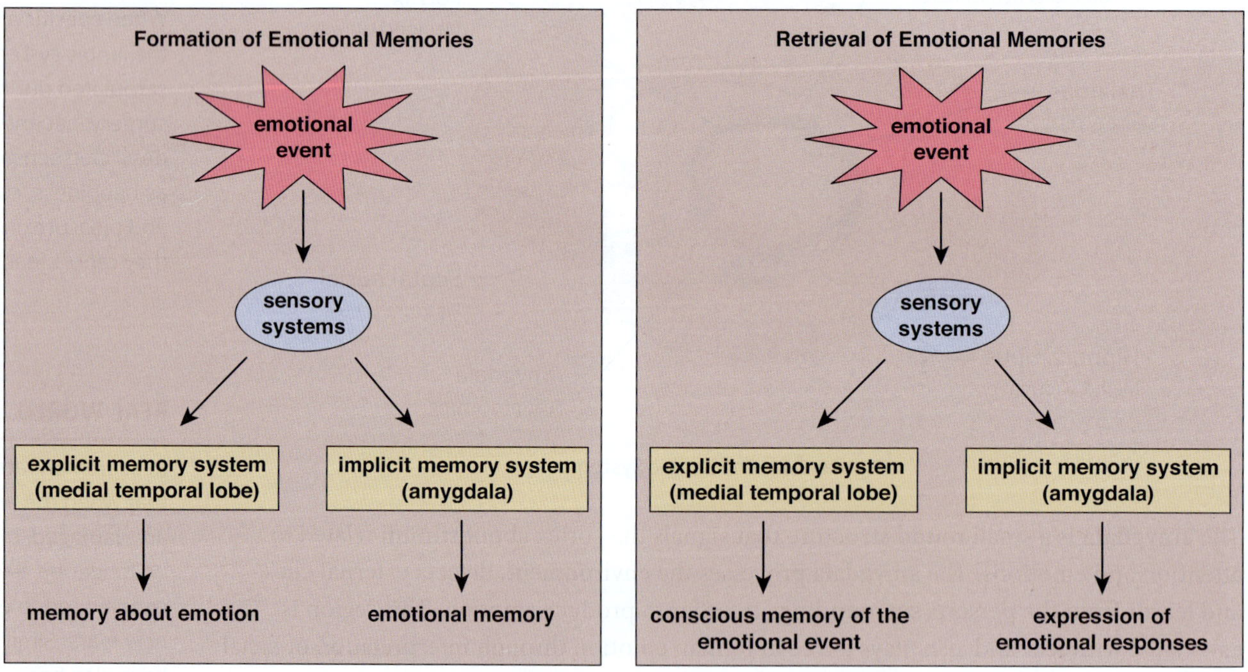

Figure 5.13 Formation and Retrieval of Emotional Memories

The ability to distinguish and interpret others' facial expressions is primarily controlled by the temporal lobe, with some input from the occipital lobe. This function is lateralized: the right hemisphere is more active when discerning facial expressions than the left. There are also gender differences: women demonstrate more activation of these brain areas than men. This ability is present but weak in children and develops into adulthood; adults are much more effective at identifying both positive and negative emotions.

The **prefrontal cortex** is the anterior portion of the frontal lobes and is associated with planning intricate cognitive functions, expressing personality, and making decisions. The prefrontal cortex also receives arousal input from the brainstem, coordinating arousal and cognitive states. It has been demonstrated that the left prefrontal cortex is associated with positive emotions and the right prefrontal cortex with negative emotions. The **dorsal prefrontal cortex** is associated with attention and cognition, while the **ventral prefrontal cortex** connects with regions of the brain responsible for experiencing emotion. Specifically, the **ventromedial prefrontal cortex**, shown in Figure 5.14, is thought to play a substantial role in decision making and controlling emotional responses from the amygdala.

REAL WORLD

One of the most notable studies on prefrontal cortex function is that of Phineas Gage. Gage was involved in an accident in which a metal rod pierced his brain, destroying the left frontal lobe. Gage's memory, speech, and motor skills were unaffected, but his personality was dramatically altered. Post-accident, Gage displayed irritable and impatient behavior, which inhibited his ability to complete simple tasks.

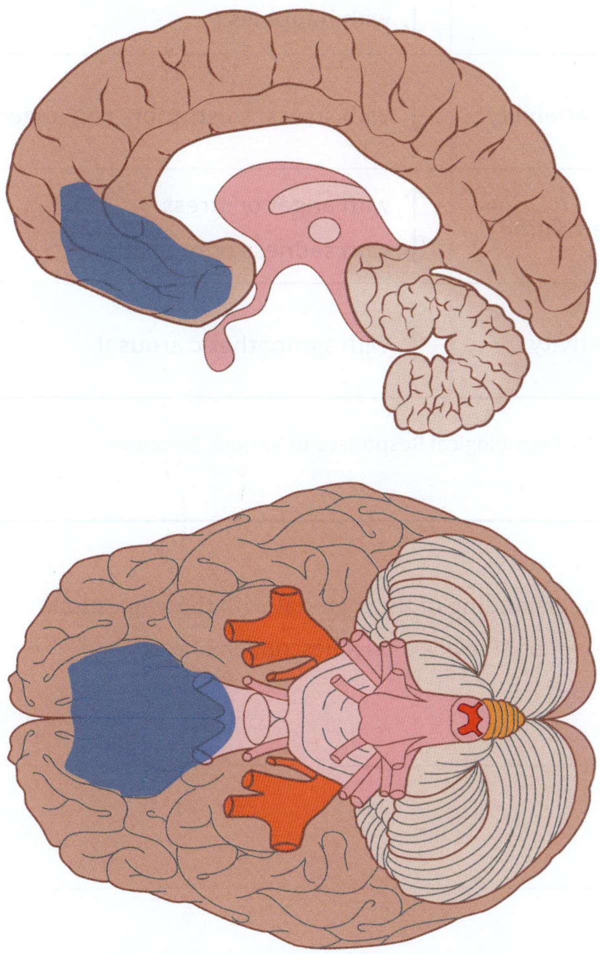

Figure 5.14 Ventromedial Prefrontal Cortex
The ventromedial prefrontal cortex is highlighted in blue.

As described earlier, the **autonomic nervous system** is also related to emotion; specific physiological reactions are associated with specific emotions. Skin temperature, heart rate, breathing rate, and blood pressure are all affected when experiencing emotion. Decreased skin temperature is detected in subjects experiencing fear, while increased skin temperature is associated with anger. Increased heart rate is observed in subjects experiencing both anger and fear, while decreased heart rate is observed in subjects who are feeling happiness. Heart rate variability is another factor used to determine emotion. Decreased heart rate variability is associated with stress, frustration, and anger. Blood pulse volume increases with anger or stress and decreases with sadness or relaxation. Skin conductivity is directly correlated with sympathetic arousal; however, a specific emotion cannot be identified by skin response. Diastolic blood pressure is increased to the greatest degree by anger, followed by fear, sadness, and happiness. See Figure 5.15 for a simplified look at all these physiological changes to different emotions.

Skin temperature	↓ with **fear** ↑ with **anger**
Heart rate	↑ with **anger** and **fear** ↓ with **happiness**
Heart rate variability	↓ with **stress, frustration**, and **anger**
Blood pulse volume	↑ with **anger** or **stress** ↓ with **sadness** or **relaxation**
Skin conductivity	↑ with **sympathetic arousal**

Figure 5.15 Physiological Responses to Various Emotions

MCAT CONCEPT CHECK 5.2

Before you move on, assess your understanding of the material with these questions.

1. What are the three elements of emotion? Provide a brief description of each.

2. What are the seven universal emotions?

-

-

-

-

-

-

3. Compare and contrast the James–Lange, Cannon–Bard, and Schachter–Singer theories of emotion:

James–Lange Theory	Cannon–Bard Theory	Schachter–Singer Theory

What is the function of each part of the limbic system listed below?

- Amygdala:
- Thalamus:
- Hypothalamus:
- Hippocampus:
- Ventromedial prefrontal cortex:

5.3 Stress High Yield

LEARNING OBJECTIVES

After Chapter 5.3, you will be able to:

- Distinguish between primary and secondary appraisals of stress
- Recall the three stages of general adaptation syndrome and the physiological changes associated with each stage
- Recognize common stressors and effective techniques for management of stress

In all aspects of life, at all times of day, we must make decisions, overcome challenges, and continue forward. While some of these decisions are small, others require planning and adaptation to new circumstances. Behavior of others and the perception of our surroundings affect our behavior and mental state, at times in a negative manner. It is our response to challenging events, be they physical, emotional, cognitive, or behavioral, that defines **stress**.

Cognitive Appraisal of Stress

Cognitive appraisal is the subjective evaluation of a situation that induces stress. This process consists of two stages, both of which are depicted in Figure 5.16. Stage 1, or **primary appraisal**, is the initial evaluation of the environment and the associated threat. This appraisal can be identified as irrelevant, benign–positive, or stressful. If primary appraisal reveals a threat, stage 2 appraisal begins. **Secondary appraisal** is directed at evaluating whether the organism can cope with the stress. This appraisal involves the evaluation of three things: harm, or damage caused by the event; threat, or the potential for future damage caused by the event; and challenge, or the potential to overcome and possibly benefit from the event. Individuals who perceive themselves as having the ability to cope with the event experience less stress than those who don't. In general, appraisal and stress level are personal, as individuals have different skills, abilities, and coping mechanisms. For example, while a spider might incite fear and stress in some, it would result in irrelevant appraisal in others. Some situations require ongoing monitoring through constant **reappraisal**, such as the perception of being followed.

MCAT EXPERTISE

The MCAT will expect you to know the two stages of stress appraisal: primary and secondary. Primary appraisal is the initial examination, which results in the identification of the stress as irrelevant, benign–positive, or stressful. If identified as a threat, secondary appraisal is an evaluation of one's ability to cope with the stress.

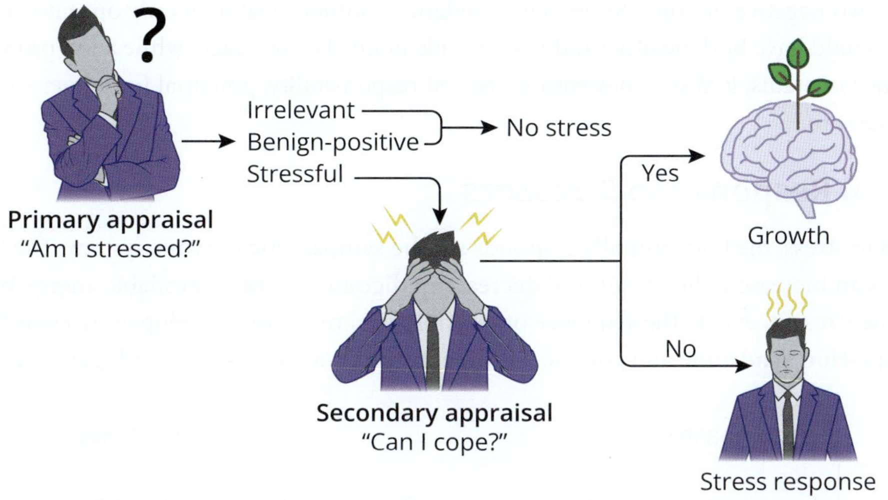

Figure 5.16 The Two Stages of Stress Appraisal

Types of Stressors

A **stressor** is a biological element, external condition, or event that leads to a stress response. The severity of stressors can range from minimal or irritating hassles, like temporarily lost keys, to catastrophic scenarios, such as an impending natural disaster. Common stressors include:

- Environmental factors: uncomfortable temperature, loud sounds, inclement weather
- Daily events: running late, losing items, unexpected occurrences
- Workplace or academic setting: assignments, hierarchical interactions, time management
- Social expectations: demands placed on oneself by society, family, and friends
- Chemical and biological stressors: diet, alcohol, drugs, viruses, allergies, medications, medical conditions

Stressors are classified as either causing distress or causing eustress. **Distress** occurs when a stressor is perceived as unpleasant (e.g., a threat), whereas **eustress** is the result of a positively-perceived stressor (e.g., a challenge). Eustress can include life events such as graduating from college, studying to achieve a high score on the MCAT, getting married, or buying a house. While these events are largely positive, any event requiring individuals to change or adapt their lifestyle leads to stress. Stress level can be measured in "life change units" in a system called the **social readjustment rating scale**.

Stressors can also be psychological. Pressure, control, predictability, frustration, and conflict are all forms of psychological stress. Pressure is experienced when expectations or demands are put in place from external sources; this produces a feeling of urgency to complete tasks, perform actions, or display particular behaviors. The ability to control one's surroundings typically reduces stress levels; the inability to control a situation or event increases stress. In a study of nursing home patients, it was observed that those who had the most control of their daily environment displayed more active, positive, and social behavior. Predictability also plays a role in stress levels. For example, firefighters and police officers who cannot predict their daily scenarios experience higher levels of stress on the job. Frustration, which occurs when attaining a goal or need is prevented, increases stress. These frustration stresses can be external, such as not getting a raise, or internal, such as a disability interfering with everyday life. Finally, conflict stresses arise from the need to make a choice. Approach–approach conflict refers to the need to choose between two desirable options. Avoidance–avoidance conflicts are choices between two negative options. Approach–avoidance conflicts deal with only one choice, goal, or event, but the outcome could have both positive and negative elements. For instance, while a job promotion might mean more money or status, it also comes with increased responsibility, potential for longer working hours, and increased pressure.

Physiological Response to Stressors

When subjected to stress, the body initially responds via the sympathetic nervous system. The "fight-or-flight" response initiates an increase in heart rate and decrease in digestion, with all available energy being reserved for reacting to the stressful event. The sequence of physiological responses developed by Hans Selye is called the **general adaptation syndrome** and consists of three distinct stages, as shown in Figure 5.17.

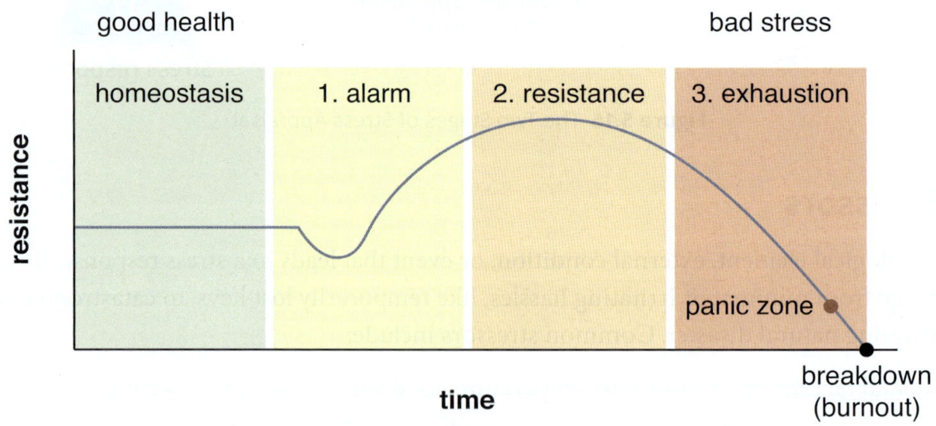

Figure 5.17 Three Stages of Stress Response

First is **alarm**, or the initial reaction to a stressor and the activation of the sympathetic nervous system. Shortly thereafter, the hypothalamus stimulates the pituitary to secrete adrenocorticotropic hormone (ACTH). This hormone stimulates the adrenal glands to produce cortisol, which maintains the steady supply of blood sugar needed to respond to stressful events. The hypothalamus also activates the adrenal medulla, which secretes epinephrine and norepinephrine to activate the sympathetic nervous system. The next stage is **resistance**, in which the continuous release of hormones allows the sympathetic nervous system to remain engaged to fight the stressor. Last, a person will experience **exhaustion** when the body can no longer maintain an elevated response with sympathetic nervous system activity. At this point, individuals become more susceptible to illnesses and medical conditions (such as ulcers and high blood pressure), organ systems can begin to deteriorate (with effects including heart disease), and in extreme cases, death can result. Some of the positive and negative effects of stress are shown in Table 5.3.

Organ System	Acute Stress	Chronic Stress
Nervous system	Increased alertness, decreased pain perception	Memory problems, heightened risk of depressive disorders
Endocrine system	Adrenals secrete cortisol and other hormones to increase available energy	Slowed recovery from stress response due to high levels of cortisol and other hormones
Immune system	Thymus and other glands and tissues primed for immune response	Diminished immune response
Circulatory system	Increased heart rate, vasoconstriction to direct more oxygen to muscle tissue	High blood pressure, heightened risk of cardiovascular disorders
Reproductive system	Temporary suppression of functions	Heightened risk of infertility or miscarriage

Table 5.3 Positive and Negative Effects of Stress

Emotional and Behavioral Responses to Stress

Beyond the effects on the human body, stress also takes a psychological toll on people who are unable to reduce their stress levels. On the emotional level, elevated stress can result in individuals feeling irritable, moody, tense, fearful, and helpless. They may also have difficulties with concentration and memory. Negative behavior responses to stress include withdrawing from others, difficulties at work or at school, substance use, aggression, and suicide. Additionally, chronic stress can lead to mental health disorders. The **diathesis-stress model** proposes that individuals have a predisposition to a set of biological or genetic traits (diatheses), and exposure to environmental conditions (stressors) may trigger disorders like schizophrenia and depression.

Coping and Stress Management

Strategies for coping with stress fall into two groups. **Problem-focused strategies** involve working to overcome a stressor, such as reaching out to family and friends for social support, confronting the issue head-on, and creating and following a plan of problem-solving actions. **Emotion-focused strategies** center on changing one's feelings about a stressor. They include taking responsibility for the issue, engaging in self-control, distancing oneself from the issue, engaging in wishful thinking, and using positive reappraisal to focus on positive outcomes instead of the stressor. Figure 5.18 provides helpful images for remembering these two coping approaches. Some coping strategies are **adaptive**, and reduce stress in a healthy way. A person who is feeling stressed could, for example, reach out to a loved one for help as a support-seeking coping strategy. However, coping strategies may also be **maladaptive** and include detrimental tactics, such as turning to drugs or alcohol.

BRIDGE

Maladaptiveness is a key factor in determining whether a behavior should be considered a disorder. Maladaptive behaviors are discussed in more detail in Chapter 7 of *MCAT Behavioral Sciences Review*.

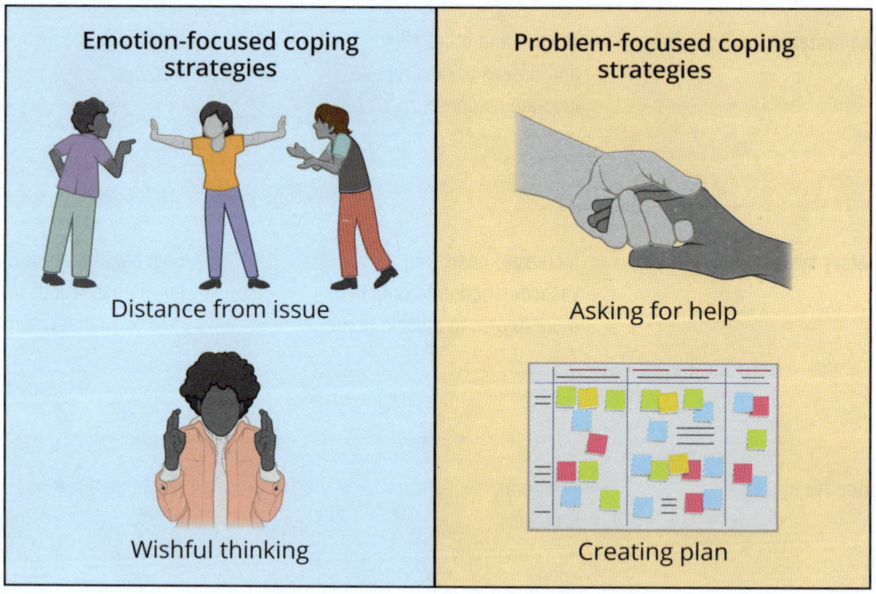

Figure 5.18 Coping Strategies

Individuals can also engage in stress management to reduce their stress levels. Exercise is a powerful stress management tool that not only improves health and well-being, but also enhances mood. Exercise releases endorphins, opioid neuropeptides that act as "feel-good" neurotransmitters. Relaxation techniques, including meditation, diaphragmatic breathing, and progressive muscle relaxation have also been found to reduce stress. Additionally, studies have shown that engaging in a spiritual practice helps to manage stress.

MCAT EXPERTISE

Use these coping and stress management techniques to boost your performance (and mood) on Test Day!

Lastly, there are two more strategies for handling stress that the MCAT wants you to know for Test Day. The first of these is **stress inoculation training**. This is a cognitive behavioral practice primarily focused on preparing people to handle stressful situations with less of an emphasis on attending to the current moment. On the other hand, **mindfulness meditation** is a practice that requires focusing attention on the present moment along with all the current thoughts, feelings, and sensations. This method would be the most effective stress reduction technique for an individual who always thinks about the past or the future.

MCAT CONCEPT CHECK 5.3

Before you move on, assess your understanding of the material with these questions.

1. What are the key features of primary and secondary cognitive appraisal of stress?
   - Primary appraisal:

   ___

   - Secondary appraisal:

   ___

2. What are the three stages of the general adaptation syndrome? What physiological changes are evident in each stage?

Stage	Physiological Changes

3. What are some common stressors? What are some effective techniques for managing stress?
   - Common stressors:

   ___

   - Stress management techniques:

   ___

   ___

   ___

Conclusion

The ability to strive for our goals and desires, be it for internal or external reasons, is an important aspect of psychology and behavior. Motivation is the mechanism used to meet our needs, act toward an end goal, and ultimately survive. While there are many factors that influence motivation, including instincts, arousal, drives, and needs, they all result in action to obtain perceived rewards, fulfill needs, or avoid perceived punishments. Emotion is a complex process resulting in physiological, cognitive, and behavioral elements, described in different fashions by the James–Lange, Cannon–Bard, and Schachter–Singer theories of emotion. Many components of the nervous system play a role in experiencing emotions, including the seven universal emotions. The response of the body and mind to challenges defines stress. Stress appraisal has phases that identify and allow the body to respond to the stressor encountered. The physical and mental response to stress can be severe, but there are many management and coping mechanisms commonly used to reduce the level of stress experienced.

Hopefully this chapter has left you motivated to keep working toward that goal of an excellent MCAT score and becoming the doctor you deserve to be. Studying for the MCAT certainly introduces a significant stress, but effective stress management techniques and a solid foundation in MCAT content and strategy will turn Test Day into eustress. Just keep your eyes on that white coat, an important garment that will someday be part of your identity—a topic we'll explore in the next chapter.

GO ONLINE

You've reviewed the content, now test your knowledge and critical thinking skills by completing a test-like passage set in your online resources!

CONCEPT SUMMARY

Motivation

- **Motivation** is the purpose, or driving force, behind our actions.
- Motivation can be **extrinsic**, based on external circumstances; or **intrinsic**, based on internal drive or perception.
- The primary factors that influence motivation are instincts, arousal, drives, and needs.
  - **Instincts** are innate, fixed patterns of behavior. In the **instinct theory** of motivation, people perform certain behaviors because of these evolutionarily programmed instincts.
  - In the **arousal theory**, people perform actions to maintain **arousal**, the state of being awake and reactive to stimuli, at an optimal level. The **Yerkes–Dodson law** shows that performance is optimal at a medium level of arousal.
  - **Drives** are internal states of tension that beget particular behaviors focused on goals. Primary drives are related to bodily processes; secondary drives stem from learning and include accomplishments and emotions. **Drive reduction theory** states that motivation arises from the desire to eliminate drives, which create uncomfortable internal states.
  - Satisfying **needs** may also motivate. **Maslow's hierarchy of needs** prioritizes needs into five categories: physiological needs (highest priority), safety and security, love and belonging, self-esteem, and self-actualization (lowest priority).
  - **Self-determination theory** emphasizes the role of three universal needs: autonomy, competence, and relatedness.
- **Incentive theory** explains motivation as the desire to pursue rewards and avoid punishments.
- **Expectancy–value theory** states that the amount of motivation for a task is based on the individual's expectation of success and the amount that success is valued.
- **Opponent-process theory** explains motivation for drug use: as drug use increases, the body counteracts its effects, leading to tolerance and uncomfortable withdrawal symptoms.
- Sexual motivation is related to hormones as well as cultural and social factors.

Emotion

- **Emotion** is a state of mind, or feeling, that is subjectively experienced based on circumstances, mood, and relationships.
- The three components of emotion are **cognitive** (subjective), **behavioral** (facial expressions and body language), and **physiological** (changes in the autonomic nervous system).
- The **seven universal emotions** are happiness, sadness, contempt, surprise, fear, disgust, and anger.
- There are multiple theories of emotion, based on the interactions of the three components of emotion.
  - In the **James–Lange theory**, nervous system arousal leads to an emotional experience.
  - In the **Cannon–Bard theory**, arousal of the nervous system and the experience of emotion occur simultaneously.
  - In the **Schachter–Singer theory**, nervous system arousal is combined with cognition to create the experience of emotion.

- The **limbic system** is the primary nervous system component involved in experiencing emotion.
  - The **amygdala** is involved with attention and fear, helps interpret facial expressions, and is part of the intrinsic memory system for emotional memory.
  - The **thalamus** is a sensory processing station.
  - The **hypothalamus** releases neurotransmitters that affect mood and arousal.
  - The **hippocampus** creates long-term explicit (episodic) memories.
  - The **prefrontal cortex** is involved with planning, expressing personality, and making decisions. The **ventral prefrontal cortex** is critical for experiencing emotion; the **ventromedial prefrontal cortex**, specifically, is involved in controlling emotional responses from the amygdala and decision making.

Stress

- The physiological and cognitive response to challenges or life changes is defined as **stress**.
- Stress appraisal has two stages:
  - **Primary appraisal** is classifying a potential stressor as irrelevant, benign–positive, or stressful.
  - **Secondary appraisal** is directed at evaluating if the organism can cope with the stress, based on harm, threat, and challenge.
- A **stressor** is anything that leads to a stress response and can include environment, daily events, workplace or academic settings, social expectations, chemicals, and biological stressors. Psychological stressors include pressure, control, predictability, frustration, and conflict.
- Stressors can lead to **distress** or **eustress**.
- The three stages of the **general adaptation syndrome** are alarm, resistance, and exhaustion.
- Stress management can include psychological, behavioral, and spiritual aspects.

ANSWERS TO CONCEPT CHECKS

5.1

1.

Theory	Factor for Motivation
Instinct theory	Instincts: innate, fixed patterns of behavior in response to stimuli
Arousal theory	Maintaining a constant level of arousal, the psychological and physiological state of being awake and reactive to stimuli
Drive reduction theory	Drives: internal states of tension or discomfort that can be relieved with a particular action
Need-based theories	Needs: factors necessary for physiological function or emotional fulfillment

2. Physiological needs, safety and security, love and belonging, self-esteem, self-actualization
3. Cocaine is a stimulant, causing euphoria, restlessness, increased heart rate, increased temperature, and anxiety. According to opponent-process theory, cocaine withdrawal should be the opposite: depressed mood, fatigue, decreased heart rate, decreased temperature, and apathy.

5.2

1. The three elements of emotion are as follows:
   - Physiological response (autonomic nervous system): heart rate, breathing rate, skin temperature, blood pressure
   - Behavioral response: facial expressions, body language
   - Cognitive response: subjective interpretation, memories of past experiences, perception of cause of emotion
2. The seven universal emotions are happiness, sadness, contempt, surprise, fear, disgust, and anger.

3.

James–Lange Theory	Cannon–Bard Theory	Schachter–Singer Theory
• Stimulus leads to physiological arousal • Arousal leads to the conscious experience of emotion • *My skin is hot and my blood pressure is high so I must be angry* • Requires connection between sympathetic nervous system and brain	• Stimulus leads to physiological arousal and feeling of emotion • Thalamus processes sensory information, sends it to cortex and sympathetic nervous system • Action is secondary response to stimulus • *I see a snake, so I am afraid and my heart is racing... Let me out of here!* • Does not explain vagus nerve	• Both arousal and labeling based on environment are required to experience an emotion • *I am excited because my heart is racing and everyone else is happy*

4. The amygdala is involved with attention and emotions (specifically fear), helps interpret facial expressions, and is part of the intrinsic memory system for emotional memory. The thalamus is a sensory processing station. The hypothalamus releases neurotransmitters that affect mood and arousal. The hippocampus creates long-term explicit memories (episodic memories). The ventromedial prefrontal cortex is involved in decision making and controlling emotional responses from the amygdala.

5.3

1. Primary appraisal is categorizing the stressor as irrelevant, benign–positive, or stressful. Secondary appraisal is the evaluation of the ability of the organism to cope with that stress.

2.

Stage	Physiological Changes
Alarm	Activation of sympathetic nervous system, release of ACTH and cortisol, stimulation of adrenal medulla to secrete epinephrine and norepinephrine
Resistance	Continuous release of hormones activates sympathetic nervous system
Exhaustion	Can no longer maintain elevated sympathetic nervous system activity, more susceptible to illness and medical conditions, organ systems deteriorate, death

3. Common stressors include environmental or physical discomfort, daily events, workplace or academic setting, social expectations, and chemical and biological stressors. Effective stress management techniques include exercise, relaxation techniques (meditation, diaphragmatic breathing, progressive muscle relaxation), spiritual practice, and many more.

SCIENCE MASTERY ASSESSMENT EXPLANATIONS

1. **A**

Due to the competitive nature of the motivation, this is considered extrinsic motivation. Extrinsic motivation is based on external conditions, including perceived reward or fear of punishment. In this case, the reward is beating the sibling. There is no suggestion of an uncomfortable internal state or tension, which is an aspect of drives, eliminating **(C)** and **(D)**.

2. **D**

The Yerkes–Dodson law states that there is an optimal level of arousal necessary to perform. If levels of arousal are too high, poor performance can result. In the case of this student performing at a recital, arousal level is very high as a result of nervousness and anxiety, resulting in a poor performance.

3. **A**

Drive reduction theory is the theory that one will act to eliminate uncomfortable internal states known as drives. The body will push toward equilibrium, or homeostasis.

4. **A**

The seven universal emotions are happiness, sadness, contempt, surprise, fear, disgust, and anger.

5. **C**

The three components of emotion are the physiological (changes in the autonomic nervous system), cognitive (subjective interpretation of an emotion), and behavioral (facial expressions and body language) responses.

6. **D**

Experiencing a physiological reaction to a stimulus and then labeling that response as emotion is in line with the James–Lange theory of emotion. In the statement, seeing the bear is the stimulus, an increase in heart rate and breathing rate is the physiological reaction, and identifying this as fear is the emotion experienced.

7. **C**

According to Darwin's theory of evolution, all species have instincts that help them survive. The instinct theory of motivation states that people are motivated to act based on instincts that they are programmed to exhibit.

8. **D**

The Cannon–Bard theory of emotion is based on the premise that conscious feelings and physiological components of emotion are experienced at exactly the same time. In this theory, this combination then leads to action. This is commonly confused with the Schachter–Singer theory, **(A)**, in which nervous system arousal occurs and then is labeled based on the context provided by the environment.

9. **C**

The amygdala, prefrontal cortex, and thalamus all play a role in the experience of emotions. The basal ganglia are involved in smooth movement and are not primarily responsible for the experience of emotions.

10. **A**

The left frontal lobe is associated with positive feelings, corresponding with joy and happiness. The right frontal lobe is associated with negative feelings, such as sadness and disgust, **(B)** and **(D)**.

11. **B**

Secondary appraisal of stress is the stage at which the ability of the organism to cope with the stressor is evaluated. This is based on the harm, threat, and challenge of the stressor, which are all correlated with its intensity. Primary appraisal is simply the initial determination of whether there is a negative association at all, not its intensity.

12. **D**

A positive stressor creates eustress. Because working out is used to relax, it is considered a eustress. Hassle, **(A)**, and frustration, **(B)**, are both types of distress, **(C)**, or negative stressors.

13. **A**

Approach–approach conflict is one in which both results are good outcomes. While one must be chosen, neither choice results in a negative outcome: for example, choosing between two desserts. Avoidance–escape conflict, **(D)**, is not a recognized form of conflict; these two terms are related to types of negative reinforcers.

14. **A**

The initial reaction to stress, which is activation of the sympathetic nervous system, is the alarm stage of stress response.

15. **C**

Progressive muscle relaxation is a relaxation technique demonstrated to help reduce stress in a manner that is beneficial to the body and psyche. The other methods described here, including avoidance of the stressor, **(D)**, serve to increase stress or merely change the source of the stress.

GO ONLINE

Consult your online resources for additional practice.

SHARED CONCEPTS

Behavioral Sciences Chapter 1
Biology and Behavior

Behavioral Sciences Chapter 3
Learning and Memory

Behavioral Sciences Chapter 7
Psychological Disorders

Biology Chapter 4
The Nervous System

Biology Chapter 5
The Endocrine System

Biology Chapter 10
Homeostasis

CHAPTER 6

IDENTITY AND PERSONALITY

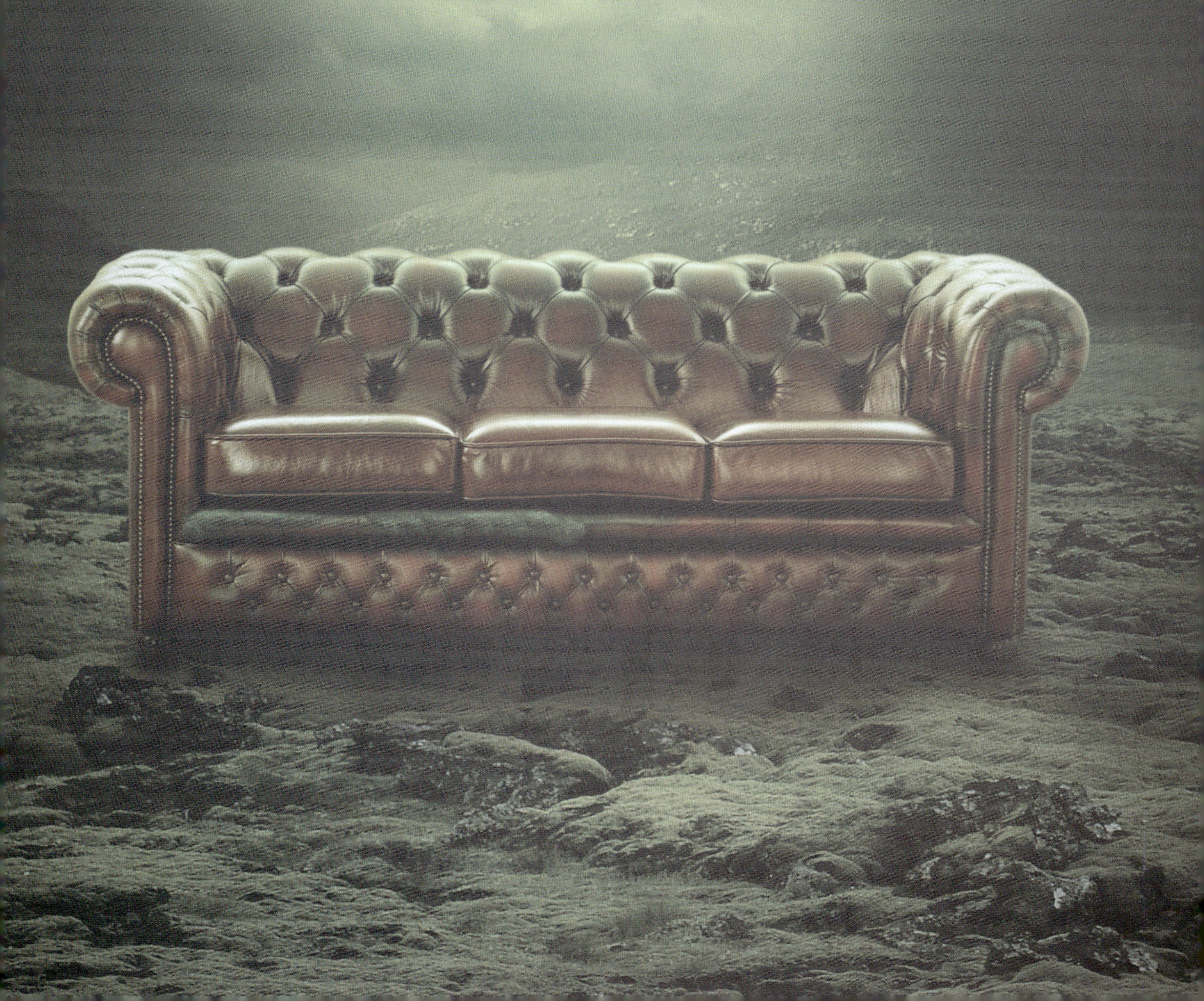

SCIENCE MASTERY ASSESSMENT

Every pre-med knows this feeling: there is so much content I have to know for the MCAT! How do I know what to do first or what's important?

While the high-yield badges throughout this book will help you identify the most important topics, this Science Mastery Assessment is another tool in your MCAT prep arsenal. This quiz (which can also be taken in your online resources) and the guidance below will help ensure that you are spending the appropriate amount of time on this chapter based on your personal strengths and weaknesses. Don't worry though—skipping something now does not mean you'll never study it. Later on in your prep, as you complete full-length tests, you'll uncover specific pieces of content that you need to review and can come back to these chapters as appropriate.

How to Use This Assessment

If you answer 0–7 questions correctly:

Spend about 1 hour to read this chapter in full and take limited notes throughout. Follow up by reviewing **all** quiz questions to ensure that you now understand how to solve each one.

If you answer 8–11 questions correctly:

Spend 20–40 minutes reviewing the quiz questions. Beginning with the questions you missed, read and take notes on the corresponding subchapters. For questions you answered correctly, ensure your thinking matches that of the explanation and you understand why each choice was correct or incorrect.

If you answer 12–15 questions correctly:

Spend less than 20 minutes reviewing all questions from the quiz. If you missed any, then include a quick read-through of the corresponding subchapters, or even just the relevant content within a subchapter, as part of your question review. For questions you answered correctly, ensure your thinking matches that of the explanation and review the Concept Summary at the end of the chapter.

1. Each of the following is considered a part of a person's self-concept EXCEPT:
   - **A.** the past self.
   - **B.** the ought self.
   - **C.** the future self.
   - **D.** self-schemata.

2. As a gender identity, androgyny is defined as:
   - **A.** low femininity, low masculinity.
   - **B.** high femininity, low masculinity.
   - **C.** low femininity, high masculinity.
   - **D.** high femininity, high masculinity.

3. A high school student struggles consistently with math and feels that no amount of studying will help because "I just don't get it." Which of the following is the most likely short-term result with respect to the student's ability to do math?
   - **A.** Low self-esteem
   - **B.** Low self-efficacy
   - **C.** Learned helplessness
   - **D.** An external locus of control

4. A district attorney with an internal locus of control wins an important court trial. Which of the following best represents the lawyer's attribution of the events?
   - **A.** "I won because I made great arguments and had more experience than the defense."
   - **B.** "I won because the jury was on my side from the beginning and believed my arguments."
   - **C.** "I won because the defense did not adequately present their side of the case."
   - **D.** "I shouldn't have won because I don't deserve to be successful."

5. A person keeps an extremely tidy desk and becomes very nervous whenever things are disorganized or out of place. In which of the following stages would a psychodynamic therapist say this person had become fixated?
   - **A.** The oral stage
   - **B.** The anal stage
   - **C.** The phallic stage
   - **D.** The genital stage

6. According to Erikson's stages of psychosocial development, which of the following would be the most important for a recent college graduate to accomplish?
   - **A.** Figuring out what identities are most important personally
   - **B.** Feeling like a contributing member of society
   - **C.** Forming an intimate relationship with a significant other
   - **D.** Finding a feeling of accomplishment in life

7. Matt and Cati discuss the reasons why they avoid driving above the speed limit. Matt cites wanting to avoid a traffic fine, while Cati says that speeding is dangerous and, if everyone did it, there would be more accidents and people would get hurt. According to Kohlberg, which of the following describes the phases of moral reasoning demonstrated by Matt and Cati, respectively?
   - **A.** Preconventional; conventional
   - **B.** Preconventional; postconventional
   - **C.** Conventional; preconventional
   - **D.** Postconventional; conventional

8. A child cannot make an origami swan alone, but is able to do so when observing and being assisted by an adult. This scenario is described in the ideas of which of the following theorists?

- **A.** Albert Bandura
- **B.** Alfred Adler
- **C.** B. F. Skinner
- **D.** Lev Vygotsky

9. Which of the following is a conclusion that can be made from research in role-taking and observational learning?

- **A.** Young children will only model actions performed by their parents.
- **B.** Celebrities and athletes are an adolescent's most important role models.
- **C.** Children who role-take identities that are not gender typical are more likely to take on those roles later in life.
- **D.** A female child is more likely to model the behavior of another female than a male.

10. A person feels extremely guilty after having an extramarital affair. According to the psychodynamic perspective, which of the following is responsible for this anxiety?

- **A.** The id
- **B.** The ego
- **C.** The superego
- **D.** The libido

11. A woman advances through the ranks of a company, eventually becoming the CEO. Which of the following Jungian archetypes reflects this woman's drive to be successful within the company?

- **A.** The persona
- **B.** The anima
- **C.** The animus
- **D.** The shadow

12. Researchers discover that polymorphisms in the *DRD2* gene can be associated with thrill-seeking behavior, and that individuals with certain forms of the gene are more likely to become extreme athletes and have more dangerous hobbies. Which of the following theories is supported by this discovery?

- **I.** The social cognitive perspective
- **II.** The behavioral perspective
- **III.** The biological perspective

- **A.** I only
- **B.** III only
- **C.** I and III only
- **D.** II and III only

13. A person who works as an EMT identifies as a bit of a rebel, but is highly sociable and is able to keep calm in an emergency. This person would likely score in the lower range of which of the following traits?

- **A.** Psychoticism
- **B.** Neuroticism
- **C.** Extraversion
- **D.** Conscientiousness

14. Stockholm syndrome is a phenomenon in which people who are kidnapped or held hostage may begin to identify with or even feel affection for their captors. A psychoanalyst might explain Stockholm syndrome by citing which of the following defense mechanisms?

- **A.** Reaction formation
- **B.** Regression
- **C.** Projection
- **D.** Displacement

15. Having struggled for years through an economic recession, a young professional begins to buy lottery tickets every Friday. "If I won the lottery," the individual reasons, "I'd finally have the life I've always wanted. All my stress would go away and I could live comfortably." These thoughts regarding winning the lottery are most representative of:

- **A.** a cardinal trait.
- **B.** fictional finalism.
- **C.** functional autonomy.
- **D.** unconditional positive regard.

Answer Key

1. **B** (See section 6.1)
2. **D** (See section 6.1)
3. **B** (See section 6.1)
4. **A** (See section 6.1)
5. **B** (See section 6.2)
6. **C** (See section 6.2)
7. **A** (See section 6.2)
8. **D** (See section 6.2)
9. **D** (See section 6.2)
10. **C** (See section 6.3)
11. **C** (See section 6.3)
12. **C** (See section 6.3)
13. **B** (See section 6.3)
14. **A** (See section 6.3)
15. **B** (See section 6.3)

The relevant section of the chapter to review for each question is given in parentheses after the correct answer. Detailed explanations can be found at the end of the chapter.

CHAPTER 6

IDENTITY AND PERSONALITY

In This Chapter

Introduction

Social psychologists are concerned with how our social lives influence the ways in which we perceive ourselves. Specifically, researchers have focused on the influence that other people's views, our social roles, and our group memberships have on our perceptions of who we are.

Who are you? If you're like most people, you could probably answer that question in many different ways. You might list your physical characteristics, your family relationships, your emotional tendencies, or your skills and talents. In fact, many introductory psychology courses include an exercise in which students are asked to make a list of answers to the question *Who am I?* Completing this list gives each student a glimpse into their identity and personality. These ideas form the core of the study of psychology, in which the central goal is explaining our thoughts and behaviors. In this chapter, we'll discuss this and review the key theorists and their approaches to answering the question of who we are.

CHAPTER PROFILE

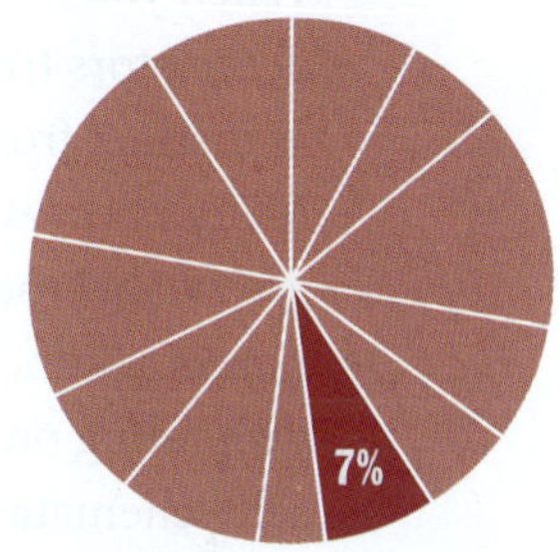

The content in this chapter should be relevant to about 7% of all questions about the behavioral sciences on the MCAT.

This chapter covers material from the following AAMC content categories:

7A: Individual influences on behavior

8A: Self-identity

6.1 Self-Concept and Identity High Yield

LEARNING OBJECTIVES

After Chapter 6.1, you will be able to:

- Distinguish between self-concept and identity
- Recall the factors that contribute to different types of identity, such as gender and ethnicity
- Predict how a person would explain an event to themselves based on their locus of control

When you look in the mirror, whom do you see? If you're studying to take the MCAT, chances are some descriptors that come to mind include *student, intelligent, future doctor*, and so on. Our awareness of ourselves as distinct from others and our own internal list of answers to the question *Who am I?* form our **self-concept**. Many of the ways in which we define ourselves fall under the classification of a **self-schema**; that is, a self-given label that carries with it a set of qualities. For example, the *athlete* self-schema usually carries the qualities of youth, physical fitness, and dressing and acting in certain ways, although these qualities may change depending on culture, socioeconomic status, and personal beliefs. The idea of self-concept goes beyond these self-schemata; it also includes our appraisal of who we used to be and who we will become. Figure 6.1 visualizes this distinction between self-concept and self-schemata.

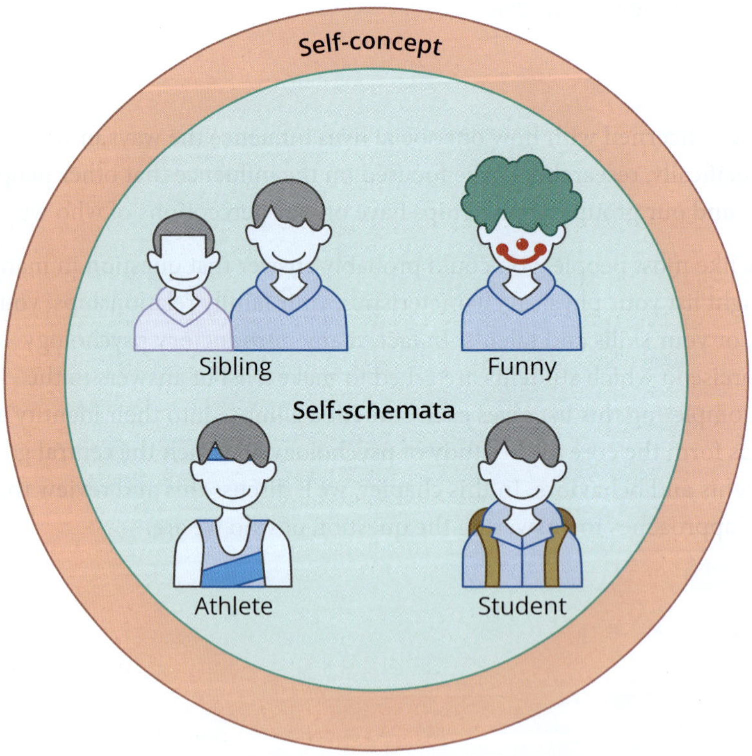

Figure 6.1 The Self-Concept Framework

Sometimes the terms *self-concept* and *identity* are used interchangeably, but psychologists generally use them to refer to two different but closely related ideas. Social scientists define **identity** as the individual components of our self-concept related to the groups to which we belong. Whereas we have one self-concept, we have multiple identities that define who we are and how we should behave within any given context. Religious affiliation, sexual orientation, personal relationships, and membership in social groups are just a few of the identities that sum to create our self-concept. In fact, our individual identities do not always need to be compatible. Are you the same person when interacting with your friends as you are when you interact with coworkers or family? For most people the answer is *no*; they take on particular identities in different social situations.

Types of Identity

While there are many different types of identity, the MCAT—for historical or social reasons—tends to focus on some forms of identity more than others.

Gender Identity

Gender identity describes people's appraisals of themselves on scales of masculinity and femininity. While these concepts were long thought to be two extremes on a single continuum, theorists have reasoned that they must be two separate dimensions because an individual can achieve high scores on scales of both masculinity and femininity. **Androgyny** is defined as the state of being simultaneously very masculine and very feminine, while those who achieve low scores on both scales are referred to as **undifferentiated**. An initial sense of gender identity is usually established by age three, although it may morph and change over time. Some theories, such as the theory of **gender schema**, hold that key components of gender identity are transmitted through cultural and societal means.

Keep in mind that gender identity is not necessarily tied to biological sex or sexual orientation, although in many cultures these concepts are seen as closely related. While it is typical of many cultures to view gender as a strictly binary concept, some cultures recognize three or more genders. For example, some peoples of Samoa refer to androgynous but phenotypically male individuals as *fa'afafine*. To these Samoans, the *fa'afafine* are seen as an important social caste and are accepted as equals, although this is not always the case for all genders across all cultures.

REAL WORLD

Individuals who are transgender are those for whom gender identity does not match sex assigned at birth. They have been a heavily stigmatized group in American culture. In fact, it was not until the publication of the DSM-5 in 2013 that gender identity disorder was formally removed as a diagnosis. The DSM-5 includes the diagnosis gender dysphoria, which is given only to individuals for whom gender identity causes significant psychological stress.

Ethnic and National Identity

Ethnic identity refers to the part of one's identity associated with membership in a particular racial/ethnic group. Members in a given ethnic group often share a common ancestry, cultural heritage, and language. Many social psychologists study the ways in which our ethnic identity influences our perspectives of ourselves. In a 1947 study, Kenneth and Mamie Clark explored ethnic self-concepts among children who were ethnically White and Black using a doll preference task: the experimenter showed each child a Black doll and a White doll and asked the child a series of questions about how the child felt about the dolls. As reflected in Figure 6.2, the majority of children, both White and Black, preferred the White doll. This study was important because it highlighted the negative effects of racism and underrepresented group status on the self-concept of Black children at the time. However, subsequent research using improved methodology (for example, randomizing the ethnicity of the experimenter), has shown that children who are Black hold more positive views of their own ethnicity; this may also represent societal changes at large.

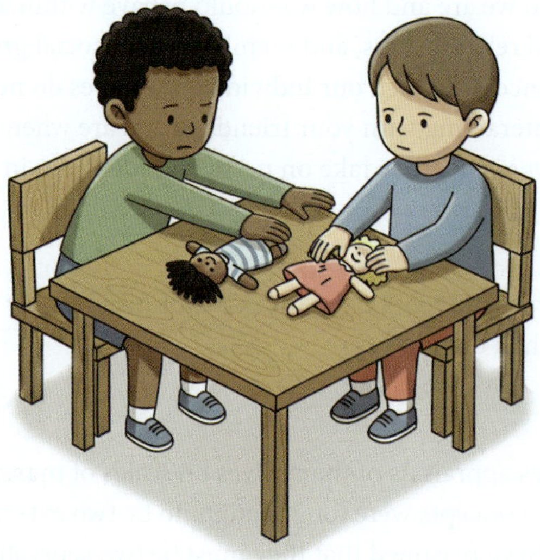

Figure 6.2 The Findings of the Clark Doll Experiment

While ethnicity is largely an identity into which we are born, **nationality** is based on political borders. National identity is the result of shared history, media, cuisine, and national symbols such as a country's flag. Nationality need not be tied to one's ethnicity or even to legal citizenship. Symbols play an important role in both ethnic and national identity. Some examples of symbols, representing American nationality, are shown in Figure 6.3.

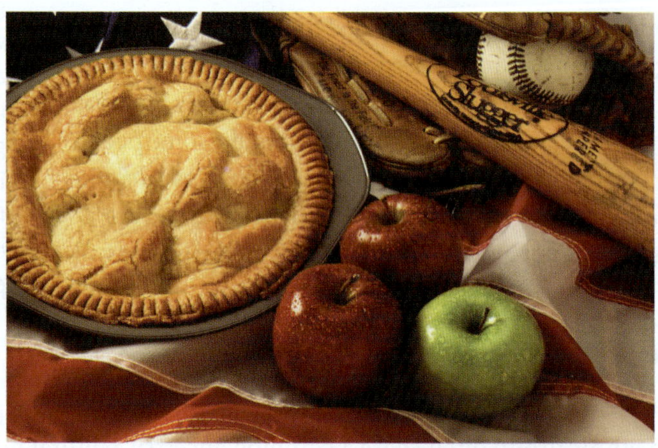

Figure 6.3 Examples of National Symbols
Symbols commonly associated with residents of the United States of America

Other Types of Identity

Of course, there are many more categories through which we evaluate our identity. We compare ourselves to others in terms of age, class, religious affiliation, sexual orientation, and so on. Aspects of these other identities are explored in other parts of *MCAT Behavioral Sciences Review*.

It is important to know that there are several factors that determine which identity will be enacted in particular situations. It is believed that our identities are organized according to a **hierarchy of salience**, such that we let the situation dictate which identity holds the most importance for us at any given moment. For instance, male and female college students in same-gender groups are less likely to list gender in their self-descriptions than students in mixed-gender groups. Furthermore, researchers have found that the more salient the identity, the more we conform to the role expectations of the identities. Salience is determined by a number of factors, including the amount of work we have invested into the identity, the rewards and gratification associated with the identity, and the amount of self-esteem we have associated with the identity.

Self-Evaluation

Our individual self-concept plays a very important role in the way we evaluate and feel about ourselves. This evaluation begins with **self-identification**, which is defined as one's ability to recognize one's own appearance. Next, **self-discrepancy theory** maintains that each of us has three selves and that perceived differences between these selves lead to negative feelings. Our self-concept makes up our **actual self**, the way we see ourselves as we currently are. Our **ideal self** is the person we would like to be, and our **ought self** is our representation of the way others think we should be. Generally, the closer these three selves are to one another, the higher our **self-esteem** or self-worth will be. Figure 6.4 depicts this relationship between esteem and the three selves.

BRIDGE

Remember that *esteem* is one of Maslow's hierarchy of needs (#4 in priority). This model is discussed in Chapter 5 of *MCAT Behavioral Sciences Review.*

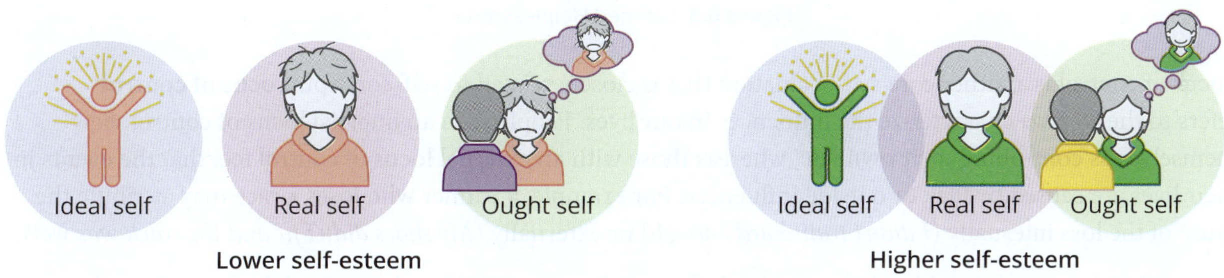

Figure 6.4 The Self-Discrepancy Theory

Those with low self-esteem don't necessarily view themselves as worthless, but they will be far more critical of themselves. As a result, they take criticism from others poorly and typically believe that people will only accept them if they are successful. Research also shows that they are more likely to use drugs, to be pessimistic, and to give up when facing frustration than their counterparts with high self-esteem.

While self-esteem is the measure of how we feel about ourselves, **self-efficacy** is our belief in our ability to succeed. Self-efficacy can vary by activity for individuals; we all can think of situations in which we hold the belief that we are able to be effective and, conversely, those in which we feel powerless. Of course, we are more motivated to pursue those tasks for which our self-efficacy is high, but we can get into trouble when it is too high. **Overconfidence** can lead us to take on tasks for which we are not ready, leading to frustration, humiliation, or sometimes even personal injury. On the other hand, self-efficacy can also be depressed; an individual can develop a perceived lack of control over the outcome of a situation, a phenomenon called **learned helplessness**. Learned helplessness has been found to be strongly related to clinical depression. Figure 6.5 presents a cartoon example of learned helplessness. Even though the cartoon is a little humorous, it expresses the struggle of an individual dealing with depression and learned helplessness. Someone without depression might not understand how a situation that looks from the outside like a minor problem with an obvious solution can seem to paralyze some people. However, for a person with depression, the little obstacles in life can feel insurmountable.

BRIDGE

Locus of control and cognitive dissonance are integral to attribution theory. In order to preserve self-esteem, we often see our successes as a direct result of our efforts and our failures as the result of uncontrollable outside influences. Attribution theory is discussed in Chapter 10 of *MCAT Behavioral Sciences Review*.

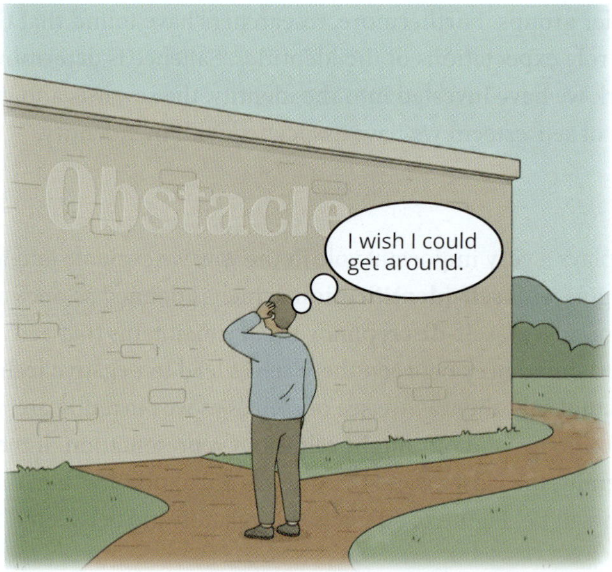

Figure 6.5 Learned Helplessness

Locus of control is another core self-evaluation that is closely related to self-concept. **Locus of control** refers to the way we characterize the influences in our lives. People with an internal locus of control view themselves as controlling their own fate, whereas those with an external locus of control feel that the events in their lives are caused by luck or outside influences. For example, a runner who loses a race may attribute the cause of the loss internally (*I didn't train hard enough*) or externally (*My shoes didn't fit and the track was wet*).

Comparison of ourselves with others can also influence the way we self-evaluate. **Social comparison theory** describes the idea that individuals evaluate themselves by comparing themselves to others. Within this theory, there are three types of social comparisons (illustrated in Figure 6.6): **upward social comparison**, where individuals compare themselves to someone they perceive as better; **lateral social comparison**, where individuals compare themselves to someone they believe to be comparable to them; and finally, **downward social comparison**, where individuals compare themselves to someone they believe is not as good as they are. This theory suggests that comparing oneself to others can affect self-esteem and our views of ourselves, either in positive or negative ways.

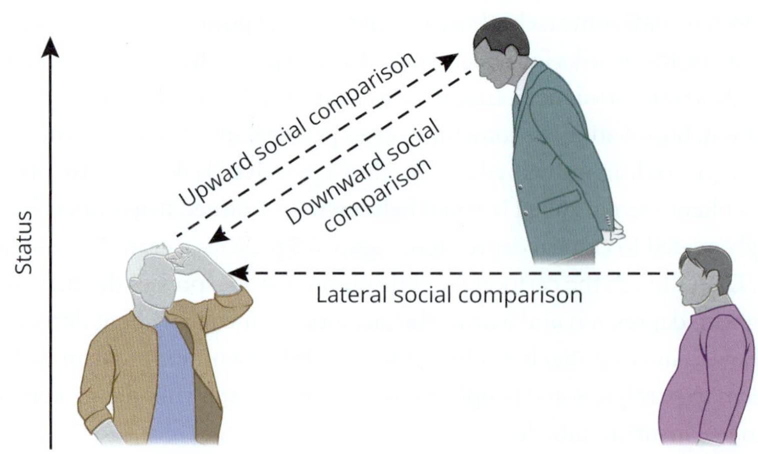

Figure 6.6 Social Comparison Theory

Another concept that relates to self-evaluation is **metacognition**, defined as the awareness of one's own thoughts and emotions. Sometimes referred to as "thinking about thinking," metacognition is an important method by which people critically analyze their own thinking and learning patterns, which can facilitate their self-improvement.

All of these ideas work hand-in-hand to influence the way we feel about ourselves. The happiest among us are those who have high self-esteem, view themselves as effective people, feel that they are in control of their destinies, and see themselves as living up to their own expectations of who they would like to be.

MCAT EXPERTISE

Effective MCAT students review full-length exams with an internal locus of control: *What can I do to prepare myself better for the next practice test?* An external locus of control prevents students from actually gaining anything from their practice: *Oh, that was just a stupid question*.

MCAT CONCEPT CHECK 6.1

Before you move on, assess your understanding of the material with these questions.

1. What is the difference between self-concept and identity?

____

2. List three factors that contribute to a person's ethnic identity. How are these factors different from those that determine national identity?

    1. ______________________________
    2. ______________________________
    3. ______________________________

    - National identity:

____

3. A high school student fails a history test. How might a student with an internal locus of control interpret this event? What about a student with an external locus of control?

    - Internal:

____

    - External:

____

6.2 Formation of Identity

High Yield

LEARNING OBJECTIVES

After Chapter 6.2, you will be able to:

- Identify the three major phases of Kohlberg's theory of moral development and their central tenets
- Explain, and distinguish between, the theories of identity of Erikson, Freud, Vygotsky, and Kohlberg

Psychologists generally agree that we are not born with our self-concept and identity in place and fully developed. As young children, our identities are largely defined by our relationship to our caregivers. As we move into adolescence, we begin to develop into unique individuals, deciding who we want to be when on our own. Several theorists have proposed stages through which we develop. They vary in scope with respect to both the aspects of our identity they describe and their time span, but they all have one thing in common: the MCAT loves to test your mastery of these theories!

Freud: Psychosexual Development

Sigmund Freud was a pioneer in charting personality and emotional growth. For Freud, human psychology and human sexuality were inextricably linked. In fact, Freud made the assertion that far from lying dormant until puberty, the **libido** (sex drive) is present at birth. Freud believed that libidinal energy and the drive to reduce libidinal tension were the underlying dynamic forces that accounted for human psychological processes.

Freud hypothesized five distinct stages of psychosexual development, summarized in Table 6.1 at the end of this section. In each stage, children are faced with a conflict between societal demands and the desire to reduce the libidinal tension associated with different erogenous zones of the body. Each stage differs in the manner in which libidinal energy is manifested and the way in which the libidinal drive is met. **Fixation** occurs when a child is overindulged or overly frustrated during a stage of development. In response to the anxiety caused by fixation, the child forms a personality pattern based on that particular stage, which persists into adulthood as a functional mental disorder known as a **neurosis**.

The first stage is the **oral stage**, spanning from 0 to 1 year of age. During this stage, gratification is obtained primarily through putting objects into the mouth, biting, and sucking. Libidinal energy is centered on the mouth. An adult who is orally fixated would be expected to exhibit excessive dependency.

Next is the **anal stage**, from 1 to 3 years, during which the libido is centered on the anus and gratification is gained through the elimination and retention of waste materials. Toilet training occurs during this stage. Fixation during this stage would lead to either excessive orderliness (*anal-retentiveness*) or sloppiness in the adult.

The **phallic stage**, sometimes known as the **Oedipal stage**, is the third of Freud's stages of psychosexual development. Generally, children aged 3 to 5 years are in this developmental stage. This stage centers on resolution of the **Oedipal conflict**

MCAT EXPERTISE

Though revolutionary at the time, Freud's theories have largely been discredited. They do, however, provide an interesting window into the history of personality theory. Expect the MCAT to test these ideas from a historical context, usually prefaced by *According to Freud's theory of psychosexual development . . .*

BRIDGE

Freud's stages of psychosexual development are based on the same principles as drive reduction theory, as discussed in Chapter 5 of *MCAT Behavioral Sciences Review:* libidinal energy creates internal tension, which we aim to reduce through certain behaviors.

for male children or the analogous **Electra conflict** for female children. In Freud's view, the male child envies his father's intimate relationship with his mother and fears castration at his father's hands. He wishes to eliminate his father and possess his mother, but the child feels guilty about these wishes. To successfully resolve the conflict, he deals with his guilty feelings by identifying with his father, establishing his sexual identity, and internalizing moral values. Also, the child to a large extent de-eroticizes, or **sublimates** his libidinal energy. This may be expressed through collecting objects or focusing on schoolwork. Freud did not elaborate much on the Electra conflict, although he theorized a similar desire. Because females cannot have castration fear (instead, they are theorized to have **penis envy**), female children are expected to exhibit less stereotypically female behavior and to be less morally developed in this theory.

Once the libido is sublimated, the child has entered the **latency stage**, which lasts until puberty is reached.

For Freud, the final stage is the **genital stage**, beginning in puberty and lasting through adulthood. According to Freud, if prior development has proceeded correctly, the person should enter into healthy heterosexual relationships at this point. Freud claimed, however, that if sexual traumas of childhood have not been resolved, such behaviors as homosexuality, asexuality, or fetishism may result.

Stage	Description
Oral	Libidinal energy centered on the mouth; fixation can lead to excessive dependency
Anal	Toilet training occurs during this time; fixation can lead to excessive orderliness or messiness
Phallic	Oedipal or Electra conflict is resolved during this stage
Latency	Libido is largely sublimated during this stage
Genital	Begins at puberty; in theory, if previous stages have been successfully resolved, the person will enter into heterosexual relationships

Table 6.1 Freud's Stages of Psychosexual Development

Erikson: Psychosocial Development

Erik **Erikson's theory of psychosocial development** theorizes that personality development is driven by the successful resolution of a series of social and emotional conflicts.For example, the first such conflict is that of **trust vs. mistrust**, which occurs during the first year of life. Newborn humans are quite helpless and unsure of their environment. A newborn depends on their caregivers for support. So, the psychosocial conflict that a newborn faces is whether or not to trust caregivers to reliably provide that support. If caregivers do reliably care for the newborn, then the newborn will learn trust, which is a social skill. In different circumstances, the newborn could fail to learn to trust. However, according to Erikson's theory, such an individual may nevertheless move on to the next stage of psychosocial development, and may even learn trust later in life.

This example illustrates three key features of Erikson's theory. First, the conflicts that Erikson describes arise because an individual lacks some critical social or emotional skill. Each conflict therefore represents an opportunity to learn a new social or emotional skill, which, according to Erikson, is the mechanism for psychosocial development. Second, each conflict has either a positive or negative resolution. For example, a newborn can learn to be mistrustful. This outcome does represent a resolution of the trust vs. mistrust conflict. However, this outcome would be a negative outcome and, in Erikson's view, would represent a failure to develop. Psychosocial development means not only resolving each conflict, but obtaining a positive resolution. However, the third key idea is that, in Erikson's theory, an individual who fails to obtain a positive resolution at one stage can still advance to later stages and, later in life, may even learn the skill that they failed to learn during the developmental conflict.

The second conflict is **autonomy vs. shame and doubt** (1 to 3 years), where children begin to explore their surroundings and develop their interests. The favorable outcome here is feeling able to exert control over the world and to exercise choice as well as self-restraint. However, if children are overly controlled and criticized, the unfavorable outcome is a sense of doubt and a persistent external locus of control.

The next conflict confronted is **initiative vs. guilt** (3 to 6 years), in which children learn basic cause and effect principles in physics, and starting and finishing out tasks for a purpose. Favorable outcomes include a sense of purpose, the ability to initiate activities, and the ability to enjoy accomplishment. If guilt wins out, children will be so overcome by the fear of punishment that they may either unduly restrict themselves or may overcompensate by showing off.

Next is the conflict of **industry vs. inferiority** (6 to 12 years), where pre-adolescents are becoming aware of themselves as individuals. If resolved favorably, children will feel competent, be able to exercise their abilities and intelligence in the world, and be able to affect the world in the way that they desire. Unfavorable resolution results in a sense of inadequacy, a sense of inability to act in a competent manner, and low self-esteem.

During adolescence (12 to 20 years), individuals experience **identity vs. role confusion**. During this conflict, adolescents explore their independence to determine who they are and what their purpose is in society. At this stage, individuals either form a single identity or become unsure about their place in society. The favorable outcome is fidelity, the ability to see oneself as a unique and integrated person with sustained loyalties. Unfavorable outcomes are confusion about one's identity and an amorphous personality that shifts from day to day.

The main crisis of young adulthood (20 to 40 years) is **intimacy vs. isolation**, where people focus on creating long-lasting bonds with others. Favorable outcomes are love, the ability to have intimate relationships with others, and the ability to commit oneself to another person and to one's own goals. If this crisis is not favorably resolved, there will be an avoidance of commitment, alienation, and distancing of oneself from others and one's ideals. Isolated individuals are either withdrawn or capable of only superficial relationships with others.

The conflict of middle age (40 to 65 years) is **generativity vs. stagnation**, where the focus is on advancing present and future society. The successful resolution of this conflict results in an individual capable of being a productive, caring, and contributing member of society. If this crisis is not overcome, one acquires a sense of stagnation and may become self-indulgent, bored, and self-centered with little care for others.

REAL WORLD

The conflict of identity vs. role confusion has some positive effects: teenagers identifying their interests, gravitating toward friends who share these interests, and creating a sense of who they want to be. On the other hand, this conflict can lead to the formation of cliques, bullying, and significant peer pressure. The increase of online and in-person bullying among adolescents has led to a number of programs to ease this crisis, such as *StopBullying.gov* and the *It Gets Better* campaign.

Finally, old age (above 65 years) brings about the crisis of **integrity vs. despair**, where the focus tends to be reflective and contemplative. If favorably resolved, we will see wisdom, which Erikson defined as detached concern with life itself, with assurance in the meaning of life, dignity, and an acceptance of the fact that one's life has been worthwhile, along with a readiness to face death. If not resolved favorably, there will be feelings of bitterness about one's life, a feeling that life has been worthless, and at the same time, fear over one's own impending death.

Erikson's Stage (Crisis)	Age	Existential Question
Trust vs. mistrust	0 to 1 year	Can I trust the world?
Autonomy vs. shame and doubt	1 to 3 years	Is it okay to be me?
Initiative vs. guilt	3 to 6 years	Is it okay for me to do, move, and act?
Industry vs. inferiority	6 to 12 years	Can I make it in the world of people and things?
Identity vs. role confusion	12 to 20 years	Who am I? What can I be?
Intimacy vs. isolation	20 to 40 years	Can I love?
Generativity vs. stagnation	40 to 65 years	Can I make my life count?
Integrity vs. despair	65 years to death	Is it okay to have been me?

Table 6.2 Erikson's Stages of Psychosocial Development

Kohlberg: Moral Reasoning

Lawrence Kohlberg's theory of personality development focuses not on urges or on resolving conflicts, but rather on the development of moral thinking. For this reason, this theory is often called **Kohlberg's theory of moral reasoning**. Kohlberg reasoned that, as our cognitive abilities grow, we are able to think about the world in more complex and nuanced ways, and this directly affects the ways in which we resolve moral dilemmas and perceive the notion of right and wrong.

Kohlberg's observations about moral reasoning were based on responses of subjects to hypothetical moral dilemmas. One often-cited example is the *Heinz dilemma* (depicted in Figure 6.7). In this scenario, a man named Heinz has a wife who is dying of a rare disease. There is a druggist in the town who invented a drug that could cure the disease. It costs him $200 to produce, yet he sells it for $2000. Heinz cannot afford this price, so he goes to the druggist and asks him if he would lower the price, a request that the druggist refuses. Desperate to save his wife, Heinz breaks into the druggist's office one night and steals the medication. Kohlberg presented dilemmas such as this one to volunteers and asked them to explain whether the characters in the story acted morally and why or why not. Kohlberg wasn't interested in the participants' appraisal of the actions as right or wrong, as he believed either answer could be justified. Instead, he was far more interested in the reasoning behind the appraisal. Based on the participants' responses, Kohlberg organized moral reasoning into six distinct stages ranging from the concrete to the abstract. He then organized these stages into three phases consisting of two stages each. Kohlberg's stages are summarized below in Figure 6.8.

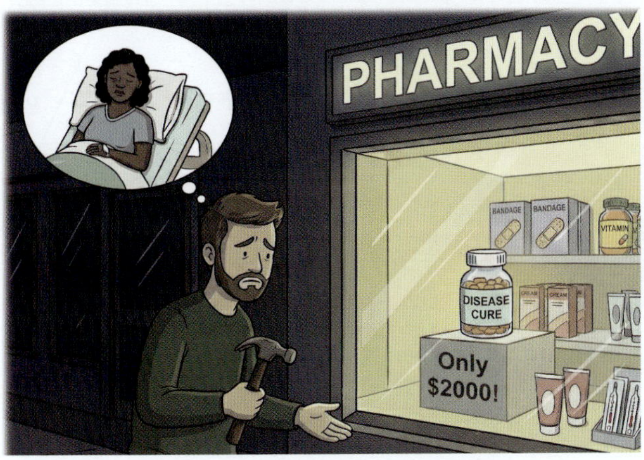

Figure 6.7 The Heinz Dilemma

Preconventional morality, the first of these phases, is typical of preadolescent thinking and places an emphasis on the consequences of the moral choice. Stage one (**obedience**) is concerned with avoiding punishment (*If I steal the drug, I'll go to jail*), while stage two (**self-interest**) is about gaining rewards (*I need to save my wife because I want to spend more of my life with her*). Stage two is often called the **instrumental relativist stage** because it is based on the concepts of reciprocity and sharing: *I'll scratch your back, you scratch mine.*

The second phase is **conventional morality**, which begins to develop in early adolescence when individuals begin to see themselves in terms of their relationships to others. This phase is based on understanding and accepting social rules. Stage three (**conformity**) places emphasis on the "nice person" orientation in which an individual seeks the approval of others (*I should not steal the drug because stealing is wrong*). Stage four (**law and order**) maintains the social order in the highest regard (*If everyone stole things they couldn't afford, people who produce those items would not be able to continue their business*).

The third phase is **postconventional morality**, which describes a level of reasoning that Kohlberg claimed not everyone was capable of and is based on social mores, which may conflict with laws. Stage five (**social contract**) views moral rules as conventions that are designed to ensure the greater good, with reasoning focused on individual rights (*Everyone has a right to live; businesses have a right to profit from their products*). Finally, stage six (**universal human ethics**) reasons that decisions should be made in consideration of abstract principles (*It is wrong for one person to hold another's life for ransom*).

KEY CONCEPT

Conventional morality corresponds to average adult moral reasoning. Preconventional is therefore expected in children, and postconventional is expected in a smaller subset of adults with more advanced moral reasoning skills than the average population.

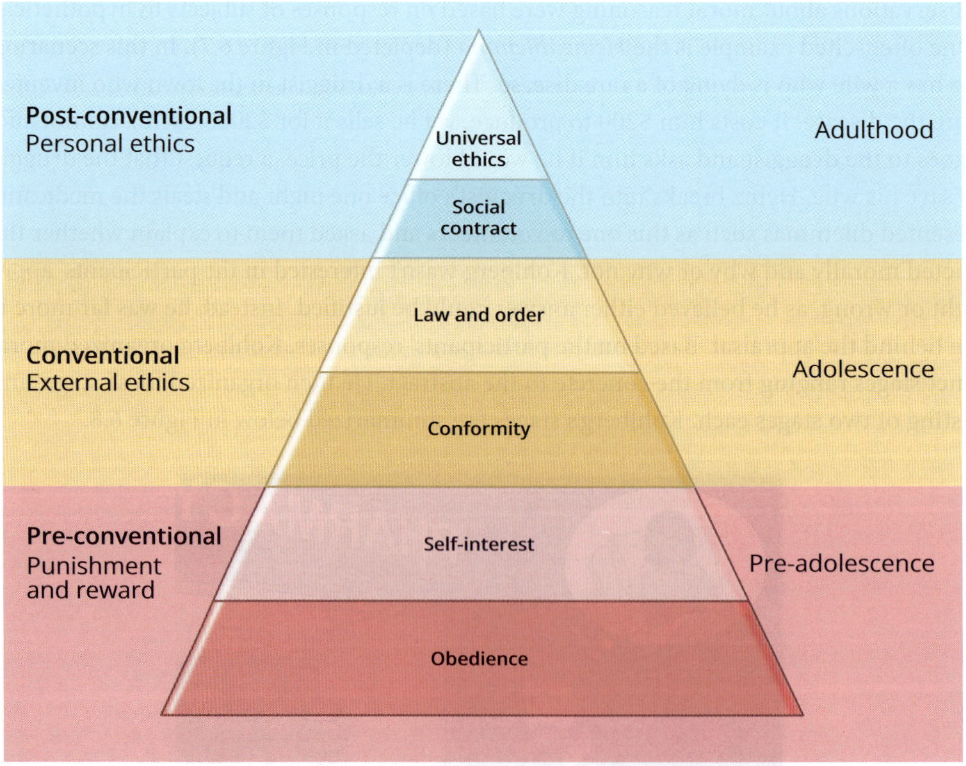

Figure 6.8 Kohlberg's Stages of Moral Development

Kohlberg viewed these stages as a progression in which each stage is adopted and then abandoned for the next as the individual progresses. In other words, we all begin in stage one and progress to varying degrees as our thinking matures.

Kohlberg is not without his critics. Some argue that postconventional morality describes views that are more prevalent in individualistic societies and is therefore biased against collectivist cultures. Similarly, Kohlberg's research was only performed using male subjects, which may cloud differences in reasoning patterns that may exist between genders.

Vygotsky: Cultural and Biosocial Development

Like Kohlberg, Lev Vygotsky's work was focused on understanding cognitive development. For Vygotsky, the engine driving cognitive development was the child's internalization of various aspects of culture: rules, symbols, language, and so on. As the child internalized these various interpersonal and cultural rules, cognitive activity developed accordingly.

Vygotsky is known for his concept of the **zone of proximal development**, referring to those skills and abilities that have not yet fully developed but are in the process of development. Gaining these skills successfully requires the help of a "more knowledgeable other," typically an adult. For example, children may struggle to ride a bicycle on their own, but with the help and guidance of an adult may be successful. Vygotsky would say that this skill is currently within the children's zone of proximal development. The zone of proximal development is visually defined in Figure 6.9.

BRIDGE

Kohlberg and Vygotsky's theories of cognitive development were both heavily influenced by Piaget's work in this area, discussed in Chapter 4 of *MCAT Behavioral Sciences Review.*

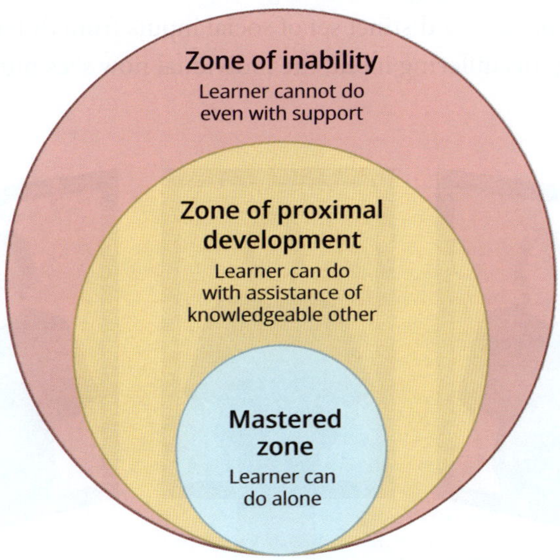

Figure 6.9 Vygotsky's Zone of Proximal Development

Vygotsky recommended a process of guided learning that would later be called **scaffolding**. Like a scaffold used in construction, scaffolding in education provides temporary support to help learners build new skills and knowledge. This support, often provided by a more knowledgeable other, enables learners to tackle tasks within their zone of proximal development. As the learner progresses, the support is gradually reduced, much like a scaffold is removed once the building is complete.

The Influence of Others on Identity

Our personalities do not form in a vacuum; we are as much a product of those around us as a product of our own internal growth and development. Albert Bandura, who was also the psychologist behind the Bobo doll experiment described in Chapter 3 of *MCAT Behavioral Sciences Review*, claimed that observational learning contributes greatly to our future behaviors.

Young children observe and encode the behaviors they see in others, and may later imitate these behaviors. Children are more likely to imitate behaviors performed by someone who is like them: for example, young children will reliably mimic behaviors performed by their same-gender siblings. Children's first models are their caregivers, but as children grow and form more relationships, other role models emerge. Siblings, teachers, and the media all play an important role in modeling behavior for a developing child, but by adolescence, peers become the most important role models in a person's life.

As children grow, they become more able to see the identities of others as different from their own. They might experiment with other identities by taking on the roles of others, such as when children play *house* or *school*. Such **role-taking** is good practice for later in life, when a child begins to understand the perspectives and roles of others. Eventually, children become able to see how others perceive them and to imagine themselves from the outside. The ability to sense how another's mind works—for example, understanding how a friend is interpreting a story while you tell it—is referred to as **theory of mind**. Once we develop a theory of mind, we begin to recognize and react to how others think about us. We become aware of judgments from the outside world and react to these judgments. Our reactions to how others perceive us can be varied—maintaining, modifying, downplaying, or accentuating different aspects of our personality. Our understanding of how others see us, which relies on perceiving a reflection of ourselves based on the words and actions of others, is appropriately called the **looking-glass self**. Figure 6.10 illustrates how this looking-glass self might be experienced. Each mirror represents a distinct set of social inputs from different groups a person has interacted with. After receiving this differing input, the individual now sees multiple versions of the self that the different groups perceive.

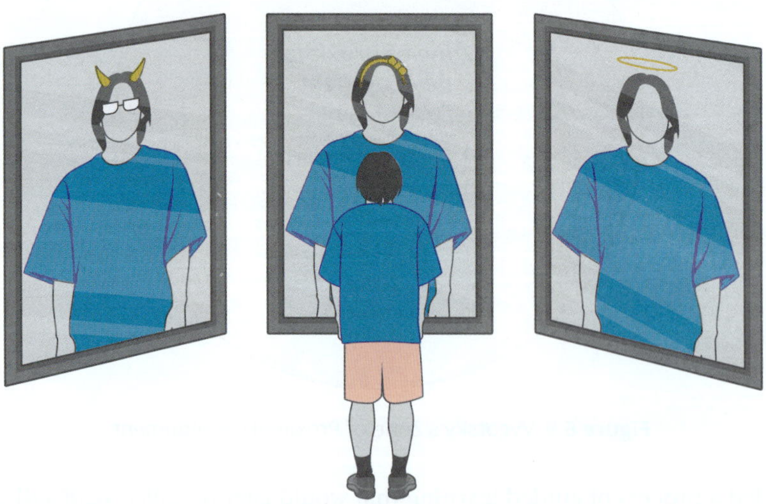

Figure 6.10 The Looking-Glass Self

A related concept is a **reference group**, the group that we use as a standard to evaluate ourselves. Our self-concept often depends on whom we are comparing ourselves to. For example, in 2012, the average annual salary for a physician in the United States was about $200,000. Compared to the national median household salary (approximately $50,000), these individuals were quite well off. However, only 11 percent considered themselves "rich." Why? Many physicians live in higher socioeconomic areas and regularly interact with other physicians, and their responses may thus be biased by comparison to those around them.

MCAT CONCEPT CHECK 6.2

Before you move on, assess your understanding of the material with these questions.

1. Each of the following theorists evaluates an individual and determines that the person has failed in completing one of the theorist's developmental stages. What would each say is the most likely outcome for this person?
   - Freud:

   ____

   - Erikson:

   ____

   - Kohlberg:

   ____

2. Name and briefly describe the three major phases of Kohlberg's theory of moral development.

Phase	Description

3. How could Vygotsky's concept of zone of proximal development be applied to standardized test preparation?

   ____

6.3 Personality High Yield

LEARNING OBJECTIVES

After Chapter 6.3, you will be able to:

- Describe how personality is defined by the psychoanalytic, humanistic, type, behaviorist, social cognitive, biological, and trait perspectives
- List the traits described by Eysenck's PEN theory
- List the Big Five personality traits
- Recall the roles of the id, ego, and superego in the psychoanalytic perspective of personality

We've seen that identity is the way we define ourselves. **Personality**, while similar, describes the set of thoughts, feelings, traits, and behaviors that are characteristic of an individual across time and location. In a way, identity describes who we are, while personality describes how we act and react to the world around us. There are many different theories of personality, and different theorists within each category espouse sometimes conflicting views in an attempt to describe behavior. Like the various theories of development discussed earlier in this chapter, some of these ideas have been discredited, and so will only be tested on the MCAT from a historical perspective.

We can categorize theories of personality into four areas: psychoanalytic (psychodynamic), humanistic (phenomenological), type and trait, and behaviorist. There are great differences between and within these divisions in how personality is defined and how abnormal personalities are explained.

MCAT EXPERTISE

The psychoanalytic perspective, much like other Freudian and Jungian theories within psychology, is not backed by more modern understandings of personality and has fallen from use in professional circles, though it remains prevalent in popular culture. However, the psychoanalytic perspective is useful as a contrast to other theories of personality, and is included within testable materials as laid out by the AAMC.

The Psychoanalytic Perspective

The **psychoanalytic** or **psychodynamic theories of personality** contain some of the most widely varying perspectives on behavior, but they all have in common the assumption of unconscious internal states that motivate the overt actions of individuals and determine personality. The most noteworthy supporter of the psychoanalytic theory is Freud.

Sigmund Freud

Freud's contribution to the study of personality was his structural model, which involved three major entities: the id, ego, and superego, illustrated in Figure 6.11.

The **id** consists of all the basic, primal, inborn urges to survive and reproduce. It functions according to the **pleasure principle**, in which the aim is to achieve immediate gratification to relieve any pent-up tension. The **primary process** is the id's response to frustration based on the pleasure principle: *obtain satisfaction now, not later*. Mental imagery, such as daydreaming or fantasy, that fulfills this need for satisfaction is termed **wish fulfillment**.

REAL WORLD

If a person is hungry and food is unavailable, wish fulfillment—fantasizing or daydreaming about food—helps relieve some of the tension created by the pleasure principle.

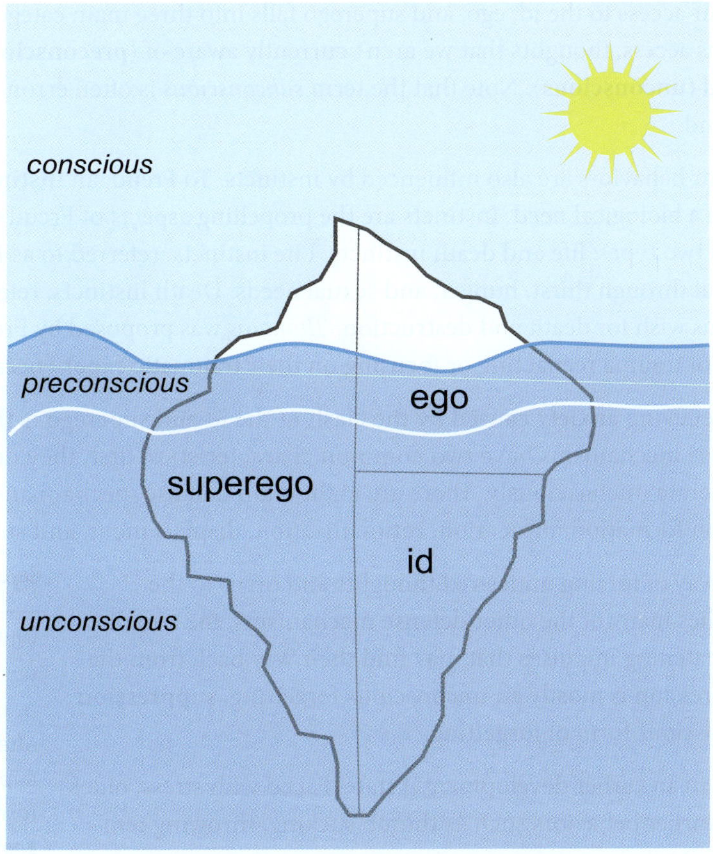

Figure 6.11 Freud's Topographic Model of the Mind

Because this mental image cannot effectively reduce tension on a permanent basis, the **ego** comes into play. The ego operates according to the **reality principle**, taking into account objective reality as it guides or inhibits the activity of the id and the id's pleasure principle. This guidance is referred to as the **secondary process**. The aim of the reality principle is to postpone the pleasure principle until satisfaction can actually be obtained. It must be emphasized that while the ego suspends the workings of the primary process, it does so only to meet the demands of objective reality. The mutual give and take of the ego and reality promotes the growth of perception, memory, problem solving, thinking, and reality testing. The ego can be understood to be the organizer of the mind: it receives its power from—and can never be fully independent of—the id.

REAL WORLD

When stuck in traffic, our id may desire to honk loudly at the cars in front of us, or to even pull over to the shoulder of the highway and drive recklessly past the congestion. Our ego knows that this would be unwise, and may advise us to breathe deeply and change the radio station to something calming instead.

The ego is also responsible for moderating the desires of the superego. Whereas the id's desires are basic needs, those of the superego are refined and focused on the ideal self. The **superego** is the personality's perfectionist, judging our actions and responding with pride at our accomplishments and guilt at our failures. The superego can be divided into two subsystems, both of which are a reflection of the morals taught to children by their caregivers. The **conscience** is a collection of the improper actions for which a child is punished, and the **ego-ideal** consists of those proper actions for which a child is rewarded. Ultimately, a system of right and wrong substitutes for caregivers' rewards and punishments.

Freud also stated that our access to the id, ego, and superego falls into three main categories: thoughts to which we have conscious access, thoughts that we aren't currently aware of (**preconscious**), and thoughts that have been repressed (**unconscious**). Note that the term *subconscious* is often erroneously used to refer to Freud's unconscious mind.

Freud postulated that our behaviors are also influenced by instincts. To Freud, an **instinct** is an innate psychological representation of a biological need. Instincts are the propelling aspects of Freud's dynamic theory of personality and fall into two types: life and death instincts. Life instincts, referred to as *Eros*, promote an individual's quest for survival through thirst, hunger, and sexual needs. Death instincts, referred to as *Thanatos*, represent an unconscious wish for death and destruction. *Thanatos* was proposed by Freud as a response to his observations of victims of trauma reenacting or focusing on their traumatic experiences.

The ego's recourse for relieving anxiety caused by the clash of the id and superego is through **defense mechanisms**. All defense mechanisms have two common characteristics: first, they deny, falsify, or distort reality; second, they operate unconsciously. There are eight main defense mechanisms: repression, suppression, regression, reaction formation, projection, rationalization, displacement, and sublimation.

Repression is the ego's way of forcing undesired thoughts and urges to the unconscious and underlies many of the other defense mechanisms, the aim of which is to disguise threatening impulses that may find their way back from the unconscious. While repression is mostly an unconscious forgetting, **suppression** is a more deliberate, conscious form of forgetting.

KEY CONCEPT

While repression is unconscious forgetting (such as that which may occur after traumatic events), suppression is a conscious form of forgetting: *I'm not going to think about that right now.*

Regression is reversion to an earlier developmental state. Faced with stress, older children may return to earlier behaviors such as thumb sucking, throwing temper tantrums, or clinging to their caregivers.

Reaction formation occurs when an individual suppresses urges by unconsciously converting these urges into their exact opposites. For example, a person pining after an inaccessible celebrity may outwardly express hatred for the celebrity as a way of reducing the stress caused by these unrequited feelings.

Projection is the defense mechanism by which individuals attribute their undesired feelings to others. *I hate my parents* might, for example, turn into *My parents hate me*. Projection is an important part of personality analysis. Tests that make use of projection to gain insight into a client's mind are common in psychoanalytic therapy. For example, the **Rorschach inkblot test**, shown in Figure 6.12, relies on the assumption that clients project their unconscious feelings onto the shape.

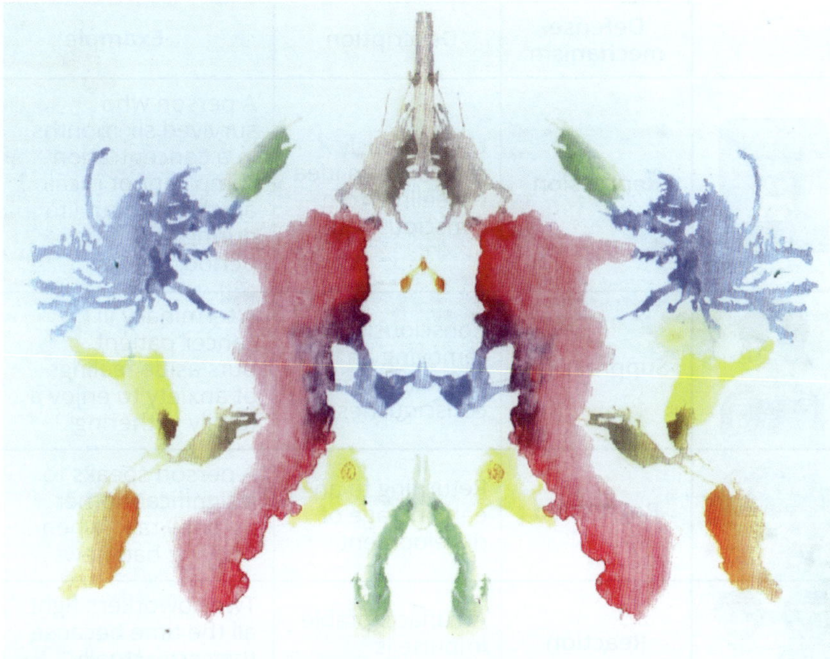

Figure 6.12 Card #10 from the Rorschach Inkblot Test

Similarly, the **thematic apperception test** consists of a series of pictures that are presented to the client, who is asked to make up a story about each one. The story, presumably, will elucidate the client's own unconscious thoughts and feelings.

Rationalization is the justification of behaviors in a manner that is acceptable to the self and society. Drivers who engage in reckless feats such as the Cannonball Run (a cross-country race from Los Angeles to New York) might justify their dangerous pursuits by saying, both to themselves and others: *I'm in complete control, and besides, there are plenty of dangerous drivers on the road. What difference will one more make?*

Displacement describes the transference of an undesired urge from one person or object to another. Someone angry at a supervisor at work may remain quiet there but snap at a family member at home.

Finally, **sublimation** is the transformation of unacceptable urges into socially acceptable behaviors. Freud might say that pent-up sexual urges may be sublimated into a drive for business success or artistic creativity.

The descriptions of the most commonly tested defense mechanisms, as well as examples, are provided in Table 6.3.

	Defense mechanism	Description	Example
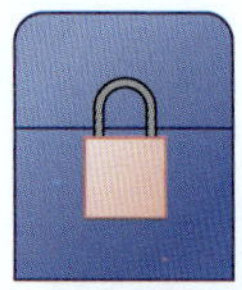	Repression	Unconsiously removing an idea or feeling from consciousness	A person who survived six months in a concentration camp cannot recall anything about life during that time period
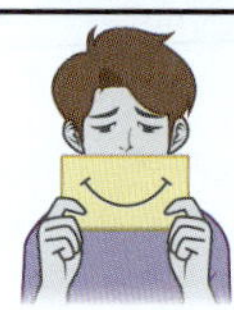	Suppression	Consciously removing an idea or feeling from consciousness	A terminally ill cancer patient puts aside feelings of anxiety to enjoy a family gathering
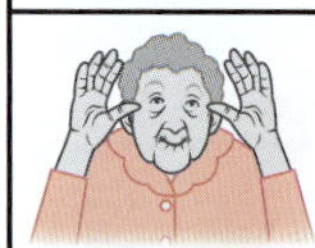	Regression	Returning to an earlier stage of development	A person speaks to a significant other in "baby talk" when relaying bad news
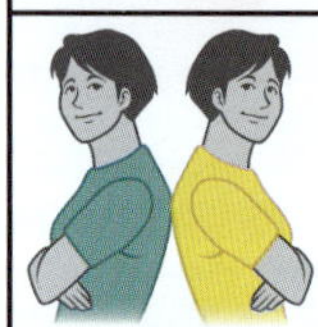	Reaction formation	An unacceptable impulse is transformed into it's opposite	Two coworkers fight all the time because they are actually attracted to each other
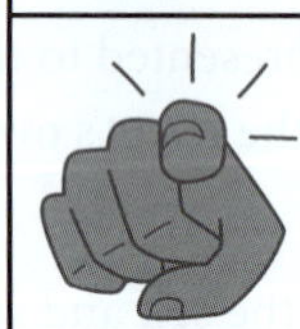	Projection	Attribution of wishes, desires, thoughts, or emotions to someone else	Someone who interrupts a lot accuses others of not being good listeners
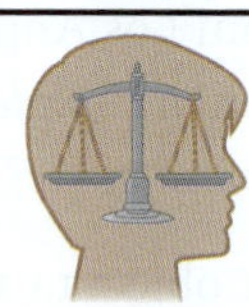	Rationalization	Justification of attitudes, beliefs, or behaviors	A murderer claims that, while killing is wrong, this particular victim "deserved it"
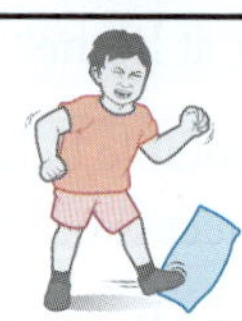	Displacement	Changing the target of an emotion, while the feelings remain the same	When sent to their room as punishment, children begin to punch and kick their pillows
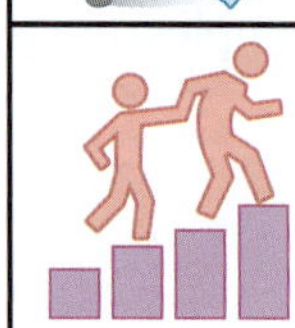	Sublimation	Channeling of unacceptable impulses in a socially acceptable direction	A boss who is attracted to an employee becomes that employee's mentor and advisor

Table 6.3 Commonly Tested Defense Mechanisms

Carl Jung

Later psychoanalytic theories have given more emphasis to interpersonal, sociological, and cultural influences, while maintaining their link with the psychoanalytic tradition. Carl Jung preferred to think of libido as psychic energy in general, not just psychic energy rooted in sexuality. Jung identified the ego as the conscious mind, and he divided the unconscious into two parts: the **personal unconscious**, similar to Freud's notion of the unconscious, and the collective unconscious. The **collective unconscious** is a powerful system that is shared among all humans and considered to be a residue of the experiences of our early ancestors. Its building blocks are images of common experiences, such as having caregivers as children. These images invariably have an emotional element, and are referred to as **archetypes** in Jung's theory. You can see an example of two archetypal images in Figure 6.13: God and the Devil.

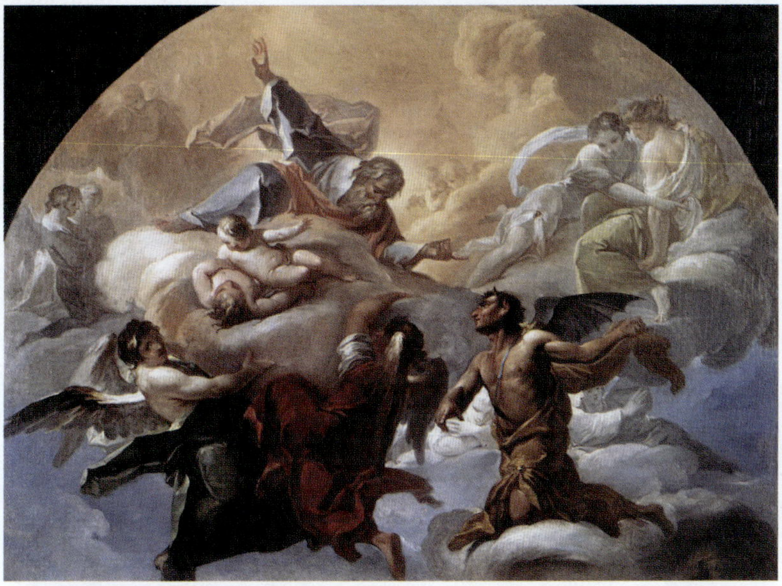

Figure 6.13 Jungian Archetypes: God and the Devil
Archetypes are underlying forms or concepts that give rise to archetypal images, which may differ somewhat between cultures.

There are several important Jungian archetypes. The **persona** is likened to a mask that we wear in public, and is the part of our personality that we present to the world. Like our identity, Jung described the persona as adaptive to our social interactions, emphasizing those qualities that improve our social standing and suppressing our other, less desirable qualities. The **anima** (feminine) and the **animus** (masculine) describe gender-inappropriate qualities—in other words, feminine behaviors in males and masculine behaviors in females. For example, in Jung's theory, the anima is the suppressed female quality in males that explains emotional behavior (described by Jung as a *man's inner woman*), while the animus is the analogous male quality of females that explains power-seeking behavior (*a woman's inner man*). The **shadow** archetype is responsible for the appearance of unpleasant and socially reprehensible thoughts, feelings, and actions experienced in the unconscious mind.

KEY CONCEPT

Important Jungian archetypes:

- Persona—the aspect of our personality we present to the world
- Anima—a "man's inner woman"
- Animus—a "woman's inner man"
- Shadow—unpleasant and socially reprehensible thoughts, feelings, and actions experienced in the unconscious mind

The **self**, to Jung, was the point of intersection between the collective unconscious, the personal unconscious, and the conscious mind. The self strives for unity. Jung symbolized the self as a *mandala* (Sanskrit: "circle"), shown in Figure 6.14. Jung saw the mandala, a symbol of the universe in Buddhism and Hinduism, as the mythic expression of the self: the reconciler of opposites and the promoter of harmony. Jung also developed **word association testing** to assess how unconscious elements may be influencing the conscious mind and thus the self. In word association testing, patients respond to a single word with the first word that comes to mind. Jung believed that patient responses, in combination with evaluating mood and speed of response, would reveal elements of the unconscious.

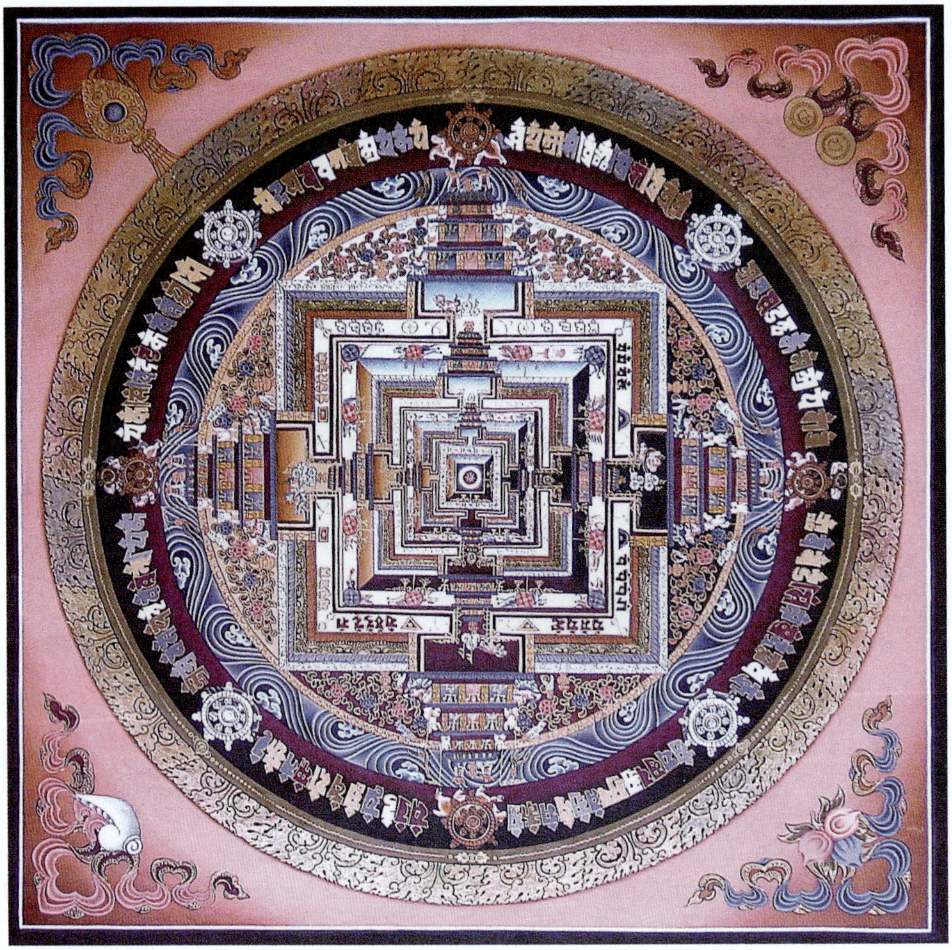

Figure 6.14 Tibetan Mandala
Jung saw the self as a mandala: the promoter of unity, balance, and harmony between the conscious mind, personal unconscious, and collective unconscious.

Jung described three dichotomies of personality:

- Extraversion (E, orientation toward the external world) vs. introversion (I, orientation toward the inner, personal world)
- Sensing (S, obtaining objective information about the world) vs. intuiting (N, working with information abstractly)
- Thinking (T, using logic and reason) vs. feeling (F, using a value system or personal beliefs)

In most individuals, both sides of each dichotomy are present to some degree, but one tends to dominate. Jung's work laid the groundwork for creation of the **Myers–Briggs Type Inventory** (**MBTI**), a classic personality test. Each of Jung's three dichotomies, and a fourth—judging (J, preferring orderliness) vs. perceiving (P, preferring spontaneity)—is labeled as a specific personality type, as shown in Figure 6.15.

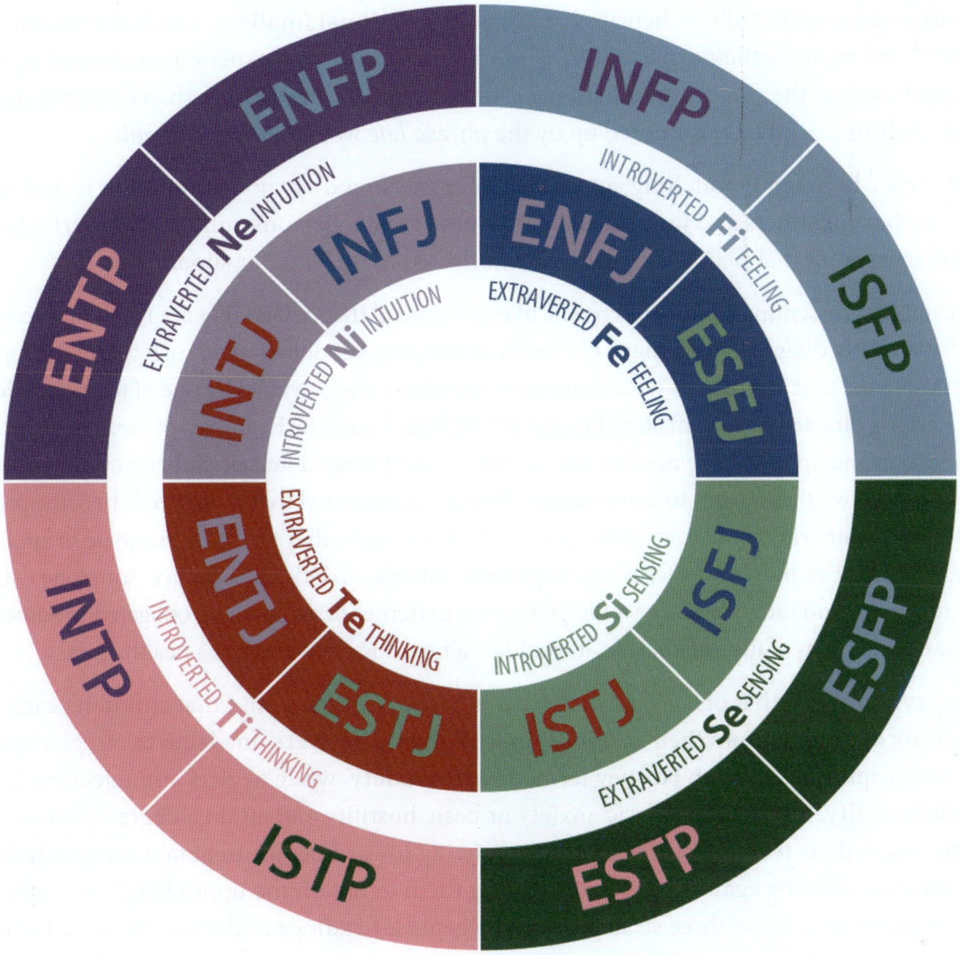

Figure 6.15 Myers–Briggs Type Inventory Personality Types

Other Psychoanalysts

As with most psychological movements, psychoanalysis gained a following of theorists who learned from and often disagreed with its original tenets. In opposition to many of Freud's key ideas, later psychoanalysts often emphasized social rather than sexual motivations for behavior. Jung can be counted among these, as can Alfred Adler, whose theory focused on the immediate social imperatives of family and society and their effects on unconscious factors.

Adler was the originator of the concept of the **inferiority complex**: an individual's sense of incompleteness, imperfection, and inferiority both physically and socially. According to Adler, striving for superiority drives the personality. This striving enhances the personality when it is oriented toward benefiting society, but yields disorder when it is selfish.

The notions of the creative self and style of life were also important to Adler's theory. The **creative self** is the force by which individuals shape their uniqueness and establish their personality. **Style of life** represents the manifestation of the creative self and describes a person's unique way of achieving superiority. The family environment is crucial in molding the person's style of life.

Another important concept in Adler's theory of personality is **fictional finalism**. This is the notion that individuals are motivated more by their expectations of the future than by past experiences. According to Adler, human goals are based on the subjective or fictional estimate of life's values rather than objective data from the past. Fictional finalism can often be summed up by the phrase *Life would be perfect if only…*

Notice the difference between Freud, Jung, and Adler. Whereas Freud's major assumption is that behavior is motivated by inborn instincts and Jung's principal axiom is that a person's conduct is governed by inborn archetypes, Adler assumes that people are primarily motivated by striving for superiority.

Karen Horney, another dissenting student of Freud's, likewise argued that personality is a result of interpersonal relationships, and adamantly disagreed with many of Freud's assumptions about women, such as the concept of penis envy. Horney postulated that individuals with neurotic personalities are governed by one of ten **neurotic needs**. Each of these needs is directed toward making life and interactions bearable. Examples of these neurotic needs are the need for affection and approval, the need to exploit others, and the need for self-sufficiency and independence. While healthy people have these needs to some degree, Horney emphasized that these needs become problematic if they fit at least one of four criteria: they are disproportionate in intensity, they are indiscriminate in application, they partially disregard reality, or they have a tendency to provoke intense anxiety. For instance, someone with a neurotic need for self-sufficiency and independence would go to great extremes to avoid being obligated to someone else in any way. As the central focus of the person's life, it would be a neurotic need and not a healthy one.

Horney's primary concept is that of basic anxiety. This is based on the premise that children's early perception of self is important and stems from their relationship with their caregivers. Inadequate caregiving can cause vulnerability and helplessness, which Horney termed **basic anxiety**, while neglect and rejection cause anger known as **basic hostility**. To overcome basic anxiety or basic hostility and attain a degree of security, children use three strategies in their relationships with others: moving toward people to obtain the goodwill of people who provide security; moving against people, or fighting them to obtain the upper hand; and moving away, or withdrawing, from people. These three strategies are the general headings under which the ten neurotic needs fall. Healthy people use all three strategies, depending on the situation. However, the highly threatened child will use one of these strategies rigidly and exclusively, and carries this strategy into adulthood.

Object relations theory also falls under the realm of psychodynamic theories of personality. In this context, *object* refers to the representation of caregivers based on subjective experiences during early infancy. These objects then persist into adulthood and impact our interactions with others, including the social bonds we create and our predictions of others' behavior.

The Humanistic Perspective

In direct contrast to the psychoanalysts, who focus on "sick" individuals and their troubling urges, **humanistic** or **phenomenological theorists** focus on the value of individuals and take a more person-centered approach, describing those ways in which healthy people strive toward self-realization. Humanism is often associated with **Gestalt therapy**, in which practitioners tend to take a holistic view of the self, seeing each individual as a complete person rather than reducing the person to individual behaviors or drives. For the humanists, our personality is the result of the conscious feelings we have for ourselves as we attempt to attain our needs and goals.

Kurt Lewin's **force field theory** puts very little stock in constraints on personalities such as fixed traits, habits, or structures such as the id, ego, and superego. Further, Lewin focused little on an individual's past or future, focusing instead on situations in the present. Lewin defined the field as one's current state of mind, which was simply the sum of the forces (influences) on the individual at that time. If the focus of humanistic psychology is exploring how an individual reaches self-realization, then these forces could be divided into two large groups: those assisting in our attainment of goals and those blocking the path to them.

Abraham Maslow, whose hierarchy of needs is discussed in Chapter 5 of *MCAT Behavioral Sciences Review*, was a humanist who studied the lives of individuals such as Ludwig van Beethoven, Albert Einstein, and Eleanor Roosevelt, who he felt were self-actualizers and had lived rich and productive lives. He identified several characteristics that these people had in common, including a nonhostile sense of humor, originality, creativity, spontaneity, and a need for some privacy. According to Maslow, self-actualized people are more likely than people who are not self-actualized to have what he called **peak experiences**: profound and deeply moving experiences in a person's life that have important and lasting effects on the individual.

George Kelly used himself as a model to theorize about human nature, and set aside the traditional concepts of motivation, unconscious emotion, and reinforcement in his descriptions of **personal construct psychology**. Kelly thought of the individual as a scientist, a person who devises and tests predictions about the behavior of significant people in the individual's life. The individual constructs a scheme of anticipation of what others will do, based on knowledge, perception, and relationships with these other people. Thus, the anxious person, rather than being the victim of inner conflicts and pent-up energy (as in psychodynamic theory), is one who is having difficulty constructing and understanding the variables in the environment. According to Kelly, psychotherapy is a process of insight whereby people acquire new constructs that will allow them to successfully predict troublesome events. Then, the individual will be able to integrate these new constructs into already existing ones.

Carl Rogers is most known for his psychotherapy technique known as **client-centered**, **person-centered**, or **non-directive** therapy. Rogers believed that people have the freedom to control their own behavior, and are neither slaves to the unconscious (as the psychoanalysts would suggest), nor subjects of faulty learning (as the behaviorists would say). Rather than providing solutions or diagnoses, the person-centered therapist helps clients reflect on problems, make choices, generate solutions, take positive action, and determine their own destiny. Rogers was the originator of the concepts of the real and ideal self discussed earlier in the chapter, and his therapeutic techniques aimed to help clients reconcile the differences between the various selves and reduce stress-inducing incongruence. Rogers also pioneered the concept of **unconditional positive regard**, a therapeutic technique by which the therapist accepts the client completely and expresses empathy in order to promote a positive therapeutic environment.

The Type and Trait Perspectives

The type and trait theorists were also borne out of dissatisfaction with psychoanalysis. **Type theorists** attempt to create a taxonomy of personality types, while **trait theorists** prefer to describe individual personality as the sum of a person's characteristic behaviors. For our purposes, we will consider them together.

Early attempts at personality types are generally discredited today. The ancient Greeks, for example, devised **personality types** based on **humors** or body fluids, an imbalance of which could lead to various personality disorders, as shown in Figure 6.16.

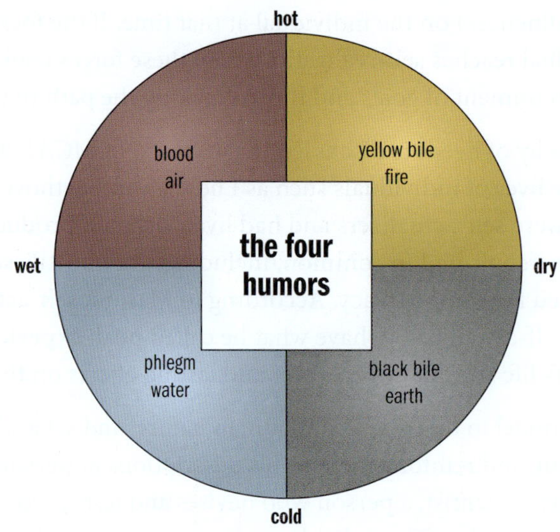

Figure 6.16 The Four Humors
Each humor was correlated with an element, an imbalance of which could lead to different personalities: blood (sanguine; impulsive and charismatic), bile (choleric; aggressive and dominant), black bile (melancholic; depressive and cautious), and phlegm (phlegmatic; relaxed and affectionate).

In the early 20th century, William Sheldon proposed personality types based on body type called **somatotypes**. Sheldon presumed that all short, stocky people were jolly, all tall people were high-strung and aloof, and people in between were strong and well-adjusted. One well-known type theory divides personalities into Types A and B. Individuals with **Type A** personalities are characterized by behavior that tends to be competitive and compulsive, while someone described as **Type B** is generally laid-back and relaxed. Not surprisingly, people with Type A personalities are more prone to heart disease than those with Type B personalities, although there is not much evidence to suggest that people with Type A personalities have a higher mortality rate. An illustration of both types in a work environment are shown in Figure 6.17.

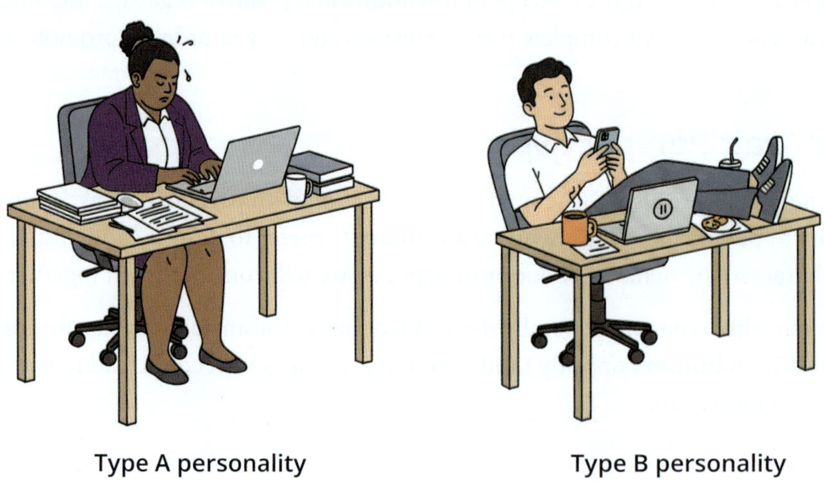

Figure 6.17 Type A and Type B in the Workplace

The Myers–Briggs Type Inventory, described earlier in this chapter, also stands as a well-known example of a type theory.

Trait theorists instead use clusters of behaviors to describe individuals. Hans and Sybil Eysenck used factor analysis to group behaviors that typically occur together and assigned labels to those groups. These groups of behaviors are often also called **traits**. For example, people who are more reserved and less outspoken in groups also tend to enjoy solitary activities and avoid overstimulation. These behaviors fall under the label of introversion. The Eysencks described three traits in the **PEN model**: **Psychoticism** is a measure of nonconformity or social deviance. **Extraversion** is a measure of tolerance for social interaction and stimulation. **Neuroticism** is a measure of emotional arousal in stressful situations. The three-dimensionality of the PEN model is depicted in Figure 6.18. In the same way a mathematical point can be placed in a three-dimensional representation of space, an individual's specific traits can be plotted at a point in the "field" of personalities.

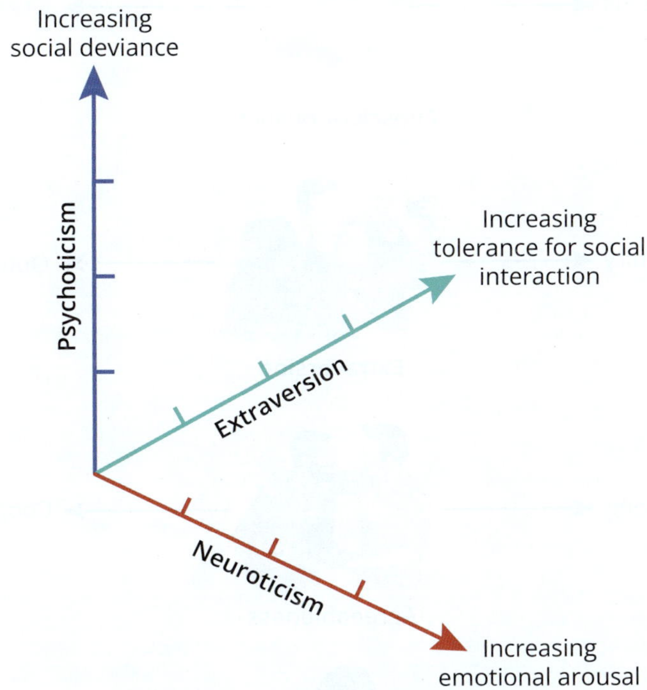

Figure 6.18 The Three-Dimensional PEN Model

Negative affect, though not directly included in the PEN model, is related to neuroticism and describes how a person thinks of themselves and experiences negative emotions. High negative affect corresponds with neuroticism and anxiety, and is associated with several mood disorders. The Eysencks reasoned that people could be distinguished from one another based on where they fell in each of these three dimensions. More recently, the PEN theory has been expanded to what is known as the Five Factor Model, the **Big Five**, which as the name would suggest, uses dimensions of five traits: openness, conscientiousness, extraversion, agreeableness, and neuroticism. Figure 6.19 summarizes and distinguishes these five traits. In this theory, **openness** describes openness to experience, or willingness to engage with the world and desire to try new things. Low openness is associated with persevering in tasks and difficulty with abstraction. **Conscientiousness** is in some ways analogous to self-control, with high conscientiousness associated with high impulse control and low conscientiousness associated with spontaneity.

MNEMONIC

The Big Five Traits of Personality: **OCEAN**

- **O**penness
- **C**onscientiousness
- **E**xtraversion
- **A**greeableness
- **N**euroticism

Agreeableness refers to the degree to which a person is concerned about maintaining peace and harmony in their interactions with others.

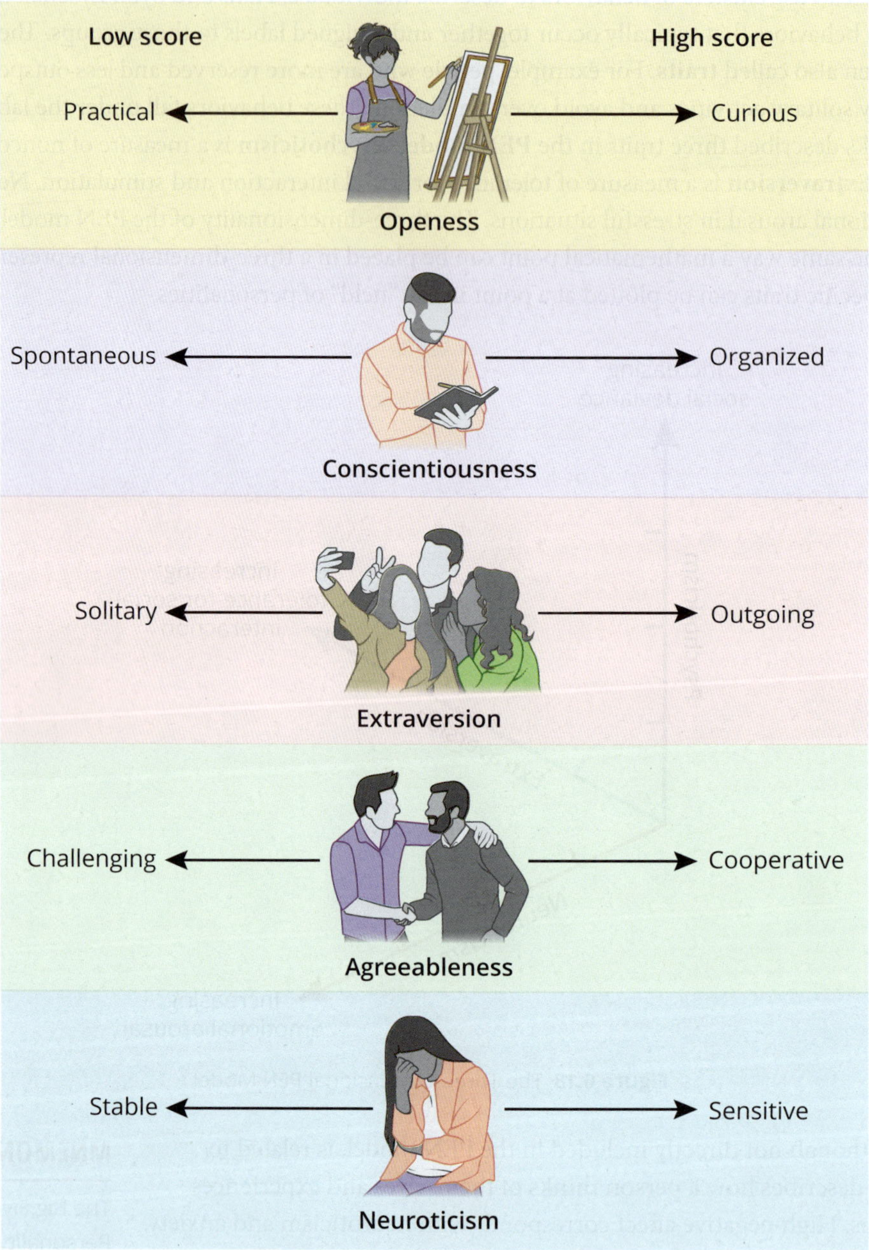

Figure 6.19 The Big Five Traits (OCEAN)

Gordon Allport, primarily a trait theorist, listed three basic types of traits or dispositions: cardinal, central, and secondary. **Cardinal traits** are traits around which people organize their lives. For instance, Mother Teresa's cardinal trait may have been self-sacrifice. While not everyone develops a cardinal trait, everyone does have central and secondary traits. **Central traits** represent major characteristics of the personality that are easy to infer, such as honesty or charisma. **Secondary traits** are other personal characteristics that are more limited in occurrence: aspects of one's personality that only appear in close groups or specific social situations. A major part of Allport's theory is the concept of **functional autonomy**, in which a behavior continues despite satisfaction of the drive that originally created the behavior. A hunter, for example, may have originally hunted to obtain food to eat. However, the hunter may continue even after there is enough food simply for the enjoyment of the hunt: that which began as a means to obtain a goal became the goal itself.

David McClelland identified a personality trait that is referred to as the need for achievement (N-Ach). People who are rated high in N-Ach tend to be concerned with achievement and have pride in their accomplishments. These individuals avoid high risks (to avoid failing) and low risks (because easy tasks will not generate a sense of achievement). Additionally, they set realistic goals, and stop striving toward a goal if success is unlikely.

BEHAVIORAL SCIENCES GUIDED EXAMPLE WITH EXPERT THINKING

Flow is a psychological state marked by high but subjectively effortless attention to a task that usually is accompanied by feelings of complete immersion, enjoyment, and loss of a sense of time. Feelings of flow are maximal in cases in which the task provides a significant challenge, but the individual's skill allows them to meet that challenge. Flow proneness, the likelihood that an individual will enter a flow state given an appropriate compatibility between skill and demand, correlates positively with psychological well-being, self-esteem, life satisfaction, coping strategies, and conscientiousness. It has also been shown that flow proneness correlates negatively with traits related to neuroticism, such as trait anxiety.

New term: flow. Challenge and task tell me this may be related to Yerkes–Dodson. I'll be on the lookout for more relationships between these concepts.

New term: flow proneness. Self-esteem stands out here as a component of identity. I also see conscientiousness and neuroticism, which opens the door for the MCAT to ask about the Big Five.

Behavioral inhibition is a temperamental trait associated with fear and avoidance of novel experience. Because behavioral inhibition is also associated with anxiety and neurotic introversion, it would be reasonable to expect that low behavioral inhibition correlates with flow proneness.

Yet another new term: behavioral inhibition (BI). I want to keep these relationships straight. BI is related to the same OCEAN traits that correspond with low flow proneness (FP), so FP should relate to low BI.

Since the feelings of happiness and enjoyment related to flow derive from intrinsic motivation and rewards, it has also been shown that flow proneness is also correlated with an internal locus of control. Indeed, those with an internal locus of control are more sensitive to differences between individual skill and task challenge but are more likely to experience flow when performing tasks in which skill and challenge are compatible. Locus of control has also been shown to relate to high conscientiousness and low neuroticism.

More relationships: locus of control (LoC) is related in several ways to FP, and one of those ways involves the OCEAN traits again. High FP = Internal LoC = Low BI

Researchers analyzed data from a web-based survey of approximately 11,000 twins registered with the Swedish Twin Registry. This survey included a flow proneness questionnaire, a locus of control scale, and a measure of behavioral inhibition. These results confirmed a low but statistically significant correlation between flow proneness, low behavioral inhibition, and internal locus of control. Analysis also showed a strong relationship between specific genetic markers and all three measures, indicating that a specific set of genes account for a significant amount of the variance in these traits between individuals, possibly through dopaminergic pathways. The data support a dominant inheritance pattern.

Twin study = genetics.

IV: genetic relationship

DV: survey results

Analyzing relationship between dependent variables (survey results). Confirms relationship that correlation is low but significant.

Genetics confirmed. Summary: a few genes related to dopamine might be behind incidence of all of these traits.

Adapted from: Mosing MA, Pedersen NL, Cesarini D, Johannesson M, Magnusson PKE, Nakamura J, et al. (2012) Genetic and Environmental Influences on the Relationship between Flow Proneness, Locus of Control and Behavioral Inhibition. *PLoS ONE* 7(11): e47958. https://doi.org/10.1371/journal.pone.0047958

Which theory of personality is most supported by this experiment, and in what way do concepts from the study of both identity and personality contribute to this support?

The question demands that we integrate the data from the study with our outside knowledge of theories of personality. This passage blends quite a few topics together, so we'll want to read strategically and identify where and when new topics are introduced and explained; any time the passage alludes to content that we've studied we want to be ready to answer at least one question about that topic, so it's worth taking a few seconds to remind ourselves of what we know. Trait theory is definitely included, since the passage makes explicit reference to two of the Big Five: conscientiousness, which is the tendency to be organized, self-disciplined, and achievement focused; and neuroticism, the tendency to be prone to psychological stress and quickness to experience unpleasant emotions such as anger and anxiety. Two more Big Five traits are hinted at in the discussion of behavioral inhibition, which mentions avoidance of novel experience (low openness to experience) and introversion (the opposite of extraversion). If we're careful to look for these types of links as we read the first time, it will save us quite a lot of time on Test Day.

The passage also mentions self-esteem and locus of control, two ideas related to self-concept, and states that they are related to the traits discussed. With all this talk of traits, it would be reasonable to think that the passage is supporting trait theory, but the phrasing of the question stem is key here. We are asked about the experiment specifically, which is only located in the last paragraph of the study. In fact, while we've included a lot of analysis for the sake of completeness, a particularly astute test taker might even avoid some of this analysis and focus solely on analyzing the experiment to answer this question. By tying genetics to personality traits, the experiment in the passage most strongly supports the biological perspective. Overall, the results demonstrate a correlation between the genes regulating dopamine and reward pathways and the traits relating to rewards such as discipline, motivation, and locus of control. Then those traits are linked to the tendency in question in the study, flow proneness.

In summary, while the passage discusses other theories of personality and does provide some support for trait theory, the experiment and data provided most directly support the biological perspective of personality theory.

Other Theories of Personality

Of course, entire textbooks can be (and in fact are) devoted to personality theorists and their ideas. The MCAT tests only the key ideas of each theory, or the concepts that overlap heavily with other topics in this text.

The **behaviorist** perspective, championed by B. F. Skinner, is based heavily on the concepts of operant conditioning, discussed in Chapter 3 of *MCAT Behavioral Sciences Review*. Skinner reasoned that personality is simply a reflection of behaviors that have been reinforced over time. Therapy, then, should focus on learning skills and changing behaviors through operant conditioning techniques. **Token economies**, for example, are often used in inpatient therapeutic settings: positive behavior is rewarded with tokens that can be exchanged for privileges, treats, or other reinforcers.

The **social cognitive** perspective takes behaviorism one step further, focusing not just on how our environment influences our behavior, but also on how we interact with that environment. Albert Bandura's concept of reciprocal determinism is a central idea to this perspective. **Reciprocal determinism** (Figure 6.20) refers to the idea that our thoughts, feelings, behaviors, and environment all interact with each other to determine our actions in a given situation. People choose environments that suit their personalities, and their personalities determine how they will feel about and react to events in those environments. Locus of control is another important concept in the social cognitive perspective: some people feel more in control of their environment while others feel that their environment controls them. For a social cognitive theorist, the best predictor of future behavior is past behavior in similar situations.

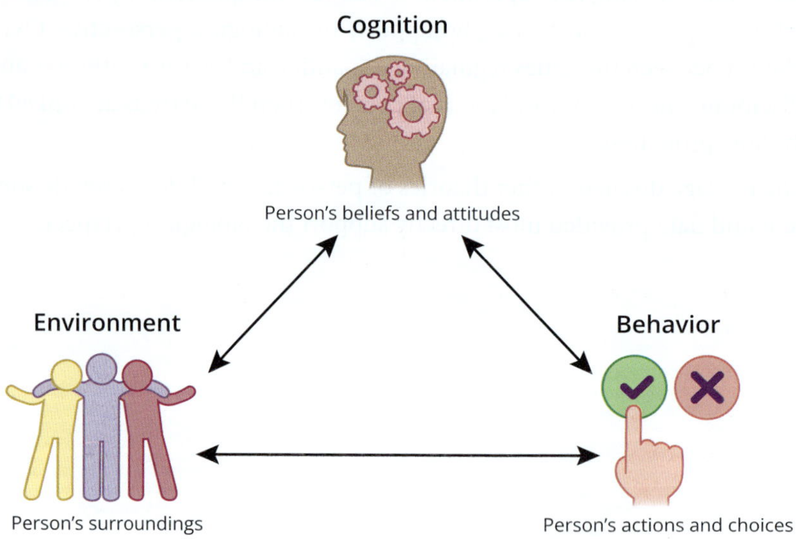

Figure 6.20 Reciprocal Determinism

On the other end of the spectrum lies the **biological** perspective, which holds that personality can be explained as a result of genetic expression in the brain. The biological and trait perspectives are closely linked, as biological theorists maintain that many traits can be shown to result from genes or differences in brain anatomy.

The dichotomy presented by the social cognitive and biological perspectives of personality is similar to another debate in psychology: whether behavior is primarily determined by an individual's personality (the **dispositional approach**) or by the environment and context (the **situational approach**). This division is investigated in depth in the section on attribution theory in Chapter 10 of *MCAT Behavioral Sciences Review*.

MCAT CONCEPT CHECK 6.3

Before you move on, assess your understanding of the material with these questions.

1. For each of the following perspectives, briefly describe how each would define personality.
   - Psychoanalytic:
   - Humanistic:
   - Type:
   - Trait:
   - Behaviorist:
   - Social cognitive:
   - Biological:
2. What are the roles of the id, ego, and superego, according to the psychoanalytic perspective?
   - Id:
   - Ego:
   - Superego:

3. What are the traits described by the Eysencks' PEN theory, and what does each describe?
   - P:

   ____

   - E:

   ____

   - N:

   ____

4. What are the Big Five personality traits?
   1. ____
   2. ____
   3. ____
   4. ____
   5. ____

Conclusion

In this chapter, we discussed two concepts that are central to the study of psychology: identity, which describes who we are, and personality, which describes the set of thoughts, feelings, traits, and behaviors that are characteristic of each of us across time and different locations. We discussed a variety of approaches to both, each with their own theorists and critics. The ideas presented in this chapter are ripe for the MCAT to test; expect questions on Test Day to ask you to identify the various perspectives and the differences between them as they apply to behavior and research.

Many of the theories of personality focus on problems in everyday life: how we cope with stresses, anxiety, and depression. In medical school, your focus will be primarily on these pathologic states of mind, or psychological disorders. It is to this extremely important topic—abnormal psychology—that we turn our attention in the next chapter.

GO ONLINE

You've reviewed the content, now test your knowledge and critical thinking skills by completing a test-like passage set in your online resources!

CONCEPT SUMMARY

Self-Concept and Identity

- **Self-concept** is the sum of the ways in which we describe ourselves: in the present, who we used to be, and who we might be in the future.
- Our **identities** are individual components of our self-concept related to the groups to which we belong. Religious affiliation, sexual orientation, and ethnic and national affiliations are examples of identities.
- **Self-esteem** describes our evaluation of ourselves. Generally, the closer our **actual self** is to our **ideal self** (who we want to be) and our **ought self** (who others want us to be), the higher our self-esteem will be.
- **Self-efficacy** is the degree to which we see ourselves as being capable at a given skill or in a given situation. When placed in a consistently hopeless scenario, self-efficacy can be diminished to the point where **learned helplessness** results.
- **Locus of control** is a self-evaluation that refers to the way we characterize the influences in our lives. People with an internal locus of control see their successes and failures as a result of their own characteristics and actions, while those with an external locus of control perceive outside factors as having more of an influence in their lives.

Formation of Identity

- Freud's psychosexual stages of personality development are based on the tensions caused by the **libido**. Failure at any given stage leads to **fixation** that causes personality disorders. Freud's phases (oral, anal, phallic [Oedipal], latent, and genital) are based on the erogenous zones that are the focus of each phase of development.
- Erikson's stages of psychosocial development stem from conflicts that occur throughout life (trust vs. mistrust, autonomy vs. shame and doubt, initiative vs. guilt, industry vs. inferiority, identity vs. role confusion, intimacy vs. isolation, generativity vs. stagnation, integrity vs. despair). These conflicts are the result of decisions we are forced to make about ourselves and the environment around us at each phase of our lives.
- Kohlberg's stages of moral development describe the approaches of individuals to resolving moral dilemmas. Kohlberg believed that we progress through six stages divided into three main phases: **preconventional**, **conventional**, and **postconventional**.
- Vygotsky described development of language, culture, and skills. He proposed the idea of the **zone of proximal development**, which describes those skills that a child has not yet mastered and require a **more knowledgeable other** to accomplish.
- **Imitation** and **role-taking** are common ways children learn from others. Children first reproduce the behaviors of role models, and later learn to see the perspectives of others and practice taking on new roles.
- Our self-concept depends in part on our **reference group**, or the group to which we compare ourselves. Two individuals with the same qualities might see themselves differently depending on how those qualities compare to their reference groups.

Personality

- The **psychoanalytic** perspective views personality as resulting from unconscious urges and desires.
    - Freud's theories are based on the **id** (base urges of survival and reproduction), the **superego** (the idealist and perfectionist), and the **ego** (the mediator between the two and the conscious mind). The ego makes use of **defense mechanisms** to reduce stress caused by the urges of the id and the superego.
    - Jung assumed a **collective unconscious** that links all humans together. He viewed the personality as being influenced by **archetypes**.
    - Other psychoanalysts such as Adler and Horney have distanced themselves from Freud's theories, claiming that the unconscious is motivated by social rather than sexual urges.
- The **humanistic** perspective emphasizes the internal feelings of healthy individuals as they strive toward happiness and self-realization. Maslow's **hierarchy of needs** and Rogers's therapeutic approach of **unconditional positive regard** flow from the humanistic view of personality.
- **Type** and **trait** theorists believe that personality can be described as a number of identifiable traits that carry characteristic behaviors.
    - Type theories of personality include the ancient Greek notion of humors, Sheldon's **somatotypes**, division into **Types A** and **B**, and the **Myers–Briggs Type Inventory**.
    - The Eysencks identified three major traits which could be used to describe all individuals. The acronym for these traits is PEN: **psychoticism** (nonconformity), **extraversion** (tolerance for social interaction and stimulation), and **neuroticism** (arousal in stressful situations). Later trait theorists expanded these traits to the **Big Five**: openness, conscientiousness, extraversion, agreeableness, and neuroticism.
    - Allport identified three basic types of traits: cardinal, central, and secondary. **Cardinal traits** are the traits around which people organize their lives; not everyone develops a cardinal trait. **Central traits** represent major characteristics of the personality and **secondary traits** are more personal characteristics and are limited in occurrence.
    - McClelland identified the personality trait of the need for achievement (N-Ach).
- The **social cognitive** perspective holds that individuals interact with their environment in a cycle called **reciprocal determinism**. People mold their environments according to their personalities, and those environments in turn shape our thoughts, feelings, and behaviors.
- The **behaviorist** perspective, based on the concept of operant conditioning, holds that personality can be described as the behaviors one has learned from prior rewards and punishments.
- **Biological** theorists claim that behavior can be explained as a result of genetic expression.

ANSWERS TO CONCEPT CHECKS

6.1

1. Self-concept describes the sum of all of the phrases that come to mind when we think of who we are, who we used to be, and who we may become in the future. Identity, on the other hand, describes a set of behaviors and labels we take on when in a specific group.
2. Ethnic identity is determined by common ancestry, cultural heritage, and language, among other similarities. Rather than being determined by birth, national identity is determined by the political borders of where one lives and the cultural identity of that nation.
3. A student with an internal locus of control will look for internal factors, such as not having studied hard enough. A student with an external locus of control will blame external factors such as bad luck or the test being too difficult.

6.2

1. Freud would say that the individual has become fixated in that stage and will display the personality traits of that fixation for life. Erikson would say that the individual will still move through subsequent phases, but will be lacking the skills and virtues granted by successful resolution of that stage. Kohlberg would say that the individual was incapable of reasoning at the level of failure, and that the individual would use the reasoning described in previous stages to resolve moral dilemmas.
2.

Phase	Description
Preconventional	Reasoning is based on individual rewards and punishments
Conventional	Reasoning is based on the relationship of the individual to society
Postconventional	Reasoning is based on abstract principles

3. Zone of proximal development does not just apply to children, but rather the acquisition of new skills and abilities at any age. Standardized tests require students to utilize many skills that they may not yet have fully developed, but are in the process of development. This is why results can be improved by getting the help of those with more knowledge about the exam, such as expert instructors and authors.

6.3

1. Psychoanalytic: Personality is the result of unconscious urges and desires.

   Humanistic: Personality comes from conscious feelings about oneself resulting from healthy striving for self-realization.

   Type: Personalities are sets of distinct qualities and dispositions into which people can be grouped.

   Trait: Personalities are assembled from having different degrees of certain qualities and dispositions.

   Behaviorist: Personality is the result of behavioral responses to stimuli based on prior rewards and punishments.

   Social cognitive: Personality comes from the interactions between individuals and their environment.

   Biological: Personality is based on genetic influences and brain anatomy.
2. The id is the sum of our basic urges to reproduce and survive, while the superego is our sense of perfectionism and idealism. The ego mediates the anxieties caused by the actions of the id and superego by using defense mechanisms.
3. Psychoticism: nonconformity or social deviance

   Extraversion: tolerance for social interaction and stimulation

   Neuroticism: emotional arousal in stressful situations
4. The Big Five personality traits are openness, conscientiousness, extraversion, agreeableness, and neuroticism.

SCIENCE MASTERY ASSESSMENT EXPLANATIONS

1. **B**

Self-concept is defined as the sum of all of the ways in which we see ourselves, including who we are, as in **(D)**, who we were in the past, **(A)**, and who we may become in the future, **(C)**. The ought self, while closely related to self-esteem, is our appraisal of how others see us and is not a part of our self-concept.

2. **D**

Androgyny is defined as scoring highly on scales of both femininity and masculinity. Achieving a low score on both scales, **(A)**, would be considered undifferentiated, while **(B)** and **(C)** would be described as feminine and masculine, respectively.

3. **B**

Because there is nothing in the question stem to suggest that this situation will fundamentally change this student's attitudes in the short term, **(A)** and **(D)** can be eliminated. **(C)** is unlikely in the short term, as learned helplessness requires a repeated inability to have any effect on a situation over a long period of time and is much more severe, usually manifesting as depression. It is far more likely that the student will simply feel ineffective when it comes to math, which is low self-efficacy.

4. **A**

Because we know the lawyer has an internal locus of control, we expect belief in being in control of the events happening in life. Both **(B)** and **(C)** attribute success to outside factors, representing an external locus of control. While **(D)** perhaps represents an attribution that could correlate to low self-esteem, it is not indicative of locus of control.

5. **B**

Both excessive organization and excessive sloppiness are indicative of fixation in the anal stage of psychosexual development—what is commonly referred to as anal-retentiveness.

6. **C**

As a postadolescent young adult, this person would be described by Erikson as experiencing the conflict of intimacy vs. isolation, and so forming significant relationships with others would be a primary goal. **(B)** and **(D)** represent the next two stages in life (generativity vs. stagnation and integrity vs. despair, respectively), while **(A)** is the conflict that Erikson would say should have been resolved in adolescence (identity vs. role confusion).

7. **A**

Matt's reasoning reflects a desire to avoid punishment, which reflects stage one in Kohlberg's preconventional phase (obedience). Cati's reasoning takes into account social order, reflecting stage four in the conventional phase (law and order).

8. **D**

This situation is best described by Lev Vygotsky's zone of proximal development theory, which holds that children are often unable to perform tasks by themselves, but can complete the task with the help of a more knowledgeable other.

9. **D**

(C) has no support from role-taking research and can be eliminated. **(A)** and **(B)** are both inaccurate; the Bobo doll experiment shows young children modeling behavior not performed by their parents, and teens are most influenced by their peers, not celebrities and athletes. The research does suggest, however, that children are more likely to engage in behavior modeled by individuals who are like themselves; thus, a female child is more likely to imitate behavior by another female.

10. **C**

The superego is responsible for moral guilt when we do not live up to our ideals. While the id and the libido, **(A)** and **(D)**, may be responsible for the urge to have an affair, the superego is responsible for the anxiety one feels afterward.

11. **C**

Jung saw the drive for power and success as typically male traits, so Jung would say this woman is exercising her "inner man." The animus is the archetype that most closely reflects this quality.

12. **C**

This research supports a link between genetic expression and behavior, which is a central tenet of the biological perspective. The social cognitive perspective also holds that people's behaviors and traits shape their environments, which in turn have an effect on their identity, so the discovery also supports this perspective. Behaviorism is not supported, as the discovery is not related to rewards and punishments.

13. **B**

As a rebel and a sociable person, this individual would score highly on both psychoticism and extraversion, respectively. Neuroticism is associated with high emotional arousal in stressful situations, so being able to keep calm in an emergency is a sign of low neuroticism. Conscientiousness, a trait associated with being hardworking and organized instead of impulsive, is not described by the question stem.

14. **A**

Reaction formation is a defense mechanism that converts unwanted feelings into their exact opposite. A psychodynamic theorist would say that the terror and hatred victims feel toward their captors might be unconsciously turned into affection in an effort to reduce the stress of the situation.

15. **B**

Fictional finalism is comprised of internal, idealistic beliefs about the future. The assumption that winning the lottery will solve all of life's problems is representative of this form of thinking. Cardinal traits, **(A),** are the traits around which individuals organize their entire life. Functional autonomy, **(C)**, is when a behavior continues after the drive behind the behavior has ceased; for example, if this young professional continued purchasing lottery tickets after winning simply for enjoyment, then this behavior would have gained functional autonomy. Unconditional positive regard, **(D)**, is used in some forms of humanistic therapy in which the therapist believes in the internal good of the client and does not judge the client negatively for any words or actions.

GO ONLINE

Consult your online resources for additional practice.

SHARED CONCEPTS

Behavioral Sciences Chapter 3
Learning and Memory

Behavioral Sciences Chapter 4
Cognition, Consciousness, and Language

Behavioral Sciences Chapter 5
Motivation, Emotion, and Stress

Behavioral Sciences Chapter 7
Psychological Disorders

Behavioral Sciences Chapter 9
Social Interaction

Behavioral Sciences Chapter 10
Social Thinking

CHAPTER 7

PSYCHOLOGICAL DISORDERS

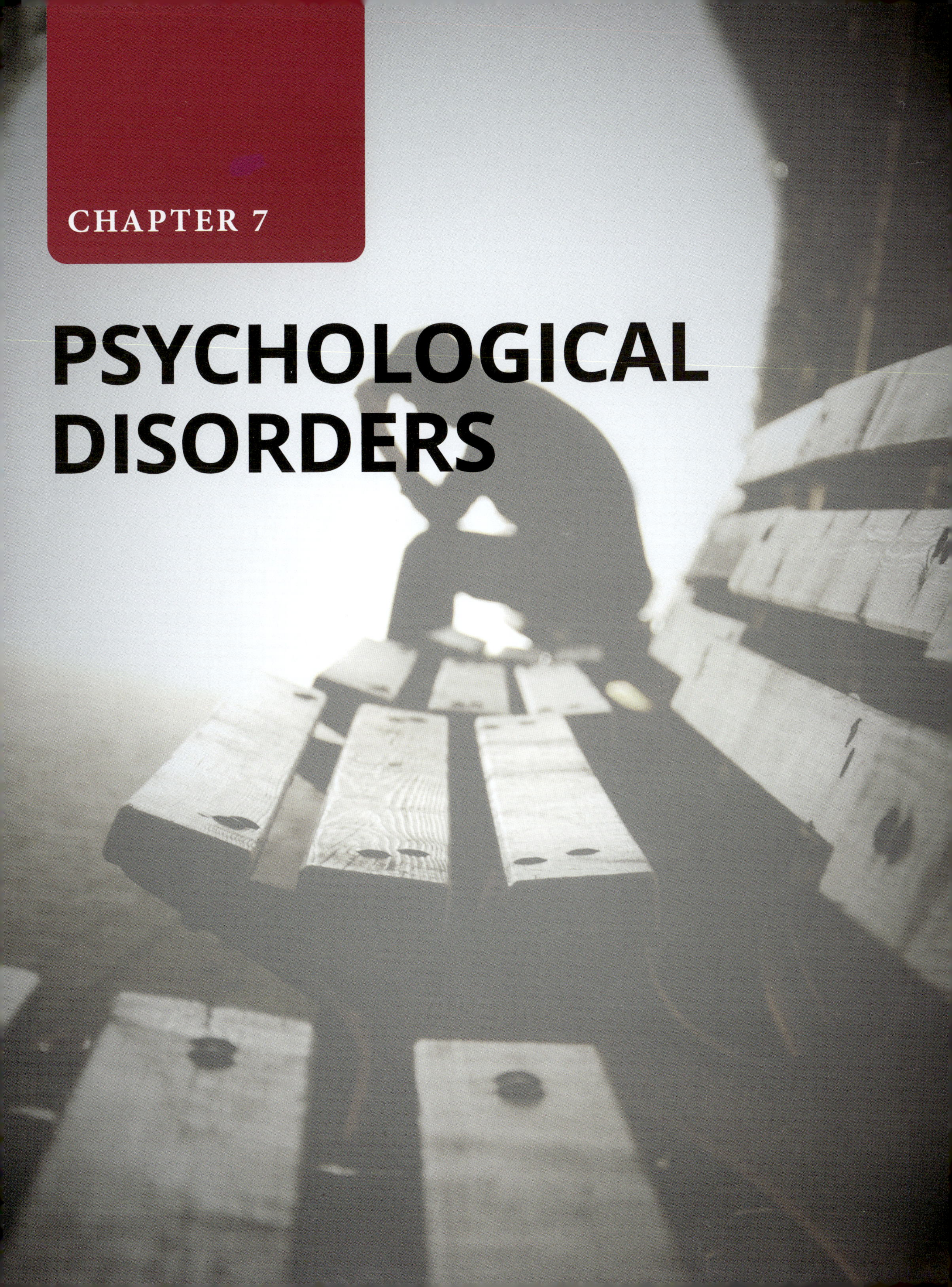

SCIENCE MASTERY ASSESSMENT

Every pre-med knows this feeling: there is so much content I have to know for the MCAT! How do I know what to do first or what's important?

While the high-yield badges throughout this book will help you identify the most important topics, this Science Mastery Assessment is another tool in your MCAT prep arsenal. This quiz (which can also be taken in your online resources) and the guidance below will help ensure that you are spending the appropriate amount of time on this chapter based on your personal strengths and weaknesses. Don't worry though—skipping something now does not mean you'll never study it. Later on in your prep, as you complete full-length tests, you'll uncover specific pieces of content that you need to review and can come back to these chapters as appropriate.

How to Use This Assessment

If you answer 0–7 questions correctly:

Spend about 1 hour to read this chapter in full and take limited notes throughout. Follow up by reviewing **all** quiz questions to ensure that you now understand how to solve each one.

If you answer 8–11 questions correctly:

Spend 20–40 minutes reviewing the quiz questions. Beginning with the questions you missed, read and take notes on the corresponding subchapters. For questions you answered correctly, ensure your thinking matches that of the explanation and you understand why each choice was correct or incorrect.

If you answer 12–15 questions correctly:

Spend less than 20 minutes reviewing all questions from the quiz. If you missed any, then include a quick read-through of the corresponding subchapters, or even just the relevant content within a subchapter, as part of your question review. For questions you answered correctly, ensure your thinking matches that of the explanation and review the Concept Summary at the end of the chapter.

1. Which of the following is an example of a negative symptom seen in schizophrenia?
   - **A.** Auditory hallucinations
   - **B.** Disorganized behavior
   - **C.** Disturbance of affect
   - **D.** Delusions

2. During an interview with a schizophrenic patient, a psychiatrist notices that the patient keeps repeating what the psychiatrist says. This phenomenon is known as:
   - **A.** echolalia.
   - **B.** echopraxia.
   - **C.** loosening of associations.
   - **D.** neologisms.

3. A 42-year-old patient has always been extremely neat and tidy. This person works as a secretary and stays long after normal working hours to check the punctuation and spelling of letters prepared during the day. The patient was referred for counseling by a supervisor after repeatedly getting into fights with coworkers. "They don't take the job to heart," the patient says. "They just joke around all day." The most likely preliminary diagnosis for this patient is:
   - **A.** obsessive–compulsive personality disorder.
   - **B.** antisocial personality disorder.
   - **C.** narcissistic personality disorder.
   - **D.** borderline personality disorder.

4. Which of the following is true with regard to a major depressive episode?
   - **A.** It may last less than two weeks.
   - **B.** It must involve thoughts of suicide or a suicide attempt.
   - **C.** It may involve a decrease in sleep.
   - **D.** It must involve feelings of sadness.

5. A young person moves to a new city to start work on an accelerated degree program. After a few months this individual visits the doctor complaining of stress and isolation and is diagnosed with depression. The doctor ascribes the cause to low levels of serotonin and prescribes an SSRI for treatment. Which of the following best describes the physician's approach to diagnosis and treatment?
   - **A.** Biomedical approach with indirect therapy
   - **B.** Biomedical approach with direct therapy
   - **C.** Biopsychosocial approach with indirect therapy
   - **D.** Biopsychosocial approach with direct therapy

6. A young person of unknown age is brought by the Philadelphia police to the local emergency department for evaluation after being found wandering in a park. The patient carries no identification and is unable to provide a first or last name or any life details, except that the name Phoenix seems familiar. The police in Arizona are contacted and find a missing persons report matching the patient's description. Based on this information, the most likely diagnosis for this patient is:
   - **A.** depersonalization/derealization disorder.
   - **B.** dissociative identity disorder.
   - **C.** somatic symptom disorder.
   - **D.** dissociative amnesia with dissociative fugue.

7. In addition to being a freestanding diagnosis, agoraphobia is most often seen in association with which other psychiatric diagnosis?
   - **A.** Obsessive–compulsive disorder
   - **B.** Avoidant personality disorder
   - **C.** Generalized anxiety disorder
   - **D.** Panic disorder

8. A researcher is interested in studying fear responses to a variety of different stimuli. To rule out potential confounding variables, the research excludes individuals with phobias from the study. In a sample of 50 participants, how many will likely be excluded from the study, assuming that the sample is representative of the overall population?
   - **A.** 45
   - **B.** 15
   - **C.** 10
   - **D.** 5

Questions 9–10 refer to the scenario described below.

A physician is attempting to diagnose a patient's mental disorder based on a set of symptoms. The confirmed symptoms currently include appetite disturbance, substantial weight change, decreased energy, a feeling of worthlessness, and excessive guilt.

9. What two disorders could these symptoms indicate?
   - **A.** Major depressive and bipolar disorders
   - **B.** Dissociative amnesia and depersonalization/derealization disorder
   - **C.** Alzheimer's disease and Parkinson's disease
   - **D.** Specific phobia and panic disorder

10. What should the physician ask about to distinguish between the two possible disorders affecting that patient?
    - **A.** Whether the patient has amnesia
    - **B.** Whether the patient has also had manic episodes
    - **C.** Whether the patient is irrationally afraid of anything
    - **D.** Whether the patient has experienced difficulty performing familiar tasks

11. All of the following are risk factors or diagnostic criteria for Alzheimer's disease EXCEPT:
    - **A.** Extra copies of the β-amyloid precursor protein gene.
    - **B.** Decreased abundance of serotonin and norepinephrine.
    - **C.** Neurofibrillary tangles of hyperphosphorylated tau protein.
    - **D.** Deficient blood flow to the parietal lobes.

12. Splitting is a defense mechanism commonly seen with which personality disorder?
    - **A.** Antisocial personality disorder
    - **B.** Borderline personality disorder
    - **C.** Histrionic personality disorder
    - **D.** Narcissistic personality disorder

13. A patient comes to the doctor with a two-week history of complete paralysis of the left arm. The patient has had no injury to the extremity, and full neurological workup fails to demonstrate any underlying cause. The patient seems surprisingly unconcerned about the paralysis, and seems more worried about an argument that happened one month ago in which the patient hit a family member. Based on this information, the patient's most likely diagnosis is:
    - **A.** conversion disorder.
    - **B.** generalized anxiety disorder.
    - **C.** illness anxiety disorder.
    - **D.** histrionic personality disorder.

14. A patient is taken to the doctor after starting to move the fingers in such a way that it looks like rolling something, despite nothing actually being there. The patient also exhibits slowed movement and a shuffling gait. Which neurotransmitter is likely to be present in decreased levels in the patient's brain?
    - **A.** Epinephrine
    - **B.** Histamine
    - **C.** Dopamine
    - **D.** Serotonin

15. Which of the following is/are true regarding bipolar disorders?
    - **I.** They have little, if any, genetic heritability.
    - **II.** They are associated with increased levels of serotonin in the brain.
    - **III.** They all require at least one depressive episode for diagnosis.
    - **A.** I only
    - **B.** II only
    - **C.** I and III only
    - **D.** II and III only

Answer Key

1. **C** (See section 7.2)
2. **A** (See section 7.2)
3. **A** (See section 7.2)
4. **C** (See section 7.2)
5. **B** (See section 7.1)
6. **D** (See section 7.2)
7. **D** (See section 7.2)
8. **D** (See section 7.1)
9. **A** (See section 7.2)
10. **B** (See section 7.2)
11. **B** (See section 7.3)
12. **B** (See section 7.2)
13. **A** (See section 7.2)
14. **C** (See section 7.3)
15. **B** (See section 7.2)

The relevant section of the chapter to review for each question is given in parentheses after the correct answer. Detailed explanations can be found at the end of the chapter.

CHAPTER 7

PSYCHOLOGICAL DISORDERS

In This Chapter

CHAPTER PROFILE

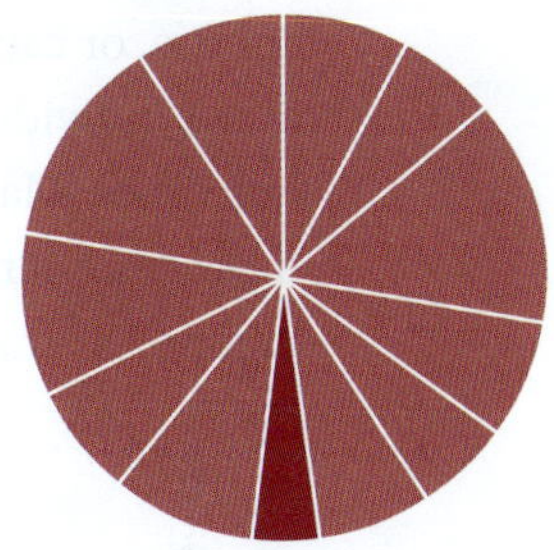

4%

The content in this chapter should be relevant to about 4% of all questions about the behavioral sciences on the MCAT.

This chapter covers material from the following AAMC content category:

7A: Individual influences on behavior

Introduction

The progress in our understanding of hysteria has come largely through the elaboration of the so-called mechanisms by which the symptoms arise. These mechanisms have been declared to reside or to have their origin in the subconsciousness or coconsciousness. The mechanisms range all the way from the conception of Janet that the personality is disintegrated owing to lowering of the psychical tension to that of Freud, who conceives all hysterical symptoms as a result of dissociation arising through conflicts between repressed sexual desires and experiences and the various censors organized by the social life.

The above is an excerpt from the *Journal of Abnormal Psychology* in 1915. Merely a century ago, our understanding of psychological disorders was in its infancy. Hysteria—the antiquated name for conversion disorder—was thought to result from marital discord and repressed sexual desires. We are now beginning to understand the underlying psychological and biological factors at play in a number of mental illnesses. In this chapter, we will focus on several different types of psychological disorders, their classification, causes, and frequencies.

MCAT EXPERTISE

If you've taken a glance at the rest of this book, you might have noticed that this chapter has a low percentage of relevant content as compared to the rest of the chapters within *MCAT Behavioral Sciences Review*. While Chapter 7 materials will be tested less often than the other materials in this book, there are so many psychology questions on the MCAT that even lower-yield topics within the behavioral sciences will get you points!

7.1 Understanding Psychological Disorders

LEARNING OBJECTIVES

After Chapter 7.1, you will be able to:

- Compare and contrast the biomedical and the biopsychosocial models of psychological disorders
- Recall the most common psychological disorders in the United States

Psychological disorders are characteristic sets of thoughts, feelings, or actions that cause noticeable distress to the sufferer, are considered deviant by the individual's culture, or cause **maladaptive** functioning in society, meaning that some aspect of the individual's behavior negatively impacts others or leads to self-defeating outcomes. Many disorders can be treated once diagnosed. The process of defining these disorders varies, and there are two main classification systems (depicted in Figure 7.1) that you'll need to know for the MCAT.

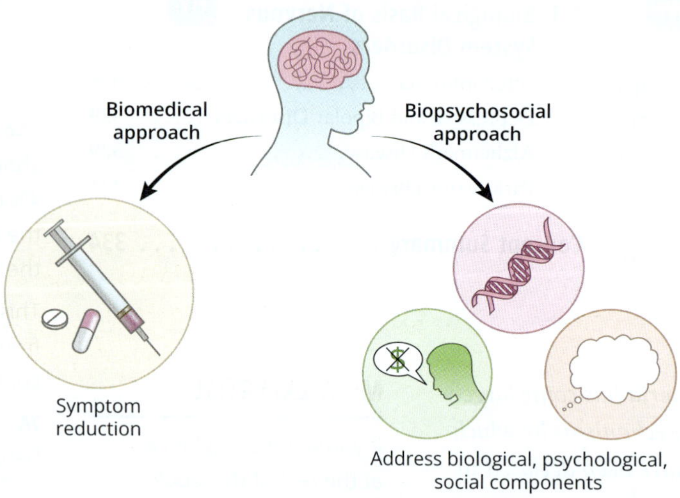

Figure 7.1 The Biomedical and Biopsychosocial Approaches

REAL WORLD

Thomas Szasz, an outspoken critic of labeling people "mentally ill," argues that most of the disorders treated by clinicians are not really illnesses. Rather, they are traits or behaviors that differ from the cultural norm. Szasz argues that labeling people as mentally ill is a way to force them to change and conform to societal norms rather than allowing them to attack the societal causes of their problems.

Biomedical vs. Biopsychosocial Approaches

The first classification system to know for the MCAT is the **biomedical approach** to psychological disorders. Biomedical therapy emphasizes interventions that rally around symptom reduction of psychological disorders. In other words, this approach assumes that any disorder has roots in biomedical disturbances, and thus the solution should also be of a biomedical nature. This view is thought of as narrower than other approaches because it fails to take into account many of the other sources of disorders, such as lifestyle and socioeconomic status. For example, heart disease clearly has roots within the mechanisms of the cardiac muscle, but the causes of these malfunctions have as much to do with biomedical causes (such as genetics) as they do with lifestyle causes (such as a diet rich in salty, fatty foods; smoking; and alcohol use). Similarly, this biomedical approach can miss some underlying sources of psychological disorders and is often more effective when supplemented with a broader approach to diagnosis and treatment.

A broader classification system commonly used for these psychological disorders is the **biopsychosocial approach**. This method assumes that there are biological, psychological, and social components to an individual's disorder. The biological component of a disorder is something in the body, like having a particular genetic syndrome. The psychological component of a disorder stems from the individual's thoughts, emotions, or behaviors. Finally, the disorder's social component results from the individual's surroundings and can include issues of perceived class in society and even discrimination or stigmatization. All three of these aspects of a disorder are considered in the biopsychosocial approach for both diagnosis and treatment.

To better understand the biopsychosocial approach, consider depression. Certain genetic factors can make an individual more or less susceptible to depressive tendencies, showing a purely biological influence on the disorder. However, from a psychological perspective, the levels of stress that the individual experiences can also contribute to the severity of the depression experienced. Finally, the social environment may provide additional stressors or support from one's career, family, and friends. Accordingly, in the biopsychosocial model, the goal is often to provide not only **direct therapy**—treatment that acts directly on the individual, such as medication or periodic meetings with a psychologist—but also **indirect therapy**, which aims to increase social support by educating and empowering family and friends of the affected individual.

MCAT EXPERTISE

The biopsychosocial model was originally theorized in a 1977 *Science* article and has grown in breadth, depth, and applicability since it was first described. In fact, the increased recognition of psychological and social factors on patient care was one of the primary drivers for the creation of the *Psychological, Social, and Biological Foundations of Behavior* section of the MCAT!

Classifying Psychological Disorders

To aid clinicians in considering these factors, the ***Diagnostic and Statistical Manual of Mental Disorders*** (**DSM**) was created. Originally, the manual was written to collect statistical data in the United States. It is now used as a diagnostic tool in the United States and various other countries. The manual is currently in its fifth edition, which was published in May 2013, so the common abbreviation seen is DSM-5. This manual is a compilation of many known psychological disorders. The DSM-5's classification scheme is not based on theories of etiology (cause) or treatments of different disorders. Rather, it is based on descriptions of symptoms. It is used by clinicians to fit lists of compiled symptoms from a patient into a category and thus to diagnose that patient. The DSM-5 has 20 diagnostic classes of mental disorders; those that will be tested on the MCAT are discussed in this chapter.

REAL WORLD

David Rosenhan studied whether it was possible to be judged sane if you are in an "insane place" (a psychiatric hospital). Rosenhan and seven other "sane" people were admitted into psychiatric hospitals by reporting auditory hallucinations. Each of these pseudopatients was diagnosed to have either schizophrenia or bipolar disorder, and each was admitted. Once admitted, they acted completely normal—but it still took an average of three weeks to be discharged, and each was still given the diagnosis of schizophrenia in remission. Once labeled, it is very hard to distance oneself from the diagnosis of mental illness.

Rates of Psychological Disorders

Suffering from a mental disorder can be a lonely experience because the disorder usually occurs only in the mind of the patient. However, the rates of these psychological disorders are higher than this experience would otherwise suggest. Table 7.1 covers these rates in detail.

MCAT EXPERTISE

The MCAT tests many, but not all, categories of mental disorder described within the DSM-5. Neurodevelopmental disorders, eating disorders, impulse control disorders, sleeping disorders, and others are not listed within the AAMC's guide to MCAT content, and as such are not included within this text.

Disorder	Percentage Affected	Number Affected (in Millions)
Any mental disorder	18.3	44.7
Specific phobia	9.1	22.2
Social anxiety disorder	7.1	17.3
Major depressive disorder	6.7	16.4
Posttraumatic stress disorder	3.6	8.8
Bipolar disorder	2.8	6.8
Generalized anxiety disorder	2.7	6.6
Panic disorder	2.7	6.6
Borderline personality disorder	1.4	3.4
Obsessive–compulsive disorder	1.2	2.9
Agoraphobia	0.9	2.2
Anorexia nervosa	0.6	1.5
Schizophrenia	0.6	1.5
All cancers*	6.1	15.1
Diabetes*	9.4	23.0

*Note: These nonpsychological conditions are included for comparison.

All data from this website: https://www.nimh.nih.gov/health/statistics/index.shtml

Table 7.1 One-Year Prevalence Rates for Psychological Disorders in the United States

Treatment of Psychological Disorders

Psychological disorders can be treated in many ways, but treatments fall under the two broad categories of **psychopharmacology**, or the use of medications, and **psychotherapy**, or the use of specialized techniques by a trained therapist. Psychotherapy can be further subdivided into **talk therapy**, which emphasizes verbal interactions and the exploration of thoughts and feelings, and **behavioral therapy**, which focuses on directly modifying maladaptive behaviors using learning principles. Figure 7.2 illustrates these approaches to treatment.

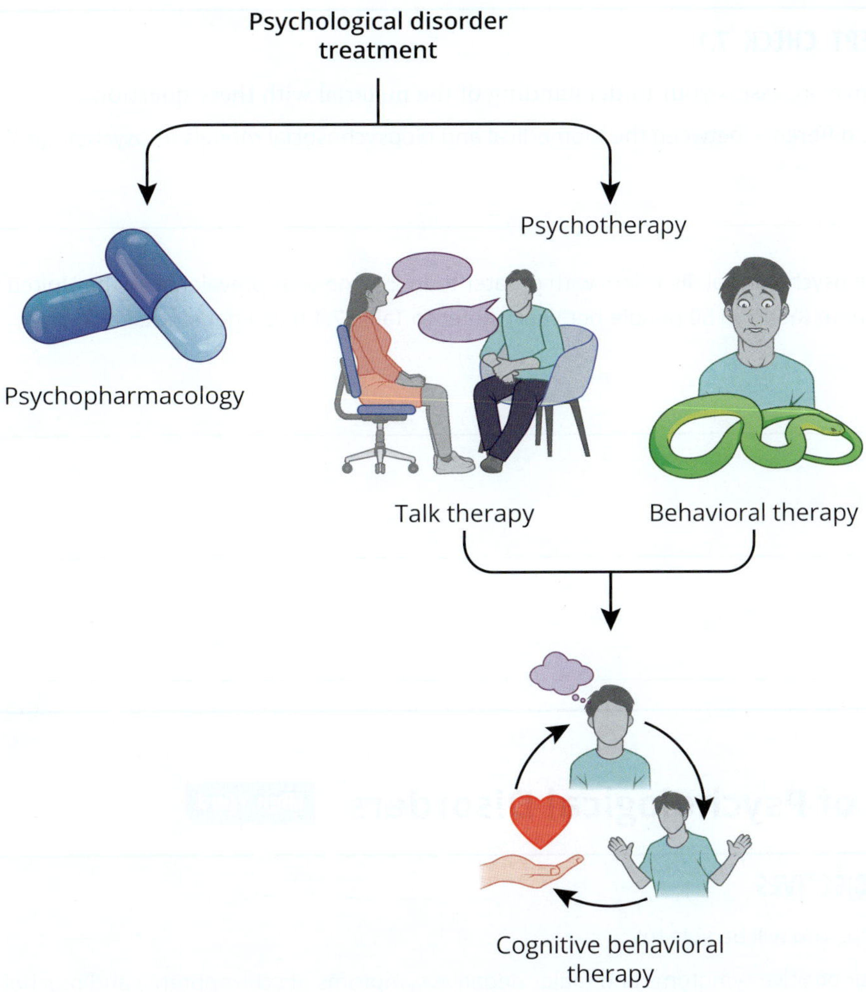

Figure 7.2 Treatment Types for Psychological Disorders

Examples of talk therapy include psychoanalysis and humanistic therapy (see Chapter 6 for more on the theories of personality these types of therapies are based upon). Behavioral therapy includes techniques like systematic desensitization, a method typically used to treat phobias. In **systematic desensitization**, a patient with a phobia is gradually exposed to the feared object or situation while being taught relaxation techniques, ultimately reducing the fear response. Some psychotherapies employ a hybrid approach with both talk and behavioral elements, like **cognitive behavioral therapy (CBT)**. CBT, which is one of the most widely practiced types of therapy today, operates on the principle that maladaptive thought patterns and behaviors contribute to psychological distress, and by identifying and modifying these patterns, individuals can experience symptom relief and improved well-being. CBT therapists help individuals challenge negative or distorted thoughts, develop healthier coping mechanisms, and gradually confront feared situations. CBT is used to treat a wide range of disorders, including depression, anxiety disorders, and post-traumatic stress disorder (PTSD).

MCAT CONCEPT CHECK 7.1

Before you move on, assess your understanding of the material with these questions.

1. What is the difference between the biomedical and biopsychosocial models of psychological disorders?

---

2. Name three psychological disorders with greater than 2% one-year prevalence in the United States (affecting more than 1 in 50 people per year). Refer to Table 7.1 if you get stuck.
   -
   -
   -

7.2 Types of Psychological Disorders High Yield

LEARNING OBJECTIVES

After Chapter 7.2, you will be able to:

- List the major positive symptoms and major negative symptoms of schizophrenia and psychotic disorders
- Recall the features of major depressive episodes, manic and hypomanic episodes
- Distinguish between the testable mood disorders
- Relate obsessions and compulsions to the symptoms of obsessive–compulsive disorder
- Describe and explain the symptoms of posttraumatic stress disorder (PTSD)
- Describe and distinguish dissociative and somatic symptom disorders
- Describe the features and individual disorders that fall under cluster A, B, and C personality disorders

As mentioned earlier, the DSM-5 categorizes common symptoms into 20 diagnostic classes. Many of these classes represent significant revisions from the DSM-5's immediate predecessor, the DSM-IV-TR. The most heavily tested diagnostic classes on the MCAT are schizophrenia spectrum and other psychotic disorders, bipolar and related disorders, depressive disorders, anxiety disorders, obsessive–compulsive and related disorders, trauma- and stressor-related disorders, dissociative disorders, somatic symptom and related disorders, and personality disorders.

Schizophrenia and Other Psychotic Disorders

According to the DSM-5, individuals with a **psychotic disorder** present with one or more of the following symptoms: delusions, hallucinations, disorganized thought, disorganized behavior, catatonia, and negative symptoms. Like most psychological categories, psychotic disorders are on a spectrum. To delineate the psychotic disorders as described in the DSM-5, psychotic symptoms must be understood.

Psychotic symptoms are divided into positive and negative types. **Positive symptoms** are behaviors, thoughts, or feelings added to normal behavior. In other words, positive symptoms are features that are experienced in individuals with psychotic disorders that are not present in the general population. Examples include delusions and hallucinations, disorganized thought, and disorganized or catatonic behavior. Positive symptoms are considered by some to be two distinct dimensions—the psychotic dimension (delusions and hallucinations) and the disorganized dimension (disorganized thought and behavior)—perhaps with different underlying causes. **Negative symptoms** are those that involve the absence of normal or desired behavior, such as disturbance of affect and avolition. Figure 7.3 summarizes these positive and negative symptoms, with a more elaborate explanation of each following.

REAL WORLD

The term schizophrenia is a relatively recent term, coined in 1911 by Eugen Bleuler. Before Bleuler, schizophrenia was called *dementia praecox*. Schizophrenia literally means "split mind" because the disorder is characterized by distortions of reality and disturbances in the content and form of thought, perception, and affect. Unfortunately, this has led to confusion with dissociative identity disorder (formerly multiple personality disorder). By *split mind*, Bleuler did not mean that the mind is split into different personalities, but that the mind is split from reality.

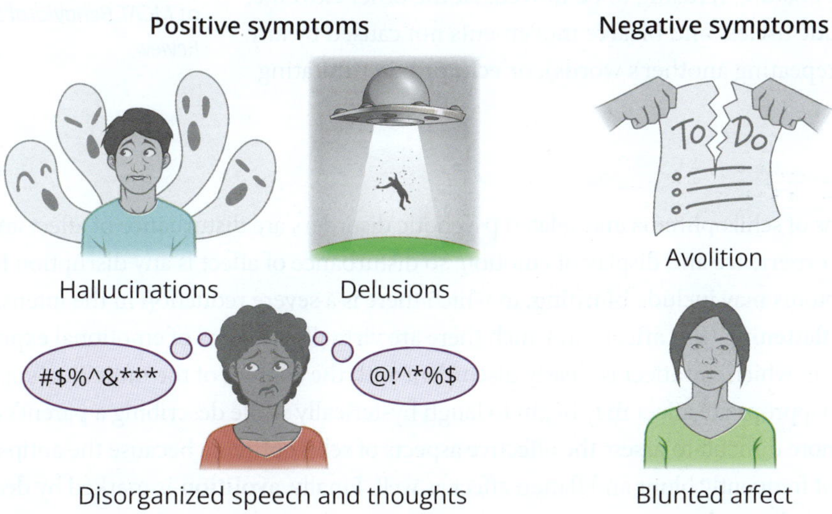

Figure 7.3 Schizophrenia's Positive and Negative Symptoms

MCAT EXPERTISE

The fact that delusions must be considered deviant from the society in which an individual lives provides an excellent opportunity for the MCAT to integrate mental illness and sociology. For example, a belief in shamanism—which is common in the Caribbean, Central and South America, Africa, and in some American Indian tribes—would not be considered a delusion within societies that endorse shamanic medicine.

Positive Symptoms

Delusions are false beliefs discordant with reality and not shared by others in the individual's culture. These delusions are maintained often in spite of strong evidence to the contrary. Common delusions include delusions of reference, persecution, and grandeur. **Delusions of reference** involve the belief that common elements in the environment are directed toward the individual. For example, people with delusions of reference may believe that characters in a TV show are talking to them directly. **Delusions of persecution** involve the belief that the person is being deliberately interfered with, discriminated against, plotted against, or threatened. **Delusions of grandeur**, also common in bipolar I disorder, involve the belief that the person is remarkable in some significant way, such as being an inventor, historical figure, or religious icon. Other common delusions involve the concept of **thought broadcasting**, which is the belief that one's thoughts are broadcast directly from one's head to the external world, **thought withdrawal**, the belief that thoughts are being removed from one's head, and **thought insertion**, the belief that thoughts are being placed in one's head.

Hallucinations are perceptions that are not due to external stimuli but which nevertheless seem real to the person perceiving them. The most common form of hallucination is auditory, involving voices that are perceived as coming from inside or outside the patient's head. Visual and tactile hallucinations are less common, but may be seen in drug use or withdrawal.

Disorganized thought is characterized by loosening of associations. This may be exhibited as speech in which ideas shift from one subject to another in such a way that a listener would be unable to follow the train of thought. A patient's speech may be so disorganized that it seems to have no structure—as though it were just words thrown together incomprehensibly. This is sometimes called **word salad**. In fact, a person with schizophrenia may even invent new words, called **neologisms**.

BRIDGE

Word salad can be seen in severe schizophrenia as well as Wernicke's (receptive) aphasia. Patients will string together unrelated words, although the prosody of the speech (its rhythm, stress, and intonation) remains intact. Aphasias are discussed in Chapter 3 of *MCAT Behavioral Sciences Review*.

Disorganized behavior refers to an inability to carry out activities of daily living, such as paying bills, maintaining hygiene, and keeping appointments. **Catatonia** refers to certain motor behaviors characteristic of some people with schizophrenia. The patient's spontaneous movement and activity may be greatly reduced or the patient may maintain a rigid posture, refusing to be moved. At the other extreme, catatonic behavior may include useless and bizarre movements not caused by any external stimuli, **echolalia** (repeating another's words), or **echopraxia** (imitating another's actions).

Negative Symptoms

The classic negative symptoms of schizophrenia and related psychotic disorders are disturbance of affect and avolition. **Affect** refers to the experience and display of emotion, so disturbance of affect is any disruption to these abilities. Affective symptoms may include **blunting**, in which there is a severe reduction in the intensity of affect expression; **emotional flattening** (**flat affect**), in which there are virtually no signs of emotional expression; or **inappropriate affect**, in which the affect is clearly discordant with the content of the individual's speech. For example, a patient with inappropriate affect may begin to laugh hysterically while describing a parent's death. Interestingly, it has become more difficult to assess the affective aspects of schizophrenia because the antipsychotic medications used in treatment frequently blunt and flatten affect as well. Finally, **avolition** is marked by decreased engagement in purposeful, goal-directed actions.

Schizophrenia

Schizophrenia is the prototypical psychotic disorder in this category of disorders. **Schizophrenia** is characterized by a break between an individual and reality. In fact, the term *schizophrenia* literally means "split mind." Eugen Bleuler coined the term in reference to the splitting of one's mind from reality. To be given the diagnosis of schizophrenia, an individual must show continuous signs of the disturbance for at least six months, and this six-month period must include at least one month of positive symptoms (delusions, hallucinations, or disorganized speech).

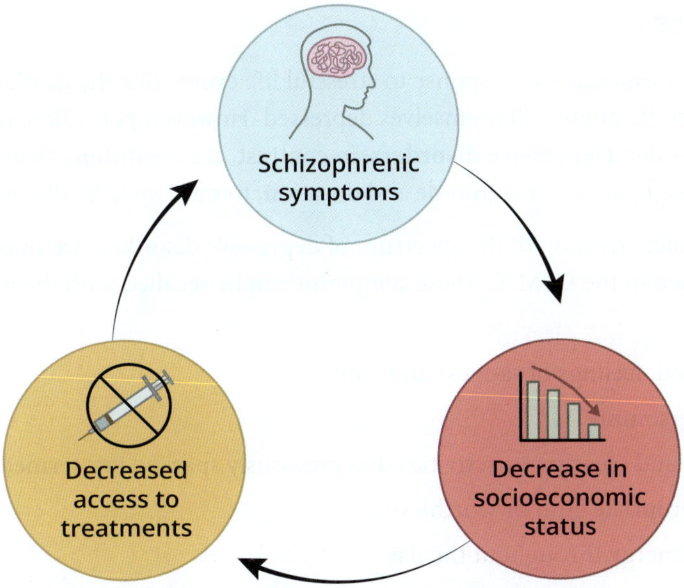

Figure 7.4 The Downward Drift of Schizophrenia

MCAT EXPERTISE

When the MCAT tests schizophrenia, it is likely to include a connection to sociology through the **downward drift hypothesis** (Figure 7.4), which states that schizophrenia causes a decline in socioeconomic status, leading to worsening symptoms, which sets up a negative spiral for the patient toward poverty and psychosis. This is why rates of schizophrenia are much, much higher among homeless and indigent people.

Phases of Schizophrenia

The diagnosis and course of schizophrenia typically follows a specific path, termed the phases of schizophrenia. Before schizophrenia is diagnosed, a patient often goes through a phase characterized by poor adjustment. This phase is called the **prodromal phase**. The prodromal phase is exemplified by clear evidence of deterioration, social withdrawal, role functioning impairment, peculiar behavior, inappropriate affect, and unusual experiences. This is followed by the **active phase** in which pronounced psychotic symptoms are displayed. If schizophrenia development is slow, correct diagnosis is difficult and the prognosis is especially poor. If the onset of symptoms is intense and sudden, the diagnosis is readily made and the prognosis is better. Diagnosis usually occurs during the active phase. The **residual phase,** also called the **recovery phase,** occurs after an active episode and is characterized by mental clarity often resulting in concern or depression as the individual becomes aware of previous behavior.

Other Psychotic Disorders

Other psychotic disorders differ from schizophrenia by the presence, severity, and duration of psychotic symptoms. As a general trend, the *other psychotic disorders* present symptoms to a lesser degree in comparison to schizophrenia.

- **Schizotypal Personality Disorder**: Include both personality disorder and psychotic symptoms, with the personality symptoms having been already established before psychotic symptoms present. This condition is covered in greater detail in *Personality Disorders.*
- **Delusion Disorder**: Psychotic symptoms are limited to delusions and are present for at least a month.
- **Brief Psychotic Disorder**: Positive psychotic symptoms are present for at least a day, but less than a month.
- **Schizophreniform Disorder**: Same diagnostic criteria as schizophrenia except in duration; the required duration for this diagnosis is only 1 month.
- **Schizoaffective Disorder**: Major mood episodes (major depressive episodes and manic episodes) while also presenting psychotic symptoms.

Depressive Disorders

Sadness is a natural part of life, especially in response to stressful life events like the death of a loved one. During periods of sadness, people might call themselves depressed. However, periodic sadness in response to life events is not a mental disorder. **Depressive disorders**, in contrast, are conditions characterized by feelings of sadness that are severe enough, in both magnitude and duration, to meet specific diagnostic criteria.

To understand the DSM-5's categorization of the spectrum of depressive disorders, we must first discuss the 9 **depressive symptoms** defined in the DSM-5. These symptoms can be recalled with the mnemonic **sadness + SIG E. CAPS**:

- **Sadness**: Depressed mood, feelings of sadness and emptiness
- **S**leep: Insomnia or hypersomnia
- **I**nterest: Loss of interest and pleasure in activities that previously sparked joy, termed **anhedonia**
- **G**uilt: A feeling of inappropriate guilt or worthlessness
- **E**nergy: Lower levels of energy throughout the day
- **C**oncentration: Decrease in ability to concentrate (self described, or observed by others)
- **A**ppetite: Pronounced change in appetite (increase or decrease) resulting in a significant change (5%+) in weight.
- **P**sychomotor symptoms: Psychomotor retardation (slowed thoughts and physical movements) and psychomotor agitation (restlessness resulting in undesired movement)
- **S**uicidal thoughts: Recurrent suicidal thoughts

In addition to depressive symptoms, the DSM-5 also categorizes depressive disorders based on duration, timing, and cause of depressive symptoms.

Major Depressive Disorder

The key diagnostic feature of **major depressive disorder (MDD)** is the presence of major depressive episodes. A **major depressive episode** is defined as a 2-week (or longer) period in which 5 of the 9 defined depressive symptoms are encountered, which must include either depressed mood or **anhedonia** (inability to feel and anticipate pleasure). In addition, the symptoms must be severe enough to impair one's daily social- or work-related activities.

Persistent Depressive Disorder

Considering the difference in naming between major depressive disorder and persistent depressive disorder, it may seem reasonable to assume that persistent depressive disorder is a lesser form of major depressive disorder. However, this is not the case. In fact, major depressive episodes can coincide with persistent depressive disorder. A diagnosis of **persistent depressive disorder (PDD)**, also known as **dysthymia**, is given when an individual experiences a period, lasting at least 2 years, in which they experience a depressed mood on the majority of days. With the primary diagnostic feature of PDD being time, a patient can receive both the PDD and MDD diagnosis if they meet both the duration and severity requirements of both disorders.

MNEMONIC

Symptoms of a major depressive episode: **SIG E. CAPS**

Sadness +

- **S**leep
- **I**nterest
- **G**uilt
- **E**nergy
- **C**oncentration
- **A**ppetite
- **P**sychomotor symptoms
- **S**uicidal thoughts

BRIDGE

The most common first-line treatment for depression is the class of medications called selective serotonin reuptake inhibitors (SSRIs). These block the reuptake of serotonin by the presynaptic neuron, resulting in higher levels of serotonin in the synapse and relief of symptoms. The nervous system is outlined in Chapter 1 of *MCAT Behavioral Sciences Review* and Chapter 4 of *MCAT Biology Review*.

Other Depressive Disorders

Whereas major depressive disorder and persistent depressive disorder are characterized by severity and duration of depressive symptoms, other depressive disorders can be characterized by their age of incidence and apparent cause.

Children often exhibit more dramatic emotional responses than adults and, in previous editions of the DSM, this led to the potential overdiagnosis of bipolar disorders in children. To address this concern the DSM-5 includes **disruptive mood dysregulation disorder**, which is typically diagnosed between the ages of 6 and 10, and has the key diagnostic feature of persistent and recurrent emotional irritability in multiple environments (school, home, etc.).

Depressive symptoms can also arise in response to specific times and situations; if these symptoms meet certain diagnostic criteria then they are considered disorders. **Premenstrual dysphoric disorder** is characterized by mood changes, often depressed mood, occurring a few days before menses and resolving after menses onset.

Although not freestanding diagnoses in the DSM-5, both seasonal affective disorder and postpartum depression are conditions that have an apparent cause. In **seasonal affective disorder** (**SAD**), the dark winter months are believed to be the source of depressive symptoms and thus the disorder is best categorized as major depressive disorder with seasonal onset, while in **postpartum depression** the rapid change in hormone levels just after giving birth is the cause of the depressive symptoms. In the case of seasonal affective disorder, depressive symptoms are present only in the winter months. This disorder may be related to abnormal melatonin metabolism; it is often treated with **bright light therapy**, where the patient is exposed to a bright light for a specified amount of time each day, as demonstrated in Figure 7.5.

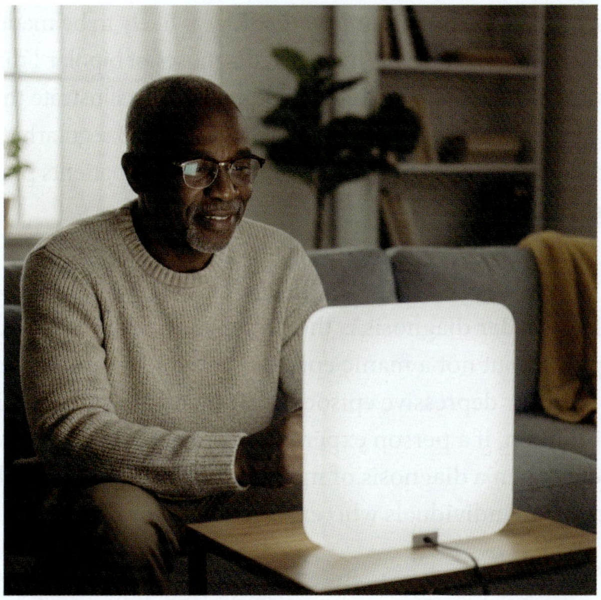

Figure 7.5 Bright Light Therapy for Seasonal Affective Disorder

Bipolar and Related Disorders

This category of disorders is characterized by the presence of manic and depressive symptoms, which if severe and persistent enough can be labelled as episodes. **Manic symptoms** are associated with an exaggerated elevation in mood, accompanied by an increase in goal-directed activity and energy. Put simply, manic symptoms can be thought of as the prolonged and exaggerated emotion of happiness or joy. According to the DSM-5, there are 7 manic symptoms. These symptoms can be recalled with the mnemonic **DIG FAST**:

- **D**istractibility: Inability to remain focused on an activity
- **I**rresponsibility: Engaging in risky activities without considering future consequences
- **G**randiosity: Exaggerated and unrealistic increase in self-esteem
- **F**light of thoughts: Racing thoughts, self-reported or revealed through rapid speech
- **A**ctivity or agitation: Increase in goal-oriented work or social activities
- **S**leep: Decreased need for sleep, e.g. sleeping for only a couple hours but feeling rested
- **T**alkative: Exaggerated desire to speak

The presence of manic symptoms are considered a **hypomanic episode** if the symptoms are present for at least 4 days and include at least 3 or more of the 7 defined manic symptoms, yet the symptoms are not severe enough to impair the person's social or work activities. However, the diagnosis progresses to a **manic episode** if the manic symptoms (3 or more of the defined 7) are severe enough to impair a person's social or work activities and persist for at least 7 days.

In addition to manic symptoms and their associated episodes, the presence or absence of depressive symptoms and their associated episodes are also used to differentiate bipolar and related disorders. Specifically, these disorders are classified by the presence or absence of manic, hypomanic, and major depressive episodes. Depressive symptoms were covered in *Depressive Disorders*.

Bipolar I Disorder

When manic episodes are present, a diagnosis of **bipolar I disorder** is likely to be made, as the key diagnostic feature of this disorder is the presence of manic episodes. While most diagnoses of bipolar I disorder also include depressive symptoms, often major depressive episodes, they are not a requirement. To illustrate this point consider two hypothetical patients: Patient A only experiences manic episodes, while Patient B regularly experiences both manic and major depressive episodes, cycling between the two regularly. Despite both patients presenting very differently, both fit the categorization of bipolar I disorder.

Bipolar II Disorder

The key feature of a **bipolar II disorder** diagnosis is the presence of both a major depressive episode and an accompanying hypomanic episode, but not a manic episode. To avoid confusion, it is worth noting that if a patient has experienced both major depressive episodes and manic episodes, a diagnosis of bipolar I disorder will likely be made. In addition, if a person experiences only major depressive symptoms (absence of hypomanic and manic episodes), then a diagnosis of major depressive disorder is likely to be made. Thus, the diagnosis of bipolar II only captures individuals who experience major depressive episodes and the lesser, hypomanic episodes.

Cyclothymic Disorder

The diagnostic features of cyclothymic disorder are the presence of both manic and depressive symptoms that are not severe enough to be considered episodes. In other words, the patient has not experienced major depressive, manic, or hypomanic episodes. Or, more specifically, the patient has never experienced *3 or more of the 7 manic symptoms in a 4 day period* (diagnostic criteria for hypomanic episode) and has never experienced *5 or more of the 9 depressive symptoms in a 2-week period* (diagnostic criteria for a major depressive episode). Considering the relatively low threshold of symptom requirements, it may seem that everyone would be diagnosed with cyclothymic disorder. However despite the relatively low symptom requirements, the duration requirements for this disorder are high. For a diagnosis of **cyclothymic disorder** to be made, a person must have experienced numerous periods of manic and depressive symptoms for the majority of time over a 2-year (or longer) period.

To more easily distinguish between bipolar I disorder, bipolar II disorder, and cyclothymic disorder, refer to Figure 7.6.

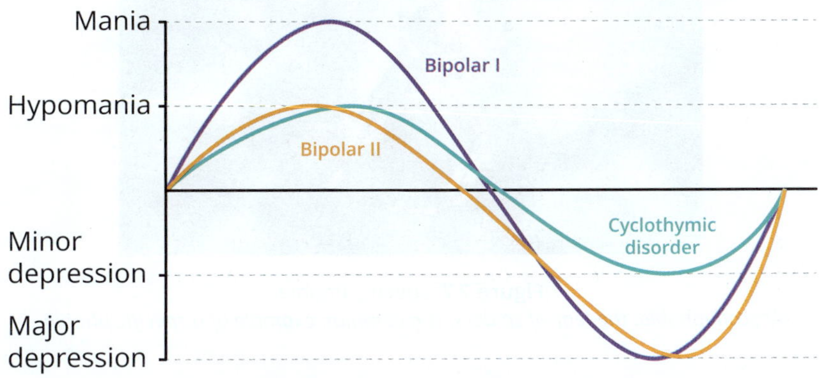

Figure 7.6 Bipolar I and II and Cyclothymic Disorders

Before moving on to anxiety disorders, a brief discussion of proposed neurological etiologies of mood disorders is warranted. The most common explanation revolves around the neurotransmitters norepinephrine and serotonin. These two are often linked together into what is called the **monoamine** or **catecholamine theory of depression**. This theory holds that too much norepinephrine and serotonin in the synapse leads to mania, while too little leads to depression. Although more recent research has shown that it is not that simple, you should be aware of this theory for the MCAT.

Anxiety Disorders

From an evolutionary perspective, emotions served to direct and modulate behavior based on environmental stimuli. As seen in bipolar and depressive disorders, when the regulation of emotions, such as happiness or sadness, are insufficient, then symptoms arise. In the case of anxiety, fear is the associated emotion. Fear is often defined as an emotional response to an immediate threat, while **anxiety** can be viewed as fear of an upcoming or future event. Like fear, anxiety is healthy and important in one's life. It is only considered an **anxiety disorder** when irrational and excessive fear or anxiety affects an individual's daily functioning.

There are more than 10 disorders listed in the anxiety disorders portion of the DSM-5. These disorders are categorized by the situation or stimulus that induces anxiety.

Specific Phobias

The most common type of anxiety disorder is a phobia. A **phobia** is an irrational fear of something that results in a compelling desire to avoid it. Most of the phobias that you are likely familiar with are what the DSM-5 calls specific phobias. A **specific phobia** is one in which fear and anxiety are produced by a specific object or situation. Unlike other sources of anxiety, specific phobias lack a specific ideation or thought pattern and instead present as

REAL WORLD

Depressive and manic episodes are essentially two sides of the same coin: Depression is associated with low norepinephrine and serotonin levels, and manic episodes are associated with high levels of these neurotransmitters. When patients are put on treatment for depression, they must be watched for signs of mania because antidepressant medications may trigger manic symptoms or episodes.

BRIDGE

For all anxiety disorders, clinicians must rule out hyperthyroidism—excessive levels of the thyroid hormones triiodothyronine (T_3) and thyroxine (T_4)—because increasing the whole body's metabolic rate will create anxiety-like symptoms. Thyroid function is discussed in Chapter 5 of *MCAT Biology Review*.

an immediate and irrational fear response to the specific object or situation. For example, *claustrophobia* is an irrational fear of closed places, *acrophobia* is an irrational fear of heights, and *arachnophobia* is an irrational fear of spiders (Figure 7.7).

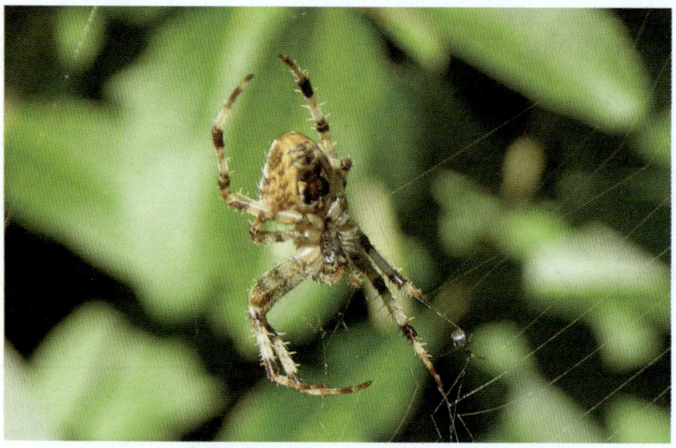

Figure 7.7 Specific Phobia
Arachnophobia, the fear of spiders, is a common example of a specific phobia.

Separation Anxiety Disorder

Separation anxiety is the excessive fear of being separated from one's caregivers or home environment. Although some separation anxiety is common and to be expected in young children, when this anxiety is excessive and persists beyond the age where it is deemed developmentally appropriate, the person may be diagnosed with **separation anxiety disorder**. This diagnosis is accompanied by the ideation that when separated, the caregiver or the individual themselves will be harmed (e.g. kidnapping, getting sick). These persistent beliefs may result in avoidant behaviors such as refusal to leave the home, shadowing the caregiver, etc.

Social Anxiety Disorder

On the surface, social anxiety disorder can be viewed as a social phobia, that is, fear and anxiety towards social situations and encounters. However, unlike previously discussed specified phobias, social anxiety disorder has an accompanying ideation in which individuals think that they will be perceived negatively by others. Thus, the key diagnostic feature of **social anxiety disorder** is fear or anxiety towards social situations with the belief that the individual will be exposed, embarrassed, or simply negatively perceived by others.

Like other anxiety disorders, avoidant behaviors are often conditioned as a means to reduce the associated anxiety. In the case of social anxiety, this can be as broad as avoiding social situations entirely or as narrow as avoiding handshakes out of fear of sweaty palms. Avoidant behavior to the point of social or occupational impairment is necessary for a social anxiety disorder diagnosis.

Selective Mutism

Although categorized as a separate anxiety disorder, **selective mutism** is heavily associated with social anxiety disorder and characterized by the consistent inability to speak in situations where speaking is expected. However, in situations that are more relaxed or when communication is not expected, speaking is unaffected. From this perspective, selective mutism may be conceptualized as a patient's fear of being negatively evaluated for what the patient might say.

Panic Disorder

The key diagnostic feature of **panic disorder** is the recurrence of unexpected panic attacks. To understand panic disorder, we must first cover panic attacks. From a physiological perspective, a panic attack is the misfiring of the sympathetic nervous system resulting in an unwanted *fight or flight* response. From a psychological perspective, a panic attack includes the associated emotions that accompany the sympathetic response, such as intense fear and *a sense of impending doom/danger*. Combining these two perspectives, a **panic attack** is the sudden surge of fear in which individuals feel that they are losing control of their body and/or that they are dying. The occurrence of an individual's attacks may be associated with specific triggers, in which case the attacks are termed **expected panic attacks**. If there is no clear trigger and the panic attacks are seemingly random, they are termed **unexpected panic attacks**.

The diagnosis of panic disorder requires the recurrence of *unexpected* panic attacks. The unexpected panic attacks themselves can produce an associated anxiety. In other words, an individual may become anxious at the thought of having an unexpected panic attack. If this anxiety impairs one's daily functions and persists for at least a month, then the diagnosis of panic disorder is made.

BRIDGE

Notice that a large number of the symptoms of panic disorder are caused by excess activation of the sympathetic nervous system (autonomic overdrive). These include trembling, sweating, hyperventilation, shortness of breath, a racing heart rate, and palpitations. The autonomic nervous system is discussed in Chapter 1 of *MCAT Behavioral Sciences Review* and Chapter 4 of *MCAT Biology Review*.

It is worth noting that panic attacks themselves are not considered a psychological disorder. They may occur in the absence of physiological disorders or may be associated with anxiety disorders in which there is a clear trigger. For instance, an individual with arachnophobia may experience expected panic attacks when encountering a spider.

Agoraphobia

Agoraphobia is an anxiety disorder characterized by a fear of being in places or situations where it might be difficult for an individual to escape. This fear may stem from the thought that the individual may experience a panic attack or similar event in which they would need to escape to avoid embarrassment. People who have agoraphobia tend to be uncomfortable leaving their homes, using public transport, being in open spaces, waiting in lines, or simply being in crowds. Due to agoraphobia's association with panic attacks and fear of being negatively evaluated by others, it is often comorbid with panic disorder, social anxiety disorder, and specific phobias.

Generalized Anxiety Disorder

As previously mentioned, the DSM-5 categorizes anxiety disorders based on the stimulus that induces fear or anxiety. For instance, anxiety towards social interactions is termed social anxiety; anxiety at the thought of separation from one's caregivers is termed separation anxiety. On the other hand, some individuals have more anxious temperaments, making them susceptible to anxiety triggered by a multitude of stimuli. It is for this reason that specific anxiety disorders are often comorbid with one another, resulting in patients having multiple diagnoses. However, a better diagnosis for some patients with many triggers for anxiety might be generalized anxiety disorder.

Generalized anxiety disorder (GAD) is defined as a disproportionate and persistent worry about many different things—making mortgage payments, doing a good job at work, returning emails, political issues, and so on—for at least six months. In addition, the worrying is difficult to control, even in cases where the individual knows that their worrying and fear is irrational. These individuals often have physical symptoms like fatigue, muscle tension, and sleep problems that accompany the worry. General anxiety disorder is relatively common in the US population, with approximately 3% of the population experiencing GAD in a 12-month period. Furthermore, over the course of a lifetime, individuals have a 1 in 10 chance of meeting the diagnostic criteria for general anxiety disorder.

Obsessive–Compulsive and Related Disorders

Formerly classified under anxiety and somatic symptom disorders, the disorders in this group were relabeled as obsessive–compulsive and related disorders in the DSM-5. The reason for this organizational change reveals the common feature among these conditions. Across all of the following disorders, individuals perceive a particular need and respond to the need by completing a particular action. Disorders in this category are differentiated by the compulsiveness of the need to be met as well as the nature of the action.

Obsessive–Compulsive Disorder

Obsessive–compulsive disorder (**OCD**) is characterized by obsessions (persistent, intrusive thoughts and impulses), which produce tension, and compulsions (repetitive tasks) that relieve tension but cause significant impairment in a person's life. The relationship between the two is key: obsessions raise the individual's stress level, and the compulsions relieve this stress. Obsessions and their compulsions are ego-dystonic, meaning that the individual knows that their behavior is irrational, but the anxiety that arises when compulsions are not performed cannot be ignored.

Obsessions are perceived needs with the accompanying ideation that if a particular need is not met, then disastrous events will follow. Actions paired with obsessions are termed **compulsions**. As individuals with OCD attempt to satisfy their obsessions, rituals or sets of rules are developed for how their compulsions must be performed. For example, individuals may need to wash their hands for a specific length of time or else the intrusive thought of getting sick occurs (see Figure 7.8). Alternatively, individuals may need to check if their door is locked a specific number of times or else worry obsessively about getting robbed. To be diagnosed with OCD, the compulsions must impair one's daily activities, for instance by taking up a lot of time during the day.

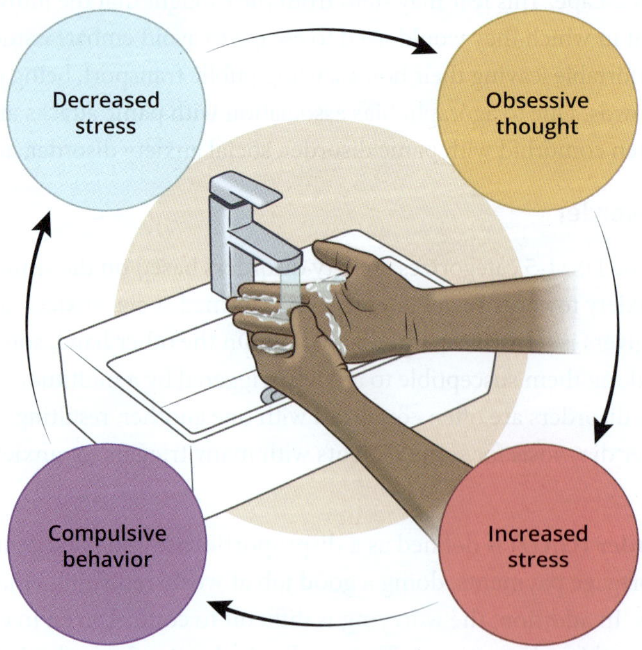

Figure 7.8 The OCD Cycle

Body Dysmorphic Disorder

In **body dysmorphic disorder**, a person has an unrealistic negative evaluation of personal appearance and attractiveness, usually directed toward a certain body part. This is known as a **preoccupation**, a type of worry which lacks the disastrous ideation that accompanies obsessions. Patients with this disorder see their nose (as in Figure 7.9), skin, or stomach as ugly or even horrific when actually ordinary in appearance. This body-focused preoccupation also disrupts day-to-day life, and the sufferer may seek multiple plastic surgeries or other extreme interventions. A common association with this disorder is **muscle dysmorphia**, in which individuals believe that their body is too small or unmuscular (a preoccupation) and respond through working out. Like body dysmorphic disorder in general, this belief persists even with clear evidence to the contrary.

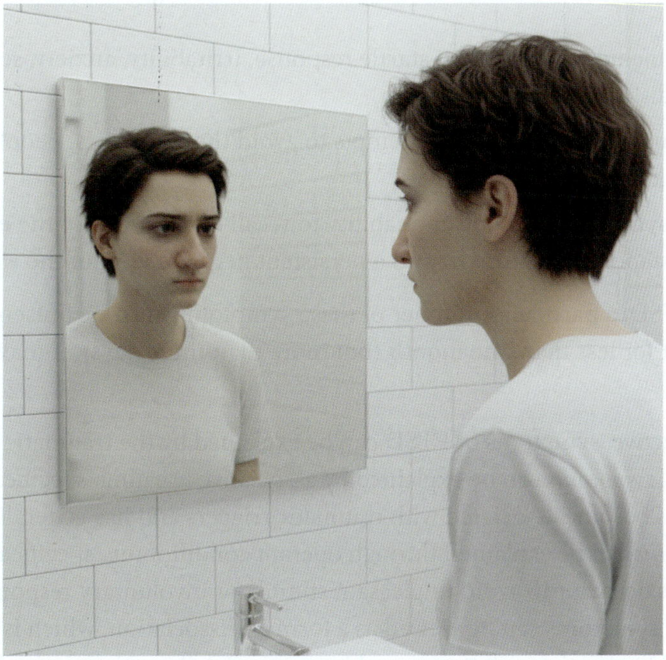

Figure 7.9 Body Dismorphic Disorder

Hoarding Disorder

Hoarding disorder presents as a need to save or keep items and is often paired with excessive acquisition of objects. This behavior stems from several possible sources, ranging from the belief that kept items will eventually be useful to the feeling that the patient has a responsibility to care for the items. As a result, individuals with hoarding disorder often fill their homes with seemingly useless items even past the point where the accumulation of belongings impairs daily life.

Obsessive–Compulsive and Related Disorders with Body-Focused Repetitive Behaviors

Trichotillomania and excoriation are two obsessive–compulsive and related disorders that both present with body-focused compulsions. In the case of **trichotillomania**, individuals are compelled to pull out their hair, while with **excoriation disorder,** individuals are compelled to pick at their skin. A required diagnostic feature in both of these disorders is that patients have previously attempted to stop their body-focused compulsions but have so far failed.

Trauma- and Stressor-Related Disorders

This category captures disorders where a traumatic event is the source of the symptoms and thus is a diagnostic requirement in these disorders. The typical response to traumatic events includes fear, helplessness, and perhaps anxiety. In trauma and stressor related disorders, however, individuals also present with maladaptive symptoms like anhedonia, dysphoria (generalized dissatisfaction with life), aggression, or dissociation.

By far, the most notable disorder in this category is **posttraumatic stress disorder** (**PTSD**). PTSD occurs after experiencing or witnessing a traumatic event, such as war, a home invasion, rape, or a natural disaster, and consists of intrusion symptoms, arousal symptoms, avoidance symptoms, and negative cognitive symptoms.

- **Intrusion symptoms** include recurrent reliving of the event, flashbacks, nightmares, and prolonged distress.
- **Arousal symptoms** include an increased startle response, irritability, anxiety, self-destructive or reckless behavior, and sleep disturbances.
- **Avoidance symptoms** include deliberate attempts to avoid the memories, people, places, activities, and objects associated with the trauma.
- **Negative cognitive symptoms** include an inability to recall key features of the event, negative mood or emotions, feeling distanced from others, and a persistent negative view of the world.

To meet the criteria of PTSD, a particular number of these symptoms must be present for at least one month. If the same symptoms last for less than one month (but more than three days), it may be called **acute stress disorder**.

From a behaviorist perspective, symptoms of PTSD can be explained by the traumatic event and one's reaction to it. *Intrusion* and *arousal symptoms* can be explained by associative learning, specifically classical conditioning, in which the event has become associated with traumatic triggers and has generalized to include everyday stimuli. *Avoidance symptoms* can be explained through operant conditioning, specifically avoidance learning, in which an individual learns behavior to avoid unpleasant stimuli, or involuntary responses in the case of PTSD. Finally, negative cognitive symptoms can be viewed as a form of dissociation, which is a defense mechanism to avoid unpleasant stimuli. Dissociation will be covered in greater detail in *Dissociative Disorders*.

Dissociative Disorders

Patients with **dissociative disorders** avoid stress by escaping from parts of their identity. Such patients otherwise still have an intact sense of reality. Examples of dissociative disorders include dissociative amnesia, dissociative identity disorder (formerly multiple personality disorder), and depersonalization/derealization disorder.

Dissociative Amnesia

Dissociative amnesia is characterized by an inability to recall past experiences. The qualifier *dissociative* simply means that the amnesia is not due to a neurological disorder. This disorder is often linked to trauma. Some individuals with this disorder may also experience **dissociative fugue**: a sudden, unexpected move or purposeless wandering away from one's home or location of usual daily activities. Individuals in a fugue state are confused about their identity and can even assume a new identity. Significantly, they may actually believe that they are someone else, with a complete backstory.

Dissociative Identity Disorder

In **dissociative identity disorder** (**DID**, formerly multiple personality disorder), there are two or more personalities that recurrently take control of the patient's behavior, as represented in Figure 7.10. This disorder results when the components of identity fail to integrate. In most cases, patients have suffered severe physical or sexual abuse as young children. After much therapy, the personalities can sometimes be integrated into one. The existence of dissociative identity disorder is justifiably debated within the medical community, but its characteristics are still important to recognize on Test Day.

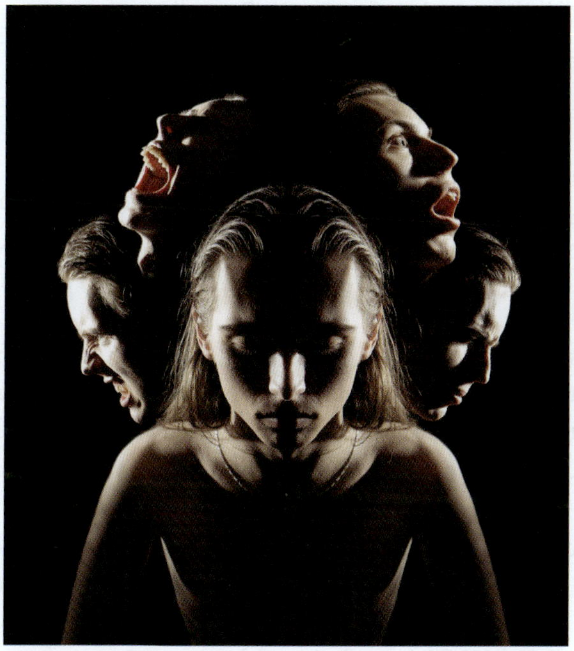

Figure 7.10 Dissociative Identity Disorder (DID)
One artist's interpretation of many personalities seen in DID.

REAL WORLD

One of the first and most famous cases of dissociative identity disorder in the media is Shirley Ardell Mason, also known as "Sybil," who claimed to have at least 13 separate personalities. Mason underwent years of therapy in an attempt to combine her personalities into a single one. Two separate TV movies, both called *Sybil*, have been produced to tell the story of Sybil's struggle with this disorder.

Depersonalization/Derealization Disorder

In **depersonalization/derealization disorder**, individuals feel detached from their own minds and bodies (**depersonalization**) or from their surroundings (**derealization**). Both of these scenarios are artistically represented in Figure 7.11. This often presents as a feeling of automation, and can include symptoms like a failure to recognize one's reflection. An out-of-body experience is an example of depersonalization. Derealization is often described as giving the world a dreamlike or insubstantial quality. Such patients may also experience depersonalization and derealization simultaneously. These feelings cause significant impairment of regular activities. However, even during these times, such patients do not display psychotic symptoms like delusions or hallucinations.

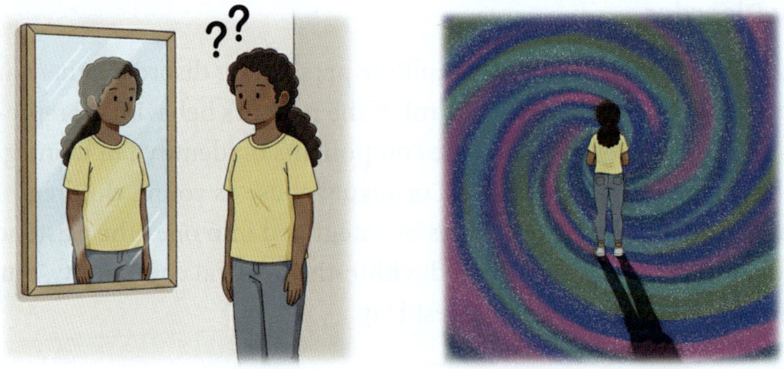

Figure 7.11 Depersonalization and Derealization

Somatic Symptom and Related Disorders

Diagnoses in this category are marked by somatic (bodily) symptoms that cause significant stress or impairment.

Somatic Symptom Disorder

Individuals with **somatic symptom disorder** have at least one somatic symptom, which may or may not be linked to an underlying medical condition, and that is accompanied by disproportionate concerns about its seriousness, devotion of an excessive amount of time and energy to it, or elevated levels of anxiety.

Illness Anxiety Disorder

Illness anxiety disorder is characterized by being consumed with thoughts about having or developing a serious medical condition. Individuals with this disorder are quick to become alarmed about their health, and either excessively check themselves for signs of illness or avoid medical appointments altogether. Most patients classified under hypochondriasis in the DSM-IV-TR now fit into either somatic symptom disorder if somatic symptoms are present, or illness anxiety disorder if they are not.

Conversion Disorder

Conversion disorder, also known as **functional neurological symptom disorder**, is characterized by symptoms affecting voluntary motor or sensory functions that are incompatible with the patient's neurophysiological condition. The symptoms generally begin soon after the individual experiences high levels of stress or a traumatic event, but may not develop until some time has passed after the initiating experience. Examples include paralysis or blindness without evidence of neurological damage. The patient may be surprisingly unconcerned by the symptom—what is called ***la belle indifférence***. Conversion disorder was historically called *hysteria*. The symptoms seen in conversion disorder may sometimes be connected with the inciting event in a literal or poetic way; for example, a parent going blind shortly after watching a child die tragically.

Personality Disorders

A **personality disorder** is a pattern of behavior that is inflexible and maladaptive, causing distress or impaired functioning in at least two of the following: cognition, emotions, interpersonal functioning, or impulse control. Personality disorders are considered **ego-syntonic**, meaning that individuals perceive their behavior as correct, normal, or in harmony with their goals. This is in contrast to the other disorders covered in this chapter that are **ego-dystonic**, meaning that individuals see the illness as something thrust upon them that is intrusive and bothersome. The scenario in Figure 7.12 contrasts these perspectives by showing two potential thought processes that could occur (one that's ego-syntonic and one that's ego-dystonic) while someone is behaving in an antisocial way, angrily attempting to enforce a minor rule. In addition to **general personality disorder** (which fits the diagnostic criteria described above), there are ten personality disorders grouped into three clusters: cluster A (paranoid, schizotypal, and schizoid), cluster B (antisocial, borderline, histrionic, and narcissistic), and cluster C (avoidant, dependent, and obsessive–compulsive). Personality disorder criteria will continue changing over time; the DSM-5 includes a section specifically devoted to research models for redefining personality disorders.

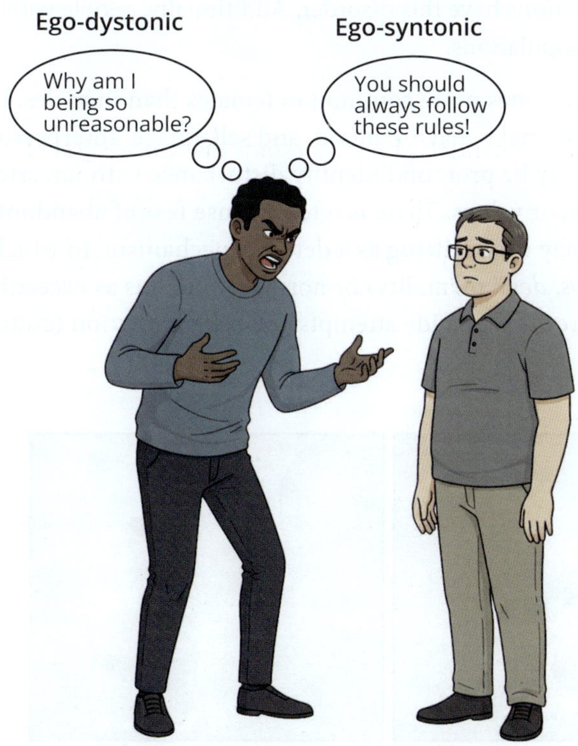
Ego-dystonic
Ego-syntonic
Why am I being so unreasonable?
You should always follow these rules!

Figure 7.12 Ego-Dystonic vs. Ego-Syntonic

REAL WORLD

The distinction between **ego-syntonic** and **ego-dystonic** symptoms is a key feature in differential diagnosis of disorders in the DSM-5. For instance, social anxiety disorder shares many of the same symptoms as avoidant personality disorder, such as anxiety directed towards social interactions and maladaptive avoidance behavior. The distinction between these disorders is that individuals with social anxiety disorder often know that their fear of being ridiculed is irrational (ego-dystonic), while individuals with avoidant personality disorder actually believe they are inferior and that their fear of ridicule is valid (ego-syntonic).

Cluster A (Paranoid, Schizotypal, and Schizoid Personality Disorders)

The **cluster A personality disorders** are all marked by behavior that is labeled as odd or eccentric by others. Its three examples include paranoid, schizotypal, and schizoid personality disorders.

Paranoid personality disorder is marked by a pervasive distrust of others and suspicion regarding their motives. In some cases, these patients may actually be in the prodromal phase of schizophrenia and are termed premorbid.

Schizotypal personality disorder refers to a pattern of odd or eccentric thinking. These individuals may have ideas of reference (similar to delusions of reference, but not as extreme in intensity) as well as magical thinking, such as superstitiousness or a belief in clairvoyance.

Finally, **schizoid personality disorder** is a pervasive pattern of detachment from social relationships and a restricted range of emotional expression. People with this disorder show little desire for social interactions, have few or no close friends, and have poor social skills. It should be noted that neither schizotypal nor schizoid personality disorder are the same as schizophrenia.

Cluster B (Antisocial, Borderline, Histrionic, and Narcissistic Personality Disorders)

The **cluster B personality disorders** are all marked by behavior that is labeled as dramatic, emotional, or erratic by others. Its four examples include antisocial, borderline, histrionic, and narcissistic personality disorders.

Antisocial personality disorder is three times more common in males than in females. The essential feature of the disorder is a pattern of disregard for and violations of the rights of others. This is evidenced by repeated illegal acts, deceitfulness, aggressiveness, or a lack of remorse for said actions. Many serial killers and career criminals who show no guilt for their actions have this disorder. Additionally, people with this disorder comprise about 20 to 40 percent of prison populations.

Borderline personality disorder is two times more common in females than in males. In this disorder, there is pervasive instability in interpersonal behavior, mood, and self-image. Interpersonal relationships are often intense and unstable. There may be profound identity disturbance with uncertainty about self-image, sexual identity, long-term goals, or values. There is often intense fear of abandonment. Individuals with borderline personality disorder may use **splitting** as a defense mechanism, in which they view others as either all good or all bad (an *angel vs. devil* mentality) or normal situations as exceedingly good or equally terrible as exemplified in Figure 7.13. Suicide attempts and self-mutilation (cutting or burning) are common.

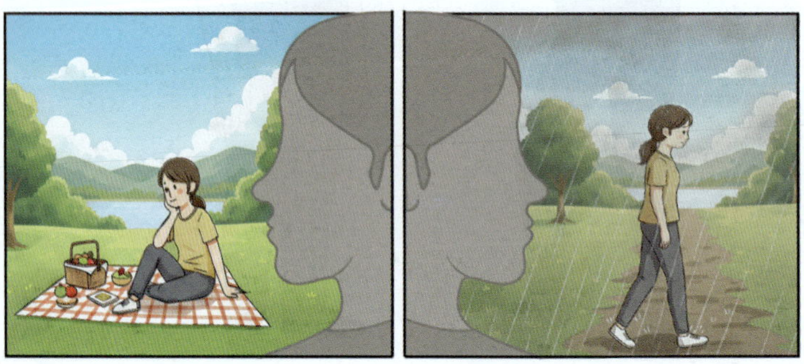

Figure 7.13 Splitting as a Result of Borderline Personality Disorder

Histrionic personality disorder is characterized by constant attention-seeking behavior. These individuals often wear colorful clothing, are dramatic, and are exceptionally extroverted. They may also use seductive behavior to gain attention.

In **narcissistic personality disorder**, the patient has a grandiose sense of self-importance or uniqueness, preoccupation with fantasies of success, a need for constant admiration and attention, and characteristic disturbances in interpersonal relationships such as feelings of entitlement. As used in everyday language, narcissism refers to those who like themselves too much. However, people with narcissistic personality disorder have very fragile self-esteem and are constantly concerned with how others view them. There may be marked feelings of rage, inferiority, shame, humiliation, or emptiness when these individuals are not viewed favorably by others.

Cluster C (Avoidant, Dependent, and Obsessive–Compulsive Personality Disorders)

The **cluster C personality disorders** are all marked by behavior that is labeled as anxious or fearful by others. Its three examples include avoidant, dependent, and obsessive–compulsive personality disorders.

In **avoidant personality disorder**, the affected individual has extreme shyness and fear of rejection. Individuals who have this disorder will see themselves as socially inept and are often socially isolated, despite an intense desire for social affection and acceptance. These individuals tend to stay in the same jobs, life situations, and relationships despite wanting to change.

Dependent personality disorder is characterized by a continuous need for reassurance. Individuals with dependent personality disorder tend to remain dependent on one specific person, such as a caregiver or significant other, to take actions and make decisions.

In **obsessive–compulsive personality disorder** (**OCPD**), the individual is perfectionistic and inflexible, tending to like rules and order. Other characteristics may include an inability to discard worn-out objects, lack of desire to change, excessive stubbornness, lack of a sense of humor, and maintenance of careful routines. Note that obsessive–compulsive personality disorder is not the same as obsessive–compulsive disorder. Whereas OCD has obsessions and compulsions that are focal and acquired, OCPD is lifelong. OCD is also ego-dystonic (*I can't stop washing my hands because of the germs!*), whereas OCPD is ego-syntonic (*I just like rules and order!*).

KEY CONCEPT

Obsessive–compulsive disorder (OCD) and obsessive–compulsive personality disorder (OCPD) are not synonymous. OCD is marked by obsessions (intrusive thoughts causing tension) and compulsions (repetitive tasks that relieve this tension but cause significant impairment). OCPD is a personality disorder in which individuals are perfectionistic and inflexible.

BEHAVIORAL SCIENCES GUIDED EXAMPLE WITH EXPERT THINKING

The following individuals are patients at an inpatient mental health facility.

Patient A's hospitalization is the result of an intense argument with a family member that involved threats of violence, which prompted the police to be called. For the first two weeks of her stay, Patient A spoke often about plans to start several online business ventures, saying that she felt she was a "business genius" and that she would be a billionaire by the end of the year. She slept very little and was irritable, often becoming angry with clinic staff when they tried to reason with her about the soundness of her plans. In the following weeks of Patient A's stay, her mood leveled and she expressed regret over her treatment of her family.

A: Elevated mood, irritable, rapid speech. Lasts 2 weeks.

Patient B arrived at the clinic as a result of complaints from his neighbors. When police entered his apartment, they found it in complete disrepair, and it was clear that he had stopped attending to his personal hygiene long ago. During the first few weeks of his stay, Patient B made no effort to speak to staff or other patients. When he did respond to questions, his answers were short phrases, sometimes unrelated to the question, and sometimes simply a repetition of a few words from the question. He spent his days isolated, often sitting, immobile and unresponsive to occurrences around him.

B: Not taking care of himself, not talking or reacting to others.

Based only on the information provided, what diagnosis from the DSM-5 is most likely for each of these patients?

If you're asked to make a diagnosis for a hypothetical patient, make a checklist of the symptoms described in the passage or question, and then match them to what you know about the disorders that are within the scope of the MCAT. It is worth taking a moment to consider the severity of the symptoms as well, since it can help to differentiate between similar disorders (depression and dysthymic disorder, for example).

Patient A exhibits grandiose self-esteem, rapid speech, a lack of need for sleep, and irritability, which are all symptoms of mania and together are sufficient to apply the label of manic episode. The described transition out of mania into a different mood state suggests bipolar disorder. Specifically, the presence of a full manic episode rules out bipolar II and would lead to a diagnosis of bipolar I, which does not require a depressive episode to follow.

Patient B is trickier, but consider that the writers of the MCAT know that you are not a trained psychiatrist and so will not require a nuanced diagnosis from you. The symptoms that they present will be straightforward and should add up to a description of a disorder that you are familiar with. For patient B, those symptoms are avolition (an inability to perform basic goal-directed activities), flat or blunted affect (lack of emotional expression), and alogia (reduction in speaking). These are all negative symptoms of schizophrenia. The description of patient B also includes echolalia (repetition of words or short phrases), which is a positive symptom and is a signal to you as a test taker that this is indeed schizophrenia, rather than a case of severe depression. While there is still the possibility that Patient B has another, related disorder, the MCAT would not present you with a choice that would require you to distinguish between, say, schizophrenia and schizoid personality disorder without substantial additional information allowing that decision to be made.

In summary, patient A is most likely experiencing bipolar I disorder, and patient B is most likely experiencing schizophrenia or a related disorder.

MCAT CONCEPT CHECK 7.2

Before you move on, assess your understanding of the material with these questions.

1. A schizophrenic patient is started on the atypical antipsychotic *risperidone*, which is effective for treatment of the positive symptoms of schizophrenia, but not the negative symptoms. Which of the patient's symptoms are likely to improve, and which are not?

____

____

____

2. What are the features of a major depressive episode? Of a manic episode?

    - Major depressive episode:

    ____

    - Manic episode:

    ____

3. For each of the following disorders, briefly describe their makeup with respect to depressive episodes, manic episodes, and other mood disturbances:

    - Major depressive disorder:

    ____

    - Bipolar I disorder:

    ____

    - Bipolar II disorder:

    ____

    - Cyclothymic disorder:

    ____

4. A patient with obsessive-compulsive disorder believes that the latch on the apartment door must be checked five times before it is okay to go to bed. Without checking the latch five times, the patient cannot sleep for fear that someone will break into the apartment. Identify the patient's obsession, the patient's compulsion, and how they are related in obsessive-compulsive disorder.

   - Obsession:

   - Compulsion:

   - Relationship:

   ---

5. What features describe each cluster of personality disorders? Which personality disorders fall into each cluster?

Cluster	Features	Personality Disorders
A		
B		
C		

7.3 Biological Basis of Nervous System Disorders

High Yield

LEARNING OBJECTIVES

After Chapter 7.3, you will be able to:

- Describe the impact of depression on hormone and neurotransmitter levels
- Recall the general features and risk factors for Alzheimer's disease
- Explain the role of dopamine in schizophrenia and Parkinson's disease

In addition to knowing the psychological and sociological components of these diagnoses, the MCAT also expects you to know the biological basis of a few mental disorders. These disorders include schizophrenia, depression, Alzheimer's disease, and Parkinson's disease. Research into how to stop the progression of the biological component of these diseases is widespread and will also be something to stay apprised of as a medical student and a physician.

Schizophrenia

Schizophrenia is an area of active research, though some biological factors have been isolated. Most potential causes are genetic, but trauma at birth, especially hypoxemia (low oxygen concentrations in the blood), is also considered to be a risk factor. Other exposures may also play a role; excessive marijuana use in adolescence is associated with increased risk. There is significant data to indicate that schizophrenia is partially inherited. If a person has this disorder, the risk that first-degree relatives will also have the disorder is ten times that of an unrelated person in the general population; this measurement controls for environmental effects.

Schizophrenia may be associated with structural changes in the brain, but more research is needed to determine their significance and prevalence within the affected population. Schizophrenia is highly associated with an excess of dopamine in the brain; many medications used to treat schizophrenia, such as neuroleptics, block dopamine receptors. The term **neuroleptic** means that these medications depress nerve function. Neuroleptics are also known as **antipsychotics**.

Depressive and Bipolar Disorders

There are a host of markers associated with depression:

- Abnormally high glucose metabolism in the amygdala
- Hippocampal atrophy after a long duration of illness
- Abnormally high levels of glucocorticoids (cortisol)
- Decreased norepinephrine, serotonin, and dopamine (monoamine theory of depression)

It has been found that both these neurotransmitters and their metabolites are decreased in depressed patients, meaning that their actual production is decreased (rather than production staying the same and their degradation increasing).

For bipolar disorders, there exists a different set of biological factors and genetic corollaries that contribute to the disease:

- Increased norepinephrine and serotonin (monoamine theory)
- Higher risk if parent has bipolar disorder
- Higher risk for persons with multiple sclerosis

Alzheimer's Disease

Alzheimer's disease is a type of dementia characterized by gradual memory loss, disorientation to time and place, problems with abstract thought, and a tendency to misplace things. Later stages of the disease are associated with changes in mood or behavior, changes in personality, difficulty with procedural memory, poor judgment, and loss of initiative. Now, each of these symptoms alone doesn't necessarily point to Alzheimer's; however, when all or almost all of these symptoms are seen in one person, and especially when the symptoms end up inhibiting normal daily function, this points to Alzheimer's disease. This disease is most common in patients older than 65, and women are at greater risk than men. Family history is a significant risk factor and, interestingly, there is a lower risk of developing the disease with higher levels of education.

There is a genetic component to Alzheimer's disease. Research shows that mutations in the *presenilin* genes on chromosomes 1 and 14 contribute to having the disease, and mutations in the *apolipoprotein E* gene on chromosome 19 can also alter the likelihood of acquiring the disease. Finally, the *β-amyloid precursor protein* gene on chromosome 21 is known to contribute to Alzheimer's disease, explaining the much higher risk of Alzheimer's in individuals with Down syndrome.

While the precise biological cause of Alzheimer's disease is unknown, there are many biological markers that are found in patients with the disease. Don't worry about understanding each of these markers in depth, but rather be able to recognize these factors if you see them on the MCAT:

- Diffuse atrophy of the brain on CT or MRI
- Flattened sulci in the cerebral cortex
- Enlarged cerebral ventricles, shown in Figure 7.14(a)
- Deficient blood flow in parietal lobes, which is correlated with cognitive decline
- Reduction in levels of acetylcholine
- Reduction in *choline acetyltransferase* (ChAT), the enzyme that produces acetylcholine
- Reduced metabolism in temporal and parietal lobes
- Senile plaques of **β-amyloid** (a misfolded protein in β-pleated sheet form), shown in Figure 7.14(b)
- Neurofibrillary tangles of hyperphosphorylated tau protein, shown in Figure 7.14(c)

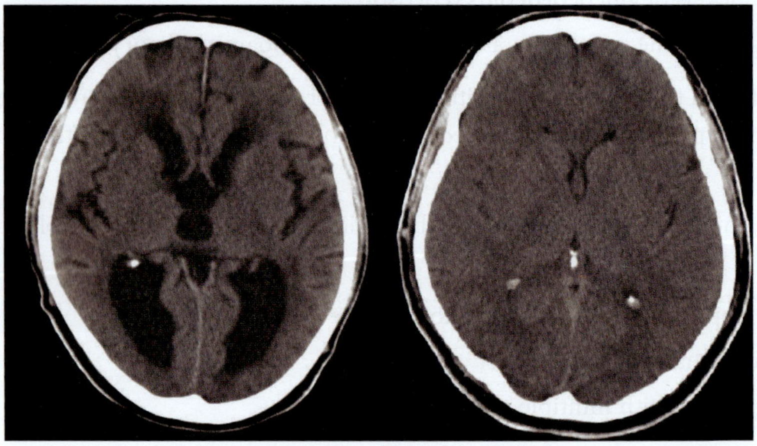

Figure 7.14(a) Symptoms of Alzheimer's Disease
Enlarged cerebral ventricles (left) vs. normal cerebral ventricles (right)

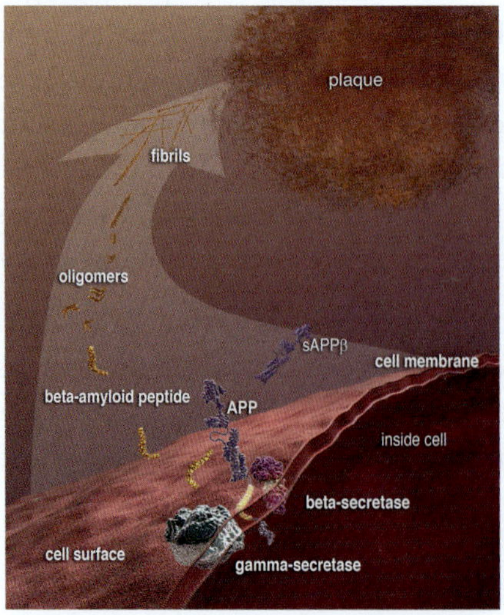

Figure 7.14(b) Symptoms of Alzheimer's Disease
Formation of senile plaques of β-amyloid

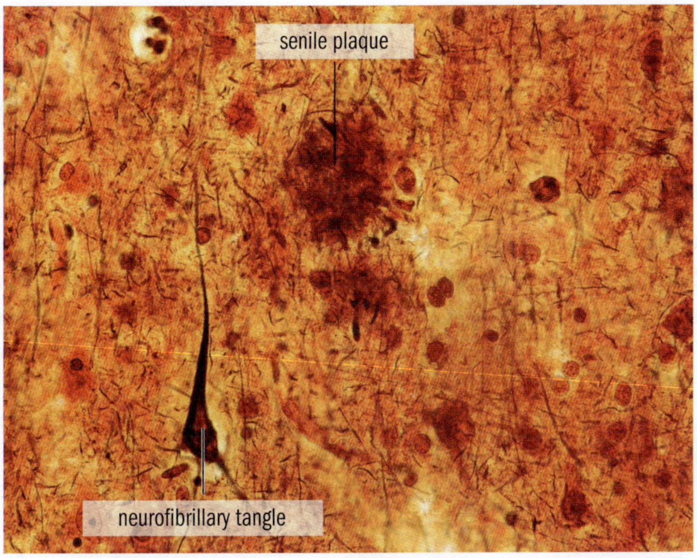

Figure 7.14(c) Symptoms of Alzheimer's Disease
Neurofibrillary tangles of hyperphosphorylated tau protein (magenta)

Parkinson's Disease

Parkinson's disease, demonstrated in Figure 7.15, is characterized by **bradykinesia** (slowness in movement), **resting tremor** (a tremor that appears when muscles are not being used), **pill-rolling tremor** (flexing and extending the fingers while moving the thumb back and forth, as if rolling something in the fingers), **masklike facies** (static and expressionless facial features, staring eyes, and a partially open mouth), **cogwheel rigidity** (muscle tension that intermittently halts movement as an examiner attempts to manipulate a limb), and a **shuffling gait** with stooped posture. A common but not characteristic symptom is depression. Dementia is also common in Parkinson's disease.

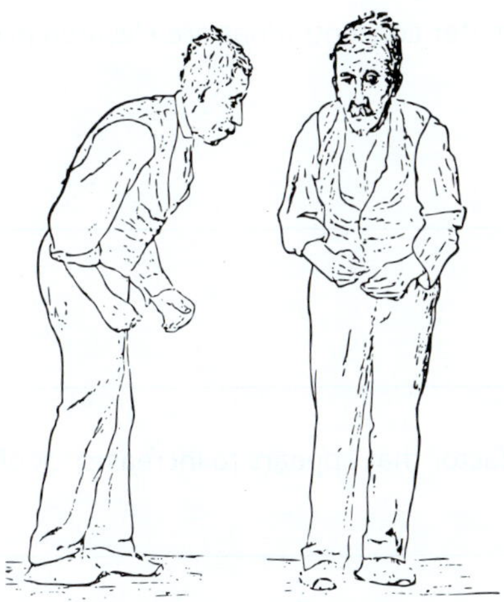

Figure 7.15 Findings of Parkinson's Disease
Note the masklike facies, shuffling gait, and stooped posture.

The biological basis of this disease is decreased dopamine production in the **substantia nigra**, a layer of cells in the brain that functions to produce dopamine to permit proper functioning of the **basal ganglia**, as shown in

Figure 7.16. The basal ganglia are critical for initiating and terminating move ments, as well as sustaining repetitive motor tasks and smoothening motions; thus, the symptoms of Parkinson's disease flow logically from its underlying cause. This condition can be partially managed, therefore, with **L-DOPA**, a precursor that is converted to dopamine once in the brain, replacing that which is lost due to Parkinson's disease. There have also been attempts to regenerate dopaminergic neurons in the substantia nigra using stem cells placed into the central nervous system. Similar stem cell-based therapies have been used in other contexts, such as after a spinal cord injury or stroke to attempt to regenerate function in the central nervous system, with limited results.

REAL WORLD

Note the connection between schizophrenia and psychosis (caused by an excess of dopamine) and Parkinson's disease (caused by a deficit of dopamine). Antipsychotic medications often lead to "parkinsonian" side effects, like muscle rigidity and flattened affect. Medications used in Parkinson's disease often lead to psychotic side effects, such as hallucinations and delusions.

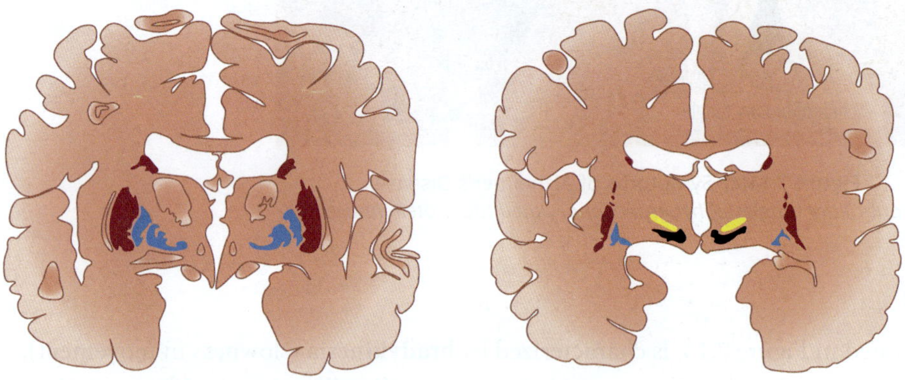

Figure 7.16 The Basal Ganglia
The substantia nigra in the midbrain (black) releases dopamine to activate the other regions of the basal ganglia (blue, red, and yellow).

MCAT CONCEPT CHECK 7.3

Before you move on, assess your understanding of the material with these questions.

1. Which hormone and neurotransmitter concentrations are elevated in depression? Which ones are reduced?
   - Elevated:

   ____

   - Reduced:

   ____

2. Provide an example of a genetic factor that appears to increase risk of Alzheimer's disease.

   ____

3. How are dopamine levels related in schizophrenia and Parkinson's disease?

   ____

Conclusion

The content covered in this chapter will allow you to score more points on the MCAT—and to prepare for your clinical clerkships in psychiatry. This chapter is unique in that it covers not how the mind normally works, as we see in the other chapters in this book, but rather how the mind works when it is functioning abnormally. The MCAT tests critical thinking; one common way to do this is to ask what happens when a system—like the mind—is not functioning normally. Thus, this chapter covered high-yield information that is likely to appear on the MCAT because it connects all three subjects of the *Psychological, Social, and Biological Foundations of Behavior* section. In the next chapter, we move away from the individual as we begin to explore social psychology; from there, we'll continue expanding outward as we move into sociology.

▶ GO ONLINE

You've reviewed the content, now test your knowledge and critical thinking skills by completing a test-like passage set in your online resources!

CONCEPT SUMMARY

Understanding Psychological Disorders

- The **biomedical approach** to psychological disorders takes into account only the physical and medical causes of a psychological disorder. Thus, treatments in this approach are of a biomedical nature.
- The **biopsychosocial approach** considers the relative contributions of biological, psychological, and social components to an individual's disorder. Treatments also fall into these three areas.
- The ***Diagnostic and Statistical Manual of Mental Disorders*** is used to diagnose psychological disorders. Its current version is DSM-5 (published May 2013). It categorizes mental disorders based on symptom patterns.
- Psychological disorders, especially anxiety, depressive, and substance use disorders, are very common in the population.
- Psychological disorders can be treated with **psychopharmacology** (medication) and/or **psychotherapy**, which includes **talk therapy** techniques like psychoanalysis and **behavioral therapy** techniques that directly modify behavior like **systematic desensitization** for treating phobias. **Cognitive behavioral therapy (CBT)** is one popular psychotherapy that uses a hybrid approach.

Types of Psychological Disorders

- **Schizophrenia** is the prototypical disorder with psychosis as a feature. It contains positive and negative symptoms.
  - **Positive symptoms** add something to behavior, cognition, or affect and include delusions, hallucinations, disorganized speech, and disorganized behavior.
  - **Negative symptoms** are the loss of something from behavior, cognition, or affect and include disturbance of affect and avolition.
- **Depressive disorders** include major depressive disorder, dysthymia, and seasonal affective disorder.
  - **Major depressive disorder** contains at least one major depressive episode.
  - **Persistent depressive disorder (dysthymia)** is the presence of depressive symptoms for at least two years that do not meet criteria for major depressive disorder.
- **Bipolar and related disorders** have manic or hypomanic episodes.
  - **Bipolar I disorder** contains at least one manic episode.
  - **Bipolar II disorder** contains at least one major depressive episode and least one hypomanic episode.
  - **Cyclothymic disorder** describes periods of manic and depressive symptoms that are not severe enough to be labeled an episode. These symptoms must persist for at least 2 years and be present the majority of that time.
- **Anxiety disorders** capture conditions in which excessive fear or anxiety impairs one's daily functions. Anxiety disorders are differentiated by the stimuli that induces anxiety.
  - **Specific phobias** are irrational fears of specific objects or situations.
  - **Separation anxiety disorder** is anxiety due to separation from one's caregivers, often with the ideation that if separated, either the caregiver or the patient will be harmed.

- **Social anxiety disorder** is anxiety due to social or performance situations with the ideation that the patient will be negatively evaluated.
- **Selective mutism** disorder is the impairment of speech in situations where speaking is expected.
- **Panic disorder** is marked by recurrent panic attacks: intense, overwhelming fear and sympathetic nervous system activity with no clear stimulus. It may lead to agoraphobia.
- **Agoraphobia** is a fear of places or situations where it is hard for an individual to escape.
- **Generalized anxiety disorder** is a disproportionate and persistent worry about many different things for at least six months.

- **Obsessive–compulsive disorder and related disorders** are characterized by perceived needs (obsessions or preoccupations) and paired actions to meet those needs (compulsions).
  - **Obsessive–compulsive disorder** is characterized by **obsessions** (persistent, intrusive thoughts and impulses) and **compulsions** (repetitive tasks that relieve tension but cause significant impairment in a person's life).
  - **Body dysmorphic disorder** is characterized by an unrealistic negative evaluation of one's appearance or a specific body part. The individual often takes extreme measures to correct the perceived imperfection.
  - **Hoarding disorder** is characterized by the reluctance of giving up one's physical possessions. Often this behavior is associated with excessive acquisition of physical items.
- **Posttraumatic stress disorder** (**PTSD**) is characterized by intrusion symptoms (reliving the event, flash-backs, nightmares), avoidance symptoms (avoidance of people, places, objects associated with trauma), negative cognitive symptoms (amnesia, negative mood and emotions), and arousal symptoms (increased startle response, irritability, anxiety). These symptoms can be explained from the behaviorist perspective.
- **Dissociative disorders** include dissociative amnesia, dissociative identity disorder, and depersonalization/derealization disorder.
  - **Dissociative amnesia** is an inability to recall past experience without an underlying neurological disorder. In severe forms, it may involve **dissociative fugue**, a sudden change in location that may involve the assumption of a new identity.
  - **Dissociative identity disorder** is the occurrence of two or more personalities that take control of a person's behavior.
  - **Depersonalization/derealization disorder** involves feelings of detachment from the mind and body or from the environment.
- **Somatic symptom and related disorders** involve significant bodily symptoms.
  - **Somatic symptom disorder** involves at least one somatic symptom, which may or may not be linked to an underlying medical condition, that causes disproportionate concern.
  - **Illness anxiety disorder** is a preoccupation with thoughts about having, or coming down with, a serious medical condition.
  - **Conversion disorder** involves unexplained symptoms affecting motor or sensory function and is associated with prior trauma.
- **Personality disorders** (**PD**) are patterns of inflexible, maladaptive behavior that cause distress or impaired functioning in at least two of the following: cognition, emotions, interpersonal functioning, or impulse control. They occur in three **clusters**: **A** (odd, eccentric), **B** (dramatic, emotional, erratic), and **C** (anxious, fearful).

- Cluster A includes paranoid, schizotypal, and schizoid PDs. Cluster B includes antisocial, borderline, histrionic, and narcissistic PDs. Cluster C includes avoidant, dependent, and obsessive–compulsive PDs.
- **Paranoid PD** involves a pervasive distrust and suspicion of others.
- **Schizotypal PD** involves ideas of reference, magical thinking, and eccentricity.
- **Schizoid PD** involves detachment from social relationships and limited emotion.
- **Antisocial PD** involves a disregard for the rights of others.
- **Borderline PD** involves instability in relationships, mood, and self-image. **Splitting** is characteristic, as are recurrent suicide attempts.
- **Histrionic PD** involves constant attention-seeking behavior.
- **Narcissistic PD** involves a grandiose sense of self-importance and need for admiration.
- **Avoidant PD** involves extreme shyness and fear of rejection.
- **Dependent PD** involves a continuous need for reassurance.
- **Obsessive–compulsive PD** involves perfectionism, inflexibility, and preoccupation with rules.

Biological Basis of Nervous System Disorders

- Schizophrenia may be associated with genetic factors, birth trauma, adolescent marijuana use, and family history. There are high levels of dopaminergic transmission.
- Depression is accompanied by high levels of glucocorticoids and low levels of norepinephrine, serotonin, and dopamine.
- Bipolar disorders are accompanied by high levels of norepinephrine and serotonin. They are also highly heritable.
- Alzheimer's disease is associated with genetic factors, brain atrophy, decreases in acetylcholine, senile plaques of **β-amyloid**, and **neurofibrillary tangles** of hyperphosphorylated tau protein.
- **Parkinson's disease** is associated with **bradykinesia**, **resting tremor**, **pill-rolling tremor**, **masklike facies**, **cogwheel rigidity**, and a **shuffling gait**. There is decreased production of dopamine by cells in the **substantia nigra**.

ANSWERS TO CONCEPT CHECKS

7.1

1. Whereas the biomedical model considers only the physical, pathological mechanisms that underlie mental illness, the biopsychosocial model considers the contributions of these biological factors along with psychology (thoughts, emotions, or behaviors) and social situation (environment, social class, discrimination, or stigmatization).
2. The following disorders occur in greater than 2 percent of the United States population per year: specific phobia, social anxiety disorder, major depressive disorder, posttraumatic stress disorder, bipolar disorder, generalized anxiety disorder, and panic disorder.

7.2

1. Positive symptoms of schizophrenia, including delusions, hallucinations (usually auditory), disorganized thought, and disorganized behavior, are likely to improve from treatment with an antipsychotic medication. Negative symptoms, including disturbance of affect and avolition, are largely unaffected by antipsychotic medications.
2. Major depressive episodes include a two-week duration of at least five of the following symptoms: depressed mood, loss of interest (anhedonia), sleep disturbance, feelings of guilt, lack of energy, difficulty concentrating, changes in appetite, psychomotor symptoms, and suicidal thoughts. At least one of the symptoms must be depressed mood or anhedonia. Manic episodes include a one-week duration of at least three of the following symptoms: elevated or expansive mood, distractibility, decreased need for sleep, grandiosity, flight of ideas or racing thoughts, agitation, pressured speech, and engagement in risky behavior.
3. Major depressive disorder contains at least one major depressive episode with no manic episodes. Bipolar I disorder has at least one manic episode with or without depressive episodes. Bipolar II disorder has at least one hypomanic episode with at least one major depressive episode. Cyclothymic disorder has hypomanic episodes and dysthymia that is not severe enough to be a major depressive episode.
4. Obsessions are persistent, intrusive thoughts and impulses that produce tension. In this case, the obsession is the patient's thought that someone will break into the apartment. Compulsions are repetitive tasks that relieve tension but cause significant impairment in a person's life. This patient's compulsion is having to check the latch on the apartment door five times before going to bed. Their relationship is that obsessions raise tension while compulsions relieve that tension.
5.

Cluster	Features	Personality Disorders
A	Odd or eccentric	Paranoid, schizotypal, schizoid
B	Dramatic, emotional, or erratic	Antisocial, borderline, histrionic, narcissistic
C	Anxious or fearful	Avoidant, dependent, obsessive–compulsive

7.3

1. In depression, levels of cortisol are increased. Many neurotransmitter levels are reduced, including norepinephrine, serotonin, and dopamine.
2. Mutations in the *presenilin* genes (chromosomes 1 and 14) and β-amyloid precursor protein gene (chromosome 21) are associated with increased risk for Alzheimer's disease.
3. Dopamine levels are elevated in schizophrenia and reduced in Parkinson's disease. Thus, treatments for one disorder may cause symptoms similar to those of the other.

SCIENCE MASTERY ASSESSMENT EXPLANATIONS

1. **C**

Negative symptoms are the absence of normal or desired behavior, which include disturbance of affect and avolition. Positive symptoms are the addition of abnormal behavior, including hallucinations, **(A)**, disorganized behavior, **(B)**, and delusions, **(D)**.

2. **A**

Echolalia is an involuntary repetition of others' words and utterances and may be seen in schizophrenia. Echopraxia, **(B)**, is imitation of others' actions. Loosening of associations, **(C)**, is a type of disordered thought in which the patient moves between remotely related ideas. Neologisms, **(D)**, are newly invented words.

3. **A**

Focusing on details, loving routine, having a sense that there is only one right way to do things, and lack of humor suggests an obsessive–compulsive personality disorder.

4. **C**

Depression is marked by a period of at least two weeks in which the patient has five of nine cardinal symptoms, one of which must be depressed mood or lack of interest (anhedonia). While decreased need for sleep is commonly seen in manic episodes, it may also appear in depression, as sleep disturbance is one of the nine cardinal symptoms. Not all depressed individuals are suicidal, as in **(B)**. In older individuals, depression may often manifest as anhedonia without feelings of sadness, invalidating **(D)**.

5. **B**

The doctor is using the biomedical approach since the focus is on only the biological cause of the patient's symptoms. Furthermore, since the treatment centers only on the patient, the doctor is using direct therapy. This combination of approach and therapy matches **(B)** as the correct answer. By contrast, a doctor using the biopsychosocial approach would likely consider the patient's recent move, stresses associated with the accelerated program, and lack of support structure as potential causes of depression. Additionally, treatment using the biopsychosocial approach includes indirect therapy which focuses on increasing social support.

6. **D**

Dissociative fugue is characterized by sudden travel or change in normal day-to-day activities and occurs in some cases of dissociative amnesia. Symptoms include an inability to recall one's past or confusion about one's identity. Thus, the described patient is most likely to be suffering dissociative amnesia accompanied by dissociative fugue.

7. **D**

Agoraphobia, or a fear of places or situations in which it would be difficult to escape, is commonly seen in panic disorder. Concern about having a panic attack in public may make these individuals fearful of leaving their home.

8. **D**

Phobias affect approximately 9% of the population, meaning that on average 9 in 100 individuals will have some sort of phobia. In a sample of 50 people, 4 or 5 people will need to be excluded, assuming that the sample is representative of the larger population. Thus, **(D)** is correct.

9. **A**

The symptoms listed indicate a major depressive episode. However, depressive episodes can be a part of bipolar disorders, which also contain manic episodes. Thus, if manic episodes have not yet been asked about, one cannot distinguish between depression or bipolar disorder as the correct diagnosis yet.

10. **B**

To determine if this patient has major depressive disorder or a bipolar disorder, the presence of manic (or hypomanic) episodes should be confirmed. Bipolar disorders contain manic (or hypomanic) episodes, while major depressive disorder does not.

11. **B**

The correct answer should be a statement that is not relevant to Alzheimer's disease. Choice **(B)**, a decreased abundance of serotonin and norepinephrine, describes the monoamine theory of depression. These neurochemical changes are not known risk factors or diagnostic criteria for Alzheimer's disease, making **(B)** the correct answer. The remaining choices are either risk factors or diagnostic criteria for Alzheimer's disease. Choice **(A)** describes the increased risk of Alzheimer's disease in individuals with Down syndrome, as the gene for β-amyloid precursor is on chromosome 21. Choices **(C)** and **(D)** both describe biological markers of Alzheimer's disease.

12. **B**

Splitting, the consideration of others as either "all good" or "all bad," is characteristic of borderline personality disorder.

13. **A**

Conversion disorder is marked by a motor or sensory symptom in the absence of an underlying physical or neurological cause. It is associated with an inciting event that, in this case, may have been the argument with the family member. The patient's lack of concern over the deficit is referred to as *la belle indifférence.*

14. **C**

The symptoms indicate that the patient likely has Parkinson's disease. This disease is caused by decreased dopamine production in the substantia nigra.

15. **B**

Bipolar disorders have been shown to be highly heritable and are associated with increased levels of norepinephrine and serotonin in the brain. Bipolar I disorder can be diagnosed with a single manic episode and does not require a major depressive episode. Bipolar II disorder requires at least one hypomanic episode and one major depressive episode. Cyclothymic disorder contains at least one hypomanic episode and dysthymia.

GO ONLINE

Consult your online resources for additional practice.

SHARED CONCEPTS

Behavioral Sciences Chapter 1
Biology and Behavior

Behavioral Sciences Chapter 3
Learning and Memory

Behavioral Sciences Chapter 12
Social Stratification

Biology Chapter 4
The Nervous System

Biology Chapter 5
The Endocrine System

Biology Chapter 12
Genetics and Evolution

CHAPTER 8

SOCIAL PROCESSES, ATTITUDES, AND BEHAVIOR

SCIENCE MASTERY ASSESSMENT

Every pre-med knows this feeling: there is so much content I have to know for the MCAT! How do I know what to do first or what's important?

While the high-yield badges throughout this book will help you identify the most important topics, this Science Mastery Assessment is another tool in your MCAT prep arsenal. This quiz (which can also be taken in your online resources) and the guidance below will help ensure that you are spending the appropriate amount of time on this chapter based on your personal strengths and weaknesses. Don't worry though—skipping something now does not mean you'll never study it. Later on in your prep, as you complete full-length tests, you'll uncover specific pieces of content that you need to review and can come back to these chapters as appropriate.

How to Use This Assessment

If you answer 0–7 questions correctly:

Spend about 1 hour to read this chapter in full and take limited notes throughout. Follow up by reviewing **all** quiz questions to ensure that you now understand how to solve each one.

If you answer 8–11 questions correctly:

Spend 20–40 minutes reviewing the quiz questions. Beginning with the questions you missed, read and take notes on the corresponding subchapters. For questions you answered correctly, ensure your thinking matches that of the explanation and you understand why each choice was correct or incorrect.

If you answer 12–15 questions correctly:

Spend less than 20 minutes reviewing all questions from the quiz. If you missed any, then include a quick read-through of the corresponding subchapters, or even just the relevant content within a subchapter, as part of your question review. For questions you answered correctly, ensure your thinking matches that of the explanation and review the Concept Summary at the end of the chapter.

1. The behavior of the individuals in the Stanford prison experiment is best explained by which of the following terms?
   I. Bystander effect
   II. Deindividuation
   III. Internalization
   IV. Social loafing
   A. I only
   B. III only
   C. II and III only
   D. II and IV only

2. A jury member who initially feels that a strict penalty should be placed on the defendant votes for an even stricter penalty after deliberation with the other jury members. This behavior is best described by which social phenomenon?
   A. Social facilitation
   B. Group polarization
   C. Assimilation
   D. Socialization

3. Which of the following would decrease the likelihood of a bystander lending aid to a victim?
   A. Increasing the number of people in the room
   B. Increasing the degree of danger experienced by the victim
   C. Making the victim an acquaintance instead of a stranger
   D. Being alone in the room with the victim

4. During groupthink, members of the group do all of the following EXCEPT:
   A. stereotype members outside of the group.
   B. withhold opposing views.
   C. ignore warnings against the ideas of the group.
   D. create a sense of negativity against risk taking.

5. Adult prison systems may attempt to change the behavior of inmates through all of the following mechanisms of socialization EXCEPT:
   A. primary socialization.
   B. secondary socialization.
   C. anticipatory socialization.
   D. resocialization.

6. Your neighbors ask you to collect their mail while they are out of town and you agree. Later that day, they ask you to water their plants as well. What technique for compliance are they using in this scenario?
   A. Lowball technique
   B. That's-not-all technique
   C. Foot-in-the-door technique
   D. Door-in-the-face technique

7. Which of the following statements represents the affective component of an attitude?
   A. "I love action movies."
   B. "I'm going to see a new action movie at the theater."
   C. "Action movies are much better than comedies."
   D. "Tomorrow, I'm going to rent an action movie."

8. After sitting in a lecture, determining that a professor is a bad teacher based on the professor's unprofessional attire and monotone speech is an example of which type of processing?
   - **A.** Knowledge route processing
   - **B.** Adaptive route processing
   - **C.** Central route processing
   - **D.** Peripheral route processing

9. In the Milgram shock experiment, many subjects were willing to give the maximal voltage shock because they were influenced by which psychological principle?
   - **A.** Deviance
   - **B.** Obedience
   - **C.** Conformity
   - **D.** Compliance

10. Each individual in a group of teenagers is asked to estimate the height of a tree. One individual estimates the height to be 25 feet, but after discussing with the group is convinced that the height is likely closer to 40 feet. Which type of conformity is seen here?
   - **A.** Normative
   - **B.** Identification
   - **C.** Internalization
   - **D.** Compliance

11. Which of the following is NOT a component of the functional attitudes theory?
   - **A.** Knowledge
   - **B.** Acceptance
   - **C.** Ego defense
   - **D.** Ego expression

12. The swimming times for all members of a swim team are tracked over a six-month period in team-only practices and at public meets. For 14 of the 16 members, top times were clocked at the meets. What social phenomenon does this evidence support?
   - **A.** Social facilitation
   - **B.** Peer pressure
   - **C.** Identification
   - **D.** Group polarization

13. An 18-year-old is completing the final months of high school and begins to wake up early each day to run five miles in preparation for joining the Army. What type of socialization is this young person experiencing?
   - **A.** Normative socialization
   - **B.** Informative socialization
   - **C.** Resocialization
   - **D.** Anticipatory socialization

14. Which of the following best reflects the difference between social action and social interaction?
   - **A.** Social action refers to positive changes one makes in their society; social interaction refers to the route by which these changes occur.
   - **B.** Social action refers to the effects of a group on an individual's behavior; social interaction refers to the effects that multiple individuals all have on each other.
   - **C.** Social action refers to changes in behavior caused by internal factors; social interaction refers to changes in behavior caused by external factors.
   - **D.** Social action refers to changes in behaviors that benefit only the individual; social interaction refers to changes in behavior that benefit others.

15. In the group setting, the mentality of "If you aren't with us, you're against us" is most representative of which factor of groupthink?
   - **A.** Illusion of invulnerability
   - **B.** Illusion of morality
   - **C.** Pressure for conformity
   - **D.** Self-censorship

Answer Key

1. **C** (See section 8.1)
2. **B** (See section 8.1)
3. **A** (See section 8.1)
4. **D** (See section 8.1)
5. **A** (See section 8.2)
6. **C** (See section 8.2)
7. **A** (See section 8.3)
8. **D** (See section 8.3)
9. **B** (See section 8.2)
10. **C** (See section 8.2)
11. **B** (See section 8.3)
12. **A** (See section 8.1)
13. **D** (See section 8.2)
14. **B** (See section 8.2)
15. **C** (See section 8.1)

The relevant section of the chapter to review for each question is given in parentheses after the correct answer. Detailed explanations can be found at the end of the chapter.

CHAPTER 8

SOCIAL PROCESSES, ATTITUDES, AND BEHAVIOR

In This Chapter

CHAPTER PROFILE

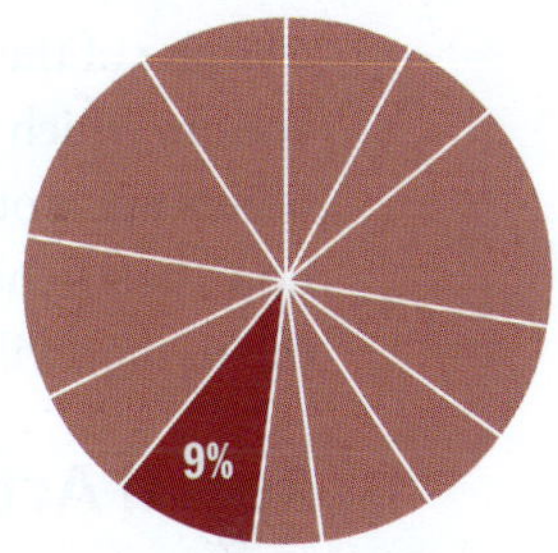

The content in this chapter should be relevant to about 9% of all questions about the behavioral sciences on the MCAT.

This chapter covers material from the following AAMC content categories:

7A: Individual influences on behavior

7B: Social processes that influence human behavior

7C: Attitude and behavior change

Introduction

The renowned Italian painter and sculptor Michelangelo Buonarroti stated that a sculptor simply releases and uncovers the ideal figures that are hidden within stone. This idea has led psychologists and sociologists to describe what is known as the **Michelangelo phenomenon**. The concept of self is made up of both the intrapersonal self, the ideas that individuals have regarding their own abilities, traits, and beliefs, and the interpersonal self, the manner in which others influence creation of the ideal self. In the Michaelangelo phenomenon, a close relationship between two individuals 'sculpts' both individuals' skills and traits. This development occurs because of each individual's perceptions of the other, and their behaviors in response to one another.

In this chapter, you will learn about the social processes and interactions that develop this self. The behavior and attitudes of individuals are highly influenced by the people with whom they interact, the society in which they live, and the culture in which they are immersed. Humans, being naturally social creatures, learn how to behave and react based on their relationships and experiences. The following pages will give us an in-depth look at the ways behavior is affected by the presence of others, group processes, culture, and socialization, as well as how attitudes are formed and how they impact behavior.

8.1 Group Psychology High Yield

LEARNING OBJECTIVES

After Chapter 8.1, you will be able to:

- Describe social facilitation, deindividuation, the bystander effect, social loafing, and peer pressure
- Compare and contrast group polarization and groupthink
- Distinguish between assimilation and multiculturalism

Understanding social processes and interaction has long been a goal of sociologists, notably Max Weber, who was one of the first sociologists to study this interaction. Weber attempted to understand and describe **social action**, which he defined as actions and behaviors that individuals are performing or modulating because others are around. The idea is that humans will behave in different ways based on their social environment and how their behavior will affect those around them. If individuals predict a negative reaction from those around them, they will often modify their behavior.

Social Action

Social action should be contrasted with social interaction. Social action considers just the individual that is surrounded by others. When examining social interaction, we will look at the behavior and actions of two or more individuals who take one another into account.

Social Facilitation

It has been observed that people tend to perform better on simple tasks when in the presence of others. This tendency is known as **social facilitation**, and it supports the idea that people naturally exhibit a performance response when they know they are being watched. Although being in the presence of others does not necessarily constitute an evaluation, the theory suggests that performance sparks a perceived evaluation in the individual performing. According to the **Yerkes–Dodson law of social facilitation**, being in the presence of others will significantly raise arousal, which enhances the ability to perform tasks one is already good at (or **simple tasks**), and hinders the performance of less familiar tasks (or **complex tasks**). For example, an expert pianist may perform better in concert than when alone in practice sessions. However, someone with very limited knowledge of music would perform worse in a social setting than when alone. This is demonstrated in Figure 8.1.

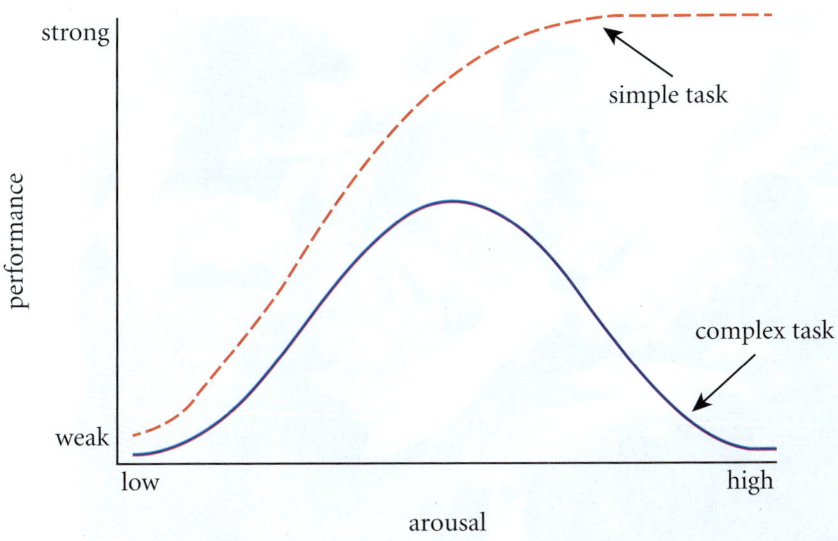

Figure 8.1 Yerkes–Dodson Law

BRIDGE

The Yerkes–Dodson law is also used to describe the relationship between stress or sympathetic arousal and performance. Just as social facilitation can enhance the ability to perform tasks, so can moderate levels of arousal. Arousal can also be an effect of being surrounded by others and feeling pressure to perform: if there's too much pressure, performance drops. Motivation and stress are discussed in Chapter 5 of *MCAT Behavioral Sciences Review*.

Note the difference between Figure 5.3 (in Chapter 5 of *MCAT Behavioral Sciences Review*) and Figure 8.1. Whereas Figure 5.3 focuses solely on new or less-familiar tasks, Figure 8.1 also includes simple tasks, which are not adversely affected by heightened arousal. Social facilitation reflects the idea that performance is not solely influenced by individual ability, but also by social environment and awareness of that environment. In contrast to social facilitation, **social inhibition** occurs when an individual has a worse performance in front of an audience. On the Yerkes-Dodson curve, this inhibition would likely occur when a person performing a complex or unfamiliar task is at the highest level of arousal.

Deindividuation

Deindividuation describes the loss of one's self-awareness in a group setting and the associated adoption of a more group oriented identity. This phenomenon is sometimes called mob mentality, as the individuals of the group lose their own sense of morals and judgment and follow along with the actions of the group. To explain this phenomenon social psychologists have cited group cohesion and individual anonymity as factors impacting deindividuation. If an individual can relate to the group, perhaps through a sports team or political affiliation, then the likelihood of that person adopting the group identity increases. In addition, group settings increase anonymity and thus diffuse the sense of individual responsibility for the actions of the group. Thus, as group anonymity increases, so does the strength of deindividuation. Applied to the real world, deindividuation often leads to **antinormative behavior**, that is, behavior not socially acceptable in most social circumstances; behavior "against the norm." A commonly cited example of antinormative behavior in the context of deindividuation is the violence seen in crowds and riots. Large, homogenous groups are postulated to increase deindividuation effects, particularly when relative anonymity is a factor due to the group's size. These factors can be further enhanced when a group is in uniform or masked, as shown in Figure 8.2.

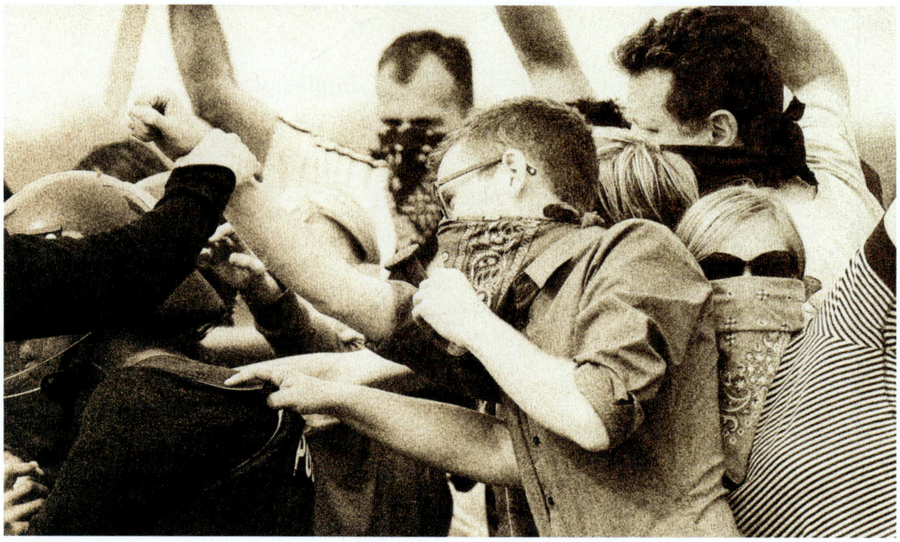

Figure 8.2 Deindividuation
Being masked or in uniform facilitates anonymity in a crowd.

Diffusion of Responsibility

When a task is presented to a group, it becomes less likely that an individual will take responsibility due to the belief that someone else in the group will take action instead. This social phenomenon is known as **diffusion of responsibility**. The greater the number of people in the group, the more likely this phenomenon is to occur. Diffusion of responsibility contributes to several social phenomena, including the bystander effect and social loafing (both discussed below) and groupthink (discussed later in this chapter).

One powerful example of diffusion of responsibility in action is the **bystander effect**. This occurs when individuals do not intervene to assist those who are in perceived need when other people are present. The likelihood and timeliness of response is inversely related to the number of bystanders. In other words, the more people standing by, the less likely any one of those people is to help. There are several factors at play in the bystander effect. First, when in groups, people are less likely to notice danger or anything out of the ordinary. Additionally, when in groups, humans take cues from others. If other people are not responding to a situation, an individual is less likely to perceive the situation as a threat or emergency. The degree of emergency or the perceived danger plays a role in response. In low-danger scenarios, bystanders are less likely to provide aid; in high-danger scenarios, bystanders are more likely to intervene. Another factor is the degree of responsibility felt by the bystanders. This is determined by the competency of the bystanders, their relationship to the at risk individual(s), and whether they consider the person(s) at risk to be deserving of aid. Finally, cohesiveness of the group has been shown to influence responsiveness. In groups made up of strangers, the likelihood of a response, and the speed of that response, is much slower than in a group of well-acquainted individuals. Such a situation is shown in Figure 8.3.

REAL WORLD

The violent 1964 murder of Kitty Genovese outside her home in Queens created interest in the bystander effect after her murder and a lack of response by neighbors were reported in the newspaper. Kitty reportedly cried out while being attacked in her apartment parking lot. One neighbor called out the window for the attacker to leave her alone. The attacker left, but returned ten minutes later and found Kitty barely conscious just outside the back door. Genovese was attacked again for over half an hour and ultimately died en route to the hospital. Of the 38 witnesses (bystanders), it was reported that no one had called the police. Later investigation determined this not to be true, but the misreported incident was nevertheless influential for promoting the idea of the bystander effect.

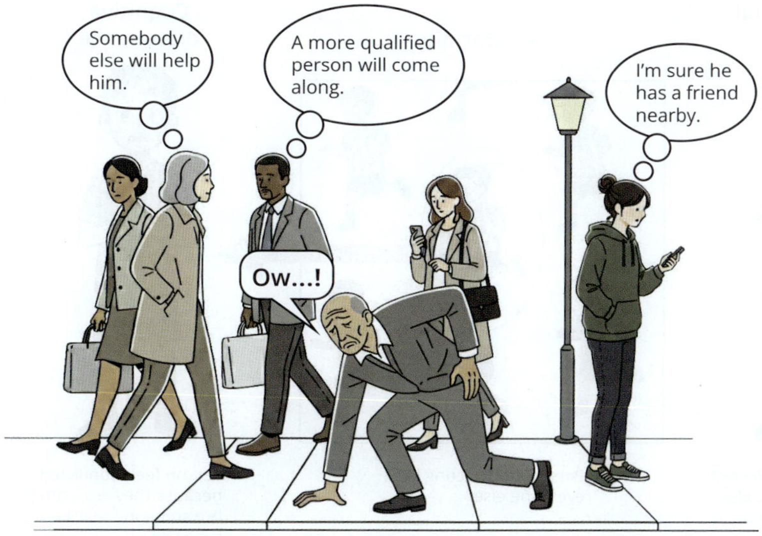
Somebody else will help him.
A more qualified person will come along.
I'm sure he has a friend nearby.
Ow...!

Figure 8.3 The Bystander Effect

Diffusion of responsibility can also lead to a phenomenon known as **social loafing**, the tendency of individuals to reduce effort when in a group setting. This phenomenon may apply in many contexts: physical effort, such as carrying a heavy object; mental effort, such as working on a group project; or initiative, such as coming up with the solution to a problem.

Peer Pressure

From a sociology perspective, **peers** are individuals who are regarded as equals within a social group. **Peer pressure** refers to the social influence placed on an individual by one's peers. Peer pressure exists at all ages. This pressure can come in many forms, including religious ideals, appearance, values, and sexual behavior. It can be positive or negative; certain types of peer pressure can benefit the individual experiencing the influence. In children, social acceptance is associated with being most like the social norm of the group, regardless of positive or negative connotations.

In adolescence, peers play an extremely important role in determining lifestyle, appearance, and social activities. While caregivers and other adults provide the foundation for development of beliefs and values, peers become very important as teenagers become independent from their parental figures. The pressure exerted by peers can cause changes in behavior, attitudes, or beliefs to conform to the norms of the group. Stress and the presence of peers can lead to poor choices and potentially facilitate **risky behaviors** such as binge eating, reckless driving, and violent activities.

Changes in beliefs or behavior due to peer pressure can be explained by the **identity shift effect**. When an individual's state of harmony is disrupted by a threat of social rejection, the individual will often conform to the norms of the group. Upon doing so, however, the individual will begin to experience internal conflict because the behavior is outside the normal character of the individual. To eliminate the sense of internal conflict, individuals experience an identify shift wherein they adopt the standards of the group as their own. The identity shift effect also highlights a larger theme in psychology: **cognitive dissonance**, the simultaneous presence of two opposing thoughts or opinions. This generally leads to an internal state of discomfort, which may manifest as anxiety, fear, anger, or confusion. Individuals will try to reduce this discomfort by changing, adding to, or minimizing one of these dissonant thoughts. Figure 8.4 illustrates this identity shift effect.

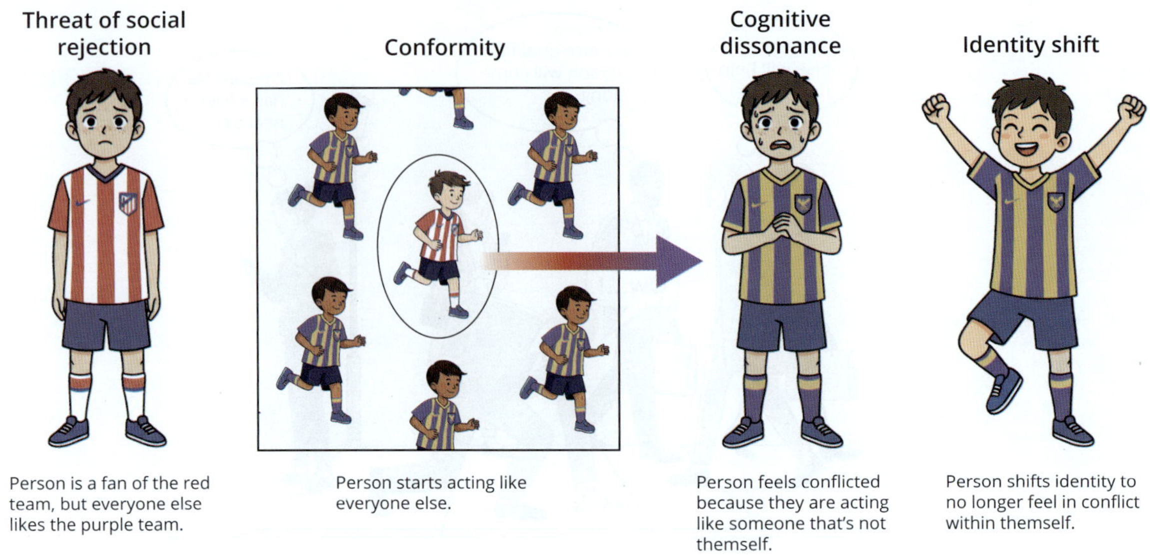

Figure 8.4 The Identity Shift Effect

Solomon Asch's conformity experiment showed that individuals will often conform to an opinion held by the group. In this experiment, male college students participated in simple tasks of perception. The study was set up to have one individual who made observations in the presence of confederates, or actors who were pretending to be a part of the experiment. The point of the study was to examine if the behavior of the individual was influenced by the confederates. The participants were shown two cards like those in Figure 8.5. They were then asked to say aloud which line on the second card, labeled A, B, or C, matched the length of the line on the first card. Prior to the experiment, the confederates were secretly told to unanimously respond correctly or incorrectly to the question. When the confederates answered correctly, the error rate for the real participants was less than 1 percent. However, when the confederates answered incorrectly, it was seen that the real participants answered incorrectly up to one-third of the time. Thus, Asch concluded, individuals will sometimes provide answers they know to be untrue if it avoids going against the group: the urge toward conformity could outweigh the desire to provide the correct answer.

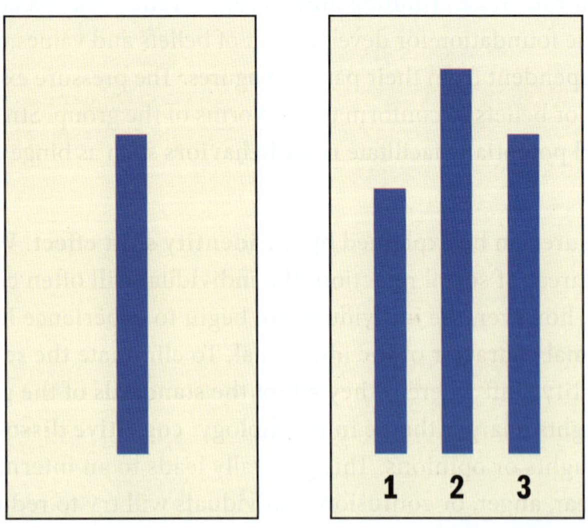

Figure 8.5 Example of Cards Used in the Asch Conformity Experiment

MCAT EXPERTISE

The MCAT can ask about psychological experiments by name, so you should be familiar with some of the landmark experiments in social psychology. For example, a question may refer to the Asch conformity experiment by name, or it may include a similar experiment without a direct reference and ask you to draw conclusions using your content knowledge.

Group Processes

In contrast to social action, **social interaction** explores the ways in which two or more individuals can both shape each other's behavior. These include group processes and establishment of culture.

Group Polarization

Group polarization describes the tendency for groups to collaboratively make decisions that are more extreme than the individual ideas and inclinations of the members within the group. Thus, polarization can lead to riskier or more cautious decisions based on the initial tendencies of the group members toward risk or caution. This phenomenon has shown that individuals in groups will form opinions that are more extreme than the opinions they would reach in isolation. The hypothesis underlying polarization is that initial ideas tend not to be extreme, but that through discussion within the group, these ideas tend to become more and more extreme. This concept was originally termed **risky shift** because it was noted that groups tended to make riskier decisions than individuals. However, when psychologists began to realize that groups could also shift toward caution, the term became **choice shift**. Choice shift and group polarization refer to very similar concepts. However, choice shift refers specifically to measured changes in decisions before and after group interaction, whereas group polarization refers more generally to the tendency of a group to move to more extreme conclusions and decisions as a result of interaction.

Group polarization explains many real-life scenarios, including policy making, violence, and terrorism. For example, members of the same political party may espouse the same ideals and opinions in the group setting, but may waver slightly on issues when alone. This kind of polarization is also seen in jury deliberation. In the case of punitive damages (monetary penalties for a certain behavior), jurors who initially favor a high punishment may deliberate and decide upon an even higher punishment after discussion. As social media has exploded in recent decades, research has shown that the group does not necessarily need to be together physically in order for polarization to occur. Simply reading others' ideas on social media sites can result in more extreme ideas from individuals.

REAL WORLD

The Bay of Pigs Invasion and Cuban Missile Crisis were used by Janis as case studies. When JFK took over the White House, the administration inherited a CIA Cuban invasion plan, and it was accepted without critique. When Senator Fulbright and Secretary Schlesinger expressed objections, they were ignored by the Kennedy team. Over time, Fulbright and Schlesinger started to perform self-censorship. After the invasion, it was revealed that there were many inaccuracies in the CIA plan, including underestimation of the Cuban air force and the assumption that Castro would not have the ability to quell uprisings.

Groupthink

Groupthink refers to a social phenomenon in which desire for harmony or conformity results in a group of people coming to an incorrect or poor decision. In an attempt to eliminate or minimize conflict among the group members, consensus decisions are reached without alternative ideas being assessed. In these cases, the desire to agree with the group causes a loss of independent critical thinking. The group also begins to isolate and ignore external viewpoints, seeing its own ideas as correct without question.

Groupthink can have a large impact on group decision making and is influenced by a variety of factors, including group cohesiveness, group structure, leadership, and situational context. Irving Janis conducted the first research on the theory in the 1970s. Janis studied the effect of extreme stress on group cohesiveness and its resulting effect on groupthink. Janis further investigated the decision making of groups that had led to disastrous American foreign policy decisions, including the Bay of Pigs invasion. Janis specifically examined eight factors that are indicative of groupthink:

- **Illusion of invulnerability:** Members encourage risks, ignore possible pitfalls and are too optimistic.
- **Collective rationalization:** Members ignore expressed concerns about group approved ideas.
- **Illusion of morality:** Members believe ideas produced by the group are morally correct, disregarding evidence to the contrary.
- **Excessive stereotyping:** Members construct stereotypes of those expressing outside opinions.
- **Pressure for conformity:** Members feel pressured not to express opinions that disagree with the group, and view opposition as disloyal.
- **Self-censorship:** Members withhold ideas and opinions that disagree with the group.
- **Illusion of unanimity:** Members believe the decisions and judgments of the group to be without disagreement, even if it does exist.
- **Mindguards:** Some members may decide to take on a role protecting the group against opposing views.

Many of these factors, including illusion of morality, excessive stereotyping, pressure for conformity, and mindguards can be seen in Figure 8.6, a propaganda poster from the United States during the McCarthy era. The poster draws on antisemitic stereotypes and fear of Communist influence to argue against public health measures like water fluoridation, polio vaccines, and mental healthcare.

At the Sign of THE UNHOLY THREE

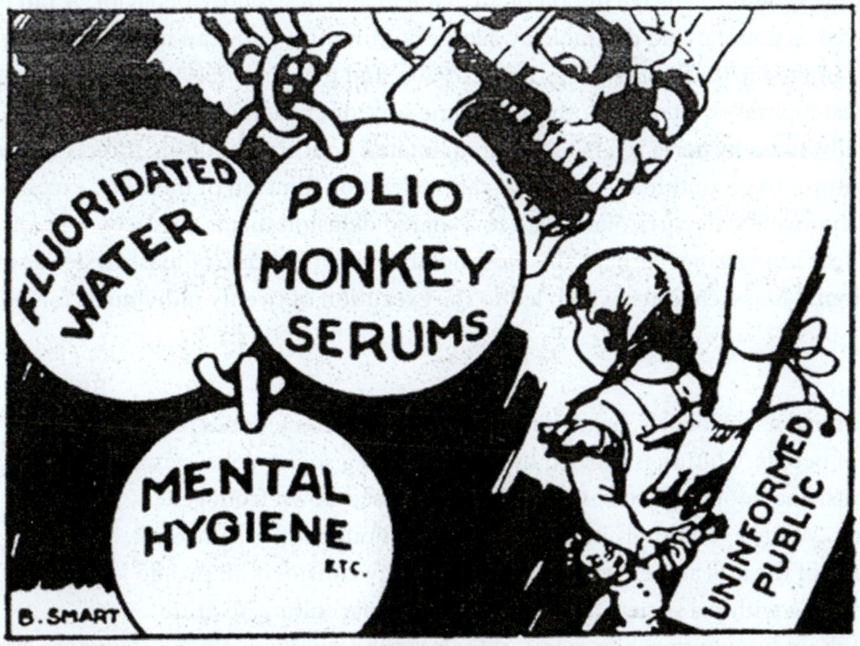

Are you willing to PUT IN PAWN to the UNHOLY THREE all of the material, mental and spiritual resources of this GREAT REPUBLIC?

FLUORIDATED WATER

1—Water containing Fluorine (rat poison—no antidote) is already the only water in many of our army camps, making it very easy for saboteurs to wipe out an entire camp personel. If this happens, every citizen will be at the mercy of the enemy—already within our gates.

POLIO SERUM

2—Polio Serum, it is reported, has already killed and maimed children; its future effect on minds and bodies cannot be guaged. This vacciné drive is the entering wedge for nation-wide socialized medicine, by the U. S. Public Health Service, (heavily infiltrated by Russian-born doctors, according to Congressman Clare Hoffman.) In enemy hands it can destroy a whole generation.

MENTAL HYGIENE

3—Mental Hygiene is a subtle and diabolical plan of the enemy to transform a free and intelligent people into a cringing horde of zombies.

Rabbi Spitz in the American Hebrew, March 1, 1946: "American Jews must come to grips with our contemporary anti-Semites; we must fil our insane asylums with anti-Semitic lunatics."

FIGHT COMMUNISTIC WORLD GOVERNMENT by destroying THE UNHOLY THREE ! ! ! It is later than you think!

KEEP AMERICA COMMITTEE
Box 3094, Los Angeles 54, Calif. H. W. Courtois, Secy. May 16, 1955

Figure 8.6 Groupthink as Seen in McCarthy-Era Propaganda

Similar patterns of thinking, in which a group arrives at a common (but often extreme) consensus also underlie many cultural phenomena, including riots, fads, and mass hysteria. Antinormative behavior in riots was described previously in the section on deindividuation. Still, like groupthink, a shared political or social motivation may urge groups to engage in potentially violent and destructive behavior. A **fad** is a behavior that is transiently viewed as popular and desirable by a large community. Fads can include owning certain objects (such as pet rocks in the 1970s, Rubik's cubes in the 1980s, and pogs in the 1990s) or engaging in certain behaviors (using catchphrases, altering clothing in some way, or engaging in particular types of media such as viral videos). Finally, **mass hysteria** refers to a shared, intense concern about the threats to society. In mass hysteria, many features of groupthink—collective rationalization, illusion of morality, excessive stereotyping, and pressure for conformity, in particular—lead to a shared delusion that is augmented by distrust, rumors, propaganda, and fear mongering. Perhaps the most notable historical case of mass hysteria was the Salem witch trials in colonial Massachusetts, which led to the execution of twenty individuals for fears of witchcraft.

Culture

Culture can be defined as the beliefs, behaviors, actions, and characteristics of a group or society of people. Culture is learned by living within a society, observing behaviors and traits, and adopting them. Culture is also passed down from generation to generation. While a "cultured" individual is often thought of as someone who has knowledge of the arts and expensive taste, sociology considers all people to be cultured by living within a society and participating in its culture. Culture is universal throughout humanity; while many animals exhibit purely instinctual behavior, humans show variable behaviors based on the cultures in which they reside. For example, while all wolf parents care for their pups in the same manner, human parents show vast differences in their caregiving. In some cultures, children are breastfed for years, while in others, infants are breastfed for mere months or not at all. Some groups have multiple caregivers who are not a parent, while others allow only a parent to care for the child. Even within a given culture, beliefs about the correct way to respond to infants crying can vary dramatically: some groups instantly comfort crying children and others let them "cry it out." The beliefs held by an individual are typically based on learned behavior, expectations, and pressure from the group one is in. Cultural differences include everything from typical jobs, common dwellings, and diet to what time of day one eats and where one travels on vacation, if at all. When traveling outside of one's own society, these cultural differences can seem quite dramatic and are often referred to as **culture shock**.

BRIDGE

A discussion of culture in the context of social structure is described in Chapter 11 of *MCAT Behavioral Sciences Review.*

Assimilation and Multiculturalism

Cultural **assimilation** is the process by which an individual's or group's behavior and culture begin to resemble that of another group. A simple example of cultural assimilation is depicted in Figure 8.7. This can also mean that groups with different cultures begin to merge. Assimilation integrates new aspects of a society and culture with old ones, transforming the culture itself. While one society melds into another, it is typically not an even blend. One group will generally have more power and influence than the other, resulting in more traits of that culture being displayed after transformation. Four primary factors are sometimes used to assess the degree of assimilation in immigrant communities: socioeconomic status, geographic distribution, language attainment, and intermarriage.

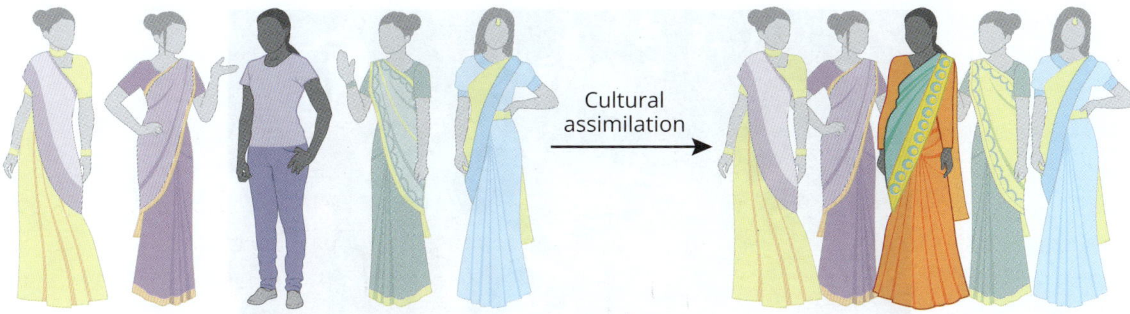

Figure 8.7 Cultural Assimilation

One alternative to assimilation is the creation of **ethnic enclaves**, which are locations (usually neighborhoods) with a high concentration of one specific ethnicity, as shown in Figure 8.8. These are most common in urban areas and often have names like Chinatown or Little Italy.

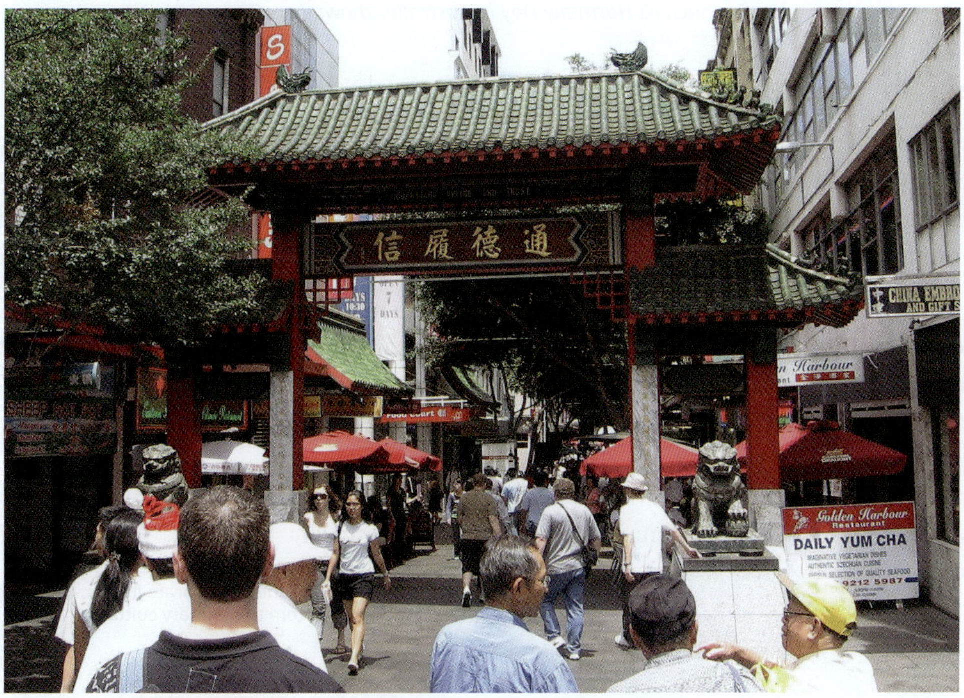

Figure 8.8 An Ethnic Enclave
Entrance to Chinatown, Sydney, Australia

Multiculturalism, also known as **cultural diversity**, refers to communities or societies containing multiple cultures or ethnic groups. From a sociology perspective, multiculturalism encourages, respects, and celebrates cultural differences, as shown in Figure 8.9. **Multicultural socialization** encourages the learning of norms and behaviors from multiple different cultures. This view can enhance acceptance of cultures within society, which contrasts with the concept of assimilation. While multiculturalism is often described as creating a *cultural mosaic*, or mixture of cultures and ethnic groups that coexist in society, assimilationism is described as creating a *melting pot*, or melting together of different elements of culture into one homogeneous culture.

KEY CONCEPT

- Assimilation—(usually uneven) merging of cultures; a melting pot
- Multiculturalism—celebration of coexisting cultures; a cultural mosaic

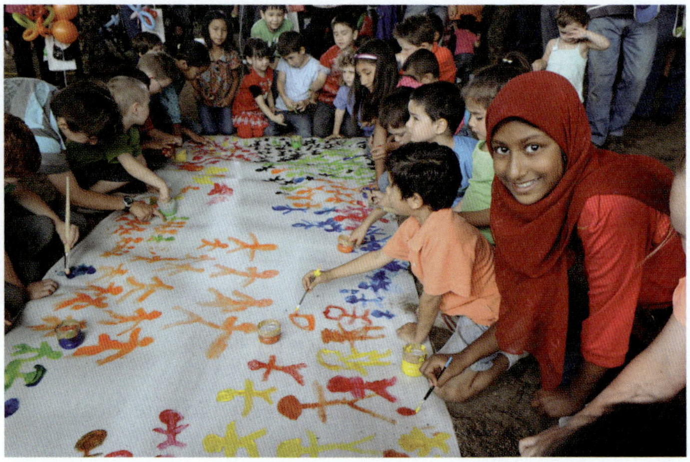

Figure 8.9 Multiculturalism
Multiculturalism may be celebrated through holidays and festivals, such as Harmony Day in Australia, shown here.

Subcultures

Subcultures refer to groups of people within a culture that distinguish themselves from the primary culture to which they belong. When studying subcultures, symbolic attachment to things such as clothing or music can differentiate the group from the majority. Subcultures can be formed based on race, gender, ethnicity, sexuality, and other differentiating factors from the whole of society.

Subcultures can be perceived as negative when they subvert the majority culture's definitions of normalcy. In the case of **counterculture**, the subculture group gravitates toward an identity that is at odds with the majority culture and deliberately opposes the prevailing social mores. A counterculture, in effect, attempts to separate itself from the primary culture and its component subcultures, as visualized in Figure 8.10.

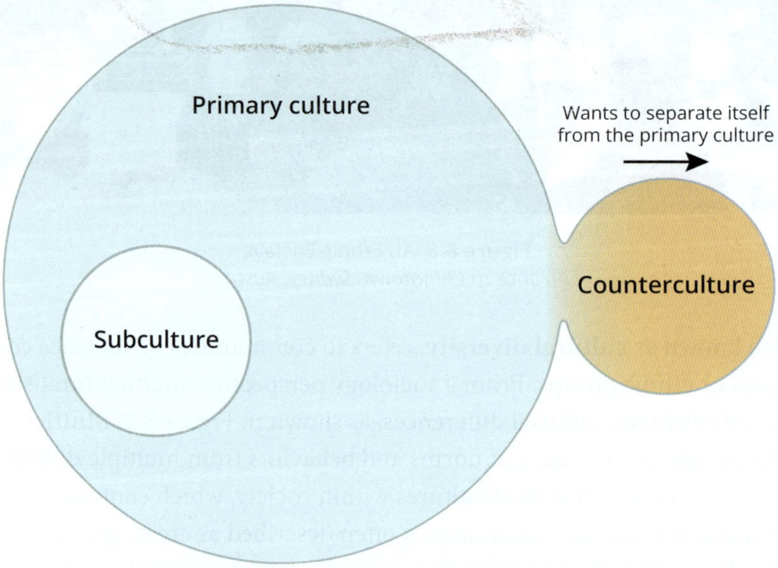

Figure 8.10 Primary Culture and Subcultures

MCAT CONCEPT CHECK 8.1

Before you move on, assess your understanding of the material with these questions.

1. Provide a brief definition for the following social phenomena:
   - Social facilitation:
   - Deindividuation:
   - Bystander effect:
   - Social loafing:
   - Peer pressure:
2. What are the similarities and differences between group polarization and groupthink?
3. What are the differences between assimilation and multiculturalism?

8.2 Socialization High Yield

LEARNING OBJECTIVES

After Chapter 8.2, you will be able to:

- Distinguish between conformity, compliance, and obedience
- Compare and contrast primary and secondary socialization
- Describe compliance techniques, such as foot-in-the-door, door-in-the-face, lowball, and that's-not-all

More than any other animal, humans use social experiences to learn acceptable behavior in the culture in which they live. Sociologists and psychologists use the term **socialization** when discussing the process of developing, inheriting, and spreading norms, customs, and beliefs. Individuals gain the knowledge, skills, habits, and behaviors that are necessary for inclusion in society. Widely held views in a society become the accepted viewpoints and are generally adopted by the majority of individuals within that society. Beliefs, customs, and cultural norms are often passed down from one generation to another within a society in a process called **cultural transmission** or **cultural learning**. Spread of norms, customs, and beliefs from one culture to another can also occur, and is called **cultural diffusion**.

Socialization can be further categorized into different types as seen in Figure 8.11. **Primary socialization** occurs during childhood when we initially learn acceptable actions and attitudes in our society, primarily through observation of our caregivers and other adults in close proximity. In children, this sets the stage for future socialization and provides the foundation for creating personal opinions. **Secondary socialization** is the process of learning appropriate behavior within smaller sections of the larger society. This type of socialization occurs outside of the home and is based on learning the rules of specific social environments. For example, the behavior necessary to thrive in school is different from that in the home setting, and also from that which is acceptable on a sports field or in a church. Secondary socialization is typically associated with adolescents and adults and includes smaller changes and refinements to behavior that were established in primary socialization. Secondary socialization can also occur when moving to a new region or changing schools or professions. **Anticipatory socialization** is the process by which a person prepares for future changes in occupations, living situations, or relationships. A premedical student shadowing physicians to assimilate and practice appropriate behaviors in expectation of one day becoming a doctor is an example of anticipatory socialization. **Resocialization** is another process by which one discards old behaviors in favor of new ones, typically through intensive retraining, and can have positive or negative connotations. The method by which members of the armed forces are trained to obey orders and commands without hesitation is a prime example of resocialization, but so is attracting and indoctrinating members into a cult.

REAL WORLD

Cults that have become a mainstay in media today are often "Doomsday cults." This term refers both to groups that prophesy catastrophe and apocalypse and to those who attempt to bring it about. In December of 2012, nearly 1000 members of the Chinese cult Church of Almighty God were arrested for broadcasting fears of apocalypse and encouraging the overthrow of the Communist Party.

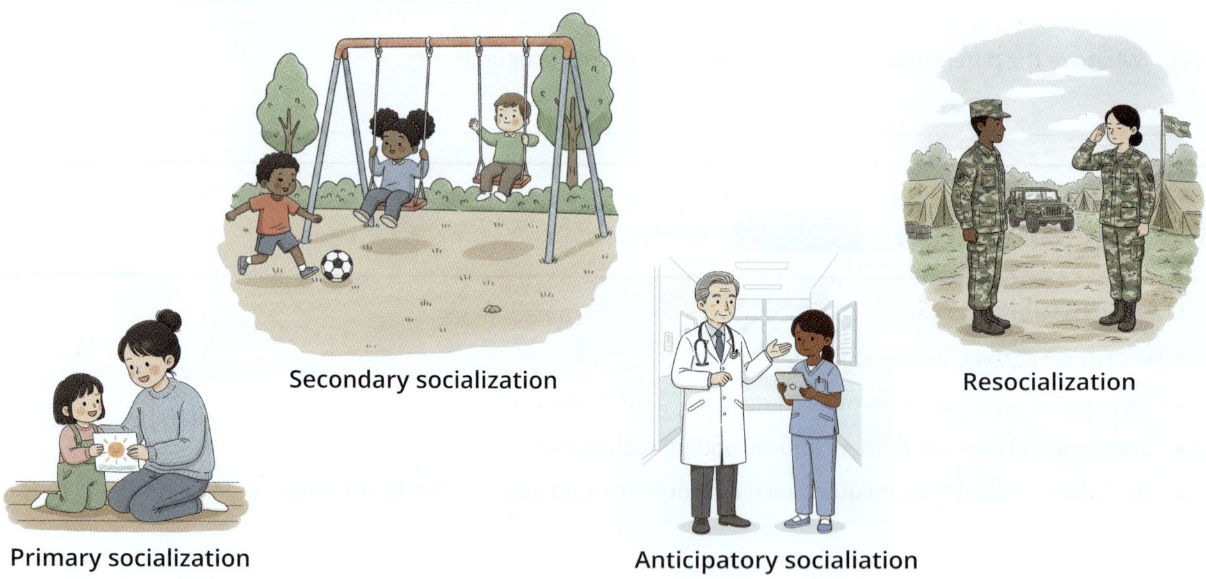

Figure 8.11 Types of Socialization

Norms

Sociologists define **norms** as societal rules that define the boundaries of acceptable behavior. **Mores** are widely observed social norms. While norms are not laws, they do provide a mechanism for regulating the behavior of individuals and groups and thereby serve as a means of **social control**. Penalties for misconduct or rewards for appropriate behavior, called **sanctions**, can also be used to maintain social control. Negative sanctions punish behaviors that deviate from norms, while positive sanctions reward behaviors that comply with norms. Sanctions can also be categorized as formal or informal. **Formal sanctions** are enforced by formal social institutions like governments or employers and can include receiving a promotion (positive) or a jail sentence (negative). By contrast, **informal sanctions** are enforced by social groups. Informal sanctions might include being allowed to sit at a particular table in the school cafeteria (positive) or exclusion from a social group (negative). Figure 8.12 presents visual examples of each of the four possible categories of sanctions.

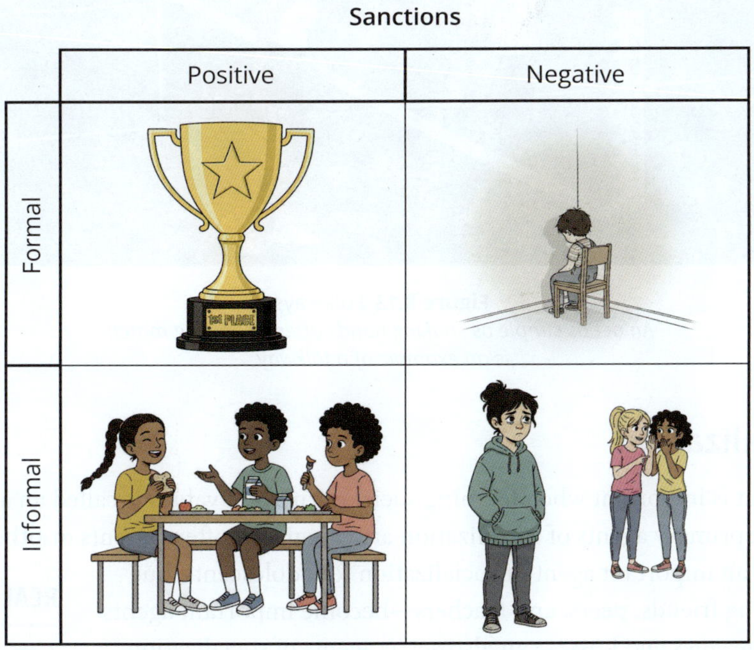

Figure 8.12 The Four Sanction Categories

Norms provide us with a sense of what is appropriate, what we should do, and what is considered **taboo**—socially unacceptable, disgusting, or reprehensible. Norms exist for behavior, speech, dress, home life, and more and can differ between groups within a society, and also between different cultures. For example, many Americans tend to be extraverted and talkative, even among strangers, while Japanese culture sometimes teaches that showing too much of oneself in a public setting is a sign of weakness. Thus, a very quiet person who does not make eye contact could seem odd in America but may fit in perfectly in Japan. **Folkways** are norms that refer to behavior that is considered polite in particular social interactions, such as shaking hands after a sports match, as seen in Figure 8.13.

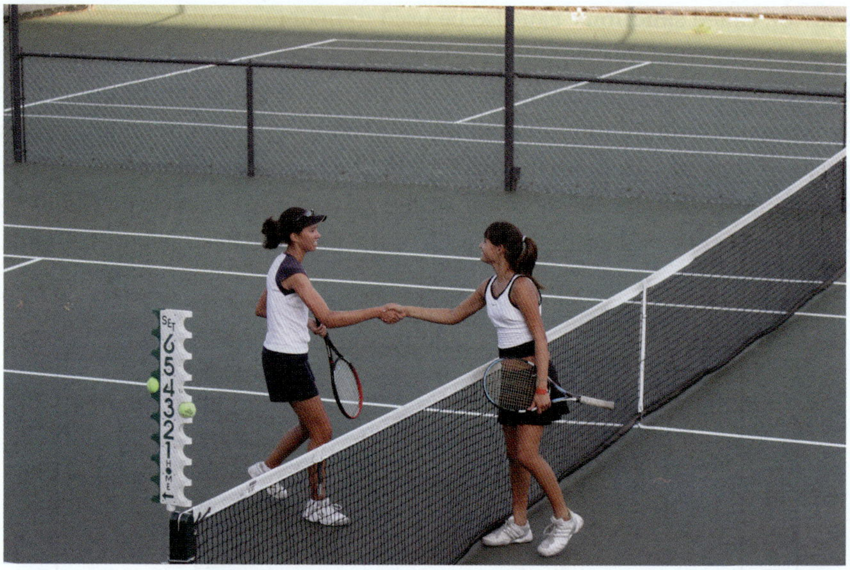

Figure 8.13 Folkways
An act as simple as shaking hands after a sporting match is an example of a folkway.

Agents of Socialization

Any part of society that is important when learning social norms and values is called an **agent of socialization**. For children, the primary agents of socialization are caregivers, often parents or other family members. Direct family remains an important agent of socialization for adolescents, but social circles—including friends, peers, and teachers—become important agents as well. For adults, colleagues and bosses can also act as agents of socialization. Aside from personal relationships, the environment is another agent of socialization. For example, when entering college, some teenagers may experience a complete lifestyle change and are in nearly constant interaction with people of their own age. This new environment creates a shift in acceptable behavior that can include late nights out with friends or all-night study sessions. When entering the workforce, another change in environment leads to socialization within the organization. Ethnic background, religion, and government also play a role in learned behavior, and are therefore also important agents of socialization. And geography at the national, regional, and neighborhood levels also dictates norms of behavior: acceptable behavior in downtown Manhattan is not identical to acceptable behavior in rural Montana.

Furthermore, the media are an important agent of socialization through their influence on what is accepted within a particular society. **Popular culture**, i.e. common trends and beliefs prevalent at a given point in time, is heavily influenced by the media. The media can determine what is considered important in a particular society. Mass media is most commonly accessed through television, radio, newspapers, and the Internet. It delivers impersonalized communication to a vast audience, and can thereby establish trends in American or international popular culture. Many of the agents of socialization are summarized in Figure 8.14.

REAL WORLD

A study published in 2002 examined the link between television and violence. In the study, the researchers followed 707 subjects for 17 years. Study subjects who watched more than one hour of TV per day were approximately four times more likely to act aggressively toward others later in life than those who watched less than one hour of TV. Of those who watched more than three hours of TV per day, nearly 30% were involved in assaults, robberies, or other aggressive behaviors. While this is an interesting link, remember that it shows correlation—not causation!

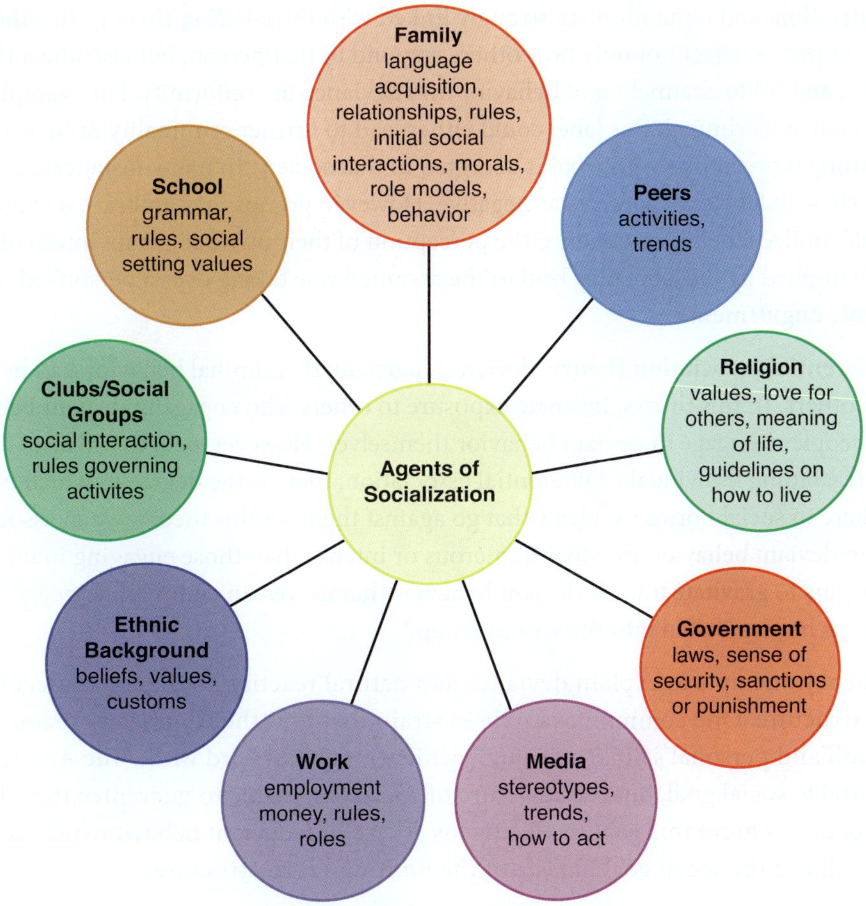

Figure 8.14 Agents of Socialization

Deviance and Stigma

Deviance refers to any violation of norms, rules, or expectations within a society. It is important to note that using the term *deviant* is often associated with strongly negative connotations; however, in the sociological context, it simply refers to any act that goes against societal norms. Deviance can vary in severity, from something as simple as jaywalking to something as serious as committing murder. Deviance also includes any act that meets with disapproval from the larger society.

Social stigma is the extreme disapproval or dislike of a person or group based on perceived differences from the rest of society. These deviations from the norm can include differences in beliefs, abilities, behaviors, and appearance. Certain medical conditions such as HIV, achondroplasia (dwarfism), and obesity can also be stigmatized. Stigma can also spread to affect others who are associated with a particular individual. For example, family members of an alleged or convicted murderer or rapist can be stigmatized. Stigma also evolves over time: whereas divorce was stigmatized in the early twentieth century, it no longer has such strong negative connotations.

BRIDGE

Mental illness has long been stigmatized in American society. While this is slowly changing, the potential stigma associated with a mental health diagnosis continues to be a hurdle to many patients seeking out or receiving care. Many common psychological disorders are discussed in Chapter 7 of *MCAT Behavioral Sciences Review*.

Deviance, stigmatization, and reputation are strongly linked with the **labeling theory**. This theory posits that the labels given to a person affect not only how others respond to that person, but also affect that person's self-image. Labels can lead to channeling of behavior into deviance or conformity. For example, if members of society label a person as a criminal, this label could either lead to further criminality or to a change in behavior toward something more in line with what is accepted in that society. In many instances, we resist being labeled, particularly with labels we perceive as negative. However, groups may embrace deviant labels. Biker gangs, for example, utilize labeling to enhance the perception of their own subgroup. Internalizing a label and assuming the role implied by the label may lead to the assumed role taking over a person's identity, a phenomenon known as **role engulfment**.

According to **differential association theory**, deviance, particularly criminal behavior, can be learned through interactions with others. In this theory, intimate exposure to others who engage in deviant behavior lays the groundwork for people to engage in deviant behavior themselves. However, people will also likely come into contact with norm-abiding individuals. Differential association, then, is the degree to which one is surrounded by ideals that adhere to social norms vs. ideals that go against them. In this theory, when associations with others engaging in deviant behavior are more numerous or intense than those engaging in normative behavior, individuals begins to gravitate toward deviant behavior themselves. In common language, we might describe someone as having "fallen into the wrong group."

Finally, **strain theory** attempts to explain deviance as a natural reaction to the disconnect between social goals and social structure. One common example in strain theory is the American dream, which refers to acquiring wealth and personal stability through achievement and hard work. The American dream is considered a desirable social goal, but the structure of society is unable to guarantee the education and opportunity needed to achieve this goal to all citizens. Therefore, deviant behavior such as theft may arise as an attempt to achieve the social goal *outside* of the limiting social structure.

While deviance is often associated with negative behavior such as crime, functional theorists argue that it is necessary for social order. These theorists argue that deviance provides a clear perception of social norms and acceptable boundaries, encourages unity within society, and can even promote social change.

Conformity, Compliance, and Obedience

While deviance is defined as going against societal norms, conformity, compliance, and obedience are manners of adhering to social expectations or others' requests.

Conformity

Conformity is matching one's attitudes, beliefs, and behaviors to group or societal norms. The pressure to conform can be real or imagined: an actual pressure from others, or a perceived pressure or expectation. Conformity is also known as **majority influence**. The Asch experiments, described earlier, showed the strength of social influence on **normative conformity**, the desire to fit into a group because of fear of rejection.

There are distinct types of conformity, including internalization and identification. **Internalization** involves changing one's behavior to fit with a group while also privately agreeing with the ideas of the group. **Identification** refers to the outward acceptance of others' ideas without personally taking on these ideas.

KEY CONCEPT

Internalization and identification both deal with accepting others' ideas, but whereas internalization also reflects a change in internal thoughts to agree with the idea, identification is acceptance of the idea on the surface level without internalizing it.

A classic experiment looking at internalization was Philip Zimbardo's Stanford Prison Experiment. Zimbardo advertised for a role-playing experiment in which he recruited 21 male college students. The study participants were randomly assigned the role of prisoner or guard. The prisoners were arrested in their homes and taken to a "prison" created in the Stanford University psychology building. Guards were issued uniforms, including whistles, handcuffs, and dark glasses to prevent eye contact. The prisoners and guards quickly fell into their roles and displayed related behaviors almost immediately. Guards began to taunt and harass prisoners, appearing to enjoy their role. Prisoners also adopted their new role, taking the prison rules very seriously, and becoming more and more dependent on the guards. As the guards became more aggressive, the prisoners became more submissive, although they also attempted to mount a revolt. The study had to be ended after six days because the guards had begun to physically abuse the prisoners so severely that ethical concerns were raised. After the study ended, Zimbardo interviewed each participant. The guards and prisoners, who had internalized their roles, were both shocked by their behavior during the experiment.

REAL WORLD

In recent years, design flaws in the Stanford Prison Experiment have come to light. These include sampling biases, ethical concerns, lack of controls, and active participation in the experiment by Zimbardo himself.

The likelihood of conformity differs among cultures. For instance, individualist cultures tend to value independent thought and unique ideas and are thus less likely to conform; in collectivist cultures, group mentality often supersedes the individual. The latter type of society tends toward conformity.

Compliance

Compliance is a change in behavior based on a direct request. The person or group that asks the individual to make the change typically has no actual power or authority to command the individual, yet will ask the individual to change behavior. There are several notable techniques used to gain compliance of others, particularly within the marketing arena. The **foot-in-the-door** technique begins with a small request, and after gaining compliance, a larger request is made. An example of this scenario could be a fellow classmate asking to borrow your notes after missing class. You agree and offer to share the notes at the next class session. Later in the day, when you see the student again, you're asked if you would be willing to make copies of your notes too. Many people will still agree at this point, as the first request opened the door to continued compliance.

The next technique is called the **door-in-the-face technique**. This is the opposite of the foot-in-the-door technique, wherein a large request is made at first and, if refused, a second, smaller request is made. Often, this smaller request is the actual goal of the requester. Using this technique, a fellow student might ask you to make a copy of your notes from class and bring them to the next class. If you deny the request, the student might follow up with a smaller request, asking to borrow your notes to make personal copies. The second, more reasonable request may be granted.

Another common method of achieving compliance is the **lowball technique**. In this technique, the requestor will get an initial commitment from an individual, and then raise the cost of the commitment. It is important to note that cost need not only include money, but can also include effort and time. An example of this technique is a scenario in which you are asked by your boss to head a committee with a time commitment of five hours per month of meetings. You agree to head the committee, but later discover that the commitment also includes written reports from each meeting and a quarterly presentation.

Yet another technique used to gain compliance is the **that's-not-all technique**. In this method, an individual is made an offer, but before making a decision, is told the deal is even better than expected. This method is frequently seen in infomercials: *We can offer you these earrings for the stunningly low price of $19.99. But wait! If you buy them, you'll also receive our matching necklace, normal retail value $49.99, absolutely free.*

Obedience

While compliance deals with requests made by people without actual authority over an individual, **obedience** is changing one's behavior in response to a direct order or expectation expressed by an authority figure. While a classmate has no authority to demand notes from you, an authority figure has social power over other individuals. For instance, if a teacher demands that you hand over your notes from class, you would be obeying rather than complying. People are far more likely to obey than comply due to the real or perceived social power of the individual.

One of the most notable obedience experiment series was conducted by Stanley Milgram. In this classic set of studies, Milgram claimed to be recruiting participants for a study to test the effects of punishment on learning behavior. Participants were told they would be randomly assigned to be the "teacher" or "learner"; however, the "learner" was actually a paid actor (confederate). The teachers were told that they would be controlling an electrical panel that would administer shocks to the learners if they made mistakes. This experimental setup is depicted in Figure 8.15. Prior to giving the first shock, the teachers were given a sample 45 V shock to make them aware of what they would be doing to the learners. The teachers were then told that they would need to increase the voltage by 15 V each time an incorrect response was given. The learners, who received no actual shock, were provided with scripts telling them to show pain, ask to stop the experiment, scream, and even feign passing out. As the learners acted more and more uncomfortable, the teachers became less willing to increase the shock voltage. However, by using increasingly demanding language (from *Please continue* to *You have no other choice, you must go on*), the researchers were able to get 65 percent of the participants to administer shocks to the maximum of 450 V, even if they showed discomfort in doing so. Milgram and other researchers were surprised at the level of obedience the participants showed during the experiment. This type of experiment has been repeated many times and has consistently shown that more than 60 percent of people will obey even if they do not wish to continue.

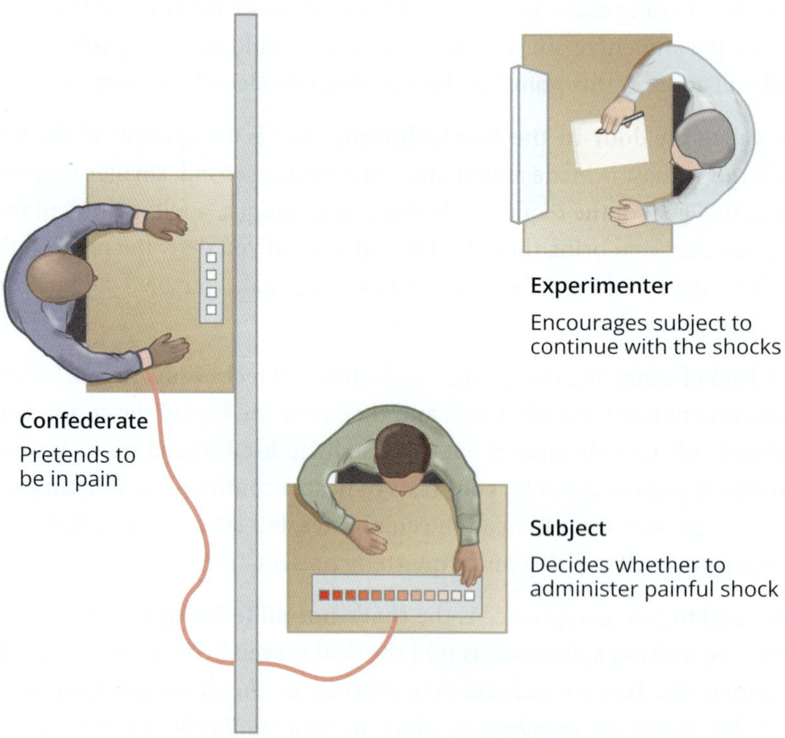

Figure 8.15 Milgram's Obedience Experiment

MCAT CONCEPT CHECK 8.2

Before you move on, assess your understanding of the material with these questions.

1. What is the difference between primary and secondary socialization?

____

2. What are conformity, compliance, and obedience?
   - Conformity:

   ____

   - Compliance:

   ____

   - Obedience:

   ____

3. For each of the compliance techniques listed below, provide a brief description:
   - Foot-in-the-door:

   ____

   - Door-in-the-face:

   ____

   - Lowball:

   ____

   - That's-not-all:

   ____

8.3 Attitudes and Behavior **High Yield**

LEARNING OBJECTIVES

After Chapter 8.3, you will be able to:

- Recall the three components of attitude
- Describe the four functional areas of the functional attitude theory
- Identify the roles of central route and peripheral route processing in the elaboration likelihood model
- Recall the three interactive factors of Bandura's triadic reciprocal causation

Social cognition focuses on the ways in which people think about others and how these ideas impact behavior. Our attitudes—the ways in which we perceive others—impact the ways we behave toward them.

Components of Attitudes

An **attitude** is the expression of positive or negative feeling toward a person, place, thing, or scenario. Attitudes develop from experiences with others who affect our opinions and behaviors. Even prior to meeting someone, past experiences and information from others can influence your attitude toward a person.

There are three primary components of attitude: affective, behavioral, and cognitive (Figure 8.16). The **affective** component of attitude refers to the way a person feels toward something, and is the emotional component of attitude. *Snakes scare me* and *I love my family* are both affective expressions of attitude. The **behavioral** component of attitude is the way a person acts with respect to something. For example, avoiding snakes and spending time with one's family would reflect the behavioral component of the attitudes described earlier. Finally, the **cognitive** component of attitude is the way an individual thinks about something, which is usually the justification for the other two components. In the snake example above, knowing that snakes can be dangerous (and sometimes venomous) provides a reason to be afraid of snakes and to avoid them.

MNEMONIC

Components of Attitude: **ABC**

- **A**ffective
- **B**ehavioral
- **C**ognitive

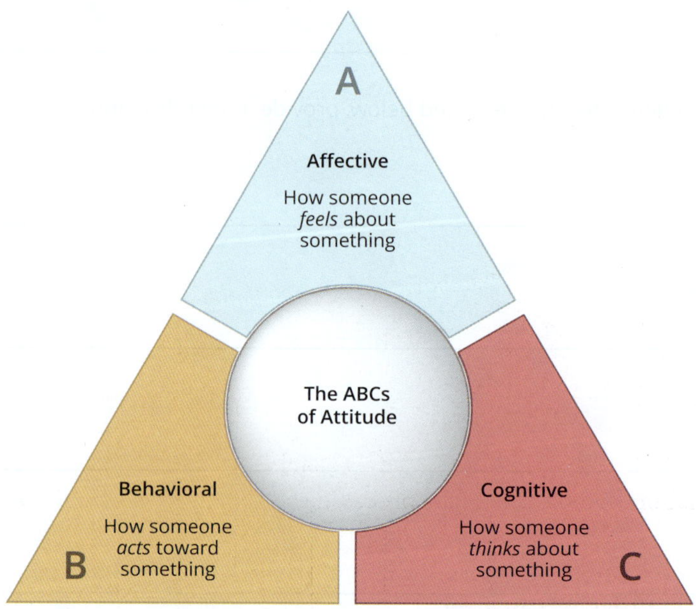

Figure 8.16 The ABCs of Attitude

Theories of Attitudes

The **functional attitudes theory** states that attitudes serve four functions: knowledge, ego expression, adaptation, and ego defense. The **knowledge function** can be summarized as follows: attitudes help provide organization to thoughts and experiences, and knowing the attitudes of others helps to predict their behavior. For example, one would predict that an individual who cares about political action would vote in an upcoming election. Attitudes facilitate being **ego-expressive**, allowing us to communicate and solidify our self-identity. For instance, if a person strongly identifies with a sports team, that person might wear a team hat to identify as having a positive attitude towards that team. **Adaptive** attitude is the idea that expressed socially acceptable attitudes will lead to acceptance. For example, a person declaring to a social group that they enjoyed a popular movie can help to build social bonds. Lastly, attitudes are **ego-defensive** if they protect our self-esteem or justify actions that we know are wrong. For example, a child who has difficulty doing math may develop a negative attitude toward the subject.

Learning theory posits that attitudes are developed through different forms of learning. Direct contact with the object of an attitude can influence attitude towards that object. For example, children form a positive attitude toward sweets almost immediately after tasting them. Direct instruction from others can also influence attitudes. For instance, a child who is taught by caregivers not to use curse words can form a negative attitude toward curse words and, indirectly, a negative attitude toward those who use curse words. Our attitudes can also be influenced by others' attitudes. For example, teenagers may begin to have a positive attitude toward smoking if they notice that all of their friends smoke. Finally, attitudes may be formed through classical conditioning, operant conditioning, or observational learning, all of which are discussed in Chapter 3 of *MCAT Behavioral Sciences Review*.

KEY CONCEPT

- Central route processing (high elaboration)—scrutinizing and analyzing the content of persuasive information
- Peripheral route processing (low elaboration)—focusing on superficial details of persuasive information, such as appearances, catchphrases and slogans, and credibility

The **elaboration likelihood model** is a theory of attitude formation and attitude change that separates individuals on a continuum based on how they process persuasive information. At one extreme are those who elaborate extensively, that is, those who think deeply about information, scrutinize its meaning and purpose, and draw conclusions or make decisions based on this analysis. Deep thinking in this manner is referred to as **central route processing** and focuses on **central message characteristics** like logical soundness, clarity, and coherence. When an attempt to influence attitudes uses information that appeals to central route processing, this attempt is said to be using the **central route to persuasion**. A scientific paper would be one example of an attempt to influence attitudes that uses the central route to processing. At the other extreme are those who do not elaborate and focus instead on **peripheral message characteristics**, including superficial details such as the appearance of the person delivering the argument, catchphrases and slogans, and credibility. This type of processing is known as **peripheral route processing**. When attempts to influence attitudes appeal to peripheral route processing, these attempts are said to be using the **peripheral route to persuasion**. An advertisement with just a logo that contains a visually appealing image is one example of an attempt to influence attitudes that uses the peripheral route to persuasion. To contrast these two types of processing, consider two voters watching a well-informed and charismatic politician speak: One voter might be swayed by the cogent arguments made by the politician, and this illustrates high elaboration, central route processing. The other voter might be swayed by the perception that the speaker is likable and a good person, illustrating low elaboration, peripheral route processing. Figure 8.17 presents another example of the contrast involving the rationale behind the purchase of an electric car. Most individuals fall in the middle of this continuum, and the degree to which we elaborate on information can vary depending on the specific situation.

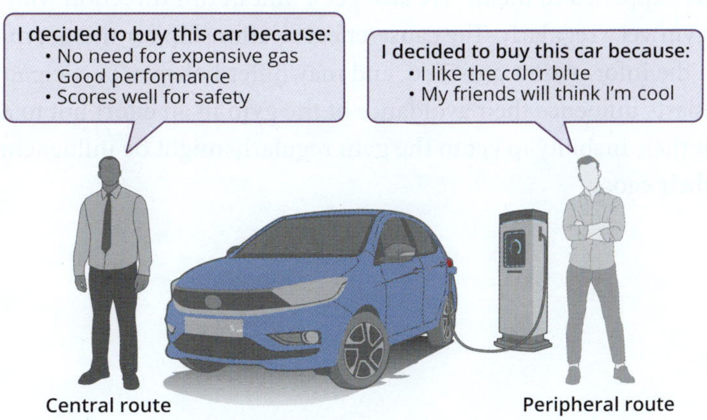

Figure 8.17 The Two Paths of the Elaboration Likelihood Model

BEHAVIORAL SCIENCES GUIDED EXAMPLE WITH EXPERT THINKING

Corporate researchers conducted a longitudinal study of gym members at ten locations in the second week of January for five consecutive years. Participants engaged in a short series of physical activities and measurements assessing physical fitness, then responded to questions about attitudes and fitness. Participants who were present for at least three of the five years and received consistent, low scores in physical fitness measures were associated with the following: lower self-reported gym attendance, lower perceived value of exercise, and low expressed regard for those who attended the gym with a frequency greater than five visits/week. These participants also reported high levels of seasonal motivation (New Year's resolutions).

This is giving me context on a specific set of beliefs involving consistent behavior over time. With a consistent social behavior (high motivation and low adherence) I'm expecting questions about social psychology.

In response to these data, gym owners established a social media group devoted to creating small local workout groups meeting 3–4 days per week with regular check-ins for their members and invited gym attendees within this demographic set to join.

Social psychology: it sounds like the gym owner is trying for positive peer pressure.

How might the group who received consistent low scores in physical fitness measures respond to the new initiative if they choose to participate? How do the results of the five year study inform predictions of their adherence to the 3–4 day per week workout plan?

The writers of the MCAT will hint at a concept in the passage or question stem and then ask us a question about recognizing or applying that concept to the situation described. We'll want to be familiar enough with the content that when the question tells a story or mentions some specific example, we can say to ourselves "Oh, that's ________!"

In order to answer this question, we're going to have to dive into the scenario and identify factors that will influence behavioral outcomes. In the first paragraph, these gym members have maintained the same low level of fitness and low gym attendance for five years, which should remind us of attribution theory: consistent behaviors tend to have dispositional rather than situational explanations. Despite the finding of high seasonal motivation to engage with exercise, it's likely that this group of individuals aren't already in shape because of their attitudes towards themselves or working out ("I'm nervous people will judge me at the gym" or "I just don't enjoy lifting weights"), rather than situational barriers ("My preferred gym is being renovated" or "I'm just super busy this year"). In other words, such attributions are about "who they are" instead of "what has happened to them." We also get a hint in this direction with the finding about low regard for people who attend the gym very regularly. The cause/effect relationship for this set of findings and past behaviors is difficult to assess with the information provided, and may differ between participants. It could be that for some, the thoughts on gym enthusiasts influence their avoidance of the gym in an effort not to adopt similar behaviors. But for others, it could also be that their inability to get to the gym regularly might be influencing their attitudes about those who do in order to protect their egos.

Things are different this year, thanks to the creation of the new fitness group by the gym owners. Some subset of this group of participants have now joined a group of people who will be going to the gym together and will hold each other accountable. We should identify a specific social phenomenon as soon as we read that sentence: peer pressure!

Now that we've identified the important information in the scenario, we should return to the question itself. The question asks how the information we already have about this group of participants might predict their behaviors, which are the three factors of social-cognitive theory. Social-cognitive theory says that all of these things influence one another. If we put together everything we've learned, we see that the attitudes expressed in this group make it less likely that they'll stick to working out, but they've also taken steps to change their environment by opting to join a new peer group for themselves, which makes it more likely that their behaviors may change. While it's impossible to tell which of these influences will win out over the other, it is possible that putting themselves into this new environment and changing their behaviors will in fact change their attitudes over time to be more accepting of those people (now including themselves!) who go to the gym often.

In short, our answer is: the data on this group indicates a possible disposition that makes it less likely they will consistently go and work out at the gym. However, there is now a competing influence to go to the gym that applies to them based on peer pressure from their new group.

Social cognitive theory postulates that people learn how to behave and shape attitudes by observing the behaviors of others. According to this theory, behavior is not learned by trial-and-error, but develops through direct observation and replication of the actions of others. This learning is influenced by personal factors (such as thoughts about the behavior) and the environment in which the behavior is observed. These three factors—behavior, personal factors, and environment—are not independent concepts, but influence each other, as shown in Bandura's triadic reciprocal causation in Figure 8.18. For example, the work ethic of employees in a company (behavior) is affected by how hard their colleagues work, their previous attitudes toward hard work (personal), and the systems and infrastructure of the company (environment). Reciprocally, this behavior may create a change in the employees' attitude toward work (personal) and the systems within the company (environment).

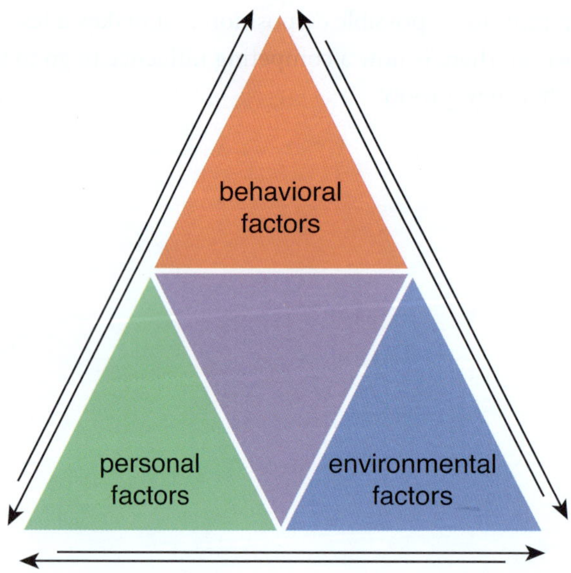

Figure 8.18 Bandura's Triadic Reciprocal Causation

MCAT EXPERTISE

MCAT passages tend to describe an experiment or a scenario and drop in sentences or even short phrases that hint at related scientific content that is then used in questions. The better you are at recognizing this content, the more ready you will be to answer these questions quickly and correctly. But don't feel like you need to scour each passage for every single concept that could appear in the question set.

MCAT CONCEPT CHECK 8.3

Before you move on, assess your understanding of the material with these questions.

1. What are the three components of attitude?
    -
    -
    -

2. What are the four functional areas of the functional attitudes theory?
    -
    -
    -
    -

3. What are the routes of processing used to explain the elaboration likelihood model? Which is associated with high elaboration?
    -
    -

4. What are the three interactive factors of Bandura's triadic reciprocal causation?
    -
    -
    -

Conclusion

Human behavior is learned and influenced by those around us. Simply being around others can lead to changes in behavior from how we act when alone. Pressure from others can also lead to changes in behavior when people crave acceptance: inclusion in a group can lead to changes in thought processes and decision making. Social norms, which are learned through experience and observation, can be rejected by individuals, leading to deviance and stigmatization. However, the need to fit in can lead to conformity, compliance, and obedience. Attitudes are also developed through observations, experiences, and interactions with others, and there are multiple theories explaining their specific methods of formation.

This chapter focused primarily on how groups influence an individual's behavior. In the next chapter, we'll look at the structure of these groups and how we present ourselves to the larger society. We'll explore methods of communication between individuals—both verbal and nonverbal—and consider how we encourage others to gain certain impressions about us.

GO ONLINE

You've reviewed the content, now test your knowledge and critical thinking skills by completing a test-like passage set in your online resources!

CONCEPT SUMMARY

Group Psychology

- **Social facilitation** describes the tendency of people to perform at a different level based on the fact that others are around.
- **Deindividuation** is a loss of self-awareness in large groups, which can lead to drastic changes in behavior.
- The **bystander effect** describes the observation that when in a group, individuals are less likely to respond to a person in need.
- **Peer pressure** refers to the social influence placed on individuals by others they consider equals.
- Group decision making may differ from individual decision making.
  - Group **polarization** is the tendency toward making decisions in a group that are more extreme than the thoughts of the individual group members.
  - **Groupthink** is the tendency for groups to make decisions based on ideas and solutions that arise within the group without considering outside ideas. Ethics may be disturbed as pressure is created to conform and remain loyal to the group.
- **Culture** describes the beliefs, ideas, behaviors, actions, and characteristics of a group or society of people.
  - **Assimilation** is the process by which a group or individual's culture begins to melt into another culture.
  - **Multiculturalism** refers to the encouragement of multiple cultures within a community to enhance diversity.
  - **Subcultures** refer to a group of people within a culture that distinguish themselves from the primary culture to which they belong.

Socialization

- **Socialization** is the process of developing and spreading norms, customs, and beliefs.
- **Norms** are what determine the boundaries of acceptable behavior within society.
- Agents of socialization include family, peers, school, religious affiliation, and other groups that promote socialization.
- **Stigma** is the extreme disapproval or dislike of a person or group based on perceived differences from the rest of society.
- **Deviance** refers to any violation of norms, rules, or expectations within a society.
- **Conformity** is changing beliefs or behaviors in order to fit into a group or society.
- **Compliance** occurs when individuals change their behavior based on the requests of others. Methods of gaining compliance include the foot-in-the-door technique, door-in-the-face technique, lowball technique, and that's-not-all technique, among others.
- **Obedience** is a change in behavior based on a command from someone seen as an authority figure.

Attitudes and Behavior

- **Attitudes** are tendencies toward expression of positive or negative feelings or evaluations of something.
- There are affective, behavioral, and cognitive components to attitudes.
- The **functional attitudes theory** states that there are four functional areas of attitudes that serve individuals in life: knowledge, ego expression, adaptability, and ego defense.
- The **learning theory** states that attitudes are developed through forms of learning: direct contact, direct interaction, direct instruction, and conditioning.
- The **elaboration likelihood model** states that attitudes are formed and changed through different routes of information processing based on the degree of elaboration (**central route processing**, **peripheral route processing**).
- The **social cognitive theory** states that attitudes are formed through observation of behavior, personal factors, and environment.

ANSWERS TO CONCEPT CHECKS

8.1

1. Social facilitation describes the tendency of people to perform at a different level based on the fact that others are around. Deindividuation is the idea that people will lose a sense of self-awareness and can act dramatically different because of the influence of a group. The bystander effect describes the observation that individuals are less likely to respond to a person in need when in a group. Social loafing refers to a decrease in effort seen when individuals are in a group. Peer pressure refers to the social influence placed on individuals by others they consider their equals.
2. Group polarization and groupthink are both social processes that occur when groups make decisions. Group polarization is the tendency toward extreme decisions in a group. Groupthink is the tendency for groups to make decisions based on ideas and solutions that arise within the group without considering outside ideas, given the pressure to conform and remain loyal to the group.
3. Societies that contain multiple cultures can exhibit multiculturalism or assimilation. Assimilation is the process by which multiple cultures begin to merge into one, typically with an unequal blending of ideas and beliefs. Multiculturalism refers to the idea that multiple cultures should be encouraged and respected without one culture becoming dominant overall.

8.2

1. Primary socialization refers to the initial learning of acceptable behaviors and societal norms during childhood, which is facilitated mostly by caregivers and other adults. Secondary socialization refers to learning the norms of specific subgroups or situations during adolescence and adulthood.
2. Conformity is changing beliefs or behaviors in order to fit into a group or society. Compliance occurs when individuals change their behavior based on the request of others who do not wield authority over the individual. Obedience is a change in behavior because of a request from an authority figure.
3. The foot-in-the-door technique refers to asking for favors that increase in size with each subsequent request. The door-in-the-face technique refers to making a large request and then, if refused, making a smaller request. The lowball technique refers to gaining compliance without revealing the full cost (money, effort, or time) of the favor. The that's-not-all technique refers to increasing the reward for a request before an individual has the chance to make a decision.

8.3

1. The three components of attitude are affective, behavioral, and cognitive.
2. The four functional areas of the functional attitudes theory are knowledge, ego expression, adaptation, and ego defense.
3. The routes of processing used to explain the elaboration likelihood model are central route processing and peripheral route processing. Central route processing is associated with high elaboration.
4. The three interactive factors of Bandura's triadic reciprocal causation are behavior, personal factors, and environment.

SCIENCE MASTERY ASSESSMENT EXPLANATIONS

1. **C**

When fulfilling particular roles, an individual's behavior can be very out of character. The changing of one's behavior (and internal ideas) to match a group is called internalization conformity. This was a key part of the experiment. The experiment also involved deindividuation, the loss of self-identity in the group setting that can lead to antinormative or violent behavior.

2. **B**

The fact that individual opinions became more extreme during group discussion is explained by group polarization. The jury member initially felt that a strict penalty should be given, but this opinion became more extreme after conversation with the rest of the group.

3. **A**

It has been observed that increasing the number of bystanders decreases the likelihood that any of them will aid a victim. Increasing the degree of danger experienced by the victim, **(B)**, making the victim an acquaintance instead of a stranger, **(C)**, and being alone in the room with the victim, **(D)**, would increase the likelihood that the bystander would help the victim.

4. **D**

With groupthink, a member would perform all of the actions described by the answer choices except create a sense of negativity against risk taking; in fact, there is optimism and encouragement toward risk taking in groupthink.

5. **A**

Primary socialization is the teaching of acceptable actions and attitudes during childhood, which would occur too early to be part of the adult prison system. Resocialization, **(D)**, is the process by which one changes behaviors by discarding old routines and patterns and transitions to new behaviors necessary for a life change. The prison environment is designed to change unlawful behavior into desired behavior, making this an incorrect choice. When entering prison, an inmate must also undergo secondary socialization, **(B)**, learning the rules of the specific social environment of the prison. Finally, if the inmate is not incarcerated for life, attempts at anticipatory socialization, **(C)**, must be made before releasing the inmate in preparation for life outside of the prison.

6. **C**

This is a prime example of the foot-in-the-door technique. The neighbors first ask for a small favor and, after receiving commitment, ask for a larger favor.

7. **A**

The affective component of attitude consists of feelings and emotions toward something.

8. **D**

Peripheral route processing deals with processing information that is not based on content, but instead on superficial parameters such as boring speech patterns or appearance of the speaker. Central route processing, **(C)**, is the processing of information through analysis of its content.

9. **B**

The Milgram shock experiment showed that individuals would obey orders from authority figures even if they were not comfortable with the task at hand. Conformity and compliance, **(C)** and **(D)**, also deal with changes in individual behavior, but are not based on the requests of an authority figure.

10. **C**

Internalization refers to the type of conformity in which individuals change their outward opinion to match the group and also personally agree with those ideas.

11. **B**

The four functional areas of the functional attitudes theory are knowledge, adaptability, ego expression, and ego defense. Acceptance into a group may influence attitudes or opinions; however, this is not a part of the functional attitudes theory.

12. **A**

For 14 out of the 16 members, the record times were obtained during public meets. The fact that the team members performed better when in front of a crowd supports the notion of social facilitation.

13. **D**

This young person is preparing to spend time in a new social setting. The process of preparing for future changes in environment is considered anticipatory socialization.

14. **B**

Social action is best described as the effects that a group has on individual behavior, including social facilitation, deindividuation, the bystander effect, social loafing, and peer pressure. Social interaction describes how two or more individuals influence each other's behavior, including group polarization and groupthink.

15. **C**

Placing spoken or unspoken expectations on individuals to agree with the ideas of the group is best described as pressure for conformity.

GO ONLINE

Consult your online resources for additional practice.

SHARED CONCEPTS

Behavioral Sciences Chapter 5
Motivation, Emotion, and Stress

Behavioral Sciences Chapter 6
Identity and Personality

Behavioral Sciences Chapter 9
Social Interaction

Behavioral Sciences Chapter 10
Social Thinking

Behavioral Sciences Chapter 11
Social Structure and Demographics

Physics and Math Chapter 11
Reasoning About the Design and Execution of Research

CHAPTER 9

SOCIAL INTERACTION

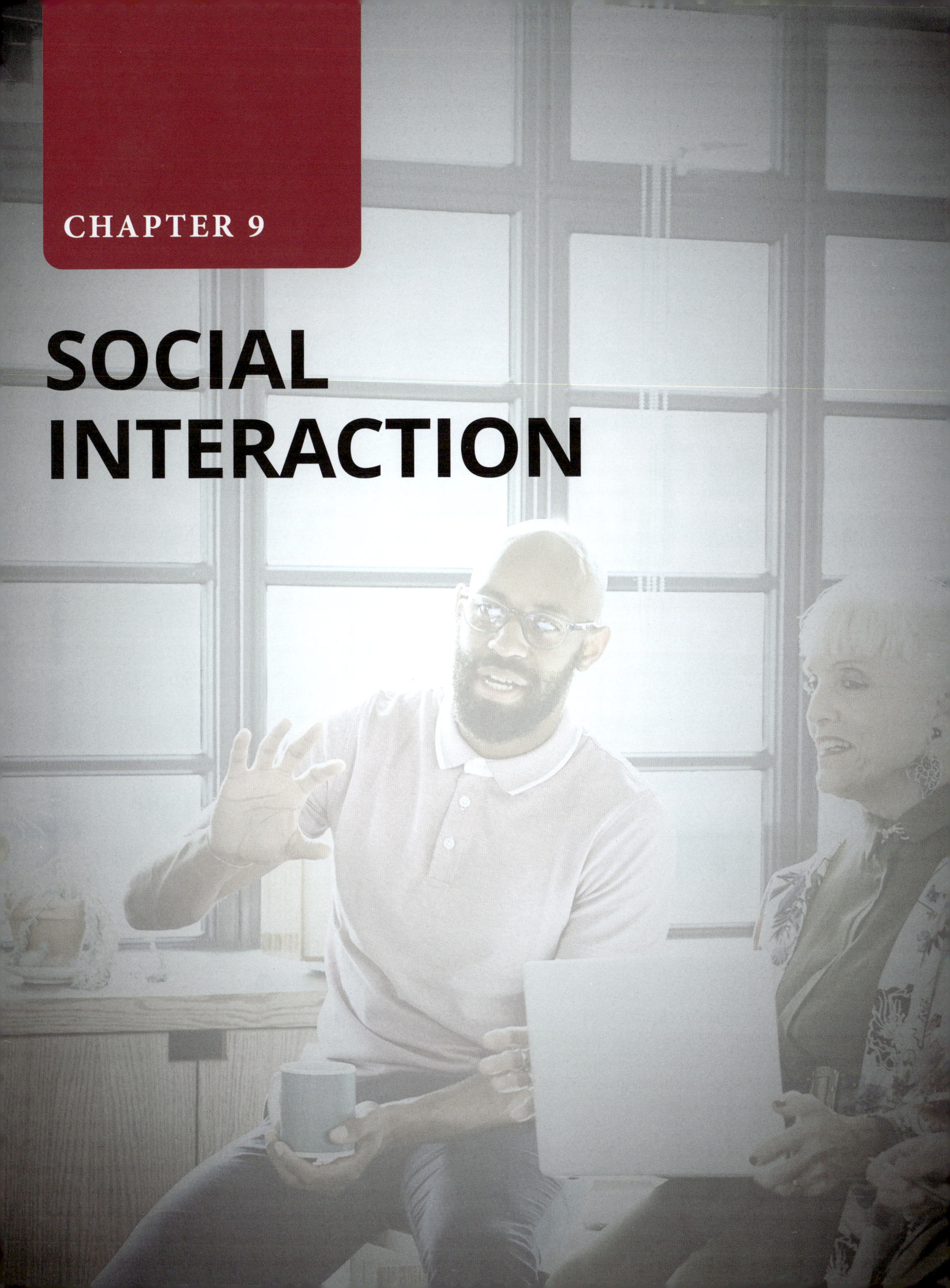

SCIENCE MASTERY ASSESSMENT

Every pre-med knows this feeling: there is so much content I have to know for the MCAT! How do I know what to do first or what's important?

While the high-yield badges throughout this book will help you identify the most important topics, this Science Mastery Assessment is another tool in your MCAT prep arsenal. This quiz (which can also be taken in your online resources) and the guidance below will help ensure that you are spending the appropriate amount of time on this chapter based on your personal strengths and weaknesses. Don't worry though—skipping something now does not mean you'll never study it. Later on in your prep, as you complete full-length tests, you'll uncover specific pieces of content that you need to review and can come back to these chapters as appropriate.

How to Use This Assessment

If you answer 0–7 questions correctly:

Spend about 1 hour to read this chapter in full and take limited notes throughout. Follow up by reviewing **all** quiz questions to ensure that you now understand how to solve each one.

If you answer 8–11 questions correctly:

Spend 20–40 minutes reviewing the quiz questions. Beginning with the questions you missed, read and take notes on the corresponding subchapters. For questions you answered correctly, ensure your thinking matches that of the explanation and you understand why each choice was correct or incorrect.

If you answer 12–15 questions correctly:

Spend less than 20 minutes reviewing all questions from the quiz. If you missed any, then include a quick read-through of the corresponding subchapters, or even just the relevant content within a subchapter, as part of your question review. For questions you answered correctly, ensure your thinking matches that of the explanation and review the Concept Summary at the end of the chapter.

1. Which of the following best describes the sociological definition of a status?
   - **A.** The emotional state of a social interaction
   - **B.** Expectations that are associated with a specific title in society
   - **C.** A position in society used to classify an individual
   - **D.** A means to describe one's peers

2. Becoming a college graduate requires hard work and diligence in academics. As such, being a college graduate could be considered a(n):
   - **A.** ascribed status.
   - **B.** achieved status.
   - **C.** master status.
   - **D.** cardinal status.

3. A bureaucracy is a specific example of a(n):
   - **A.** immediate network.
   - **B.** primary group.
   - **C.** organization.
   - **D.** reference group.

4. Which of the following is NOT characteristic of a bureaucracy?
   - **A.** Rigidly defined work procedures
   - **B.** Requirement for officials to hold an advanced degree
   - **C.** Regular salary increases
   - **D.** Election by constituents

5. Which of the following is a form of verbal communication?
   - **A.** Facial expressions
   - **B.** Eye contact
   - **C.** Written text
   - **D.** Body language

6. Which of the following best describes the impression management strategy of aligning actions?
   - **A.** Adhering to the behaviors that are expected for a given role in society
   - **B.** Relieving tension brought about by holding conflicting views in one's head
   - **C.** Providing socially acceptable reasons to explain unexpected behavior
   - **D.** Dictating that members of a group should follow similar practices to one another

7. While on the phone, a friend says: "A good friend would let me borrow the bike." This friend is using which impression management strategy?
   - **A.** Managing appearances
   - **B.** Alter-casting
   - **C.** Ingratiation
   - **D.** Self-disclosure

8. Which of the following is an example of a *Gesellschaft*?
   - **A.** A large corporation
   - **B.** A small rural neighborhood
   - **C.** Members of the same family
   - **D.** An ethnic enclave in a large city

9. In some cultures, it is considered taboo for one to show too much sadness at a funeral. In other cultures, wailing and crying loudly is expected. These cultures differ in their:
   - **A.** characteristic institutions.
   - **B.** display rules.
   - **C.** authentic selves.
   - **D.** peer groups.

10. Which of the following is NOT a dimension of the system for multiple level observation of groups (SYMLOG)?

- **A.** Friendliness vs. unfriendliness
- **B.** Dominance vs. submission
- **C.** Conformity vs. contrast
- **D.** Instrumentally controlled vs. emotionally expressive

11. Political campaign ads often focus on "exposing" an opposing candidate's negative characteristics. In the dramaturgical approach, one would describe this as:

- **A.** bringing the front stage self to the back stage.
- **B.** bringing the back stage self to the front stage.
- **C.** removing the front stage self.
- **D.** removing the back stage self.

12. In the context of impression management, which of the following selves is most similar to the ought self?

- **A.** The ideal self
- **B.** The tactical self
- **C.** The authentic self
- **D.** The presented self

13. The evolutionary role of emotions has been used as support for which model(s) of emotional expression?

- **A.** The basic model only
- **B.** The social construction model only
- **C.** Both the basic model and social construction model
- **D.** Neither the basic model nor the social construction model

14. Which of the following is an example of intraspecific animal communication?

- **A.** A dog who barks when a stranger enters the house
- **B.** An anglerfish that uses a bioluminescent appendage to attract prey
- **C.** Bats using echolocation to detect the surrounding environment
- **D.** A cat who uses scent glands to mark his territory for other cats

15. Primary groups differ from secondary groups in that:

- **A.** primary groups are shorter-lived than secondary groups.
- **B.** primary groups are larger than secondary groups.
- **C.** primary groups are formed of stronger bonds than secondary groups.
- **D.** primary groups are assigned while secondary groups are chosen.

Answer Key

1. **C** (See section 9.1)
2. **B** (See section 9.1)
3. **C** (See section 9.1)
4. **D** (See section 9.1)
5. **C** (See section 9.2)
6. **C** (See section 9.2)
7. **B** (See section 9.2)
8. **A** (See section 9.1)
9. **B** (See section 9.2)
10. **C** (See section 9.1)
11. **B** (See section 9.2)
12. **B** (See section 9.2)
13. **A** (See section 9.2)
14. **D** (See section 9.2)
15. **C** (See section 9.1)

The relevant section of the chapter to review for each question is given in parentheses after the correct answer. Detailed explanations can be found at the end of the chapter.

CHAPTER 9

SOCIAL INTERACTION

In This Chapter

CHAPTER PROFILE

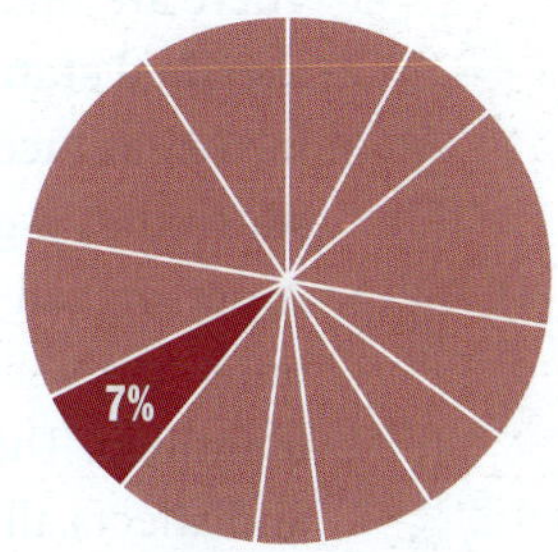

The content in this chapter should be relevant to about 7% of all questions about the behavioral sciences on the MCAT.

This chapter covers material from the following AAMC content categories:

7B: Social processes that influence human behavior

8C: Social interactions

Introduction

Every day, you present yourself to others and interact with society. You interact with others in a number of ways, using emotional expression, verbal communication, and cultural norms. You may also interact with nonhuman animals on a day-to-day basis. This interaction can be just as complex and meaningful to your emotional state and life experience. What shapes and molds your interactions? How do you know the appropriate way to connect with other members of society?

9.1 Elements of Social Interaction High Yield

LEARNING OBJECTIVES

After Chapter 9.1, you will be able to:

- Identify the meaning of social interaction terms such as status, role, group, network, and organization
- List the three types of status and provide an example of each

Society has developed out of necessity for human beings to survive and develop. Social interaction is the basis of social life and helps humans reach their full potential. Social interaction is facilitated by preexisting commonalities between individuals and shared understanding or experiences, such as a shared language. Through our social interactions, we develop culture.

Statuses

In most human societies, people do not view every individual as an equal. Instead, we create a hierarchical structure with inequalities of material goods, social opportunities, social acceptance, and skills. Some are wealthy, and some are impoverished; some are talented in sports, while others are not. Some are admired by others, most are liked, and some are disliked or even stigmatized. **Social statuses** are perceived positions in society that are used to classify individuals. Being a premed student, for example, is considered a status. Most statuses exist in relation to other statuses: being a premed student does not have meaning unless there are other statuses with which to compare it, such as *medical student* or *resident*. It is important to note that not all personal characteristics are considered to be social statuses. For example, being left-handed is not considered a status.

There are three key types of statuses: ascribed, achieved, and master statuses. An **ascribed status** is one that is given involuntarily (usually at birth), due to such factors as race, ethnicity, sex, and family background. An **achieved status** is a status that is gained as a result of one's efforts or choices, such as being a doctor. A person can hold multiple statuses at the same time (collectively known as one's status set), but one's **master status** is the status by which a person is most identified. This status is typically the most important status the individual holds and affects all aspects of that person's life. It is also generally how people view themselves and often holds a symbolic value. Master statuses can also cause pigeonholing: we may view individuals only through the lens of their master status, without regard to any other personal characteristics (such as with a president or other major political figure). Finally, **status inconsistency** refers to when an individual has multiple social positions that are of varying prestige. An example of status inconsistency would be a lawyer who also works as a low-wage employee at a fast-food company.

KEY CONCEPT

Types of statuses:

- Ascribed—given involuntarily, based on race, ethnicity, sex, family background, and so on
- Achieved—gained as a result of one's efforts or choices
- Master—status by which one is most identified; is pervasive in that person's life

Roles

Each status is associated with **roles**, or sets of beliefs, values, attitudes, and norms that define expectations for those who hold the status. **Role performance** is the carrying out of behaviors associated with a given role. Individuals can vary in how successful they are at performing a role. For example, part of a doctor's role is to translate medical information into language their patients can understand; however, some doctors are far better at this skill than others. Role performance can also change depending on the social situation and context of the interaction. When doctors interact with each other, the pertinent parts of their roles are quite different than when interacting with patients. Behaviors and expectations thus change as a result of the **role partner**—the person with whom one is interacting. Doctors have many role partners: patients, nurses, patients' relatives, other doctors, residents, and hospital administration. The various roles associated with a status are referred to as a **role set**.

Through our lives, we each take on numerous statuses, each of which may contain a variety of roles. Additionally, we are often playing several roles at one time. Due to the complex nature of statuses and role sets, it is not surprising that conflict, challenges, uncertainty, and ambivalence arise as we try to navigate the many expectations of day-to-day life. **Role conflict** is the difficulty in satisfying the requirements or expectations of multiple roles, whereas **role strain** is the difficulty in satisfying multiple requirements of the same role. Figure 9.1 contrasts these commonly confused terms. **Role exit** is the dropping of one identity for another.

REAL WORLD

A great example of role conflict is a single parent who also works a full-time job. Both of these roles carry a very large set of expectations, which are often at odds with each other.

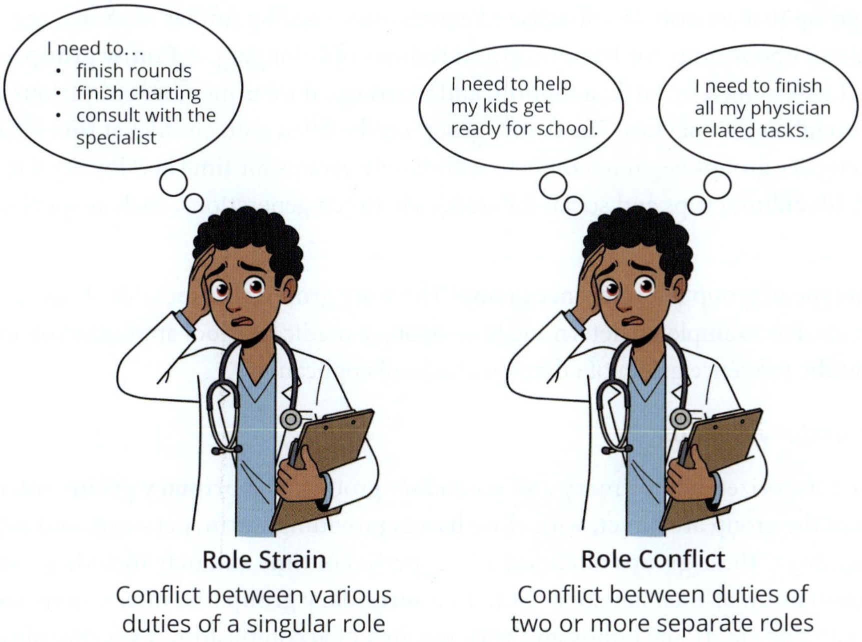
I need to...
• finish rounds
• finish charting
• consult with the specialist
I need to help my kids get ready for school.
I need to finish all my physician related tasks.
Role Strain
Conflict between various duties of a singular role
Role Conflict
Conflict between duties of two or more separate roles

Figure 9.1 Role Strain vs. Role Conflict

Groups

Another major component of social interaction involves groups. In sociological terms, a **group** (also known as a **social group**) consists of two or more people who share any number of similar characteristics as well as a sense of unity. The simplest of social groups is called a **dyad** (two people), followed by a **triad** (three people). As group size increases, the group trades intimacy for stability. Social groups are more complex than a group of individuals who happen to be in the same physical space. For example, people waiting to cross the street at a crosswalk do not constitute a social group. Common characteristics shared by social groups include values, interests, ethnicity, social background, family ties, and political representation. Many sociologists see social interaction as the most important characteristic that strengthens a social group.

We center most of our lives around social groups, from the camaraderie of teammates to the complexity of governments. Social groups also meet many of the needs we have; these groups provide an opportunity to belong and be accepted and they offer protection, safety, and support. Many people also learn, earn a living, and practice religion in groups. Groups can also be a source of conflict, including discrimination, persecution, oppression, and war. These conflicts sprout from the relationships within and between groups.

An **in-group** is a social group with which a person experiences a sense of belonging or identifies as a member. An **out-group**, on the other hand, refers to a social group with which an individual does not identify. An in-group can form based on a variety of identifying characteristics, including but not limited to race, culture, gender, religion, profession, or education. Out-groups can sometimes compete with or oppose in-groups, creating **group conflict**. Notably, negative feelings toward an out-group are not necessarily based on a sense of dislike toward the characteristics of the out-group; rather, they can be based on favoritism for the in-group and the absence of favoritism for the out-group.

A **peer group** is a group that consists of self-selected equals associated by similar interests, ages, or statuses. Peer groups provide an opportunity for friendship and feelings of belonging. A **family group**, by contrast, is not self-selected but determined by birth, adoption, and marriage. It joins members of various ages, genders, and generations through emotional ties. The family group can be filled with conflict at times; this is often true in adolescence when peer groups begin to compete with family groups for time and loyalty. Family groups may also struggle with cultural gaps and social differences between generations, such as speaking in different languages.

Another important type of group is a **reference group**. These are groups that individuals use as a standard for evaluating themselves. For example, to determine how strong a medical school applicant you are, you might compare yourself to the reference group of all medical school applicants.

Primary and Secondary Groups

Groups can also be categorized into primary and secondary groups. In a **primary group**, interactions between members of the group are direct, with close bonds providing warm, personal, and intimate relationships to members. These groups often last a long period of time and may include a core circle of friends, a tightly knit family, or members of a team. In a **secondary group**, the interactions are impersonal and businesslike, with few emotional bonds and with the goal of accomplishing a specific purpose. Secondary groups typically last for a short period of time, and they form and dissolve without any special significance to those involved, an example being students working together on a group project. Figure 9.2 distinguishes between these types of groups.

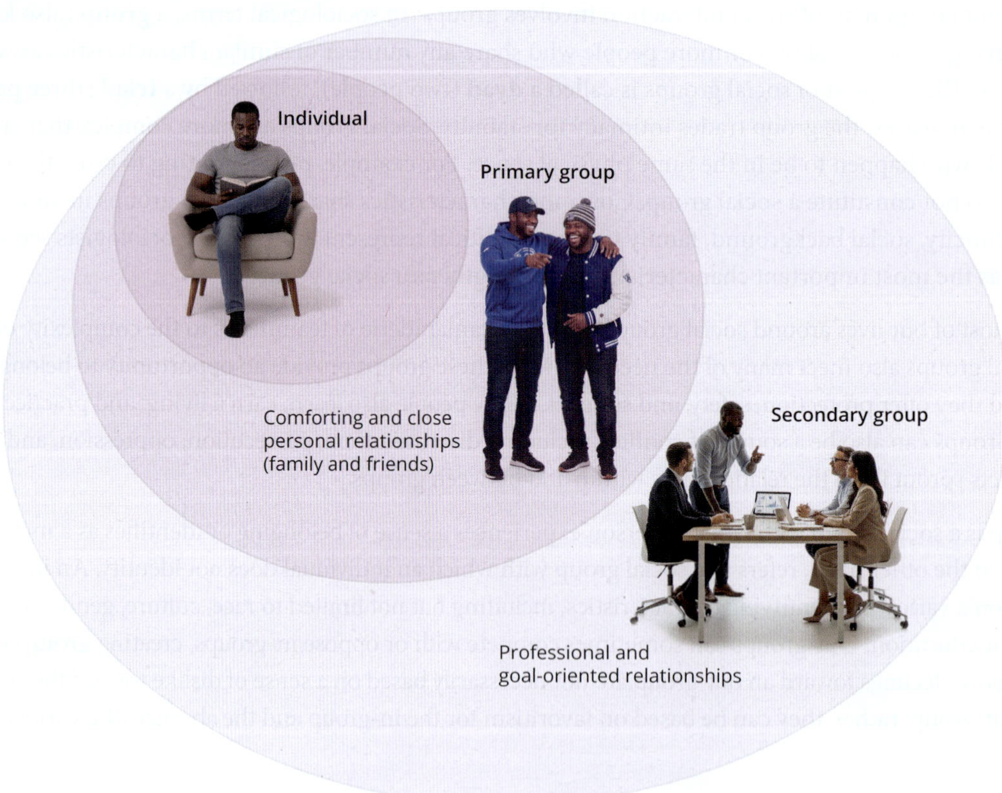

Figure 9.2 Primary and Secondary Groups

Community and Society

The German sociologist Ferdinand Tönnies distinguished two major types of groups. His theory is known as ***Gemeinschaft und Gesellschaft***, which translates to *community and society*. *Gemeinschaft* (community) refers to groups unified by feelings of togetherness due to shared beliefs, ancestry, or geography. Families and neighborhoods are examples of *Gemeinschaften*. *Gesellschaft* (society) refers to less personal groups that are formed out of mutual self-interests working together toward the same goal. Companies and countries are examples of *Gesellschaften*.

Observing and Analyzing Groups

Group size may vary; the smallest size a group can be is two people. Smaller group sizes, like dyads or triads, allow individuals to present more of themselves to the group. **Interaction process analysis** is a technique for observing, classifying, and measuring the interactions within small groups. In the 1970s, it was revised to the **system for multiple level observation of groups** (**SYMLOG**), which is based on the belief that there are three fundamental dimensions of interaction: dominance vs. submission, friendliness vs. unfriendliness, and instrumentally controlled vs. emotionally expressive.

Extensive research on groups has revealed that a group holds power over its members, creating group pressure that can ultimately shape members' behaviors. This is called **group conformity**; individuals are compliant with the group's goals, even when the group's goals may be in direct contrast to the individual's goal. Individuals conform in an attempt to fit in and be accepted by the group. Individuals will often participate in behaviors they normally would not.

Groupthink is related to group conformity and occurs when members focus on reaching a consensus at the cost of critical evaluation of relevant information. This can lead to groups not exploring all sides of an issue and may limit the group's options or views; further, group members may self-censor by not expressing their beliefs. Figure 9.3 depicts a classic groupthink scenario. A more extensive discussion of the effects of groups on individual behavior (social action) and group dynamics is explored in Chapter 8 of *MCAT Behavioral Sciences Review*.

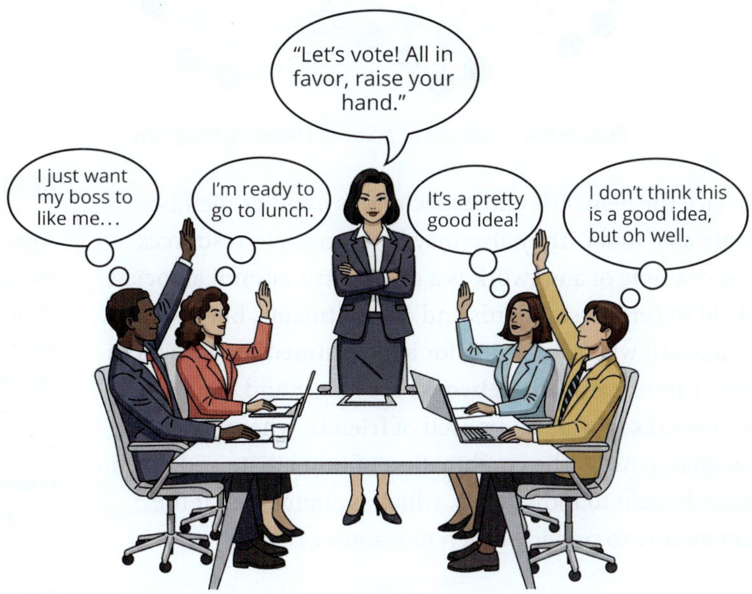
"Let's vote! All in favor, raise your hand."
I just want my boss to like me...
I'm ready to go to lunch.
It's a pretty good idea!
I don't think this is a good idea, but oh well.

Figure 9.3 Groupthink

Networks

The term **network** is used to describe the observable pattern of social relationships among individuals or groups. Patterns of relationship can be determined by mapping the interactions between individual units, the nature of which can be highly variable. For example, a sociologist may look at the patterns in the interactions between friends, family members, or societal institutions. Researchers often display networks with maps containing a series of points, with each point representing a unit in the network. They connect the points with lines to display the interactions between units, as shown in Figure 9.4. Not all contact points within a network are necessarily unique. If there are overlapping connections with the same individual, it is referred to as **network redundancy**. Network analysis can be used to gain understanding of the actions of individuals and groups and to study the broader social structure.

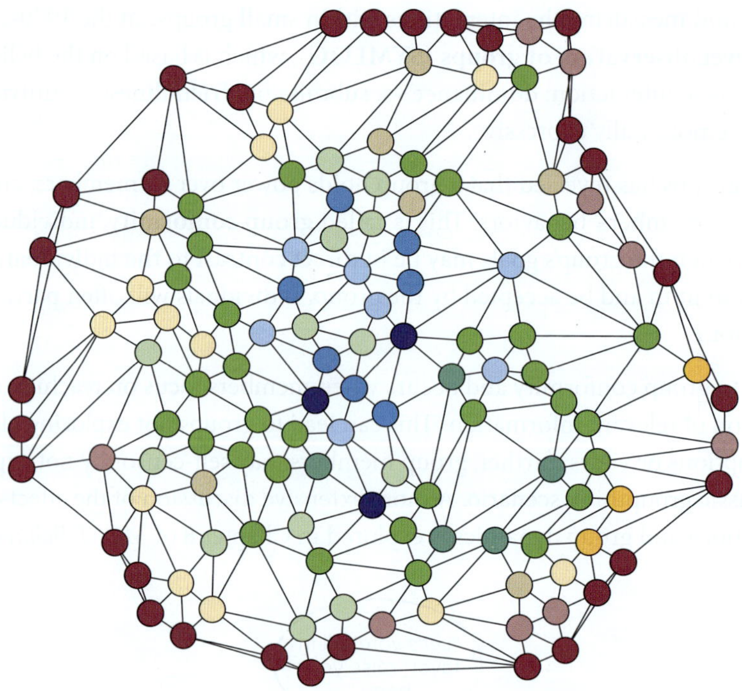

Figure 9.4 Example of a Social Network Diagram

Individuals in networks face the demands and expectations of other members, constraining what they are able to do. They also may have access to resources through the network. An example of a network is a university's alumni association: the members are held to certain standards and commitments, but also may reap the benefits of the network when searching for a job. **Immediate networks** are dense with strong ties, whereas **distant networks** are looser and contain weaker ties; immediate networks may be composed of friends, whereas distant networks may include acquaintances. The combination of immediate and distant networks provide the most benefit to individuals, which is augmented if the networks work complementarily to provide different resources.

BRIDGE

A genetic pedigree can be thought of as a specific type of network map, in which geneticists can track genetic patterns. The lines in genetic pedigrees represent mating patterns, parent–child relationships, and other familial structures. While pedigree analysis does not appear on the MCAT, the related topic of genetics is discussed in Chapter 12 of *MCAT Biology Review*.

Organizations

In sociology, **organizations** are complex secondary groups that are set up to achieve specific goals and are characterized by having a structure and a culture. We have all been members of multiple organizations, such as schools, companies, music groups, sports teams, fraternities and sororities, political organizations, community action committees, and so on. The study of organizations is at the heart of sociology because of the importance that organizations have throughout a person's life.

The modern **formal organization** developed during the Industrial Revolution as a way to maximize efficiency. The formal aspect derives from the explicit goals that guide the members and their activities. Furthermore, formal organizations have enforcement procedures that seek to control the activities of their members. Lastly, these organizations are characterized by the hierarchical allotment of formal roles or duties to members. Formal organizations can be quite large.

The basic organization of society is found in its **characteristic institution**. Throughout history this has changed. In prehistoric times, the characteristic institution was primarily the kin, clan, or sib. In modern times, as we have transformed our cities into urban centers of trade and commerce, we have moved to bureaucracy as the characteristic institution. A **bureaucracy** is a rational system of political organization, administration, discipline, and control. Generally, a bureaucracy has these six characteristics: paid, nonelected officials on a fixed salary; officials who are provided rights and privileges as a result of making their careers out of holding office; regular salary increases, seniority rights, and promotions upon passing exams or milestones; officials who enter the organization by holding an advanced degree or training; responsibilities, obligations, privileges, and work procedures rigidly defined by the organization; and responsibility for meeting the demands of one's position. Due to these characteristics, bureaucracies are often slow to change and less efficient than other organizations.

Bureaucracies have been criticized over time. The **iron law of oligarchy** (Figure 9.5) states that democratic or bureaucratic systems naturally shift to being ruled by an elite group. This shift is due to a number of factors, including the necessity of a core body of individuals to carry out the day-to-day activities of the organization, increased need for specialization, and leadership characteristics of certain members of the group. Thus, even a group established with democratic principles and complete egalitarianism will ultimately centralize, placing power in the hands of a few key leaders.

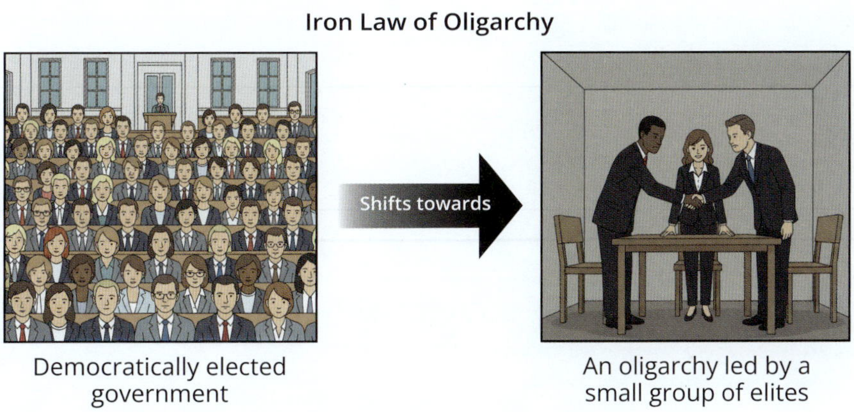

Figure 9.5 The Iron Law of Oligarchy

McDonaldization is commonly used to refer to a shift in focus toward efficiency, predictability, calculability, and control in societal practices. While the original model for McDonaldization was, of course, the fast-food restaurant and its push towards efficiency, examples of these same characteristics can be seen in many other institutions. For example, 24-hour news channels, which feature running footers of the latest news stories as "bite-size" headlines, demonstrate efficient and predictable sources of information. Corporations may mine "big data" to make business decisions using controlled, standardized methods, allowing the business to focus on the calculable outcomes of a choice such as profit and loss analysis and market share.

MCAT CONCEPT CHECK 9.1

Before you move on, assess your understanding of the material with these questions.

1. List the three types of statuses and provide an example of each:

Status	Example

2. For each of the sociological terms below, provide a brief definition:
   - Status:
   - Role:
   - Group:
   - Network:
   - Organization:

9.2 Self-Presentation and Interacting with Others

High Yield

LEARNING OBJECTIVES

After Chapter 9.2, you will be able to:

- Classify forms of communication as verbal or nonverbal
- Distinguish between front-stage self and back-stage self
- Identify examples of body language, facial expression, visual display, scent, and vocalization in communication

To Erving Goffman, the sociologist who developed the dramaturgical perspective, every interaction we have with other people is a theatrical performance in which we consciously or unconsciously use the "scene," our "costume," and the role that we "perform" to influence the way others think or feel. Whenever we try to influence others' perception with respect to a person, object, or event, we are engaging in impression management. One form of impression management is **self-presentation**, the process of displaying ourselves to society both visually (through clothing, grooming, etc.) and through our actions, often to make sure others see us in the best possible light.

Expressing and Detecting Emotions

Expressed emotions include both verbal and nonverbal behaviors that communicate internal states. We can express emotions with or without conscious awareness. There are two main theories about the development of emotional expression in humans, visualized in Figure 9.6: the basic model and the social construction model.

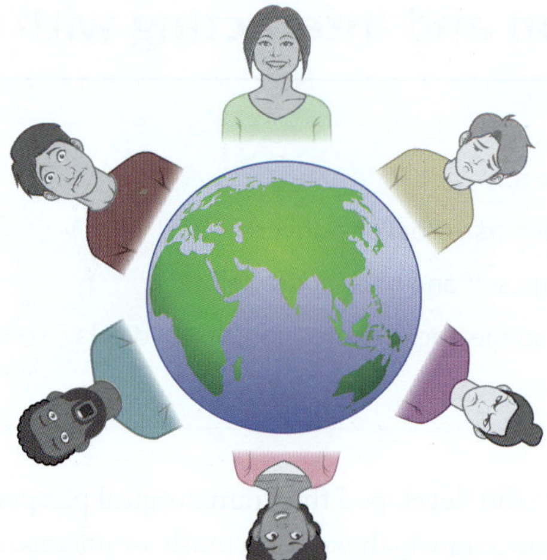

Basic model: universal emotions

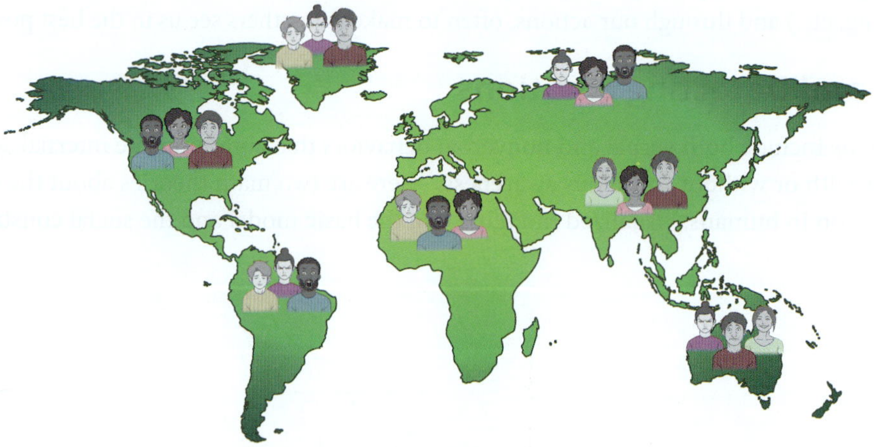

Social construction model of emotions

Figure 9.6 Basic Model vs. Social Construction Model

The **basic model of emotional expression** was first established by Charles Darwin. Darwin stated that emotional expression involves a number of components: facial expressions, behaviors, postures, vocal changes, and physiological changes. Darwin claimed that expression is consistent with his theories on evolution and should be similar across cultures. Darwin also stated that primates and animals exhibit rudimentary muscle actions that are similar to those used by humans for facial expressions. Since Darwin, many researchers have found that a number of basic human emotions are universally experienced and that their corresponding facial expressions are universally recognized. The **appraisal model** is closely related, and accepts that there are biologically predetermined expressions once an emotion is experienced, but that there is a cognitive antecedent to emotional expression.

BRIDGE

Paul Ekman's work with universal emotions, as detailed in Chapter 5 of *MCAT Behavioral Sciences Review*, was a key development in the basic model of emotional expression. Individuals knowledgeable about Ekman's work are capable of detecting very subtle and transient facial expressions that may indicate that an individual is trying to be deceptive about the emotions being conveyed.

Three of the primary models that describe individual emotion (James–Lange, Cannon–Bard, and Schachter–Singer) were discussed in Chapter 5 of *MCAT Behavioral Sciences Review*. In this chapter, we will look at how emotions are shaped by social context and culture.

The **social construction model** assumes that there is no biological basis for emotions. Instead, emotions are based on experiences and the situational context alone. It also suggests that certain emotions can only exist within social encounters and that emotions are expressed differently—and thus play different roles—across cultures. In this model, one must be familiar with social norms for a certain emotion to perform the corresponding emotional behaviors in a given social situation.

Culture provides the foundation to understand and interpret behaviors. Studies have suggested that cultural differences can lead to very different social consequences when emotions are expressed. Cultural expectations of emotions are often referred to as **display rules**. For example, in Utkuhikhalik Inuit society, anger is rarely expressed; individuals who demonstrate anger are considered social pariahs. Display rules govern which emotions can be expressed and to what degree. They may differ as a function of the culture, gender, or family background of an individual. Emotional expressions can be managed in several different ways: by simulating feelings one does not actually feel; by qualifying, amplifying, or deamplifying feelings; by masking an emotion with another emotion; or by neutralizing any emotional expression whatsoever.

A **cultural syndrome** is a shared set of beliefs, attitudes, norms, values, and behaviors among members of the same culture that are organized around a central theme. Cultural syndromes influence the rules for expressing or suppressing emotions and can even influence the ways emotions are experienced. For example, happiness is generally considered a positive emotion across cultures. However, in countries with more individualistic cultural syndromes, like the United States, happiness is viewed as infinite, attainable, and internally experienced. In contrast, in countries with a more collectivist cultural syndrome, such as Japan, happiness is a very rational emotion and generally applied to collective experiences more than to individual successes or experiences. This difference is illustrated in the contrast between the phrases *I am happy* and *I am sharing happiness with others*.

Gender can also play an important role in emotional expression. Research on the expression of emotion in the United States has shown that women are expected to express anger in public less often than men, while men are expected to repress the expression of sadness. Research also supports the conclusion that women are better at detecting subtle differences in emotional expression than men.

Impression Management

Impression management refers to our attempts to influence how others perceive us. This is done by regulating or controlling information we present about ourselves in social interactions. Impression management is often used synonymously with self-presentation. When describing impression management, theorists describe three "selves": the authentic self, the ideal self, and the tactical self. The **authentic self** describes who the person actually is, including both positive and negative attributes. The **ideal self**, as described in Chapter 6 of *MCAT Behavioral Sciences Review*, refers to who we would like to be under optimal circumstances. The **tactical self** refers to who we market ourselves to be when we adhere to others' expectations of us. This is similar to the ought self described in Chapter 6 of *MCAT Behavioral Sciences Review*.

People use a number of impression management strategies when in the presence of others. Some common strategies are summarized in Table 9.1, with examples of each.

Strategy	Definition	Example(s)
Self-disclosure	Giving information about oneself to establish an identity	Disclosing that you are a premedical student
Managing appearances	Using props, appearance, emotional expression, or associations with others to create a positive image	Wearing a white coat, keeping calm while dealing with a difficult patient, mentioning associations with important researchers during an interview
Ingratiation	Using flattery or conforming to expectations to win someone over	Blindly agreeing to someone else's opinion, complimenting a friend before asking for a favor
Aligning actions	Making questionable behavior acceptable through excuses	Justifications for missing deadlines, blaming a bad grade on too little sleep
Alter-casting	Imposing an identity onto another person	Any example in this course that says *As a good MCAT student, you should*... in which Kaplan is assigning *you* the role of *good MCAT student*

Table 9.1 Impression Management Strategies

MCAT EXPERTISE

Many of the sociological theories tested on the MCAT are far more extensive than the knowledge base the AAMC expects of test takers. The dramaturgical approach, for example, describes over twenty sociological concepts in theatrical terms; however, the MCAT only expects you to know front stage vs. back stage self.

Erving Goffman described impression management through the **dramaturgical approach**, using the metaphor of a theatrical performance to describe how individuals create images of themselves in various situations. In this analogy, Goffman relates a person's attempts to manage the impressions of others to an actor's performance in a play. A person's **front stage self** is the persona they present to an audience. A person will adapt their front stage self depending on the social situation, similar to an actor on stage in front of an audience performing according to the setting, role, and script of the play. In contrast, when an actor is back stage, the actor is hidden from the audience and is free to act in ways that may not be congruent with the actor's character in the play. According to Goffman, the **back stage self** is the persona adopted when not in a social situation and there is no concern about upholding the performance of a desired public image. The central distinction of the dramaturgical approach is depicted in Figure 9.7.

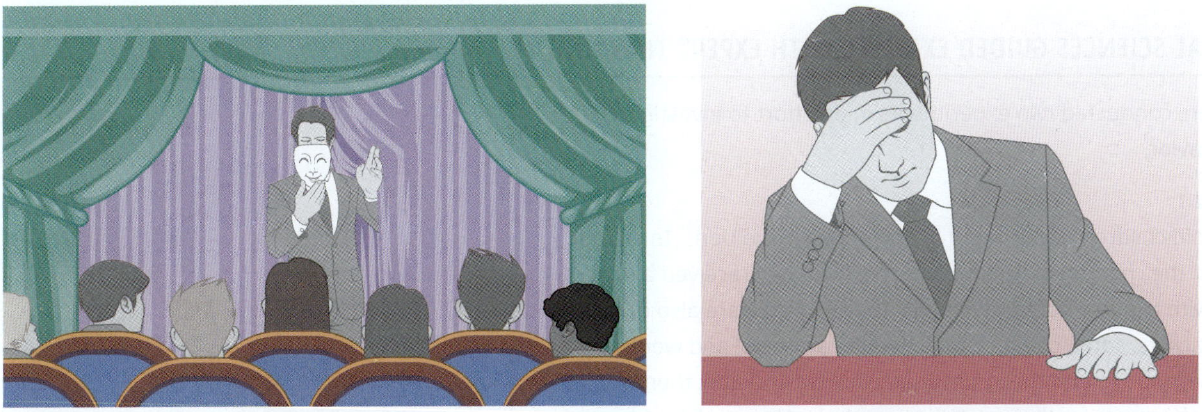
Front stage self
How people present themselves to others
Back stage self
How people act when they are not in front of others

Figure 9.7 The Dramaturgical Approach

Another theory comes from George Herbert Mead, who described the self in two parts called the *Me* and the *I*. The part of self that is developed through interaction with society is the ***Me***. The development of the *Me* comes from considering the **generalized other**, which is based on a person's established perceptions of the expectations of society. Any time that a person tries to imagine what is expected of them in a social situation, they are taking on the perspective of the generalized other. And by considering the perspective of the generalized other and adapting one's behavior appropriately, the *Me* develops. By contrast, the ***I*** is the individual's own impulses. However, the *I* is not totally independent of the *Me*. Rather, a person's impulses are shaped by their interpretation of society's expectations. In short, the *Me* shapes the *I*.

BRIDGE

Mead's description of *Me* and *I* formed the foundation for the sociological theory of symbolic interactionism, which is described in Chapter 11 of *MCAT Behavioral Science Review.*

BEHAVIORAL SCIENCES GUIDED EXAMPLE WITH EXPERT THINKING

Researchers conducted two experiments in an effort to investigate social behavior.

Experiment 1:
Five-year-old children participated in one of four conditions. In all four conditions, the children played a game in which they received a sheet of paper with five symbols drawn on it. The children were also given a sheet of stickers, some of which matched the symbols, and were given 90 seconds to find the appropriate stickers and affix them to the sheet of paper over their matching symbols. Also on the table was a second set of materials, which the children were told was for another child who would be playing the game later.

Exp. 1: Sticker matching game

In the stealing condition, the participant's sticker sheet was missing one of the five symbols necessary to complete the game, while the sticker could be found on the second sheet. In the helping condition, the second sheet was conspicuously missing one of the stickers needed to complete the game, and the participant's sheet included an extra of those stickers, which participants were told they could keep or give to the next child. In some trials, the experimenter left the child alone while the child completed the task (the unobserved case), and in others, another child who was participating in the study but not part of the same experimental group was seated near the child during the task (the observed case).

Two conditions: children need to steal to complete their task; children can give to another child who is missing stickers.

IVs: steal or help condition; observation

DV: behavior

In the stealing condition, 4% of subjects stole in the observed case and 24% stole in the unobserved case ($p = .02$). In the helping condition, 28% of subjects helped in the observed case and 11% helped in the unobserved case ($p = .07$). Results are summarized in Figure 1.

The percentages are stated here, but are summarized in the figure. Missing from the figure are the p-values. Looks like the stealing condition was significant and the helping condition wasn't, but we could call it a trend.

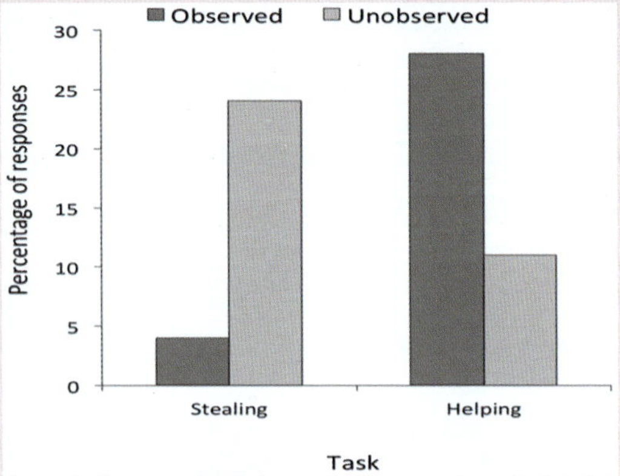

Figure 1 Stealing and helping behavior for children in their respective conditions.

Children helped when people were watching and stole when no one was.

Experiment 2:

Two chimpanzees were placed in separate cages. One of the chimps had access to a rope attached to a tray that contained food. In the stealing condition, the food was placed such that the other chimp could reach it, but pulling the rope moved the tray out of reach of both chimps. In the helping condition, the food was placed out of reach of both chimps, but pulling the rope moved the tray within reach of the second chimp. The subject chimps were not able to see the recipient chimps during the experiment, but were taught what the rope mechanism did prior to testing. Just as in Experiment 1, each of these conditions was carried out in one of two cases: either the chimps were alone in the experimental room, or a third dominant male chimp was present, observing the interaction. It is known that in chimpanzees, fitness improves with relationships to dominant group members. Results are summarized in Figure 2.

Similar conditions here. IVs: help or hurt, observation; DV: behavior.

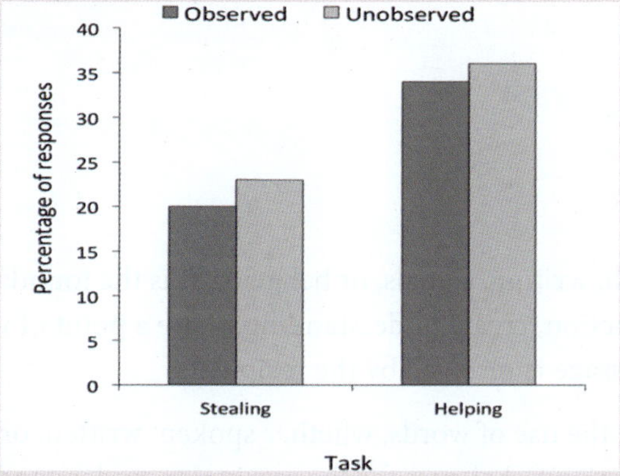

Figure 2 Stealing and helping behavior for chimps in their respective conditions.

This is different from the children. Observation didn't seem to matter.

Adapted from: Engelmann JM, Herrmann E, Tomasello M (2012) Five-Year Olds, but Not Chimpanzees, Attempt to Manage Their Reputations. *PLoS ONE* 7(10): e48433. https://doi.org/10.1371/journal.pone.0048433

What conclusion can be drawn based on these studies about the differences between human children and chimpanzees in social settings?

The question asks for a conclusion, so our plan should be to summarize the results of the studies and relate them to outside knowledge. Fortunately, once we understand the design of the two studies, the results aren't difficult to interpret. In Experiment 1, it looks like the children were more likely to steal when they were alone and more likely to help when they were being observed. From the *p*-values, it looks like that first result is statistically significant and the second result would count as merely a trend. Chimpanzees, on the other hand, showed no such concern for the presence of others. If this were a multiple-choice question, we would look for an answer that explained both results.

Knowing exactly what bit of content to tie these results to might be tricky without answer choices, but the passage does provide a clue. In Experiment 2, we're told that it is adaptive for chimpanzees to gain the favor of dominant group members, so these researchers are likely interested in the way individuals may change their behavior in order to gain the favor of others. This could be called self-presentation, reputation management, or impression management.

Applying this concept to the results of the study, we can conclude that children have at least some capacity for acting in a prosocial manner to manage impressions, but chimpanzees in the given situation are incapable of or unconcerned with doing the same.

Verbal and Nonverbal Communication

Communication is the ability to convey information by speech, writing, signals, or behavior. It is the foundation of social interaction and is often used to elicit changes, generate action, create understanding, share a point of view, or inform. Effective communication occurs when the desired message is received by the recipient.

Verbal communication is the transmission of information via the use of words, whether spoken, written, or signed. It is tied to nonverbal communication and is often dependent on nonverbal cues for the receiver to understand the sender's full meaning. While face-to-face conversations are rich with nonverbal communication, even phone conversations include nonverbal means of communication, such as pauses and changes in tone.

Nonverbal communication refers to how people communicate, intentionally or unintentionally, without words. Some examples of nonverbal communication are facial expressions, tone of voice, body position and movement, touches, and eye positioning. Gestures involving the hands and other parts of the body are often nonverbal, but the formal signs of a sign language count as verbal communication. Nonverbal cues serve a number of functions in communication, including expression of emotions, as shown in Figure 9.8, conveyance of attitudes and personality traits, and facilitation of verbal communication. Nonverbal communication is often dictated by culture. For example, in US culture, people can be suspicious of someone who does not make eye contact, as this is sometimes considered to be a sign of lying. However, in many other cultures, direct eye contact is used far less often than in the United States. For example, many children in Thailand are taught not to make eye contact with teachers and adults in order to show respect. Some types of verbal and nonverbal communication are listed in Table 9.2.

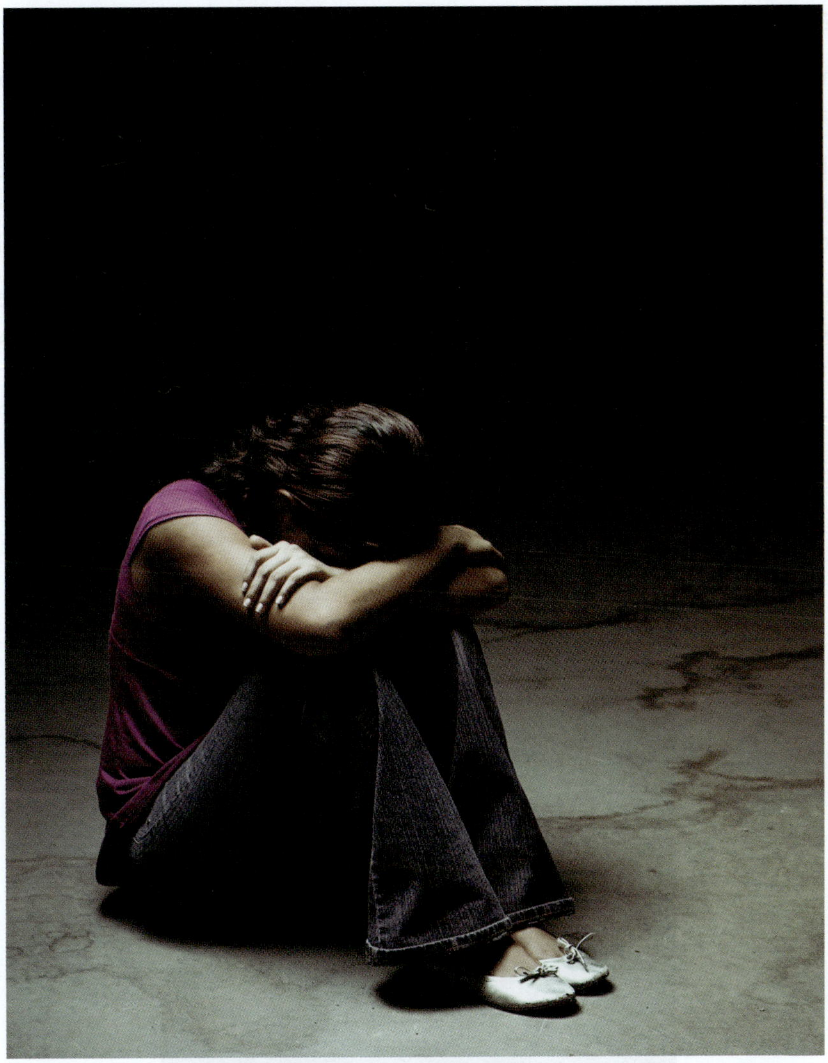

Figure 9.8 Human Body Language
The individual in this image sits in a way that suggests sadness or exhaustion.

Verbal	Nonverbal
Spoken language	Facial expressions
Written language (print and electronic)	Body language (posture)
Sign languages (American Sign Language)	Gestures
Tactile languages (Braille alphabet)	Tone of voice (prosody)
	Eye contact
	Amount of personal space

Table 9.2 Verbal and Nonverbal Communication

Animal Signals and Communication

We not only communicate with other people, but also with other living creatures. **Animal communication** is defined as any behavior of one animal that affects the behavior of another.

Nonhuman animals communicate with one another in order to convey information such as emotions, intent, status, health, and the location of resources. They communicate with one another through a variety of nonverbal means, including body language, rudimentary facial expressions, visual displays, scents, and vocalizations.

The use of body language is common across a number of species. Body language can indicate that an animal is frightened, as shown in Figure 9.9, aggressive, relaxed, or even embarrassed; dogs often tuck their tails between their legs when scolded or fearful. Body language can also have significance for reproduction, as many animals will get into certain positions to signify readiness to mate.

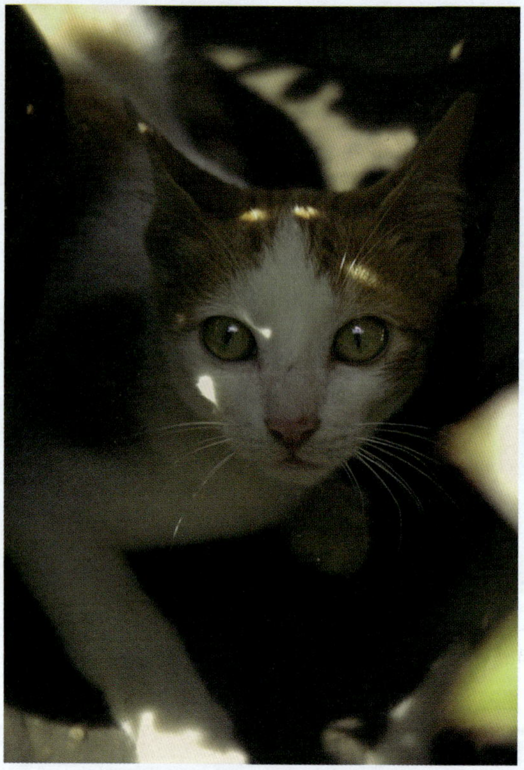

Figure 9.9 Animal Body Language
When surprised or scared, cats will recoil, crouch, and remain relatively motionless.

While humans possess far finer motor control of the muscles of facial expression, many animals (especially mammals) use facial expressions to indicate similar emotions to body language. It is noteworthy, however, that facial expressions appear to be more highly conserved between species than body language. For example, baring teeth and lunging forward, as shown in Figure 9.10, are perceived almost universally as signs of aggression or readiness to attack.

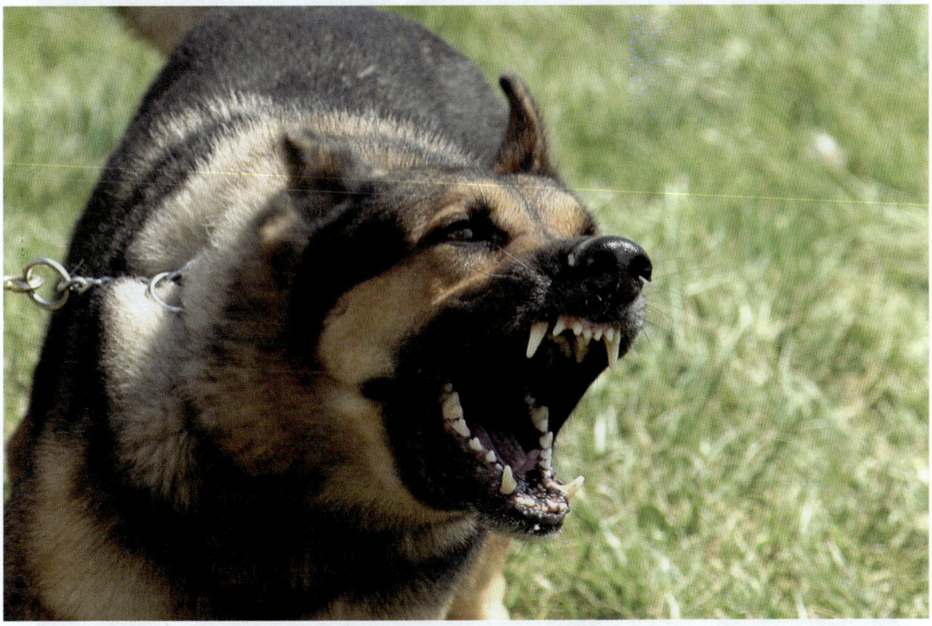

Figure 9.10 Animal Facial Expressions
Baring teeth and lunging forward are recognized by many animals as signs that an attack is imminent.

Animals may also use visual displays for communication. This is common for sex discrimination in birds; females are often less colorful than males because it permits them a greater degree of camouflage and protection when caring for their young. However, this also serves as communication between birds, as sex is readily apparent from the bird's appearance. Other visual displays include bioluminescence (the production of light), colorful plumage (as in peacocks), and dancing. Bees are well-known for communicating through dancing, as shown in Figure 9.11.

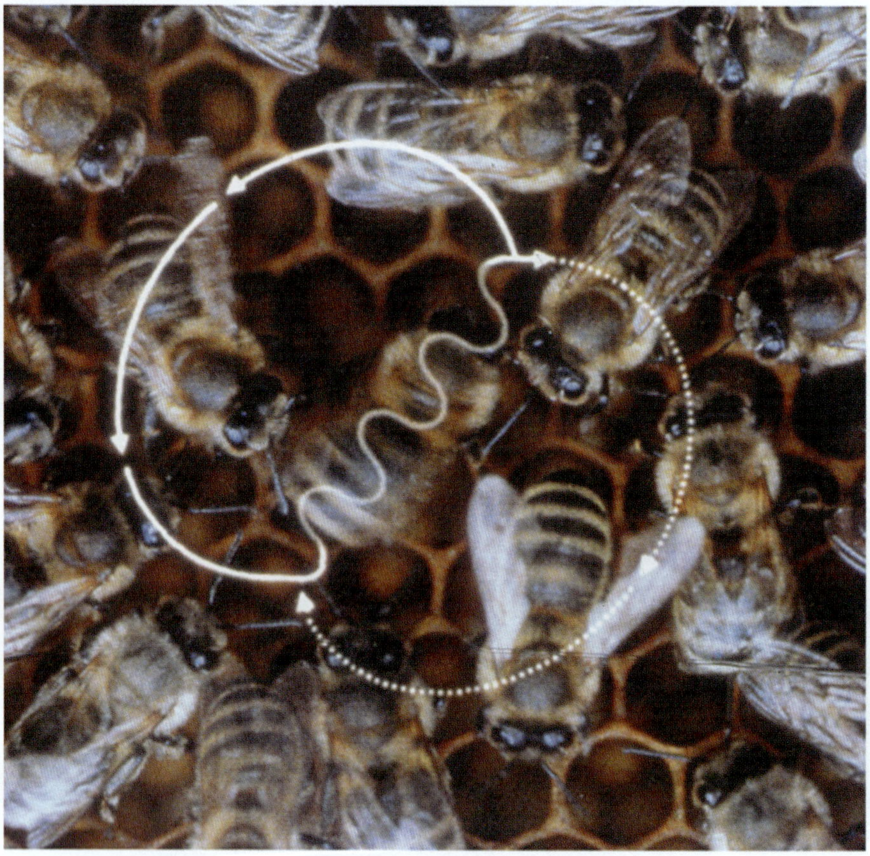

Figure 9.11 Bee Communication through Movement
The "waggle dance," illustrated here, indicates the location of food relative to the hive.

Many animals use scents to communicate both intraspecifically (between members of the same species) and interspecifically (between members of different species). Pheromones are a common example and are given off by members of a species to attract a mate. Scents can be used to mark an animal's territory or as a method of defense, such as in skunks.

Finally, animals also communicate through vocalizations with various levels of sophistication. For example, research has shown that prairie dogs have different "words" for specific predators, and can even create new words for novel objects. Bird calls are species specific and are used to attract a mate or warn of a threat.

In addition to interacting in the wild, humans use both verbal and nonverbal communication when interacting with domesticated animals, as is often seen between owners and their pets. Dog owners may use vocal commands to tell their pets to come, stay, or sit. Additionally, just as tone of voice can express joy or anger to a person, it can communicate the same information to a pet. Pets can be scolded with a look or a gesture. Communication works in the opposite direction as well, as a pet's body language and expressions convey information to its owner.

BRIDGE

It is debatable if pheromones actually have an effect on humans because we lack many of the genes necessary for function of the vomeronasal organ, an accessory olfactory organ seen in other animals. Olfaction and scent detection is discussed in Chapter 2 of *MCAT Behavioral Sciences Review*.

Communication between humans and animals is not confined strictly to pets. One of the most famous examples of animal communication is Koko, a gorilla who was able to communicate with humans through the use of American Sign Language. Koko's vocabulary included more than one thousand words.

MCAT CONCEPT CHECK 9.2

Before you move on, assess your understanding of the material with these questions.

1. Classify the following forms of communication as verbal or nonverbal:

• American Sign Language	Verbal	Nonverbal
• Turning your body away from another person	Verbal	Nonverbal
• Text messages	Verbal	Nonverbal
• Giving a "high five"	Verbal	Nonverbal
• Frowning	Verbal	Nonverbal

2. What is the front stage self? The back stage self?

   - Front stage self:

   ____

   ____

   - Back stage self:

   ____

   ____

3. For each of the methods of animal communication below, provide one example:

Method of Communication	Example
Body language	
Facial expressions	
Visual displays	
Scents	
Vocalizations	

Conclusion

Skunks are unique in how they communicate with other animals they perceive as threats. Their anal glands are capable of producing high concentrations of thiol-containing compounds, which create a distinctive malodorous scent. But it is noteworthy that skunks only carry five or six sprays' worth of material at a time—thus, they tend to use other forms of animal communication, such as body language, hissing, and foot stamping before resorting to spraying. The spray, however, is an ultimate defense: intense, caustic, and very sticky. Animals who are sprayed quickly learn that the skunk is not an animal to mess with.

Humans also use many methods of communication. While they may certainly not follow the same patterns as skunks, humans use combinations of vocalization, body language, facial expressions, and gestures to interact with each other socially. The field of sociology flows from these interactions as we create groups, networks, and organizations; organize our society into hierarchies with statuses; and fulfill the roles dictated by our statuses. We put much of our energy into controlling how we communicate with others, trying to create the optimal image of ourselves through impression management.

The content of this chapter plays a large role in your day-to-day life. Every day you interact with other people, and how you interact is largely determined by the culture and society in which you live. In the next chapter, we begin to analyze specific types of interactions, like attraction and altruism, and then examine the dark side of human society: bias, prejudice, discrimination, and stereotypes.

GO ONLINE

You've reviewed the content, now test your knowledge and critical thinking skills by completing a test-like passage set in your online resources!

CONCEPT SUMMARY

Elements of Social Interaction

- A **status** is a perceived position in society used to classify individuals.
  - An **ascribed status** is involuntarily assigned to an individual based on race, ethnicity, gender, family background, and so on.
  - An **achieved status** is voluntarily earned by an individual.
  - A **master status** is the status by which an individual is primarily identified.
- A **role** is a set of beliefs, values, and norms that define the expectations of a certain status in a social situation.
  - **Role performance** refers to carrying out the behaviors of a given role.
  - A **role partner** is a person with whom one is interacting who helps define the roles within the relationship.
  - A **role set** contains all of the different roles associated with a status.
  - **Role conflict** occurs when one has difficulty in satisfying the requirements of multiple roles simultaneously; **role strain** occurs when one has difficulty satisfying multiple requirements of the same role simultaneously.
- **Groups** are made up of two or more individuals with similar characteristics that share a sense of unity.
  - A **peer group** is a self-selected group formed around similar interests, ages, or statuses.
  - A **family group** is the group into which an individual is born, adopted, or married.
  - An **in-group** is a social group with which a person experiences a sense of belonging or identifies as a member.
  - An **out-group** is a social group with which an individual does not identify.
  - **Group conflict** occurs when an out-group competes with or opposes an in-group.
  - A **reference group** is a group to which individuals compare themselves.
  - **Primary groups** are those that contain strong, emotional bonds.
  - **Secondary groups** are often temporary and contain fewer emotional bonds and weaker bonds overall.
  - ***Gemeinschaft*** **(community)** is a group unified by feelings of togetherness due to shared beliefs, ancestry, or geography.
  - ***Gesellschaft*** **(society)** is a group unified by mutual self-interests in achieving a goal.
  - **Groupthink** occurs when members begin to conform to one another's views without critical evaluation.
- A **network** is an observable pattern of social relationships between individuals or groups.
- **Organizations** are bodies of people with a structure and culture designed to achieve specific goals.

Self-Presentation and Interacting with Others

- Various models have been proposed for how we express emotion in social situations.
  - The **basic model** states that there are universal emotions, along with corresponding expressions that can be understood across cultures.
  - The **social construction model** states that emotions are solely based on the situational context of social interactions.
- **Display rules** are unspoken rules that govern the expression of emotion.
- A **cultural syndrome** is a shared set of beliefs, norms, values, and behaviors organized around a central theme, as is found among people sharing the same language and geography.
- **Impression management** refers to the maintenance of a public image, which is accomplished through various strategies.
  - **Self-disclosure** is sharing factual information.
  - **Managing appearances** refers to using props, appearance, emotional expression, or associations to create a positive image.
  - **Ingratiation** is using flattery or conformity to win over someone else.
  - **Aligning actions** is the use of excuses to account for questionable behavior.
  - **Alter-casting** is imposing an identity onto another person.
- The **dramaturgical approach** says that individuals create images of themselves in the same way that actors perform a role in front of an audience.
  - The **front stage** is where individuals are seen by the audience and where they strive to preserve their desired image.
  - The **back stage** is where individuals are not in front of an audience and where they are free to act outside of their desired image.
- Communication includes both verbal and nonverbal elements.
  - **Verbal communication** is the conveyance of information through spoken, written, or signed words.
  - **Nonverbal communication** is the conveyance of information by means other than the use of words, such as body language, prosody, facial expressions, and gestures.
  - **Animal communication** takes place not only between nonhuman animals, but between humans and other animals as well. Animals use body language, rudimentary facial expressions, visual displays, scents, and vocalizations to communicate.

ANSWERS TO CONCEPT CHECKS

9.1

1.

Status	Example
Ascribed	Any status given involuntarily, due to factors such as race, ethnicity, gender, and family background
Achieved	Any status that is gained as a result of one's efforts or choices
Master	Any status by which a person would be most readily identified and that pervades all aspects of an individual's life

2. Statuses are perceived positions in society used to classify individuals. Roles are the behaviors and expectations associated with a status in a particular context. A group is a collection of at least two individuals. A network is a more formal illustration of the relationships between individuals, usually through graphic representation. An organization is a body with a specific set of goals, a structure, and a culture; organizations are complex secondary groups that are set up to achieve specific goals.

9.2

1. Verbal: American Sign Language, text messages

   Nonverbal: turning your body away (body language), giving a "high five" (gesture), frowning (facial expression)

2. The front stage self refers to when we are on stage and performing. This requires us to live up to the roles and expectations assumed by our status. The back stage self is when we are away from others and may include behaviors that would not be appropriate or consistent with the front stage self.

3. Examples may vary.

Method of Communication	Example
Body language	Dogs: tail between the legs
Facial expressions	Various animals: baring teeth
Visual displays	Peacocks: colorful plumage
Scents	Insects (and others): pheromones
Vocalizations	Birds: birdcalls

SCIENCE MASTERY ASSESSMENT EXPLANATIONS

1. **C**

A status is a position in society used to classify a person and exists in relation to other statuses. The specific behaviors associated with this status, **(B)**, best describe a role.

2. **B**

An achieved status is one that is acquired through personal efforts. This is in contrast to an ascribed status, **(A)**, in which the status is involuntarily given based on race, ethnicity, gender, family background, and so on. A master status, **(C)**, is one that influences all aspects of an individual's life. While being a college graduate is an important aspect of day-to-day life, it does not usually pervade every part of one's life.

3. **C**

A bureaucracy is an example of an organization, specifically one with the goal of performing complex tasks as efficiently as possible. Immediate networks and primary groups, **(A)** and **(B)**, are characterized by strong, intimate bonds, which are not commonly seen in bureaucracies. Reference groups, **(D)**, are those groups to which we compare ourselves for various characteristics.

4. **D**

Generally, bureaucracies are marked by six characteristics: paid officials on a fixed salary; nonelected officials who are provided rights and privileges as a result of making their career out of holding office; regular salary increases, seniority rights, and promotions upon passing exams or milestones, **(C)**; officials who enter the organization by holding an advanced degree or training, **(B)**; responsibilities, obligations, privileges, and work procedures rigidly defined by the organization, **(A)**; and responsibility for meeting the obligations of the office one holds.

5. **C**

Verbal communication uses words (whether spoken, written, or signed). Nonverbal communication uses other means of signaling emotions or ideas, such as body language, **(D)**, facial expressions, **(A)**, eye contact, **(B)**, prosody, and personal space. Hand gestures and other bodily movements are also often nonverbal communication, but can be verbal when used as part of a sign language.

6. **C**

Aligning actions is an impression management technique in which one provides socially acceptable reasons for unexpected behavior. This may manifest as providing an excuse for poor performance or laughing off an inappropriate comment as a joke. Tension created from having conflicting thoughts or opinions, as mentioned in **(B)**, refers to cognitive dissonance.

7. **B**

Imposing a role on another person (in this case, "good friend") is the hallmark of alter-casting. This example is also the opposite of ingratiation, **(C)**, because the implication behind the statement is that not lending the bike makes one a "bad friend"; ingratiation is the use of flattery or conformity to win over someone else.

8. **A**

A *Gesellschaft* (society) is one in which individuals are working toward the same goal, such as a company or country. *Gemeinschaften* (communities), on the other hand, are those that are bonded together by beliefs, ancestry, or geography.

9. **B**

Display rules are those that dictate cultural expectations of emotion. In some cultures, sadness is considered personal and internal; in others, sadness is shared externally with the community.

10. **C**

SYMLOG is a method for analyzing group dynamics and considers groups along three dimensions: dominant vs. submissive, friendliness vs. unfriendliness, and instrumentally controlled vs. emotionally expressive.

11. **B**

If a candidate is "exposed," then personal characteristics that are usually shielded from public view have been brought in front of the public. This would be pulling aspects of the back stage self to the front stage. It would not be considered removing the front stage self, **(C)**, because the candidate still has a public image, even if it has been tarnished.

12. **B**

The ought self is who others think we should be: the expectations imposed by others on us. This is most similar to the tactical self, which is the self we present to others when we adhere to their expectations. The presented self, **(D)**, is a combination of the authentic, ideal, and tactical selves.

13. **A**

The basic model of emotion, as proposed by Charles Darwin, states that emotions serve an evolutionary purpose and thus are similar across cultures. The seven universal emotions have also been used as support for this theory. The social construction model states that emotions are always a product of the current social situation and does not posit any biological basis for emotions, implying a lack of a role for emotions in evolution.

14. **D**

Intraspecific communication refers to communication between members of the same species. Interspecific communication, on the other hand, refers to communication between members of different species. Echolocation, **(C)**, is not an example of intraspecific communication because the sender of the signal and the recipient are the same organism; this would be considered autocommunication.

15. **C**

Primary groups have direct and close bonds between members, providing warm, personal, and intimate relationships to its members. Secondary groups, in contrast, form superficial bonds and tend to last for a shorter period of time.

GO ONLINE
Consult your online resources for additional practice.

SHARED CONCEPTS

Behavioral Sciences Chapter 3
Learning and Memory

Behavioral Sciences Chapter 5
Motivation, Emotion, and Stress

Behavioral Sciences Chapter 6
Identity and Personality

Behavioral Sciences Chapter 8
Social Processes, Attitudes, and Behavior

Behavioral Sciences Chapter 10
Social Thinking

Behavioral Sciences Chapter 11
Social Structure and Demographics

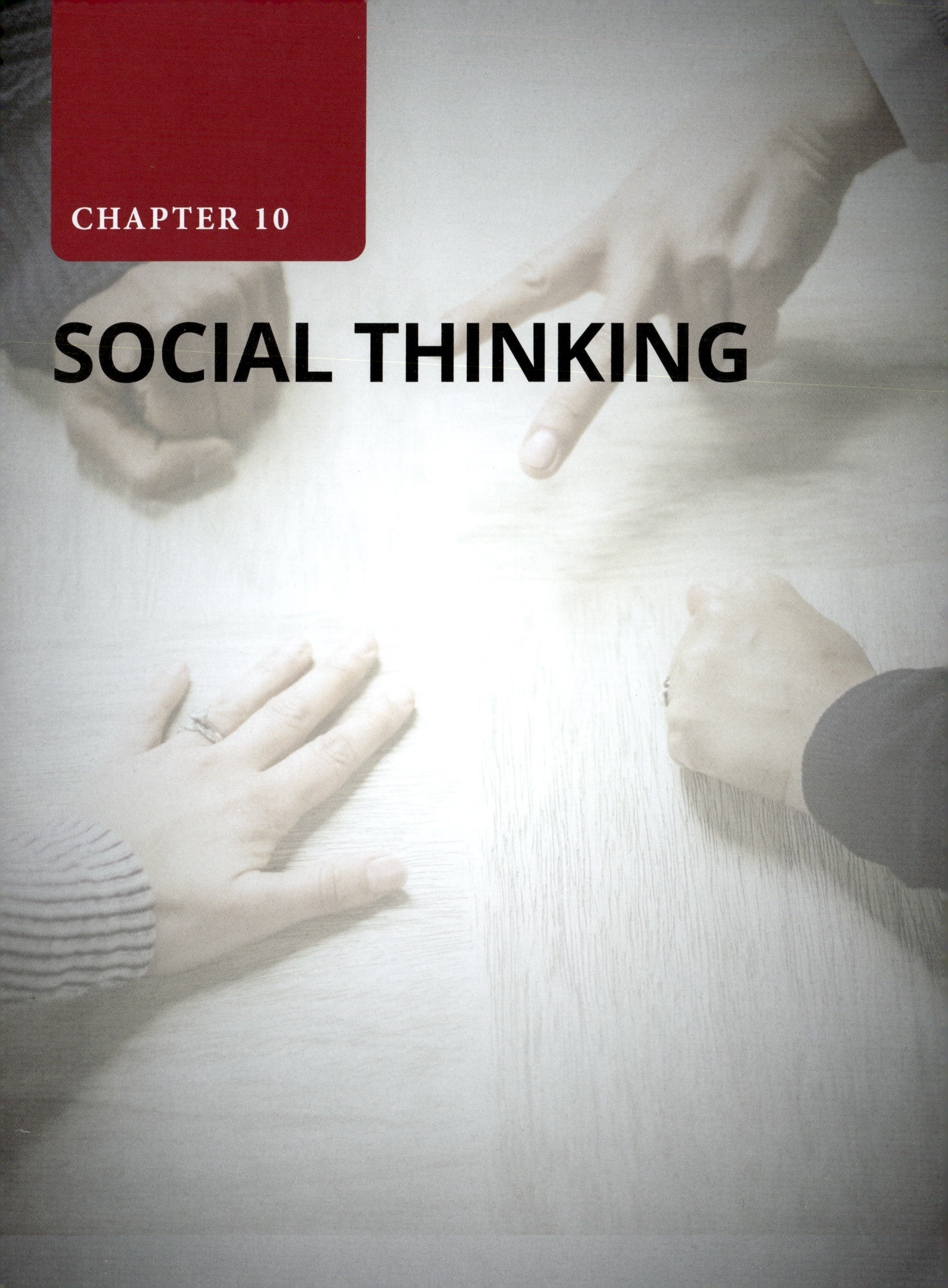

CHAPTER 10

SOCIAL THINKING

SCIENCE MASTERY ASSESSMENT

Every pre-med knows this feeling: there is so much content I have to know for the MCAT! How do I know what to do first or what's important?

While the high-yield badges throughout this book will help you identify the most important topics, this Science Mastery Assessment is another tool in your MCAT prep arsenal. This quiz (which can also be taken in your online resources) and the guidance below will help ensure that you are spending the appropriate amount of time on this chapter based on your personal strengths and weaknesses. Don't worry though—skipping something now does not mean you'll never study it. Later on in your prep, as you complete full-length tests, you'll uncover specific pieces of content that you need to review and can come back to these chapters as appropriate.

How to Use This Assessment

If you answer 0–7 questions correctly:

Spend about 1 hour to read this chapter in full and take limited notes throughout. Follow up by reviewing **all** quiz questions to ensure that you now understand how to solve each one.

If you answer 8–11 questions correctly:

Spend 20–40 minutes reviewing the quiz questions. Beginning with the questions you missed, read and take notes on the corresponding subchapters. For questions you answered correctly, ensure your thinking matches that of the explanation and you understand why each choice was correct or incorrect.

If you answer 12–15 questions correctly:

Spend less than 20 minutes reviewing all questions from the quiz. If you missed any, then include a quick read-through of the corresponding subchapters, or even just the relevant content within a subchapter, as part of your question review. For questions you answered correctly, ensure your thinking matches that of the explanation and review the Concept Summary at the end of the chapter.

1. The tendency to become close friends with neighbors rather than people in other neighborhoods is most strongly related to which of the following factors?
   - **A.** Proximity
   - **B.** Reciprocity
   - **C.** Self-disclosure
   - **D.** Similarity

2. Which of the following would be associated with high levels of aggression?
   - **I.** Increased amygdala activity
   - **II.** Decreased amygdala activity
   - **III.** Increased prefrontal cortex activity
   - **IV.** Decreased prefrontal cortex activity
   - **A.** I and III only
   - **B.** I and IV only
   - **C.** II and III only
   - **D.** II and IV only

3. A child who cries when a caregiver departs and smiles and runs to the caregiver upon return is displaying which type of attachment pattern?
   - **A.** Avoidant attachment
   - **B.** Ambivalent attachment
   - **C.** Disorganized attachment
   - **D.** Secure attachment

4. Elephant seal males mate with multiple females each mating season, while females only have one mate each. What type of mating system is this?
   - **A.** Polyandry
   - **B.** Polygyny
   - **C.** Monogamy
   - **D.** Promiscuity

5. A person with a ventromedial hypothalamus injury will likely show which behavior?
   - **A.** Increased empathy
   - **B.** Decreased empathy
   - **C.** Increased food intake
   - **D.** Decreased food intake

6. Female great reed warblers are attracted to males with larger song repertoires because they tend to produce offspring with higher viability. This is an example of which of the following?
   - **A.** Runaway selection
   - **B.** Sensory bias
   - **C.** Direct phenotypic benefits
   - **D.** Indirect phenotypic benefits

7. In several species of shrimp, the larger adults will sacrifice themselves to protect the younger, smaller shrimp. How is this behavior best explained?
   - **A.** Inclusive fitness
   - **B.** Direct benefit
   - **C.** Sensory bias
   - **D.** Foraging

8. Which of the following is NOT a component of social perception?
   - **A.** The target
   - **B.** The situation
   - **C.** The perceiver
   - **D.** The process

9. When you first meet Dustin, he is very rude to you. You run into him twice more and he is very friendly, but you still dislike him because of your first meeting. What impression bias does this describe?

A. Primacy effect
B. Recency effect
C. Reliance on central traits
D. Proximity

10. Mei brings cookies to work. Although you have not yet tasted them, you say to another coworker, "Mei is such a great person; I'm sure these cookies are fantastic!" What type of bias is this?

A. Reliance on central traits
B. Direct benefits
C. Halo effect
D. Similarity

11. A friend wins a tennis game and says, "I trained so hard—that was a great win!" After losing a subsequent match, the friend says, "My baby brother kept me up all night crying; I was tired for the match." These statements reflect which of the following principles?

A. Just-world hypothesis
B. Fundamental attribution error
C. Self-serving bias
D. Esteem bias

12. Carlos is always happy and smiling. Today, you notice he seems down and think something must have happened to upset him. What types of attribution are you making?

I. Internal
II. External
III. Situational
IV. Dispositional

A. I and III only
B. I and IV only
C. II and III only
D. II and IV only

13. A group of men and women are going to be rated on their driving abilities. The role of gender is emphasized in the experiment and the women perform worse than the men. In another experiment, the role of gender is not mentioned and the ratings are comparable between the two groups. Which principle do these results support?

A. Institutional discrimination
B. Stereotype threat
C. Prejudice
D. The just-world hypothesis

14. The behavior that accompanies the negative attitudes a person has toward a group or individual is referred to as:

A. stereotyping.
B. cultural relativism.
C. prejudice.
D. discrimination.

15. Game theory is designed to study:

A. reliance on central traits.
B. behavior attribution.
C. decision-making behavior.
D. self-enhancement.

Answer Key

1. **A** (See section 10.1)
2. **B** (See section 10.1)
3. **D** (See section 10.1)
4. **B** (See section 10.1)
5. **C** (See section 10.1)
6. **D** (See section 10.1)
7. **A** (See section 10.1)
8. **D** (See section 10.2)
9. **A** (See section 10.2)
10. **C** (See section 10.2)
11. **C** (See section 10.2)
12. **C** (See section 10.2)
13. **B** (See section 10.3)
14. **D** (See section 10.3)
15. **C** (See section 10.1)

The relevant section of the chapter to review for each question is given in parentheses after the correct answer. Detailed explanations can be found at the end of the chapter.

CHAPTER 10

SOCIAL THINKING

In This Chapter

Introduction

Social psychology is concerned with social behavior, including the ways people influence each other's attitudes and behavior. It looks at the impact that individuals have on one another, that social groups have on individual group members, that individual group members have upon the social group, and that social groups have on other social groups. In this chapter, we will continue our discussion of social psychology, highlighting its close relationship to sociology and the other fields within psychology, theoretical perspectives on human behavior within the social environment, and key concepts and classical studies in the field of social psychology. But whereas the last two chapters focused on how individuals are affected by groups and how individuals interact within groups, we will turn our attention in this chapter to specific behaviors seen across human beings, including attraction, aggression, attachment, and the need for social support. We'll also take a look at the dark side of social psychology as we look at patterns of blame in attribution theory and the misappropriation of social structure for prejudice and discrimination. This will be highly relevant for you as a physician, as many patients face prejudice based on their diagnoses or are discriminated against because of personal characteristics, including age, sex, race, ethnicity, socioeconomic status, sexual orientation, gender identity, and more.

CHAPTER PROFILE

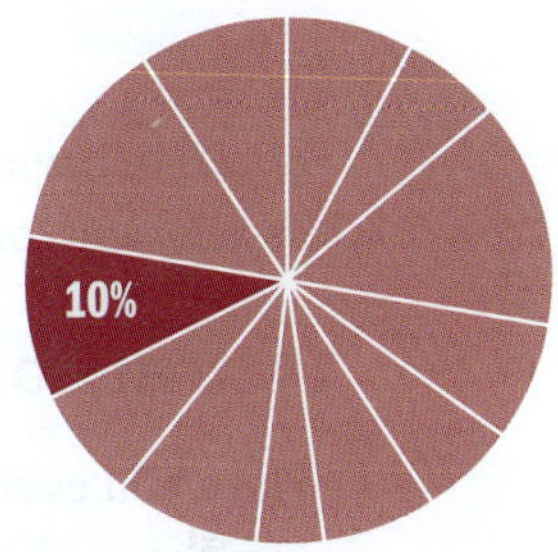

The content in this chapter should be relevant to about 10% of all questions about the behavioral sciences on the MCAT.

This chapter covers material from the following AAMC content categories:

8B: Social thinking

8C: Social interactions

10.1 Social Behavior High Yield

LEARNING OBJECTIVES

After Chapter 10.1, you will be able to:

- Describe interpersonal attraction, including the factors that influence interpersonal attraction
- Recall the meaning of the term *aggression*, including examples of aggressive behaviors
- List the four types of attachment and how they affect childhood behavior
- Identify the common types of social support
- Explain the relationship between altruism and inclusive fitness

Social behaviors involve interactions with others. These may flow from positive feelings, such as attraction or attachment, or they may flow from negative feelings, such as aggression.

Attraction

Have you ever wondered what makes some people friends and others enemies? How second graders choose their best friends? Why you keep eyeing that attractive person in your physics class? Social psychologists call this phenomenon of individuals liking each other **interpersonal attraction**. Researchers have found several factors that affect attraction, including similarity, self-disclosure, reciprocity, and proximity. Outward appearance also plays a role; the more symmetric someone's face is, the more physically attractive people tend to perceive that person to be. Humans are also attracted to individuals with certain body proportions approximating the **golden ratio** (1.618:1).

KEY CONCEPT

Interpersonal attraction is influenced by many factors, including physical characteristics, similarity, self-disclosure, reciprocity, and proximity.

We tend to be attracted to people who are similar to us in attitudes, intelligence, education, height, age, religion, appearance, and socioeconomic status. One reason for this may be convenience: it's easier to spend time together if you both want to go on a bike ride or if you both enjoy Thai food. Also, people are drawn to having their values and choices validated by another person. So why is there a cliché about opposites attracting? Social psychologists find that attraction also occurs if opposing qualities match up with each other; for example, a nurturer is attracted to someone who craves being nurtured. Notably, successful complementary relationships still have fundamental similarities in some attitudes that make the complementary aspects of the relationship work.

Another component of attraction lies in the opportunity for **self-disclosure**, or sharing one's fears, thoughts, and goals with another person and being met with nonjudgmental empathy. Engaging in this behavior deepens attraction and friendship. This must be a reciprocal behavior, however. Revealing one's innermost secrets creates a sense of vulnerability that, if not met by the other person, can be interpreted as being taken advantage of. Reciprocity is important in other aspects of interpersonal attraction as well. **Reciprocal liking** is the phenomenon whereby people like others better when they believe the other person likes them. Researchers have shown that even if we disagree with others on important issues, we will have increased interest in them if we have indications that they like us.

Finally, **proximity**, or just being physically close to someone, plays a factor in attraction to a person. Studies have shown that we are more likely to form friendships with people in the same dorm as us or with the people who sit closest to us in class. Part of this is convenience; it's easier to have conversations and make plans with people in the same area. Another explanation is the **mere exposure effect** or **familiarity effect**, the tendency for people to prefer stimuli that they have been exposed to more frequently. You may have observed this in your everyday life: Have you disliked a song the first time you heard it, only to find yourself singing along and saying, *I like this song!* after hearing it many more times? This principle is also used in marketing: the more people hear the name of a product, the more likely they are to be attracted to and purchase that product.

Aggression

Aggression is defined as a behavior that intends to cause harm or increase social dominance. Aggression can take the form of physical actions as well as verbal or nonverbal communication. Ethologists study aggression in terms of the interactions between animals in natural settings. Aggression in these settings can include bodily contact, as seen in Figure 10.1, but most displays of aggression are settled by threat and withdrawal without actual bodily harm. Threat displays are common in both animals and humans. Before a fight, someone might puff up the chest or pull back a fist to threaten another person. This display may or may not result in physical harm or violence. Other examples of aggression include a bully hurling insults at another child or a gang member making threatening gestures to a member of another gang.

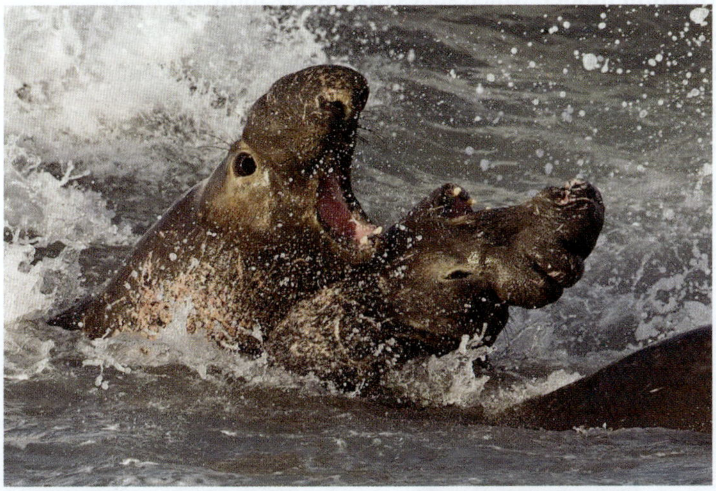

Figure 10.1 Aggression Following Threat Displays of Elephant Seals
While threat displays may lead to violence, as seen here, threat displays commonly lead to withdrawal to prevent fights.

What is the purpose of aggressive behavior if it causes so much destruction? Evolutionarily, aggression offers protection against perceived and real threats. Aggression helped our ancestors fight off predators. It also helps organisms gain access to resources such as food, additional territory, or mates. In cases of limited resources, aggression could be the deciding factor that allows one to pass on genes.

From a biological perspective, multiple parts of the brain contribute to violent behavior. The **amygdala** is the part of the brain responsible for associating stimuli and their corresponding rewards or punishments. In short, it is responsible for telling us whether or not something is a threat. If the amygdala is activated, this increases aggression. However, higher-order brain structures, such as the prefrontal cortex, can hit the brakes on a revved-up amygdala, reducing emotional reactivity and impulsiveness. Reduced activity in the prefrontal cortex has been linked to increased aggressive behavior.

Aggression is also under hormonal control. Higher levels of testosterone have been linked to more aggressive behavior in humans irrespective of sex or gender. Some speculate that the higher levels of testosterone in phenotypical males compared to phenotypical females may explain the trend that males are generally more aggressive than females across cultures and that males commit a disproportionate majority of violent crimes.

Beyond the biological contributions to aggressive behavior, studies have found many psychological and situational predictors of aggression. Do you find yourself snapping at people more when you're in pain? Have you ever gotten annoyed with a waiter when you were extremely hungry? Such responses are accounted for by the **cognitive neoassociation model**, which states that we are more likely to respond to others aggressively whenever we are feeling negative emotions, such as being tired, sick, frustrated, or in pain. Figure 10.2 pictures a common scenario representative of the cognitive neoassociation model. This can also be seen on a large scale: riots are more likely to happen on hot days than cool ones; drivers without air conditioning are more likely to honk at other drivers than those with air conditioning.

BRIDGE

The prefrontal cortex is critically important to managing the limbic system, which is important in managing emotion and stress. These roles of the prefrontal cortex are discussed in Chapter 5 of *MCAT Behavioral Sciences Review.*

REAL WORLD

Alcohol has been shown to increase aggressive behavior. Alcohol impairs judgment and limits one's ability to control aggressive reactions. It also makes one feel less inhibited by social mores that would normally restrict aggressive behavior.

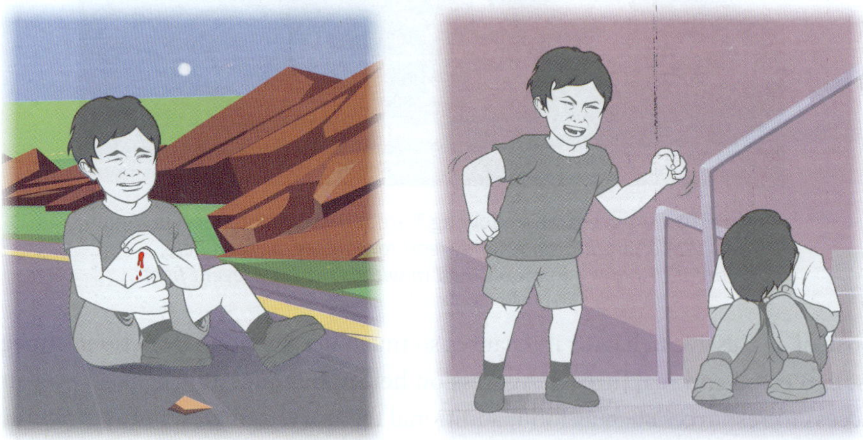

Figure 10.2 The Cognitive Neoassociation Model

Another factor that contributes to aggressive behavior is exposure to violent behavior. The effects on children of media portrayals of violence continue to be a hot topic. Research findings are mixed but tend to show that viewing violent behavior indeed correlates to an increase in aggressive behavior. The contribution of modeling to violence in children was also explored in Albert Bandura's Bobo doll experiment, described in Chapter 3 of *MCAT Behavioral Sciences Review.*

Attachment

Attachment is an emotional bond between a caregiver and a child that begins to develop during infancy. While parental figures are most common, emotional bonds can occur with any caregiver who is sensitive and responsive during social interaction. After World War II, psychiatrist John Bowlby noticed the negative effects of isolation on social and emotional development in orphaned children and started the study of attachment. In the 1970s, psychologist Mary Ainsworth expounded on this theory, saying that infants need a secure base, in the form of a consistent caregiver during the first six months to two years of life, from which to explore the world and develop appropriately. Four main types of attachment styles have been described and are illustrated in Figure 10.3: secure, avoidant, ambivalent, and disorganized.

KEY CONCEPT

In attachment, a secure base is a caregiver who is consistent, available, comforting, and responsive.

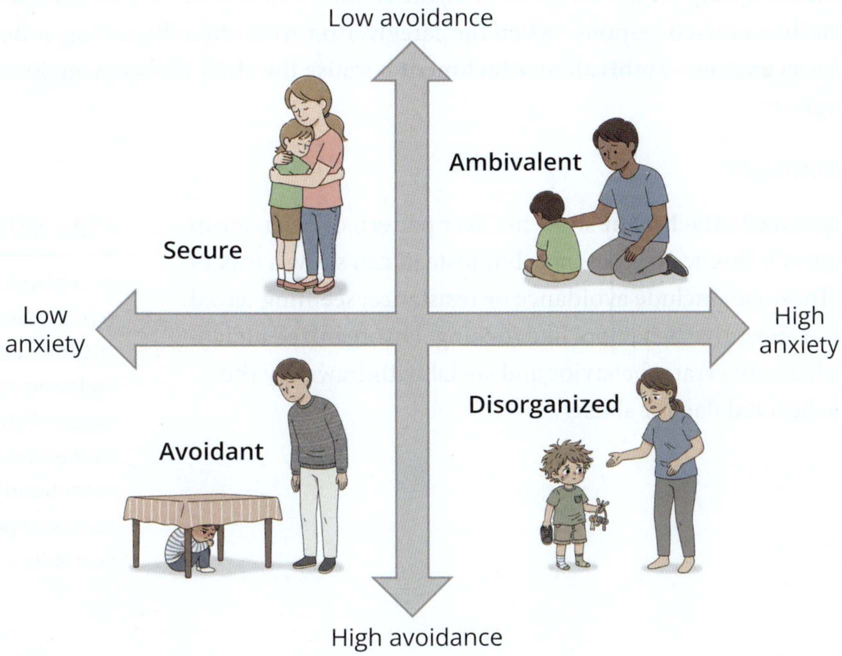

Figure 10.3 Attachment Styles

Secure Attachment

Secure attachment is seen when a child has a consistent caregiver and is able to go out and explore, knowing that there is a secure base to return to. The child will be upset at the departure of the caregiver and will be comforted by the return of the caregiver. The child trusts that the caregiver will be there for comfort, and while the child can be comforted by a stranger, the child will clearly prefer the caregiver. Having a secure attachment pattern is thought to be a vital aspect of a child's social development. Children with avoidant, ambivalent, or disorganized attachment can have deficits in social skills. Collectively, these attachment types are known as **insecure attachment**.

Avoidant Attachment

Avoidant attachment results when the caregiver has little or no response to a distressed child. Given the choice, these children will show no preference between a stranger and the caregiver. They show little or no distress when the caregiver leaves and little or no relief when the caregiver returns.

Ambivalent Attachment

Ambivalent attachment occurs when a caregiver has an inconsistent response to a child's distress, sometimes responding appropriately, sometimes neglectfully. As such, the child is unable to form a secure base because the child cannot consistently rely on the caregiver's response. The child will be very distressed on separation from the caregiver but has a mixed response when the caregiver returns, often displaying ambivalence. This is sometimes referred to as **anxious–ambivalent attachment** because the child is always anxious about the reliability of the caregiver.

Disorganized Attachment

Children with **disorganized attachment** show no clear pattern of behavior in response to the caregiver's absence or presence, but instead can show a mix of different behaviors. These can include avoidance or resistance; seeming dazed, frozen, or confused; or repetitive behaviors like rocking. Disorganized attachment is often associated with erratic behavior and social withdrawal by the caregiver. It may also be a red flag for abuse.

REAL WORLD

As a physician, you will be a mandated reporter. This means that you are required by law to report suspected cases of child abuse. Remember: It is better to report and be incorrect than to miss a potentially fatal scenario.

Parenting Styles

Flipping the perspective from child to caregiver, the ways in which parents and other caregivers interact with their children can also be characterized as particular parenting styles. There are four parenting styles from the work of clinical and developmental psychologist Diana Baumrind: authoritarian, authoritative, permissive, and rejecting. Figure 10.4 summarizes the differences between them. Note that parenting styles differ along two axes. The first is high vs. low control. This describes to what extent a parent is personally involved in structuring the child's life. The other axis is how accepting a parent is of their child. Acceptance in this context refers to how much warmth and care a parent extends toward their child. The four parenting styles are a result of dividing the two axes of variation into four quadrants, like the quadrants in a standard coordinate graph.

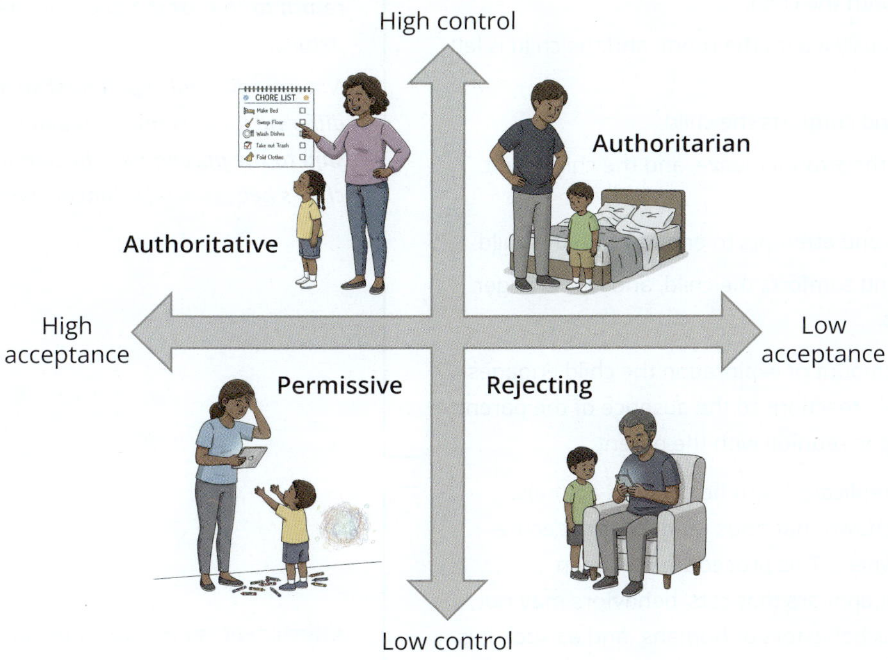

Figure 10.4 The Four Parenting Styles

BEHAVIORAL SCIENCES GUIDED EXAMPLE WITH EXPERT THINKING

The Strange Situation is an experimental procedure used to assess attachment in infants who are between 9 and 18 months old. The procedure occurs over the course of twenty-one minutes and progresses as follows:

1. The parent and child are introduced to the experimental room.
2. The parent and child are left alone in the room. The infant is allowed to explore the room. The parent does not participate.
3. A stranger enters the room, converses with the parent, and attempts to engage with the child.
4. The parent conspicuously leaves the room, and the child is left with the stranger.
5. The parent returns and comforts the child.
6. Both the parent and the stranger leave, and the child is left alone.
7. The stranger returns and attempts to engage with the child.
8. The parent returns and comforts the child, and the stranger conspicuously leaves.

Researchers observe the amount of exploration the child engages in, reactions to the stranger, reactions to the absence of the parent, and the child's behavior upon reunion with the parent.

Experimental procedure. I'll take a brief moment to picture each step, but I'll have to return to this list if a question asks for details.

Not a traditional experiment so no real IV, the differing input is the child and the relationship to the parent, and the output is the child's behavior/attachment style.

This procedure has been replicated with nonhuman animals. In particular, it has been shown that dogs tend to form secure attachments with their owners. This procedure has been attempted with cats, but it appears that cats' behaviors may not serve the same function as behaviors of humans, and as such it is difficult to use procedures developed for humans to assess cat attachment. Furthermore, individual cats' behaviors are inconsistent throughout the procedure, possibly because the experimental procedure is a scenario that cats do not frequently encounter outside the laboratory.

Attachment in nonhuman animals.

Dogs are secure and cats are complicated.

Adapted from: Potter A, Mills DS (2015) Domestic Cats (*Felis silvestris catus*) Do Not Show Signs of Secure Attachment to Their Owners. *PLoS ONE* 10(9): e0135109. https://doi.org/10.1371/journal.pone.0135109

A child exposed to the Strange Situation was uninterested in exploring the room in the presence of either parent or stranger, and did not emotionally engage with either individual. In what ways do dogs' attachment behaviors and style differ from those of the child? What experimental limitations do the researchers point out regarding assessing attachment in cats?

The beginning of the question stem presents a scenario in which a child was reluctant to explore the surroundings, regardless of who was present. This description will have to be matched to our outside content knowledge regarding attachment. The different attachment styles are content we should know for the MCAT, and avoidant attachment is characterized by children who show no substantial behavioral change based on the presence or absence of a parent. Behaviorally, we can conclude the child described is displaying an avoidant attachment style. Dogs were described in the article as demonstrating secure attachment, so we'll want to recall the characteristics of a secure attachment and apply them to this situation. In secure attachment, the subject may or may not show distress when left with a stranger, but will definitely prefer the caregiver. The dogs must have displayed distress when left alone but were easily comforted when the caregiver returned. Specifically, then, the difference between the child and a typical dog should be twofold: the dogs should show greater engagement and positive response with their caregiver as compared to this child, and the dogs should show more distress when left alone without the caregiver as compared to the child.

The answer to the second question requires that we approach the problem in a similar way, this time applied to experimental design. We'll need to consider the description we were given and attempt to match the description to a vocabulary word or concept we've studied. Here, the researchers noted two issues. The first was that the behaviors measured in cats did not serve a function with respect to attachment. Since cats aren't social animals, trying to evaluate their behavior in a social context might be inappropriate. The experiment might not actually be measuring what it seeks to measure, which is a problem with internal validity. The author also mentions that the scenario presented in the experiment might not have a real-world analogue. When an experimental procedure might not actually apply to situations outside the lab, the experiment can be said to lack external validity.

In sum, the dog displayed secure attachment, while the infant displayed avoidant attachment. The application of this methodology to cats potentially lacks both internal (not measuring the targeted variable) and external (not bearing relevance to real-world analogues) validity.

Social Support

In psychology, **social support** is the perception or reality that one is cared for by a social network. Social support can be divided into many different categories: emotional, esteem, material, informational, and network support (Figure 10.5). While social support is present at all times, it is often most pronounced—and necessary—when someone suffers a personal or family tragedy.

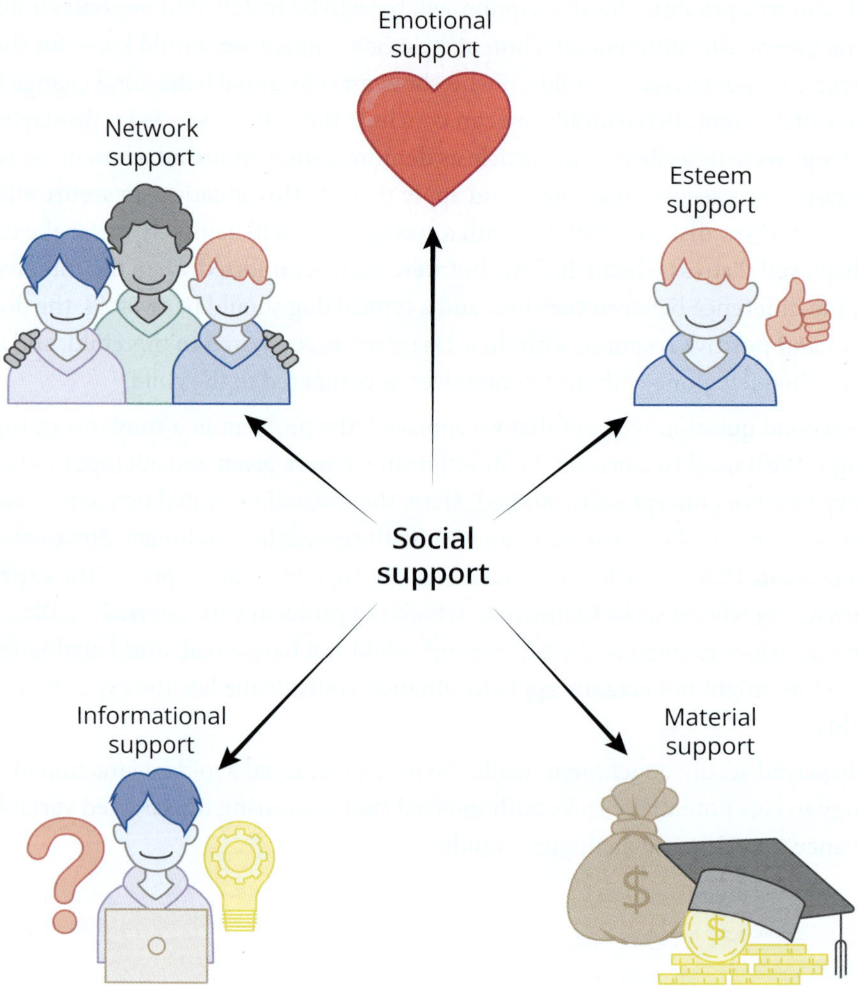

Figure 10.5 Social Support Types

Emotional support is listening, affirming, and empathizing with someone's feelings. It's the *I'm sorry for your loss* condolence card or a trip to the hospital to visit a sick relative. Many people equate social support with emotional support, but other forms of support exist as well.

Esteem support is similar, but touches more directly on affirming the qualities and skills of a person. Reminding others of the skills they possess to tackle a problem can bolster their confidence. For example, consider a friend who has missed a significant amount of school due to illness. Calling that friend a smart and efficient worker who should have no problem making up the work would be providing esteem support.

Material support, also called **tangible support**, is any type of financial or material contribution to another person. It can come in the form of making a meal for friends after they have lost a loved one or donating money to a person in need.

Informational support refers to providing information that will help someone. You will spend much of your career providing informational support to patients as you explain their diagnoses, potential treatment options, and risks and benefits of those treatment options.

Network support is the type of social support that gives a person a sense of belonging. This can be shown physically, as demonstrated in Figure 10.6, or can be accomplished through gestures, group activities, and shared experiences.

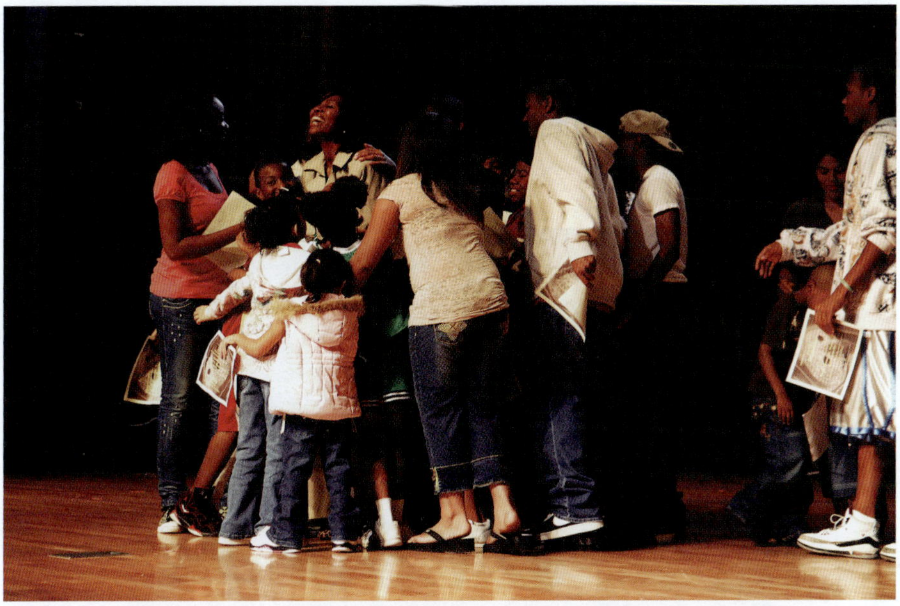

Figure 10.6 Network Support
A group hug creates a sense of belonging.

No matter the form, all of these social supports offer many different types of health benefits. Social support helps reduce psychological distress such as anxiety and depression. People with low social support show higher levels of major mental disorders, alcohol and drug use, and suicidal ideation. Beyond these intuitive improvements in mental health, there are also improvements to our physical health. Studies have found that people with low social support have a higher mortality risk from many different diseases, including diabetes, cardiovascular disease, and cancer. Strong social support appears to correlate with immunological health, too: those with higher social support are less likely to get colds and recover faster when they do.

Social Behaviors and Evolutionary Fitness

Many behaviors have neurological corollaries. Here, we will look at some specific behaviors and the brain regions that are implicated in causing them.

Foraging

The behavior of **foraging**, or seeking out and eating food, is driven by biological, psychological, and social influences. Biologically, hunger is driven by a complex pathway involving both neurotransmitters and hormones. The sensation of hunger is controlled by the **hypothalamus**. Specifically, the lateral hypothalamus promotes hunger, while the ventromedial hypothalamus responds to cues that we are full and promotes satiety. Thus, damage to the lateral hypothalamus will cause a person to lose all interest in eating; meanwhile, damage to the ventromedial hypothalamus will result in obesity because the individual never feels satiated. Foraging is also impacted by genetics. Certain genes play a role in the onset of foraging behavior and the division of tasks between members of the same group. Some species forage together while others engage in solitary foraging.

Cognitive skills play a role in the success of both solitary and group foraging. These skills include spatial awareness, memory, and decision making. In species that forage as a group, foraging is primarily a learned behavior. Young individuals learn through observing how to find and consume food and how to determine what is safe to eat, as shown in Figure 10.7. Animals also learn how to hunt by watching others. Some animals, such as wolves, hunt in packs that have strict rules regarding the order in which individuals are allowed to eat after a successful hunt.

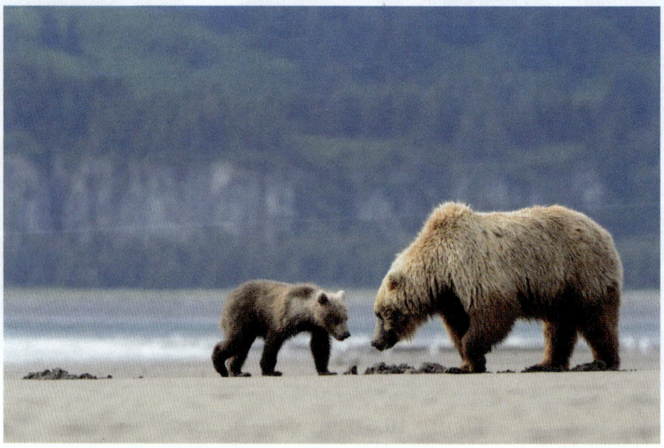

Figure 10.7 Foraging Is Learned through Observational Learning

Mating and Mate Choice

A **mating system** describes the organization of a group's sexual behavior. Mating systems seen among animals include monogamy, polygamy, and promiscuity. **Monogamy** refers to an exclusive mating relationship. **Polygamy** means having exclusive relationships with multiple partners. Having exclusive relationships with multiple females is called **polygyny** and with multiple males is called **polyandry**. Figure 10.8 contrasts these two forms of polygamy with one form of monogamy. **Promiscuity** refers to a member of one sex mating with others without exclusivity. In most animal species, there is one dominant mating system; however, humans exhibit more flexibility. In humans, mating behavior is highly influenced by both biological and social factors. Humans also differ from animals by having formal relationships to correspond with mate choice. Mating may or may not be associated with these social relationships, such as marriage or dating.

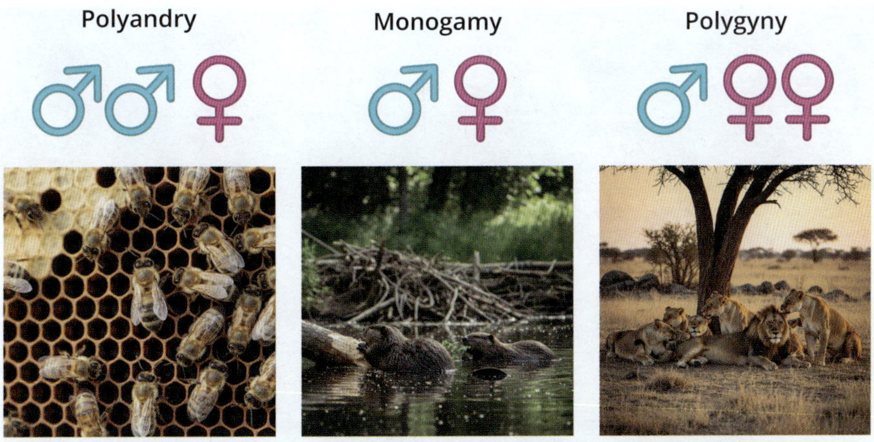

Bees have a queen who reproduces with the many males.

Beavers tend to have a single mating partner for life.

Lions form prides consisting of one male and many females.

Figure 10.8 Mating Systems

Mate choice, or **intersexual selection**, is the selection of a mate based on attraction. **Mate bias** refers to how choosy members of the species are while choosing a mate. This bias is an evolutionary mechanism aimed at increasing the fitness of the species. It may carry **direct benefits** by providing material advantages, protection, or emotional support, or **indirect benefits** by promoting better survival in offspring.

There are five recognized mechanisms of mate choice:

- **Phenotypic benefits:** observable traits that make a potential mate more attractive to the opposite sex. Usually, these traits indicate increased production and survival of offspring. For example, males that appear more nurturing are more likely to care for, and promote the survival of, their offspring.
- **Sensory bias:** development of a trait to match a preexisting preference that exists in the population. For example, fiddler crabs are naturally attracted to structures that break up the level horizon because they may indicate a food source; male crabs take advantage of this fact by building pillars around their territory to attract mates.
- **Fisherian** or **runaway selection:** a positive feedback mechanism in which a particular trait that has no effect or a negative effect on survival becomes more and more exaggerated over time. In this model, a trait is deemed sexually desirable and thus is more likely to be passed on. This increases the attractiveness of the trait, which in turn increases the likelihood that it continues to be passed on. The bright plumage of the peacock, shown in Figure 10.9, is the prototypical example of Fisherian selection.

KEY CONCEPT

Direct benefits provide advantages to the mate. Indirect benefits provide advantages to offspring.

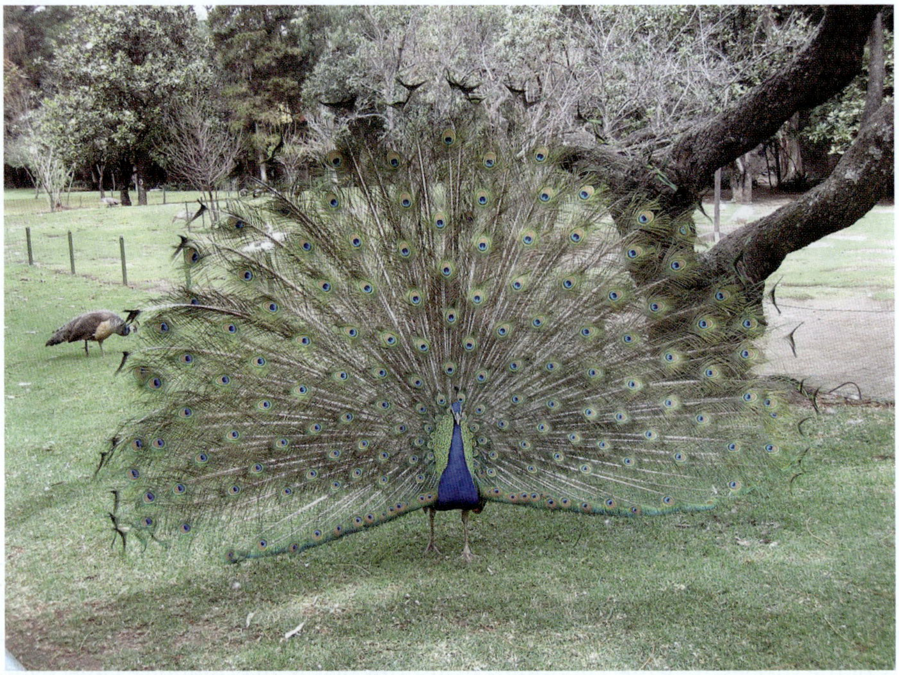

Figure 10.9 Fisherian Selection
The exaggerated plumage of the peacock is the prototypical example of Fisherian selection, in which the attractiveness of a trait that imparts a survival disadvantage leads to its continuation and exaggeration within the species.

- **Indicator traits:** traits that signify overall good health and well-being of an organism, increasing its attractiveness to mates. Notably, these traits may or may not be genetic in origin. For example, female cats are more attracted to male cats with clean and shiny coats; a dirty and dull coat may be related to an underlying genetic problem, or to malnutrition or infection.
- **Genetic compatibility:** the creation of mate pairs that, when combined, have complementary genetics. This theory provides a mechanism for the reduced frequency of recessive genetic disorders in the population: attraction to others who have starkly different genetic makeups reduces the probability of offspring being homozygotic for a disease-carrying allele.

Altruism

Altruism is a form of helping behavior in which the individual's intent is to benefit another at some cost to the self. Helping behavior can be motivated by selflessness, but can also be motivated by egoism or ulterior motives, such as public recognition. **Empathy** is the ability to vicariously experience the emotions of another, and it is thought by some social psychologists to be a strong influence on helping behavior. The **empathy–altruism hypothesis** is one explanation for the relationship between empathy and helping behavior. According to this theory, one individual helps another person when feeling empathy for the other person, regardless of the cost. This theory has been heavily debated, and more recent conceptions of altruism posit that an individual will help another person only when the benefits outweigh the costs for the individual.

REAL WORLD

Altruism creates a bit of a problem for the traditional Darwinist model of evolution. Why would an organism sacrifice its own fitness for the fitness of another? Evolutionary biologists still wrestle with this question, but inclusive fitness offers at least one potential solution.

Game Theory

Game theory attempts to explain decision-making behavior. The theory was originally used in economics and mathematics to predict interaction based on game characteristics, including strategy, winning and losing, rewards and punishments, and profits and cost. A game is defined by its players, the information and actions available to each player at decision points, and the payoffs associated with each outcome.

In the context of biology, game payoffs refer to fitness. Game theorists studying sex ratios in various species developed the concept of the **evolutionary stable strategy** (**ESS**). When an ESS is adopted by a given population in a specific environment, natural selection will prevent alternative strategies from arising. The strategies are thus inherited traits passed along with the population, with the object of the game being becoming more fit than competitors.

One of the classic evolutionary games is the Hawk–Dove game. The game focuses on access to shared food resources. In each round, a player chooses one of two strategies: hawk or dove. The hawk exhibits a fighter strategy, displaying aggression and fighting until he wins or is injured. The dove exhibits a fight avoidance strategy, displaying aggression at first but retreating if the fight escalates. If not faced with a fight, the dove will attempt to share the food resources. There are three potential outcomes. If two hawks compete, one will win and one will lose. If a hawk and a dove compete, the hawk will invariably win. If two doves compete, they will share the food resources. The payoff in this case is based on both the value of the reward and the cost of fighting: If the reward is significantly larger than the cost of fighting, then hawks have an advantage. If the cost of fighting is significantly larger, doves have an advantage. There thus exists an equilibrium point where, based on the magnitude of the reward and the cost of fighting, the hawk and dove strategies can coexist as evolutionary stable strategies.

The Hawk–Dove game represents pure competition between individuals. However, social influences apply in nature and can result in four possible alternatives for competitors when dealing with strategic interactions. The four alternatives are shown in Figure 10.10 and are:

- **Altruism:** the donor provides a benefit to the recipient at a cost to the donor
- **Cooperation:** both the donor and recipient benefit by cooperating
- **Spite:** both the donor and recipient are negatively impacted
- **Selfishness:** the donor benefits while the recipient is negatively impacted

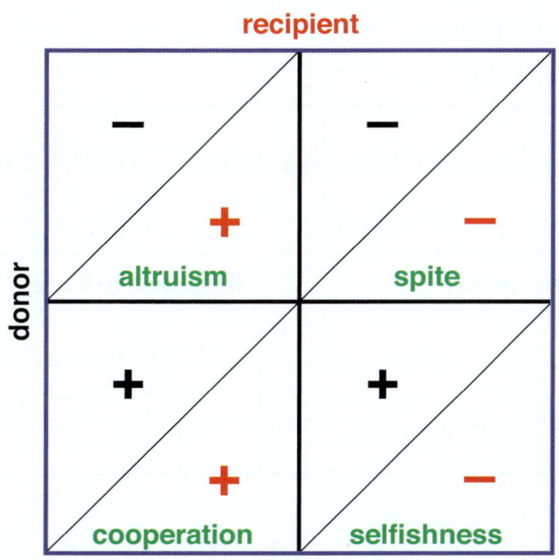

Figure 10.10 Strategic Alternatives for Socially Influenced Competitors

Other common strategy games, like rock–paper–scissors and chicken, can also be explained by game theory.

Inclusive Fitness

In evolutionary psychology, **inclusive fitness** is a measure of an organism's success in the population. This is based on the number of offspring, success in supporting offspring, and the ability of the offspring to then support others. Early descriptions of evolutionary success were based solely on the number of viable offspring of an organism. However, contemporary theories take into account the benefits of certain behaviors on the population at large. For example, the existence of altruism could be supported by the observation that close relatives of an individual will share many of the same genes; thus, promoting the reproduction and survival of related or similar individuals can also lead to genetic success. Other species show examples of inclusive fitness by protecting the offspring of the group at large. By sacrificing themselves to protect the young, these organisms ensure the passing of genes to future generations. Inclusive fitness therefore promotes the idea that altruistic behavior can improve the fitness and success of a species as a whole.

MCAT CONCEPT CHECK 10.1

Before you move on, assess your understanding of the material with these questions.

1. What is interpersonal attraction, and what are three factors that influence this attraction?

    ____

    - ______________________________
    - ______________________________
    - ______________________________

2. For a behavior to be considered aggressive, is it necessary to have the intent to do harm? Does the behavior have to be physical in nature?

    ____

3. What are the four types of attachment? How does a child with each form of attachment act with regard to the caregiver?

Type of Attachment	Response to Caregiver

4. What is social support? List three of the common types of social support.

____

____

- ____
- ____
- ____

5. What is altruism?

____

____

10.2 Social Perception and Behavior High Yield

LEARNING OBJECTIVES

After Chapter 10.2, you will be able to:

- Describe the primacy effect, recency effect, halo effect, fundamental attribution error, attribute substitution, just-world hypothesis, and self-serving bias
- Contrast dispositional and situational attributions, and what factors can make each one more likely
- Identify examples of attribution and attribution biases in real-world examples

Social perception is the name social psychologists give to how we form impressions about the characteristics of individuals and groups of people. We form impressions of others through observation of their behavior, past experiences, and personal beliefs and attitudes. We also feel the need to be able to explain and understand the behavior of others, a process we perform through attribution.

BRIDGE

Social perception is highly linked to attitudes; social perception focuses on how we form attitudes about specific characteristics of individuals and groups. Attitudes are discussed in detail in Chapter 8 of *MCAT Behavioral Sciences Review.*

Social Perception

Social perception is also referred to as **social cognition**, and provides the tools to make judgments and impressions regarding other people. These judgments and impressions include assessments of social roles, relationships, characteristics such as trustworthiness or friendliness, and **attributions**, which are explanations for the causes of a person's actions.

Components of Social Perception

There are three primary components of social perception: the perceiver, the target, and the situation. The **perceiver** is influenced by experience, motives, and emotional state. Past experiences affect our attitudes toward current and future experiences and can lead to particular expectations of events. Our motives influence what information we deem important and what we choose to ignore. Finally, emotional state can flavor our interpretation of an event. The **target** refers to the person about which the perception is made. Knowledge of the target can include past experiences or specific information that affect perception. When little information is available, there is a need for greater observation and interpretation by the perceiver. Finally, the **situation** is also important in developing perception. A given social context can determine what information is available to the perceiver.

Impression Bias

One model of social perception focuses on our selection of cues to form interpretations of others that are consistent over time. When coming into contact with an unfamiliar target, a perceiver takes in all cues from the target and environment, unfiltered. After becoming more familiar with a given target, the perceiver uses these cues to categorize the target: friend vs. enemy, caring vs. standoffish, open-minded vs. bigoted, and so on. Additional time spent with the target in the situational context will lead the perceiver to confirm the categorization. After this point, the perception of additional cues becomes selective in order to paint a picture of the target that is consistent with the perceptions the perceiver has already made. This theory is consistent with the **primacy effect**, which is the idea that first impressions are often more important than subsequent impressions. Sometimes, however, it is actually the most recent information we have about an individual that is the most important in forming our impressions; this is called the **recency effect**.

Individuals tend to organize the perception of others based on traits and personal characteristics of the target that are most relevant to the perceiver. This idea is referred to as the **reliance on central traits**. People may also project their own beliefs, opinions, ideas, and actions onto others. The categories we place others in during impression formation is based on **implicit personality theory**. This theory states that there are sets of assumptions people make about how different types of people, their traits, and their behavior are related. Making assumptions about people based on the category in which they are placed is known as **stereotyping**, and will be discussed in detail in the next section.

Halo Effect

The **halo effect** is a cognitive bias in which judgments about a specific aspect of an individual can be affected by one's overall impression of the individual. It is the tendency to allow a general impression about a person (*I like Jin*) to influence other, more specific evaluations about a person (*Jin is a good person, Jin is trustworthy, Jin can do no wrong*). The halo effect explains why people are often inaccurate when evaluating people that they either believe to be generally good or those that they believe to be generally bad. An individual's attractiveness has also been seen to produce the halo effect. As described earlier, attractiveness can be determined by a variety of traits, and the perception of these traits can impact the view of an individual's personality. It has been shown that people who are perceived as attractive are also more likely to be perceived as trustworthy and friendly. The halo effect can also be seen in professional settings for a lot of the same reasons. People may be tempted to assume that a professional with an accomplished resume is also talented outside of the office. This is artistically represented in Figure 10.11.

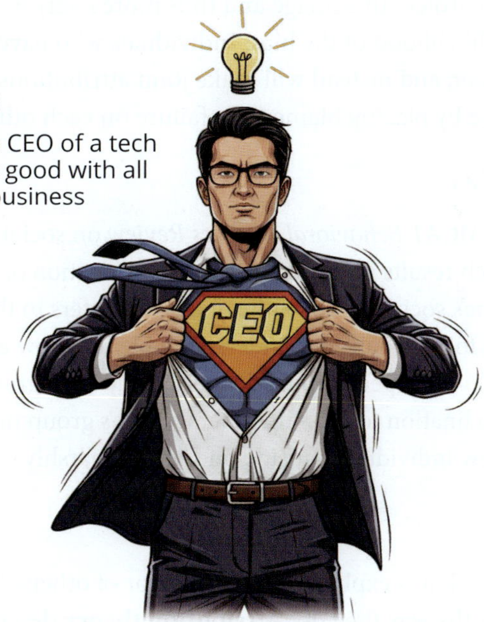
Halo Effect
Assuming a CEO of a tech company is good with all unrelated business ventures
CEO

Figure 10.11 The Halo Effect

Just-World Hypothesis

Another cognitive bias during impression formation is the **just-world hypothesis**. In a so-called just world, good things happen to good people and bad things happen to bad people; noble actions are rewarded and evil actions are punished. Consequences may be attributed to a universal restoring force; in some religions and cultures, this force is referred to as *karma*. A strong belief in a just world increases the likelihood of "blaming the victim" or stating that victims *get what they deserve* because such a worldview denies the possibility of innocent victims.

Self-Serving Bias

Self-identity and perception can be skewed through **self-serving bias**, also known as **self-serving attributional bias**, which refers to the fact that individuals credit their own successes to internal factors and blame their failures on external factors. The tendency to attribute good outcomes to our good traits or behaviors and to attribute bad outcomes to situational factors is used to protect our self-esteem. For example, students who earn a good grade on a test may attribute their success to their intelligence or to how intensely they studied. However, if they received a bad grade, they might attribute this outcome to poor teaching by the professor, unfair questions, or too long a test for the allotted time. These types of attributions have been found to occur in many settings including the workplace, school, interpersonal relationships, and athletics. Self-serving bias is influenced by motivational processes, like self-enhancement and self-verification. **Self-enhancement** focuses on the need to maintain self-worth, which can be accomplished in part by the self-serving bias. **Self-verification** suggests people will seek the companionship of others who see them as they see themselves, thereby validating a person's self-serving bias. Self-serving bias is also influenced by cognitive processes. For example, emotion is a factor in self-serving bias because emotion can impact self-esteem, which influences the need to protect one's self-identity. Individuals with higher

REAL WORLD

People with depression often have a reversed attributional bias, viewing their successes as caused by external factors (*I got lucky this time*) and failures as caused by internal factors (*It was all my fault*).

self-esteem are more likely to protect this image and thus more likely to exhibit self-serving bias. Relationships to others also determine the likelihood of the bias: Individuals who have close relationships are less likely to attribute failures to one another, and instead will make joint attributions. On the other hand, strangers are much more likely to self-serve by placing blame for a failure on each other.

In-group vs. Out-group Bias

As suggested in Chapter 9 of *MCAT Behavioral Sciences Review* on social interaction, humans naturally come together to form groups, which results in the subjective categorization of in-group and out-group. In-group refers to other members of one's social group, while out-group refers to those who are not in the group. Given the propensity for humans to form groups, it's understandable that how an individual perceives members within their group (in-group) versus people outside their group (out-group) is heavily biased. Specifically, **in-group bias** refers to the inclination to view members in one's group more favorably, while **out-group bias** refers to the inclination to view individuals outside one's group harshly.

Attribution Theory

Another aspect of social cognition is explaining the behavior of others. It is human nature to observe and try to understand why others act the way they do. **Attribution theory** describes how individuals infer the causes of other people's behavior.

Dispositional and Situational Causes

Fritz Heider, one of the founders of attribution theory, divided the causes for attribution into two main categories: dispositional (internal) and situational (external). **Dispositional (internal)** attributions are those that relate to the person whose behavior is being considered, including beliefs, attitudes, and personality characteristics. **Situational (external)** attributions are those that relate to features of the surroundings, such as threats, money, social norms, and peer pressure. For instance, suppose you hear that a friend has been nominated for an academic award. Believing that the friend has been nominated because of hard work and personal effort would be a dispositional attribution. Contrarily, chalking up the nomination to luck would be a situational attribution. Situational attributions, therefore, consider the characteristics of the social context rather than the characteristics of the individual as the primary cause.

Cues

In order to understand the behavior of others, a variety of cues are used. These include consistency cues, consensus cues, and distinctiveness cues. **Consistency cues** refer to the behavior of a person over time. The more regular the behavior, the more we associate that behavior with the motives of the person. **Consensus cues** relate to the extent to which a person's behavior differs from others. If a person deviates from socially expected behavior, we are likely to form a dispositional attribution about the person's behavior. **Distinctiveness cues** refer to the extent to which a person engages in similar behavior across a series of scenarios. If a person's behavior varies in different scenarios, we are more likely to form a situational attribution to explain it.

KEY CONCEPT

- Consistency cues—has consistent behavior over time
- Consensus cues—matches others' behavior
- Distinctiveness cues—uses similar behavior in similar situations

The **correspondent inference theory** takes this concept one step further by focusing on the intentionality of others' behavior. When an individual unexpectedly performs a behavior that helps or hurts us, we tend to explain the behavior by dispositional attribution. Thus, we may correlate these unexpected actions with the person's personality.

Fundamental Attribution Error

The **fundamental attribution error** posits that we are generally biased toward making dispositional attributions rather than situational attributions when judging the actions of others. For example, suppose that on a team project, other team members were unable to complete their assignments. According to the fundamental attribution error, our immediate response might be to assume that these team members are lazy or unreliable—both of which are dispositional attributions. We may ignore the possibility that the team members got ill, had too many concurrent assignments, or suffered a personal tragedy—all of which are situational attributions. Figure 10.12 presents another common situation in which this error can be observed. The fundamental attribution error can present itself in positive contexts as well. Imagine if you observed someone getting out of their car to help an older adult across the road. According to the fundamental attribution error, you would likely make a dispositional attribution like, "What a kind stranger!" rather than a situational attribution like, "Oh, maybe that's their grandparent." Notice that in these examples, the dispositional attributions often provide simpler explanations than the situational attributions. This difference in complexity is actually the source of the fundamental attribution error: Assuming that a person's behaviors accurately portray who they are as a person is easier than speculating about what circumstances might have caused the observed behavior.

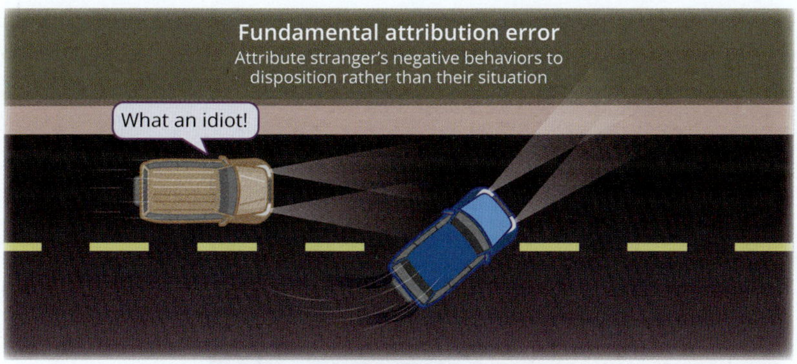

Figure 10.12 The Fundamental Attribution Error

MCAT EXPERTISE

Actor-observer asymmetry (or **bias**) results from the self-serving bias (by the actor) and the fundamental attribution error (by the observer). Actor-observer bias holds that, due to our unique knowledge about our own actions, we are more likely to make situational attributions for the self as compared to others. If you, rather than another person, failed to complete an assignment, for example, you would be far more likely to consider the situational factors involved in your behavior because you are intimately aware of them. This effect is most commonly seen with negative behaviors.

Attribute Substitution

Attribute substitution occurs when individuals must make judgments that are complex, but instead they substitute a simpler solution or apply a heuristic. When making automatic or intuitive judgments on difficult questions or scenarios, an individual may address a different question or scenario without even realizing a substitution has been made. In one study, individuals were asked to envision a sphere that could just fit inside a cube. They were then asked what percentage of the volume of the cube would be taken up by the sphere. This is challenging to envision, so most individuals likely simplified the problem in their minds to imagine a circle inside a square. The answers given in this study averaged around 74 percent, which is approximately the area of a square taken up by a circumscribed circle (79%), but significantly higher than the volume of a cube taken up by a circumscribed sphere (52%).

Attribute substitution can take place in far simpler setups as well. A classic example used in many psychology classes is the following question: *A pencil and an eraser cost $1.10 together. If the pencil costs one dollar more than the eraser, how much does the eraser cost?* Most individuals respond instinctively with the answer *ten* *cents*. It is easy to recognize that the pencil costs more, and to integrate the information given in the question stem (*$1.10* and *one dollar*) incorrectly.

This process is also common when dealing with size and color in optical illusions. For instance, when judging the size of figures in an image with perspective, the apparent sizes shown in the image can be distorted by three-dimensional context, as shown in Figure 10.13. The expected three-dimensional size of the figure, based on perspective cues, substitutes for the actual two-dimensional size of the birds within the image. It is interesting to note that painters and photographers with experience in two-dimensional images are less likely to substitute due to the fact that two-dimensional size is more understandable to their perception.

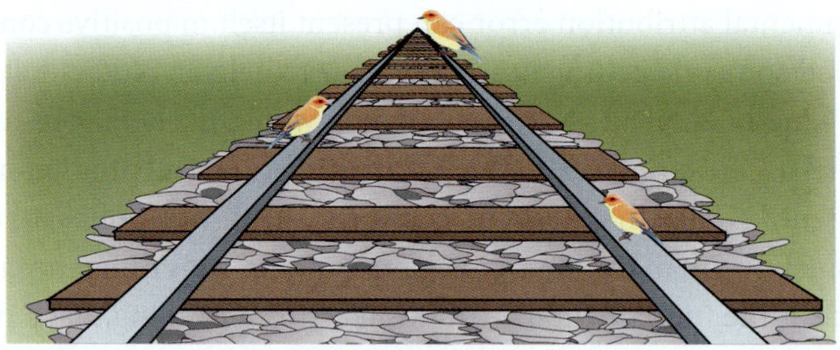

Figure 10.13 Attribute Substitution for Size in Optical Illusions
The birds are of identical size, but three-dimensional cues affect our interpretation of the image.

Shadows, patterns, the position of the sun, and other visual cues can also cause attribute substitution for color, as shown in Figure 10.14.

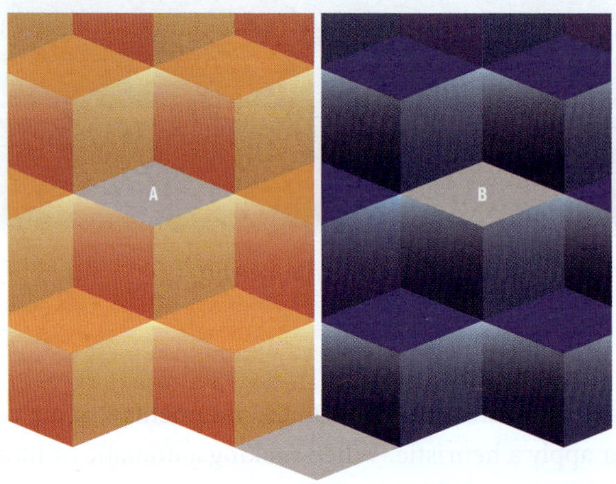

Figure 10.14 Attribute Substitution for Color in Optical Illusions
The central boxes labeled A and B are of identical color, but shadow cues affect our interpretation of the image.

Cultural Attribution

Another important factor in attribution is culture. The type of culture an individual belongs to plays a major role in the types of attributions the individual makes. Individualist cultures put high value on the individual, personal goals, and independence. Collectivist cultures view individuals as members of a group and place high value on conformity and interdependence. Individualists tend to make more fundamental attribution errors than those in collectivist cultures. Individualists are also more likely to attribute behavior to dispositional factors, whereas collectivists are more likely to attribute behavior to situational factors.

MCAT CONCEPT CHECK 10.2

Before you move on, assess your understanding of the material with these questions.

1. For each of the social cognitive biases below, provide a brief description:
   - Primacy effect:

     ___

   - Recency effect:

     ___

   - Halo effect:

     ___

   - Just-world hypothesis:

     ___

   - Self-serving bias:

     ___

2. What is attribution theory? What are the two types of attribution?

   ___

   ___

   - ___
   - ___

3. What is the fundamental attribution error?

   ___

   ___

4. What is attribute substitution?

   ___

   ___

10.3 Stereotypes, Prejudice, and Discrimination High Yield

LEARNING OBJECTIVES

After Chapter 10.3, you will be able to:

- Distinguish between stereotypes, prejudice, and discrimination
- List the types of social inequality that can influence prejudice
- Compare and contrast ethnocentrism and cultural relativism

While stereotypes, prejudice, and discrimination are terms that are related and often used together, they are very different concepts. Stereotypes are viewed as cognitive, prejudice as affective, and discrimination as behavioral. **Stereotypes** refer to the expectations, impressions, and opinions about the characteristics of members of a group. Prejudice reflects the overall attitude and emotional response to a group. Discrimination refers to differences in actions toward different groups.

KEY CONCEPT

- Stereotypes are cognitive
- Prejudices are affective
- Discrimination is behavioral

Note: Kaplan Test Prep does not endorse or encourage any of the stereotypes mentioned in this chapter; they are included only as examples.

Stereotypes

Despite their negative connotations, stereotypes often appear in everyday life, and can be beneficial when not directed toward other human beings. In a psychological sense, the purpose of a stereotype is to make sense of a complex world by categorizing and systematizing information in order to better identify items, predict their behavior, and react. In the context of stereotyping what different items of furniture look like, how different types of stores operate, or how different cuisines taste, stereotypes are extremely useful in defining categories and determining what does or does not fit into that category. However, when stereotypes are used to develop prejudices toward others and to discriminate, they are being appropriated for negative uses.

In the context of sociology, **stereotypes** occur when attitudes and impressions are based on limited and superficial information about a person or a group of individuals. The content of stereotypes are the attributes that people believe define and characterize a group. The **stereotype content model** attempts to classify stereotypes with respect to a hypothetical in-group using two dimensions: warmth and competence. Warm groups are those that are not in direct competition with the in-group for resources; competent groups are those that have high status within society. The four possible combinations of warmth and competence are shown in Table 10.1 and are associated with distinct emotions.

		Competence	
		low	high
Warmth	high	**paternalistic stereotype** low status, not competitive	**admiration stereotype** high status, not competitive
	low	**contemptuous stereotype** low status, competitive	**envious stereotype** high status, competitive

Table 10.1 Classifications of Stereotypes in the Stereotype Content Model
Adapted from Fiske et al. (2002)

Paternalistic stereotypes are those in which the group is looked down upon as inferior, dismissed, or ignored. **Contemptuous** stereotypes are those in which the group is viewed with resentment, annoyance, or anger. **Envious** stereotypes are those in which the group is viewed with jealousy, bitterness, or distrust. **Admiration** stereotypes are those in which the group is viewed with pride and other positive feelings.

Self-Fulfilling Prophecy

Stereotypes can lead to expectations of certain groups of individuals. These expectations can create conditions that then cause the expectations to become reality, a process referred to as **self-fulfilling prophecy**. For example, some medical students experience a self-fulfilling prophecy during their first days of surgery clerkship in medical school: During their first year in the wards, new students are stereotyped as being unable to quickly and efficiently throw knots during a surgery. With this knowledge in mind, these students are nervous to suture for the first time and may struggle with every step of the knot-tying process. This struggle validates the stereotype and thus completes the self-fulfilling prophecy.

Stereotype Threat

In some social situations, a person might be concerned or anxious about inadvertently confirming a negative stereotype about their social group. This concern is known as **stereotype threat**. Unfortunately, the feeling of stereotype threat often results in a self-fulfilling prophesy: People experiencing stereotype threat often exhibit stress arousal and are preoccupied by monitoring their own performance on a task, and these distractions can then lead to reduced performance on the task. An example of a well-studied group that often experiences stereotype threat is women in mathematics. A study showed that women taking a math exam scored lower when the only other test takers in the room were men. The researchers concluded that when taking an exam with only men present, women test subjects were more concerned about stereotype threat, and performed more poorly as a result of their concerns. Researchers theorize that stereotype threat may be a contributing factor to long-standing racial and gender gaps in certain careers and in academic performance.

KEY CONCEPT

Stereotype threat is concern or anxiety about confirming a negative stereotype about one's group. This may hinder performance, which may actually create a self-fulfilling prophecy.

Prejudice

From a social psychology approach, **prejudice** is defined as an irrational positive or negative attitude toward a person, group, or thing, prior to an actual experience with that entity. The process of socialization results in the formation of attitudes regarding our own groups and a sense of identity as an individual and a group member. Prejudice can form in response to dissimilarities among groups, races, ethnicities, or even environments. While racial and ethnic prejudices against individuals are at the forefront of most people's minds, prejudices exist against objects and places as well. For instance, people have attitudes toward different regions of the country based on culture, weather, and history; which car manufacturers are the most reliable; what types of food are considered unhealthy; and even what types of animals make good pets. Prejudicial attitudes can run the gamut from hate to love, contempt to admiration, and indifference to loyalty.

Prejudices may be kept internally or shared with the larger community. **Propaganda** is a common way by which large organizations and political groups attempt to create prejudices in others. Propaganda posters often invoke messages of fear, and depictions of the target group are often exaggerated to an absurd degree.

Power, Prestige, and Class

There are a variety of social factors that influence prejudice. Three of the most important are power, prestige, and class. **Power** refers to the ability of people or groups to achieve their goals despite any obstacles, and their ability to control resources. **Prestige** is the level of respect shown to a person by others. **Class** refers to socioeconomic status. Social inequality, or the unequal distribution of power, resources, money, or prestige, can result in the grouping of *haves* and *have-nots*. *Have-nots* may develop a negative attitude toward *haves* based on envy. *Haves* may develop a negative attitude toward *have-nots* as a defense mechanism to justify the fact that they have more.

Ethnocentrism

Ethnocentrism refers to the practice of making judgments about other cultures based on the values and beliefs of one's own culture, especially when it comes to language, customs, and religion. Ethnocentrism can manifest in many ways, from innocent displays of ethnic pride to violent supremacy groups. Because of this, ethnocentrism is closely tied to the previously discussed concepts of in-group vs. out-group biases and group conflict.

Cultural Relativism

In order to avoid ethnocentrism, the concept of cultural relativism has been employed by sociologists to compare and understand other cultures. **Cultural relativism** is the recognition that social groups and cultures should be studied on their own terms. When studying a culture, social relativism acknowledges that the values, mores, and rules make sense in the context of that culture, and should not be judged against the norms of another culture. In other words, while one group may follow a given set of rules (say, the dietary rules of *kashrut* or *halal*), cultural relativism holds that those rules should not be perceived as superior or inferior to those of other cultures—just different.

Discrimination

Discrimination occurs when prejudicial attitudes cause individuals of a particular group to be treated differently from others. While prejudice is an attitude, discrimination is a behavior. As prejudice typically refers to a negative attitude, discrimination typically refers to a negative behavior. It is also important to note that prejudice does not always result in discrimination. For instance, a person might have strong feelings against a particular race (prejudice), but may not express those feelings or act on them. As social inequality influences prejudice, the same idea applies to discrimination. The unequal distribution of power, prestige, and class influence discrimination.

Individual vs. Institutional Discrimination

Discrimination can be either individual or institutional. **Individual discrimination** refers to one person discriminating against a particular person or group, whereas **institutional discrimination** refers to the discrimination against a particular person or group by an entire institution. Individual discrimination is considered to be conscious and obvious, and can be eliminated by removing the person who is displaying the behavior. Sociologists have begun to stress the need to focus on institutional discrimination, as it is discrimination built into the structure of society, so it is far more covert and harder to extricate. Because it is part of society, it is perpetuated by simply maintaining the status quo.

The United States has a long history of institutional discrimination against myriad groups. Perhaps the most overt example was that of racial segregation that existed in the early to mid-twentieth century. Even today, there are still concerns of institutional discrimination against individuals based on their race, ethnicity, gender identity, sexual orientation, religion, and other characteristics.

MCAT CONCEPT CHECK 10.3

Before you move on, assess your understanding of the material with these questions.

1. What are the distinctions between stereotypes, prejudice, and discrimination?
   - Stereotypes:

   ____

   - Prejudice:

   ____

   - Discrimination:

   ____

2. List three types of social inequality that can influence prejudice:
   -

   ____

   -

   ____

   -

   ____

3. What is the difference between ethnocentrism and cultural relativism?

   ____

Conclusion

Social psychology focuses on social behavior and the attitudes, perceptions, and influences of others that impact behavior. In this chapter, we first looked at social behaviors, including attraction, aggression, attachment, and social support. We also looked at the biological explanations of specific social behaviors, including foraging, mate choice, altruism, game theory, and inclusive fitness. We further defined the components of social perception and impression biases. The way we view ourselves also influences the way we view others and how we attribute behavior to others. Finally, we took a look at stereotypes, prejudice, and discrimination.

These last few topics demonstrate a negative side of classifying individuals. We can use classification to create hierarchies, inequities in opportunity and finances, as well as to silence or suppress communities. But classification can also serve a positive purpose. In social science, we often classify populations to study interactions between groups, changes in population makeup over time, and to track migration patterns. These classifications are considered in the field of demographics, which we will explore in the next chapter.

GO ONLINE

You've reviewed the content, now test your knowledge and critical thinking skills by completing a test-like passage set in your online resources!

CONCEPT SUMMARY

Social Behavior

- **Interpersonal attraction** is what makes people like each other and is influenced by multiple factors:
    - Physical attractiveness, which is increased with symmetry and proportions close to the **golden ratio**
    - Similarity of attitudes, intelligence, education, height, age, religion, appearance, and socioeconomic status
    - **Self-disclosure**, which includes sharing fears, thoughts, and goals with another person and being met with empathy and nonjudgment
    - **Reciprocity**, in which we like people who we think like us
    - **Proximity**, or being physically close to someone
- **Aggression** is a physical, verbal, or nonverbal behavior with the intention to cause harm or increase social dominance.
- **Attachment** is an emotional bond to another person, and usually refers to the bond between a child and a caregiver. There are four types of attachment:
    - **Secure attachment** requires a consistent caregiver so the child is able to go out and explore, knowing there is a secure base to return to; the child will show strong preference for the caregiver.
    - **Avoidant attachment** occurs when a caregiver has little or no response to a distressed, crying child; the child shows no preference for the caregiver compared to strangers.
    - **Ambivalent attachment** occurs when a caregiver has an inconsistent response to a child's distress, sometimes responding appropriately, sometimes neglectfully; the child will become distressed when the caregiver leaves and is ambivalent when the caregiver returns.
    - **Disorganized attachment** occurs when a caregiver is erratic or abusive; the child shows no clear pattern of behavior in response to the caregiver's absence or presence and may show repetitive behaviors.
- **Social support** is the perception or reality that one is cared for by a social network.
    - **Emotional support** includes listening to, affirming, and empathizing with someone's feelings.
    - **Esteem support** affirms the qualities and skills of the person.
    - **Material support** is providing physical or monetary resources to aid a person.
    - **Informational support** is providing useful information to a person.
    - **Network support** is providing a sense of belonging to a person.
- **Foraging** is searching for and exploiting food resources.
- A **mating system** describes the way in which a group is organized in terms of sexual behavior.
    - **Monogamy** consists of exclusive mating relationships.
    - **Polygamy** consists of multiple exclusive relationships, including **polygyny** (with multiple females) and **polyandry** (with multiple males).
    - **Promiscuity** means mating without exclusivity.

- **Mate choice**, or **intersexual selection**, is the selection of a mate based on attraction and traits.
- **Altruism** is a form of helping behavior in which people's intent is to benefit someone else at some cost to themselves.
- **Game theory** attempts to explain decision making between individuals as if they are participating in a game.
- **Inclusive fitness** is a measure of an organism's success in the population. This is based on the number of offspring, success in supporting offspring, and the ability of the offspring to then support others.

Social Perception and Behavior

- **Social perception** or **social cognition** is the way by which we generate impressions about people in our social environment. It contains a **perceiver**, a **target**, and the **situation** or social context of the scenario.
- **Implicit personality theory** states that people make assumptions about how different types of people, their traits, and their behavior are related.
- Certain cognitive biases impact our perceptions of others.
    - The **primacy effect** refers to when first impressions are more important than subsequent impressions.
    - The **recency effect** is when the most recent information we have about an individual is most important in forming our impressions.
    - A **reliance on central traits** is the tendency to organize the perception of others based on traits and personal characteristics that matter to the perceiver.
    - The **halo effect** is when judgments of an individual's character can be affected by the overall impression of the individual.
    - The **just-world hypothesis** is the tendency of individuals to believe that good things happen to good people and bad things happen to bad people.
    - **Self-serving bias** refers to the fact that individuals will view their own successes as being based on internal factors, while viewing failures as being based on external factors.
- **Attribution theory** focuses on the tendency for individuals to infer the causes of other people's behavior.
    - **Dispositional (internal)** causes are those that relate to the features of the person whose behavior is being considered.
    - **Situational (external)** causes are related to features of the surroundings or social context.
- **Correspondent inference theory** is used to describe attributions made by observing the intentional (especially unexpected) behaviors performed by another person.
- **Fundamental attribution error** is the bias toward making dispositional attributions rather than situational attributions in regard to the actions of others.
- **Attribute substitution** occurs when individuals must make judgments that are complex but instead substitute a simpler solution or heuristic.
- Attributions are highly influenced by the culture in which one resides.

Stereotypes, Prejudice, and Discrimination

- **Stereotypes** occur when attitudes and impressions are made based on limited and superficial information about a person or a group of individuals.
- Stereotypes can lead to expectations of certain groups, which can create conditions that lead to confirmation of the stereotype, a process referred to as **self-fulfilling prophecy**.
- **Stereotype threat** is concern or anxiety about confirming a negative stereotype about one's social group.
- **Prejudice** is defined as an irrational positive or negative attitude toward a person, group, or thing prior to an actual experience.
- **Ethnocentrism** refers to the practice of making judgments about other cultures based on the values and beliefs of one's own culture.
- **Cultural relativism** refers to the recognition that social groups and cultures should be studied on their own terms.
- **Discrimination** is when prejudicial attitudes cause individuals of a particular group to be treated differently from others.
  - **Individual discrimination** refers to one person discriminating against a particular person or group.
  - **Institutional discrimination** refers to the discrimination against a particular person or group by an entire institution.

ANSWERS TO CONCEPT CHECKS

10.1

1. Interpersonal attraction is what makes people like each other and is influenced by at least five factors discussed in the chapter: physical attractiveness, similarity, self-disclosure, reciprocity, and proximity.
2. No, in addition to behavior with the intent to cause harm, aggression can also be a behavior that increases relative social dominance. Aggression can be physical, verbal, or nonverbal.
3.

Type of Attachment	Response to Caregiver
Secure	Upset at departure of caregiver, comforted by return; trusts caregiver, who is viewed as a secure base
Avoidant	Shows no preference for a stranger or caregiver; shows little distress at departure and little relief by return of caregiver
Ambivalent	Distressed by departure of caregiver with mixed reactions at return
Disorganized	No clear pattern of behavior; sometimes exhibits repetitive behaviors or seems dazed, frozen, or confused

4. Social support is the perception or reality that one is cared for by a social network. There are five types discussed in this chapter: emotional support, esteem support, material support, informational support, and network support.
5. Altruism is a form of helping behavior in which people's intent is to benefit someone else at some cost to themselves.

10.2

1. The primacy effect is the power of first impressions over later impressions of an individual. The recency effect is weighing the most recent information of a person as the most important. The halo effect occurs when one applies general feelings about a person (usually, "good" or "bad") to specific characteristics of that person. The just-world hypothesis is the belief that good things happen to good people and bad things happen to bad people. Self-serving bias is the tendency to attribute our successes to internal factors and our failures to external factors.
2. Attribution theory focuses on the tendency of individuals to infer the causes of other people's behavior. Attributions are divided into two types: dispositional (internal) causes, which relate to the features of the target, and situational (external) causes, which relate to features of the surroundings or context.
3. Fundamental attribution error is the general bias toward making dispositional attributions rather than situational attributions about the behavior of others, especially in negative contexts.
4. Attribute substitution occurs when individuals must make judgments that are complex but instead substitute a simpler solution or heuristic.

10.3

1. Stereotypes occur when attitudes and impressions are made based on limited and superficial information about a person or a group of individuals and are cognitive. Prejudice is defined as an irrational negative, or occasionally positive, attitude toward a person, group, or thing, which is formed prior to an actual experience and is affective. Discrimination is when prejudicial attitudes cause individuals of a particular group to be treated differently than others and is behavioral.
2. Power, prestige, and class all influence prejudice through unequal distribution of wealth, influence, and resources.
3. Ethnocentrism refers to the practice of making judgments about other cultures based on the values and beliefs of one's own culture. Cultural relativism refers to the recognition that social groups and cultures must be studied on their own terms. In both cases, an individual perceives another group to which that individual does not belong; however, it is the reaction to that other group that determines which paradigm is being used.

SCIENCE MASTERY ASSESSMENT EXPLANATIONS

1. **A**

Each of the answer choices influences social attraction; however, proximity deals with the tendency to be attracted to those who are physically close by.

2. **B**

Aggression is influenced both by the amygdala and prefrontal cortex activity. Activity of the amygdala increases aggression. The prefrontal cortex should control aggression; decreased activity in the prefrontal cortex, therefore, is associated with increased aggression.

3. **D**

This attachment pattern is representative of secure attachment. Secure attachment is seen when a child has a consistent caregiver and is able to go out and explore, knowing there is a secure base to return to. The child will be upset at the departure of the caregiver and will be comforted and resume exploring upon the return of the caregiver.

4. **B**

Polygamy involves having exclusive relationships with several partners, several females (polygyny), or several males (polyandry), **(A)**. Monogamy, **(C)**, consists of exclusive mating relationships. Promiscuity, **(D)**, refers to mating with others without exclusivity.

5. **C**

A person with a ventromedial hypothalamus injury will never feel satiated when eating and will therefore never feel the sensation to stop eating. A person with a lateral hypothalamus injury will never feel hunger and will have decreased food intake, **(D)**.

6. **D**

Phenotypic benefits refer to observed traits in an individual that make them more attractive to other members of their species. Benefits associated with increased fitness through direct material advantages are direct benefits, **(C)**, while indirect benefits involve increased genetic fitness for offspring.

7. **A**

In evolutionary psychology, inclusive fitness is a measure of the number of offspring an individual has, how they support their offspring, and how their offspring can support others. Inclusive fitness promotes the idea that altruistic behavior can improve the fitness and success of a species; the behavior in this scenario can be described as altruism: benefiting another at one's own expense.

8. **D**

There are three primary components of perception: the perceiver, the target, and the situation.

9. **A**

The impressions we form when meeting others are influenced by a number of perceptual biases. The primacy effect refers to those occasions when first impressions are more important than subsequent impressions.

10. **C**

The halo effect is a cognitive bias in which judgments of an individual's character can be affected by the overall impression of the individual.

11. **C**

Self-serving bias refers to the fact that individuals will view their own successes as being based on internal factors, while viewing their failures as being based on external factors.

12. **C**

Types of attribution fall into two main categories: dispositional (internal) and situational (external). Dispositional (internal) causes are related to the features of the person whose behavior is being considered. Situational (external) causes are related to features of the surroundings.

13. **B**

Stereotype threat refers to the phenomenon of people being concerned or anxious about confirming a negative stereotype of their social group. Stereotype threat can hinder performance, creating a self-fulfilling prophecy.

14. **D**

Discrimination is when prejudicial attitudes cause individuals of a particular group to be treated differently than others. While prejudice is an attitude, discrimination is a behavior.

15. **C**

Game theory was originally designed to study decision-making behavior in economics and mathematics; it has since been used to describe decision making in politics, biology, philosophy, and other fields.

GO ONLINE

Consult your online resources for additional practice.

SHARED CONCEPTS

Behavioral Sciences Chapter 5
Motivation, Emotion, and Stress

Behavioral Sciences Chapter 6
Identity and Personality

Behavioral Sciences Chapter 8
Social Processes, Attitudes, and Behavior

Behavioral Sciences Chapter 9
Social Interaction

Behavioral Sciences Chapter 11
Social Structure and Demographics

Behavioral Sciences Chapter 12
Social Stratification

CHAPTER 11

SOCIAL STRUCTURE AND DEMOGRAPHICS

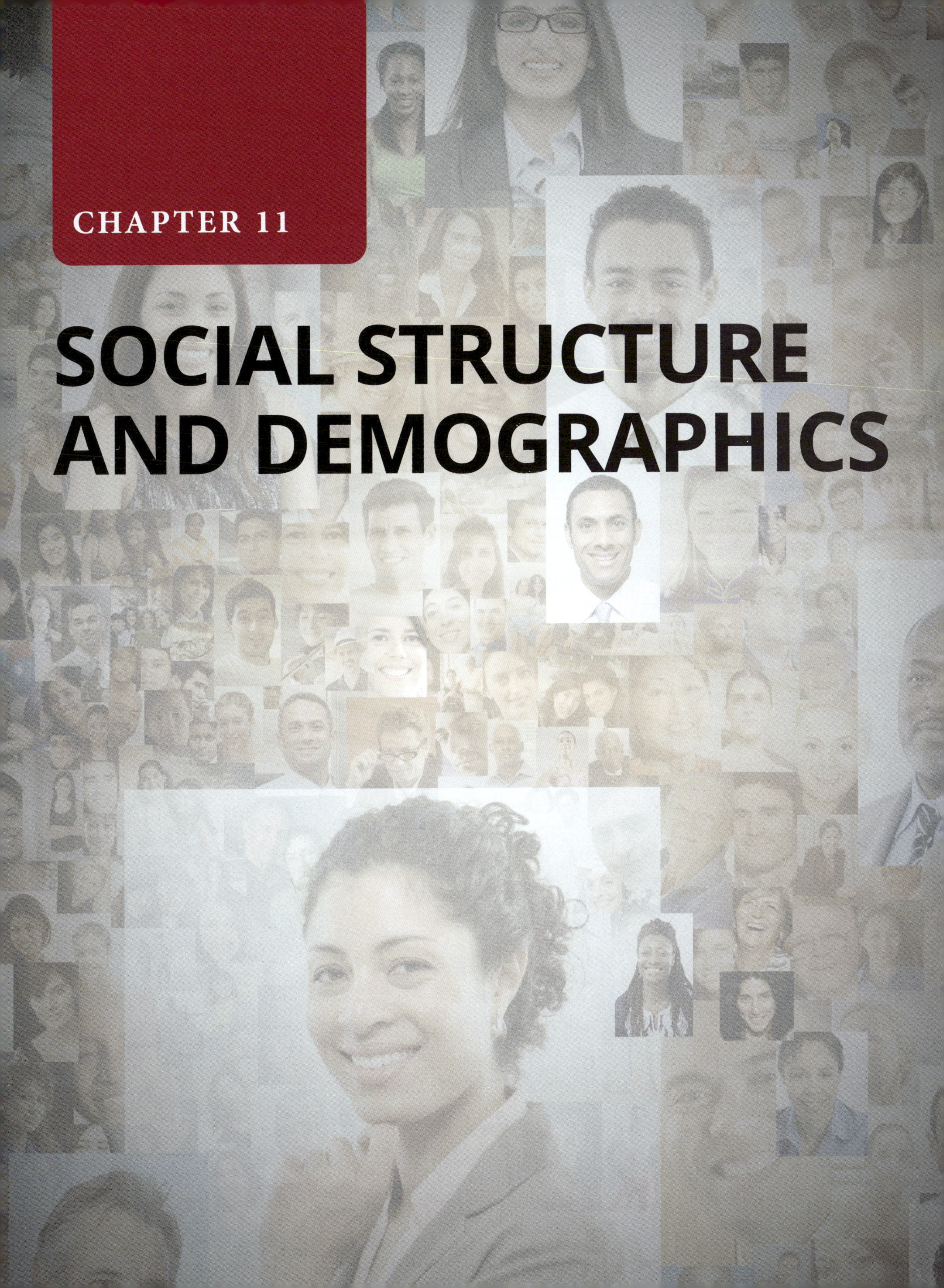

SCIENCE MASTERY ASSESSMENT

Every pre-med knows this feeling: there is so much content I have to know for the MCAT! How do I know what to do first or what's important?

While the high-yield badges throughout this book will help you identify the most important topics, this Science Mastery Assessment is another tool in your MCAT prep arsenal. This quiz (which can also be taken in your online resources) and the guidance below will help ensure that you are spending the appropriate amount of time on this chapter based on your personal strengths and weaknesses. Don't worry though—skipping something now does not mean you'll never study it. Later on in your prep, as you complete full-length tests, you'll uncover specific pieces of content that you need to review and can come back to these chapters as appropriate.

How to Use This Assessment

If you answer 0–7 questions correctly:

Spend about 1 hour to read this chapter in full and take limited notes throughout. Follow up by reviewing **all** quiz questions to ensure that you now understand how to solve each one.

If you answer 8–11 questions correctly:

Spend 20–40 minutes reviewing the quiz questions. Beginning with the questions you missed, read and take notes on the corresponding subchapters. For questions you answered correctly, ensure your thinking matches that of the explanation and you understand why each choice was correct or incorrect.

If you answer 12–15 questions correctly:

Spend less than 20 minutes reviewing all questions from the quiz. If you missed any, then include a quick read-through of the corresponding subchapters, or even just the relevant content within a subchapter, as part of your question review. For questions you answered correctly, ensure your thinking matches that of the explanation and review the Concept Summary at the end of the chapter.

1. Which of the following best describes a manifest function?
   - **A.** An intended positive effect on a system
   - **B.** An intended negative effect on a system
   - **C.** An unintended positive effect on a system
   - **D.** An unintended negative effect on a system

2. Studying why a nod means "yes" in many cultures is most representative of which of the following sociological concepts?
   - **A.** Demographic transition
   - **B.** Expectancy theory
   - **C.** Symbolic interactionism
   - **D.** Demographic shift

3. Which of the following ethical principles states that physicians should avoid using treatments with greater potential for harm than benefit?
   - **A.** Autonomy
   - **B.** Beneficence
   - **C.** Justice
   - **D.** Nonmaleficence

4. A Cuban-American man living in the United States has the dominant physical features of a Black man. He speaks Spanish, prefers Latin foods, and listens to Latin music. His preferences are best defined through which of the following attributes?
   - **I.** Race
   - **II.** Ethnicity
   - **III.** Culture
   - **A.** I only
   - **B.** II only
   - **C.** II and III only
   - **D.** I, II, and III

5. A patient who resides in the United States says, "I love you," and hugs the doctor after every routine visit. This behavior violates:
   - **A.** personal beliefs.
   - **B.** patient autonomy.
   - **C.** social values.
   - **D.** social norms.

6. Which of the following demographics can be measured in events per 1000 people per year?
   - **I.** Birth rate
   - **II.** Fertility rate
   - **III.** Mortality rate
   - **A.** I only
   - **B.** I and III only
   - **C.** II and III only
   - **D.** I, II, and III

7. Because there are more than 500 American Indian tribes, there are several different healing practices among them. Some tribes may have ceremonies that include chanting, singing, body painting, dancing, and even use of mind-altering substances to persuade the spirits to heal the sick person. These ceremonies are examples of:
   - **A.** latent functions.
   - **B.** rituals.
   - **C.** cultural barriers.
   - **D.** social movements.

8. Over the last few decades, the United States population has become:
   - **A.** bigger, older, and more diverse.
   - **B.** bigger, younger, and more diverse.
   - **C.** smaller, older, and less diverse.
   - **D.** smaller, older, and more diverse.

9. Which of the following is NOT an example of material culture?
   - A. Traditional Kenyan clothing
   - B. Japanese cuisine
   - C. American values
   - D. American Indian sand paintings

10. During which stage of demographic transition are both birth rates and mortality rates low?
    - A. Stage 1
    - B. Stage 2
    - C. Stage 3
    - D. Stage 4

11. Shortly after a state legalizes gambling in casinos, a formal coalition forms to oppose the building of any casinos in the major cities of the state. This scenario includes:
    - I. conflict theory.
    - II. social institutions.
    - III. a social movement.
    - A. I only
    - B. I and III only
    - C. II and III only
    - D. I, II, and III

12. A young adult male claims to have had sexual relationships mostly with other men, although he has been attracted to women at times. What would be his most likely score on the Kinsey scale?
    - A. 0
    - B. 1
    - C. 5
    - D. 6

13. Which of the following demographic variables is known to be biologically determined?
    - A. Gender
    - B. Sex
    - C. Ethnicity
    - D. Sexual orientation

14. Which of the following would contribute to increasing population growth over time?
    - A. A fertility rate less than 2
    - B. An immigration rate larger than emigration rate
    - C. An increase in mortality rate
    - D. A decrease in birth rate

15. Urbanization can cause all of the following negative effects EXCEPT:
    - A. decreased opportunity for social interaction.
    - B. increased transmission of infectious disease.
    - C. decreased air quality and sanitation.
    - D. increased rates of violent crime.

Answer Key

1. **A** (See section 11.1)
2. **C** (See section 11.1)
3. **D** (See section 11.1)
4. **C** (See section 11.3)
5. **D** (See section 11.2)
6. **B** (See section 11.3)
7. **B** (See section 11.2)
8. **A** (See section 11.3)
9. **C** (See section 11.2)
10. **D** (See section 11.3)
11. **D** (See section 11.1)
12. **C** (See section 11.3)
13. **B** (See section 11.3)
14. **B** (See section 11.3)
15. **A** (See section 11.3)

The relevant section of the chapter to review for each question is given in parentheses after the correct answer. Detailed explanations can be found at the end of the chapter.

CHAPTER 11

SOCIAL STRUCTURE AND DEMOGRAPHICS

In This Chapter

CHAPTER PROFILE

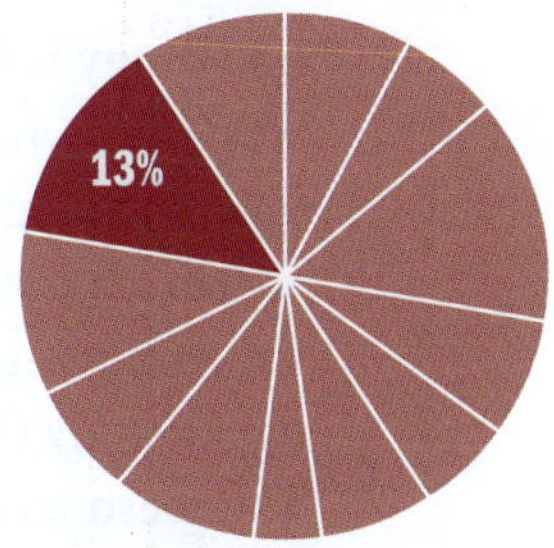

The content in this chapter should be relevant to about 13% of all questions about the behavioral sciences on the MCAT.

This chapter covers material from the following AAMC content categories:

7B: Social processes that influence human behavior

9A: Understanding social structure

9B: Demographic characteristics and processes

Introduction

A frail, older man is admitted to the Intensive Care Unit at a local hospital. He is gaunt, weighing just over 100 pounds, in severe respiratory distress, and nearing circulatory collapse. The intensive care team works to stabilize the patient by starting intravenous lines and pumping fluids. The patient screams statements in a language the team doesn't speak and is eventually sedated so they can intubate and ventilate him. They begin to run tests and discover that the man has widespread metastatic lung cancer that is unlikely to be cured or even controlled through chemotherapy or radiation. The patient's wife and children visit the next morning and are told of the bad news. After crying for some time, they turn to the intensive care team and ask them not to inform the patient of this grave diagnosis. They explain that in their culture family members are expected to make healthcare decisions for the ill to avoid burdening them with such matters. The members of the medical team, however, feel that they must adhere to the tenets of local medical ethics—and their country's laws—and allow the patient to make his own healthcare decisions. As the head of the hospital ethics committee, you get a call from the team to help them make this decision. What would you do?

Ethicists and sociologists alike wrestle with medical dilemmas like these. As a clinician in an ever-diversifying society, you will certainly run into challenging situations like these, where you must try to balance a patient's cultural beliefs with the processes and protocols of the healthcare system in which you work. In this chapter, we'll explore some of the sociological topics on the MCAT, focusing on theoretical models and the key institutions on which you are likely to be tested. We'll then explore culture itself. Finally, we'll describe demographics, the mathematical and statistical modeling of sociological concepts.

11.1 Sociology: Theories and Institutions High Yield

LEARNING OBJECTIVES

After Chapter 11.1, you will be able to:

- Recall the primary theses of major sociological theories, including functionalism, conflict theory, symbolic interactionism, social constructionism, rational choice theory, and feminist theory
- Contrast manifest and latent functions of given elements of a sociological system
- List the four key tenets of American medical ethics

Sociology is the study of society: how we create society, how we interact within and change society, and how we define what is normal and abnormal in society. Whereas psychologists focus on the behaviors of individuals, sociologists focus on the way groups organize and interact. Of course, it would be difficult to describe society as a whole since human society is not completely uniform and is instead made up of distinct cultures, subcultures, groups, and institutions, each with its own structure, patterns, and interests. As a result, sociologists study the subject at different levels: The **micro** level consists of family groups and local communities. The **meso** level consists of organizations, institutions, and ethnic subcultures. And the **macro** level consists of national and international systems.

Theoretical Approaches

Because human interaction is so complex, sociologists have proposed many models, called **theoretical approaches to sociology**, to help analyze and explain aspects of human social behavior. Sociologists don't necessarily disagree about which model is "best." Rather, each model was created to explain certain aspects of sociology, and is inadequate for explaining other aspects. For example, one theoretical approach we will examine is symbolic interactionism, which studies how humans interact and communicate using language, writing, and other symbols. By contrast, another approach, called conflict theory, examines how groups with little power in society can rise up and create more equality. These two models are not necessarily competing explanations. Rather, they examine such vastly different aspects of human interaction that both models are necessary!

As you read this section, keep track of which aspects of human behavior each model explains, and what the weaknesses of each model are. For example, approaches such as symbolic interactionism, social constructionism, and rational choice (exchange) theory tend to focus on society at the micro- and meso-levels. On the other hand, conflict theory, structural-functionalism, and feminist theory are more applicable at the macro-level.

Symbolic Interactionism

Communication among humans stretches far beyond just language, spoken, signed, or written. Our bodies are tools of communication through our posture, facial expressions, and informal hand gestures. We recognize and put meaning into images like the smiley face, traffic signs, or corporate logos. Sacred emblems like the cross, the Star of David, or the star and crescent communicate deep religious significance. Even our clothing can communicate meaning. Any object, image, sound, or action that carries meaning to humans is a **symbol**. Importantly, according to this definition, while many physical objects are symbols, a symbol need not be a physical object. For example, spoken words are symbols, and so are meaningful grunts. Body language and hand gestures are symbols. Anything that carries meaning beyond its own existence is a symbol.

Symbolic interactionism is an approach to sociology pioneered by influential sociologist George Herbert Mead that attempts to understand human action and interaction by studying the symbols we use to communicate. This theoretical approach makes three main assumptions about human behavior:

- Humans act toward symbols based on the meanings that these symbols carry.
- The meanings symbols carry come from social interaction.
- Humans interpret the meaning of symbols, and this interpretation influences action.

Therefore, according to symbolic interactionism, humans are different from lower animals in that lower animals simply respond to stimuli, while humans have the capability to interpret the stimulus first, then react. For example, a dog might bare its teeth, which is a gesture that other dogs always interpret as a symbol of aggression. Lower animals are not able to conceive of alternative meanings to gestures. By contrast, the thumbs up gesture in American culture generally signifies approval. In a different context, however, it could be used sarcastically to communicate disapproval. And in some Middle Eastern countries, it is an offensive gesture. The meaning of the thumbs up symbol therefore depends not only on social and cultural understanding, but also on a person's interpretation.

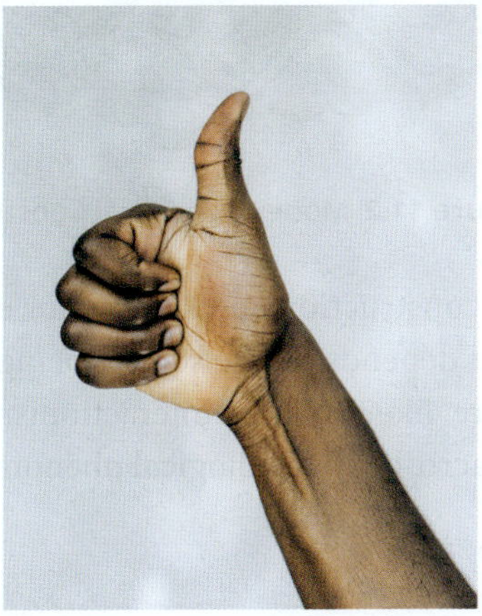

Figure 11.1 Symbolic Interactionism
Hand gestures do not always carry the same meaning across cultures. The thumbs-up is a sign of approval in American culture; in some Middle Eastern countries, it is an offensive gesture.

Not only do hand gestures carry different meanings in different cultures, but different cultures have unique languages and slang, alphabets and number systems, traffic signs, and so on. In fact, the meaning of a symbol might differ even from group to group within a culture. The shared understanding of symbols is therefore a micro- or meso-level phenomenon. One major limitation to the symbolic interactionist approach is that it overlooks macro-level structures, like cultural norms or class interactions.

Social Constructionism

The agreed-upon meaning of symbols can change. For example, the peace sign, which today is a symbol signifying peace and freedom in general, originally was used to indicate support for nuclear disarmament specifically. Society's interpretation of the peace sign has therefore broadened over time. This example shows that the meaning of a symbol does not come from the symbol itself, but from implicit social agreement. Symbols are therefore examples of social constructs.

KEY CONCEPT

Symbolic interactionism reflects on how we use symbols to interact with each other. Social constructionism reflects on how we, as a society, construct concepts and principles.

A **social construct** is any idea that has been created and accepted by the people in a society. **Social constructionism** is the attempt to understand a society through the study of the society's social constructs.

Symbols are not the only type of social construct. Abstract ideas might also be social constructs. For example, the definitions of concepts like honor and justice rely on group agreement among individuals within a given society, and these concepts are therefore social constructs. Sociologists also apply social constructionism to physical objects, such as money. Paper money and coinage do not inherently have significant value; it is only because we, as a society, imbue these objects with value that they can be used to trade for goods and services (Figure 11.2). Other examples of social constructs include work ethic, acceptable dress, and gender roles.

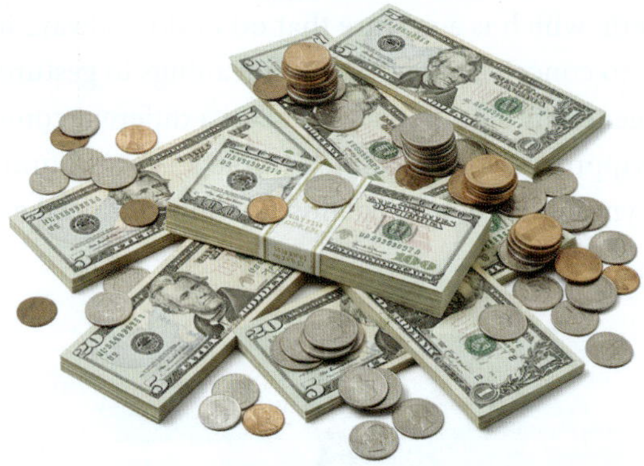

Figure 11.2 Money as a Social Construct

As with symbolic interactionism, social constructionism is useful for explaining micro- and meso-level sociological phenomena. Any social construct depends on the society being studied, and different societies will have different social constructs. Therefore, like symbolic interactionism, a limitation of social constructionism is that this theory cannot account for macro-level sociological phenomena.

Rational Choice (Exchange) Theory

Rational choice theory is one more micro- to meso-level approach to sociology. This theory focuses on individual decision making. According to rational choice theorists, humans will make rational choices to further their own self-interests. This theory claims that people weigh the costs and benefits when making choices, ranking their options based on maximizing perceived benefit. For example, when deciding to purchase a new laptop, rational choice theory claims that a person will gather information about characteristics such as cost, performance, brand recognition, and so on, and then will rank their options and choose the best one.

This laptop example illustrates that rational choice theory is influenced by the study of economics. Rational choice theory becomes a model of sociology when this idea of rational transactions is applied to the social interaction. The rational choice perspective views all social interactions as transactions that take into consideration the benefits and harms to the individual. Every outcome in a given social interaction can be associated with particular social rewards (such as accolades, honor, prestige, or social approval) and with particular punishments (such as embarrassment, humiliation, sanctions, or stigmatization). From the rational choice perspective, an individual carefully considers all of the possible rewards and punishments of each social action and chooses the option that results in the greatest social benefit.

Moreover, according to rational choice theorists, people evaluate whether there is reciprocity and balance in social relationships: People stay in relationships because they get something from the exchange, and they leave relationships when there are more social costs than benefits. Due to this view of relationships as exchanges of social value, rational choice theory is sometimes called **social exchange theory**, or just **exchange theory** for short.

Rational choice (exchange) theory is acceptable for explaining some micro- and meso-level sociological phenomena. However, rational choice (exchange) theory does not easily explain charitable, illogical, unselfish, or altruistic behavior.

Conflict Theory

Conflict theory is a macro theory that attempts to understand society by examining the inevitable conflicts between groups in society. Conflict theory has its origins in the writings of Karl Marx, a 19th century social philosopher who examined the influence of capitalism on 19th century society. **Capitalism** is an economic system in which individuals and corporations, rather than governments, own and control what Marx called the means of production, meaning property, machinery, factories, or any other means of creating a saleable good or service. According to Marx, such private ownership naturally leads to a small, wealthy **capitalist (bourgeoisie) class**, who control the means of production. In Marx's model, the rest of society is relegated to a lower **worker (proletariat) class** that performs manual labor. Because the capitalist class owns the means of production, this class has power over the worker class, and the disparity in power and resources between these two groups leads to conflict. This hierarchy is depicted in Figure 11.3. According to Marx, the conflict in such a society would be a physical one: Eventually, the worker class would rise up and overthrow the capitalist class and form a new, classless society.

REAL WORLD

Conflict theory can be applied to healthcare and medicine. Conflict theorists would not deny that modern healthcare can help people maintain or restore their health; however, they may ask who holds the power in the healthcare system. Is it the patient? The doctor? Hospitals? Pharmaceutical companies? Insurance companies? The government? This is an issue the United States continues to grapple with.

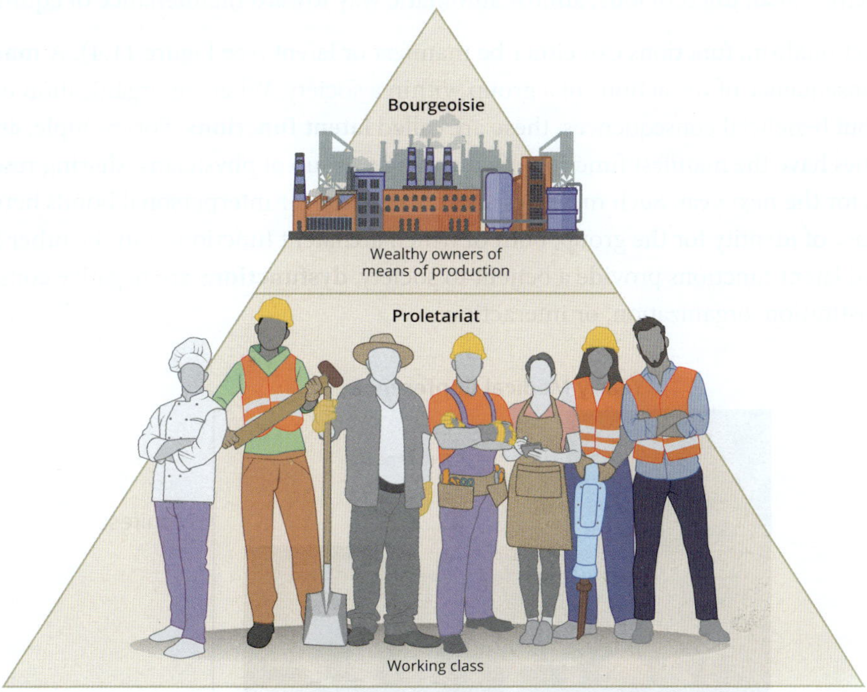
Bourgeoisie
Wealthy owners of
means of production
Proletariat
Working class

Figure 11.3 Bourgeoisie vs. Proletariat

Where Marx focused specifically on conflict between capitalists and workers, modern conflict theory expands this idea to examine any conflict between groups with more power and those with less. For example, conflict might exist between people of different generations, different religions, or different regions of a country. According to conflict theory, in any such conflict, individuals in the group with more power attempt to preserve their power by shaping the structure of society itself. The group with more power uses their influence to dictate the laws, customs, and cultural norms of the society. However, according to conflict theorists, if people in lower-status positions recognize this power differential and see that others share a common dissatisfaction, then these individuals can organize to form **interest groups**, through which they can use tools such as protesting or voting to enact change and equalize power. In short, according to conflict theory, for the more powerful in society, maintenance of the status quo is usually desirable, and for the less powerful, change comes through disruption and revolution.

While conflict theory is a useful model for describing many large-scale changes and other macro-level societal phenomena, it is not very effective for explaining the choices of individuals in society. Also, conflict theorists tend to focus on social stress and disharmony, so conflict theory is less effective than some other models at explaining social cohesion, cooperation, and altruism.

Structural-Functionalism

In some ways, **structural-functionalism** is the inverse of conflict theory. The founder of structural-functionalism, Émile Durkheim, was interested in how large societies survive over long time periods, and was therefore concerned with social cohesion and stability. Durkheim compared society to an organism and proposed that each group in society has a role to play in the overall health and operation of society. These roles might be very different, in the same way that different organs or even different cells have very different functions within an organism, but each is important. Durkheim called each social group's role its **function**: the contribution made by that group to the system. According to structural-functionalist theory, the different groups of society work together in an unconscious, almost automatic way toward maintenance of equilibrium.

In structural-functionalism, functions can either be manifest or latent (see Figure 11.4). A **manifest function** is an intended consequence of the actions of a group within a society. When an organization or institution has unintended but beneficial consequences, these are called **latent functions**. For example, annual meetings of medical societies have the manifest function of educating a group of physicians, sharing research findings, and setting goals for the next year. Such meetings also create stronger interpersonal bonds between physicians and provide a sense of identity for the group, both of which are latent functions. On the other hand, while both manifest and latent functions provide a benefit to society, **dysfunctions** are negative consequences of the existence of an institution, organization, or interaction.

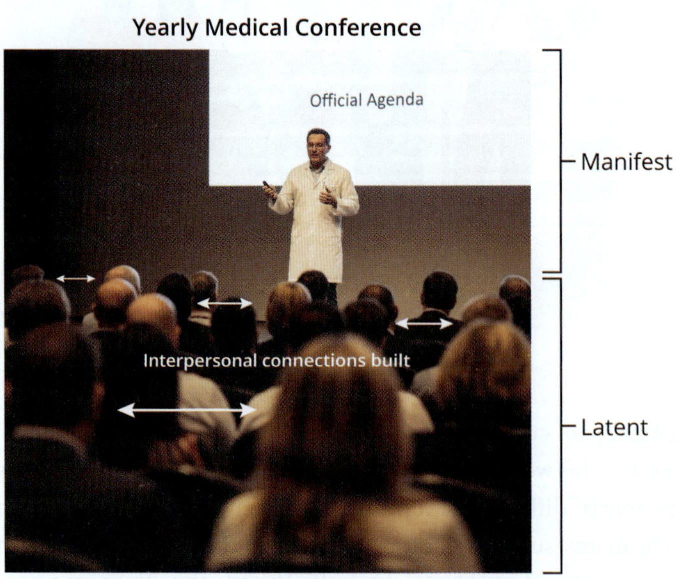

Figure 11.4 Manifest and Latent Functions

Because structural-functionalism focuses on social cohesion and equilibrium, this approach is not well suited for explaining social change. Additionally, while structural-functionalism attempts to explain how groups interact with other groups, it does not explain how individuals interact *within* a group. To understand those kinds of micro-level interactions, other models are better suited.

Feminist Theory

Feminist theory critiques the institutional power structures that disadvantage women in society. Feminist theory was originally an offshoot of conflict theory. From a conflict theory perspective, feminist theory describes society as inherently **patriarchal**, with men seeking to preserve their position of power over women through societal privilege and institutional discrimination. For example, some feminist theorists argue that the study of sociology itself has been historically dominated by a male perspective.

In developed countries, gender stratification and inequality typically lessens, often as a result of the activism of feminist interest groups. However, imbalances of power still exist. In the workplace, for example, the term **glass ceiling** refers to processes that limit the progress of women to the highest job positions because of invisible social barriers to promotion. In contrast, even in cases where men do not seek to climb the job ladder, invisible social forces sometimes push men up to higher positions, a phenomenon called the **glass escalator**. The glass escalator is especially prevalent for men working in traditionally female occupations. Both the glass ceiling and the glass escalator are depicted in Figure 11.5.

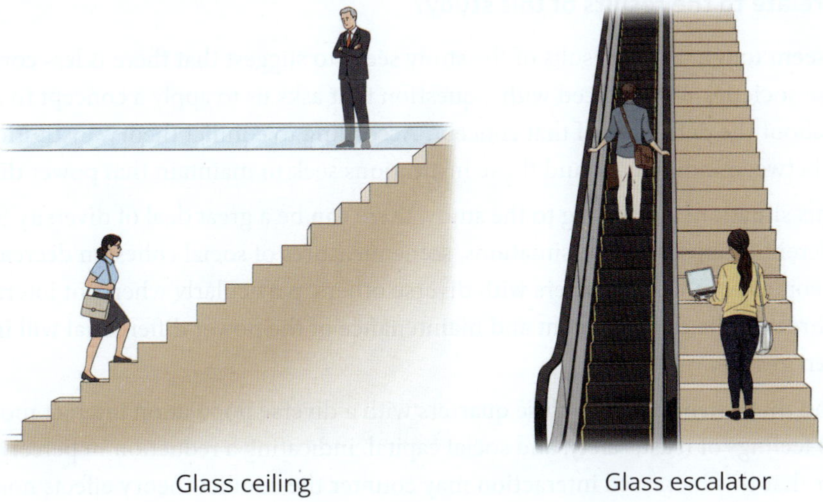

Figure 11.5 The Glass Ceiling and Escalator

BEHAVIORAL SCIENCES GUIDED EXAMPLE WITH EXPERT THINKING

In societies facing increasing amounts of migration and ethnic integration, concerns about intergroup conflicts have prompted research into the effects of diversity on a society as a whole. Previous studies suggest that ethnic diversity negatively impacts social cohesion, but critics have pointed out that historic measures of social cohesion have focused on single indicators such as trust or volunteering.

Older studies demonstrated a negative relationship between diversity and social cohesion, but those are in doubt.

The current study sought to operationalize social cohesion across a more comprehensive set of indicators. Ethnic diversity was found to be associated with lower social cohesion with respect to some indicators, particularly volunteering and feelings of safety, but this trend could not be generalized when including a larger scope of indicators of social cohesion, such as neighborhood social capital or belonging. When heterogeneous groups showed increased contact with one another, subject assessment via survey showed a significant increase in feelings of trust, safety, and social capital.

Several results here. Not only were previous studies possibly wrong, but new results show that integration increases *cohesion. Not an experiment so no experimenter-controlled IV, looking at association only.*

Adapted from: McKenna S, Lee E, Klik KA, Markus A, Hewstone M, Reynolds KJ (2018) Are diverse societies less cohesive? Testing contact and mediated contact theories. *PLoS ONE* 13(3): e0193337. https://doi.org/10.1371/journal.pone.0193337

How does conflict theory relate to the results of this study?

This question at first might seem tough, as the results of the study seem to suggest that there is less conflict than one would expect in more diverse societies. When faced with a question that asks us to apply a concept to a new situation, it's useful to think critically about the definition of that concept. According to conflict theory, institutions arise as a result of power differentials between individuals, and those institutions seek to maintain that power differential.

So where is the conflict in this situation? According to the study, there can be a great deal of diversity in an area that has low interaction between different groups. In those situations, some measures of social cohesion decrease, including feelings of safety. So when people are in close quarters with diverse others, particularly when not interacting with those others regularly, perceived threat to the establishment and maintenance of the power differential will increase, which increases the conflict between groups.

However, the study also found that when people in close quarters with a diverse population interact more with diverse others, they report increased feelings of trust, safety, and social capital, indicating a reduction in perceived threat from other groups. We could infer that this increased interaction may counter the conflict theory effects noted earlier: increased trust and safety reduces fear of others, generally, and fear of loss of power, specifically. With a reduction in perceived threat and increased social cohesion, motivation for conflict should decrease, as power differentials are less threatened or groups are actively integrated into the existing power structure.

So, in summary, conflict theory provides some explanation as to why those who are not interacting with their diverse society may experience more perceived threat and conflict motivation. The study further indicates the perceived threat effect, and possibly societal conflict overall, can be countered by increased social interaction.

Social Institutions

Social institutions are well-established social structures that dictate certain patterns of behavior or relationships and are accepted as a fundamental part of culture. Social institutions regulate the behavior of individuals in core areas of society. For example, family is a social institution that encourages learning of acceptable behavior, socialization, and bonding.

Institutions exist at the meso-level of sociological analysis because they are a part of society, but are not dependent upon the individuals involved—in the United States, the idea of "government" stays basically the same even as the president, senators, representatives, and other officials change. The exact nature of each institution differs from culture to culture, although each institution performs a similar role regardless of culture. Often, institutions are dependent upon and support one another, though competition over resources can bring institutions into conflict. A summary of six of the major social institutions is provided in Table 11.1 at the end of this section.

Family

The definition of **family** differs greatly from culture to culture. For some, the term means "those people to whom I maintain close ties and who are related to me by blood." For others, family is simply "the people who live in my house." In fact, even terms for different family members (such as *sister*, *father*, *cousin*, and so on) are not conserved across time and culture; different **patterns of kinship** may be reflected by these terms. For example, it is common in Hawaiian culture to refer to all family members as *cousins*, while this term would not be used by many other Americans to describe one's mother's brother (the term *uncle* being preferred by many continental Americans). Different patterns of kinship between societies have bearing on responsibility for child rearing, familial loyalty, and even the boundaries of what is considered incest.

Regardless of the definition, family is the most basic of institutions. It is the institution most closely tied to the individual and helps to meet many of our most basic needs, especially when we are young, providing food, shelter, emotional and physical security, and intimacy. Additionally, many life rituals and rites of passage, such as marriage, funerals, and graduations occur in the context of family.

BRIDGE

Families help to meet many of the basic needs at the base of Maslow's hierarchy pyramid. Maslow's hierarchy of needs is discussed in chapter 5 of *MCAT Behavioral Science Review*.

Sociologists studying family relationships may examine the stages of coupling (courtship, cohabitation, engagement, and marriage), changes in relationships between spouses through time, or parenting. Parenting is a complex topic that involves socialization of children; varied definitions of the role of father, mother, and child; and single parenting, same-sex parenting, adoption, and foster parenting. Not all families are composed of a mother, a father, and children. Alternative forms exist, including single-parent families; families that cohabitate with other family members beyond the nuclear family, such as grandparents, aunts, uncles, cousins, godparents, and surrogate kin; and families with marital disunions (divorce). A number of different family structures are illustrated in Figure 11.6.

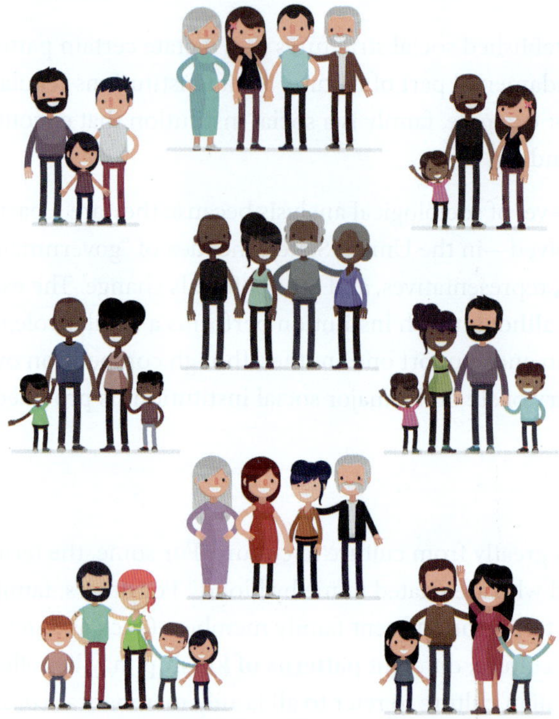

Figure 11.6 Various Family Structures

Divorce rates in the United States rose significantly in the second half of the twentieth century but have started to drop over the last two decades.

While the family can be a source of joy and support, it can also be a source of violence. Spousal abuse (**domestic violence**) is seen across all social classes and genders and can include not only physical violence, but sexual abuse, emotional abuse, and financial abuse. Domestic violence is the #1 cause of injury to American women, and is most common in families with drug abuse, especially alcoholism. Victims of domestic violence may find it challenging to leave the abusive relationship for a variety of reasons, including lack of a safe haven to escape to, financial restrictions, and psychological disorders (consider the connection to learned helplessness, described in Chapter 6 of *MCAT Behavioral Sciences Review*). **Elder abuse** is also seen across all socioeconomic classes, and most commonly manifests as neglect of an older relative—although physical, psychological, and financial abuse may occur as well. The caretaker of the individual is most commonly the source of abuse. Finally, **child abuse** also most commonly manifests as neglect, although physical, sexual, and psychological abuse are also common. During medical school, you will be trained to recognize certain signs suggestive of nonaccidental trauma, such as a broken femur in a child who is too young to have begun walking or burn marks on the buttocks from placing a child in scalding water. As a physician, you will be considered a **mandated reporter**, which means that you are legally required to report suspected cases of elder or child abuse. Domestic abuse does not fall under mandated reporting laws, but counseling and information about shelters for victims of intimate partner violence should be provided.

MCAT EXPERTISE

The MCAT will not expect you to know any specific demographic numbers for the exam, but you should be familiar with some of the recent trends seen in the United States population.

Education

Education, as an institution, aims to provide a population with a set of skills that will be useful to them or to society. In many societies, education is formal—in other words, it takes place in a setting designated for educational purposes using a prescribed curriculum. The function of formal education is to teach skills, facts, and mental processes, but the system also has a social latent function, providing opportunities for peer socialization and reinforcing social stratification, both within individual schools and through comparisons between schools. Education, therefore, includes not only the information and cognitive skills students learn but also the **hidden curriculum** of transmitting social norms, attitudes, and beliefs to students. Sociological investigations into education may focus on the ethics, morals, practices, political influence, finances, and values of an education system. Sociologists also explore educational trends, including grade inflation and deflation, adult education, online education, and accessibility of education.

Performance in the education system depends not only on a student's intrinsic abilities, but also on the education system itself. **Teacher expectancy** refers to the idea that teachers tend to get what they expect from students. Thus, a teacher who places high demands on students—but who also believes that students can rise to the challenge—will more often see students succeed than a teacher who places the same demands but doubts that the students can achieve them. This is an example of a self-fulfilling prophecy, discussed in Chapter 10 of *MCAT Behavioral Sciences Review*, and may be due to differences in how teachers motivate, interact, and offer feedback to their students.

Education is susceptible to inequalities across socioeconomic class. Lower socioeconomic status is associated with decreased accessibility to and quality of education. This is not an easy trend to reverse. Low funding, deprioritization of education, and poor historical performance can make it challenging for a failing school district to acquire resources and improve education to its students.

As mentioned earlier, institutions are intentionally or unintentionally connected, and there is a well-known, persistent association between education and medicine. Health disparities between more educated and less educated individuals are significant, and lack of education may be a hurdle to accessing or trusting healthcare providers.

Religion

As an institution, **religion** is a pattern of social activities organized around a set of beliefs and practices that seek to address the meaning of existence. **Religiosity** refers to how religious one considers oneself to be, and includes strength of religious beliefs, engagement in religious practices, and attitudes about religion itself.

More than 80% of the global population identifies with a religion. Most follow either Christianity or Islam; other world religions include Hinduism, Buddhism, Sikhism, and Judaism. These religions are generally divided into multiple **denominations** or **sects** that may share certain beliefs and practices but not others. A denomination is simply a part of a **church**, a term which can refer both to a large, universal religious group and to the building in which the congregation of such a group meets. Orthodox and Reform are examples of Jewish denominations, and the Sunni and Shia are examples of Islamic denominations. Denominations often coexist, but can come into conflict when their religious beliefs promote opposing values. Whereas the word *sect* was historically a pejorative term, it now refers more properly to a religious group that has chosen to break off from the parent religion. The Amish would be considered a sect of Christianity. In rare cases, a religious sect may take on extreme or deviant philosophies and transform into a **cult**.

As the twenty-first century continues, religious groups—many of which have existed in more or less the same form for thousands of years—grapple with finding a place in contemporary society. For many religious groups, this is reflected by a shift toward modernization within the religion and relaxing historical practices. For others, there is a shift away from religion as society **secularizes**, or moves from a world dominated by religion toward rationality and scientific thinking. For other groups, maintenance of strict adherence to religious code, or **fundamentalism**, predominates.

While spirituality and religion are not equivalent terms, they are often linked to each other because they both seek to understand the meaning of existence and to identify what is sacred. Spirituality and religion may play a role in a patient's understanding of disease, may impact healthcare decisions, and can be an essential component of the patient's coping mechanisms.

Government and Economy

Government and **economy** can be defined as systematic arrangements of political and capital relationships, activities, and social structures that affect rule making, representation of the individual in society, rights and privileges, division of labor, and production of goods and services. Notably, political and economic institutions impact all other institutions to some extent. That is, the government may sanction or define specific family structures, may finance and regulate education, may recognize some religions but not others, and may play a key role in funding and certifying healthcare and medicine. The effects of the economy on institutions can also be viewed from the individual level. For example, when the economy takes a downturn, large swaths of the population may have trouble supporting their families and paying for health insurance. Note that this institutional influence is bidirectional: because of the economic downturn and changes in family, education, or health, an individual may choose to vote a new political candidate into office, or to support or oppose a particular piece of legislation.

While an in-depth exploration of the American (or any other) government is outside the scope of the MCAT, you could be asked to distinguish between different types of government. A **democracy** allows every citizen a political voice, usually through electing representatives to office (i.e., a representative democracy). **Monarchies** include a royal ruler (a king or queen), although the ruler's powers may be significantly limited by the presence of a constitution, a parliamentary system, or some other legislative body. A **dictatorship** is a system where a single person holds power, and usually includes mechanisms to quell threats to this power. A **theocracy** is a system where power is held by religious leaders. Many of these systems of leadership are based around a **charismatic authority** (a leader with a compelling personality).

In comparative economics, the largest division is between capitalist and socialist economies. **Capitalist** economies focus on free market trade and laissez-faire policies, where success or failure in business is primarily driven by consumerism with as little intervention from central governing bodies as possible. In capitalism, a private owner or corporation maintains and profits from the success of the business. Capitalist societies encourage **division of labor**, where specific components of a larger task (say, developing, manufacturing, quality testing, and marketing goods) are separated and assigned to skilled and trained individuals. This promotes specialization and efficiency. **Socialist** economies, on the other hand, treats large industries as collective, shared businesses, and compensation is provided based on the work contribution of each individual into the system. Profit, then, is distributed equally to the workforce. There are many other forms of government and economy, but these would be defined and explained if necessary on Test Day.

Healthcare and Medicine

The institutions of **healthcare** and **medicine** are aimed at maintaining or improving the health status of the individual, family, community, and society as a whole. Healthcare is an ever-changing field, but some of the key goals in American healthcare over the past few decades include:

- Increased access to care
- Decreased costs of healthcare
- Prevention of disease before it occurs
- Association of patients with a primary care physician or a patient-centered medical home
- Increased education for the public with public health outreach
- Decreased paternalism (*doctor knows best* mentality)
- Reduced economic conflicts of interest for physicians
- **Life course approach to health** (maintaining and considering a comprehensive view of the patient's history beyond the immediate presenting symptoms)

There has also been a shift in the role of the patient in the medical system. In the mid-twentieth century, sociologists believed that a patient who is ill takes on what was called the **sick role**. These sociologists believed that such patients are not responsible for their illness and are exempt from normal social roles. But on the other hand, these sociologists also believed that a patient had the obligation to want to become well and to seek out competent help. While this paradigm still exists, patients are now expected to take more ownership of their health through diet, exercise, seeking help before it is needed (through annual primary care visits and screenings), and so on. Modern sociologists also recognize that the notion that patients should feel an obligation to want to become better does not fit patients with chronic, long-term, or permanent conditions.

Even our understanding of disease has shifted over time. On the one hand, many ordinary parts of the human condition, including the full range of sexual orientations and gender identities, are no longer defined as medical conditions, as they misguidedly were in earlier editions of the DSM. On the other hand, other types of behaviors have become **medicalized**, meaning that they are now defined and treated as medical conditions. This latter shift can be seen in the addition of a number of diagnostic entities to the DSM-5, such as hoarding disorder and binge eating disorder.

The medical community also now recognizes that health is not only characterized by physiological wellness or disease, but also by a person's subjective experience of their health. The phrase **illness experience** refers to the ways in which people, rather than doctors, define and adjust to changes in their health. For example, people can experience disease without illness, as is the case for someone living a full and productive life with a manageable condition such as HIV. People can also experience illness without disease, such as when a person experiences somatic symptoms as a result of psychological stress.

Sociologists studying healthcare are often interested in **social epidemiology**. Epidemiology is the study of health and its determinants within a society (discussed in detail in Chapter 12 of *MCAT Behavioral Sciences Review*); social epidemiology is specifically the study of the effects of institutions, social structures, and relationships on health. Social epidemiologists study the effects of racial and economic inequality or government safety net legislation on health and access to healthcare. They might also be interested in how social conditions early in life affect healthcare outcomes later.

In addition, many sociologists investigate medical ethics. In the United States, physicians are expected to adhere to four key tenets of medical ethics:

- **Beneficence:** the physician has a responsibility to act in the patient's best interest.
- **Nonmaleficence:** *do no harm*; the physician has a responsibility to avoid treatments or interventions in which the potential for harm outweighs the potential for benefit.
- **Respect for patient autonomy:** the physician has a responsibility to respect patients' decisions and choices about their own healthcare. While there are exceptions to this rule (significant psychiatric illness interfering with decision-making capacity, children, public health threats), patients do have the right to refuse life-saving therapies.
- **Justice:** the physician has a responsibility to treat similar patients with similar care, and to distribute healthcare resources fairly.

Social Institution	Needs Met by Institution	Statuses	Values	Norms
Education	Transmit knowledge and skills across generations	Teacher, student, dean, principal	Academic honesty, good grades	Doing homework, preparing for lectures, being kind to other students
Family	Regulate reproduction, socialize and protect children	Father, mother, son, daughter, brother, sister, uncle, aunt, grandparent	Sexual fidelity, providing for children, keeping a clean home, respect for caregivers	Having as many children as one desires, being faithful to one's spouse
Religion	Concerns about life and death, the meaning of suffering and loss, desire to connect with a creator	Clergy, worshipper, teacher, disciple, missionary, prophet, convert	God and holy texts should be honored	Going to services, following teachings of the religion, applying beliefs outside of worship
Government	Maintain social order, enforce laws	President, senator, lobbyist, voter, candidate	Transparency, accountability, professionalism	Acting in the best interest of constituents, debating political issues
Economy	Organize money, goods, and services	Worker, boss, buyer, seller, creditor, debtor, advertiser	Making money, paying bills on time, producing efficiently	Maximizing profits, *the customer is always right*, working hard
Medicine	Heal the sick and injured, care for the dying	Doctor, nurse, pharmacist, insurer, patient	Hippocratic oath, staying in good health, following care providers' recommendations	Beneficence, nonmaleficence, respect for autonomy, justice

Table 11.1 Social Institutions

MCAT CONCEPT CHECK 11.1

Before you move on, assess your understanding of the material with these questions.

1. What are manifest and latent functions?

   - Manifest functions:

   ____

   - Latent functions:

   ____

2. For each of the theoretical approaches listed below, what is the primary thesis or idea of the theory?

Theoretical Approach	Primary Thesis or Idea
Functionalism	
Conflict theory	
Symbolic interactionism	
Social constructionism	
Rational choice-exchange theory	
Feminist theory	

3. What are the four key tenets of American medical ethics? Provide a short description of each.

Ethical Principle	Description

11.2 Culture

LEARNING OBJECTIVES

After Chapter 11.2, you will be able to:

- Distinguish between material and symbolic culture
- Recall the definitions of, and the differences between, the values, beliefs, norms, and rituals of a culture

The study of culture is likely the most diverse and complex dimension within sociology. **Culture** can be defined as encompassing the entire lifestyle for a given group. It binds our nation-states, political institutions, marketplaces, religions, and ideologies. Culture flavors our interpretations of the world, and is generally passed through familial lines. In short, culture is what makes human societies unique from one another.

BRIDGE

A description of culture in the context of group processes is described in Chapter 8 of *MCAT Behavioral Sciences Review.*

MCAT EXPERTISE

Ethnography is the study of cultures and customs, and **ethnographic methods** are experimental methods used to study the ethnicity or culture of a group.

Material and Symbolic Culture

Sociologists view culture according to two different categories: material culture and symbolic culture.

BRIDGE

Symbols are also discussed in Chapter 6 of *MCAT Behavioral Sciences Review.*

Material Culture

One can discern a lot about people by looking at their **artifacts**: material items that they make, possess, and value. This examination surrounds **material culture**, which includes the physical items one associates with a given group, such as artwork, emblems, clothing, jewelry, foods, buildings, and tools. Sociologists explore the meaning of these objects to a given society.

An example of material culture in the United States is the American flag. This item is used to reinforce a sense of belonging via shared American citizenship. Other symbols that are considered traditionally American include barbecue, baseball, apple pie, and rock and roll.

Material culture is often most visible during ceremonies, such as birthdays, weddings, and funerals. Some artifacts of traditional Indian material culture are shown in Figure 11.7.

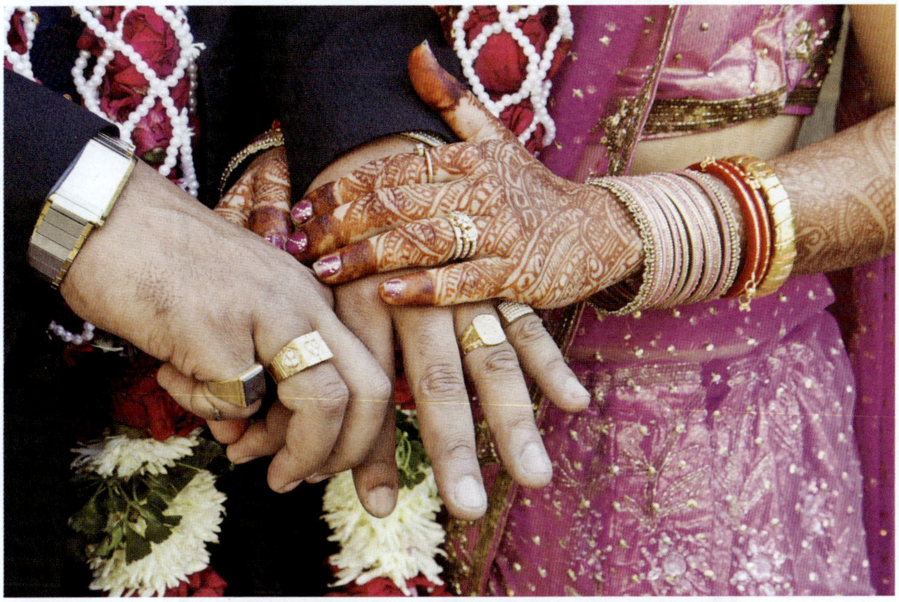

Figure 11.7 Material Culture
Material culture includes objects important to a group, including clothing, jewelry, cuisine, ceremonial objects, and so on.

Symbolic Culture

Symbolic culture, also called **nonmaterial culture**, focuses on the ideas that represent a group of people. These may be encoded in mottos, songs, or catchphrases, or may simply be themes that are pervasive in the culture. Phrases like *free enterprise* and *life, liberty, and the pursuit of happiness* are examples of American symbolic culture. Material culture is often the tangible embodiment of the underlying ideas of symbolic culture.

KEY CONCEPT

Material culture is associated with artifacts (objects). Symbolic culture is associated with ideas.

For any social group to remain connected over time, there must be a culture that binds its members together. In times of war and crisis, governments often draw upon symbolic culture to rally people to action, using songs, parades, discussion of heroes past, and so on, as shown in Figure 11.8. It is not a coincidence that most high schools have a school mascot, school colors, and a school song. Such cultural artifacts are in place to help create a shared sense of identity, loyalty, and belonging. Symbolic culture includes both cognitive and behavioral components; that is, it informs cultural values and beliefs, as well as cultural norms and communication styles.

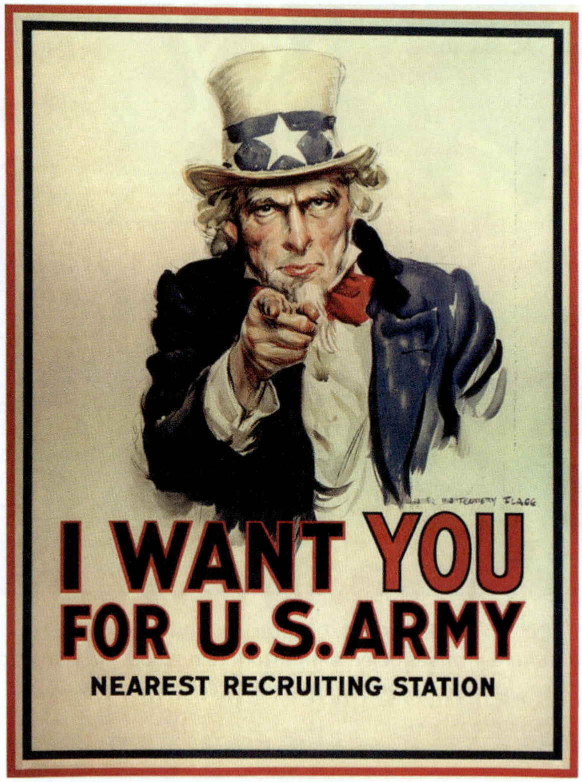

Figure 11.8 Symbolic Culture
Symbolic culture includes ideas that identify a culture; it may be drawn upon to encourage loyalty or patriotism, as shown here.

Symbolic culture is usually slower to change than material culture, which can lead to the phenomenon of **culture lag**. The expansion of devices and technology in contemporary times are prototypical examples of culture lag: whereas American culture still prizes individuality and privacy, the development of smartphones and social media push toward a more community-oriented and less private world. Still, there is evidence that symbolic culture is beginning to change in response to these technological (material) innovations: younger generations appear to be less concerned about what personal information is publicly accessible than older generations.

Language

Language is the most highly developed and complex symbol system used by most cultures. Language consists of spoken, written, or signed symbols, which are regulated according to certain rules of grammar and syntax. Language enables us to share our ideas, thoughts, experiences, discoveries, fears, plans, and desires with others. Written language extends our capacity to communicate across both spatial and temporal boundaries. Without language, it would be difficult to transmit culture. Understanding a group's language is critical to understanding its culture.

BRIDGE

Language is critically important in the transmission of culture. It requires a complex interplay of multiple brain circuits, which are discussed in Chapter 4 of *MCAT Behavioral Sciences Review*.

Values, Beliefs, Norms, and Rituals

An important component of culture are the rules that structure society. **Values** are what a person deems important in life, which dictates one's ethical principles and standards of behavior. A **belief** is something that an individual accepts to be truth. Every culture has its own beliefs and value systems. This will be important in your future career, as patients tend to carry their beliefs into the healthcare system. For example, as described in the chapter introduction, some Asian cultures believe that healthcare decisions should be the responsibility of a patient's family, which avoids burdening the patient (who is already ill) with having to make such a decision. This belief is in direct contrast to the American belief that patient autonomy should be prized and that healthcare decisions should be made by a patient whenever possible. These conflicts can prove challenging to healthcare professionals, and there is not always one correct answer to such dilemmas. Such situations—when a cultural difference impedes interaction with others—are called **cultural barriers**.

As described in Chapter 8 of *MCAT Behavioral Sciences Review*, **norms** are societal rules that define the boundaries of acceptable behavior. While norms are not laws, they do govern the behavior of many individuals in society and provide a sense of social control. Norms are what provide us with a sense of what is appropriate, what we should do, and what we should not do. Norms exist for behavior, speech, dress, home life, and more.

A **ritual** is a formalized ceremony that usually involves specific material objects, symbolism, and additional mandates on acceptable behavior. Rituals tend to have a prescribed order of events or routine. These rituals can be associated with specific milestones, such as a baby-naming, graduation ceremony, wedding, or funeral; with holidays, such as a Thanksgiving dinner, trick-or-treating on Halloween, or a Passover seder, shown in Figure 11.9; or with regular activities, such as a Catholic mass, a pregame pep rally, or even just getting ready in the morning (showering, brushing teeth, eating breakfast, and so on).

REAL WORLD

Many health systems have an ethics board to deal with conflicts that may arise from differences in belief systems between patient and practitioner, among other ethical issues. These committees tend to facilitate discussion, rather than simply issuing a decision.

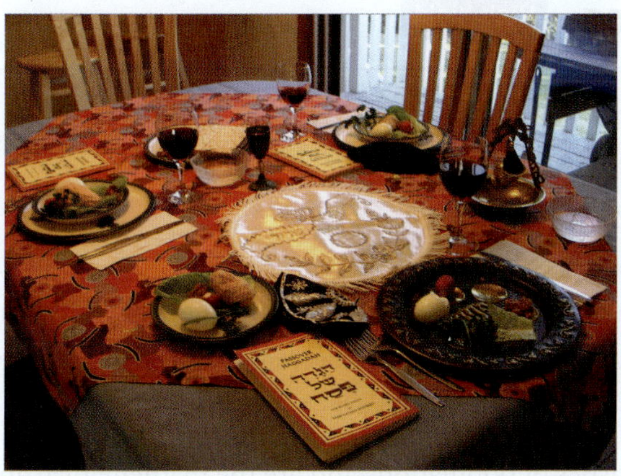

Figure 11.9 A Passover Seder Is an Example of a Ritual
Seder means "order" in Hebrew; most rituals have a specific order of events.

Evolution and Human Culture

Evolution may have selected for the development of culture. Culture serves as a method of passing down information from generation to generation; in prehistoric times, the transmission of information through culture served to teach future generations how to create tools, hunt, domesticate animals, and grow crops.

Culture also creates a sense of loyalty and allegiance, which, as described in Chapter 10 of *MCAT Behavioral Sciences Review*, may help explain altruistic behavior. Finally, culture creates a sense of *us vs. them*, which presumably served a role in the dispersion of populations across the globe in different environmental niches.

Culture, in turn, may also influence evolution. There is evidence that some genetic traits may have been favored because of cultural values and beliefs. For example, human beings—at least those who are not lactose intolerant—are the only animals that are able to digest milk after adolescence; they are also the only animals that ingest another animal's milk. These evolutionary adaptations may have arisen out of Northern European cultures, which relied heavily on cattle farming for sustenance. A mutation permitting digestion of milk into adulthood presumably imparted a nutritional and survival advantage to certain individuals, and would thus be retained within the population.

MCAT CONCEPT CHECK 11.2

Before you move on, assess your understanding of the material with these questions.

1. What are material and symbolic culture?
   - Material culture:

   ____

   - Symbolic culture:

   ____

2. What is the difference between a value and a belief?

   ____

11.3 Demographics **High Yield**

LEARNING OBJECTIVES

After Chapter 11.3, you will be able to:

- Distinguish between race and ethnicity
- Describe symbolic ethnicity
- Describe fertility rate, birth rate, and mortality rate and how they shift during a demographic transition
- Recall examples of proactive and reactive social movements and how the two types of movements differ

Demographics refer to the statistics of populations and are the mathematical applications of sociology. Demographics can be gathered informally, such as a professor asking how many freshmen, sophomores, juniors, and seniors are in a given course, or may be gathered formally. For example, the United States Census Bureau gathers demographic data about every individual in the country every ten years.

Common Demographic Categories

Demographers can classify individuals based on hundreds of different criteria. The MCAT will not expect you to know advanced topics within demographics, but familiarity with some of the common demographic categories as well as their implications on society and healthcare are important. In this section, we'll explore age, gender, race and ethnicity, sexual orientation, and immigration status.

Age

Aging is a inevitable process experienced by all people around the world. In this section we will explore the implications of an individual's age on healthcare, then dive deeper into its implications on society.

Considering an individual's age and cumulative life experiences when analyzing their personality, social status, health, and other social metrics is known as the **life course perspective** (sometimes referred to as the **life course approach**). Figure 11.10 visualizes the stages of life commonly delineated in this perspective. For example, in healthcare, a psychiatrist may consider a patient's early life events and how those events continue to impact a patient's condition. Or perhaps a general practitioner chooses to conduct additional lung screenings on a patient who previously worked in a coal mine. In both these examples, the physician is incorporating the life course perspective into the treatment of the patient.

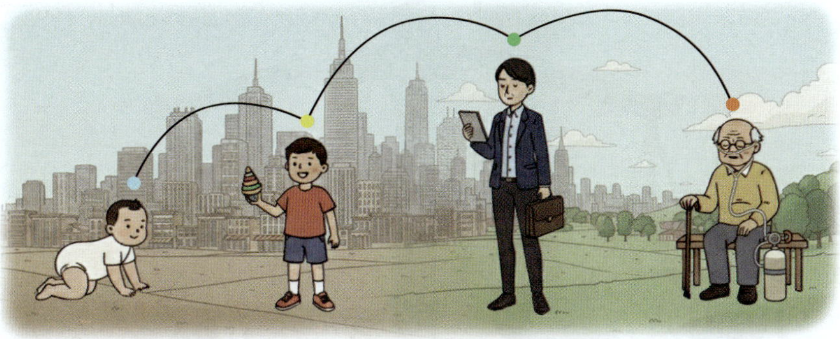

Figure 11.10 The Life Course Perspective

With the potentially large difference in the experiences between age cohorts, prejudice or discrimination based on a person's age can arise. This is known as **ageism** and can be seen at all ages. For example, young professionals entering the workplace are often viewed as being inexperienced, and their opinions and ideas may therefore be ignored or downplayed. Older individuals may be perceived as frail, vulnerable, or less intelligent, and may thus be treated with less respect.

In order to understand and analyze age-related differences, researchers can group individuals based on their age or birth year; these groupings are known as **age cohorts** (sometimes called generational cohorts). The utility of age cohorts goes beyond understanding the differences of an individual's life course, as they allow researchers to look at a population at a macroscopic level. An analysis of a population's distribution among its age cohorts can predict demographic shifts, such as an aging population, the shift from a developing to developed economy, or a stable population. We'll explore examples of each below.

In the United States, many sociologists document a "graying of America" as the Baby Boomer generation ages. The term Baby Boomer stems from the large spike in fertility rates (birth rates) after World War II, or in other words, a "boom of babies." Due to the baby boom spanning from the 1940s to 1960s, over 70 million Americans will be 65 or older by 2030, representing nearly 20 percent of the population. Thus, the fastest-growing age cohort in the United States is the 85-or-older group. This has profound effects on healthcare: more than 40 percent of adult patients in acute care hospital beds are 65 or older. Considering this shift in demographics, government programs such as Medicare and Social Security will experience increased demand, which may pose challenges for these programs.

This situation is an application of the **dependency ratio**, which is the ratio of the number of members of a population that are not in the workforce to the number of members that are in the workforce. This ratio depends on two components, the youth ratio and age dependency ratio. The **youth ratio** is defined by the number of people under the age of 15 divided by the number of people aged 15–65. The **age dependency ratio** is defined by the number of people over 65 divided by the number of people aged 15–65. Applied to societies, the dependency ratio quantifies the economic burden felt by the working age population (15–65) in order to support the portion of the population outside of the workforce (under 15 and over 65). The dependency ratio is represented in Figure 11.11.

REAL WORLD

The demographic tool of age cohorts has woven its way into our everyday language. If you've heard terms like the Silent Generation, Baby Boomers, Generation X, Millennial (Generation Y), and Generation Z, then you've encountered age cohorts. These generational terms group individuals by their birth year. However, age cohorts can be used to group individuals based on their current age, such as 0–14, 15–30, etc.

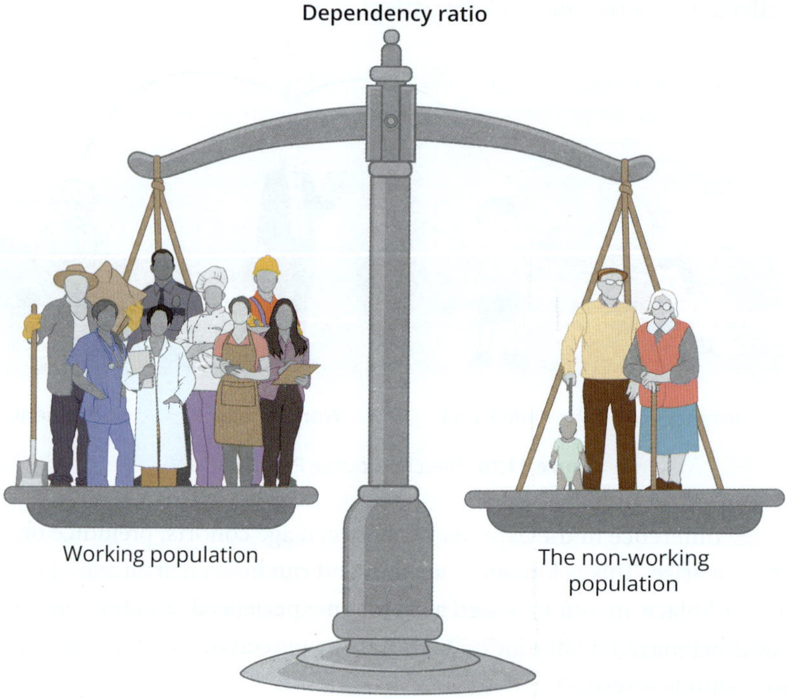

Figure 11.11 The Dependency Ratio

In contrast to the United States, developing countries, such as Uganda, see the reverse trend with 48% of the population being under the age of 15 years old, resulting in a dependency ratio of about 1 (2% of the population is 65 years and over, which means the dependent population roughly equals the working age population). This can be explained by the country's steadily dropping infant mortality rate over the last several decades. Forecasting the next 10 to 20 years for Uganda would predict a large proportion of the population entering the working-age age cohort. Although this may lead to an increase in the country's economic productivity, this demographic shift must be matched with job growth. If that does not occur, unemployment rates will increase, which could lead to civil unrest or other negative outcomes. This shift from developing to developed country is explained by demographic transition theory, covered later in this chapter.

Finally, when a population's fertility rate and mortality rate remain relatively consistent over a long period of time, the distribution of the population among the age cohorts remains fairly constant. This is known as a **stable population**.

Gender

Sex and gender are not synonymous terms. **Sex** is a biological category. In many species, including humans, a phenotypical female is an individual that produces the larger gamete (the ovum) and carries offspring. **Gender** refers to a society's notions of femininity, masculinity, and other sexual identities. Gender is therefore a socially constructed set of ideas about what it means to be male, female, or otherwise in a given culture. A culture's ideas about gender usually include expected behavioral traits associated with a particular sex. These expected behavioral traits are known as **gender roles**. As such, gender roles are also social constructs. Once an individual understands these socially constructed behavioral expectations, an individual can adopt behaviors that project the gender that individual wishes to portray, which is known as the individual's **gender identity**.

Gender segregation is the separation of individuals based on perceived gender. Such segregation includes divisions of male, female, and gender-neutral bathrooms, or separating male and female sports teams. Differences between genders and the phenomenon of gender segregation do not necessarily imply inequality, although inequality can occur. **Gender inequality** is the intentional or unintentional empowerment of one gender to the detriment of others. In the presence of gender inequality, gender stratification may occur. **Gender stratification** is defined as any inequality in access to social resources that is based on gender, and is an example of social stratification in general, which will be studied in Chapter 12 of *MCAT Behavioral Sciences Review*. To illustrate the difference between gender segregation and gender stratification: Single-gender schools are an example of gender segregation. Children enrolled in such schools do not necessarily receive unequal qualities of education. However, if there is a systemic difference in resource allocation between single-gender schools, the result is uneven access to resources, leading to gender stratification.

REAL WORLD

Certain racial and ethnic groups have a higher incidence of specific health problems. For example, the Chinese population accounts for a disproportionate number of chronic hepatitis B infections and liver cancer. Mediterranean and African populations have a significantly higher rate of hemoglobinopathies (diseases related to hemoglobin). The Ashkenazi Jewish population has a higher rate of autoimmune diseases. Some American Indian populations are associated with gallbladder and biliary tree diseases. Being of a particular race or ethnicity is not necessary for the development of any disease, but may certainly be associated with increased risk.

Race and Ethnicity

The definition of race has changed through recent history, and continues to change. The term originally referred to speakers of a common language, and later indicated national origin. However, the term has also historically been used to denote certain shared phenotypic similarities between people. The five racial categories currently recognized by the U.S. Census exemplify these shifting definitions of race. These categories are: White, Black, Asian, American Indian or Alaskan native, and Native Hawaiian/Pacific Islander. Observe that some of these racial categories, like White and Black, describe phenotypic similarities, while other categories, like American Indian and Pacific Islander, are based on national origin. Furthermore, no other country uses these same five racial labels, and in fact the officially recognized races differ in each country. So, there is no uniform agreement about racial categories; rather each society generates its own racial labels, making race a social construct. The social process by which racial groups are associated with specific attributes or characteristics is called **racialization**.

If race is not consistently defined, then why do sociologists concern themselves with this concept? The answer is that racial labels, though socially constructed, do materially affect the lives of people through institutionalized practices of preference and discrimination. In order to define race more scientifically, sociologists specify that the term **race** refers to socially constructed groupings of people based specifically on inherited phenotypic characteristics. Note that the human history of migration and mixing of populations means that there are few if any genetically isolated people left on earth. So sociologists recognize that scientifically categorizing people by genetic differences is not possible. Nevertheless, societies continue to generate racial labels based on perceived phenotypic differences, and so sociologists study how each society treats its socially defined racial groups.

An important takeaway from the above discussion is that sociologists narrow the definition of the term race to refer specifically to attempts to group people by phenotypic difference. However, sociologists recognize that societies also group people by shared language, cultural heritage, religion, and/or national origin. The term sociologists use for these types of groupings is **ethnicity**. While certain ethnicities are often associated with certain racial labels, race and ethnicity are distinct. Here is an illustration of the difference: African American individuals, African immigrants, and West Indian immigrants speak different languages and express different cultural norms. These three groups represent three different ethnicities. However, due to some phenotypic similarities shared by some members of these groups, individuals in these groups would generally be given the same racial label. Like race, ethnicity is also a social construct, in that ethnic labels and the criteria for inclusion in a certain ethnic group change from society to society and change over time.

Symbolic ethnicity describes a specific connection to one's ethnicity in which ethnic symbols and identity remain important, even when ethnic identity does not play a significant role in everyday life. For example, many Irish Americans in the United States celebrate their heritage only one day per year: St. Patrick's Day. In all other facets of life, these individuals' Irish-American ethnicity does not play a significant role. Other examples include attending folk festivals, visiting specific cultural locales for holidays, or participating in an ethnic celebration.

It is important to consider how race and ethnicity may affect one's ability to receive proper healthcare. The Agency for Healthcare Research and Quality (AHRQ), a government agency, reports that race and ethnicity influence a patient's chance of receiving many specific procedures and treatments. Whether due to conscious or unconscious bias, there is evidence that different races are not always offered the same level of care escalation in a medical emergency.

BRIDGE

Many public health outreach efforts are aimed at closing the gap in health disparities between populations. Health and healthcare disparities are discussed in Chapter 12 of *MCAT Behavioral Sciences Review.*

On the other hand, there are a number of public health outreach projects that target at-risk racial or ethnic populations through education, screening, and treatment. These specific strategies are geared to close gaps in health disparities. Many large university health systems run free clinics in local neighborhoods and may target specific populations; for example, some of these clinics will staff Spanish-speaking doctors and medical students to cater to the Hispanic immigrant population.

Sexual Orientation

Sexual orientation can be defined as the direction of one's sexual interest. In scientific and healthcare communities, sexual orientation has historically been divided into three categories:

- **Heterosexual**: attraction to individuals of a different sex
- **Bisexual** (or pansexual): attraction to members of multiple sexes
- **Homosexual**: attraction to individuals of the same sex

Sexual orientation involves a person's sexual feelings and may or may not be a significant contributor to that person's sense of identity. It may or may not be evident in the person's appearance or behavior. Disclosure of minority sexual orientations, sometimes called *coming out of the closet*, can be a major milestone in the absorption of sexuality into one's identity. This disclosure has also been shown sometimes to have therapeutic effects: coming out is associated with decreases in depressive and anxious symptoms linked to cortisol levels and stress.

Human sexuality continues to be an important area of research for psychologists, sociologists, and biologists alike, but evidence shows that sexuality is likely more fluid than previously believed. Alfred Kinsey was a pioneer in this area, and—in addition to a number of other models and publications—described sexuality on a zero to six scale, with zero representing exclusive heterosexuality and six representing exclusive homosexuality. When ranked on this **Kinsey scale**, few people actually fell into the categories of zero and six, with a significant proportion of the population falling somewhere between the two.

Sexual and gender identity minorities are often grouped together under the umbrella term **LGBTQ** (lesbian, gay, bisexual, transgender, and queer or questioning). In some cases, this acronym has been expanded to include other self-definitions of sexuality and sexual identity, including I (intersex) or A (asexual).

Several health disparities have been recognized within the LGBTQ community. The most significant historical disparity is HIV, which disproportionately affected individuals who are gay in urban environments during the early 1980s. While the prevalence of HIV is still slightly higher in men who have sex with men (MSM), it exists in all populations. Efforts to encourage safe sex and increase screening have helped to slow the epidemic of HIV, as has increased awareness of those with HIV/AIDS with projects like the AIDS Memorial Quilt, shown in Figure 11.12. Within the healthcare system, individuals who are lesbian receive less screening for cervical cancer and may not be screened for other sexually transmitted infections. Individuals who are transgender have multiple areas of increased risk, including off-label or unsupervised use of "street hormones" without proper counseling on their side effects.

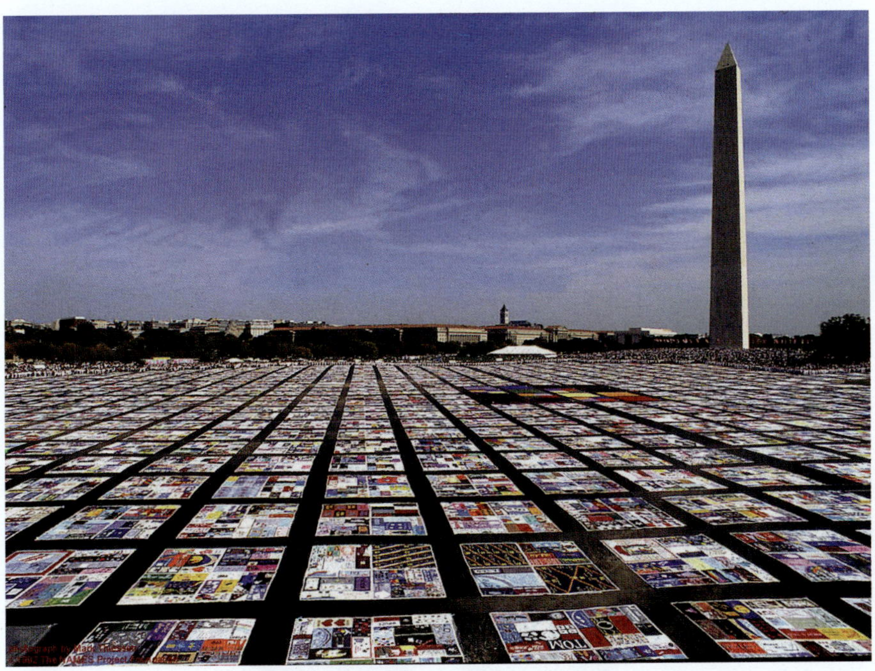

Figure 11.12 The AIDS Memorial Quilt

Mental health disparities are also common in the LGBTQ community. LGBTQ youth are at significantly higher risk for bullying, victimization, and violence, and have higher rates of suicide. In adults, the LGBTQ population has a higher prevalence of depression and anxiety than their heterosexual and cisgender counterparts. In addition, men who are gay have an increased rate of eating disorders as compared to men who are heterosexual. A host of campaigns and outreach efforts have begun to target these disparities.

Immigration Status

According to the US Census Bureau, the nation's total recent immigrant population is growing rapidly; it was quantified at 40.4 million in 2011 and is expected to increase by roughly 20 million in the next two decades. This tells us that immigrants, whether documented or undocumented, are interwoven into every social structure and institution in the United States. The nativity of immigrant populations changes over time; in the most recent census, the largest proportions of immigrants had emigrated from Mexico, the Caribbean, and India. **Generational status** refers to the place of birth of a specific person or that person's parents. For instance, first generation refers to someone who is born outside of their place of residence. Second generation refers to a person that has at least one parent that is foreign-born.

Considering the number of immigrant communities, there are often barriers that affect interactions with social structures and institutions. The complex organization of the United States healthcare system is starkly different from those of most other nations, and this may present a barrier to use for immigrants. Language barriers may also make it difficult for immigrants to access healthcare or to take control of their healthcare decisions; telephone translation services have been created to help facilitate the conversation between clinician and patient. Racial and ethnic identity may be more apparent in first-generation immigrants, and the biases and prejudices against certain racial and ethnic groups might be compounded by the individual's immigrant status; this interplay between multiple demographic factors—especially when it leads to discrimination or oppression—is termed **intersectionality** (Figure 11.13). Finally, undocumented status presents a major barrier for many immigrants to access healthcare for fear of reporting and deportation.

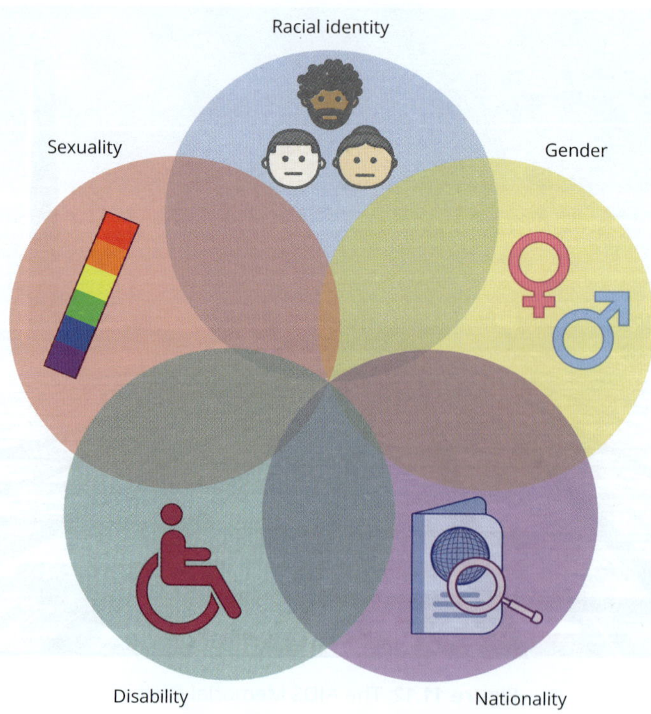

Figure 11.13 Intersectionality

Demographic Shifts and Social Change

Since 1950, the United States population has roughly doubled. In addition to increasing in size, the makeup of the American population has changed significantly. The average age in the United States has increased, and the population is continuing to become more racially and ethnically diverse. These are examples of **demographic shifts**: changes in the makeup of a population over time. These shifts can be measured by considering the **population density**, which counts the number of people per square kilometer of land area.

Population projections attempt to predict changes in population size over time, and can be assisted by historical measures of growth, understanding of changes in social structure, and analysis of other demographic information. To aid in the construction of population projections, **population pyramids** provide a histogram of the population size of various age cohorts, as shown in Figure 11.14.

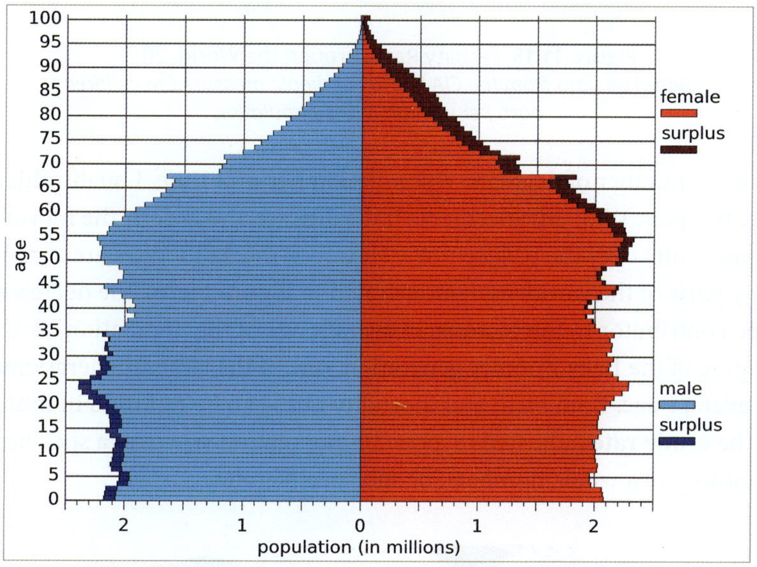

Figure 11.14 U.S. Population Pyramid, 2014
Surplus occurs when one gender has a larger population than another.

Fertility, Mortality, and Migration

The increased population of the United States is due to a number of factors that center around fertility, mortality, and migration. **Fertility rate** refers to the average number of children born to a woman over a lifetime in a population. In many parts of the world, fertility rate is the primary driver of population expansion; for example, in some parts of Africa, the average fertility rate is between four and eight children per woman, as seen in Figure 11.15. In the United States, fertility rates have trended downward over time; in 2013, the rate was still above two, indicating that fertility rates were still contributing to population growth.

KEY CONCEPT

Demographic statistics:

- Fertility rate = children per woman per lifetime
- Birth rate = children per 1000 people per year
- Mortality rate = deaths per 1000 people per year
- Migration rate = immigration rate minus emigration rate

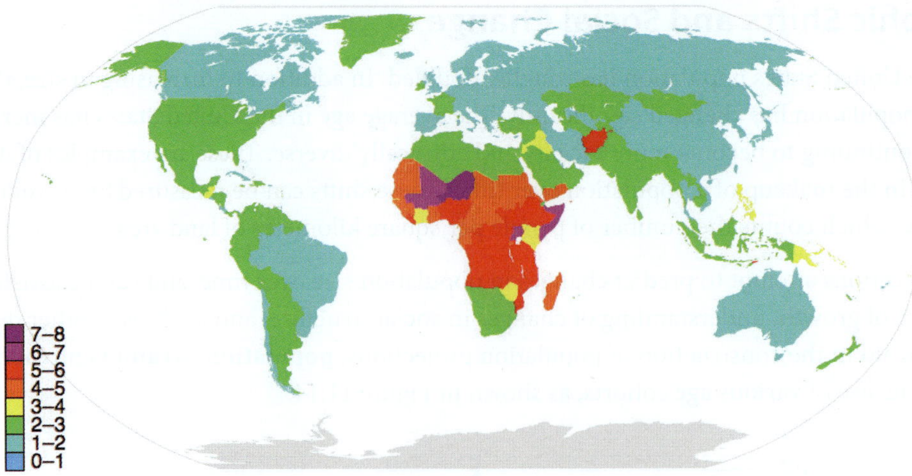

Figure 11.15 Fertility Rates around the World, 2013
Based on data from the CIA World Factbook; measured in children born per woman in the population

Mortality rates refer to the number of deaths in a population per unit time. Usually, this rate is measured in deaths per 1000 people per year. With advancements in healthcare and access, the mortality rate in the United States has dropped significantly over the past century. However, mortality rates are a significant brake on population growth in many parts of the world, as demonstrated in Figure 11.16. The decreased mortality rate in the United States is one contributor to the increase in average age of the population, as is a decreased fertility rate. In addition, the aging of the Baby Boomer generation, one of the largest generations in United States history, increases this average age. Both birth and mortality rates can be reported in multiple forms: the total rate for a population, the **crude rate** (adjusted to a certain population size over a specific period of time and multiplied by a constant to give a whole number), or age-specific rates.

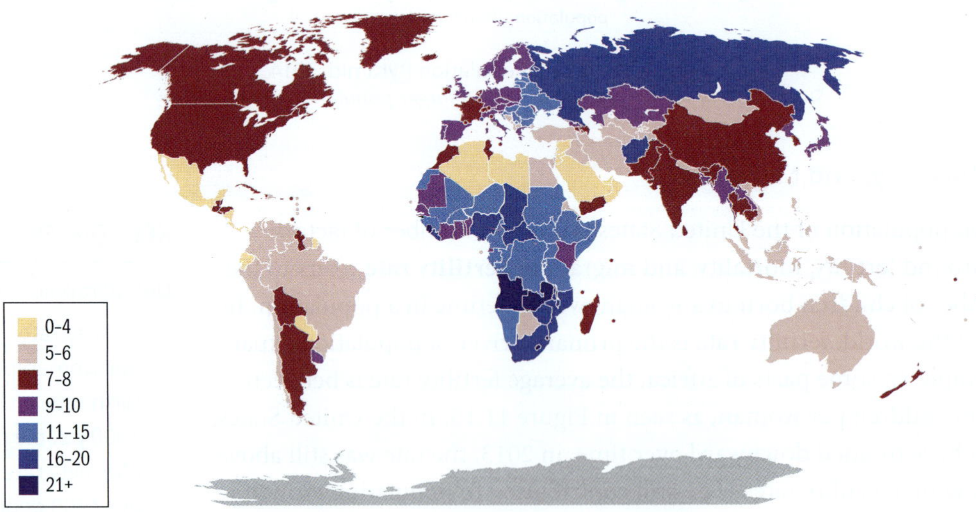

Figure 11.16 Mortality Rates around the World, 2009
Based on data from the CIA World Factbook; measured in deaths per 1000 individuals per year

Finally, **migration** is a contributor to population growth. **Immigration** is defined as movement into a new geographic space, whereas **emigration** is movement away from a geographic space. As described earlier, the United States continues to have larger net immigration than emigration, driving an increase in the population size. Immigration also increases the racial and ethnic diversity of the United States, as do increased mobility within the country and increases in intermarriage between different races and ethnicities. Migration can be motivated by both **pull factors**, which are positive attributes of the new location that attract new residents (for example, education and economic opportunity), and **push factors**, which are negative attributes of the old location that encourage existing residents to leave (for example, war and famine). Both pull factors and push factors are visualized in Figure 11.17.

KEY CONCEPT

The United States population is getting bigger, older (average age has increased), and more diverse (through immigration, mobility, and intermarriage).

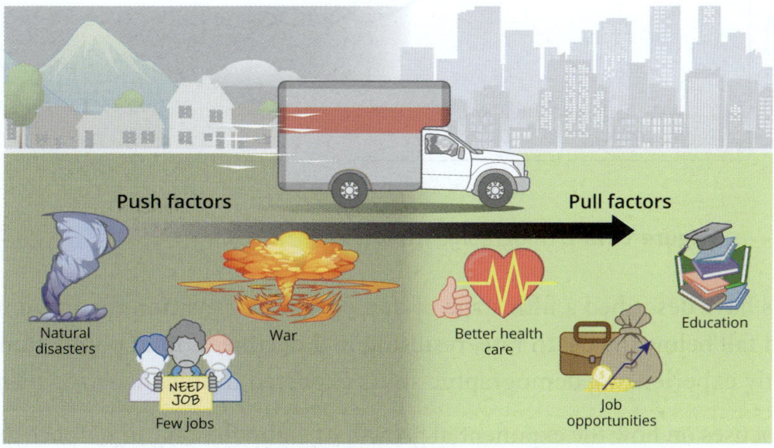

Figure 11.17 The Push and Pull Factors of Migration

Demographic Transition Theory

While demographic shift refers to general changes in population makeup over time, **demographic transition** is a specific example of a demographic shift that occurs as a country develops from a preindustrial, or agrarian, society to an economy that is more centered on manufacturing, which is termed **industrialization**. Demographic transition has been seen in the United States since the Industrial Revolution and is currently occurring in many developing countries. **Demographic transition theory** explains this link between economic development and demographic shift in four stages:

- **Stage 1**: Preindustrial society; birth and death rates are both high, resulting in a stable population.
- **Stage 2**: Economic progress leads to improvements to healthcare, nutrition, sanitation, and wages, causing a decrease in death rates. Thus, total population increases.
- **Stage 3**: Improvements in contraception, women's rights, and a shift from an agricultural to an industrial economy cause birth rates to drop. For example, with an industrializing society, children must go to school for many years to be productive in society and may need to be supported by parents for a longer period of time than was formerly the case. Thus families have fewer children, and birth rates drop. As birth and death rates equalize, population growth hits an inflection point and begins to level off.
- **Stage 4**: An industrialized society; birth and death rates are both low, resulting in a relative constant total population.

A model of demographic transition can be seen in Figure 11.18.

KEY CONCEPT

During demographic transition, mortality rate drops before birth rate. Therefore, the population grows at first while mortality rate is dropping, and then plateaus as the birth rate decreases as well.

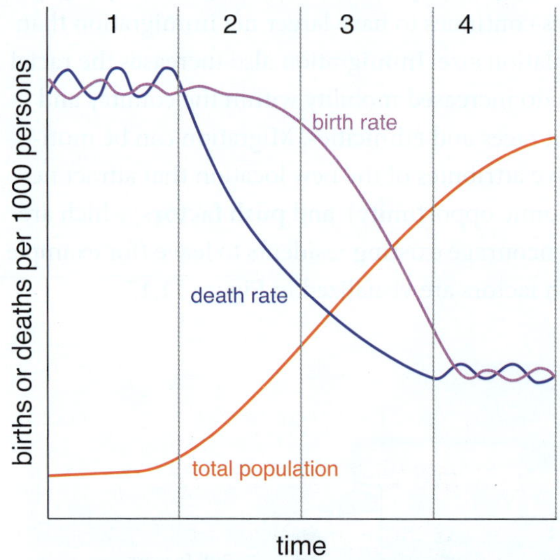

Figure 11.18 Demographic Transition

Recently, sociologists have described a fifth stage of demographic transition theory in which birth rates continue to drop and fall below the death rate, resulting in a decline of total population. Japan and Germany are currently experiencing demographic shifts expected in this theorized fifth stage.

Malthusian theory focuses on how the exponential growth of a population can outpace growth of the food supply and lead to social degradation and disorder. For example, some theorists predict that demographic transition among developing nations might cause growth in the world's population to outpace the world's ability to generate food. The resulting hypothetical mass starvation is called the Malthusian catastrophe (Figure 11.19). This result is similar to the death phase of bacterial growth, when resources in the environment have been depleted, as described in Chapter 1 of *MCAT Biology Review*.

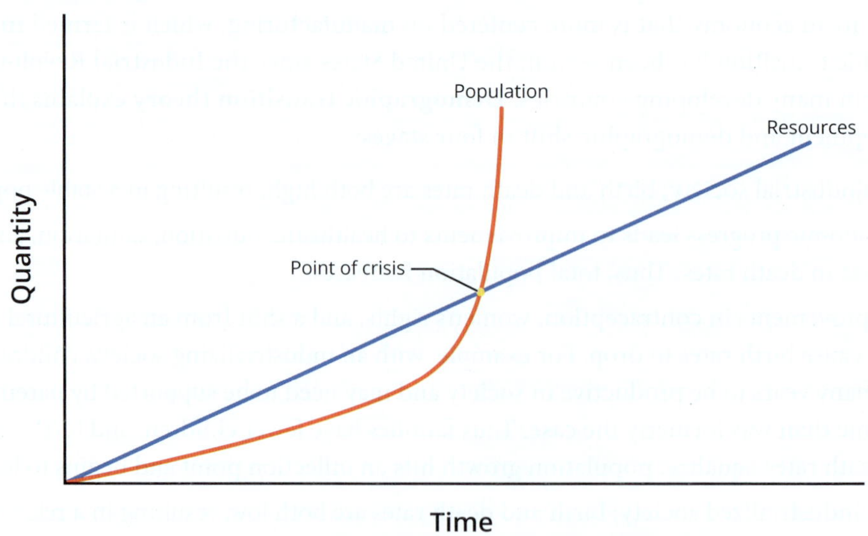

Figure 11.19 Malthusian Catastrophe

Social Movements

Social movements are organized either to promote or to resist social change. These movements are often motivated by a group's perceived **relative deprivation**, which is a decrease in resources, representation, or agency relative to the whole of society, or relative to what the group is accustomed to from the past. Social movements that promote social change are termed **proactive**; those that resist social change are **reactive**. Members of social movements work to correct what they perceive as social injustices. Some examples of proactive movements include the civil rights movement, women's rights movement, gay rights movement, animal rights movement, and environmentalism movement. Some examples of reactive movements include the White supremacist movement, counterculture movement, antiglobalization movement, and anti-immigration movement. To further their goals, social movements may establish coordinated organizations. Social movements may also seek to use different methods for driving forward their goals. The theory of **resource mobilization** considers how groups involved in social movements successfully achieve their objectives through the utilization and collection of resources, such as money, attention, skills, or materials. For example, in addition to coordinating cooperation between different groups, social movements may also seek to increase their audience by sharing their message through social media, which in turn can lead to increased support and more donations. Political involvement is also common through lobbying and donations, where the hope is to gain political favor that aids in the support of the group and their goals.

Globalization

Globalization is the process of merging of the separate nations of the world into a single sociocultural entity, and is a relatively recent phenomenon spurred on by improvements in global communication technology and economic interdependence. Globalization leads to a decrease in the geographical constraints on social and cultural exchanges and can lead to both positive and negative effects. For example, the availability of foods (especially produce) from around the world during the entire calendar year can only be accomplished through trade with an extremely large number of world markets. However, significant worldwide unemployment, rising prices, increased pollution, civil unrest (particularly in unindustrialized or undemocratic nations), and global terrorism are negative effects of globalization.

Traditionally, the health sector has been organized at the national, state, or local level, but this is beginning to change. Groups such as the World Health Organization (WHO), the American Red Cross, and Doctors Without Borders supply aid to populations in need around the globe. Many medical schools are also increasing opportunities for medical students to complete rotations in other countries.

Urbanization

Urbanization refers to dense areas of population creating a pull for migration. In other words, cities are formed as individuals move into and establish residency in these new urban centers. Urbanization is not a new phenomenon; ancient populations established cities in Jerusalem, Athens, Timbuktu, and other locations. The economic opportunities offered in cities and creation of a large number of "world cities" has fueled an increase in urbanization during the last few decades. Currently, more than half of the world's populations live in what are considered urban areas. Sociologists and other professionals have found links between urban societies and health challenges related to water sanitation, air quality, environmental hazards, violence and injuries, infectious diseases, unhealthy diets, and physical inactivity.

Cities are rarely homogenous with respect to their population makeup. Most cities have areas that are more socioeconomically well-off and others that are more impoverished. Sometimes, members of specific racial, ethnic, or religious groups are concentrated in particular areas, usually due to social or economic inequities. In the most extreme cases, as shown in Figure 11.20, there arises an extremely densely populated area of a city with low-quality, often informal housing and poor sanitation.

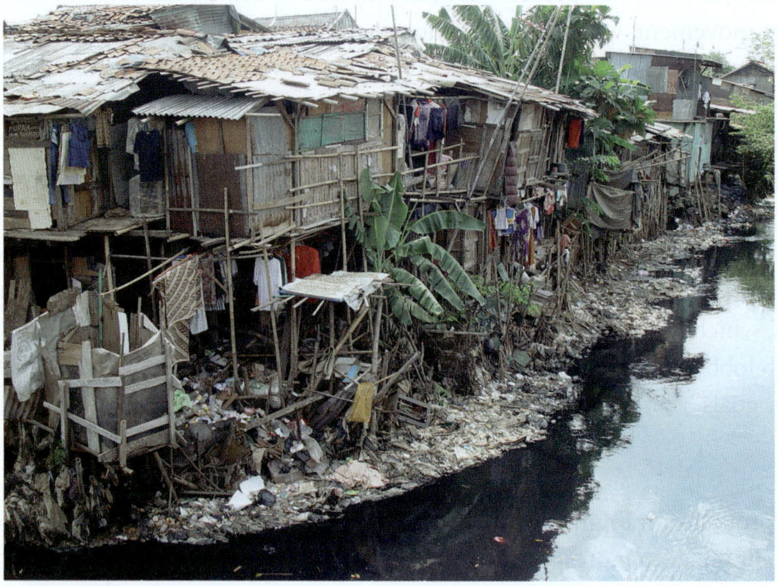

Figure 11.20 A Disadvantaged Area in Jakarta, Indonesia

MCAT CONCEPT CHECK 11.3

Before you move on, assess your understanding of the material with these questions.

1. What is the difference between race and ethnicity?

____

2. What is symbolic ethnicity?

____

3. Define the following demographic statistics:

   - Fertility rate:

____

   - Birth rate:

____

   - Mortality rate:

____

4. During demographic transition, what happens to the mortality rate? To the birth rate?
   - Mortality rate:

   ____

   - Birth rate:

   ____

5. What are the two types of social movements? How do they differ?
   - ______________________________
   - ______________________________

Conclusion

There are three major trends that are changing our nation's healthcare needs and our patient population. First, the increased diversity in the American population as a whole (from immigration, increased social and academic mobility, and interconnectedness through technology) puts us in front of patients whose thoughts and beliefs about health and well-being may be starkly different from our own. Second, increased access to healthcare through reform legislation has allowed millions of Americans to reach providers for the first time. Finally, our successes in medicine and public health have increased survival rates of many formerly fatal conditions and have enabled us to live longer. This leaves us with an aging population, in which individuals may be coping with multiple illnesses simultaneously.

To arm physicians of the future with the skills needed to take care of this population, many medical schools are increasing their coursework in interpersonal skills (*Doctor–Patient Relationship*; *Doctoring*; or *Physician, Patient, and Society* are such courses at various schools), as well as **cultural sensitivity**, the recognition and respect of differences between cultures, and research ethics. This is part of the biopsychosocial model of medicine described in Chapter 7 of *MCAT Behavioral Sciences Review*. Knowledge of the structure of society and how it shifts over time, as explained in this chapter, will enhance your ability to communicate with patients. Unlike the old model of *doctor knows best* (often referred to as the paternalistic approach to medicine), today's doctors must work together with patients to find solutions to their health problems. By working with patients on their own terms, you will be able to help maintain and improve their health status and begin to correct the health inequities that exist in today's population. In the next chapter—the last of *MCAT Behavioral Sciences Review*—we will explore these inequities in resources, health status, and healthcare.

GO ONLINE

You've reviewed the content, now test your knowledge and critical thinking skills by completing a test-like passage set in your online resources!

CONCEPT SUMMARY

Sociology: Theories and Institutions

- Theoretical approaches provide frameworks for the interactions we observe within society.
  - **Functionalism** focuses on the function of each component of society and how those components fit together. **Manifest functions** are deliberate actions that serve to help a given system; **latent functions** are unexpected, unintended, or unrecognized positive consequences of manifest functions.
  - **Conflict theory** focuses on how power differentials are created and how these differentials contribute to the maintenance of social order.
  - **Symbolic interactionism** is the study of the ways individuals interact through a shared understanding of words, gestures, and other symbols.
  - **Social constructionism** explores the ways in which individuals and groups make decisions to agree upon a given social reality.
  - **Rational choice theory** states that individuals will make decisions that maximize potential benefit and minimize potential harm; **exchange theory** applies rational choice theory within social groups.
  - **Feminist theory** critiques the institutional power structures that disadvantage women in society.
- **Social institutions** are well-established social structures that dictate certain patterns of behavior or relationships and are accepted as a fundamental part of culture. Common social institutions include the family, education, religion, government and the economy, and health and medicine.
- There are four key ethical tenets of American medicine.
  - **Beneficence** refers to acting in the patient's best interest.
  - **Nonmaleficence** refers to avoiding treatments for which risk is larger than benefit.
  - **Respect for autonomy** refers to respecting patients' rights to make decisions about their own health-care.
  - **Justice** refers to treating similar patients similarly and distributing healthcare resources fairly.

Culture

- **Culture** encompasses the lifestyle of a group of people and includes both material and symbolic elements.
  - **Material culture** includes the physical items one associates with a given group, such as artwork, emblems, clothing, jewelry, foods, buildings, and tools.
  - **Symbolic culture** includes the ideas associated with a cultural group.
- **Cultural lag** refers to the idea that material culture changes more quickly than symbolic culture.
- A **cultural barrier** is a social difference that impedes interaction.
- **Language** consists of spoken, signed, or written symbols combined into a system and governed by rules.
- A **value** is what a person deems important in life.
- A **belief** is something a person considers to be true.
- A **ritual** is a formalized ceremonial behavior in which members of a group or community regularly engage. It is governed by specific rules, including appropriate behavior and a predetermined order of events.

- **Norms** are societal rules that define the boundaries of acceptable behavior.
- There is evidence that culture flows from evolutionary principles, and that culture can also influence evolution.

Demographics

- **Demographics** refer to the statistics of populations and are the mathematical applications of sociology. One can analyze hundreds of demographic variables; some of the most common are age, gender, race and ethnicity, sexual orientation, and immigration status.
  - **Ageism** is prejudice or discrimination on the basis of a person's age.
  - **Gender** is the set of behavioral, cultural, or psychological traits typically associated with a biological sex. **Gender inequality** is the intentional or unintentional empowerment of one gender to the detriment of the other.
  - **Race** is a social construct based on phenotypic differences between groups of people; these may be either real or perceived differences.
  - **Ethnicity** is also a social construct that sorts people by cultural factors, including language, nationality, religion, and other factors. **Symbolic ethnicity** is recognition of an ethnic identity that is only relevant on special occasions or in specific circumstances and does not specifically impact everyday life.
  - **Sexual orientation** can be defined by one's sexual interest toward members of same or different genders.
  - **Immigration** is the movement into a new geographic area. **Emigration** is the movement away from a geographic area.
- A **fertility rate** is the average number of children born to a woman over a lifetime in a population. A **birth rate** is relative to a population size over time, usually measured as the number of births per 1000 people per year.
- A **mortality rate** is the average number of deaths per population size over time, usually measured as the number of deaths per 1000 people per year.
- **Migration** refers to the movement of people from one geographic location to another.
- **Demographic transition** is a model used to represent drops in birth and death rates as a result of industrialization.
- **Social movements** are organized to either promote (**proactive**) or resist (**reactive**) social change.
- **Globalization** is the process of integrating a global economy with free trade and tapping of foreign labor markets.
- **Urbanization** refers to the process of dense areas of population creating a pull for migration or, in other words, creating cities.

ANSWERS TO CONCEPT CHECKS

11.1

1. Manifest functions are actions that are intended to help some part of a system. Latent functions are unintended, unstated, or unrecognized positive consequences of these actions on society.

2.

Theoretical Approach	Primary Thesis or Idea
Functionalism	Each part of society serves a function; when these functions work together correctly, society overall can function normally
Conflict theory	Power differentials are created when groups compete for economic, social, and political resources; these differentials contribute to the maintenance of social order
Symbolic interactionism	Humans communicate through words, gestures, and other symbols to which we attach meaning
Social constructionism	Individuals and groups make decisions to agree upon a given social reality
Rational choice theory	Individuals will make decisions that maximize potential benefit and minimize potential harm
Feminist theory	Critiques the institutional power structures that disadvantage women in society

3.

Ethical Principle	Description
Beneficence	Act in the patient's best interest
Nonmaleficence	*Do no harm*; avoid interventions where the potential for harm outweighs the potential for benefit
Respect for autonomy	Respect patients' decisions and choices about their own healthcare
Justice	Treat similar patients with similar care; distribute healthcare resources fairly

11.2

1. Material culture focuses on the artifacts associated with a group: the physical objects, such as artwork, emblems, clothing, jewelry, foods, buildings, and tools. Symbolic culture focuses on the ideas and principles that belong to a particular group.
2. A value is what a person deems to be important; a belief is what a person deems to be true. While these terms are often used interchangeably in everyday life, they have specific definitions in the social sciences.

11.3

1. Race is based on phenotypic differences between groups of people. Ethnicity is based on common language, religion, nationality, or other cultural factors.
2. Symbolic ethnicity is recognition of an ethnic identity on special occasions or in specific circumstances, but not during everyday life.
3. Fertility rate is the average number of children a woman has over a lifetime in a population. Birth rate is the number of births in a population per unit time, usually measured as births per 1000 people per year. Mortality rate is the number of deaths in a population per unit time, usually measured as deaths per 1000 people per year.
4. During demographic transition, both the mortality and birth rates decrease.
5. Proactive social movements are in favor of a specific social change. Reactive social movements run against a specific social change.

SCIENCE MASTERY ASSESSMENT EXPLANATIONS

1. **A**

A manifest function is an intended positive effect on a system. A latent function is an unintended positive effect on a system, **(C)**. A negative effect on a system, **(B)** and **(D)**, is termed a dysfunction.

2. **C**

Symbolic interactionism studies how individuals interact through a shared understanding of words, gestures, and other symbols. A nod is thus a symbol in many cultures that signifies "yes."

3. **D**

The principle of nonmaleficence states that physicians must not only act in their patient's best interest (beneficence, **(B)**), but must also avoid treatments where the potential for harm outweighs the potential for benefit.

4. **C**

Although one's dominant physical features are associated with race, this man's preferences are those of Latino ethnicity and culture. Ethnicity is a social construct that considers language, religion, nationality, and cultural factors. Culture relates to a group's way of life; the preferences listed in the question are examples of material and symbolic culture.

5. **D**

In the United States, it is not a common practice to say, "I love you," and hug one's physician after each routine checkup; therefore, this behavior could be considered deviant, going against the social norm. Values, **(C)**, are what an individual deems to be important.

6. **B**

Both birth rate and mortality rate can be measured per 1000 people per year. Fertility rate is measured in number of children per woman over a lifetime.

7. **B**

Rituals are formalized ceremonial behaviors in which members of a group or community regularly engage. Therefore, these activities are examples of rituals performed for healing.

8. **A**

With a decrease in mortality rate and a higher immigration rate than emigration rate, the United States population continues to grow, with an increasing average age and increasing racial and ethnic diversity.

9. **C**

Material culture includes any cultural artifact—an object to which meaning is assigned. Values are ideas, which are associated with symbolic culture.

10. **D**

During demographic transition, both birth rates and mortality rates are high in stage 1, **(A)**. Mortality rates drop during stage 2, **(B)**, and then birth rates drop during stage 3, **(C)**. In stage 4, both birth rates and mortality rates are low.

11. **D**

In this scenario, a group is fighting for social power, which is an aspect of conflict theory. Further, this group is an example of a reactive social movement because it is running counter to social change. The fact that gambling had been legalized implies the involvement of the government, a social institution.

12. **C**

This man is describing his sexuality as mostly homosexual, although he has also had some heterosexual attractions. The Kinsey scale scores a 6, **(D)**, as exclusively homosexual. A score of 3 would equate to bisexuality. Thus, this man would likely score a 4 or 5.

13. **B**

Sex is determined by one's genotype, and therefore is biologically determined. Gender, **(A)**, may or may not match biological sex and therefore is not biologically determined. Ethnicity, **(C)**, is a social construct that sorts people by cultural factors, and therefore is not biologically determined. Sexual orientation, **(D)**, may have some biological component, but the relative role of biology and environment is not yet known.

14. **B**

If the immigration rate in a geographic area is larger than the emigration rate, then there is a larger influx than efflux of people. This will increase the population of that area.

15. **A**

Urbanization is the migration of people into urban centers to create cities. The increased population density should provide additional opportunities for social interaction, not decreased opportunities.

GO ONLINE

Consult your online resources for additional practice.

SHARED CONCEPTS

Behavioral Sciences Chapter 6
Identity and Personality

Behavioral Sciences Chapter 8
Social Processes, Attitudes, and Behavior

Behavioral Sciences Chapter 9
Social Interaction

Behavioral Sciences Chapter 10
Social Thinking

Behavioral Sciences Chapter 12
Social Stratification

Biology Chapter 12
Genetics and Evolution

CHAPTER 12

SOCIAL STRATIFICATION

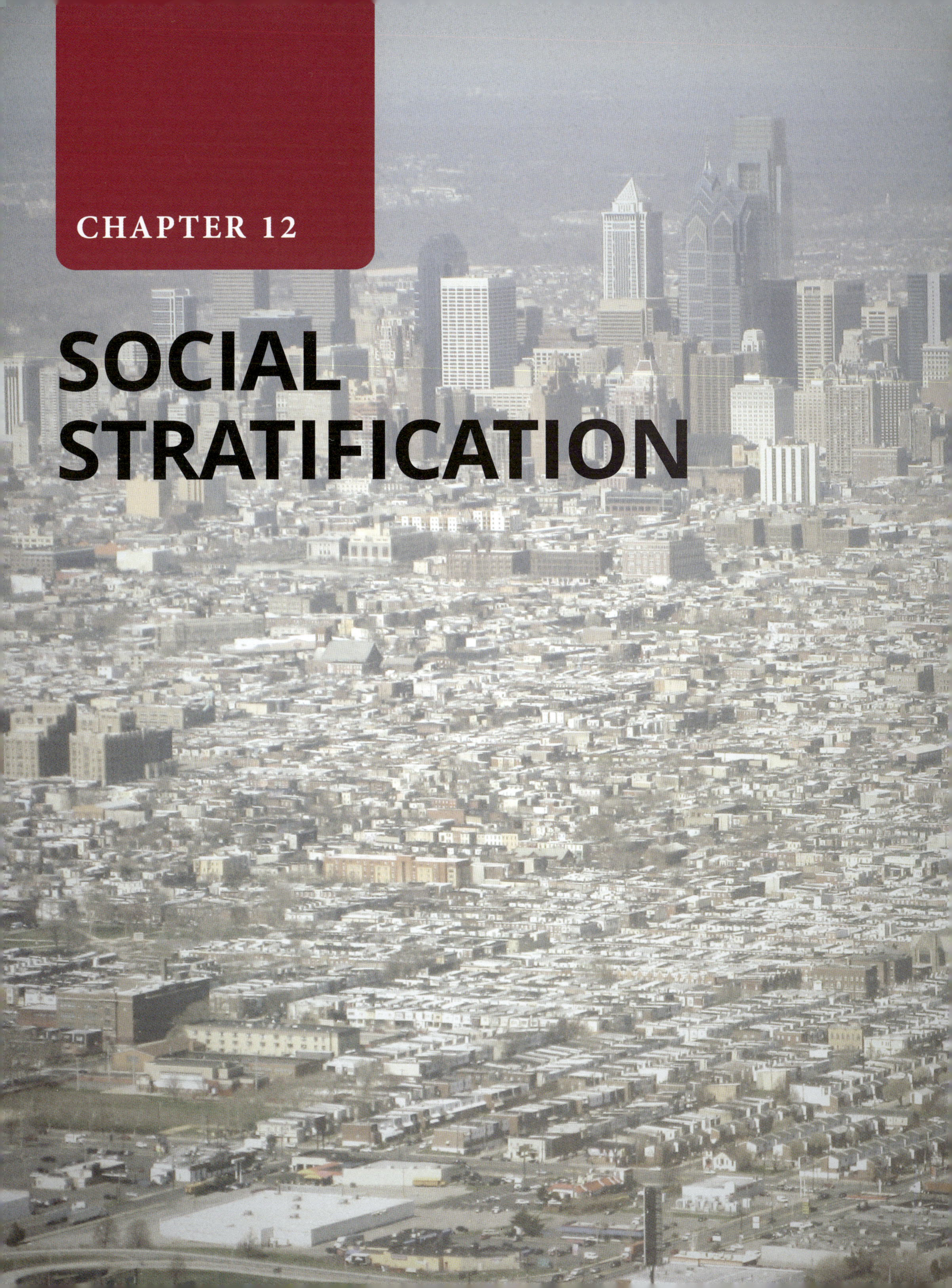

SCIENCE MASTERY ASSESSMENT

Every pre-med knows this feeling: there is so much content I have to know for the MCAT! How do I know what to do first or what's important?

While the high-yield badges throughout this book will help you identify the most important topics, this Science Mastery Assessment is another tool in your MCAT prep arsenal. This quiz (which can also be taken in your online resources) and the guidance below will help ensure that you are spending the appropriate amount of time on this chapter based on your personal strengths and weaknesses. Don't worry though—skipping something now does not mean you'll never study it. Later on in your prep, as you complete full-length tests, you'll uncover specific pieces of content that you need to review and can come back to these chapters as appropriate.

How to Use This Assessment

If you answer 0–7 questions correctly:

Spend about 1 hour to read this chapter in full and take limited notes throughout. Follow up by reviewing **all** quiz questions to ensure that you now understand how to solve each one.

If you answer 8–11 questions correctly:

Spend 20–40 minutes reviewing the quiz questions. Beginning with the questions you missed, read and take notes on the corresponding subchapters. For questions you answered correctly, ensure your thinking matches that of the explanation and you understand why each choice was correct or incorrect.

If you answer 12–15 questions correctly:

Spend less than 20 minutes reviewing all questions from the quiz. If you missed any, then include a quick read-through of the corresponding subchapters, or even just the relevant content within a subchapter, as part of your question review. For questions you answered correctly, ensure your thinking matches that of the explanation and review the Concept Summary at the end of the chapter.

1. Which of the following best describes the component of socioeconomic status attributable to direct individual efforts?
   A. Ascribed status
   B. Meritocratic competition
   C. Anomic condition
   D. Achieved status

2. Which of the following displays a correct association?
   A. High social networking and low social capital
   B. High social mobility and low social capital
   C. Low social class and low social capital
   D. Low social networking and high social capital

3. Which of the following phenomena are LEAST likely to coincide?
   A. Hazardous waste facilities and low-income neighborhoods
   B. Tuberculosis and poor living conditions
   C. Environmental pollution and populations of underrepresented groups
   D. Globalization and global equality

4. Which of the following trends is most likely FALSE?
   A. Mortality rates are increased in groups with low income.
   B. Life expectancy is decreased in groups with high income.
   C. Birth weights are decreased in children of low-income women.
   D. Rates of lung cancer are increased in low-income groups.

Questions 5–6 refer to the scenario described below.

A small town has 1000 residents, including 500 males and 500 females. In this town, 20 of the males have prostate cancer. During a calendar year, 10 more males are diagnosed with prostate cancer. Assume none of the males are cured or die during the year.

5. What is the prevalence of prostate cancer in the population that can develop the condition at the end of the year?
   A. $10 \div 480$
   B. $10 \div 1000$
   C. $20 \div 500$
   D. $30 \div 500$

6. What is the incidence of prostate cancer in this population during the year?
   A. $10 \div 480$
   B. $10 \div 1000$
   C. $20 \div 500$
   D. $30 \div 1000$

7. A low-income single parent works a part-time job and lives in a small apartment in the city. When the single parent's children grow up, they take similar jobs and live in similar housing. This is an example of:
   A. upward social mobility.
   B. downward social mobility.
   C. social exclusion.
   D. social reproduction.

8. Which of the following is true with regard to relative poverty?
- **A.** Individuals in relative poverty have incomes below the poverty line.
- **B.** Individuals in relative poverty exhibit downward social mobility.
- **C.** Individuals in relative poverty may be in the upper class.
- **D.** Individuals in relative poverty exhibit upward social mobility.

9. In comparison to urban centers, suburbs tend to have:
- **A.** larger racially and ethnically underrepresented populations.
- **B.** higher rates of poverty.
- **C.** larger upper- and middle-class populations.
- **D.** higher rates of crime and homicide.

10. Which of the following terms refers to the burden or degree of disease associated with a given illness?
- **A.** Morbidity
- **B.** Mortality
- **C.** Second sickness
- **D.** Chronicity

11. Compared to White Americans, which of the following racial or ethnic groups tends to have a better overall health profile?
- **A.** African Americans
- **B.** Asian Americans
- **C.** Hispanic Americans
- **D.** American Indians

12. Which of the following best describes the populations targeted by Medicare and Medicaid, respectively?
- **A.** Medicare: mostly patients without employer-guaranteed healthcare; Medicaid: mostly patients who have recently immigrated
- **B.** Medicare: mostly patients who have recently immigrated; Medicaid: mostly patients without employer-guaranteed healthcare
- **C.** Medicare: mostly patients in older age groups; Medicaid: mostly patients with low socioeconomic status
- **D.** Medicare: mostly patients with low socioeconomic status; Medicaid: mostly patients in older age groups

13. Morbidity is increased in low-income groups because of all of the following EXCEPT:
- **A.** higher rates of obesity.
- **B.** less access to healthcare.
- **C.** higher rates of homicide.
- **D.** lower rates of physical activity.

14. Hypertension (high blood pressure) can be diagnosed by having two or more blood pressure readings higher than 140/90 on two different occasions, separated by a week. Suppose that the criteria were changed to include anyone with a reading higher than 130/80 on at least one occasion. How would this change the prevalence of diagnosed hypertension in the population?
- **A.** The prevalence would increase.
- **B.** The prevalence would decrease.
- **C.** The prevalence would remain the same.
- **D.** There is not enough information to determine the change in prevalence.

15. Which of the following trends regarding healthcare disparities has NOT been documented?
- **A.** Females are more likely to be insured than males.
- **B.** Primary care use is more likely among males than females.
- **C.** Low-income individuals have more difficulty accessing care than high-income individuals.
- **D.** LGBTQ individuals have more barriers to healthcare than other individuals.

Answer Key

1. **D** (See section 12.1)
2. **C** (See section 12.1)
3. **D** (See section 12.1)
4. **B** (See section 12.2)
5. **D** (See section 12.2)
6. **A** (See section 12.2)
7. **D** (See section 12.1)
8. **C** (See section 12.1)
9. **C** (See section 12.1)
10. **A** (See section 12.2)
11. **B** (See section 12.2)
12. **C** (See section 12.2)
13. **C** (See section 12.2)
14. **A** (See section 12.2)
15. **B** (See section 12.2)

The relevant section of the chapter to review for each question is given in parentheses after the correct answer. Detailed explanations can be found at the end of the chapter.

CHAPTER 12

SOCIAL STRATIFICATION

In This Chapter

CHAPTER PROFILE

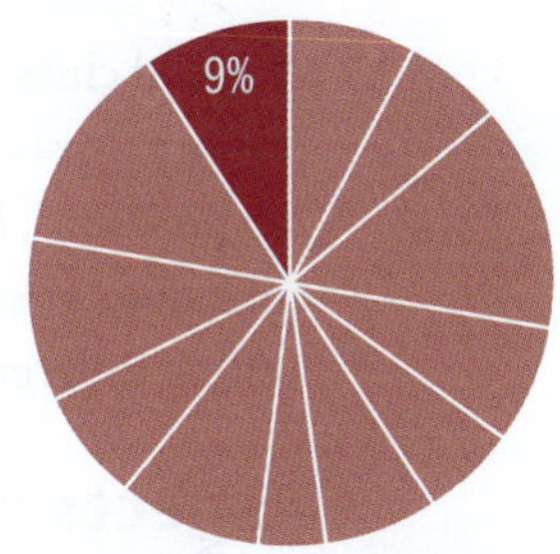

The content in this chapter should be relevant to about 9% of all questions about the behavioral sciences on the MCAT.

This chapter covers material from the following AAMC content categories:

8B: Social thinking

8C: Social interactions

10A: Social inequality

Introduction

The wonderfully witty Oscar Wilde once said, "Work is the curse of the drinking classes." While this quote is intended to be humorous, it does speak to the stereotypical characteristics associated with socioeconomic class. Some Americans think that class and social stratification are nonissues in our society. Unlike earlier feudal societies, most Americans are not royals or gentry, possessing inherited titles, land, or palaces; we're often considered to be a much more equality-oriented society, in keeping with our constitutional ideals. Yet how do we explain such differences in wealth, power, and privilege as a Manhattan lawyer driving a shiny Porsche past a homeless person rooting through a trash can? Such scenes make it hard to ignore the uneven distributions of material wealth and the overall social inequality in the United States.

To understand social inequalities in America and how such disparities impact health and healthcare services, we will examine several aspects of social stratification in terms of class, status, and social capital and how these intersect with race, gender, and age. We will also focus on patterns of social mobility and how poverty and location play major roles in health and illness. Later, we will connect how race, gender, and socioeconomic inequalities impact health profiles and access to quality healthcare.

12.1 Social Class

High Yield

LEARNING OBJECTIVES

After Chapter 12.1, you will be able to:

- Explain how socioeconomic status of an individual or a community is determined
- Define social capital and social cohesion
- Identify groups that suffer disproportionate social inequality
- Describe the relationship between social mobility and merit

A **social class** is defined as a category of people who share a similar socioeconomic position in society, and can be identified by looking at the economic opportunities, job positions, lifestyles, attitudes, and behaviors of a given slice of society. **Social cohesion**, or social integration, refers to the solidarity and sense of connectedness among different social groups and social classes in society.

KEY CONCEPT

It's important to keep in mind that socioeconomic status is not only determined by merit (achieved status), but also external characteristics or outward appearances like skin color and gender (ascribed status).

Aspects of Social Stratification

Social stratification focuses on social inequalities and studies the basic question of who gets what and why. Social stratification is thus related to one's **socioeconomic status (SES)**, which may depend on ascribed or achieved status, and causes the emergence of status hierarchies. **Ascribed status** derives from clearly identifiable characteristics, such as age, gender, and skin color; **achieved status** is acquired via direct, individual efforts. In other words, ascribed status is involuntary, while achieved status is obtained through hard work or merit. An important factor in achieved status is **educational attainment**, which is the highest degree obtained, or number of years of education completed. Caste and estate systems stratify by ascribed SES, while class systems stratify by achieved SES. After breaking free from British colonial rule, the United States moved toward a class-based system of social stratification.

BRIDGE

There are three major types of status: ascribed, achieved, and master status. While ascribed and achieved statuses are described here, remember that a master status is one that pervades all aspects of an individual's life. The role of statuses in social interaction is discussed in Chapter 9 of *MCAT Behavioral Sciences Review*.

Class, Status, and Power

There are three major classes—upper, middle, and lower—although these vary to different degrees in different locations. The upper class consists of those who have great wealth, along with recognized reputations and lifestyles, and have a larger influence on society's political and economic systems. In other words, the upper class has a high concentration of prestige and power. The middle class can be further divided into three levels: upper-middle, middle-middle, and lower-middle class. The middle class includes successful business and professional people (upper-middle), those who have been unable to achieve the upper-middle lifestyle because of educational and economic shortcomings (middle-middle), and those who are skilled and semiskilled workers with fewer luxuries (lower-middle). The lower class includes people who have lower incomes, and has a greatly reduced amount of sociopolitical power. The proportional improvement in healthcare as one moves up in socioeconomic status is called the **socioeconomic gradient** in health and development.

Prestige refers to the amount of positive regard society has for a given person or idea. Certain occupations, such as physicians, are broadly viewed with high levels of status, respect, and importance. Particular educational institutions, organizations, awards, and accolades may also be considered prestigious.

Power can be described as the ability to affect others' behavior through real or perceived rewards and punishments, and is based on the unequal distribution of valued resources. At its core, power defines the relationship between individuals, groups, and social institutions. Power relationships function to maintain order, organize economic systems, conduct warfare, and rule over and exploit people. As a result, power creates worldwide social inequalities as people tend to fall somewhere within the *haves* and the *have-nots*.

You may recall from Chapter 11 of *MCAT Behavioral Sciences Review* that Marxist theory, also called conflict theory, proposes that the *have-nots*, called the proletariat, could overthrow the *haves*, called the bourgeoisie, as well as the entire capitalist economy by developing class consciousness. **Class consciousness** refers to the organization of the working class around shared goals and recognition of a need for collective political action. By working together as one unit, the proletariat could revolt and take control of the political and economic system, laying the groundwork for a socialist state. The one major barrier to class consciousness, however, is **false consciousness**, a misperception of one's actual position within society. Members of the proletariat either do not see just how bad conditions are, do not recognize the commonalities between their own experiences and others, or otherwise are too clouded to assemble into the revolutionaries Marx envisioned.

Even in developed countries of the modern, globalized world, social inequality persists. Early sociologists explained that social inequality is further accelerated by what is called **anomie**, which refers to a lack of widely accepted social norms and the breakdown of social bonds between an individual and society. **Strain theory** focuses on how anomic conditions can lead to deviance. Anomic conditions include excessive individualism, social inequality, and isolation; these all erode **social solidarity**, which is the sense of community and social cohesion. Other sociologists have focused on the importance of social trust in the proper functioning of civil society. Social trust comes from two primary sources: social norms of reciprocity (*I'll scratch your back if you scratch mine*) and social networks. In the past several decades, as some societies have become more urbanized, self-oriented, and materialistic, associational ties have diminished and consequently have led to a decline in social capital. But what is the relationship between social stratification, social capital, and power?

KEY CONCEPT

Anomic conditions in postindustrial modern life have accelerated the decline of social inclusion and, as a result, have further obstructed opportunities to acquire social capital.

Social Capital

Essentially, **social capital** is the investment people make in their society in return for economic or collective rewards; the greater the investment, the higher the level of **social integration**, which is the movement of new or underrepresented populations into a larger culture while maintaining their ethnic identities. One of the main forms of social capital is the social network. Social networks can create two types of social inequality: situational (socioeconomic advantage) and positional (based on how connected one is within a network and one's centrality within that network). Inequality in networks creates and reinforces **privilege**, which is inequality in opportunity. Moreover, low social capital leads to greater social inequality. As social capital refers to the benefits one receives from group association, **cultural capital** refers to the benefits one receives from knowledge, abilities, and skills.

Communities are joined together through what are called strong and weak ties. **Strong ties** refer to peer group and kinship contacts, which are quantitatively small but qualitatively powerful. **Weak ties** refer to social connections that are personally superficial, such as associates, but that are large in number and provide connections to a wide range of other individuals. Social networking websites—especially those focusing on professional relationships—are examples of groups of weak ties. People without multiple weak ties, such as disadvantaged groups, may find accessing and contributing to social capital extremely difficult.

REAL WORLD

People who experience poor mental health are one of the largest disadvantaged groups to lack both strong and weak ties. Due to repercussions of social exclusion, these individuals may find that social capital is out of their reach. Consequently, this group is personally and socially disempowered, further propelling a cycle of exclusion. Social exclusion has huge financial repercussions on healthcare, with greater morbidity rates.

Intersections with Race, Gender, and Age

Social stratification, or, more properly, social inequality, remains higher among certain disadvantaged groups than others, including groups who are racially and ethnically underrepresented (especially Hispanic and African American people), households headed by women, and older adults. Think about who you know that may fall into these underprivileged or underserved groups. Your friends? Your relatives? Yourself? Socioeconomic inequalities remain in the United States. As described in Chapter 11 of *MCAT Behavioral Sciences Review*, this continued socioeconomic inequality is partially due to **intersectionality**—the compounding of disadvantage seen in individuals who belong to more than one underserved group.

Patterns of Social Mobility

Unlike a caste-based or estate-based system of social stratification, people in North America generally have the ability to move up or down from one class to another. In a class system, **social mobility**, also known as **structural mobility**, is typically the result of an economic and occupational structure that allows one to acquire higher-level employment opportunities given proper credentials and experience requirements. In the United States, the class system encourages this type of ambition through dedication and hard work, an ethos embodied in the phrase *The American Dream*.

MCAT EXPERTISE

For the guided example that follows, we were able to answer part of the question very quickly. On Test Day, all questions are multiple choice, so as soon as you have even part of the answer to a question, you can look at the answers and eliminate any that aren't a match.

Intergenerational and Intragenerational Mobility

As shown in Figure 12.1, social mobility can either occur within a generation or across generations. **Intragenerational mobility** refers to changes in social status that happen within a person's lifetime, while **intergenerational mobility** refers to changes in social status from parents to children. Many people consider the United States to be *the land of opportunity*, where intragenerational and intergenerational mobility can easily occur. However, others argue that opportunities for social mobility are diminishing because the gap between the upper class and the middle and lower classes continues to widen.

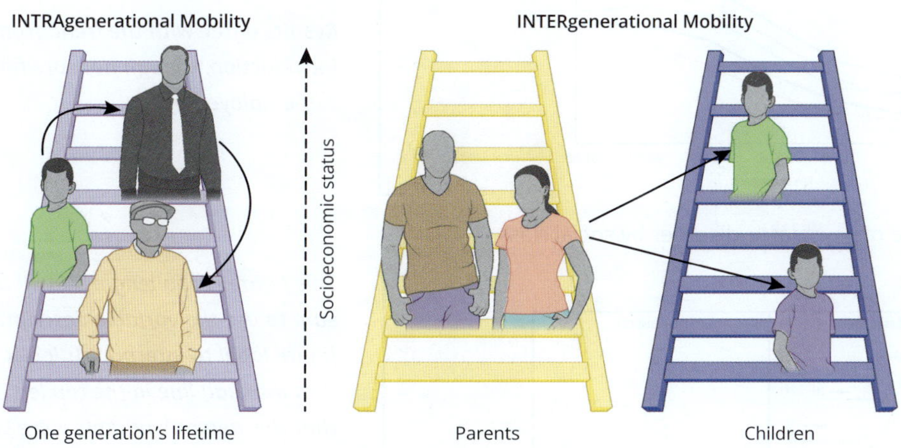

Figure 12.1 Generational Mobility

BEHAVIORAL SCIENCES GUIDED EXAMPLE WITH EXPERT THINKING

Social class differences are related to health and mortality outcomes as a result of differences in stress, financial strain, and working conditions, among others. The present study focused on incidence of psychiatric disorder and its relation to social class, and social mobility as compared to parental social status in predicting mental health outcomes.

Purpose: evaluate relationship between psych disorders and socioeconomic status/social mobility

Researchers conducted a longitudinal study to target this relationship. Participants were adults born between 1949 and 1959. Participants' adult social class between 1980 and 1990 was coded by occupation type and compared to parental social class at participants' birth. Researchers then noted participants' psychiatric admissions between 1990 and 2005. Results are summarized in Figures 1 and 2.

Standard longitudinal study: collected outcome data over 15 years.

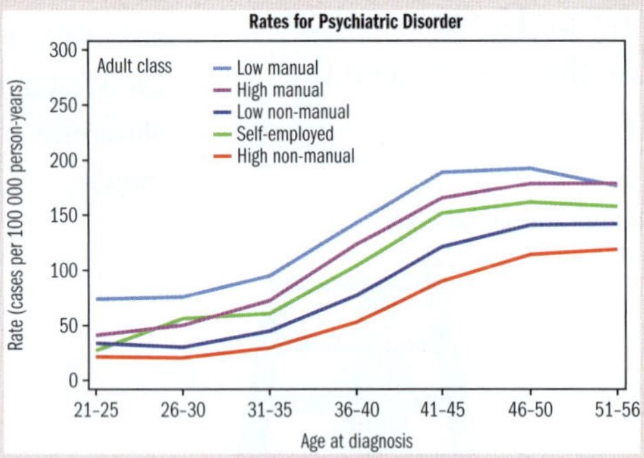

Figure 1 Incidence of psychiatric disorder by social class

IV: age, class

DV: rate of psychiatric cases

Results agree with the trend from the introduction, though not sure how self-employed fits.

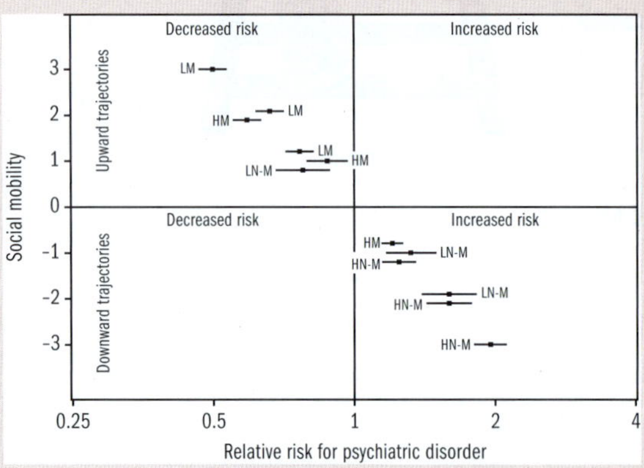

This figure is challenging, I will have to make sure to use the variable descriptions from the figure label to interpret. It looks like the LM (low manual) line in the top left corner means that this person's parents were LM and their own mobility is +3, which would put them at HN-M (high non-manual). These individuals have a 0.5 relative risk compared to LM individuals whose parents were LM, meaning that they're half as likely to develop mental health issues. The overall trend is linear and seems strong: higher upward mobility means lower risk.

Figure 2 Risk for psychiatric disorder resulting from social mobility compared to that of subjects who were socially stable. Social mobility scale and labels for confidence intervals are based on parental status, in order from high to low: high non-manual, low non-manual, high manual, low manual.

Figure label defines the variables, but I'll have to identify the relationship between them. The first letter of each word is the label in the graph.

Adapted from: Tiikkaja S, Sandin S, Malki N, Modin B, Sparén P, Hultman CM (2013) Social Class, Social Mobility and Risk of Psychiatric Disorder—A Population-Based Longitudinal Study. *PLoS ONE* 8(11): e77975. https://doi.org/10.1371/journal.pone.0077975

Researchers examined the records of three individuals: Person A (HM, parental class HN-M), Person B (LM, parental class LN-M), and Person C (HM, parental class HM). What can be predicted about the comparative risk of psychiatric disorder for A, B, and C?

This question is asking for a direct application of the results of the study, so the first thing to do to answer the question is to take a deeper look at the figures and determine what can be learned about these three individuals. Figure 1 gives overall incidence of mental health diagnoses for each class, and it looks like risk is inversely proportional to social class: people in lower social classes have a higher risk for psychiatric disorder. We can use this information alone to answer part of the question: Because the social class of person A is HM, i.e. "high manual," and the social class of person B is LM, i.e. "low manual," person B is in a lower social class and is therefore overall more likely to develop a psychiatric disorder.

Figure 2 is a little tougher to interpret, but we can start by finding the region of the graph where persons A and B would be located. Person A has parents in the HN-M class, but is in the HM class, for a mobility of −2. Person B has the same mobility, −2, from LN-M to LM. Looking at the data for individuals at −2 mobility, both persons A and B are about 1.75 times more likely to develop a psychiatric disorder than members of their respective social class with stable mobility. So, although person A will have a lower overall risk compared to person B due to social class, both persons A and B will have an elevated risk compared to socially stable members of their respective social class.

By contrast, person C shares a social class with their parents, meaning no additional risk is conferred to person C by downward social mobility. Given that persons A and C are in the same social class, but person C did not experience intergenerational downward mobility, person C would be expected to have a lower risk of disorder than person A.

Therefore, in order of risk, person C is at the lowest risk for psychiatric disorder based on the results of this study, followed by person A, with person B at the highest risk for psychiatric disorder based on both social status and downward social mobility.

Meritocracy

One of the largest factors driving American social mobility has been meritocratic competition or a merit-based system of social mobility. **Meritocracy** is a social structure in which intellectual talent and achievement are means for a person to advance up the social ladder. Given the rising levels of social inequality and concentration of wealth in the United States, some argue that motivation, a strong work ethic, a conscientious drive, and mastery of skills no longer offer the same opportunities for advancement. Some fear that the US meritocratic system is quickly becoming a **plutocracy**, or a rule by the upper classes. Nonetheless, merit still plays a key role in many segments of society, but merit does not always guarantee positive social mobility.

Upward and Downward Mobility

Social mobility usually occurs in one of two directions: up or down. Upward and downward mobility both refer to patterns of **vertical mobility**, or movement from one social class to another. **Upward mobility** is a positive change in a person's social status, resulting in a higher position. **Downward mobility** is the opposite: a negative change in a person's social status, wherein they fall to a lower position. Social mobility is often directly correlated with education, although other factors can contribute to upward mobility as well. Some of the best examples of upward mobility are seen with professional athletes, professional musicians, and entrepreneurs. So, in addition to education, athletics, music, and greater opportunities for small businesses may offer disadvantaged individuals more potential ladders to a higher social status.

Horizontal Mobility

Horizontal mobility is a change in occupation or lifestyle by an individual that keeps that individual within the same social class. For example, a construction worker who switches jobs to work in custodial services or mechanical maintenance has made a shift in occupation but typically remains in the lower-middle class.

Poverty

Poverty is defined by low socioeconomic status and a lack of possessions or financial resources. Poverty can be handed down from generation to generation, and can be defined on its own terms or in comparison to the rest of the population.

Social Reproduction

Social inequality, especially poverty (but also inherited wealth), can be reproduced or passed on from one generation to the next. This idea is referred to as **social reproduction** and is represented in Figure 12.2. Some consider social reproduction to be a cycle-of-poverty explanation for social inequality. In other words, the lifestyle of poverty, powerlessness, isolation, and even apathy is handed down from one generation to another as a feature of the society. However, there are many other factors that contribute to poverty, including where one lives and an emphasis on present orientation, in which people do not plan for the future. One theory, that of **structural poverty**, is based on the concept of "holes" in the structure of society being more responsible for poverty than the actions of any individual. Proponents of structural poverty argue that the same individuals do not by necessity occupy these "holes" from year to year, but the percentage of a society that falls under the poverty line stays relatively constant due to their existence. To understand how poverty is reproduced, it may be helpful to examine what types of poverty exist.

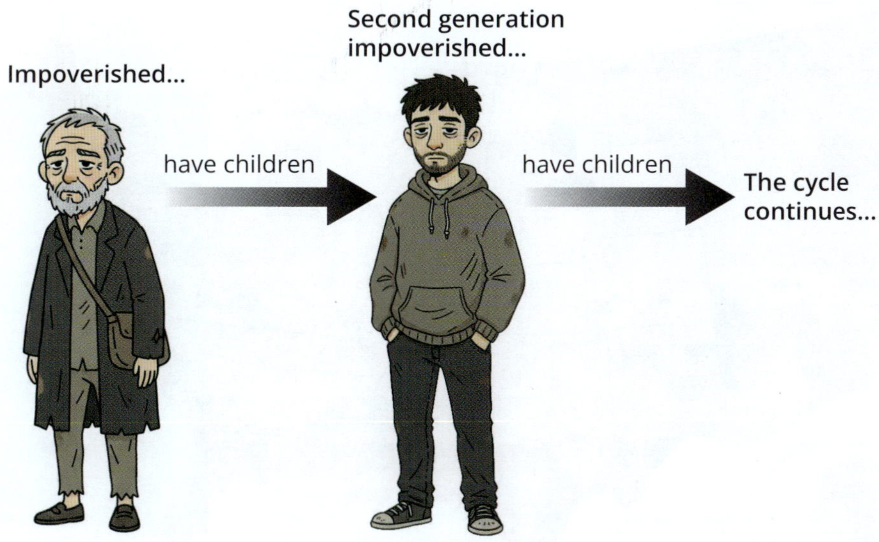

Figure 12.2 Social Reproduction

Absolute and Relative

On an **absolute** level, poverty is a socioeconomic condition in which people do not have enough money or resources to maintain a quality of living that includes basic life necessities such as shelter, food, clothing, and water. This absolute poverty view applies across locations, countries, and cultures. Poverty can also be defined as **relative**, in which people have less income and wealth in comparison to the larger population in which they live. For example, surviving on a low teaching salary while living in the Upper East Side of Manhattan may very well be considered poor relative to the other, far wealthier residents of that neighborhood.

In the United States, the official definition of the **poverty line** is derived from the government's calculation of the minimum income requirements for families to acquire the minimum necessities of life. Poverty is highly related to geography, as can be seen in Figure 12.3. One of the main problems with the official poverty line is that it is not contextualized according to geographic location and, as a result, does not take into account the cost of living in different communities. For example, the price of renting an apartment in a major urban center is much higher than the cost of rent in a rural small town. Some conceive of poverty as a form of powerlessness or a sociological and psychological condition of hopelessness, indifference, and distrust. In other words, poverty can be the result of the inability to control events that shape a person's life, often leading to a large degree of dependency on others.

KEY CONCEPT

In the United States, poverty is determined by the government's estimation of the minimum income requirements for families to acquire their minimum needs, such as shelter, food, water, and clothing. The problem with this official definition is that it fails to take into account geographical variables that impact the value of money in different locations. Certain areas are more costly to live in than others.

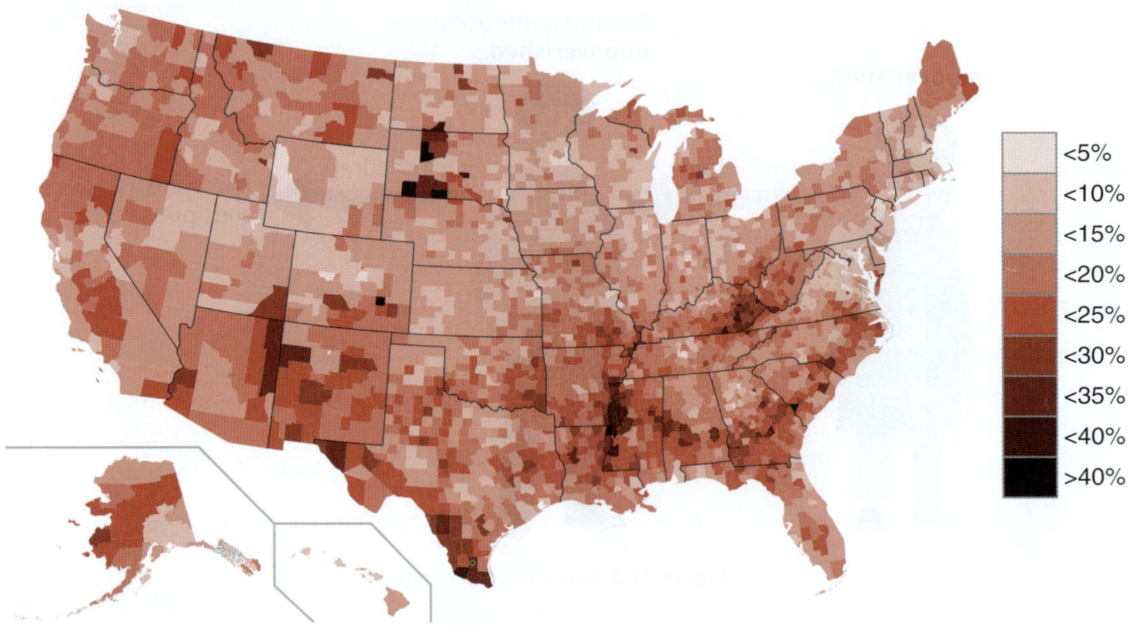

Figure 12.3 Percentage of Population Living below the Poverty Line by County, 2009

Social Exclusion

Social exclusion can arise from a sense of powerlessness when individuals who are poor or otherwise disadvantaged feel segregated and isolated from society. This feeling can create further obstacles to achieving self-help, independence, and self-respect. Disadvantaged groups, such as the racially and ethnically underrepresented, can experience magnified feelings of alienation and powerlessness when living in an affluent community. These feelings are similar to anomic conditions, which tend to further accelerate social inequality.

Spatial Inequality

Another important factor influencing poverty is the spatial setting of one's social life. In other words, where one lives plays a major role in the distribution of valuable resources. Does a person living in a low-income neighborhood in Mumbai have the same access to clean water and electricity as someone living in the posh neighborhood of London's West End? **Spatial inequality** focuses on social stratification across territories and their populations. Examining space helps to illuminate social inequalities because it attends to how geography influences social processes. Social categories such as gender, ethnicity and race, and class are distributed across spaces differently, as shown in Figure 12.4. In turn, these groups use spaces differently. For example, some cultures consider the home the center of family life, culture, and entertainment, while other cultures may view the home as merely a stop-off point for eating and sleeping while spending most of their time outside of the home.

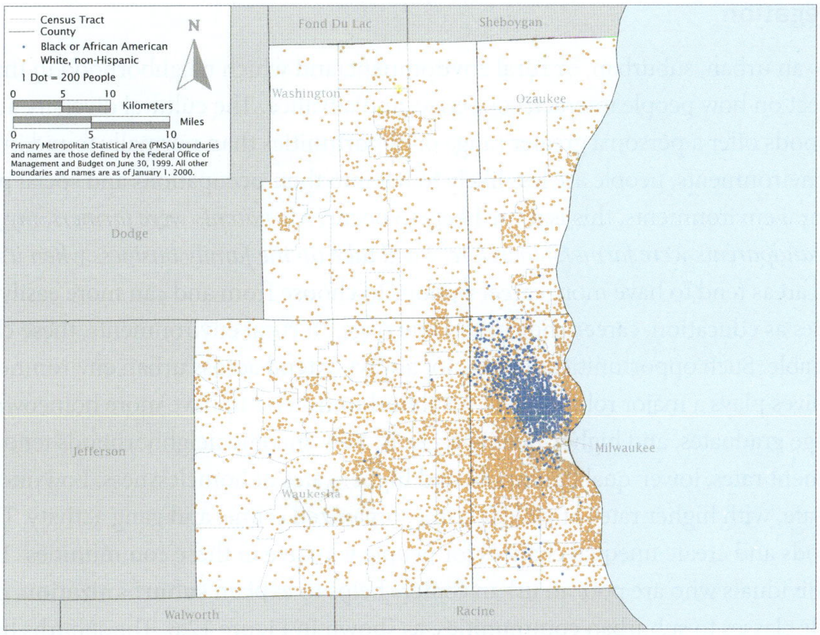

Figure 12.4 White and Black Population Distribution in Milwaukee County, WI

Space can be used to reinforce existing inequalities and can even amplify their effects, particularly poverty, leading to population segregation and the formation or expansion of destitute neighborhoods. Space can also be used to create social inequalities. In other words, social relationships between different agents, such as capitalists, laborers, the government, and citizens, result in spatially-varied social structures, built environments, and unequal regional development. For example, poorer neighborhoods tend to have less political and social influence than more affluent neighborhoods; as a result, "undesirable" buildings, like water refineries, trash-smoldering plants, and chemical manufacturers, tend to be placed in low-income areas, as shown in Figure 12.5. Citizens of these areas may lack the social resources to fight government and industry. To further understand spatial inequality, we must explore this idea on three levels: residential, environmental, and global.

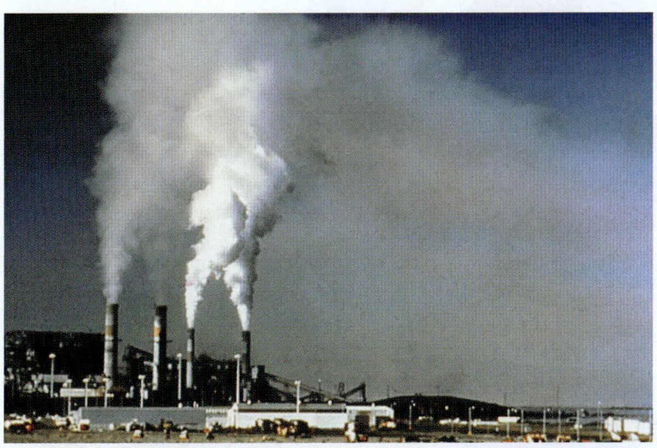

Figure 12.5 Industrial Park in a Low Socioeconomic Area

Residential Segregation

Where one resides—an urban, suburban, or rural environment, and which neighborhood in that environment—has a substantial effect on how people interact, cooperate, and advance. The cultural diversity and anonymity of urban neighborhoods offer a person a greater range of opportunities than normally found in rural areas. For example, in urban environments, people are less likely to fall into their occupations and social positions because of familial ties. In rural environments, this is more likely to occur: *My parents were farmers, my grandparents were farmers, my great-grandparents were farmers; therefore, I will take up the family business when it's handed down to me.* People in urban areas tend to have more career options to choose from and can more easily improve their SES through such avenues as education, career choice, and marriage. In rural environments, these choices exist, but are less universally available. Such opportunities also do not always extend across urban environments. The neighborhood in which one lives plays a major role: affluent neighborhoods tend to have more homeowners, professionals and managers, college graduates, and higher-quality schools. Low-income neighborhoods tend to have greater poverty, unemployment rates, lower-quality schools, and higher rates of homelessness. Low-income neighborhoods are also less safe, with higher rates of violent crime, organized crime, and gang activity. These key attributes stratify neighborhoods and create unequal chances for people who live in these communities. The overall greater concentration of individuals who are poor in urban centers helps to explain **suburbanization**, or the migration pattern of the middle classes to suburban communities, as shown in Figure 12.6. The suburbs have become more attractive as they are generally cleaner and less crowded, have lower crime rates, and often have better school systems.

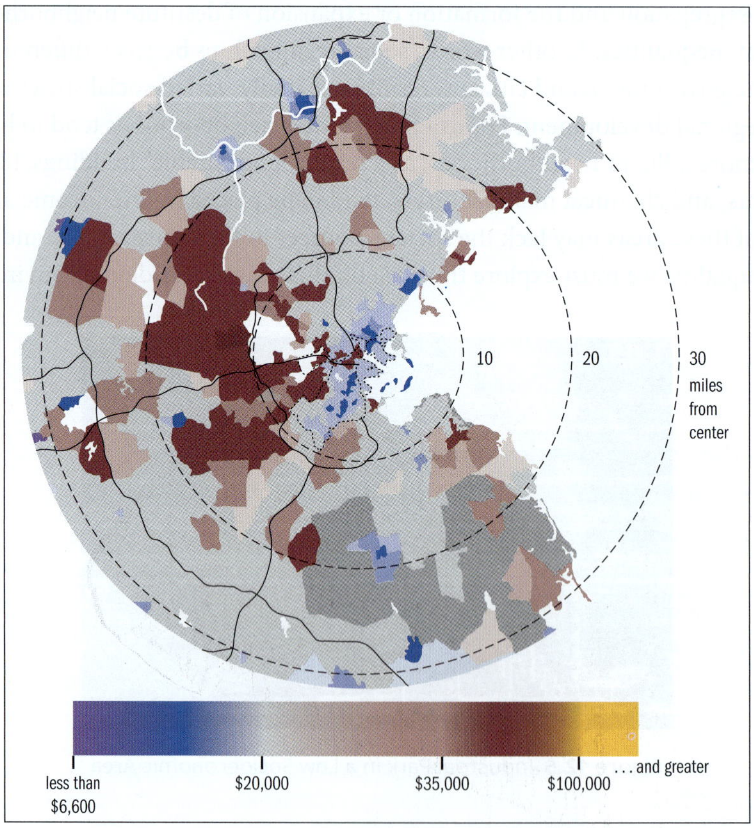

Figure 12.6 The Boston "Doughnut" of Income and Socioeconomic Status
Urban centers tend to contain lower-SES communities, surrounded by a ring of middle- to upper-SES suburbs. Further out are lower-SES exurbs and rural areas.

Unlike the middle or upper classes, members of the lower class are often less able to relocate to areas that might offer them better opportunities. Many disadvantaged groups therefore remain in urban centers under poor living conditions. To make matters worse, this type of environment can easily expose low-income groups to illness and disease. Suburbanization can also lead to **urban decay**, in which a previously functional portion of a city deteriorates and becomes decrepit over time. Interestingly, this process can spontaneously reverse in the process of **urban renewal**, in which city land is reclaimed and renovated for public or private use. Urban renewal is often fueled by **gentrification**, when upper- and middle-class populations begin to purchase and renovate neighborhoods in deteriorated areas, displacing the low-SES population (Figure 12.7).

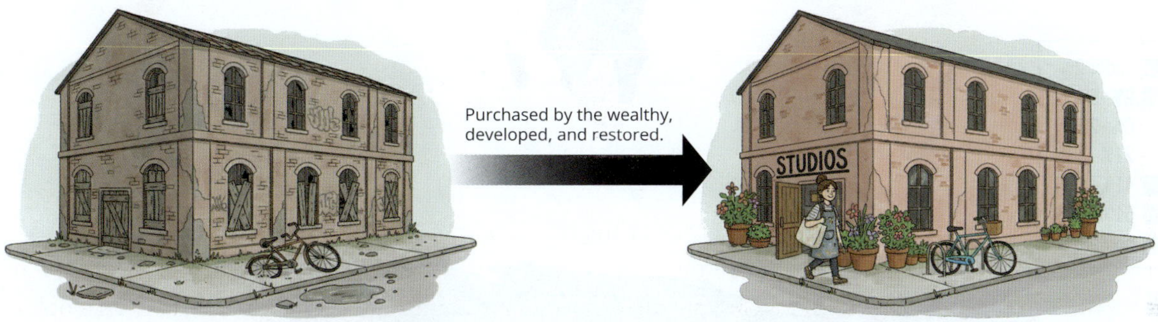

Figure 12.7 The Process of Gentrification

Environmental Justice

Poor living conditions and dangerous environmental conditions can result in an increase in illness and disease. Many low-income and underrepresented groups tend to reside closer to sites of environmental pollution because these areas are usually cheaper housing markets. Environmental risks, such as hazardous waste-producing plants and toxic waste dumps, tend to be located in low-income areas with a high concentration of groups who are racially and ethnically underrepresented. It is no surprise that inadequate housing, heating, and sanitation, in concert with toxin exposure, can contribute to acute medical problems. Illnesses such as influenza, pneumonia, substance use disorders, tuberculosis, and whooping cough are much more common among people living in poor-quality conditions. As mentioned earlier, these low-income areas also may lack the social and political power to prevent environmental risks from encroaching on their communities.

Global Inequalities

Poverty and social inequalities are not limited to hierarchies within a country. The **world system theory** categorizes countries and emphasizes the inequalities of the division of labor at the global level. **Core nations** focus on higher skills and higher paying productions while exploiting **peripheral nations** for their lower-skilled productions. **Semi-peripheral nations** are midway between the two—these nations work toward becoming core nations, while having many characteristics of peripheral nations. Much of the world, especially within semi-peripheral and peripheral nations, lives on less than the equivalent of $1.25 per day. Such rates of poverty are especially prevalent in parts of India, sub-Saharan Africa, and South Central Asia, as shown in Figure 12.8.

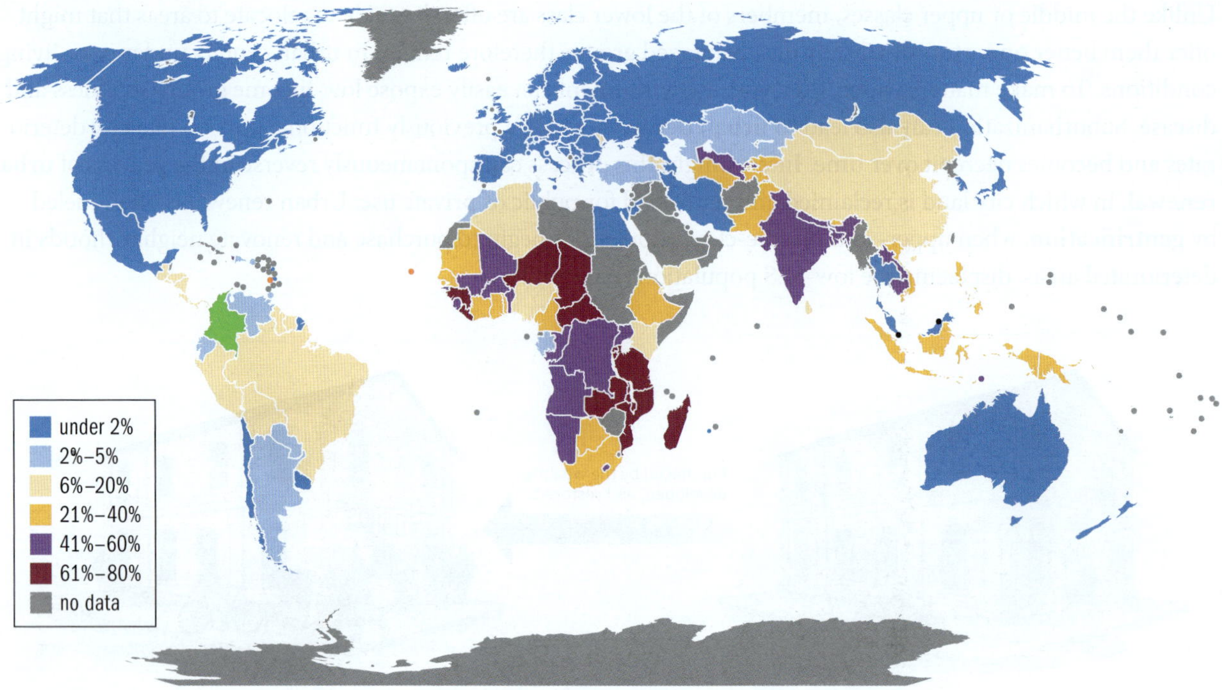

Figure 12.8 Percentage of Population Living on Less than $1.25 per Day, 2008

Largely due to the effects of globalization, massive restructuring of industry and trade patterns have had a major impact on local communities, specifically because of the production of cheap goods at suppressed rates for the global market. This reconfiguration obstructs or limits access to power and resources as the production of goods constantly shifts from location to location. Social inequalities have increased on a worldwide level as local communities become more and more subject to the ebb and flow of the global market. Since the advent of globalization, with the development of world cities, international communication chains, and global immigration, interaction between industrialized and developing nations has had more of an impact on peoples and regions within the state, and has thereby led to further inequalities in space, food and water, energy, housing, and education. Global inequality has been further exacerbated by an unprecedented large population spike, placing strain on the world's resources. The majority of the world also has limited access to healthcare. Consequently, many people around the globe suffer from malnutrition and parasitic and infectious diseases, and have higher rates of morbidity and mortality.

MCAT CONCEPT CHECK 12.1

Before you move on, assess your understanding of the material with these questions.

1. How is socioeconomic status (SES) determined?

2. How does social capital affect social cohesion?

3. What are some groups that suffer disproportionate social inequality?

4. What is the relationship between merit and social mobility?

5. With regard to health, which groups are most often affected by environmental hazards?

12.2 Epidemiology and Disparities

LEARNING OBJECTIVES

After Chapter 12.2, you will be able to:

- Identify the causes of Waitzkin's "second sickness"
- Explain why women are more likely to have better health profiles than men
- Describe the links between class, ethnicity, and healthcare disparities

An old saying intones that *Your health is your wealth*. This same correlation certainly holds true in reverse: the wealthier tend to have better health and better access to healthcare. Wherever there is low social capital, high urban degradation, interpersonal violence, and low social trust, the social environment is poor, and there is less protection against disease. As a result, class gradients often increase. Poor health conditions and lower life expectancy, as shown in Figure 12.9, are some of the many consequences of social stratification. Low-income groups are significantly worse off than the middle or upper classes when it comes to health disparities, meaning they tend to be sicker than others. **Social epidemiology** is a branch of epidemiology that studies the ways in which health and disease correlate to social advantages and disadvantages.

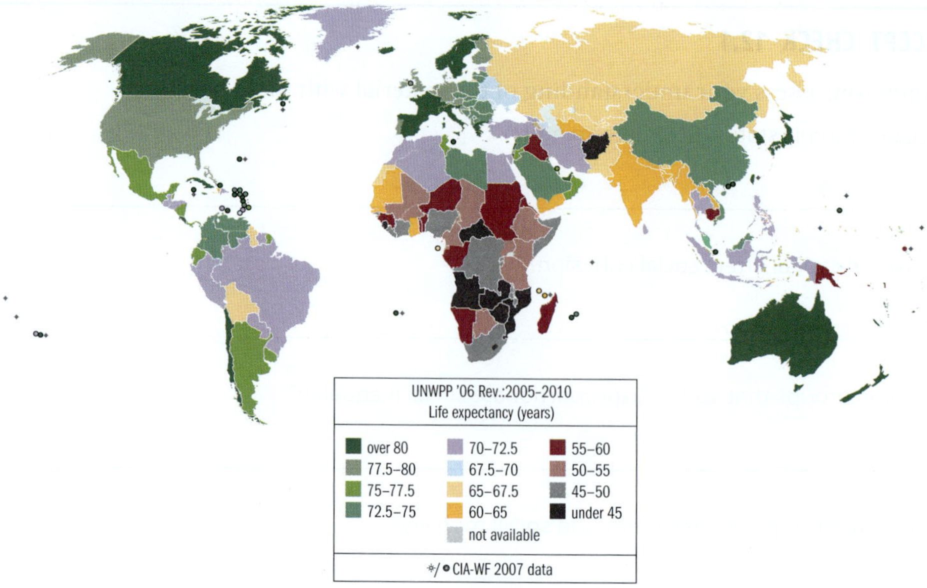

Figure 12.9 Life Expectancy at Birth, 2005–2010

To understand health statistics, it is important to define a few epidemiological terms. **Incidence** is defined as the number of new cases of an illness per population at risk in a given amount of time; for example, the number of new cases of lung cancer per 1000 at-risk people per year. **Prevalence** is a measure of the number of cases of an illness overall—whether new or chronic—per population in a given amount of time; for example, the number of people with new or chronic lung cancer per 1000 people per year. Health statistics are also given in terms of morbidity and mortality. **Morbidity** is the burden or degree of illness associated with a given disease, while **mortality** refers to deaths caused by a given disease.

KEY CONCEPT

Epidemiology statistics:

- Incidence = new cases/population at risk/time
- Prevalence = total cases/total population/time

Note that incidence is relative to the population at risk, not the total population; if you already have the illness, you are no longer at risk!

Inequities in Health

Science has clearly demonstrated that there are many non-medical factors that influence health outcomes, which are termed **social determinants of health**. These determinants include environmental factors such as where one is born or raised, or social factors such as culture or social class. Such a correlation was first demonstrated in the nineteenth century, when John Snow's investigation of a cholera outbreak in London in 1854 demonstrated a link between location and the outbreak. Snow tracked cases of cholera on a map, as shown in Figure 12.10, and was able to deduce that a water pump in the neighborhood was causing the spread of the infectious agent (a bacterium called *Vibrio cholerae*).

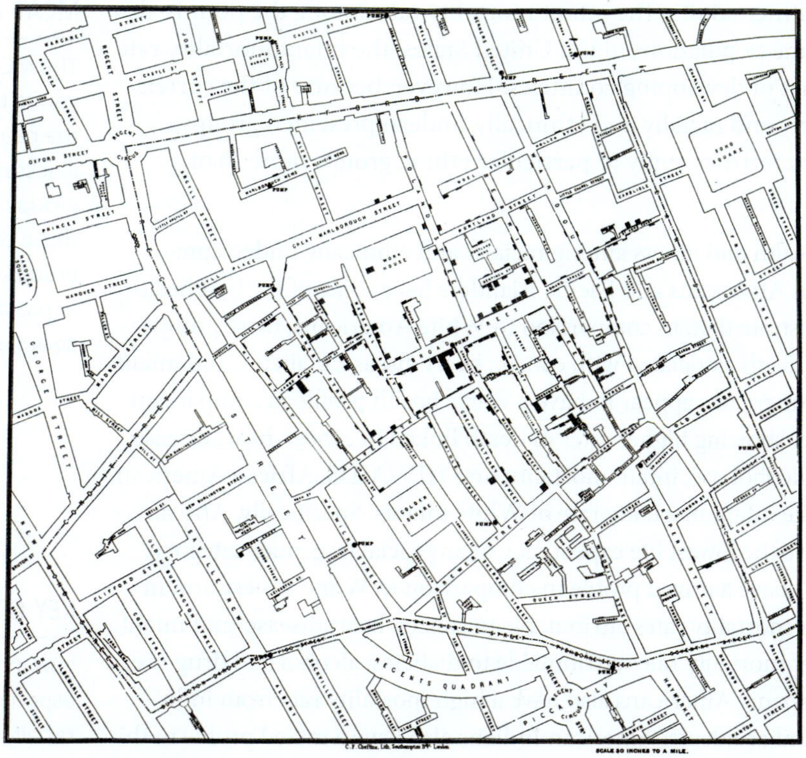

Figure 12.10 John Snow's Map of Disease Cases during the 1854 Cholera Outbreak in London
By tracing the geography of the disease, Snow deduced that a water pump was responsible for cholera transmission.

Health is dependent not only on geography, but also on social and economic factors. Over time, socioeconomic improvements lead to greater general health in the population, and the best health outcomes are generally seen in egalitarian societies. However, despite the ambitions of the modern **welfare state** (the system of government that protects the health and well-being of its citizens), the Black Report of 1980 showed that class differences in health still exist, with professional groups having longer life expectancies than working-class people. Howard Waitzkin described this outcome as the **second sickness**, which is an exacerbation of health outcomes caused by social injustice. As the Centers for Disease Control and Prevention (CDC) have shown, low-income groups are more likely to have poorer health, be uninsured, and die younger than middle- or upper-class adults. Poverty, in combination with a culture of inequality, leads to worse health outcomes, and this effect runs across gender, age, and racial and ethnic boundaries. For example, low-income women are more likely to deliver babies with low birth weights, thereby placing these babies at risk for numerous physical and cognitive problems in life. Similarly, impoverished members of racially and ethnically underrepresented groups have lower life expectancies. Members of the lower class, overall, are four times more likely to view themselves in worse health compared with affluent groups. Low-income groups are much more likely to develop life-shortening diseases such as lung cancer, diabetes, heart disease, and other degenerative illnesses. These groups are also more likely to commit suicide and die from homicide in comparison to wealthier adults. The infant mortality rate among the poor is also much higher; in some populations of the United States, the infant mortality rate can approximate that of developing countries. However, because of the correlation between poverty and racially and ethnically underrepresented groups, many of these characteristics apply to particular ethnic groups more than others.

MCAT EXPERTISE

The MCAT will not expect you to be able to rattle off the relative rates of these illnesses across racial groups, but a sensitivity to these differences between groups may be important in passages related to sociology and public health.

When it comes to health and illness among racially and ethnically underrepresented groups, Asian Americans and Pacific Islanders have some of the best health profiles. Reports illustrate that, in comparison to White Americans, these groups have a lower rate of death associated with cancer, heart disease, diabetes, and infant mortality. African Americans appear to have a worse health profile in comparison to White Americans, showing higher rates of death linked to cancer, heart disease, diabetes, drug and alcohol use, infant mortality, and HIV/AIDS. African American infants have twice the infant mortality rate of White infants. Specifically, African American males have the lowest life expectancy of any racial or gender category. Hispanic Americans have a mixed profile in comparison to White Americans, in that they have lower mortality rates attributable to cancer, heart disease, and infant mortality, but higher mortality rates attributable to diabetes, alcohol and drug use, and HIV/AIDS. Hispanic Americans also have a high mortality rate from influenza, pneumonia, and accidents. American Indians also have a mixed profile in this regard, showing higher rates of death from diabetes, alcohol and drug use, and infant mortality, but lower mortality rates compared to White Americans from cancer, heart disease, and HIV/AIDS. American Indians also show some of the highest rates of death by suicide in comparison to the general population. This group also has some of the highest mortality rates linked to diabetes compared to any racial category.

KEY CONCEPT

Low-income groups, especially those who are racially and ethnically underrepresented, have an overall worse health profile in terms of morbidity and mortality rates.

When it comes to gender-related health disparities, most statistical information shows that women have better health profiles than men. This trend is true throughout the world. Female life expectancy has been consistently higher than male life expectancy since records began. While the gap in life expectancy is beginning to narrow in the United States, most countries still have higher life expectancies for female citizens than male citizens, as shown in Figure 12.11.

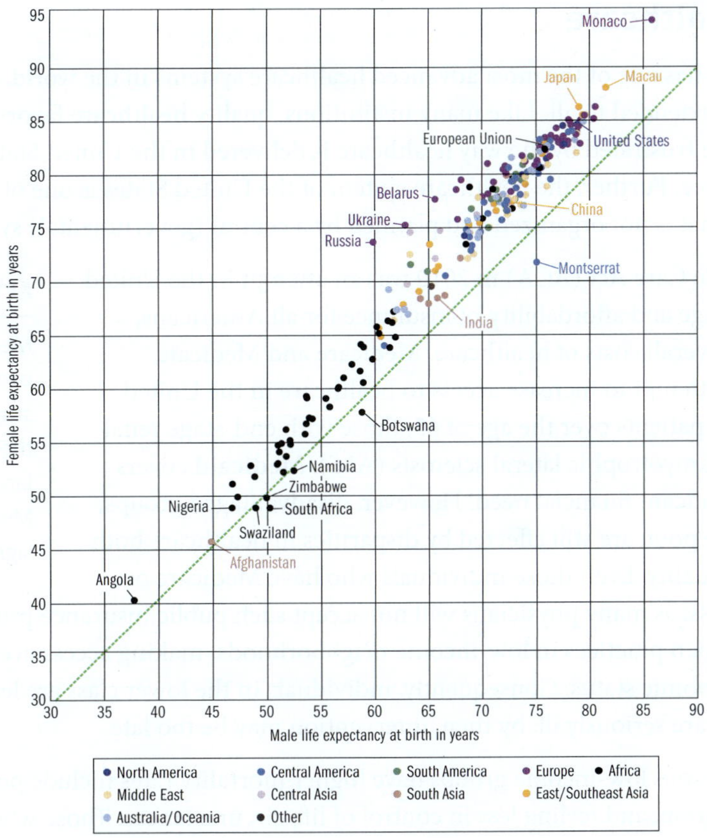

Figure 12.11 Male and Female Life Expectancies by Region and Country
Note that female life expectancies are almost universally higher than male life expectancies. Based on data from the CIA World Factbook.

Mortality rates from heart disease, cancer, chronic lower respiratory diseases, and diabetes are higher for men than women. Men are also three times more likely than women to die from accidents, suicide, and homicide. Men are far less likely to seek medical attention than women. Men, especially those raised to have hypermasculine behaviors, may try to "tough it out" rather than go to a doctor. When men do seek healthcare, they are less likely to comply with medical instructions or adhere to medical advice.

While women show better mortality rates, this is not the case when it comes to morbidity rates for certain acute and chronic diseases. More women than men suffer from infectious and parasitic diseases, digestive problems, respiratory conditions, high blood pressure (hypertension), arthritis, diabetes, and inflammatory bowel diseases (colitis). Women tend to suffer more from illnesses and disabilities than men, but their conditions are less often life threatening.

The reasons that men tend to have lower life expectancy rates are both sociological and biological. Sociologically, men are considered to be bigger risk takers, and therefore more likely to expose themselves to accidents and unintentional injuries. This is especially true of young men. Men are also more likely to be employed in dangerous jobs, such as the police force, steel industry, and coal mining. Men also have higher rates of alcohol use, speeding, and participation in potentially violent sports. Biologically speaking, men are at a disadvantage from infancy onward. Throughout life, men are more likely to come down with diseases that are life threatening.

KEY CONCEPT

In comparison to women, men tend to have worse mortality rates. However, women have higher morbidity rates. Differences in male and female health profiles are both biologically and sociologically determined, the latter being the result of factors like risk-taking behavior, hypermasculinity, and dangerous employment.

Inequities in Healthcare

While the United States has one of the most advanced healthcare systems in the world, quality healthcare and services are not always extended to all. Like many institutions, quality healthcare favors those in higher social classes. Many people are frustrated by the way healthcare is delivered in the United States, especially with regard to health insurance. Further, the healthcare system of the United States is one of the few among industrialized nations that is not organized and planned by a central (governmental) system.

Passage of the Affordable Care Act (ACA) in 2010 was an attempt in the United States to increase coverage and affordability of insurance for all Americans, and also to reduce the overall costs of healthcare. Medicare and Medicaid are also programs that attempt to increase access to healthcare in the United States. **Medicare** covers patients over the age of 65, those with end-stage renal disease, and those with amyotrophic lateral sclerosis (ALS). **Medicaid** covers patients who are in significant financial need. However, disadvantaged groups, especially those who are poor, are still affected by disparities in healthcare both in terms of access and quality. Even those individuals who have Medicare or Medicaid may lack access, as many physicians will not accept such public insurance programs. Additionally, some doctors will not open practices in low-income neighborhoods, making access even harder for populations with low socioeconomic status. Consequently, individuals in the lower class are less likely to seek medical assistance until they are seriously ill; by then, intervention may be too late.

KEY CONCEPT

Medicare covers patients over 65, those with end-stage renal disease, and those with amyotrophic lateral sclerosis (ALS). Medicaid covers patients in significant financial need.

Some of the primary reasons low-income groups have higher mortality rates include poor access to quality medical care, poor nutrition, and feeling less in control of life circumstances. Those who are poor are more likely to smoke and be overweight or obese; they are less likely to engage in physical activity. In addition to socioeconomic status, race and ethnicity can create barriers to care. In race-concordant patient-physician relationships, the patient and physician are of the same race, whereas they are of different races in race-discordant relationships. Sometimes, culture and non-native language are viewed as contributors to pathology because they can act as obstacles to diagnosis and treatment. Also, despite efforts to systemically address unequal treatment of underrepresented populations by physicians, there are still inequalities and disparities in treatment relative to race and ethnicity over a wide range of medical specialties. In other words, underrepresented and low-income groups tend to face greater barriers to care, and poorer quality of care when they receive it. To be specific, it has been demonstrated that African Americans, Asian Americans, American Indians, and Hispanic Americans receive worse care than White Americans.

Quality of preventative care, acute treatment, and chronic disease management also differ regionally. States in New England and the Mid-Atlantic are shown to be in the top quartile of healthcare quality while states in the South are in the bottom quartile.

Outside of race and ethnicity, other identifiable characteristics may have a large impact on how patients are treated by their providers. One of the most common biases is discrimination against overweight and obese patients. This bias can apply to any individual who is overweight, regardless of socioeconomic status, gender, age, and racial and ethnic background, although there is a higher prevalence of obesity in low-income groups. Doctors may assume that being overweight or obese is the only cause of a patient's health problems, which can sometimes lead to misdiagnoses and ineffective treatments. This, in turn, damages the trust necessary to form a strong doctor–patient relationship. As a result, patients who are overweight or obese are more likely than other patients to switch doctors repeatedly. When one does not have a consistent primary care doctor, continuity of care is nearly nonexistent. Additionally, patients who are overweight or obese are less likely to have quality preventative care and screenings, including screenings for breast and colon cancer.

In terms of gender, women tend to be favored by the healthcare system. As a whole, women tend to fare better when it comes to accessing healthcare, largely because women are more likely to be insured. Women tend to utilize healthcare services more than men, with more examinations, blood pressure checks, lab tests, drug prescriptions, and physician visits per year. Women also receive more services per visit than men do. Healthcare use is likely more common among women due to higher morbidity rates among women for many illnesses, thereby facilitating the need to seek medical attention. On the other hand, women are more likely to be delayed or unable to obtain necessary medical care, dental care, and prescription medicines. Also, for LGBTQ individuals, discrimination and decreased access to healthcare are quite common, often due to homophobia and other prejudices.

MCAT CONCEPT CHECK 12.2

Before you move on, assess your understanding of the material with these questions.

1. What is Waitzkin's second sickness?

____

2. What is the relationship between class, ethnicity, and health?

____

3. Why are women more likely to have better health profiles than men?

____

4. What are some of the factors that contribute to healthcare disparities between classes?

____

Conclusion

So what have we learned? We do not live in a perfect world where valuable materials and resources are unlimited and evenly distributed. In the United States and on a worldwide level, social stratification is an unfortunate reality. In a class-based economic system such as ours, status and power are inextricably linked, which can either facilitate or hinder access to social capital and its associated rewards. This is especially the case for certain disadvantaged groups based on categories of class, race, gender, and age. While not perfect, our class system does tend to allow for upward social mobility either in one's lifetime or across generations. At the heart of America's socioeconomic values is the principle of meritocracy, which means that through hard work, credentials, and dedication, one can move up in society. However, many people in the United States remain impoverished. Social inequality and social exclusion make it increasingly difficult for low-income groups to improve their socioeconomic condition. Some hold that social inequalities such as poverty remain because these inequalities are passed down from one generation to another. While there is some truth to the social reproduction of poverty, one's situational context also plays a role through spatial inequality. Where one lives in this world has an impact on one's position in life, especially in terms of accessing key resources and prosperous opportunities. Spatial inequality remains at the residential, environmental, and global level.

But how do such social inequalities influence health and healthcare disparities? Well, as is the case with many facets of life, wealth matters. Those with greater income typically have access to better quality healthcare. This is especially the case in the U.S. healthcare system because of uneven levels of coverage and high healthcare costs. Socioeconomic status or class greatly impacts one's ability to navigate the system and procure healthcare in the United States. Low-income racially and ethnically underrepresented groups tend to be worse off, having both poorer health and poorer access to healthcare. Women, despite being more prone to chronic and degenerative diseases, tend to fare better than men when it comes to overall health and accessing and utilizing healthcare resources.

While the U.S. healthcare system is undergoing a significant reorientation and taking on a more preventative approach, it is more important now than ever to place a greater emphasis on sociological issues to understand the relationship between social stratification and health and healthcare disparities. Illness and disease are a product of social as well as psychological and physiological issues. This chapter is the last chapter in *MCAT Behavioral Sciences Review*; you have therefore covered all of the psychology and sociology content required for the MCAT. This is a fitting chapter to finish this discussion, and we leave you with a charge: as you prepare for the MCAT, medical school, and life as the physician you deserve to be, think about the changes that are needed in the U.S. healthcare system. Serve your local, national, and international community and improve the health status of those around you, while contributing to a future where everyone can access quality healthcare.

GO ONLINE

You've reviewed the content, now test your knowledge and critical thinking skills by completing a test-like passage set in your online resources!

CONCEPT SUMMARY

Social Class

- Social stratification is based on **socioeconomic status** (**SES**). Socioeconomic status depends on ascribed status and achieved status.
  - **Ascribed status** is involuntary and derives from clearly identifiable characteristics, such as age, gender, and skin color.
  - **Achieved status** is acquired through direct, individual efforts.
- A **social class** is a category of people with shared socioeconomic characteristics. The three main social classes are upper, middle, and lower class. These groups also have similar lifestyles, job opportunities, attitudes, and behaviors.
- **Prestige** is the respect and importance tied to specific occupations or associations.
- **Power** is the capacity to influence people through real or perceived rewards and punishments. It often depends on the unequal distribution of valued resources. Power differentials create social inequality.
- **Anomie** is a state of normlessness. Anomic conditions erode social solidarity by means of excessive individualism, social inequality, and isolation.
- **Social capital** is the investment people make in their society in return for economic or collective rewards. Social networks, either situational or positional, are one of the most powerful forms of social capital and can be achieved through establishing strong and weak social ties.
- **Meritocracy** refers to a society in which advancement up the social ladder is based on intellectual talent and achievement.
- **Social mobility** allows one to acquire higher-level employment opportunities by achieving required credentials and experience. Social mobility can either occur in a positive upward direction or a negative downward direction depending on whether one is promoted or demoted in status.
- **Poverty** is a socioeconomic condition. In the United States, the poverty line is determined by the government's calculation of the minimum income requirements for families to acquire the minimum necessities of life.
- **Social reproduction** refers to the passing on of social inequality, especially poverty, from one generation to the next.
- Poverty can either be absolute or relative.
  - **Absolute poverty** is when people do not have enough resources to acquire basic life necessities, such as shelter, food, clothing, and water.
  - **Relative poverty** is when one is poor in comparison to a larger population.
- **Social exclusion** is a sense of powerlessness when individuals feel alienated from society.
- **Spatial inequality** is a form of social stratification across territories and their populations, and can occur along residential, environmental, and global lines.
  - Urban areas tend to have more diverse economic opportunities and more ability for social mobility than rural areas. Urban areas also tend to have more neighborhoods that are low-income and racially and ethnically underrepresented than do rural areas.
  - Formation of higher-income suburbs is a common occurrence, and is due in part to the limited mobility of lower-income groups in urban centers.

- **Environmental injustice** refers to an uneven distribution of environmental hazards in communities. Lower-income neighborhoods may lack the social and political power to prevent the placement of environmental hazards in their neighborhoods.
- **Globalization** has led to further inequalities in space, food and water, energy, housing, and education as the production of goods shifts to cheaper and cheaper labor markets. This has led to significant economic hardship in industrializing nations.

Epidemiology and Disparities

- **Incidence** is calculated as the number of new cases of a disease per population at risk in a given period of time: for example, new cases per 1000 at-risk people per year.
- **Prevalence** is calculated as the number of cases of a disease per population in a given period of time: for example, cases per 1000 people per year.
- **Morbidity** is the burden or degree of illness associated with a given disease.
- **Mortality** refers to deaths caused by a given disease.
- Health is dependent on geographic, social, and economic factors.
    - The **second sickness** refers to an exacerbation of health outcomes caused by social injustice.
    - Poverty is associated with worse health outcomes, including decreased life expectancy, higher rates of life-shortening diseases, higher rates of suicide and homicide, and higher infant mortality rates.
    - Certain racially and ethnically underrepresented groups have worse health profiles than others. African Americans have the worst health profiles; White Americans, American Indians, and Hispanic Americans have health profiles in the middle; and Asian Americans and Pacific Islanders have the best health profiles.
    - Females have better health profiles than males, including higher life expectancy, lower rates of life-threatening illnesses, and higher rates of accessing and utilizing health resources. However, females have higher rates of chronic diseases and higher morbidity rates.
- Efforts to improve healthcare for underserved populations include the **Affordable Care Act** (**ACA**) and the **Medicare** and **Medicaid** programs.
- Healthcare access and quality differ across the population.
    - Low-income groups and racially and ethnically underrepresented groups (specifically, African Americans, Asian Americans, American Indians, and Hispanic Americans) receive worse care than high-income groups and White Americans, respectively.
    - Biases against overweight or obese patients are associated with lower-quality treatment, including less preventative care and fewer screenings.
    - Women tend to have better access to healthcare and utilize more healthcare resources than men.
    - LGBTQ individuals may have barriers to care due to prejudices, discrimination, homophobia, and transphobia.

ANSWERS TO CONCEPT CHECKS

12.1

1. SES is determined by two factors: it can be ascribed according to physical or external characteristics such as age, gender, or skin color, or acquired through direct efforts such as hard work or merit.
2. The less social capital a person has (reduced network equality and equality of opportunity), the more social inequality. This, in turn, decreases social cohesion.
3. Social inequality is highest among racially and ethnically underrepresented groups (especially African Americans and Hispanic Americans), households headed by women, and older adults. It is also most prevalent among those living in poverty.
4. Social mobility can be dependent on intellectual talent and achievement (meritocratic competition) but can also be obstructed by concentrated power as well as discrimination based on ethnicity, gender, age, or other identifiable characteristics.
5. Environmental hazards tend to be located in low-income areas with a higher population of racially and ethnically underrepresented groups. Poor living conditions can result in increased illness and disease among these groups of people.

12.2

1. The second sickness refers to the fact that health outcomes are exacerbated by social inequalities and social injustice. As a result, higher-income groups have longer life expectancies than lower-income groups.
2. Low-income racially and ethnically underrepresented groups have higher morbidity rates and overall worse health compared to the middle and upper classes. The lower class also has higher infant mortality rates, homicide rates, and suicide rates in comparison to wealthier classes.
3. Women typically have longer life expectancies and an overall better health profile in comparison to men. This can be attributed to both biological and sociological causes: women are less likely to have life-threatening conditions, although they do have higher morbidity rates. Women are also more likely to seek care and to utilize healthcare services than men.
4. Low-income groups have less access to healthcare services and often experience lower quality healthcare. Poor Americans are less likely to be insured and consequently are less likely to seek medical attention until conditions have become extremely serious, thereby limiting available interventions. As a result, morbidity and mortality rates are highest among low-income groups.

SCIENCE MASTERY ASSESSMENT EXPLANATIONS

1. **D**

Social stratification based on direct efforts, such as merit, is a form of achieved socioeconomic status. Ascribed socioeconomic status, **(A)**, is based on identifiable external characteristics. Achieved status may be due to meritocratic competition, **(B)**, but other individual efforts can also be associated with achieved status. Anomic conditions, **(C)**, are those that cause a breakdown between the individual and society and erode social solidarity.

2. **C**

Low social class may lead to low social capital. Members of the lower class often have smaller numbers of weak ties in social networks, and therefore have less opportunity to invest in society and reap its benefits.

3. **D**

Globalization does not typically lead to global equality; rather, globalization tends to create further global inequalities. In regard to environmental justice, higher numbers of hazardous waste facilities tend to be found in low-income neighborhoods, **(A)**. Poor living conditions tend to be associated with greater health problems, including tuberculosis, **(B)**. Finally, environmental pollution is more prevalent in areas with larger populations of underrepresented groups, especially when low-income, **(C)**.

4. **B**

Groups with high income tend to have increased life expectancy rates, not decreased. People with low income have higher mortality rates than those with high income, **(A)**. Low-income women tend to have children with lower birth weights, **(C)**. Finally, rates of various diseases, including lung cancer, are increased among low-income groups, **(D)**.

5. **D**

Prevalence is defined as the total number of cases divided by the possibly affected population during a period of time. Here, the period of time is defined as one point: the end of the year. At the end of the year, there are 30 total cases in a population of 1000 individuals, but only 500 of those individuals can develop prostate cancer, meaning the prevalence is $30 \div 500$.

6. **A**

Incidence is defined as the total number of new cases divided by the at-risk population during a period of time. Here, the period of time is one year. There were 10 new cases in this year, and the at-risk population will be only the males who do not already have prostate cancer; the 20 males already diagnosed and the 500 females should not be included in the at-risk population. Therefore, the incidence in this population is $10 \div 480$.

7. **D**

In this scenario, the children remain in the same socioeconomic class as their parent, indicating a lack of social mobility, **(A)** and **(B)**. Rather, this is an example of social reproduction, in which social inequality, especially poverty, is passed from one generation to the next.

8. **C**

Relative poverty is a comparative term: it describes being poorer than those in the surrounding population. Members of the upper class can live in relative poverty compared to others in their neighborhood if they are not as well-off as their neighbors. Relative poverty is not directly associated with upward or downward social mobility, eliminating **(B)** and **(D)**; individuals living in relative poverty could exhibit mobility in either direction or no social mobility at all.

9. **C**

Suburbs tend to have larger upper- and middle-class populations than urban centers; urban centers tend to have larger low-socioeconomic status populations than suburbs. This is due, in part, to the increased mobility seen in upper- and middle-class populations, which permits their migration into the suburbs.

10. **A**

Morbidity refers to the burden of illness, or the severity or degree of illness. Mortality, **(B)**, refers to deaths caused by a given illness. Second sickness, **(C)**, is a term used to describe the exacerbation of health outcomes due to social injustice. Chronicity, **(D)**, refers to the duration of a disease, not its severity or significance for the patient.

11. **B**

In comparison to White Americans, Asian Americans tend to have better overall health profiles. African Americans, **(A)**, tend to have worse overall health profiles. Hispanic Americans and American Indians, **(C)** and **(D)**, both have mixed health profiles in comparison to White Americans: they are better off in some categories and worse off in others. However, Hispanic Americans and American Indians do not have better overall health profiles than White Americans.

12. **C**

Medicare covers patients over the age of 65 (older age groups), those with end-stage renal disease, and those with amyotrophic lateral sclerosis (ALS). Medicaid covers patients below a certain socioeconomic level.

13. **C**

Morbidity refers to the burden or severity of disease. All of the factors listed are true with regard to low-socioeconomic status populations; however, high homicide rates cause increases in mortality, not morbidity.

14. **A**

If the threshold for hypertension (high blood pressure) were lowered, more individuals would be fit the criteria for the disease. If the number of individuals with the disease increases and the population stays the same overall, there will be an increased prevalence of the disease.

15. **B**

In comparison to females, males visit primary care doctors less frequently. All of the other trends listed here have been documented.

GO ONLINE

Consult your online resources for additional practice.

SHARED CONCEPTS

Behavioral Sciences Chapter 5
Motivation, Emotion, and Stress

Behavioral Sciences Chapter 6
Identity and Personality

Behavioral Sciences Chapter 7
Psychological Disorders

Behavioral Sciences Chapter 8
Social Processes, Attitudes, and Behavior

Behavioral Sciences Chapter 10
Social Thinking

Behavioral Sciences Chapter 11
Social Structure and Demographics

GLOSSARY

Absolute poverty–Poverty wherein people do not have enough resources to acquire basic life necessities such as shelter, food, clothing, and water.

Absolute threshold–The minimum stimulus energy needed to activate a sensory system.

Accommodation–Process by which existing schemata are modified to encompass new information.

Acetylcholine–A neurotransmitter associated with voluntary muscle control.

Achieved status–A status gained as a result of direct, individual action.

Acquisition–In classical conditioning, the process of taking advantage of reflexive responses to turn a neutral stimulus into a conditioned stimulus.

Actor-observer bias–The tendency to make situational attributions about the self, but dispositional attributions about others, regarding similar behaviors.

Adaptation–In perception, a decrease in stimulus perception after a long duration of exposure; in learning, the process by which new information is processed; consists of assimilation and accommodation.

Adaptive coping–Healthy and effective strategies that a person uses to manage stressful situations in a way that reduces distress and promotes well-being.

Adaptive value–The extent to which a trait benefits a species by influencing the evolutionary fitness of the species.

Affect–The experience and display of emotion. Can be described as a scale, with both positive and negative affect having separate scales.

Afferent neuron–Sensory neurons which transmit information to the brain from the body in response to sensory input.

Ageism–Prejudice or discrimination on the basis of a person's age.

Agent of socialization–Any part of society that is important when learning social norms and values.

Aggression–A behavior with the intention to cause harm or increase relative social dominance; can be physical or verbal.

Agnosia–The loss of the ability to recognize objects, people, or sounds, though typically just one of the three.

Alcohol myopia–The inability to think about consequences and possible outcomes of one's actions due to alcohol intoxication.

Alertness–State of consciousness in which one is aware, able to think, and able to respond to the environment; nearly synonymous with arousal.

Algorithm–A formula or procedure for solving a certain type of problem.

Aligning actions–An impression management strategy in which one makes questionable behavior acceptable through excuses.

Alter-casting–An impression management strategy in which one imposes an identity onto another person.

Altruism–A form of helping behavior in which people's intent is to benefit someone else at a cost to themselves.

Alzheimer's disease–Degenerative brain disorder that is characterized by dementia and memory loss. Neurofibrillary tangles and β-amyloid plaques are phenomena found in the brains of Alzheimer's patients.

Amphetamine–A central nervous system stimulant that increases activity of both dopamine and norepinephrine in the brain.

Amygdala–A portion of the limbic system that is important for memory and emotion, especially fear.

Anomie–A state of normlessness; anomic conditions erode social solidarity by means of excessive individualism, social inequality, and isolation.

Anterograde amnesia–Form of memory loss in which new long-term memories cannot be established.

Anxiety disorders–Disorders that involve worry, unease, fear, and apprehension about future uncertainties based on real or imagined events that can impair physical and psychological health.

Aphasia–Deficit of language production or comprehension.

Appetitive conditioning–A type of classical conditioning in which the unconditioned stimulus is desirable, increasing the frequency of a response.

Appetitive stimulus–A pleasant or desirable stimulus that functions to increase the frequency of a response.

Appraisal model–A similar theory to the basic model, accepting that there are biologically predetermined expressions once an emotion is experienced; accepts that there is a cognitive antecedent to emotional expression.

Archetype–In Jungian psychoanalysis, a thought or image that has an emotional element and is a part of the collective unconsciousness.

Arcuate fasciculus–A bundle of axons that connects Wernicke's area (language comprehension) with Broca's area (motor function of speech).

Arousal–A psychological and physiological state of being awake or reactive to stimuli; nearly synonymous with alertness.

Arousal theory–A theory of motivation that states there is a particular level of arousal required in order to perform actions optimally; summarized by the Yerkes–Dodson law.

Ascribed status–A status that one is given at birth, such as race, ethnicity, or sex.

Assimilation–In psychology, the process by which new information is interpreted in terms of existing schemata; in sociology, the process by which the behavior and culture of a group or an individual begins to merge with that of another group.

Associative learning–The process by which a connection is made between two stimuli or a stimulus and a response; examples include classical conditioning and operant conditioning.

Attachment–An emotional bond to another person, particularly a parent or caregiver. The four main attachment styles are: secure, avoidant, ambivalent, and disorganized.

Attitude–A tendency toward expression of positive or negative feelings or evaluations of a person, place, thing, or situation.

Attribute substitution–A phenomenon observed when individuals must make judgments that are complex but instead substitute a simpler solution or perception.

Attribution theory–A theory that focuses on the tendency for individuals to infer the causes of other people's behavior.

Auditory cortex–Region of the temporal lobe devoted to sound processing.

Auditory pathway–After entering the brain, sound is processed by several regions, including the MGN, auditory cortex, superior olive, and inferior colliculus.

Authentic self–Who someone actually is, including both positive and negative attributes.

Automatic processing–The brain process most closely resembling autopilot, enabling performance of multiple activities at the same time.

Autonomic nervous system–The involuntary branch of the peripheral nervous system that controls involuntary functions such as heart rate, bronchial dilation, temperature, and digestion.

Autonomy–The ethical tenet that the physician has the responsibility to respect patients' choices about their own healthcare.

Availability heuristic–A shortcut in decision making that relies on the information that is most readily available, rather than the total body of information on a subject.

Avoidance learning–A form of negative reinforcement in which one avoids the unpleasantness of something that has yet to happen.

Babbling–Precursor to language known to spontaneously occur in children.

Back stage–In the dramaturgical approach, the setting where players are free from their role requirements and not in front of the audience; back stage behaviors may not be deemed appropriate or acceptable and are thus kept invisible from the audience.

Barbiturate–A drug that acts as a central nervous system depressant; often used for anxiety, for insomnia, and as an antiseizure medication.

Basal ganglia–A portion of the forebrain that coordinates muscle movement and routes information from the cortex to the brain and spinal cord.

Base-rate fallacy–Using prototypical or stereotypical factors while ignoring actual numerical information when making a decision.

Basic model–First established by Charles Darwin, a theory that states that emotional expression involves a number of systems: facial expression as well as behavioral and physical responses; claims that emotions are universal and should be similar across cultures.

Behavioral therapy–A type of psychotherapy that focuses on directly modifying maladaptive behaviors using learning principles.

Behaviorism–B. F. Skinner's theory that all behaviors are conditioned. Behaviorism can be applied across many bodies of psychological thought, including theories of development, of identity, and of personality.

Belief–An acceptance that a statement is true or that something exists.

Belief perseverance–The inability to reject a particular belief despite clear evidence to the contrary.

Beneficence–The ethical tenet that the physician has a responsibility to act in the patient's best interest.

Benzodiazepine–A central nervous system depressant that is often used to reduce anxiety or promote sleep.

Biomedical approach–An approach to psychological disorders that considers only pathophysiological causes and offers pharmaceutical and medical solutions for symptom alleviation.

Biopsychosocial approach–An approach to psychological disorders that considers conditions and treatments to be dependent on biological, psychological, and social causes. Treatment under this approach includes both direct and indirect therapy.

Bipolar disorders–Class of mood disorders characterized by both depression and mania.

Birth rate–The number of births per population in a period of time; usually the number of births per 1000 people per year.

Bisexual–A sexual orientation wherein individuals are attracted to members of multiple sexes.

Blindsight–A rare phenomenon in which a person who is cortically blind can respond to visual stimuli in their blind field without any conscious awareness of seeing them.

Bottom-up processing–Object recognition by parallel processing and feature detection in response to sensory stimuli.

Brainstem–The most primitive portion of the brain, which includes the midbrain and hindbrain; controls the autonomic nervous system and communication between the spinal cord, cranial nerves, and brain.

Broca's aphasia–Loss of the motor function of speech, resulting in intact understanding with an inability to correctly produce spoken language.

Broca's area–A brain region located in the inferior frontal gyrus of the frontal lobe (usually in the left hemisphere); largely responsible for the motor function of speech.

Bureaucracy–A formal organization with the goal of performing complex tasks as efficiently as possible by dividing work among a number of bureaus.

Bystander effect–The observation that, when in a group, individuals are less likely to respond to a person in need.

Cannon–Bard theory–A theory of emotion that states that a stimulus is first received and is then simultaneously processed physiologically and cognitively, allowing for the conscious emotion to be experienced.

Cataplexy–Loss of muscle control with intrusion of REM sleep during waking hours, usually caused by an emotional trigger.

Catatonia–Disorganized motor behavior characterized by various unusual physical movements or stillness.

Central nervous system (CNS)–The portion of the nervous system composed of the brain and spinal cord.

Central route processing–According to the elaboration likelihood model, the process of making a judgment by deeply thinking about information, scrutinizing its meaning and purpose, and drawing conclusions from it.

Cerebellum–A portion of the hindbrain that maintains posture and balance and coordinates body movements.

Cerebral cortex–The outermost layer of the cerebrum, responsible for complex perceptual, behavioral, and cognitive processes.

Cerebrospinal fluid (CSF)–An aqueous solution in which the brain and spinal cord rest; produced by cells lining the ventricles of the brain.

Cerebrum–A portion of the brain that contains the cerebral cortex, limbic system, and basal ganglia.

Characteristic institution–The social structure or institution about which societies are organized.

Chemoreceptors–Sensory neurons that respond to chemical stimuli.

Choice shift–This term is analogous to group polarization, but describes the behavior change of the group as a whole rather than the individual.

Circadian rhythm–The alignment of physiological processes with the 24-hour day, including sleep–wake cycles and some elements of the endocrine system.

Circular reaction–A repetitive action that achieves a desired response; seen during Piaget's sensorimotor stage.

Class consciousness–In Marxist theory, the organization of the working class around shared goals and recognition of a need for collective political action.

Classical conditioning–A form of associative learning in which a neutral stimulus becomes associated with an unconditioned stimulus such that the neutral stimulus alone produces the same response as the unconditioned stimulus; the neutral stimulus thus becomes a conditioned stimulus.

Cocaine–Drug that decreases reuptake of dopamine, norepinephrine, and serotonin, with effects similar to amphetamines.

Cognition–The process of acquiring knowledge and understanding through thought, experiences, and the senses; how we think and respond to the world.

Cognitive appraisal–The subjective evaluation of a situation that induces stress, consisting of both an initial primary appraisal and a potential secondary appraisal if a threat is revealed during primary appraisal.

Cognitive behavioral therapy (CBT)–A type of psychotherapy that focuses on identifying and modifying maladaptive thought patterns and behaviors to treat psychological disorders.

Cognitive development–The development of one's ability to think and solve problems across the life span.

Cognitive dissonance–The simultaneous presence of two opposing thoughts or opinions.

Cognitive reassociation model–A model of aggression which states that we are more likely to respond aggressively when experiencing negative emotions.

Collective unconscious–In Jungian psychoanalysis, the part of the unconscious mind that is shared among all humans and is a result of our common ancestry.

Colliculi–Two structures in the midbrain involved in sensorimotor reflexes; the superior colliculus receives visual sensory input, and the inferior colliculus receives auditory sensory input.

Compliance–A change of behavior of an individual at the request of another.

Concordance rates–In twin studies, the presence of a trait in both twins.

Conditioned response–In classical conditioning paradigms, the reflexive response caused by a conditioned stimulus.

Conditioned stimulus–In classical conditioning paradigms, this is an initially neutral stimulus that is paired with an unconditioned stimulus to train a behavioral response, rendering the previously neutral stimulus a conditioned stimulus.

Conduction aphasia–A speech disorder characterized by the inability to repeat words with intact spontaneous speech production and comprehension; usually due to injury to the arcuate fasciculus.

Confirmation bias–A cognitive bias in which one focuses on information that supports a given solution, belief, or hypothesis and ignores evidence against it.

Conflict theory–A theoretical framework that emphasizes the role of power differentials in producing social order.

Conformity–The changing of beliefs or behaviors in order to fit into a group or society.

Consciousness–Awareness of oneself; can be used to describe varying levels of awareness that occur with wakefulness, sleep, dreaming, and drug-induced states.

Conservation–Concept seen in quantitative analysis performed by a child; develops when a child is able to identify the difference between quantity by number and actual amount, especially when faced with identical quantities separated into varying pieces.

Constancy–In sensory perception, perceiving certain characteristics of object to remain the same despite differences in the environment.

Context effect–A retrieval cue by which memory is aided when a person is in the location where encoding took place.

Contralateral–On the opposite side of the body, relative to something else (usually a side of the brain).

Controlled (conscious) processing–Processing method used when a task requires complete attention.

Correspondent inference theory–A theory that states that people pay closer attention to intentional behavior than accidental behavior when making attributions, especially if the behavior is unexpected.

Cortical homunculus–A "map" that relates regions of the brain to the anatomical regions of the body.

Critical period–A time during development during which exposure to language is essential for eventual development of the effective use of language; occurs between two years of age and puberty.

Crystallized intelligence–Cognitive capacity to understand relationships or solve problems using information acquired during schooling and other experiences.

Cues–In understanding the behavior of others, indicators of the underlying cause of a behavior. This includes consistency cues, consensus cues, and difference cues.

Cultural capital–The benefits one receives from knowledge, abilities, and skills.

Cultural diffusion–The spread of norms, cultures, and beliefs throughout a culture.

Cultural relativism–The theory that social groups and cultures must be studied on their own terms to be understood.

Cultural sensitivity–Recognizing and respecting the differences between cultures.

Cultural syndrome–A shared set of beliefs, attitudes, norms, values, and behaviors organized around a central theme and found among people who speak the same language and share a geographic region.

Cultural transmission–The means by which a society socializes its members.

Culture–The beliefs, behaviors, actions, and characteristics of a group or society of people.

Culture shock–Cultural differences that are seen as quite dramatic when travelling outside of one's own society.

Deductive reasoning–A form of cognition that starts with general information and narrows down that information to create a conclusion.

Defense mechanism–In Freudian psychoanalysis, a technique used by the ego that denies, falsifies, or distorts reality in order to resolve anxiety caused by undesirable urges of the id and superego.

Deindividuation–The idea that people will lose a sense of self-awareness and can act dramatically differently based on the influence of a group.

Delayed reinforcement–A reward that is given after an extended period of time following the desired behavior.

Delirium–Rapid fluctuation in cognitive function that is reversible and has a nonpsychological cause.

Delusions–Fixed, false beliefs that are discordant with reality and not shared by one's culture, and are maintained in spite of strong evidence to the contrary.

Dementia–Intellectual decline starting with impaired memory and progressing to impaired judgment and confusion.

Demographic shift–A change in the makeup of a population over time.

Demographic transition–The transition from high birth and mortality rates to lower birth and mortality rates, seen as a country develops from a preindustrial to an industrialized economic system.

Demographics–The statistical arm of sociology, which attempts to characterize and explain populations by quantitative analysis.

Depressant–Any substance that reduces nervous system function.

Depressive disorder–Sadness meeting certain conditions of severity and duration such that a diagnosis of a mental health issue is warranted. Depressive disorders include, among others: major depression, dysthymic disorder, and seasonal affective disorder.

Depressive episode–A period of at least two weeks in which there is a prominent and persistent depressed mood or lack of interest and at least four other depressive symptoms.

Deviance–The violation of norms, rules, or expectations within a society.

***Diagnostic and Statistical Manual of Mental Disorders* (DSM)**–The guide by which most psychological disorders are characterized, described, and diagnosed; currently in its fifth edition (DSM-5, published May 2013).

Diathesis-stress model–A theory that predisposition to certain biological traits (diatheses), coupled with exposure to environmental stressors, may trigger psychological disorders.

Diencephalon–A portion of the prosencephalon that becomes the thalamus, hypothalamus, posterior pituitary gland, and pineal gland.

Differential association theory–Theory that deviance can be learned through interactions with others who engage in deviant behavior, provided those interactions outnumber interactions with those who conform to social norms in number and/or importance.

Diffusion of responsibility–The phenomenon in which individuals are less likely to take responsibility for a task when in a group, due to the expectation that others will take action.

Disconfirmation principle–The idea that states that if evidence obtained during testing does not confirm a hypothesis, then the hypothesis is discarded or revised.

Discrimination–In classical conditioning, the process by which two similar but distinct conditioned stimuli produce different responses; in sociology, when individuals of a particular group are treated differently than others based on their group.

Discriminative stimulus–In behavioral conditioning, a stimulus whose presence indicates the opportunity for reward.

Dishabituation–A sudden increase in response to a stimulus, usually due to a change in the stimulus or addition of another stimulus; sometimes called resensitization.

Displacement–A defense mechanism by which undesired urges are transferred from one target to another, more acceptable one.

Display rules–Cultural expectations of how emotions can be expressed.

Dispositional (internal) attributions–Attributions that relate to the decisions or personality of the person whose behavior is being considered.

Dissociative disorders–Disorders that involve a perceived separation from identity or the environment.

Distal stimulus–Part of the outside world that serves as a source for stimuli that reach the sensory neurons.

Distant networks–Networks that are looser and composed of weaker ties.

Distress–The stress response to unpleasant stressors.

Divided attention–The ability to attend to multiple stimuli simultaneously and to perform multiple tasks at the same time.

Dizygotic twins–Fraternal twins who share approximately 50% of their genes, as with most siblings.

Dominant hemisphere–The side of the brain that provides analytic, language, logic, and math skills; in most individuals, the left hemisphere.

Dopamine–A neurotransmitter associated with smooth movements, steady posture, the reward pathway, and psychosis.

Downward drift hypothesis–A hypothesis that proposes that individuals with disorders like schizophrenia tend to "drift down" the socioeconomic ladder as a consequence of their illness.

Downward social comparison–Comparing oneself to someone perceived as inferior.

Dramaturgical approach–An impression management theory that represents the world as a stage and individuals as actors performing to an audience.

Dreaming–Phenomenon which mostly occurs during REM sleep. Theories proposed to explain this phenomenon include activation-synthesis theory, problem-solving dream theory, and cognitive process dream theory.

Drive reduction theory–A theory that explains motivation as being based on the goal of eliminating uncomfortable internal states.

Drives–Deficiencies that activate particular behaviors focused on a goal, which can be further subdivided into either primary (body-sustaining) or secondary (not biologically necessary) drives.

Dual-coding theory–A cognitive theory that states that both visual and verbal associations are used to encode and retrieve information.

Duplicity theory of vision–A theory which holds that the retina contains two types of specialized photoreceptors: rods specialized for light and dark perception and cones specialized for color perception.

Dyssomnia–A sleep disorder in which one has difficulty falling asleep, staying asleep, or avoiding sleep.

Ecstasy–Common name for MDMA (3,4-methylenedioxy-*N*-methylamphetamine); a central nervous system stimulant with effects similar to both amphetamines and hallucinogens.

Efferent neurons–Motor neurons that transmit information from the central nervous system to the periphery.

Ego–In Freudian psychoanalysis, the part of the unconscious mind that mediates the urges of the id and superego; operates under the reality principle.

Egocentrism–Self-centered view of the world in which one is not necessarily able to understand the experience of another person; seen in Piaget's preoperational stage.

Elaboration likelihood model–A theory in which attitudes are formed and changed through different routes of information processing based on the degree of deep thought given to persuasive information. There are two possible processing routes within this model: central route processing (deep thinking or elaborative) and peripheral route processing (non-elaborative).

Elaborative rehearsal–The association of information in short-term memory to information already stored in long-term memory; aids in long-term storage.

Electroencephalography (EEG)–A test used to study the electrical patterns of the brain under varying conditions; consists of multiple electrodes placed on the scalp. Characteristic EEG patterns include beta, alpha, theta, and delta waves, as well as patterns associated with REM sleep.

Emotion–A feeling and state of mind derived from circumstances, mood, or relationships.

Emotion-focused coping–A coping strategy that aims to reduce the negative emotional responses associated with stress.

Emotional support–Listening to, affirming, and empathizing with someone's feelings as part of social support.

Empathy–The ability to vicariously experience the emotions of another.

Empathy-altruism hypothesis–Theory that one individual helps another when they feel empathy for the other person.

Encoding–The process of receiving information and preparing it for storage; can be automatic or effortful.

Encoding specificity–A phenomenon in which recall is improved when the conditions present during encoding are also present during retrieval.

Endorphins–Natural painkillers produced by the brain.

Epinephrine–A neurotransmitter associated with the fight-or-flight response.

Errors of growth–Misuse of grammar characterized by universal application of a rule, regardless of exceptions; seen in children during language development.

Escape learning–A form of negative reinforcement in which one reduces the unpleasantness of something that already exists.

Esteem support–Affirming qualities and skills of the person as part of social support.

Ethnic enclave–Locations with a high concentration of one specific ethnicity that can often slow assimilation.

Ethnicity–A social construct that sorts people by cultural factors, including language, nationality, religion, and other factors.

Ethnocentrism–The practice of making judgments about other cultures based on the values and beliefs of one's own culture.

Eustress–The stress response to positive conditions.

Evolutionary stable strategy–A strategy that, once adopted, will use natural selective pressure to prevent alternate strategies from arising.

Exchange theory–In social structure, an extension of rational choice theory that focuses on interactions in groups. Exchange theory holds that behavior is engaged in based on expectancy of future rewards and/or punishments.

Expectancy-value theory–The amount of motivation needed to reach a goal is the result of both expectation of success in reaching the goal and degree to which reaching the goal is valued.

Explicit memory–Memory that requires conscious recall, divided into facts (semantic memory) and experiences (episodic memory); also known as declarative memory.

Extinction–In classical conditioning, the decrease in response resulting from repeated presentation of the conditioned stimulus without the presence of the unconditioned stimulus.

Extrapyramidal system–Part of the basal ganglia that modulates motor activity.

Extraversion–In trait theory, the degree to which an individual is able to tolerate social interaction and stimulation.

Extrinsic motivation–Motivation that is external, or outside the self, including rewards and punishments.

Facial-feedback effect–A theory that certain facial expressions can influence emotions; also called the facial-feedback hypothesis.

False consciousness–In Marxist theory, a misperception of one's actual position within society.

Family group–A group determined by birth, adoption, and marriage rather than self-selection (as in a peer group).

Fertility rate–The average number of children born to a woman during her lifetime in a population.

Fisherian selection–Also called runaway selection, this is a positive feedback mechanism in which a trait with no impact (or a negative impact) on survival becomes more and more exaggerated over time, especially if the trait is deemed sexually desirable.

Fixation–In Freudian psychoanalysis, the result of overindulgence or frustration during a psychosexual stage causing a neurotic pattern of personality based on that stage.

Flat affect–Behavior characterized by showing virtually no signs of emotion or affective expression.

Fluid intelligence–Ability to quickly identify relationships and connections, and then use those relationships and connections to make correct deductions.

Foraging–The act of searching for and exploiting food resources.

Forebrain–A portion of the brain that is associated with complex perceptual, cognitive, and behavioral processes such as emotion and memory.

Fornix–A long projection from the hippocampus that connects to other nuclei in the limbic system.

Front stage–In the dramaturgical approach, the setting where players are in front of an audience and perform roles that are in keeping with the image they hope to project about themselves.

Frontal lobe–A portion of the cerebral cortex that includes the prefrontal cortex and the motor cortex; it controls motor processing, executive function, and the integration of cognitive and behavioral processes.

Functional attitudes theory–Theory that attitudes serve four functions: knowledge, ego expression, adaptation, and ego defense.

Functional fixedness–The inability to identify uses for an object beyond its usual purpose.

Functionalism–A theoretical framework that explains how parts of society fit together to create a cohesive whole, via both manifest (intended to help some part of the system) and latent (unintended positive) functions.

Fundamental attribution error–The general bias toward making dispositional attributions rather than situational attributions when analyzing another person's behavior.

Game theory–A model that explains social interaction and decision making as a game, including strategies, incentives, and punishments.

γ-aminobutyric acid (GABA)–A neurotransmitter associated with stabilizing and quelling brain activity.

Ganglia–Collections of neuron cell bodies found outside the central nervous system.

Gemeinschaft und Gesellschaft–Theory that distinguishes between two major types of groups: communities (*Gemeinschaften*), which share beliefs, ancestry, or geography; and societies (*Gesellschaften*), which work together toward a common goal.

Gender–The set of behavioral, cultural, or psychological traits typically associated with a biological sex.

Gender inequality–The intentional or unintentional empowerment of one gender to the detriment of others.

Gender segregation–The separation of individuals based on perceived gender.

General adaptation syndrome–Sequence of physiological responses developed by Selye in response to stress, initiating with alarm, followed by resistance, and finally exhaustion.

Generalization–In classical conditioning, the process by which two distinct but similar stimuli come to produce the same response.

Genotype–The genetic makeup of an individual.

Gentrification–The process of renewal of low income areas by upper-class populations, ultimately displacing the lower income residents.

Gestalt principles–Governed by the law of prägnanz, ways for the brain to infer missing parts of a picture when a picture is incomplete.

Globalization–The process of integrating the global economy with free trade and tapping of foreign labor markets.

Glutamate–An excitatory neurotransmitter in the central nervous system.

Glycine–An inhibitory neurotransmitter in the central nervous system.

Group–A social entity that involves at least two people, usually those sharing common characteristics.

Group conformity–Compliance with a group's goals, even when the group's goals may be in direct contrast to an individual's goals.

Group polarization–The tendency toward decisions that are more extreme than the individual inclinations of the group members.

Groupthink–The tendency for groups to make decisions based on ideas and solutions that arise within the group without considering outside ideas and ethics; based on pressure to conform and remain loyal to the group.

Gyrus–A ridge of the cerebral cortex.

Habituation–A decrease in response caused by repeated exposure to a stimulus.

Hallucinations–Perceptions that are not due to external stimuli but have a compelling sense of reality.

Hallucinogens–A group of drugs that cause distortions of reality in users, including lysergic acid diethylamide (LSD) and psilocybin-containing mushrooms.

Halo effect–A cognitive bias in which judgments of an individual's character can be affected by the overall impression of the individual.

Heterosexual–A sexual orientation wherein individuals are attracted to members of a different sex.

Heuristic–A rule of thumb or shortcut that is used to make decisions.

Hidden curriculum–In education, the transmission to students of social norms, attitudes, and beliefs.

Hierarchy of salience–Theory of identity organization that posits that we let situations dictate which identity holds the most importance at any given moment.

Hindbrain–A portion of the brain that controls balance, motor coordination, breathing, digestion, and general arousal processes.

Hippocampus–A portion of the limbic system that is important for memory and learning.

Homosexual–A sexual orientation wherein individuals are attracted to members of the same sex.

Humanistic theory–The set of theories that hold that personality is the result of the conscious feelings we have for ourselves as we attempt to attain our needs and goals. The theories of Kelly, Maslow, Lewin, and others fall into this category.

Hypnagogic hallucinations–Hallucinations that occur when going to sleep; seen in narcolepsy.

Hypnopompic hallucinations–Hallucinations that occur when awakening from sleep; seen in narcolepsy.

Hypnosis–An altered state of consciousness in which a person appears to be awake but is, in fact, in a highly suggestible state in which another person or event may trigger action by the person.

Hypothalamus–A portion of the forebrain that controls homeostatic and endocrine functions by controlling the release of pituitary hormones.

Id–In Freudian psychoanalysis, the part of the unconscious resulting from basic, instinctual urges for sexuality and survival; operates under the pleasure principle and seeks instant gratification.

Ideal self–The person one would optimally like to be.

Identity–A piece of an individual's self-concept based on the groups to which that person belongs and relationships to others.

Identity shift effect–When an individual's state of harmony is disrupted by a threat of social rejection, the individual will often conform to the norms of the group, followed by a corresponding identity shift to reduce cognitive dissonance.

Immediate networks–Networks that are dense with strong ties; generally overlap with distant networks.

Implicit memory–Memory that does not require conscious recall; consists of skills and conditioned behaviors.

Implicit personality theory–A theory that states that people tend to associate traits and behavior in others, and that people have the tendency to attribute their own beliefs, opinions, and ideas onto others.

Impression management–Behaviors that are intended to influence the perceptions of other people about a person, object, or event.

Incentive–A reward intended to motivate particular behaviors.

Incentive theory–Theory that behavior is motivated by the desire to pursue rewards and avoid punishments.

Incidence–The number of new cases of a disease per population at risk in a given period of time; usually, new cases per 1000 at-risk people per year.

Inclusive fitness–A measure of reproductive success; depends on the number of offspring an individual has, how well they support their offspring, and how well their offspring can support others.

Individual discrimination–One person discriminating against a particular person or group.

Inductive reasoning–A form of cognition that utilizes generalizations to develop a theory.

Industrialization–The process by which an economy transitions from a preindustrial or agrarian society to one centered on manufacturing.

Inferior colliculus–Region of the midbrain that receives and integrates sensory input from the auditory system, and is involved in reflexive reactions to auditory input.

Information processing model–Model of human cognition containing four key components: information intake, information analysis, situational modification, and content/complexity of problem.

Informational support–Support given by providing information to help another person.

Ingratiation–An impression management strategy that uses flattery to increase social acceptance.

In-group–A social group to which people experience a sense of belonging or one in which they identify as a member.

Innate behavior–A behavior that is genetically programmed or instinctive.

Insomnia–Sleep disorder characterized by either an inability to fall asleep or difficulty staying asleep.

Instinct–An innate behavioral response to stimuli.

Instinct theory–In motivation, the theory that people are driven to engage in behaviors based on evolutionarily preprogrammed instincts.

Instinctive drift–The tendency of animals to resist learning when a conditioned behavior conflicts with the animal's instinctive behaviors.

Institutional discrimination–Discrimination against a particular person or group by an entire institution.

Intelligence quotient–Numerical measurement of intelligence, usually accomplished by some form of standardized testing.

Interaction process analysis–A technique of observing and immediately classifying the activities of small groups.

Interference–A retrieval error caused by the learning of information; can be proactive (old information causes difficulty learning new information) or retroactive (new information interferes with older learning).

Internalization–Changing one's behavior to fit with a group while also privately agreeing with the ideas of the group.

Interneuron–A neuron found between sensory and motor neurons; involved in the reflex arc.

Interpersonal attraction–The force that makes people like each other.

Intersectionality–The interconnected nature of social categorizations as they apply to a given individual/group, especially when they lead to discrimination or oppression.

Intrinsic motivation–Motivation that is internal or that comes from within.

Intuition–Perceptions about a situation that may or may not be supported by available evidence, but are nonetheless perceived as information that may be used to make a decision.

Ipsilateral–On the same side of the body, relative to something else (usually a side of the brain).

Iron law of oligarchy–Democratic or bureaucratic systems naturally shift to being ruled by an elite group.

James–Lange theory–A theory of emotion that states that a stimulus results in physiological arousal, which then leads to a secondary response in which emotion is consciously experienced.

Justice–In medical ethics, the tenet that the physician has a responsibility to treat similar patients with similar care and to distribute healthcare resources fairly.

Just-noticeable difference (jnd)–The minimum difference in magnitude between two stimuli before one can perceive this difference; also called a difference threshold.

Just-world hypothesis–The cognitive bias that good things happen to good people, and bad things happen to bad people.

Labeling theory–Theory that labels given to people affect not only how others respond to that person, but also the person's self-image.

Language–Spoken or written symbols (verbal and nonverbal symbols), which are regulated according to certain rules of conduct or social norms and used for communication.

Language acquisition device (LAD)–An innate capacity for language acquisition that is triggered by exposure to language; part of the nativist (biological) perspective of language acquisition.

Latent learning–Learning that occurs without a reward but that is spontaneously demonstrated once a reward is introduced.

Lateral social comparison–Comparing oneself to someone perceived as similar.

Law of effect–The principle that behaviors followed by desirable outcomes are more likely to be repeated.

Learned helplessness–A state of hopelessness and resignation resulting from being unable to avoid repeated negative stimuli; often used as a model of depression.

Learning–In psychology, the way in which new behaviors are acquired.

Learning (behaviorist) theory–A theory that attitudes are developed through forms of learning (direct contact, direct interaction, direct instruction, and conditioning).

Libido–In Freudian psychoanalysis, the sex or life drive.

Life course approach to health–An analysis of health and probable outcomes that includes consideration of the patient's entire history.

Limbic system–A portion of the cerebrum that is associated with emotion and memory and includes the amygdala and hippocampus.

Linguistic relativity hypothesis–A hypothesis suggesting that one's perception of reality is largely determined by the content, form, and structure of language; also known as the Whorfian hypothesis.

Locus of control–The characterization of the source of influences on the events in one's life; can be internal or external.

Long-term memory–The relatively limitless form of memory reserved for information that is sufficiently rehearsed or of sufficient impact. There are both implicit and explicit forms of long-term memory.

Long-term potentiation–The strengthening of neural connections due to rehearsal or relearning; thought to be the neurophysiological basis of long-term memory.

Looking-glass self–Social psychological construct stating that the self is developed through interpersonal reactions, specifically through a person's understanding of the perception others have of them.

Magnocellular cells–In vision processing, cells that have high temporal resolution and detect motion.

Maintenance rehearsal–Repetition of a piece of information either to keep it within working memory or to store it.

Maladaptive coping–When coping temporarily reduces the distress of a stressful situation but ultimately causes more harm and prevents a healthy adjustment to the stressor in the long term.

Malthusian theory–Theory of demographic transition that focuses on how population growth can outpace food supply growth and lead to social degradation and disorder.

Managing appearances–An impression management strategy in which one uses props, appearance, emotional expression, or associations with others to create a positive image.

Manic episode–A period of at least one week with prominent and persistent elevated or expansive mood and at least two other manic symptoms.

Maslow's hierarchy of needs–Abraham Maslow's theory that certain needs will yield a greater influence on motivation. Maslow's hierarchy consists of five "levels" of need.

Mass hysteria–A shared, intense concern about the threats to society.

Master status–A status with which a person is most identified.

Mate bias–A measure of how choosy members of a species are in choosing a mate, based upon both direct and indirect benefits of mate selection.

Mate choice–The selection of a mate based on attraction and traits.

Material culture–The physical items one associates with a given cultural group.

Material support–Providing economic or other physical resources to aid a person as part of social support.

Mating system–The way in which a group organizes its sexual behavior and sexual relationships.

McDonaldization–A shift in focus toward efficiency, predictability, calculability, and control in societies.

Meditation–A state of consciousness entered voluntarily, characterized by a decreased level of physiological arousal and a quieting of the mind.

Medulla oblongata–A portion of the brainstem that regulates vital functions, including breathing, heart rate, and blood pressure.

Melatonin–A serotonin derivative secreted by the pineal gland that is associated with sleepiness.

Meninges–A thick layer of connective tissue that covers and protects the brain; composed of the dura mater, arachnoid mater, and pia mater.

Mental set–A tendency to repeat solutions that have yielded positive results at some time in the past.

Mere exposure effect–An explanation of attraction, also called the familiarity effect, which holds that people prefer stimuli that they have been exposed to more frequently.

Meritocracy–A society in which advancement up the social ladder is based on intellectual talent and achievement.

Mesencephalon–The embryonic portion of the brain that becomes the midbrain.

Mesolimbic reward pathway–Dopaminergic pathway in the brain including the nucleus accumbens, ventral tegmental area, and the medial forebrain bundle. This pathway is normally involved in motivation and emotional response, and is involved in drug addiction.

Metacognition–The awareness of one's own thoughts and emotions; also known as "thinking about thinking."

Metencephalon–The embryonic portion of the brain that becomes the pons and cerebellum.

Midbrain–A portion of the brainstem that manages sensorimotor reflexes to visual and auditory stimuli and gives rise to some cranial nerves.

Migration–The movement of people from one population to another, including immigration and emigration.

Mindfulness meditation–A stress reduction practice that encourages individuals to focus on the present moment and their active thoughts, feelings, and sensations.

Mirror neurons–Neurons located in the frontal and parietal lobes and which fire both when an individual performs an action and when an individual sees that action performed.

Misinformation effect–A phenomenon in which memories are altered by misleading information provided at the point of encoding or recall.

Mnemonic–A technique that aids in memory recall.

Monogamy–An exclusive mating relationship.

Monozygotic twins–Identical twins, sharing the same genetic material.

Mood disorder–A mental health diagnosis category containing disorders primarily characterized by disturbance in mood. This includes depressive disorders, substance-induced, and bipolar disorders.

Moral reasoning–Kohlberg's theory of personality evelopment, which is focused on the development of moral thinking through preconventional, conventional, and postconventional stages.

Morbidity–The burden or degree of illness associated with a given disease.

Morphology–The structure of words, including their building blocks (prefixes, suffixes, and so on).

Mortality rate–The number of deaths in a population per unit time.

Motivation–The process of psychological and physical requirements, goals, or desires causing behavior.

Motor neuron–A neuron that transmits motor information from the spinal cord and brain to the periphery.

Multicultural socialization–The process of learning the norms and behaviors of multiple different cultures.

Multiculturalism–The encouragement of multiple cultures in a society to enhance diversity; also referred to as cultural diversity.

Multiple intelligences–The idea that intelligence may exist in multiple areas, not just in the areas typically assessed by traditional intelligence quotient tests.

Myelencephalon–The embryonic portion of the brain that becomes the medulla oblongata.

Narcolepsy–A sleep disorder characterized by a lack of voluntary control over the onset of sleep; also involves cataplexy and hypnagogic and hypnopompic hallucinations.

Nativist theory (of language)–Theory credited to Noam Chomsky that posits the existence of an innate capacity for language, referred to as the language acquisition device.

Needs–Physiological and psychological requirements that motivate and influence behavior.

Negative symptoms–In mental illness, symptoms characterized by the absence of normal or desired behaviors.

Neologism–Coining a new word; seen in schizophrenia.

Network–A term used to describe the observable pattern of social relationships among individual units of analysis.

Network redundancy–Overlapping contact points within a social network.

Network support–Providing a sense of belonging as part of social support.

Neurocognitive models of dreaming–Models of dreaming that correlate subjective, cognitive experiences of dreaming with measurable physiological changes.

Neuroleptics (antipsychotics)–A class of drugs used to treat schizophrenia by blocking dopamine receptors.

Neuromodulator–Peptides that act as signaling molecules in the central nervous system; they are slower to act and longer lasting than neurotransmitters.

Neuroplasticity–Change in neural connections caused by learning or a response to injury.

Neuropsychology–The study of functions and behaviors associated with specific regions of the brain.

Neurosis–In Freudian theory, a disorder that occurs in response to the anxiety of a fixation during childhood that impacts personality development.

Neuroticism–In trait theory, the degree to which an individual is prone to emotional arousal in stressful situations.

Neurotransmitter–A chemical that transmits signals from a neuron to a target cell across a synapse.

Neurulation–Stage in development in which the ectoderm furrows over the notochord, forming the neural crest and neural tube.

Night terror–An experience of intense anxiety during sleep, causing the sleeper to scream in terror with no recall of the event in the morning; occurs during slow-wave sleep.

Nondominant hemisphere–The side of the brain associated with sensitivity to the emotional tone of language, intuition, creativity, music, and spatial processing; in most individuals, the right hemisphere.

Nonmaleficence–The ethical tenet that the physician has a responsibility to avoid interventions in which the potential for harm outweighs the potential for benefit.

Non-rapid eye movement (NREM) sleep–Stages 1 through 4 of sleep; contains ever-slowing brain waves as one gets deeper into sleep.

Nonverbal communication–How people communicate, intentionally or unintentionally, without using words; examples include body language, gestures, and facial expressions.

Norepinephrine–A neurotransmitter associated with wakefulness and alertness.

Norms–Societal rules that define the boundaries of acceptable behavior.

Obedience–The changing of behavior of an individual based on a command from someone seen as an authority figure.

Object permanence–Knowledge that an object does not cease to exist even when the object cannot be seen; a milestone in cognitive development.

Observational learning–A form of learning in which behavior is modified as a result of watching others.

Obsessive–compulsive disorders–This category, which also includes related disorders, describes the set of disorders where people feel the need to check things repeatedly or have certain thoughts repeatedly, without the ability to control these thoughts or activities.

Occipital lobe–A portion of the cerebral cortex that controls visual processing.

Olfactory chemoreceptors–Receptors in the olfactory epithelium in the upper part of the nasal cavity that respond to volatile or aerosolized compounds by binding to chemical stimuli; also known as olfactory nerves.

Onlooker–A stage of development in which a child actively watches other children play, often talking to them and asking questions, but does not join in the activity.

Operant conditioning–A form of associative learning in which the frequency of a behavior is modified using reinforcement or punishment.

Opiates–A drug family consisting of naturally occurring, highly addictive, pain-reducing drugs used in both medical and recreational settings; opioids are synthetic versions of these drugs.

Opponent-process theory (color)–This theory states that the ability to perceive color is controlled by three opposing receptor systems: a red-green channel, a blue-yellow channel, and a black-white (luminance) channel.

Opponent-process theory (motivation)–A theory that states that the body will adapt to counteract repeated exposure to stimuli, such as seeing afterimages or ramping up the sympathetic nervous system in response to a depressant.

Organization–A specific type of group characterized by five traits: formality, hierarchy of ranked positions, large size, complex division of labor, and continuity beyond its members.

Ought self–The representation of the way others think one should be.

Out-group–A social group with which an individual does not identify.

Overconfidence–A tendency to interpret one's decisions, knowledge, or beliefs as infallible.

Parallel play–Play style in which children can play alongside each other without interfering in each other's behavior.

Parallel processing–The ability to simultaneously analyze and combine information regarding multiple aspects of a stimulus, such as color, shape, and motion.

Parasomnia–A sleep disorder characterized by abnormal movements or behaviors during sleep.

Parasympathetic nervous system–A branch of the autonomic nervous system that promotes resting and digesting; associated with relaxed states, reductions in heart and respiration rates, and promotion of digestion.

Parietal lobe–A portion of the cerebral cortex that controls somatosensory and spatial processing.

Parkinson's disease–A disease characterized by slowness in movement, resting tremor, pill-rolling tremor, masklike facies, cogwheel rigidity, and a shuffling gait; caused by destruction of dopaminergic neurons in the substantia nigra.

Parvocellular cells–In visual processing, cells which have very high spatial resolution and detect shape.

Peer group–A group of self-selected equals that forms around common interests, ideas, preferences, and beliefs.

Peer pressure–The social influence placed on an individual by other individuals who are perceived as equals.

Perception–Processing of incoming information to comprehend and respond to the current incoming stimuli.

Perceptual learning–The long-lasting improvement in the ability to perceive and differentiate sensory stimuli as a direct result of practice and experience.

Peripheral nervous system (PNS)–The portion of the nervous system composed of nerve tissue and fibers outside the central nervous system.

Peripheral retina–The region of the retina outside the fovea, where the concentration of rods is higher and the concentration of cones is lower.

Peripheral route processing–According to the elaboration likelihood model, the process of making a judgment by focusing on superficial details, such as the appearance of the person delivering the argument or the use of slogans, rather than the content of the argument.

Personality–The set of thoughts, feelings, traits, and behaviors that are characteristic of an individual across time and different locations.

Personality disorders–Disorders that involve patterns of behavior that are inflexible and maladaptive, causing distress or impaired function in at least two of the following: cognition, emotion, interpersonal functioning, or impulse control.

Phenotype–The expressed traits of an individual based on their genotype.

Phoneme–Individual speech sound associated with a language.

Phonology–The set of sounds that compose a language.

Piaget's theory–Piaget's theory of cognitive development divided the life span into sensorimotor, preoperational, concrete operational, and formal operational stages.

Pineal gland–A brain structure located near the thalamus that secretes melatonin.

Pituitary gland–The "master gland" of the endocrine system that triggers hormone release in other endocrine glands.

Place theory–Theory of sound conduction in the ear that holds that vibration on particular areas of the basilar membrane determines perception of pitch, also referred to as tonotopical organization.

Polyandry–A mating system in which an individual has exclusive relationships with several males.

Polygamy–A mating system in which an individual has multiple exclusive relationships.

Polygyny–A mating system in which an individual has exclusive relationships with several females.

Pons–A portion of the brainstem that relays information between the cortex and medulla, regulates sleep, and carries some motor and sensory information from the face and neck.

Positive symptoms–Behaviors, thoughts, or feelings added to normal behavior.

Poverty–A socioeconomic condition of low resource availability; in the United States, the poverty line is determined by the government's calculation of the minimum income requirements for families to acquire the minimum necessities of life.

Power–The capacity to influence people through the real or threatened use of rewards and punishments; often based on unequal distribution of valued resources.

Pragmatics–The ways in which use of language can be altered, depending on social context.

Prejudice–An irrational positive or negative attitude toward a person, group, or thing, formed prior to actual experience.

Prestige–In sociology, the amount of positive regard society has for a given person or idea.

Prevalence–The number of cases of a disease per population in a given period of time; usually, cases per 1000 people per year.

Primacy effect–The phenomenon of first impressions of a person being more important than subsequent impressions.

Primary group–A group wherein the interactions are direct, with close bonds, providing relationships to members that are very warm, personal, and intimate.

Primary stress appraisal–An initial evaluation of the environment to determine if there is an associated threat.

Priming–A retrieval cue by which recall is aided by a word or phrase that is semantically related to the desired memory.

Primitive reflexes–Reflexes present in infants that disappear with age.

Problem-focused coping–A coping strategy that targets the causes of stress by directly addressing and attempting to solve the underlying problem.

Prodromal phase–A phase of poor adjustment that precedes the full onset of schizophrenia.

Projection–A defense mechanism by which individuals attribute their undesired feelings to others.

Projection area–A portion of the cerebral cortex that analyzes sensory input.

Promiscuity–A mating system in which an individual mates with others without exclusivity.

Proprioception–The ability to tell where one's body is in space.

Prosencephalon–The embryonic portion of the brain that becomes the forebrain.

Prosody–The rhythm, cadence, and inflection of speech.

Prospective memory–Remembering to perform a task at some point in a future.

Proximal stimulus–A stimulus that directly interacts with and affects sensory receptors.

Proximity–An aspect of interpersonal attraction based on being physically close to someone.

Psychoanalytic theory–In personality theory, the set of theories based on the assumption that unconscious internal states motivate overt actions and determine personality. The theories of several psychologists, including both Freud and Jung, fall into this category.

Psychological disorder–A set of thoughts, feelings, or actions that are considered deviant by the culture at hand and that cause noticeable distress to the sufferer.

Psychopharmacology–The use of prescribed medications to treat psychological disorders.

Psychophysics–The study of the relationship between the physical nature of stimuli and the sensations/perceptions they evoke.

Psychosocial development–Erikson's theory of personality development, which is based in the concept that personality is developed based on a series of crises deriving from conflicts between needs and social demands.

Psychotherapy–The use of specialized techniques by a trained therapist to treat psychological disorders.

Psychoticism–In trait theory, the measure of nonconformity or social deviance of an individual.

Punishment–In operant conditioning, the use of an aversive stimulus designed to decrease the frequency of an undesired behavior.

Race–A social construct based on phenotypic differences between groups of people; these may be either real or perceived differences.

Racial formation theory–Theory that racial identity is fluid and dependent on political, economic, and social factors.

Racialization–The social process by which racial groups are associated with specific characteristics in a society.

Rapid eye movement (REM) sleep–Sleep stage in which the eyes move rapidly back and forth and physiological arousal levels are more similar to wakefulness than sleep; dreaming occurs during this stage.

Rational choice theory–In social structure, the theory that individuals consider benefits and harms to themselves in any given social interaction and choose the best possible action.

Rationalization–A defense mechanism by which individuals explain undesirable behaviors in a way that is self-justifying and socially acceptable.

Reaction formation–A defense mechanism by which individuals suppress urges by unconsciously converting them into their exact opposites.

Reappraisal–Process for ongoing monitoring of a continuing source of stress that cannot be dealt with via the normal 2-step appraisal method.

Recency effect–The phenomenon in which the most recent information we have about an individual is most important in forming our impressions.

Reciprocal determinism–In the social cognitive perspective, the notion that thoughts, feelings, behaviors, and environment interact to determine behavior in a given situation.

Reciprocal liking–The phenomenon whereby people like others better when they believe the other person likes them.

Reciprocity–An aspect of interpersonal attraction based on the idea that we like people who we think like us.

Recognition-primed decision model–A decision-making model in which experience and recognition of similar situations one has already experienced play a large role in decision making and actions; also one of the explanations for the experience of intuition.

Reference group–The group to which individuals compare themselves for a given identity.

Reflex–A behavior that occurs in response to a given stimulus without higher cognitive input.

Reflex arc–A neural pathway that controls reflex actions.

Regional cerebral blood flow (rCBF)–A technique used to record patterns of neural activity based on blood flow to different areas of the brain measured using detection of inhaled radioactive markers.

Regression–A defense mechanism by which an individual deals with stress by reverting to an earlier developmental state.

Reinforcement–In operant conditioning, the use of a stimulus designed to increase the frequency of a desired behavior.

Reinforcement schedule–The schedule by which reinforcement is administered for behavior in operant conditioning; reinforcement schedules can be fixed or variable, and can be based on a ratio or an interval between rewards.

Relative poverty–Poverty in comparison to the larger surrounding population.

Reliance on central traits–The tendency to organize the perception of others based on traits and personal characteristics of the target that matter to the perceiver.

REM rebound–Phenomenon in which one spends an increased time in REM sleep following a period of sleep deprivation.

Representativeness heuristic–A shortcut in decision making that relies on categorizing items on the basis of whether they fit the prototypical, stereotypical, or representative image of the category.

Repression–A defense mechanism by which the ego forces undesired thoughts and urges to the unconscious mind.

Resource mobilization–A theory that considers how groups involved in social movements achieve their objectives through the collection and utilization of money, attention, skills, materials, and other resources.

Response bias–The tendency of subjects to respond systematically to a stimulus in a particular way due to nonsensory factors.

Reticular formation–A structure in the brainstem that is responsible for alertness.

Retrieval–The process of demonstrating that information has been retained in memory; includes recall, recognition, and relearning.

Retrograde amnesia–A form of memory loss that impacts long-term memories of events prior to the time of injury.

Rhombencephalon–The embryonic portion of the brain that becomes the hindbrain.

Ritual–A formalized ceremony that usually involves specific material objects, symbolism, and additional mandates on acceptable behavior.

Role–A set of beliefs, values, attitudes, and norms that define expectations for behavior associated with a particular status.

Role conflict–A difficulty in satisfying role requirements or expectations among various roles.

Role engulfment–Internalizing a label and assuming the role implied by the label leads to the assumed role taking over a person's identity.

Role partner–The person with whom one interacts while playing a particular role; each role partner provides a different set of behavioral expectations.

Role performance–Carrying out the behaviors associated with a given role.

Role set–A group of role partners relative to a given status.

Role strain–Difficulty in satisfying multiple requirements of the same role.

Role-taking–Roleplaying, by which children come to understand the perspectives of others and the ways in which these perspectives may differ from their own.

Sanction–A societally enforced punishment or reward for behavior. Formal sanctions are those enforced by social institutions (laws), and informal sanctions are enforced by social behaviors (ostracization, etc.).

Scaffolding–Temporary support that helps learners build new skills and knowledge, enabling them to tackle tasks within their zone of proximal development.

Schachter–Singer theory–A theory of emotion that states that both physiological arousal and cognitive appraisal must occur before an emotion is consciously experienced.

Schema–An organized pattern of thought and behavior; one of the central concepts of Piaget's stages of cognitive development.

Schizophrenia–A psychotic disorder characterized by gross distortions of reality and disturbances in the content and form of thought, perception, and behavior.

Second sickness–The concept proposed by Howard Waitzkin that poor health outcomes are exacerbated by social injustice.

Secondary group–Groups wherein interactions are based on weaker, impersonal bonds.

Secondary stress appraisal–The interpretation of primary stress appraisal to determine emotional response to a given threat.

Selective attention–The ability to focus on a single stimulus even while other stimuli are occurring simultaneously.

Self-concept–The sum of the thoughts and feelings about oneself; includes self-schemata and appraisal of one's past and future self.

Self-determination theory–Need-based motivational theory that emphasizes the importance of autonomy, competence, and relatedness.

Self-disclosure–An aspect of interpersonal attraction or impression management in which one shares fears, thoughts, and goals with another person in the hopes of being met with empathy and nonjudgment.

Self-discrepancy theory–Theory that each of us has three selves: the actual self, the ideal self, and the ought self.

Self-efficacy–The degree to which individuals see themselves as being capable at a given skill or in a particular situation.

Self-enhancement–In self-serving bias, the need to maintain self worth through internal attribution of success and external attribution of failure.

Self-esteem–An individual's feelings of self-worth.

Self-fulfilling prophecy–The phenomenon of a stereotype creating an expectation of a particular group, which creates conditions that lead to confirmation of this stereotype.

Self-handicapping–An impression management strategy wherein people create obstacles to avoid self-blame when they do not meet expectations.

Self-identification–The ability to recognize one's own appearance.

Self-presentation–The process of displaying oneself to society through culturally accepted actions and behaviors.

Self-reference effect–The tendency for individuals to best recall information that they can relate to their own experiences.

Self-schema–A self-given label that carries with it a set of qualities.

Self-serving bias–The idea that individuals will view their own success as being based on internal factors, while viewing failures as being based on external factors.

Semantic network–Organization of information in the brain by linking concepts with similar characteristics and meaning.

Semantics–The association of meaning with a word.

Sensation–Transduction of physical stimuli into neurologic signals.

Sensitive period–A time during which environmental input has a maximal impact on the development of a particular ability.

Sensory memory–Visual (iconic) and auditory (echoic) stimuli briefly stored in memory; fades very quickly unless attention is paid to the information.

Sensory neuron–A neuron that transmits information from sensory receptors to the central nervous system.

Septal nuclei–Part of the limbic system and one of the pleasure centers of the brain.

Serial position effect–The tendency to better remember items presented at the beginning or end of a list; related to the primacy and recency effects.

Serial processing–The execution of cognitive processes in a sequential, step-by-step manner.

Serotonin–A neurotransmitter associated with mood, sleep, eating, and dreaming.

Sexual orientation–The direction of one's sexual interest.

Shadowing–An experimental technique in which participants recite speech immediately after hearing it.

Shaping–In operant conditioning, the process of conditioning a complicated behavior by rewarding successive approximations of the behavior.

Short-term memory–Memory which fades quickly, over about 30 seconds without rehearsal, and which is limited in capacity by the 7 ± 2 rule.

Sick role–Theory that a person who is ill enters a role of "sanctioned deviance," in which they are not responsible for the illness and are exempt from social norms.

Signal detection theory–A theory of perception in which internal (psychological) and external (environmental) context both play a role in the perception of stimuli.

Similarity–An aspect of interpersonal attraction based on being alike in attitudes, intelligence, education, height, age, religion, appearance, or socioeconomic status.

Situational (external) attributions–Attributions that relate to features of the surroundings, such as threats, money, social norms, and peer pressure, rather than to features of the individual.

Sleep apnea–Sleep disorder in which a person may cease to breathe while sleeping; may be due to obstruction or a central (neurological) cause.

Sleep cycle–A single complete progression through each stage of sleep.

Slow-wave sleep–Consists of NREM sleep stages 3 and 4; also called delta-wave sleep.

Social action–Actions and behaviors that individuals are conscious of and performing because others are around.

Social capital–The investment people make in their society in return for economic or collective rewards.

Social class–A category of people with a shared socioeconomic background that exhibit similar lifestyles, job opportunities, attitudes, and behaviors.

Social cognitive theory–A theory that attitudes are formed through observation of behavior, cognition, and the environment.

Social comparison theory–The idea that individuals evaluate themselves by comparing themselves to others.

Social construction model–A theory of emotional expression that assumes there are no biologically wired emotions; rather, they are based on experiences and situational context alone.

Social constructionism–A theoretical approach that uncovers the ways in which individuals and groups participate in the formation of their perceived social reality.

Social control–Regulating the behavior of individuals and groups within a society.

Social determinants of health–Non-medical factors, such as where one is born or raised, or social factors such as culture or social class, that influence health outcomes.

Social exclusion–The sense of being separated from and powerless in society when impoverished.

Social facilitation–The tendency of people to perform at a different level based on the fact that others are around.

Social inhibition–A decrease in performance in front of an audience, often occurring at high levels of arousal when performing a complex or unfamiliar task.

Social institutions–Well-established, structured patterns of behavior or relationships that are accepted as a fundamental part of a culture.

Social interaction–The ways in which two or more individuals can shape each other's behavior.

Social interactionist theory–In language development, the theory that language acquisition is driven by the desire to communicate. This theory includes both biological and social processes.

Social loafing–The tendency of individuals to put in less effort in group settings as compared to an individual setting.

Social mobility–The movement of individuals in the social hierarchy through changes in income, education, or occupation.

Social movements–Philosophies that drive large numbers of people to organize to promote or resist social change.

Social perception–Understanding the thoughts and motives of other people present in the social world; also referred to as social cognition.

Social reproduction–The concept that social inequality, especially poverty, can be reproduced and passed on from one generation to the next.

Social stratification–Organization of societies into a hierarchical system, usually based on socioeconomic status and social class.

Social structure–A system of people within a society organized by a characteristic pattern of relationships.

Social support–The perception or reality that one is cared for by a social network.

Socialization–The process of developing and spreading norms, customs, and beliefs.

Socioeconomic status–Social standing or class of an individual or group, determined as a combination of education, income, and occupation.

Sociology–The study of society, including how it is created, interacted with, defined, and institutionalized.

Solitary play–A stage of early childhood development in which a child plays alone, seemingly uninterested in the activities of other children nearby.

Somatic nervous system–The voluntary branch of the peripheral nervous system, which consists of sensory and motor neurons used to control bodily movements.

Somatic symptom disorders–Mental health disorders marked by bodily symptoms that cause significant stress or impairment. This category of disorder also includes related disorders, such as illness anxiety and conversion disorders.

Somatosensation–The sense of touch, which contains multiple modalities: pressure, vibration, pain, and temperature.

Somatosensory cortex–Region of the parietal lobe located on the postcentral gyrus and involved in somatosensory information processing.

Somnambulism–Sleep disorder in which one carries out actions while asleep; also called sleepwalking.

Source-monitoring error–A memory error by which a person remembers the details of an event but confuses the context by which the details were gained; often causes people to remember events that happened to someone else as having happened to themselves.

Spacing effect–The phenomenon of retaining larger amounts of information when the amount of time between sessions of relearning is increased.

Spatial inequality–A form of social stratification across territories and their populations that can involve residential, environmental, or global components.

Spontaneous recovery–The reappearance of a conditioned response previously determined to be extinct.

Spreading activation–The unconscious activation of closely linked nodes of a semantic network.

State-dependent memory–A retrieval cue by which memory is aided when a person is in the same state of emotion or intoxication as when encoding took place.

Status–A position in society used to classify individuals.

Status inconsistency–A situation in which an individual occupies multiple social positions with different levels of prestige.

Stereocilia–Structures on hair cells in the ear that sway with the movement of endolymph, causing receptor potential in the hair cells and ultimately leading to detection of incoming sound.

Stereotype content model–A model that classifies stereotypes using two dimensions: warmth and competence.

Stereotype threat–A feeling of anxiety about confirming a negative stereotype about one's social group.

Stereotypes–Attitudes and impressions that are made based on limited and superficial information about a person or a group of individuals.

Stigma–The extreme disapproval or dislike of a person or group based on perceived differences in social characteristics from the rest of society.

Stimulant–A drug that causes an increase in central nervous system arousal.

Stimulus–Any energy pattern that is sensed in some way by the body; includes visual, auditory, and physical sensations, among others.

Storage–The retention of encoded information; divided into sensory, short-term, and long-term memory.

Strain theory–Theory that explains deviance as a natural reaction to the disconnect between social goals and social structure.

Stress–The response to significant events, challenges, and decisions.

Stress inoculation training–A cognitive behavioral technique that manages stress by encouraging individuals to pay less attention to the present stress they are experiencing.

Stressors–Biological elements, external conditions, or events that lead to a stress response.

Structural poverty–Theory that poverty is due to inadequacies in societal and economic structure.

Subcultures–Groups of people within a culture that distinguish themselves from the primary culture to which they belong.

Sublimation–A defense mechanism by which unacceptable urges are transformed into socially acceptable behaviors.

Subliminal perception–Perception of a stimulus below a threshold (usually the threshold of conscious perception).

Substantia nigra–Part of the basal ganglia responsible for dopamine release that permits proper functioning of the rest of the basal ganglia.

Sulcus–A fold in the cerebral cortex.

Superego–In Freudian psychoanalysis, the part of the unconscious mind focused on idealism, perfectionism, and societal norms.

Superior colliculus–Structure in the midbrain that receives visual input and impacts eye movements and object oriented behaviors.

Symbolic culture–The nonmaterial culture that represents a group of people; expressed through ideas and concepts.

Symbolic ethnicity–An ethnic identity that is only relevant on special occasions or in specific circumstances and that does not impact everyday life.

Symbolic interactionism–A theoretical framework that studies the way individuals interact through a shared understanding of words, gestures, and other symbols.

Sympathetic nervous system–The branch of the autonomic nervous system that controls the fight-or-flight response; associated with stressful situations that increase heart and respiration rates and decrease digestion.

Synaptic pruning–Adjustment of neural connections throughout life, involving breaking of weak neural connections and bolstering of strong neural connections.

Synesthesia–A neurological phenomenon in which the stimulation of one sensory pathway automatically and involuntarily leads to experiences in a second, different sensory pathway.

Syntax–The way in which words are organized to create meaning.

System for multiple level observation of groups (SYMLOG)–A method of studying group dynamics; focuses on three fundamental dimensions of interaction: dominance vs. submission, friendliness vs. unfriendliness, and instrumentally controlled vs. emotionally expressive.

Systematic desensitization–A behavioral therapy technique in which a patient is gradually exposed to a feared object or situation while practicing relaxation techniques.

Tactical self–In impression management, the person one markets oneself to be when adhering to others' expectations.

Talk therapy–A type of psychotherapy that emphasizes verbal interactions and the exploration of thoughts and feelings.

Telencephalon–A portion of the prosencephalon that becomes the cerebrum.

Temporal lobe–A portion of the cerebral cortex that controls auditory processing, memory processing, emotional control, and language.

Tetrahydrocannabinol (THC)–The main active ingredient in marijuana.

Thalamus–A portion of the forebrain that serves as a relay and sorting station for sensory information, and then transmits the information to the cerebral cortex.

Theory of mind–The ability to sense how another's mind works.

Threshold–Also called limina; the minimum amount of a stimulus that renders a difference in perception.

Tolerance–Decreased response to a drug after physiological adaptation.

Top-down processing–Object recognition driven by memories and expectations that allow the brain to first recognize the whole object, and then recognize components based on existing expectations.

Trait theory–Personality theory that is focused on describing individual personalities as the sum of characteristic behaviors.

Transduction–Conversion of physical, electromagnetic, auditory, and other stimuli to electrical signals in the nervous system.

Transformational grammar–A linguistic theory that focuses on how changes in word order affect meaning.

Two-point threshold–The minimum distance necessary between two points of stimulation on the skin such that the points will be felt as two distinct stimuli.

Type theory–Theorifes of personality that are focused on creating taxonomies, or finite lists, of personality types.

Unconditioned response–In classical conditioning paradigms, the innate response brought about by an unconditioned stimulus prior to any conditioning.

Unconditioned stimulus–In classical conditioning paradigms, a stimulus that brings about an innate response.

Universal emotions–Emotions that are recognized by all cultures; include happiness, sadness, contempt, surprise, fear, disgust, and anger.

Upward social comparison–Comparing oneself to someone perceived as superior.

Urbanization–The process whereby large numbers of people migrate to and establish residence in relatively dense areas of population.

Value–What one deems important in life.

Ventricle–An internal cavity within the brain; cells lining the ventricles produce cerebrospinal fluid.

Verbal communication–The use of spoken or signed language.

Vestibular sense–One of the functions of the ear, the detection of rotational and linear acceleration to maintain awareness of body rotation and movement.

Visual cortex–Region of the occipital lobe devoted to processing visual information.

Visual pathways–Term which refers to both anatomical connections between eyes and brain and the flow of information from eyes to brain. The visual pathway contains several brain regions including the LGN, the visual cortex, and the superior colliculus.

Vygotsky theory–In cognitive development, the theory that the engine driving cognitive development is childhood internalization of culture.

Weber's law–A theory of perception that states that there is a constant ratio between the change in stimulus magnitude needed to produce a just noticeable difference and the magnitude of the original stimulus.

Wernicke-Korsakoff Syndrome–A condition resulting from chronic thiamine (vitamin B_1) deficiency, which is common in individuals who have alcoholism; characterized by severe memory impairment with changes in mental status and loss of coordination.

Wernicke's aphasia–Loss of language comprehension, resulting in fluid production of language without meaning.

Wernicke's area–A brain region located in the superior temporal gyrus of the temporal lobe (usually in the left hemisphere); largely responsible for language comprehension.

Working memory–Form of memory that allows limited amounts of information in short-term memory to be manipulated.

World system theory–World system theory argues there are global level inequalities in the division of labor between core, semi-peripheral, and peripheral nations.

Yerkes-Dodson law–A theory that there is a U shaped function relating arousal level and performance, dictating that performance is worst at the extreme high and low ends of arousal and optimal at intermediate arousal levels. This law is the basis of the Yerkes-Dodson law of social facilitation, a specific application of the Yerkes-Dodson law.

Zone of proximal development–Those skills that a child has not yet mastered but can accomplish with the help of a more knowledgeable other.

INDEX

R

S

T

ART CREDITS

Chapter 1 Cover—Image credited to nobeastsofierce. From Shutterstock.

Figure 1.4—Image credited to Alila Medical Media. From Shutterstock.

Figure 1.5—Image credited to Alila Medical Media. From Shutterstock.

Figure 1.9—Image credited to User: _moep_. From Wikimedia Commons.

Figure 1.26—From Shutterstock.

Chapter 2 Cover—Image credited to Phatic Photography. From Shutterstock.

Chapter 3 Cover—Image credited to Fer Gregory. From Shutterstock.

Figure 3.8—Image credited to Public Library of Science. From Wikimedia Commons. Copyright © 2006. Used under license: CC-BY-2.5.

Chapter 4 Cover—Image credited to Igor Zh. From Shutterstock.

Figure 4.16—Image credited to User: Nitramas. From Wikimedia Commons.

Figure 4.20—Image credited to William Rafti. From Wikimedia Commons. Copyright © 2006. Used under license: CC-BY-2.5.

Figure 4.21—Image credited to User: Saxo. From Wikimedia Commons.

Chapter 5 Cover—Image credited to A.B.G. From Shutterstock.

Figure 5.2—Image credited to Mohd Fuad Salleh/EyeEm. From Getty Images.

Chapter 6 Cover—Image credited to Kanea. From Shutterstock.

Chapter 7 Cover—Image credited to hikrcn. From Shutterstock.

Figure 7.10—Image credited to User: Stepan Kapl. From Shutterstock.

Figure 7.14(c)—Image credited to Jose Luis Calvo. From Shutterstock.

Chapter 8 Cover—Image credited to file404. From Shutterstock.

Figure 8.2—Image credited to RonTech2000. From Getty Images.

Figure 8.8—Image credited to Newhoggy-commonswiki. From Wikimedia Commons.

Figure 8.9—Image credited to User: russavia. From Wikimedia Commons. Copyright © 2013. Used under license: CC-BY-2.0.

Figure 8.13—Image credited to User: kance. From Wikimedia Commons. Copyright © 2006. Used under license: CC-BY-2.0.

Chapter 9 Cover—Image credited to 10'000 Hours. From Getty Images.

Figure 9.8—Image credited to aldomurillo. From Getty Images.

Figure 9.9—Image credited to Tobertz Chavez. From Wikimedia Commons. Copyright © 2006. Used under license: CC-BY-2.0.

Figure 9.10—Image credited to Josh Plueger. From Wikimedia Commons.

Figure 9.11—Image credited to J. Tautz and M. Kleinheinz. From the Public Library of Science. Copyright © 2004. Used under license: CC-BY-2.5.

Chapter 10 Cover—Image credited to eyecrave productions. From Getty Images.

Figure 10.1—Image credited to Michael L. Baird. From Wikimedia Commons. Copyright © 2008. Used under license: CC-BY-2.0.

Figure 10.7—Image credited to AndreAnita. From Shutterstock.

Figure 10.9—Image credited to Alex Pronove. From Wikimedia Commons. Copyright © 2011. Used under license: CC-BY-2.5.

Chapter 11 Cover—Image credited to John M Lund Photography Inc. From Getty Images.

Figure 11.1—Image credited to Yana Iskayeva. From Getty Images.

Figure 11.6—Image credited to Baluchis. From Getty Images.

Figure 11.7—Image credited to arfabita. From Shutterstock.

Figure 11.18—Image credited to User: NikNaks93. From Wikimedia Commons.

Figure 11.20—Image credited to User: Jonathan McIntosh. From Wikimedia Commons.

Chapter 12 Cover—Image credited to Olivier Le Queinec. From Shutterstock.

Figure 12.3—Image credited to User: TastyCakes. From Wikimedia Commons. Copyright © 2009. Used under license: CC-BY-3.0.

Figure 12.5—Image credited to the National Park Service. From Wikimedia Commons.

Notes

Notes

Notes

Notes

Notes

Notes

Notes

Notes

Notes

Notes

Notes

Notes

Examples :

(i) She will return *in* a week.

(ii) I shall finish my work *within* a weak.

5. On, Upon

'**On**' is used for things at rest; '**Upon**' is used for things in motion.

Examples :

(i) He is sitting *on* the floor.

(ii) The dog sprang *upon* the table.

6. By, With

'**By**' denotes the agent or doer, '**With**' denotes the instrument with which anything is done.

Examples :

(i) The bird was killed *by* the hunter with an arrow.

(ii) He beat the dog *with* a stick.

(iii) I shall reach here *by* five o'clock.

7. After, In

'**After**' means at the end of a period of time in the past. '**In**' means at the end of a period of time in future.

Examples :

(i) I shall return your book *in* a week.

(ii) He returned the book *after* a week.

8. For, From, Since

'**For**' is used before a noun denoting a period of time with all the tenses. '**From**' is used before a noun or phrase denoting a point of time, it is used in all the tenses. '**Since**' is used before a noun or phrase denoting some point of time and is always produced by a verb in the perfect continuous tense or third form of a verb.

Examples :

(i) We have been playing cards *for* two hours.

(ii) She stayed with her uncle *from* the 15th of March to the 15th of May.

(iii) I have been reading this book *since* morning.

9. Above, Over

'Above' means 'higher from', **Over** is used in the following four senses :

(i) In the sense of 'above' :
At noon, the sun is *over* our heads.

(ii) In the sense of 'beyond' :
I cannot get *over* my disappointment.

(iii) In the sense of 'Superiority' :
God *over* all blesses for ever more.

(iv) In the sense of 'Conclusion' :
It is all *over* with me.

10. At, Towards

'**At**' denotes the idea of aim, '**Towards**' denotes the idea of destination.

Examples :

(i) He threw the stone *at* the cat.

(ii) He went *towards* the house.

11. At, In, On

'At' is used as follows :

(i) '**At**' is used with small towns and villages.

Examples :

(a) He was born *at* Sonepat.

(b) He lives *at* village Bangra. (Bangra is a village)

(ii) **'At'** is used before a noun denoting a definite point of time.

Example :

He called on me *at* 9 p.m. yesterday.

'In' is used as follows :

(iii) '**In**' is used with the names of big cities, provinces and countries.

Examples :

(a) His father lives *in* England.

(b) His younger brother lives *in* Calcutta.

(iv) '**In**' is used before the names of months and years.

Example :

His elder sister was born *in* 1972 *in* the month of May.

'On' is used with dates and names of days.

Examples :

(a) I joined college *on* the 26th April.

(b) He will leave for Kolkata *on* Wednesday next.

Important Information

1. '**In**' is also used in the following phrases :
In the morning; In the evening, In winter, In summer.

2. '**In**' also denotes a place inside anything.
He travelled *in* a crowded bus.
3. '**At**' is used in the following phrases :
At home, *At* the station, *At* work, *At* play.

12. Below, Beneath

Below means 'of lower level in position, dignity and expectation' etc. *Beneath* means 'under'.

Examples :

(i) It is *below* my dignity to talk to her.
(ii) They rested *beneath* the shade of a tree.

13. In, Into, To

'**In**' expresses Rest or Motion inside anything. '**Into**' expresses Motion towards the inside of anything or change from one medium to another. '**To**' denotes motion from one place to another.

Examples :

(i) The boys are *in* the room.
(ii) Translate this passage from English *into* Hindi.
(iii) Every morning he goes *to* the temple.

14. Till, By, Of, Off

- 'Till' means upto or not earlier than.
- 'By' means not later than.
- 'Of' shows cause, source, separation, quality, contents, possession, apposition, point of reference, space in time etc.
- 'Off' shows separation at a near distance, and detached condition.

Consider the following examples:

(i) I shall work *till* 5 a.m.
(ii) Madhu died *of* cancer.
(iii) The nib *of* the pen is made *of* gold.
(iv) He presented me a bottle *of* perfume.
(v) Our principal is a man *of* principle.
(vi) He lived in the house *of* his friend.
(vii) *By* this time tomorrow, I'll have finished my job.
(viii) My house is *off* the road.
(ix) The book fell *off* the table.

MULTIPLE CHOICE QUESTIONS

Directions: *Tick the correct preposition for the blank in each of the following sentences.*

1. He applied ...... the manager.
A. for B. to
C. with D. by

2. Trust ...... God and do the right.
A. in B. for
C. to D. with

3. She is worthy ...... a prize.
A. with B. for
C. to D. of

4. Mr. Gomes has no taste ...... music.
A. of B. for
C. with D. to

5. You are hard ...... hearing.
A. at B. of
C. with D. for

6. He is sure ...... his success
A. for B. with
C. on D. of

7. Preeti was warned ...... the danger ahead.
A. for B. at
C. of D. about

8. I am thankful ...... you for a good advice.
A. for B. with
C. to D. of

9. Deepak would not surrender ...... the police.
A. with B. to
C. for D. on

10. The small plant in your lawn is very sensitive ...... touch.
A. on B. with
C. to D. about

11. Divya was sure to succeed ..... the examination.
A. for B. in
C. to D. with

12. Geeta was jealous ...... Ravina's beauty.
A. to B. with
C. for D. of

13. He was ignorant ..... what was happening there.
A. for B. of
C. to D. with

14. Your pen is inferior ...... mine.
A. than B. with
C. from D. to

15. Reenu is no match ...... Meenu.
A. to B. for
C. with D. upon

16. It is necessary ...... you to apply for this job.
A. on B. with
C. for D. to

17. Be loyal ...... your country.
A. for B. to
C. on D. with

18. Mukesh is junior ...... me.
A. than B. to
C. from D. of

19. Deepika was innocent ...... the crime.
A. of B. with
C. from D. to

20. I am desirous.... joining the Indian cricket team.
A. for B. of
C. to D. on

ANSWERS

1	2	3	4	5	6	7	8	9	10
B	A	D	B	B	D	D	D	B	D
11	**12**	**13**	**14**	**15**	**16**	**17**	**18**	**19**	**20**
B	D	B	D	B	D	B	B	A	B

SYNONYMS

A synonym is a word which conveys a meaning similar to the given word.

REMEMBER

Words	*Synonyms*
Add	Increase
Adequate	Enough
Adjust	Adapt
All	Aggregate
Allow	Permit
Abode	Dwelling
Apt	Proper
Assess	Appraise
Accuse	Calumniate
Abashed	Timid
Annoy	Displease
Ample	Enough, Sufficient
Amplify	Increase
Apathetic	Unenthusiastic
Accost	Address
Authentic	True
Adjust	Fit
Approve	Assent, Allow, Accept
Adapt	Conform
Adversary	Opponent, Rival, Competitor
Beat	Whack
Benign	Kind
Breeze	Zephyr
Baffle	Puzzle
Booty	Spoil
Beauty	Charm
Beast	Animal
Bandit	Robber
Blaze	Shine
Bond	Tie
Bend	Twist
Bate	Diminish
Beg	Plead
Barbaric	Wild, Savage
Bashful	Shy, Reserved

Words	*Synonyms*
Begin	Start
Blend	Mix, Mingle
Bizarre	Funny
Below	Under
Bedevil	Confuse
Bemoan	Lament
Babble	Nonsense
Blame	Fault
Behaviour	Demeanour
Call	Accost
Copy	Imitate
Close	Shut
Caress	Love
Camp	Stay
Connect	Attach
Cut	Injure, Curtail
Cling	Stick
Conical	Funny
Convey	Carry
Conspicuous	Prominent
Cheerful	Happy, Pleasant
Curtail	Decrease
Cheerless	Sad, Dejected
Curious	Strange
Circumstance	Factor, Situation, Condition
Competent	Capable
Congruent	Overlapping
Cope	Deal, Endure
Confident	Sure
Complex	Intricate
Cajole	Coax, Flatter
Cunning	Crafty
Delectable	Joyful, Delightful
Devilish	Diabolical
Delicate	Soft
Devil	Fiend
Delay	Postpone
Dislike	Repugnance
Destroy	Ruin

Words	*Synonyms*
Dwell	Live, Dilate
Declare	Pronounce
Drunk	Flushed
Deficient	Lacking
Damn	Condemn, Curse
Decrease	Diminish
Destruction	Devastation
Efficient	Competent
Ethnic	Racial
Enthral	Enslave
Earnest	Serious
Envious	Jealous
Ending	Final
Egg	Incite
Extempore	At once
Extensive	Far-ranging
Extra	Surplus
Existence	Life
Exceed	Overstep
Enormous	Vast
Excessive	Superfluous
Free	Unhindered
Frigid	Cold
Feed	Cater
Fame	Reputation
Frame	Make
First	Initial
Frighten	Terrorise, Intimidate
Fervent	Fervid
Fall	Decline
Feeble	Frail
Fickle	Changeable
Finish	Conclude
Fraud	Deception
Forgiving	Placable
Grow	Develop
Greed	Avidity
Greet	Welcome
Grave	Serious
Group	Constellation

Words	*Synonyms*
Given	Bestowed
Gratitude	Thankfulness
Have	Possess
Hire	Rent
Hit	Strike
Handsome	Beautiful
Hinder	Prevent
Heap	Pile
Hope	Expect
Hard	Harsh
Help	Aid
Hymn	Song
Henpecked	Enslaved
Hoodwink	Mystify, Cheat
Humble	Polite, Urbane, Modest
Harass	Vex, Trouble
Impart	Instil
Intact	Untouched
Instal	Establish
Indict	Impeach
Imitate	Ape
Instigate	Incite
Initiate	Start, Introduce
Inimical	Unfriendly
Insufferable	Intolerable
Impartiality	Justice
Jolly	Merry
Joyful	Delectable
Join	Conjoin
Kind	Benign
Kill	Murder
Kindred	Similar
Kinship	Relationship
Keen	Sharp
Knowledge	Scholarship
Lazy	Slothful
Large	Substantial, Gargantuan
Listless	Careless, Lackadaisical
Lax	Loose
Little	Small
Lifelike	Realistic

Words	*Synonyms*
Lofty	High
Lenient	Soft, Gentle
Lacking	Deficient, Wanting
Lessen	Decrease
Middleclass	Bourgeois
Mitigate	Lessen, Abate
Modesty	Humility, Lowliness
Mix	Mingle, Blend
Mixture	Mingling
Mixed	Assorted
Modify	Decrease
Mean	Imply
Multifarious	Varied
Miscarry	Abort
Note	Notice
Noble	Stately
Native	Indigenous
Needful	Necessary
Notify	Declare
Nervous	Shaky, Tremulous, Timid
Natural	Spontaneous
Near	Close
Normal	Natural
Offend	Displease
Oppress	Persecute, Tyrannize
Opponent	Adversary
Obstruct	Hinder, Check
Offence	Fault
Offender	Villain
Overstep	Exceed
Overlapping	Congruent
Occult	Mystic
Profane	Unholy
Patience	Forbearance
Pornographic	Obscene
Plenitude	Abundance
Prominent	Important
Prodigal	Spender
Procrastinate	Postpone
Promote	Develop, Honour
Persecute	Tyrannise

Words	*Synonyms*
Profess	Claim
Pliant	Flexible
Plebian	Common
Polished	Sophisticated
Quake	Shake
Quit	Leave
Queer	Eccentric
Quell	Suppress
Quantify	Allot
Reply	Answer
Relinquish	Retire
Read	Peruse
Relation	Reference
Render	Do
Remainder	Residuals
Repeat	Reiterate
Repentant	Contrite
Retaliative	Retaliatory
Rumour	Hearsay
Reveal	Divulge
Ritualistic	Ceremonious
Soft	Delicate
Sort	Kind, Choose, Select
Selfish	Egoistic
Sensual	Earthly
Suppress	Quell, Check
Stimulate	Provoke
Tasteless	Insipid
Travel	Journey
True	Authentic, Faithful, Truthful
Turbulence	Turmoil
Tragedy	Calamity
Tasteful	Tasty, Delicious
Touching	Painful
Thankful	Grateful
Tremendous	Great, Huge
Tough	Strong
Terminate	Conclude, End
Theory	Doctrine
Tell	Relate
Tremble	Shake, Shiver
Urge	Spur

Words	*Synonyms*
Unbeaten	Unsubdued
Use	Utilize, Practise
Underhand	Unfair, Undue
Unfair	Unjust
Unravel	Reveal, Divulge
Unimportant	Common
Unconcerned	Apathetic
Unimitated	Inimitable
Unfortunate	Unlucky
Understand	Perceive, Comprehend
Vain	Proud, Haughty, Conceited, Shameless
Vale	Valley, Dale, Dell
Vice	Fault
Virtue	Quality
Veracity	Reality
Value	Price, Prize
Vex	Tease
Vibrate	Quiver, Shake
Violent	Excessive
Vivid	Clear, Lucid
Victory	Triumph
Vulgar	Indecent
Virtuous	Honest
Variegated	Varied, Multifarious
Well	Good
Yell	Cry, Shout
Yonder	There
Yearn	Wish, Desire
Yoke	Slavery
Zest	Earnestness, Enthusiasm
Zealous	Earnest

ANTONYMS

A antonym is a word which conveys a meaning opposite to the given word.

REMEMBER

Words	*Antonyms*
Abhor	Love
Abnormal	Normal
Able	Unable
Acceptable	Unacceptable
Adequate	Inadequate
Amusing	Boring

Words	Antonyms
Angry	Calm
Apex	Bottom
Attract	Repel
Bad	Good
Barren	Fertile
Beautiful	Ugly
Bitter	Sweet
Brave	Cowardly
Brief	Lengthy
Bright	Dull
Calm	Violent
Careful	Careless
Clear	Vague, Cloudy
Cold	Hot
Cruel	Kind
Dear	Cheap
Deep	Shallow
Difficult	Easy
Direct	Indirect
Dishonest	Honest
Disobey	Obey
Encourage	Discourage
Enormous	Tiny
Excellent	Bad
Expensive	Cheap
Eat	Fast
Fair	Unfair
Fake	Authentic
False	True
Famous	Notorious
Fool	Genius
Generous	Miserly
Genius	Fool
Genuine	Unauthentic
Gigantic	Tiny
Glad	Depressed
Good	Bad
Great	Little
Happy	Sad

Words	Antonyms
Hard	Soft
Hate	Love
Honest	Dishonest
Idle	Busy
Immoral	Moral
Include	Exclude
Incorrect	Correct
Intelligent	Unintelligent
Kind	Cruel
Like	Dislike
Long	Short
Lucid	Vague
Major	Minor
Naive	Experienced
Nadir	Apex
Neat	Clumsy
Obedient	Disobedient
Obscure	Clear
Oppose	Support
Optimistic	Pessimistic
Out	In
Patience	Impatience
Peaceful	Belligerent
Pious	Impious
Polite	Impolite
Potent	Impotent
Prominent	Unimportant
Proper	Improper
Pure	Impure
Quick	Slow
Quiet	Disturbance
Real	False, Unreal
Reject	Select, Choose
Reliable	Unreliable
Respect	Disrespect
Right	Wrong
Robust	Feeble, Weak
Sad	Happy

Words	Antonyms
Secret	Open
Sensible	Insensible
Severe	Mild
Sharp	Blunt
Simple	Complex
Sociable	Unsociable
Tall	Short
Tidy	Untidy
Uncanny	Canny
Violent	Calm
Vivid	Vague

Words	Antonyms
Strong	Weak
Big	Small
Easy	Difficult
Fast	Slow
High	Low
Catchy	Unattractive
Ugly	Handsome, Beautiful, Tidy
Tasty	Insipid
Sonorous	Harsh

MULTIPLE CHOICE QUESTIONS

Directions (Qs. 1 to 20): *In the following questions choose the word which best expresses the meaning of the given word.*

1. ABSURD
A. Foolish B. Simple
C. Courageous D. Silly

2. ABANDON
A. Lose B. Profit
C. Vacate D. Foil

3. CAJOLE
A. Pause B. Lenient
C. Blast D. Lure

4. COMBAT
A. Fight B. Conflict
C. Shoot D. Quarrel

5. LAMENT
A. Condone B. Console
C. Complain D. Contribution

6. DEBACLE
A. Disgrace B. Defeat
C. Collapse D. Decline

7. SHIVER
A. Fear B. Tremble
C. Shake D. Ache

8. TORTURE
A. Terror B. Harassment
C. Torment D. Tranquility

9. LAUDABLE
A. Lovable B. Commendable
C. Profitable D. Oblivious

10. FIXED
A. Sterile B. Static
C. Stubborn D. Parennial

11. QUEER
A. Unfamiliar B. Cute
C. Curious D. Strange

12. SUFFICIENT
A. Fit B. Proper
C. Adequate D. Vast

13. GLOSS
A. Brightness B. Soothing
C. Rubbing D. Miracle

14. LONGING
A. Prune B. Apathy
C. Curtail D. Craving

15. JEER
A. Applaud B. Magnanimity
C. Avoid D. Scoff

16. ZENITH
A. Minimum B. Nadir
C. Plant D. Peak

17. GARB
A. Distort B. Dress
C. Trivial D. Rage

18. ABHOR
A. Rude B. Reconcile
C. Crave D. Detest

19. YIELD
A. Shum B. Incisive
C. Retain D. Surrender

20. YOKE
A. Twist B. Release
C. Link D. Extra

Directions (Qs. 21 to 38): *In the following questions choose the word which best expresses the opposite of the given word.*

21. TRAGIC
A. Dramatic B. Strong
C. Gentle D. Comic

22. ORAL
A. Verbal B. Sane
C. Minor D. Written

23. ADMIRE
A. Hate B. Unlike
C. Dislike D. Enough

24. VIOLENT
A. Gentle B. Savage
C. Haughty D. Decline

25. ADVERSITY
A. Windfall B. Inprosperity
C. Prosperity D. Slave

26. GENUINE
A. Spurious B. Obscure
C. Countless D. Apathetic

27. GRUDGE
A. Essence B. Guile
C. Goodwill D. Ill-will

28. STIFF
A. Soft B. Courteous
C. Lively D. Flexible

29. VANITY
A. Conceit B. Pride
C. Ostentious D. Humility

30. FRONT
A. Upper B. Unusual
C. Back D. Rear

31. ATTRACT
A. Lured B. Longing
C. Repel D. Disguise

32. COMFORT
A. Discomfort B. Discontent
C. Uncomfort D. Miscomfort

33. WELCOME
A. Repel B. Accept
C. Resist D. Fight

34. TACTFUL
A. Naive B. Loose
C. Strict D. Uncivilized

35. DUTIFUL
A. Harmful B. Watchful
C. Forgetful D. Remiss

36. RIGID
A. Flux B. Adoptable
C. Yielding D. Adaptable

37. RARE
A. Petty B. Poor
C. Small D. Common

38. ZEAL
A. Despair B. Calmness
C. Passiveness D. Indifference

ANSWERS

1	**2**	**3**	**4**	**5**	**6**	**7**	**8**	**9**	**10**
D	C	D	A	C	C	B	C	B	B
11	**12**	**13**	**14**	**15**	**16**	**17**	**18**	**19**	**20**
D	C	A	D	D	D	B	D	D	C
21	**22**	**23**	**24**	**25**	**26**	**27**	**28**	**29**	**30**
D	D	C	A	C	A	C	D	D	D
31	**32**	**33**	**34**	**35**	**36**	**37**	**38**		
C	A	C	A	D	D	D	D		

3. Sentence Completion

It is such an exercise which starts with the primary schools and continues in the highest level of competitive examinations. One must practise it regularly to score well.

Directions (Qs. 1 to 15): *Pick out the most effective word(s) from the given words to fill in the blanks to make the sentence meaningfully complete.*

1. The student ...... that book from the library to study at home.
A. issued B. borrowed
C. hired D. lent

2. I wish I ...... a king.
A. was B. am
C. should be D. were

3. He ...... to listen to my arguments and walked away.
A. denied B. disliked
C. objected D. refused

4. The flow of blood was so ...... that the patient died.
A. intense B. adequate
C. profuse D. extensive

5. When I met her yesterday, it was the first time I ...... her since Christmas.
A. saw B. have seen
C. had seen D. have been seing

6. Can you pay ...... all these articles?
A. for B. of
C. off D. out

7. I ...... you to be at the party this evening.
A. expect B. hope
C. look forward to D. desire

8. ...... being a handicapped person, he is very cooperative and self-reliant.
A. Because B. Although
C. Since D. Despite

9. The child broke ...... from his mother and ran towards the painting.
A. away B. after
C. down D. with

10. With his ...... income, he finds it difficult to live a comfortable life.
A. brief B. sufficient
C. meagre D. huge

11. He could ...... a lot of money in such a short time by using his intelligence and working hard.
A. spend B. spoil
C. exchange D. accumulate

12. Though the brothers are twins, they look ......
A. alike B. handsome
C. indifferent D. different

13. Unfavourable weather conditions can ..... illness.
A. cure B. detect
C. treat D. enhance

14. No sooner did the bell ring, ... the actor started singing.
A. when B. than
C. after D. before

15. If I ...... realised it, I would not have acted on his advice.
A. was B. had
C. were D. have

Directions (Qs. 16 to 25): *In each question, an incomplete statement (Stem) followed by four fillers* *is given. Pick out the best one which can complete the incomplete stem correctly and meaningfully.*

16. Unless you work harder you will fail, means .....
A. if you fail you will work harder.
B. you must at least plan well than you will not fail.
C. hardly you will fail if you do not desire so.
D. if you do not put more efforts, then you will fail.

17. Even if it rains I shall come, means .....
A. if I come it will not rain.
B. if it rains I shall not come.
C. I will certainly come whether it rains or not.
D. whenever there is rain I shall come.

18. Dinesh is as stupid as he is lazy means .....
A. Dinesh is stupid because he is lazy.
B. Dinesh is lazy because he is stupid.
C. Dinesh is either stupid or lazy.
D. Dinesh is equally stupid and lazy.

19. He is so lazy that he .....
A. cannot depend on others for getting his work done.
B. cannot delay the schedule of completing the work.
C. can seldom complete his work on time.
D. dislike to postpone the work that he undertakes to do.

20. He always stammers in public meetings, but his today's speech .....
A. was fairly audible to everyone present in the hall.
B. was not received satisfactorily.
C. could not be understood properly.
D. was free from that defect.

21. In order to raise the company's profit, the employees .....
A. demanded two additional increments.
B. decided to go on paid holidays.
C. requested the management to implement new welfare schemes.
D. offered to work overtime without any compensation.

22. Although, he is reputed for making very candid statements, ...
A. his today's speech was not fairly audible.
B. his promises had always been realistic.
C. his speech was very interesting.
D. his today's statements were very ambiguous.

23. I felt somewhat more relaxed .....
A. but tense as compared to earlier.
B. and tense as compared to earlier.
C. as there was already no tension at all.
D. and tension-free as compared to earlier.

24. With great efforts his son succeeded in convincing him not to donate his entire wealth to an orphanage .....
A. and lead the life of a wealthy merchant.
B. but to a home for the forsaken children.
C. and make an orphan of himself.
D. as the orphanage needed a lot of donations.

25. Even though it is a very large house, ...
A. there is a lot of space available in it for children.
B. there is hardly any space available for children.
C. there is no dearth of space for children.
D. the servants take a long time to clean it.

ANSWERS

1	**2**	**3**	**4**	**5**	**6**	**7**	**8**	**9**	**10**
B	D	D	C	C	A	A	D	A	C
11	**12**	**13**	**14**	**15**	**16**	**17**	**18**	**19**	**20**
D	D	D	B	B	D	C	D	C	D
21	**22**	**23**	**24**	**25**					
D	D	D	C	B					

4. Spotting Errors

The most common errors in English are of spellings, grammar and usage of words. By regular practice, the errors can be easily spotted and minimised.

MULTIPLE CHOICE QUESTIONS

Directions: *In the following questions some of the sentences have errors and some are correct. Find out which part of a sentence has an error, the number of that part is your answer. If a sentence is free from errors, then your answer is D i.e., No error.*

1. (A) Either Ram or/(B) you is responsible/(C) for this action./(D) No error.

2. (A) The student flatly denied/(B) that he had copied/(C) in the examination hall./(D) No error.

3. (A) By the time you arrive tomorrow/(B) I have finished/(C) my work./(D) No error.

4. (A) The captain with the members of his team/ (B) are returning/(C) after a fortnight./(D) No error.

5. (A) After returning from/(B) an all-India tour/ (C) I had to describe about it./(D) No error.

6. (A) The teacher asked his students/(B) if they had gone through/(C) either of the three chapters included in the prescribed text./(D) No error.

7. (A) Do you know/(B) how old were you/(C) when you came here?/(D) No error.

8. (A) Beware of/(B) a fair-weather friend/(C) who is neither a friend in need nor a friend indeed./ (D) No error.

9. (A) Copernicus proved/(B) that Earth/(C) moves round the Sun./(D) No error.

10. (A) The property/(B) was divided/(C) among the two brothers./(D) No error.

11. (A) I am quite certain/(B) that the lady is not only greedy/(C) but miserly./(D) No error.

12. (A) The brilliant success in the examination/ (B) as well as his record in sports/(C) deserves high praise./(D) No error.

13. (A) I cannot find/(B) where has he gone/(C) though I have tried may best./(D) No error.

14. (A) If I was/(B) the Prime Minister of India/(C) I would work wonders/(D) No error.

15. (A) If it weren't/(B) for you,/(C) I wouldn't be alive today./(D) No error.

16. (A) He looked like a lion/(B) baulked from/ (C) its prey./(D) No error.

17. (A) Widespread flooding/(B) is affecting/(C) large areas of the villages./(D) No error.

18. (A) If we really set to/(B) we can get the whole house/(C) cleaned in an afternoon./(D) No error.

19. (A) It's arrogant for you/(B) to assume you'll/ (C)win every time./(D) No error.

20. (A) The two books are the same/(B) except for the fact that this/(C) has an answer in the back./(D) No error.

21. (A) Your husband doesn't/(B) believe that you are older/(C) than I./(D) No error.

22. (A) I could not/(B) answer to/(C) the question./(D) No error.

23. (A) Two years passed/(B) since/(C) my cousin died./(D) No error.

24. (A) I am learning English/(B) for ten years/(C) without much effect./(D) No error.

25. (A) Ramesh has agreed/(B) to marry with the girl/(C) of his parent's choice./ (D) No error.

26. (A) When he was arriving./(B) the party was/(C) in full swing./(D) No error.

27. (A) The most studious boy/(B) in the class/(C) was made as the captain./(D) No error.

28. (A) I am participating/(B) in the two-miles race/(C) tomorrow morning./(D) No error.

29. (A) When the boy committed a mistake/(B) the teacher made him to do/(C) the sum again./(D) No error.

30. (A) Whenever a person lost anything/(B) the poor folk around/(C) are suspected./(D) No error.

ANSWERS

1	**2**	**3**	**4**	**5**	**6**	**7**	**8**	**9**	**10**
B	D	B	B	C	C	D	D	B	C
11	**12**	**13**	**14**	**15**	**16**	**17**	**18**	**19**	**20**
C	D	B	A	C	C	C	A	A	C
21	**22**	**23**	**24**	**25**	**26**	**27**	**28**	**29**	**30**
C	B	A	A	B	A	C	B	B	A

EXPLANATORY ANSWERS

1. Replace 'is' by 'are'.
2. No error.
3. Replace 'have' by 'would have'.
4. Replace 'are' by 'is'.
5. Replace 'had to describe' by 'described'.
6. Replace 'either' by 'any'.
7. No error.
8. No error.
9. Omit 'that'.
10. Replace 'among' by 'between'.
11. Add 'also'.
12. No error.
13. Replace 'has he' by 'he has'.
14. Replace 'was' by 'were'.
15. Replace 'wouldn't be' by 'would not have been'.
16. Replace 'its' by 'his'.
17. Replace 'areas' by 'area'.
18. Replace 'set to' by 'set on'.
19. Replace 'for' by 'of'.
20. Replace 'in' by 'on'.
21. Replace 'I' by 'me'.
22. Omit 'to'.
23. Replace 'passed' by 'have passed'.
24. Replace 'am' by 'have been'.
25. Omit 'with'.
26. Replace 'was arriving' by 'arrived'.
27. Omit 'as'.
28. Replace 'in' by 'at'.
29. Omit 'to'.
30. Replace 'lost' by 'loses'.

5. One Word Substitution

There are many single words in English language which can be perfectly used for a number of words. These words help in expressing ideas in a short and correct manner for the right occasion. Such words not only increase the vocabulary but also enable you to economise in the use of words to a great extent.

Multiple Word Expression	*Substitution*
One who always looks towards the bright side of things	Optimist
One who always looks towards the dark side of things	Pessimist
The time when one develops from a child into an adult	Adolescence
The process of growing more plants in order to form a forest.	Afforestation
The science which deals with farming	Agriculture
From some other country or place etc.	Alien
A term, etc. giving more than one meaning	Ambiguous
A vehicle which is used to carry sick persons	Ambulance
An animal which can live both in water and on land	Amphibian
A lawless situation when there is no government	Anarchy
Belonging to the history of thousands of years old	Ancient
Once a year	Annual
A very old object but still valuable	Antique
Words of opposite meanings	Antonyms
Words of similar meanings	Synonyms
Signatures of a famous person	Autograph
A government led by one person with absolute authority	Autocracy
A written work of one's own life history	Autobiography
A person who has never been married	Bachelor
A person usually having no hair on his head	Bald
A place where one can deposit money and get interest	Bank
A person who cuts our hair	Barber
A building/group of buildings where soldiers live	Barracks
A person who makes buns and biscuits	Baker
A person who lives by asking people for food and money without doing any useful job	Beggar
The crime of having married to two persons at the same time	Bigamy
The branch of science which deals with the study of plants	Botany
Able to speak two languages	Bilingual

Multiple Word Expression	*Substitution*
Able to speak more than two languages	Polyglot
The branch of science which deals with the living organisms	Biology
A powerful snow storm	Blizzard
A great successful book or movie	Blockbuster
A short news on the radio or TV	Bulletin
A system in which the most important works are organised by the government officials	Bureaucracy
A person who has no vision in his eyes	Blind
A page or a series of pages on which the information of days, weeks, months, etc. is given	Calendar
A person who eats human flesh	Cannibal
A complete list of items often arranged alphabetically	Catalogue
A sudden disaster	Catastrophe
A period of 100 years	Century
A branch of science which deals with chemicals	Chemistry
A printed leaf usually issued by banks that we sign to carry certain financial deal	Cheque
A person who makes or mends shoes	Cobbler
A group of people who has been chosen by others to make decisions on their own	Committee
A building in which nuns live	Convent
An animal which feeds on other animals	Carnivorous
A person who does criticism	Critic
A person who cannot hear	Deaf
A condition in which one loses a lot of water from one's body because of vomiting, etc.	Dehydration
A system of government in which the people cast their votes to elect their leaders	Democracy
The study of skin problems	Dermatology
A long piece of land covered with sand	Desert
The art of managing relationships between countries	Diplomacy
A piece of information about the words in a book form	Dictionary
A piece of information about the telephone numbers of the people in a book from	Directory
A person in charge of a newspapers, magazine etc.	Editor
A person who thinks he is better than the others	Egoist
To leave your country and settle in some other country	Emigrate
A book or series of books giving almost all knowledge about an area or some persons etc.	Encyclopaedia
Study of insects	Entomology
Time when day and night are of the same duration	Equinox
To sell things out of the country	Export
To purchase things from some other country	Import
A plant or animal no longer in existence	Extinct
A situation when there is a shortage of food for a long period of time	Famine
An amount of money that we pay for some action or services	Fee
Related to women	Feminine
An animal strong and aggressive	Ferocious

Multiple Word Expression	*Substitution*
A piece of land where plants grow easily from the soil that is favourable to them	Fertile
A work of literature having some imaginary events	Fiction
A large amount of water covering certain area	Flood
A person who sells flowers	Florist
A religious ceremony for burying or cremating a dead person	Funeral
A substance which kills fungus	Fungicide
A person studying or having studied the diseases and the related things of female reproductory system	Gynaecologist
The murder of the person of the same group race or country	Genocide
A substance which kills germs	Germicide
A situation in which many people die because of fire during war	Holocaust
The act of killing a person deliberately	Homicide
A word having the pronunciation as the other one does but it differs in meaning	Homophone
A word having the same spelling as the other one does but it is pronounced in some other way	Homonym
A person who is attracted towards the person of the same sex	Homosexual
Go across and parallel to the ground	Horizontal
A substance which kills the insects	Insecticide
That cannot be corrected	Incorrigible
That cannot be defeated	Invincible
That cannot be eaten	Inedible
That cannot be seen	Invisible
A place in a school or college where books are kept for the benefit of students, teachers etc.	Library
A place in a school or college where scientific experiments are performed	Laboratory
An official who is a judge in the lowest court	Magistrate
A piece of music or a book before it is printed	Manuscript
Related to men	Masculine
One who believes in the existence of God	A theist
One who does not believe in the existence of good	An atheist
That can be believed	Credible
That cannot be believed	Incredible
That which dissolves in a solvent	Soluble
That which does not dissolves in a solvent	Insoluble
Hard writing that can be read	Legible
Hard writing that cannot be read	Illegible
A person who does jobs beneficial to mankind	Philanthropist
A person who goes on foot	Pedestrian
A person who fights for his own country	Patriot
An act of killing oneself	Suicide
A woman whose husband is dead	Widow
A man whose wife is dead	Widower
A person who eats vegetarian and non-vegetarian diets	Omnivorous

Multiple Word Expression	*Substitution*
Something which is everywhere at the same time	Omnipresent
One who knows everything	Omniscient
A child who does not have parents	Orphan
An award etc. given after the death of the person	Posthumous
The place where animals are kept for amusement and to increase the knowledge of the public	Zoo
The science which deals with the study of animals	Zoology

MULTIPLE CHOICE QUESTIONS

Directions: *In questions given below, out of the four alternatives, choose the one which can be substituted for the given words/sentences.*

1. Something that relates to everyone in the world
A. General B. Common
C. Usual D. Universal

2. An expression of mild disapproval
A. Warning B. Denigration
C. Impertinence D. Reproof

3. One who is not easily pleased by anything
A. Maiden B. Medieval
C. Precarious D. Fastidious

4. Murder of a king
A. Infanticide B. Matricide
C. Genocide D. Regicide

5. A remedy for all diseases
A. Stoic B. Marvel
C. Panacea D. Recompense

6. A dramatic performance
A. Mask B. Mosque
C. Masque D. Mascot

7. Study of birds
A. Orology B. Optology
C. Ophthalmology D. Ornithology

8. Ready to believe
A. Credulous B. Credible
C. Creditable D. Incredible

9. Incapable of being seen through
A. Ductile B. Opaque
C. Obsolete D. Potable

10. One who eats everything
A. Omnivorous B. Omniscient
C. Irresistible D. Insolvent

11. A place where bees are kept is called
A. An apiary B. A mole
C. A hive D. A sanctuary

12. One who cannot be corrected
A. Incurable B. Incorrigible
C. Hardened D. Invulnerable

13. One who is in charge of a museum
A. Curator B. Supervisor
C. Caretaker D. Warden

14. Continuing fight between parties, families, clans, etc.
A. Enmity B. Feud
C. Quarrel D. Skirmish

15. A voice loud enough to be heard
A. Audible B. Applaudable
C. Laudable D. Oral

16. A paper written by hand
A. Handicraft B. Manuscript
C. Handiwork D. Thesis

17. Habitually silent or talking little
A. Serville B. Unequivocal
C. Taciturn D. Synoptic

18. To slap with a flat object
A. Chop B. Hew
C. Gnaw D. Swat

19. A person who speaks many languages
A. Linguist B. Monolingual
C. Polyglot D. Bilingual

20. A light sailing-boat built specially for racing
A. Canoe B. Yacht
C. Frigate D. Dinghy

21. A fixed orbit in space in relation to earth
A. Geological B. Geo-synchronous
C. Geo-centric D. Geo-stationary

22. A style in which a writer makes a display of his knowledge
A. Pedantic B. Verbose
C. Pompous D. Ornate

23. A religious discourse
A. Preach B. Stanza
C. Sanctorum D. Sermon

24. A place that provides refuge
A. Asylum B. Sanatorium
C. Shelter D. Orphanage

25. Detailed plan of a journey
A. Travelogue B. Travelkit
C. Schedule D. Itinerary

26. A person who insists on something
A. Disciplinarian B. Stickler
C. Instantaneous D. Boaster

27. A drawing on transparent paper
A. Red print B. Blue print
C. Negative D. Transparency

28. One who believes that all things and events in life are predetermined is a
A. Fatalist B. Puritan
C. Egoist D. Tyrant

29. A school boy who cuts classes frequently is a
A. Defeatist B. Sycophant
C. Truant D. Martinet

30. The act of violating the sanctity of the church is
A. Blasphemy B. Heresy
C. Sacrilege D. Desecration

31. A place where monks live as a secluded community
A. Cathedral B. Diocese
C. Convent D. Monastery

32. One who is fond of fighting
A. Bellicose B. Aggressive
C. Belligerent D. Militant

33. Tending to move away from the centre or axis
A. Centrifugal B. Centripetal
C. Axiomatic D. Awry

34. Words inscribed on tomb
A. Epitome B. Epistle
C. Epilogue D. Epitaph

35. Leave or remove from a place considered dangerous
A. Evade B. Evacuate
C. Avoid D. Exterminate

36. Original inhabitants of a country
A. Abroge B. Aborger
C. Aborgory D. Aborigins

37. Government by the officials
A. Theocracy B. Plutocracy
C. Bureaucracy D. Democracy

38. Incapable of being exhausted
A. Inexhaustible B. Inaexhaustible
C. Exhaustable D. Non-tired

39. A person of good understanding, knowledge and reasoning power
A. Expert B. Intellectual
C. Snob D. Literate

40. One absorbed in his own thoughts and feelings rather than in things outside
A. Scholar B. Recluse
C. Introvert D. Intellectual

ANSWERS

1	**2**	**3**	**4**	**5**	**6**	**7**	**8**	**9**	**10**
D	D	D	D	C	C	D	A	B	A
11	**12**	**13**	**14**	**15**	**16**	**17**	**18**	**19**	**20**
A	B	A	B	A	B	C	D	A	B
21	**22**	**23**	**24**	**25**	**26**	**27**	**28**	**29**	**30**
D	A	D	A	D	B	D	A	C	C
31	**32**	**33**	**34**	**35**	**36**	**37**	**38**	**39**	**40**
D	A	A	D	B	B	C	A	B	C

6. Spelling Errors

There are thousands of words in English language. It is difficult to remember the spellings and meanings of all at once. Try to learn as many as you can. Use a dictionary regularly.

Directions: *Find the correctly spelt words.*

1. A. Damage B. Dammage C. Damaige D. Dammege

2. A. Efficiant B. Effecient C. Efficient D. Eficient

3. A. Schedule B. Schdule C. Schedale D. Schedeule

4. A. Occurad B. Occurred C. Ocurred D. Occured

5. A. Grieff B. Grief C. Grieef D. Grrief

6. A. Guarantee B. Garuntee C. Guaruntee D. Gaurantee

7. A. Meddicine B. Medicine C. Medicene D. Medicinne

8. A. Benefeted B. Benefitted C. Benifited D. Benefited

9. A. Acommodation B. Acomodation C. Accomodation D. Accommodation

10. A. Querrelsome B. Quarrelsame C. Quarrelsome D. Querralsome

11. A. Sympathetic B. Smypathetic C. Sympothetic D. Sympethetic

12. A. Prograssive B. Progressive C. Progresive D. Prograsive

13. A. Uncivilized B. Uncevilized C. Uncivillized D. Uncevelized

14. A. Extravagant B. Extreragent C. Extreregant D. Extravegent

15. A. Missunderstood B. Miesunderstood C. Misunderstood D. Misunderstod

16. A. Belligerent B. Beligirent C. Belligarant D. Belligerrent

17. A. Astonished B. Astronished C. Astoneshed D. Asstonished

18. A. Sincerely B. Sencerely C. Sincerelly D. Sincerrely

19. A. Rigourous B. Rigerous C. Rigorous D. Regerous

20. A. Satellite B. Sattellite C. Satelite D. Sattelite

21. A. Pesanger B. Passenger C. Pessenger D. Pasanger

22. A. Humurous B. Humorous C. Humoreus D. Humorrous

23. A. Exeggerate B. Exaggerate C. Exadgerate D. Exagerate

24. A. Fariegn B. Forein C. Foriegn D. Foreign

25. A. Excesive B. Excessive C. Exccessive D. Exccesive

26. A. Forcaust B. Forcast C. Forecast D. Forecaste

27. A. Paralleted B. Paralelled C. Parralleled D. Parallelled

28. A. Ocasion B. Occassion
C. Occasion D. Ocassion

29. A. Boquet B. Bouquet
C. Bouquete D. Bouquette

30. A. Chettering B. Chaterring
C. Chattering D. Chatering

31. A. Discourage B. Disscourage
C. Discourege D. Discaurage

32. A. Curageous B. Courageous
C. Courrageous D. Couregeous

33. A. Abandon B. Abanddon
C. Abendon D. Abbandon

34. A. Embarassment
B. Emberrassement
C. Embarrassment
D. Embbaresment

35. A. Eccintric B. Eccentrie
C. Eccentric D. Eccintrie

36. A. Occasional B. Occassional
C. Occesional D. Occessional

37. A. Querrel B. Querral
C. Quarrel D. Quarel

38. A. Contrebution B. Contribution
C. Contributtion D. Conterbution

39. A. Desgrace B. Disgrece
C. Disgrice D. Disgrace

40. A. Harassment B. Herassment
C. Harasment D. Harassmient

41. A. Imaginative B. Imeginative
C. Imagenative D. Imaginetive

42. A. Suficient B. Suficiant
C. Sufficient D. Sufficiant

43. A. Adequate B. Edequate
C. Adaquete D. Edaquete

44. A. Exparienced B. Experianced
C. Experienced D. Experrienced

45. A. Flatering B. Fletering
C. Flattering D. Fletaring

46. A. Cuttiveted B. Culltrivated
C. Cultivated D. Caltivated

47. A. Praiceworthy B. Peiseworthy
C. Praiseworthy D. Praisaworthy

48. A. Profesional B. Professionel
C. Professional D. Profissional

49. A. Ameteur B. Amateur
C. Amataur D. Amateor

50. A. Unfevourable B. Unfevaurable
C. Unfavourable D. Unfivourable

ANSWERS

1	**2**	**3**	**4**	**5**	**6**	**7**	**8**	**9**	**10**
A	C	A	B	B	A	B	B	D	C
11	**12**	**13**	**14**	**15**	**16**	**17**	**18**	**19**	**20**
A	B	A	A	C	A	A	A	C	A
21	**22**	**23**	**24**	**25**	**26**	**27**	**28**	**29**	**30**
B	B	B	D	B	C	A	C	B	C
31	**32**	**33**	**34**	**35**	**36**	**37**	**38**	**39**	**40**
A	B	A	C	C	A	C	B	D	A
41	**42**	**43**	**44**	**45**	**46**	**47**	**48**	**49**	**50**
A	C	A	C	A	C	C	C	B	C

संख्यात्मक अभियोग्यता एवं आंकड़ों का निर्वचन
(Numerical Ability and Data Analysis)

1 संख्याएँ (Numbers)

एक संख्या हमें बताती है कि दी हुई मात्रा में कितनी इकाइयां हैं। अतः यह एक या एक से अधिक इकाइयों को प्रकट करती है। या एक ही प्रकार की एक या अधिक भिन्न वस्तुओं को प्रकट करती है। जैसे–दो गाय, चार बकरी, आठ भैंस आदि। वे शब्द जो काले दर्शाये गये हैं, संख्याओं को प्रदर्शित करते हैं।

1. **पूर्ण संख्याएं :** संख्याएं 0, 1, 2, 3, 4, 5, 6, 7, 8, 9,.....आदि संख्याओं को **"पूर्ण संख्याएं"** या **"पूर्णांक कहते** हैं। जैसे 84 एक पूर्णांक है। जबकि $\frac{61}{4}$ पूर्णांक नहीं है।
2. **सम संख्याएं :** वे संख्याएं जो 2 से पूर्णतः विभाजित हो जाती हैं उन्हें **"सम संख्याएं"** कहते हैं। जैसे–2, 4, 32, 64, 108.... आदि "सम संख्याएं" हैं।
3. **विषम संख्याएं :** वे संख्याएं जो 2 से पूर्णतः विभाजित नहीं होती हैं उन्हें **"विषम संख्याएं"** कहते हैं। जैसे–1, 3, 5, 7, 11, 17, 21, 23.... आदि "विषम संख्याएं" हैं।
4. **अभाज्य संख्याएं :** वे संख्याएं जो स्वयं और 1 के अतिरिक्त किसी अन्य संख्याओं से पूर्णतः विभाजित न हों, उन्हें **"अभाज्य संख्याएं"** कहते हैं। जैसे–2, 3, 7, 11, 13, 17.... आदि "अभाज्य संख्याएं" हैं।
5. **भाज्य संख्याएं :** वे संख्याएं जो स्वयं और 1 के अतिरिक्त किसी अन्य संख्याओं से पूर्णतः विभाजित हो जाती हों तो उन्हें **"भाज्य संख्याएं"** कहते हैं। जैसे–4, 6, 9, 10, 12, 15.... आदि "भाज्य संख्याएं" हैं।

नोट :

1. संख्या 1 न तो भाज्य है और न ही अभाज्य।

2. वह संख्या जो सम भी हो और अभाज्य भी, केवल 2 है।

आरोही क्रम (Ascending Order) : बाईं ओर से दायीं ओर लिखने पर प्राकृतिक संख्याएं मान के अनुसार बढ़ते हुए क्रम में हों तो इस क्रम को **"आरोही क्रम"** कहते हैं। जैसे–25, 30, 41, 50 आदि संख्याएं आरोही क्रम में होंगी।

अवरोही क्रम (Descending Order): बाईं ओर से दाईं ओर लिखने पर प्राकृतिक संख्याएं मान के अनुसार घटते हुए क्रम में हों, तो इस क्रम को **"अवरोही क्रम"** कहते हैं। जैसे–50, 41, 30, 25 आदि संख्याएं अवरोही क्रम में होंगी।

स्थानीय मान और जातीय (वास्तविक) मान

स्थानीय मान : किसी अंक (Number) का जो मान (Value) उसके स्थान के कारण होता है, उसे उस अंक का **स्थानीय मान** कहते हैं। जैसे–32 में इकाई के स्थान पर 2 तथा दहाई के स्थान पर 3 है। इसमें 3 का स्थानीय मान $= 3 \times 10 = 30$ तथा 2 का स्थानीय मान $= 2 \times 1 = 2$ होगा।

जातीय (वास्तविक) मान : हर अंक का अपना जातीय मान होता है। जैसे– 2 का 2, 5 का 5, 7 का 7, 9 का 9 आदि। जैसा कि हम ऊपर बता चुके हैं कि 32 में 3 का **स्थानीय मान** 30 है। परन्तु 32 में 3 का **जातीय मान** 3 होगा। इस प्रकार 32 में 3 के स्थानीय मान तथा जातीय मान के बीच अन्तर $= 30 - 3 = 27$ होगा। अतः किसी संख्या में किसी अंक का स्थानीय मान प्राप्त करने के लिए सरल तरीका यह है कि पहले उस अंक को लिख लें और उसके बाद उसमें उतने शून्य लगा दें, जितने कि उस अंक के बाद अंक हों।

उदाहरण 1 : 35011 में से 5 का स्थानीय मान क्या होगा?

हल : सबसे पहले 5 लिखें फिर देखें कि संख्या 5 के बाद कितने अंक हैं। अतः उपरोक्त दी हुई संख्या से स्पष्ट है कि 5 के बाद तीन अंक हैं। फिर 5 के बाद तीन शून्य लिख दें। 5000, इस प्रकार 35011 में 5 का **स्थानीय मान** = 5000 हुआ।

उदाहरण 2 : 751 में 7 के स्थानीय मान और जातीय मान में क्या अन्तर है?

हल : दी हुई संख्या 751 में 7 सैंकड़ा वाले स्थान पर है। अतः 7 का **स्थानीय मान** $= 7 \times 100 = 700$ होगा तथा 7 का **जातीय मान** 7 ही होगा।

$\therefore$ 7 के स्थानीय मान तथा जातीय मान के बीच अन्तर $= 700 - 7 = 693$ होगा।

नोट : प्रत्येक पूर्ण संख्या को अभाज्य संख्याओं के गुणनफल के रूप में लिखा जा सकता है।

एक संख्या के अभाज्य गुणनखण्ड किस प्रकार लिख सकते हैं :

(*i*) संख्या को 2 से भाग करो, यदि सम्भव हो, और 2 से भाग करते रहो जब तक कि ऐसा गुणनखण्ड न आ जाए जो 2 से विभाजित न हो।

(*ii*) प्राप्त परिणाम (*i*) को 3 से भाग करो, यदि सम्भव हो और 3 से भाग करते रहो जब तक कि ऐसा गुणनखण्ड न आ जाए जो 3 से विभाजित न हो।

(*iii*) प्राप्त परिणाम (*ii*) को 5 से भाग करो, यदि सम्भव हो और 5 से भाग करते रहो जब तक कि ऐसा गुणनखण्ड न आ जाए जो 5 से विभाजित न हो।

(*iv*) प्राप्त परिणामों में इसी प्रकार 7, 11, 13 आदि संख्याओं से भाग करते रहो जब तक कि सारे गुणनखण्ड अभाज्य गुणनखण्ड न हो जाएं।

उदाहरण 3 : 2310 को अभाज्य गुणनखण्डों की गुणा के रूप में प्रकट कीजिए।

हल :

2	2310
3	1155
5	385
7	77
	11

∴ 2310 के अभाज्य गुणनखण्ड $= 2 \times 3 \times 5 \times 7 \times 11$ होंगे।

संख्याओं के सम्बन्ध में मौलिक तथ्य

(*a*) दो अंकों वाली संख्याओं के सन्दर्भ में

(*i*) दो अंकों वाली कुल संख्याओं की गिनती 90 है।

(*ii*) दो अंकों की सबसे बड़ी संख्या 99 है।

(*iii*) दो अंकों की सबसे छोटी संख्या 10 है।

(*iv*) दो अंकों की सबसे छोटी और सबसे बड़ी संख्या का योग 109 होता है।

(*v*) दो अंकों की सबसे बड़ी और सबसे छोटी संख्या का अन्तर 89 होता है।

(*b*) तीन अंकों वाली संख्याओं के सन्दर्भ में

(*i*) तीन अंकों वाली कुल संख्याओं की गिनती 900 है।

(*ii*) तीन अंकों की सबसे बड़ी संख्या 999 है।

(*iii*) तीन अंकों की सबसे छोटी संख्या 100 है।

(*iv*) तीन अंकों की सबसे छोटी और सबसे बड़ी संख्या का योग 1099 होता है।

(*v*) तीन अंकों की सबसे बड़ी और सबसे छोटी संख्या का अन्तर 899 होता है।

(*c*) चार अंकों वाली संख्याओं के सन्दर्भ में

(*i*) चार अंकों वाली कुल संख्याओं की गिनती 9000 है।

(*ii*) चार अंकों की सबसे बड़ी संख्या 9999 है।

(*iii*) चार अंकों की सबसे छोटी संख्या 1000 है।

(*iv*) चार अंकों की सबसे छोटी और सबसे बड़ी संख्या का योग 10999 होता है।

(*v*) चार अंकों की सबसे बड़ी और सबसे छोटी संख्या का अन्तर 8999 होता है।

(*d*) पाँच अंकों वाली संख्याओं के सन्दर्भ में

(*i*) पाँच अंकों वाली कुल संख्याओं की गिनती 90000 है।

(*ii*) पाँच अंकों की सबसे बड़ी संख्या 99999 है।

(*iii*) पाँच अंकों की सबसे छोटी संख्या 10000 है।

(*iv*) पाँच अंकों की सबसे छोटी और सबसे बड़ी संख्या का योग 109999 होता है।

(*v*) पाँच अंकों की सबसे बड़ी और सबसे छोटी संख्या का अन्तर 89999 होता है।

(*e*) प्राकृतिक संख्याओं के सन्दर्भ में

(*i*) 1 से लेकर 10 तक की प्राकृतिक संख्याओं का योग = 55 होता है।

(*ii*) 11 से लेकर 20 तक की प्राकृतिक संख्याओं का योग = 155 होता है।

(*iii*) 21 से लेकर 30 तक की प्राकृतिक संख्याओं का योग = 255 होता है।

(*iv*) 31 से लेकर 40 तक की प्राकृतिक संख्याओं का योग = 355 होता है।

(*v*) 41 से लेकर 50 तक की प्राकृतिक संख्याओं का योग = 455 होता है।

संख्याओं में 2, 3, 4, 5, 6, 8, 9, 10 व 11 से विभाज्यता की जाँच

(A) **2 से विभाज्यता :** ऐसी संख्याएं जिनके इकाई के स्थान पर 0, 2, 4, 6 या 8 का अंक हों, तो वे संख्याएं 2 से पूर्णतः विभाजित होंगी।

(B) **3 से विभाज्यता :** ऐसी संख्याएं जिनके अंकों का योग 3 से विभाज्य हों, तो वे संख्याएं भी 3 से विभाज्य होंगी।

(C) **4 से विभाज्यता :** यदि किसी संख्या के अन्तिम दो अंक 4 से पूर्णतः विभाजित हों, तो वे संख्याएं भी 4 से विभाजित होंगी।

(D) **5 से विभाज्यता :** जिन संख्याओं के इकाई के स्थान पर 0 या 5 का अंक हो, तो वे संख्याएं 5 से विभाजित होंगी।

(E) **6 से विभाज्यता :** ऐसी संख्याएं जो 2 और 3 से अलग-अलग पूर्णतः विभाजित हों, तो वे संख्याएं भी 6 से विभाजित होंगी।

(F) **8 से विभाज्यता :** वे संख्याएं जिनके अन्तिम तीन अंक 8 से विभाज्य हों, तो वे संख्याएं भी 8 से विभाजित होंगी।

(G) **9 से विभाज्यता :** ऐसी संख्याएं जिनके अंकों का योग 9 से विभाज्य हों, तो वे संख्याएं भी 9 से विभाजित होंगी।

(H) **10 से विभाज्यता :** जिन संख्याओं के इकाई के स्थान पर 0 का अंक हो, तो वे संख्याएं 10 से विभाजित होंगी।

(I) **11 से विभाज्यता :** ऐसी संख्याएं जिनके सम तथा विषम स्थानों के अंकों के योगफलों का अन्तर 0 तथा 11 का गुणज हों, तो वे संख्याएं 11 से विभाजित होंगी।

ध्यान रखिये :

(*i*) **भाज्य = भाजक × भागफल + शेष**

(*ii*) $$\textbf{भाजक} = \frac{\textbf{भाज्यें} - \textbf{शेष}}{\textbf{भागफल}}$$

(*iii*) $$\textbf{भागफल} = \frac{\textbf{भाज्य} - \textbf{शेष}}{\textbf{भाजक}}$$

उदाहरण 1 : भाग के एक प्रश्न में भाजक 9, भागफल 114 तथा शेष 5 है, तो बताइये भाज्य कितना होगा ?

हल : ∵ **भाज्य** = भाजक × भागफल + शेष

∴ भाज्य = 9 × 114 + 5 = 1026 + 5 = 1031

अतः भाज्य = 1031 होगा।

उदाहरण 2 : यदि भाग के किसी प्रश्न में भाज्य 1031, शेष 5 तथा भाजक 9 हो तो बताइये भागफल कितना होगा?

हल : $$\textbf{भागफल} = \frac{\text{भाज्य} - \text{शेष}}{\text{भाजक}}$$

$$= \frac{1031-5}{9} = \frac{1026}{9} = 114$$

अतः भागफल = 114 होगा।

उदाहरण 3 : निम्न प्रश्न में रिक्त स्थान की पूर्ति करो?

$$63\overline{)\,7518\,}(11\otimes$$
$$\underline{\;\;\dots\;\;}$$
$$21$$

हल : उपरोक्त प्रश्न में यदि हमें भागफल प्राप्त हो जाए तो ⊗ रिक्त स्थान के मान का पता लग जायेगा।

$$\because \text{ भागफल} = \frac{\text{भाज्य} - \text{शेष}}{\text{भाजक}}$$

$$= \frac{7518-21}{63} = \frac{7497}{63} = 119$$

अतः ⊗ रिक्त स्थान पर मान 9 होगा।

उदाहरण 4 : निम्न प्रश्न में (?) चिन्ह् के स्थान पर कौन-सी संख्या होगी?

$$10?\overline{)\,37522\,}(364$$
$$\underline{\;\;\dots\dots\;\;}$$
$$30$$

हल : उपरोक्त प्रश्न में (?) चिन्ह् के स्थान पर आने वाली संख्या का मान पता लगाने के लिए भाजक का पता लगाना होगा।

$$\therefore \text{ भाजक} = \frac{\text{भाज्य} - \text{शेष}}{\text{भागफल}}$$

$$= \frac{37522-30}{364} = \frac{37492}{364} = 103$$

अतः (?) चिह्न के स्थान पर आने वाली संख्या का मान 3 होगा।

उदाहरण 5 : पांच अंकों की वह छोटी-से-छोटी संख्या क्या होगी जो 23 से पूर्णतः विभाजित हो जाए?

हल : चूंकि पांच अंकों की छोटी-से-छोटी संख्या = 10000

∵ 10000 को 23 से भाग देने पर शेष = 18

अतः 23 से पूर्णतः विभाजित होने वाली पांच अंकों की छोटी-से-छोटी संख्या

= 10000 + (23 – 18)

= 10000 + 5 = 10005 होगी।

प्रश्नमाला

1. 1 से 100 के बीच अभाज्य संख्याएं होंगीः
A. 20 B. 30
C. 22 D. 25

2. ऐसी संख्या जो अभाज्य भी है और सम भीः
A. 1 B. 2
C. 98 D. 79

3. निम्न में से कौन-सी संख्या अभाज्य संख्या होगी?
A. 149 B. 159
C. 117 D. 147

4. चार अंकों की छोटी-से-छोटी संख्या होगी?
A. 1002 B. 1001
C. 9999 D. 1000

5. 43014 में 3 का स्थानीय मान क्या होगा?
A. 3 B. 3000
C. 300 D. 30

6. 81752 में 2 के स्थानीय मान और जातीय मान में अन्तर क्या होगा?
A. 2 B. 0
C. 1 D. 20

7. संख्या 3125 में से क्या घटाया जाए ताकि शेष संख्या 13 से पूर्णतः विभाजित हो सके?
A. 5 B. 8
C. 10 D. 12

8. निम्नलिखित में से कौन-सी संख्या 3 से पूर्णतः विभाजित होगी?
A. 491 B. 371
C. 591 D. 571

9. भाग के प्रश्न में भाजक 16, भागफल 9 तथा शेष 1 हो, तो भाज्य कितना होगा?
A. 145 B. 136
C. 144 D. 152

10. 1 से 50 तक पूर्णांकों का योग कितना होगा?
A. 1275 B. 1375
C. 1225 D. 1365

11. संख्या 30, 70, 584 में अंक 7 के स्थानीय मान लिखो।
A. 700 B. 7000
C. 70,000 D. 700,000

12. 3589 में क्या जोड़ें कि यह पांच अंकों की सबसे छोटी संख्या बन जाए?
A. 6413 B. 6412
C. 6411 D. 6311

13. 2756 और तीन अंकों की सबसे बड़ी संख्या का योगफल ज्ञात करो।
A. 3655 B. 3755
C. 3756 D. 3656

14. पांच अंकों की सबसे बड़ी और छः अंकों की सबसे छोटी संख्याओं का अन्तर ज्ञात करो।
A. 1 B. 3
C. 3 D. 4

15. संख्या 36795 में अंक 6 के स्थान पर 9 तथा 9 के स्थान पर 6 बदल देने से इन संख्याओं के मान में कितना अन्तर हो जाएगा।
A. 2970 B. 3071
C. 2971 D. 3071

16. चार अंकों की बड़ी-से-बड़ी व छोटी-से-छोटी संख्याओं का योग ज्ञात करो।
A. 10990 B. 11999
C. 10909 D. 10999

17. 1 और 20 के बीच में कितनी अभाज्य संख्याएं हैं?
A. 8 B. 9
C. 7 D. 6

18. दो अंकों की कितनी ऐसी संख्याएं हैं जो 13 से पूर्णतः विभाजित हो जाती हैं?
A. 6 B. 7
C. 8 D. 5

19. 0, 2, 3, 6 और 7 अंकों से बनने वाली 5 अंकों की बड़ी से बड़ी और छोटी से छोटी संख्या का अन्तर क्या है?
A. 55955 B. 55954
C. 55853 D. 55953

20. 34 * 7 में पुष्पांकित स्थान पर क्या अंक होना चाहिए जिससे यह संख्या 11 से पूर्णतः विभाजित हो जाए?
A. 6 B. 7
C. 8 D. 9

उत्तरमाला

1	2	3	4	5	6	7	8	9	10
D	B	A	D	B	B	A	C	A	A
11	**12**	**13**	**14**	**15**	**16**	**17**	**18**	**19**	**20**
C	C	B	A	A	D	A	B	D	C

व्याख्यात्मक उत्तर

1. चूंकि 1 से 100 के बीच अभाज्य संख्याएं क्रमशः 2, 3, 5, 7, 11, 13, 17, 19, 23, 29, 31, 37, 41, 43, 47, 53, 59, 61, 67, 71, 73, 79, 83, 89 तथा 97 होंगी। अतः स्पष्ट है कि 1 से 100 तक के बीच अभाज्य संख्याओं की गिनती = 25 हैं।

2. ऐसी संख्या जो अभाज्य भी है और सम भी, केवल 2 है।

3. दिये गये विकल्प A. में 149 एक अभाज्य है, क्योंकि यह किसी अन्य संख्या से पूर्णतः विभाजित नहीं है।

4. चार अंकों की छोटी-से-छोटी संख्या = 1000 होगी। अतः आपका उत्तर विकल्प D. है।

5. $\because$ संख्या 43014 में 3 का अंक हजार के स्थान पर है
$\therefore$ संख्या में 3 का स्थानीय मान = 3 × 1000 = 3000 होगा।

6. $\because$ संख्या 81752 में 2 का अंक इकाई के स्थान पर है।
$\therefore$ संख्या में 2 का स्थानीय मान = 2 × 1 = 2 तथा संख्या में 2 का जातीय मान = 2 होगा। 2 के स्थानीय मान तथा जातीय मान के बीच अन्तर = 2 – 2 = 0 होगा।

7. चूंकि संख्या 3125 में 13 से भाग देने पर शेष 5 बचता है।
$\therefore$ संख्या 3125 को 13 से पूर्णतः विभाजित होने के लिए इसमें से 5 घटाया जाये।

8. विकल्प C. में दी गई संख्या 591, 3 से पूर्णतः विभाजित होगी, क्योंकि संख्या के अंकों का योग 3 से विभाजित हैं।

9. $\because$ भाज्य = भाजक × भागफल + शेष
= 16 × 9 + 1 = 144 + 1 = 145.

10. 1 से 50 तक के पूर्णांकों का योग

$$= \frac{n(n+1)}{2}$$ जहां n पदों की संख्या हैं।

$$= \frac{50(50+1)}{2} = \frac{50\times 51}{2} = 1275$$

11. संख्या 3070584 में
अंक 7 का स्थानीय मान = 7 दस हजार = 70,000

12. 6411

13. 3755

14. 1

15. 39765; मान में अंतर 2970

16. चार अंकों की सबसे बड़ी संख्या = 9999
चार अंकों की सबसे छोटी संख्या = 1000
$\therefore$ अभीष्ट योग = 9999 + 1000 = 10999

17. 1 और 20 के बीच अभाज्य संख्याएं 2, 3, 5, 7, 11, 13, 17 और 19 हैं।

18. 13 से विभाजित होनेवाली दो अंकों की संख्याएं = 13, 26, 39, 52, 65, 78 तथा 91 है।

19. 0, 2, 3, 6 और 7 अंकों से बनने वाली पांच अंकों की बड़ी से बड़ी संख्या = 76320 तथा 0, 2, 3, 6 और 7 अंकों से बनने वाली पांच अंकों की छोटी-से-छोटी संख्या = 20367
$\therefore$ अन्तर = 76320 – 20367 = 55953

20. दी हुई संख्या 11 से पूर्णतः विभाजित होने के लिए यह आवश्यक है कि 7 और 4 का योग वही होना चाहिए जो 3 व छूटे हुए अंक का योग है। अतः छूटा हुआ अंक 8 होना चाहिए।

☆☆☆☆☆☆

2 दशमलव (Decimals)

दशमलव बिन्दु के अंकों के समूह को **दशमलव भिन्न** कहते है। जैसे– 0.513, 0.317, 0.219, 0.6 आदि। प्रत्येक दशमलव एक भिन्न को दर्शाता है।

दशमलव भिन्न को साधारण भिन्न में बदलनाः

(*i*) एक ऐसी भिन्न लो जिसका हर 10 हो तथा अंश दशमलव के बाद दायीं ओर का पहला अंक हो।

(*ii*) एक ऐसी भिन्न लो जिसका हर 100 हो तथा अंश दशमलव के बाद दायीं ओर का दूसरा अंक हो।

(*iii*) इस प्रक्रिया को दोहराइये जब तक दशमलव के बाद के अंक समाप्त नहीं हो जाते। प्रत्येक दशा में हर, पहले हर का दस गुणा होगा।

(*iv*) इस प्रकार प्राप्त भिन्नों का योग जो परिणाम (*i*), (*ii*) और (*iii*) के योग से प्राप्त होता है, दशमलव भिन्न को प्रकट करता है।

जैसे : $0.317 = \frac{3}{10} + \frac{1}{100} + \frac{7}{1000}$

$$= \frac{300}{1000} + \frac{10}{1000} + \frac{7}{1000} = \frac{317}{1000}$$

नोटः शून्यों से बनी कोई संख्या दशमलव के दाईं ओर बिना परिवर्तन किये लिखी जाती है।

प्रश्नमाला

1. कौन-सी भिन्न $\frac{15}{25}$ के समान है?

A. $\frac{150}{25}$ B. $\frac{15}{250}$
C. $\frac{3}{5}$ D. $\frac{60}{75}$

2. कौन-सी भिन्न $\frac{13}{20}$ के समान नहीं है?

A. $\frac{26}{40}$ B. $\frac{130}{200}$
C. $\frac{39}{60}$ D. $\frac{52}{60}$

3. एक घंटे के $\frac{5}{6}$ भाग का मान है:

A. आधा घण्टा B. 40 मिनट
C. 50 मिनट D. 55 मिनट

4. एक वायुयान 1250 कि.मी. यात्रा में 2/5 भाग ईंधन खपत करता है। शेष ईंधन में यात्रा पूरी करेगाः

A. 1875 कि.मी. B. 2125 कि.मी.
C. 250 कि.मी. D. 475 कि.मी.

5. निम्नलिखित में से कौन-सी भिन्न सबसे बड़ी है?

A. $\frac{3}{15}$ B. $\frac{5}{20}$
C. $\frac{8}{64}$ D. $\frac{25}{1000}$

6. निम्नलिखित में से कौन-सी भिन्न सबसे छोटी है?

A. $\frac{1}{10}$ B. $\frac{1}{100}$
C. $\frac{9}{1000}$ D. $\frac{500}{10,000}$

7. $.001 \times 1000 = ?$

A. .1 B. 1
C. .01 D. 10

8. $1.01 \times .1 = ?$

A. 1.01 B. 10.1

C. .101 D. .0101

9. $\frac{20+8\times0.5}{20-?}=12$

A. 12 B. 4

C. 18 D. 2

10. $.01\times100\div2.5=?$

A. 4 B. .4

C. .04 D. 5

11. दी हुई भिन्नों $\frac{5}{8},\frac{21}{35},\frac{9}{16},\frac{6}{7}$ में सबसे बड़ी और सबसे छोटी भिन्न के बीच अन्तर है?

A. $\frac{33}{112}$ B. $\frac{112}{33}$

C. $\frac{32}{112}$ D. $\frac{112}{32}$

12. यदि किसी संख्या तथा उसके $\frac{1}{5}$ भाग में अन्तर 20 है तो वह संख्या क्या है?

A. 23 B. 25

C. 24 D. 26

13. एक मनुष्य के पास एक मकान का $\frac{3}{5}$ भाग था। अपने भाग का $\frac{1}{3}$ भाग उसने 250 रुपए में बेचा तो उस मकान का मूल्य क्या था?

A. 1150 रु. B. 1250 रु.

C. 1205 रु. D. 1105 रु.

14. एक धनराशि का सातवां भाग उनके नौवें भाग से 192 रुपए अधिक है। वह धनराशि बताओ।

A. 4860 रु. B. 6050 रु.

C. 6048 रु. D. 5060 रु.

15. एक मनुष्य ने अपनी जायदाद को तीन बच्चों में इस प्रकार बांटा कि पहले को कुल जायदाद का $\frac{2}{5}$ भाग मिला, दूसरे को शेष का $\frac{1}{3}$ भाग मिला और शेष तीसरे को मिला। यदि तीसरे को, दूसरे से 750 रुपए अधिक मिले हो तो कुल जायदाद का मूल्य क्या था?

A. 3720 रु. B. 3760 रु.

C. 3740 रु. D. 3750 रु.

उत्तरमाला

1	2	3	4	5	6	7	8	9	10
C	D	C	A	B	C	B	C	C	B
11	**12**	**13**	**14**	**15**					
A	B	B	C	D					

व्याख्यात्मक उत्तर

1. $\frac{15}{25}=\frac{3\times5}{5\times5}=\frac{3}{5}$

2. $\frac{26}{40}=\frac{2\times13}{2\times20}=\frac{13}{20},\ \frac{39}{60}=\frac{13\times3}{20\times3}=\frac{13}{20}$

$\frac{130}{200}=\frac{13\times10}{20\times10}=\frac{13}{20},$

$\frac{52}{60}=\frac{13\times4}{20\times3}=\frac{13}{20}\times\frac{4}{3}$

अतः $\frac{52}{60}\neq\frac{13}{20}$

3. 1 घण्टे का $\frac{5}{6}$ भाग $=\frac{5}{6}\times60$ मिनट = 50 मिनट।

4. शेष ईंधन $=1-\frac{2}{5}=\frac{5-2}{5}=\frac{3}{5}$

$\frac{2}{5}$ ईंधन में तय की गई दूरी = 1250 कि.मी.

पूरे ईंधन में तय की गई दूरी

$$= \frac{1250}{2/5} = \frac{1250 \times 5}{2} \text{ कि.मी.}$$

$\frac{3}{5}$ ईंधन में तय की गई दूरी

$$= \frac{1250 \times 5}{2} \times \frac{3}{5} = 1875 \text{ कि.मी.}$$

5. $\frac{3}{15} = \frac{1}{5}, \; \frac{8}{64} = \frac{1}{8}$

$\frac{5}{20} = \frac{1}{4}, \; \frac{25}{1000} = \frac{1}{40}$

$\frac{1}{5}, \frac{1}{4}, \frac{1}{8}, \frac{1}{40}$

$\frac{8, 10, 5, 1}{40}$

$\therefore$ सबसे बड़ी भिन्न $= \frac{1}{4} = \frac{5}{20}$

6. $\frac{1}{10} = .1, \; \frac{9}{1000} = .009$

$\frac{1}{100} = .01, \; \frac{500}{10{,}000} = \frac{5}{100} = .05$

$\therefore$ सबसे छोटी भिन्न $= 0.09 = \frac{9}{1000}$

7. $.001 \times 1000 = 001.000 = 1$

8. $1.01 \times .1 = \frac{101 \times 1}{100 \times 10} = \frac{101}{1000} = .101$

9. $\because \; \frac{20 + 8 \times 0.5}{20 - ?} \Rightarrow \frac{20 + 4}{20 - ?} = 12 \Rightarrow \frac{24}{12} = 2$

$\Rightarrow 2 = 20 - ? \Rightarrow ? = 20 - 2 = 18$

10. $.01 \times 100 \div 2.5 \quad = .01 \times \frac{100}{2.5} = .01 \times 40 = .4$

11. 8, 35, 16 और 7 का लघुत्तम **समापवर्तक** = 560

$\therefore \quad \frac{5}{8} = \frac{5 \times 70}{8 \times 70} = \frac{350}{560}$

$\frac{21}{35} = \frac{21 \times 16}{35 \times 16} = \frac{336}{560}$

$\frac{9}{16} = \frac{9 \times 35}{16 \times 35} = \frac{315}{560}$

$\frac{6}{7} = \frac{6 \times 80}{7 \times 80} = \frac{480}{560}$

$\therefore$ सबसे बड़ी भिन्न $= \frac{6}{7}$

तथा सबसे छोटी भिन्न $= \frac{9}{16}$

$\therefore$ अन्तर $= \frac{6}{7} - \frac{9}{16} = \frac{96 - 63}{112} = \frac{33}{112}$

12. माना संख्या 1 है।

$\therefore$ 1 का $\frac{1}{5} = \frac{1}{5}$

$\therefore \; 1 - \frac{1}{5} = \frac{4}{5}$

$\therefore$ संख्या $= 20 \div \frac{4}{5} = 20 \times \frac{5}{4} = 25$

13. भाग जो बेचा गया $= \frac{3}{5}$ का $\frac{1}{3} = \frac{3}{5} \times \frac{1}{3} = \frac{1}{5}$

$\because \; \frac{1}{5}$ भाग का मूल्य = 250 रुपए

$\therefore$ सम्पूर्ण भाग का मूल्य $= 250 \times \frac{5}{1} = 1250$ रुपए

14. $\because \; \frac{1}{7} - \frac{1}{9} = \frac{2}{63}$

$\because$ धन का $\frac{2}{63} = 192$ रुपए

$\therefore$ वह धन $= 192 \times \frac{63}{2} = 6048$ रुपए

15. पहले बच्चे का भाग = कुल सम्पति का $\frac{2}{5}$

$\therefore$ शेष $= 1 - \frac{2}{5} = \frac{3}{5}$

दूसरे बच्चे का भाग $= \frac{3}{5}$ का $\frac{1}{3} = \frac{1}{5}$

अब शेष बचा $= \frac{3}{5} - \frac{1}{5} = \frac{2}{5}$ जो कि तीसरे बच्चे को दिया गया।

$\therefore$ तीसरे बच्चे को दूसरे बच्चे से अधिक मिला

$= \frac{2}{5} - \frac{1}{5} = \frac{1}{5}$

$\therefore$ कुल सम्पति के $\frac{1}{5}$ भाग का मूल्य = 750 रुपए

$\therefore$ कुल संपत्ति का मूल्य $= 750 \times \frac{5}{1} = 3750$ रुपए।

☆☆☆☆☆☆

3 सरलीकरण
(Simplification)

साधारण या दशमलव भिन्नों के जटिल व्यंजक को एक साधारण भिन्न या दशमलव भिन्न में बदलने की क्रिया को ''सरलीकरण'' कहते हैं। इस प्रकार के व्यंजक में ''कोष्ठक'', ''का'', (÷), (×), (+) तथा (–) आदि चिह्न अलग-अलग या एक साथ प्रदर्शित होते हैं। अतः ऐसे व्यंजक का ''सरलीकरण'' करने में **"BODMAS"** शब्द का प्रयोग किया जाता है। **"BODMAS"** शब्द का क्रमानुसार आशय निम्नलिखित है।

"BODMAS"

B	ब्रैकेट (कोष्ठक)	$\left[\left\{\left(\overline{\ }\right)\right\}\right]$
O	ऑफ (का)	का
D	डिवीजन (भाग)	÷
M	मल्टीप्लिकेशन (गुणा)	×
A	ऐडीशन (जोड़)	+
S	सब्ट्रेक्शन (घटाना)	–

अतः किसी भी जटिल व्यंजक को **"BODMAS"** शब्द के क्रमानुसार सरल किया जाता है। अर्थात् सबसे पहले ''कोष्ठक'' उसके बाद ''का'' फिर ''भाग'' फिर ''गुणा'' उसके बाद ''जोड़'' और अन्त में ''घटाना'' सरल होता है। इस क्रम को याद रखना परम आवश्यक हैं क्योंकि ऐसा न करने पर सरलीकरण की क्रियाएं गलत हो जाती हैं।

महत्वपूर्ण नोट :

(i) **कोष्ठक चार प्रकार के होते हैं : 1. रेखा कोष्ठक जिसे बन्धनी रेखा (–) भी कहते हैं। 2. छोटा कोष्ठक(()), 3. मझला कोष्ठक ({}), 4. बड़ा कोष्ठक ([]), अतः कोष्ठक के प्रश्नों में सबसे पहले रेखा कोष्ठक (–), उसके बाद छोटा कोष्ठक (()), उसके बाद मझला कोष्ठक ({}), और अन्त में बड़े कोष्ठक ([]) को सरल करना चाहिए।**

(ii) **O (का) का सामान्य अर्थ गुणा होता है।**

नीचे कुछ उदाहरण दिये गये हैं जिनका अभ्यास करके आप भली-भाँति समझ सकेंगेः

उदाहरण 1 : $6+5\times3$ को सरल कीजिए।

हल : $\therefore$ उपरोक्त प्रश्न में + और × के चिह्न प्रदर्शित हैं।

$\therefore$ "BODMAS" नियम के अनुसार पहले गुणा उसके बाद जोड़ होगा।

$\therefore\ 6+5\times3=6+15=21$

उदाहरण 2 : $\frac{3}{4}\div\frac{1}{2}+\frac{1}{4}-\frac{1}{8}$ को सरल कीजिए।

हल : $\therefore$ उपरोक्त प्रश्न में ÷, + और – चिह्न प्रदर्शित हैं।

$\therefore$ "BODMAS" नियम के अनुसार पहले भाग, फिर जोड़ उसके बाद घटाव करें।

$$\therefore\ \frac{3}{4}\div\frac{1}{2}+\frac{1}{4}-\frac{1}{8}$$

$$=\frac{3}{4}\times\frac{2}{1}+\frac{1}{4}-\frac{1}{8}=\frac{3}{2}+\frac{1}{4}-\frac{1}{8}$$

$$=\frac{12+2-1}{8}=\frac{13}{8}=1\frac{5}{8}$$

ध्यान दें : + और – चिह्न को एक साथ हल करने पर कोई अन्तर नहीं पड़ता है।

उदाहरण 3 : $\frac{1}{2}$ का $\frac{4}{3}\times3\frac{1}{2}\div\frac{7}{4}-1$ को सरल करो।

हल : "BODMAS" नियम के अनुसार सबसे पहले 'का' फिर ÷, फिर ×, अन्त में – को सरल करें।

$$\therefore\ \frac{1}{2}\text{ का }\frac{4}{3}\times3\frac{1}{2}\div\frac{7}{4}-1$$

$$=\frac{2}{3}\times3\frac{1}{2}\div\frac{7}{4}-1=\frac{2}{3}\times\frac{7}{2}\times\frac{4}{7}-1=\frac{2}{3}\times2-1$$

$$=\frac{4}{3}-1=\frac{4-3}{3}=\frac{1}{3}$$

उदाहरण 4: $\frac{4}{15} \div \frac{4}{5} - \frac{1}{5} \times \frac{3}{5}$ का $\frac{5}{6}$ को सरल करो।

हल : "BODMAS" नियम के अनुसार सबसे पहले 'का' फिर '÷' उसके बाद × और बाद में – को सरल करें।

$\therefore \frac{4}{15} \div \frac{4}{5} - \frac{1}{5} \times \frac{3}{5}$ का $\frac{5}{6}$

$= \frac{4}{15} \div \frac{4}{5} - \frac{1}{5} \times \frac{1}{2}$

$= \frac{4}{15} \times \frac{5}{4} - \frac{1}{5} \times \frac{1}{2} = \frac{1}{3} - \frac{1}{5} \times \frac{1}{2}$

$= \frac{1}{3} - \frac{1}{10} = \frac{10-3}{30} = \frac{7}{30}$

प्रश्नमाला

1. $\frac{7}{4} - \frac{4}{7} = \frac{5}{28} + ?$

A. 2 B. $\frac{1}{7}$

C. $\frac{2}{9}$ D. 1

2. $22 \times 5 = 22$ का ?%

A. 4500 B. 5000

C. 500 D. 750

3. 200 का $\frac{1}{25} \div 8 = ?$

A. 1 B. 3

C. 8 D. 5

4. $\frac{40 \times 0.4 \times 0.04}{4 + 4 \div 4} = ?$

A. .128 B. .148

C. .15 D. .248

5. $50 \div 5 \div 5 = ?$

A. 2 B. 10

C. 1/5 D. 4

6. $\frac{40 \times 15 + 25}{26 + 4 \div 4 - 2} = ?$

A. 25 B. 30

C. 31 D. 42

7. $\frac{1.4 \times 3.6 - 1.2}{0.4 \times 1.2} = ?$

A. 8 B. 2

C. 4 D. 3

8. $14 \times 3.2 - 2 \times 2.1 + 0.8 = ?$

A. 1.08 B. 2.18

C. 1.18 D. 2.08

9. $5 \div \frac{3}{4} + \frac{2}{3} \times \frac{3}{4} - \frac{2}{3}$ का $\frac{13}{7} = ?$

A. $4\frac{12}{11}$ B. $5\frac{13}{14}$

C. $5\frac{13}{17}$ D. $6\frac{13}{14}$

10. $(9+9+9) \div 9 \times 9 = ?$

A. 27 B. 24

C. 21 D. 32

11. $2 - \left[3 - \left\{6 - \left(5 - \overline{4-3}\right)\right\}\right]$ को सरल करो।

A. 1 B. 2

C. 3 D. इनमें से कोई नहीं

12. सरल करो—

$\frac{3}{11} + \frac{4}{3} \div \frac{10}{11} \times \frac{5}{11} - \frac{28}{33}$ का $1\frac{2}{7}$

A. $\frac{5}{13}$ B. $\frac{-5}{33}$

C. $\frac{5}{33}$ D. $\frac{-5}{13}$

13. $4.51 \times \frac{2}{5} + \frac{3}{5} \times 4.51 + 4.51$ को सरल करो।

A. 9.02 B. 90.2

C. 0.902 D. 902

14. $\frac{15.72 \times 15.72 - 5.72 \times 5.72}{15.72 + 5.72}$ को सरल करो।

A. 9 B. 10

C. 8 D. 11

15. $7.55 \times 7.55 - 2 \times 7.55 \times 2.55 + 2.55 \times 2.55$

A. 16 B. 9

C. 25 D. 36

उत्तरमाला

1	2	3	4	5	6	7	8	9	10
D	C	A	A	A	A	A	A	B	A
11	**12**	**13**	**14**	**15**					
A	B	A	B	C					

व्याख्यात्मक उत्तर

1. $\frac{7}{4} - \frac{4}{7} = \frac{5}{28} + ? \Rightarrow \frac{7 \times 7 - 4 \times 4}{4 \times 7} = \frac{5}{28} + ?$

$\Rightarrow \frac{49 - 16}{28} = \frac{5}{28} + ?$

$\Rightarrow \frac{33}{28} = \frac{5}{28} + ?$

$\Rightarrow 1\frac{5}{28} = \frac{5}{28} + ?$

$\Rightarrow 1 + \frac{5}{28} = \frac{5}{28} + ? \therefore ? = 1$

2. $\because$ $22 \times 5 = 22$ का $?\%$ $\Rightarrow 110 = 22 \times \frac{?}{100}$

$\Rightarrow \frac{110 \times 100}{22} = ?$ $\therefore$ $? = 500$

3. $\because$ 200 का $\frac{1}{25} \div 8 = ? \Rightarrow 8 \div 8 = ?$

$\Rightarrow \frac{8}{8} = ? \Rightarrow 1 = ?$

4. $\because$ $\frac{40 \times 0.4 \times 0.04}{4 + 4 \div 4} = ? \Rightarrow \frac{.64}{4 + \frac{4}{4}} = ?$

$\Rightarrow \frac{.64}{4 + 1} = ? \Rightarrow \frac{.64}{5} = ? \Rightarrow .128 = ?$

5. $\because$ $50 \div 5 \div 5 = ? \Rightarrow \frac{50}{5} \div 5 = ?$

$\Rightarrow 10 \div 5 = ? \Rightarrow \frac{10}{5} = ?$ $\Rightarrow 2 = ?$

6. $\because$ $\frac{40 \times 15 + 25}{26 + 4 \div 4 - 2} = ? \Rightarrow \frac{600 + 25}{26 + \frac{4}{4} - 2} = ?$

$\Rightarrow \frac{625}{26 + 1 - 2} = ?$ $\Rightarrow$ $\frac{625}{25} = ? \Rightarrow 25 = ?$

7. $\frac{1.4 \times 3.6 - 1.2}{0.4 \times 1.2} = \frac{5.04 - 1.2}{.48} = \frac{3.84}{.48} = 8.$

8. "BODMAS" नियम के अनुसार पहले गुणा उसके बाद जोड़ और अन्त में घटाव की क्रिया करें।

$\therefore$ $1.4 \times 3.2 - 2 \times 2.1 + 0.8$

$= 4.48 - 4.2 + 0.8 = 1.08$

9. "BODMAS" नियम के अनुसार सबसे पहले का, फिर भाग, उसके बाद गुणा, फिर जोड़ और अन्त में घटाव की क्रिया करें।

$\therefore$ $5 \div \frac{3}{4} + \frac{2}{3} \times \frac{3}{4} - \frac{2}{3}$ का $\frac{13}{7}$

$= 5 \div \frac{3}{4} + \frac{2}{3} \times \frac{3}{4} - \frac{26}{21}$

$$= \frac{20}{3}+\frac{2}{3}\times\frac{3}{4}-\frac{26}{21}=\frac{20}{3}+\frac{1}{2}-\frac{26}{21}$$

$$= \frac{280+21-52}{42}=\frac{249}{42}=5\frac{39}{42}=5\frac{13}{14}$$

10. "BODMAS" नियम के अनुसार पहले कोष्ठक के अन्दर की संख्याओं को सरल करें फिर भाग, उसके बाद गुणा करें।

$\therefore \quad (9+9+9)\div 9\times 9 = 27\div 9\times 9$

$$= \frac{27}{9}\times 9 = 27.$$

11. $2-\left[3-\left\{6-\left(5-\overline{4-3}\right)\right\}\right]$

$= 2 - [3 - \{6 - (5 - 1)\}]$
$= 2 - [3 - \{6 - 4\}]$
$= 2 - [3 - 2]$
$= 2 - 1$
$= 1$

12. दिया गया व्यजंक $= \frac{3}{11}+\frac{4}{3}\div\frac{10}{11}\times\frac{5}{11}-\frac{28}{33}$ का $1\frac{2}{7}$

$$= \frac{3}{11}+\frac{4}{3}\div\frac{10}{11}\times\frac{5}{11}-\frac{28}{33}\times\frac{9}{7}$$

$$= \frac{3}{11}+\frac{4}{3}\times\frac{11}{10}\times\frac{5}{11}-\frac{28}{33}\times\frac{9}{7}$$

$$= \frac{3}{11}+\frac{2}{3}-\frac{12}{11}=\frac{9+22-36}{33}$$

$$= \frac{-5}{33}$$

13. व्यंजक $= 4.51\times\frac{2}{5}+\frac{3}{5}\times 4.51+4.51$

$$= 4.51\left(\frac{2}{5}+\frac{3}{5}+1\right)$$

$$= 4.51\left(\frac{2+3+5}{5}\right)$$

$$= 4.51\times\frac{10}{5}$$

$= 4.51 \times 2 = 9.02$

14. $\frac{15.72\times 15.72-5.72\times 5.72}{15.72+5.72}$

$$= \frac{(15.72+5.72)\,(15.72-5.72)}{(15.72+5.72)}$$

$= 15.72 - 5.72 = 10$

15. $7.55 \times 7.55 - 2 \times 7.55 \times 2.55 + 2.55 \times 2.55$
$= (7.55)^2 - 2\,(7.55)\,(2.55) + (2.55)^2$
$= (7.55 - 2.55)^2 = (5)^2 = 25$

☆☆☆☆☆☆

4 महत्तम समापवर्तक और लघुत्तम समापवर्त्य
(H.C.F. and L.C.M.)

महत्तम समापवर्तक : किन्हीं दो या दो से अधिक दी हुई संख्याओं का महत्तम समापवर्तक (म. स. प.) वह बड़ी-से-बड़ी संख्या है जो प्रत्येक दी हुई संख्याओं को पूरा-पूरा विभाजित करे।

लघुत्तम समापवर्त्य : किन्हीं दो या दो से अधिक दी हुई संख्याओं का लघुत्तम समापवर्त्य (ल. स. व.) वह छोटी-से-छोटी संख्या है जो प्रत्येक दी हुई संख्या से पूरी-पूरी विभाजित हो।

प्रश्नों से संबंधित समस्याओं को हल करने के लिए निम्नलिखित सूत्रों को ध्यान में रखिये :

(*i*) भिन्नों का महत्तम समापवर्तक (म. स. प.) = अंशों का महत्तम समापवर्तक / हरों का लघुत्तम समापवर्त्य

(*ii*) भिन्नों का लघुत्तम समापवर्त्य (ल. स. व.) = अंशों का लघुत्तम समापवर्त्य / हरों का महत्तम समापवर्तक

(*iii*) दो संख्याओं का गुणनफल = म. स. प. × ल. स. व.

उदाहरण 1 : 18, 24 तथा 60 का महत्तम समापवर्तक निकालिए।

हल : $\because$ $18 = \underline{2} \times 3 \times \underline{3}$

$24 = \underline{2} \times 2 \times 2 \times 3$ तथा $60 = 2 \times 2 \times \underline{3} \times 5$

$\because$ उपरोक्त दी हुई संख्याओं के अभाज्य गुणनखण्डों से स्पष्ट है कि तीनों संख्याओं के अभाज्य गुणनखण्डों में 2×3 उभयनिष्ठ है।

$\therefore$ अभीष्ट महत्तम समापवर्तक = 6 होगा।

उदाहरण 2 : 40, 30, 25 तथा 20 का लघुत्तम समापवर्त्य ज्ञात कीजिए।

हल : $\because$ $40 = 2 \times 2 \times 2 \times 5$

$30 = 2 \times 3 \times 5$

$25 = 5 \times 5$ तथा $20 = 2 \times 2 \times 5$

$\because$ उपरोक्त चारों संख्याओं के अभाज्य गुणनखण्डों को देखकर आसानी से ज्ञात किया जा सकता है कि कौन-सा अभाज्य गुणनखण्ड सबसे अधिक बार आया है। अतः स्पष्ट है कि अभाज्य गुणनखण्ड 2 सबसे अधिक 3 बार और 3 एक बार तथा 5 दो बार आया है।

$\therefore$ अभीष्ट लघुत्तम समापवर्त्य (ल. स. व.)

$= 2 \times 2 \times 2 \times 3 \times 5 \times 5 = 600$.

प्रश्नमाला

1. 12, 24 व 36 का महत्तम समापवर्तक कितना होगा?
A. 16 B. 18
C. 12 D. 36

2. 70, 20 व 14 का लघुत्तम समापवर्त्य क्या है?
A. 120 B. 140
C. 280 D. 70

3. दो संख्याओं का अनुपात 11 : 15 है। यदि उनका म॰स॰प॰ 13 हो, तो वे संख्याएं क्रमशः क्या होगी?
A. 143 व 195 B. 195 व 143
C. 110 व 150 D. 121 व 165

4. वह छोटी-से-छोटी पूर्ण वर्ग संख्या क्या होगी जो 56, 21 तथा 36 से पूर्णतः विभाजित हो सके?
A. 7056 B. 8056
C. 7040 D. 8100

5. वह बड़ी-से-बड़ी संख्या क्या होगी, जिससे यदि 27, 33 तथा 39 को भाग दें तो क्रमशः 2, 3 तथा 4 शेष बचे?
A. 4 B. 5
C. 3 D. 7

6. 5 अंकों की वह छोटी-से-छोटी संख्या क्या होगी जो 12, 15 तथा 18 से पूर्णतः विभाजित हो?
A. 10080 B. 10800
C. 11820 D. 12080

7. दो संख्याओं का गुणनफल 27 है। उनका महत्तम समापवर्तक 3 है, तो उनका लघुत्तम समापवर्त्य क्या होगा?
A. 81 B. 54
C. 9 D. 6

8. चार अंकों की वह बड़ी-से-बड़ी संख्या क्या है जो 2, 3, 4, 5, 6 और 7 से पूरी-पूरी विभाजित हो जाती है?
A. 9729 B. 9760
C. 9579 D. 9660

9. दो संख्याओं का गुणनफल 54 है। उनका महत्तम समापवर्तक 3 है, तो उनका लघुत्तम समापवर्त्य क्या होगा?
A. 18 B. 21
C. 9 D. 24

10. $\frac{10}{21}, \frac{25}{27}$ और $\frac{35}{24}$ का महत्तम समापवर्तक क्या है?
A. $\frac{5}{216}$ B. $\frac{5}{1080}$
C. $\frac{5}{1512}$ D. $\frac{5}{638}$

11. 27, 15, 72 का लघुत्तम ज्ञात करो।
A. 1020 B. 1080
C. 1050 D. 1060

12. 77, 88, 132 का लघुत्तम ज्ञात करो।
A. 1860 B. 1858
C. 1850 D. 1848

13. 135, 120, 90 का लघुत्तम ज्ञात करो।
A. 1050 B. 1020
C. 1080 D. 1060

14. 4, 6, 9, 12 का लघुत्तम ज्ञात करो।
A. 36 B. 38
C. 34 D. 40

उत्तरमाला

1	2	3	4	5	6	7	8	9	10
C	B	A	A	B	A	C	D	A	C
11	**12**	**13**	**14**						
B	D	C	A						

व्याख्यात्मक उत्तर

1. $\because$ $12 = \underline{2 \times 2 \times 3}$
$24 = 2 \times \underline{2 \times 2 \times 3}$
तथा $36 = \underline{2 \times 2 \times 3} \times 3$
$\therefore$ अभीष्ट महत्तम समापवर्तक $= 2 \times 2 \times 3 = 12$ होगा।

2. $\because$ $70 = 2 \times 5 \times 7$
$20 = 2 \times 2 \times 5$
तथा $14 = 2 \times 7$
$\therefore$ अभीष्ट लघुत्तम समापवर्त्य $= 2 \times 2 \times 5 \times 7 = 140$

3. माना कि वे संख्याएं क्रमशः $11x$ व $15x$ हैं।
प्रश्नानुसार, दोनों संख्याओं का म॰स॰प॰ = 13 (दिया हुआ है) अतः स्पष्ट होता है कि x के स्थान पर मान 13 होगा, क्योंकि 11×13 तथा 15×13 का म॰स॰प॰ 13 है। अतः वे संख्याएं क्रमशः $11 \times 13 = 143$ तथा $15 \times 13 = 195$ होंगी।

4. सबसे पहले 56, 21 तथा 36 का ल॰स॰व॰ ज्ञात करना है।
$\because$ $56 = 2 \times 2 \times 2 \times 7$
$21 = 3 \times 7$
तथा $36 = 2 \times 2 \times 3 \times 3$
$\therefore$ अभीष्ट ल॰स॰व॰ $= 2 \times 2 \times 2 \times 3 \times 3 \times 7$
चूंकि यह पूर्ण वर्ग संख्या नही है। अतः अभीष्ट ल॰स॰व॰ को पूर्ण वर्ग बनाने के लिए इसमें कम-से-कम 2×7 अर्थात् 14 से गुणा करना होगा।
$\therefore$ वह छोटी-से-छोटी पूर्ण वर्ग संख्या
$= 2 \times 2 \times 2 \times 3 \times 3 \times 7 \times 2 \times 7 = 7056$ होगी।

5. इस प्रकार के प्रश्नों में पहले शेषफल को संख्याओं में से घटाया जाता है फिर उन संख्याओं का म॰स॰प॰ ज्ञात किया जाता है।

$\therefore$ $27 - 2 = 25, 33 - 3 = 30$ तथा $39 - 4 = 35$

अतः 25, 30 तथा 35 का म॰स॰प॰ ज्ञात करना है।

$\because$ $25 = 5 \times 5, 30 = 2 \times 3 \times 5$ तथा $35 = 5 \times 7$

$\therefore$ अभीष्ट म॰स॰प॰ = 5

$\therefore$ वह-बड़ी-से बड़ी संख्या = 5 होगी।

6. सबसे पहले 12, 15 तथा 18 का ल॰स॰व॰ ज्ञात करना है।

$\because$ $12 = 2 \times 2 \times 3, 15 = 3 \times 5$ तथा $18 = 2 \times 3 \times 3$

$\therefore$ अभीष्ट ल॰स॰व॰ $= 2 \times 2 \times 3 \times 3 \times 5 = 180$

तथा 5 अंकों की छोटी-से-छोटी संख्या = 10000

$= 180 \times 55 + 100$

तथा स्पष्ट है कि 5 अंकों की छोटी-से-छोटी संख्या जो 12, 15 तथा 18 से पूर्णतः विभाजित होगी

$= 180 \times 56 = 10080$

7. लघुत्तम समापवर्त्य

$$= \frac{\text{दोनों संख्याओं का गुणनफल}}{\text{उनका महत्तम समापवर्तक}} = \frac{27}{3} = 9$$

8. 2, 3, 4, 5, 6 और 7 का लघुत्तम समापवर्त्य

$= 2 \times 2 \times 3 \times 5 \times 7 = 420$

चार अंकों की सबसे बड़ी संख्या = 9999

9999 को 420 से विभाजित करें तो शेष = 339

$\therefore$ अभीष्ट संख्या $= 9999 - 339 = 9660$

9. उनका लघुत्तम समापवर्त्य

$$= \frac{\text{दोनों संख्याओं का गुणनफल}}{\text{उनका महत्तम समापवर्तक}} = \frac{54}{3} = 18$$

10. भिन्नों का महत्तम समापवर्तक

$$= \frac{\text{अंशों का महत्तम समापवर्तक}}{\text{हरों का लघुत्तम समापवर्त्य}}$$

$$= \frac{\text{10, 25 और 35 का महत्तम समापवर्तक}}{\text{21, 27 और 24 का लघुत्तम समापवर्त्य}}$$

$$= \frac{5}{1512}$$

11. ल. स.

2	27,	15,	72
2	27,	15,	36
2	27,	15,	18
3	27,	15,	9
3	9,	5,	3
3	3,	5,	1
5	1,	5,	1
	1,	1,	1

अतः दी गई संख्याओं का लघुत्तम समापवर्त्य

$2 \times 2 \times 2 \times 3 \times 3 \times 3 \times 5 = 1080$

12. ल. स.

2	77,	88,	132
2	77,	44,	66
2	77,	22,	33
3	77,	11,	33
7	77,	11,	11
11	11,	11,	11
	1,	1,	1

अतः दी गई संख्याओं का लघुत्तम समापवर्त्य

$2 \times 2 \times 2 \times 3 \times 7 \times 11 = 1848$

13. ल. स.

2	135,	120,	90
2	135,	60,	45
2	135,	30,	45
3	135,	15,	45
3	45,	5,	15
3	15,	5,	5
5	5,	5,	5
	1,	1,	1

अतः दी गई संख्याओं का लघुत्तम समापवर्त्य

$2 \times 2 \times 2 \times 3 \times 3 \times 3 \times 5 = 1080$

14. ल. स.

2	4,	6,	9,	12
2	2,	3,	9,	6
3	1,	3,	9,	3
3	1,	1,	3,	1
	1,	1,	1,	1

अतः दी गई संख्याओं का लघुत्तम समापवर्त्य

$2 \times 2 \times 3 \times 3 = 36$

☆☆☆☆☆☆

5 घातांक
(Indices)

हम जानते हैं कि $x \times x = x^2$, $x \times x \times x = x^3$, $x \times x \times x \times x = x^4$ ...., $x \times x \times x \times x \times x$ .... n गुणनखण्डों तक $= x^n$ को "x की घात n" पढ़ा जाता है। इस प्रकार हम कह सकते हैं कि

2 की घात $3 = 2^3 = 2 \times 2 \times 2 = 8$

3 की घात $3 = 3^3 = 3 \times 3 \times 3 = 27$

5 की घात $4 = 5^4 = 5 \times 5 \times 5 \times 5 = 625$

8 की घात $2 = 8^2 = 8 \times 8 = 64$.

$\left(\frac{x}{y}\right)$ की घात $3 = \left(\frac{x}{y}\right)^3 = \frac{x \times x \times x}{y \times y \times y} = \frac{x^3}{y^3}$

x^2 की घात $5 = (x^2)^5 = x^2 \times x^2 \times x^2 \times x^2 \times x^2 = x^{10}$

घातांक से सम्बन्धित आवश्यक नियम

नियम 1. यदि m और n धन पूर्णांक हों तथा x, y कोई भी संख्याएं हैं तो $x^m \times x^n = x^{m+n}$

नियम 2. यदि m और n धन पूर्णांक हों तथा x, y कोई भी संख्याएं हैं तो,

$$x^m \div x^n = \frac{x^m}{x^n} = x^{m-n} \text{ जबकि } m > n$$

या

$$x^m \div x^n = \frac{x^m}{x^n} = \frac{1}{x^{n-m}} \text{ जबकि } n > m$$

नियम 3. यदि m और n धन पूर्णांक हों तथा x, y कोई भी संख्याएं हैं तो $(x^m)^n = x^{mn}$

नियम 4. यदि m और n धन पूर्णांक हों तथा x, y कोई भी संख्याएं हैं तो $(xy)^m = x^m \times y^m$

मूल : यदि कोई संख्या 'x की घात n' है तथा इसका परिणाम a अर्थात् $x^n = a$ है तो इसका अर्थ यह होता है कि a का n वां मूल x है। जिसे प्राय: इस प्रकार लिखा जाता है

$$x^n = a \Rightarrow x = \sqrt[n]{a} = (a)^{1/n}$$

इसी प्रकार यदि भिन्नात्मक घातांक $x^{p/q} = a$ है तो इसका अर्थ यह होगा कि x का q वां मूल बराबर है a का p वां मूल के, अर्थात्

$$x^{p/q} = a \Rightarrow \left(x^{1/q}\right)^p = a \Rightarrow x^{1/q} = a^{1/p} \Rightarrow \sqrt[q]{x} = \sqrt[p]{a}$$

अत: दूसरे मूल को हम वर्गमूल तथा तीसरे मूल को घनमूल भी कहते हैं।

महत्त्वपूर्ण नोट : यदि किसी संख्या या राशि की घात ''शून्य'' है तो उस संख्या या राशि का मान सदैव 1 के बराबर होगा। अर्थात् $x^0 = y^0 = z^0 = 2^0 = 5^0 = 8^0 = 1$ होगा।

प्रश्नमाला

1. $a^5 \times a^7$ का मान कितना होगा?

A. a^{35} B. a^2

C. a^{12} D. $a^{5/7}$

2. $(x^{2/3})^{-3/4}$ का मान कितना होगा?

A. $\frac{1}{x}$ B. $\frac{1}{\sqrt{x}}$

C. $\frac{1}{x^2}$ D. $\frac{1}{x^{-2}}$

3. 4 की घात 3 निम्न में से किस संख्या के बराबर होगी?

A. 64

B. 81

C. 12

D. 49

4. 2 की घात 3 तथा 3 की घात 2 में कितना अन्तर होगा?

A. 2 B. 5

C. 3 D. 1

5. $\left(-\frac{1}{125}\right)^{-\frac{2}{3}}$ का मान कितना होगा?

A. $\frac{1}{25}$ B. 25

C. 5 D. $\frac{1}{5}$

6. $(8)^{-(2^{-2})}$ का मान कितना होगा?

A. $2^{-1/4}$ B. $2^{-3/4}$

C. $2^{3/4}$ D. $2^{-1/2}$

7. यदि $\sqrt{2^n} = 64$ है, तो n का मान क्या होगा?

A. 8 B. 4

C. 12 D. 16

8. $(100)^0$ का मान कितना होगा?

A. 0 B. 10

C. 1 D. 100

9. यदि $10^{2/5} \times 10^{8/5} = 10^n$ है तो n का मान क्या होगा?

A. 2 B. 3

C. 6 D. 4

10. $27^3 \times 3^4 \div 3^{10}$ का मान कितना होगा?

A. 9 B. 27

C. 81 D. $\frac{1}{27}$

11. व्यंजक $\frac{(-1)^{132}}{5^{-1}+3^{-1}}$ का मान कितना होगा?

A. $\frac{16}{9}$ B. $-\frac{15}{8}$

C. $\frac{15}{8}$ D. $\frac{17}{8}$

12. $6a^3b^3c^2 \div 2ab^2c$ का मान कितना होगा?

A. $3a^2bc$ B. $3ab^2c$

C. $3a^2b^2c^2$ D. $3a^3b^3c^3$

13. $\sqrt{\frac{1}{\left(\frac{3}{4}\right)^{-2}}} + \sqrt[3]{\frac{27}{64}}$ का मान क्या होगा?

A. $\frac{2}{3}$ B. $\frac{4}{5}$

C. $\frac{13}{12}$ D. $\frac{3}{2}$

14. $\frac{a^{-3}.a^{-4}}{a^{-5}}$ का धन घातांकीय रूप में मान क्या होगा?

A. a^2 B. $\frac{1}{a^3}$

C. $\frac{1}{a^4}$ D. $\frac{1}{a^2}$

15. $\sqrt[3]{x^6} \div \sqrt[6]{x^{12}} \times x^{-3} \times \sqrt[3]{x^9}$ का मान कितना होगा?

A. $2x$ B. 1

C. $\frac{1}{3x^2}$ D. $\frac{1}{x}$

उत्तरमाला

1	2	3	4	5	6	7	8	9	10
C	B	A	D	B	B	C	C	A	B
11	**12**	**13**	**14**	**15**					
C	A	D	D	B					

व्याख्यात्मक उत्तर

1. $\because a^5 \times a^7 = a^{5+7} = a^{12}.$ $[\because x^m \times x^n = x^{m+n}]$

2. $\because \left(x^{\frac{2}{3}}\right)^{-\frac{3}{4}} = x^{\frac{2}{3}\times -\frac{3}{4}} = x^{-\frac{1}{2}}$

$= \frac{1}{x^{\frac{1}{2}}} = \frac{1}{\sqrt{x}}.[\because (x^m)^n = x^{mn}]$

3. $\because$ 4 की घात 3 $= 4^3 = 4 \times 4 \times 4 = 64.$

4. $\because$ 2 की घात 3 $= 2^3 = 2 \times 2 \times 2 = 8.$

तथा 3 की घात 2 $= 3^2 = 3 \times 3 = 9$

$\therefore$ अन्तर $= 9 - 8 = 1.$

5. $\left(-\frac{1}{125}\right)^{-\frac{2}{3}} = \frac{1}{\left(-\frac{1}{125}\right)^{\frac{2}{3}}}$

$= (-125)^{\frac{2}{3}}$

$= [(-125)^{1/3}]^2 = [(-5 \times -5 \times -5)^{1/3}]^2$

$= (-5^2) = -5 \times -5 = 25.$

6. $\because 8^{-(2^{-2})} = 8^{-\left(\frac{1}{2^2}\right)} = 8^{-\frac{1}{4}} = \frac{1}{8^{\frac{1}{4}}}$

$= \frac{1}{(2\times2\times2)^{\frac{1}{4}}} = \frac{1}{(2)^{\frac{3}{4}}} = 2^{-\frac{3}{4}}.$

7. $\because \sqrt{2^n} = 64 \Rightarrow 2^n = (64)^2$

$\Rightarrow 2^n$

$= (2\times2\times2\times2\times2\times2)^2 \Rightarrow 2^n = (2^6)^2$

$\Rightarrow 2^n = 2^{6\times2} = 2^{12} \Rightarrow n = 12$

अत: n का मान 12 होगा।

8. यहां विद्यार्थियों को स्मरण रखना चाहिए कि यदि किसी संख्या या राशि की घात ''शून्य'' हो तो उस संख्या या राशि का मान हमेशा 1 के बराबर होगा।

अत: स्पष्ट है कि $(100)^0$ का मान = 1 होगा।

9. $\because 10^{2/5} \times 10^{8/5} = 10^n \Rightarrow 10^{2/5+8/5} = 10^n$

$\Rightarrow 10^{10/5} = 10^n \Rightarrow 10^2 = 10^n \Rightarrow n = 2$

अत: n का मान 2 होगा।

10. $\because 27^3 \times 3^4 \div 3^{10} = 27^3 \times \frac{3^4}{3^{10}}$

$\frac{(3\times3\times3)^3 \times 3^4}{3^{10}} = \frac{(3^3)^3 \times 3^4}{3^{10}}$

$= \frac{3^9 \times 3^4}{3^{10}} = \frac{3^{9+4}}{3^{10}} = \frac{3^{13}}{3^{10}}$

$= 3^{13-10} = 3^3 = 3\times3\times3 = 27.$

11. $\because \frac{(-1)^{132}}{5^{-1}+3^{-1}} = \frac{\left((-1)^2\right)^{66}}{5^{-1}+3^{-1}}$

$= \frac{(1)^{66}}{5^{-1}+3^{-1}} = \frac{1}{\frac{1}{5}+\frac{1}{3}} = \frac{1}{\frac{3+5}{15}}$

$= \frac{1}{\frac{8}{15}} = \frac{15}{8}.$

12. $\because 6a^3b^3c^2 \div 2ab^2c$

$= \frac{6a^3b^3c^2}{2ab^2c} = 3a^{3-1}b^{3-2}c^{2-1} = 3a^2bc.$

13. $\because \sqrt{\frac{1}{\left(\frac{3}{4}\right)^{-2}}} + \sqrt[3]{\frac{27}{64}} = \sqrt{\left(\frac{3}{4}\right)^2} + \sqrt[3]{\frac{3\times3\times3}{4\times4\times4}}$

$= \sqrt{\left(\frac{3}{4}\right)^2} + \sqrt[3]{\left(\frac{3}{4}\right)^3} = \frac{3}{4}+\frac{3}{4} = \frac{6}{4} = \frac{3}{2}.$

14. $\because \frac{a^{-3}.a^{-4}}{a^{-5}} = \frac{a^5}{a^3.a^4} = \frac{a^5}{a^7} = \frac{1}{a^{7-5}} = \frac{1}{a^2}$

अत: $\frac{a^{-3}.a^{-4}}{a^{-5}}$ का धन घातांकीय रूप में मान $\frac{1}{a^2}$ होगा।

15. $\because \sqrt[3]{x^6} \div \sqrt[6]{x^{12}} \times x^{-3} \times \sqrt[3]{x^9}$

$= \frac{(x^6)^{\frac{1}{3}}}{(x^{12})^{\frac{1}{6}}} \times x^{-3} \times (x^9)^{\frac{1}{3}}$

[$\because$ BODMAS शब्द के अनुसार पहले ''भाग'' फिर ''गुणा'']

$= \frac{x^{6\times\frac{1}{3}} \times x^{-3} \times x^{9\times\frac{1}{3}}}{x^{12\times\frac{1}{6}}}$

$= \frac{x^2 \times x^{-3} \times x^3}{x^2} = x^0 = 1.$

☆☆☆☆☆☆

6 करणी (Surds)

प्राय: सभी संख्याओं के वर्गमूल सदैव पूर्ण संख्या नहीं होते, जैसे– $\sqrt{9} = 3$ परन्तु $\sqrt{15} = 3.873$, जो कि पूर्ण संख्या नहीं है, अर्थात् 15 का वर्गमूल पूर्ण संख्या नहीं है। अत: ऐसी संख्यायें जिनके वर्गमूल पूर्ण संख्या नहीं होते, जैसे– $\sqrt{3}$, $\sqrt{7}$, $2+\sqrt{11}$, $4+\sqrt{13}$ .... इत्यादि संख्यायें **करणी** कहलाती हैं।

प्रश्नों को हल करने के लिए निम्नलिखित सूत्रों का प्रयोग कीजिए :

1. $\sqrt{a} \times \sqrt{a} = a$
2. $\sqrt{a} \times \sqrt{b} = \sqrt{ab}$
3. $\left(\sqrt{a}+\sqrt{b}\right)^2 = a+b+2\sqrt{ab}$
4. $\left(\sqrt{a}-\sqrt{b}\right)^2 = a+b-2\sqrt{ab}$
5. $x\sqrt{a}+x\sqrt{b} = x\left(\sqrt{a}+\sqrt{b}\right)$
6. $\frac{1}{\sqrt{a}+\sqrt{b}} = \frac{1}{\sqrt{a}+\sqrt{b}} \times \frac{\sqrt{a}-\sqrt{b}}{\sqrt{a}-\sqrt{b}}$ $= \frac{\sqrt{a}-\sqrt{b}}{a-b}$
7. $\frac{1}{\sqrt{a}-\sqrt{b}} = \frac{1}{\sqrt{a}-\sqrt{b}} \times \frac{\sqrt{a}+\sqrt{b}}{\sqrt{a}+\sqrt{b}}$ $= \frac{\sqrt{a}+\sqrt{b}}{a-b}$
8. $a+\sqrt{b} = c+\sqrt{d} \Rightarrow a = c$ तथा $b = d$
9. $\sqrt{2} = 1.41421$, $\sqrt{3} = 1.73205$, $\sqrt{5} = 2.23607$, $\sqrt{6} = 2.4494$, $\sqrt{7} = 2.64575$, $\sqrt{8} = 2.82842$, $\sqrt{10} = 3.16227$, $\sqrt{11} = 3.31662$

प्रश्नमाला

1. $\frac{1}{\sqrt{3}}$ का मान दशमलव के तीन स्थानों तक होगा—

A. 0.577 B. 0.477
C. 0.673 D. 0.575

2. यदि $\sqrt{2} = 1.4142$ हो, तो $\frac{1}{2}\left(\frac{\sqrt{2}-1}{\sqrt{2}+1}\right)$ का मान कितना होगा?

A. .0768 B. .0658
C. .0858 D. .0458

3. यदि $\sqrt{1936} = 44$, हो तो $\sqrt{19.36}+\sqrt{0.1936}+\sqrt{.001936}$ का मान दशमलव के तीन स्थानों तक होगा—

A. 5.679 B. 4.884
C. 9.884 D. 6.778

4. $\sqrt{\left(5+\frac{4}{9}\right)}$ का मान होगा?

A. $3\frac{1}{3}$ B. $2\frac{1}{6}$
C. $4\frac{1}{3}$ D. $2\frac{1}{3}$

5. $\frac{\sqrt{2}-1}{\sqrt{2}+1}$ का मान दशमलव के तीन स्थानों तक होगा—

A. 0.172 B. 0.158
C. 0.176 D. 0.188

6. $\sqrt[3]{8^4}$ का मान कितना होगा?

A. 15 B. 9
C. 16 D. 25

7. यदि $\sqrt{6} = 2.45$, तो $\sqrt{\frac{2}{3}} + 3\sqrt{\frac{3}{2}}$ का मान किसके बराबर होगा?

A. 3.942 B. 4.492
C. 4.942 D. 9.345

8. $\sqrt{72}$ का मान किसके बराबर होगा?

A. $3\sqrt{5}$ B. $6\sqrt{2}$
C. $8\sqrt{2}$ D. $7\sqrt{3}$

9. हर के परिमेयीकरण के पश्चात व्यंजक $\frac{\sqrt{2}}{\sqrt{2}+\sqrt{3}-\sqrt{5}}$ का रूप होगा—

A. $\frac{3+\sqrt{6}+\sqrt{15}}{6}$ B. $\frac{3-\sqrt{6}-\sqrt{5}}{6}$
C. $\frac{3+\sqrt{6}+\sqrt{5}}{3}$ D. $\frac{2+\sqrt{6}-\sqrt{15}}{6}$

10. $\left(\sqrt{80} + 3 \times \sqrt{245} - \sqrt{125}\right)$ का मान कितना होगा?

A. $18\sqrt{5}$ B. $20\sqrt{5}$
C. $22\sqrt{5}$ D. $28\sqrt{2}$

11. $\left(\frac{\sqrt{5}+\sqrt{3}}{\sqrt{5}-\sqrt{3}}\right)$ का मान कितना होगा?

A. $4+\sqrt{15}$ B. $3-\sqrt{15}$
C. $2+\sqrt{15}$ D. $4-\sqrt{15}$

12. $3^{\frac{1}{5}}, 5^{\frac{3}{5}}, 7^{\frac{4}{5}}$ को आरोही क्रम में किस प्रकार से लिखा जा सकता है?

A. $5^{\frac{3}{5}} < 3^{\frac{1}{5}} < 7^{\frac{4}{5}}$ B. $3^{\frac{1}{5}} < 5^{\frac{3}{5}} < 7^{\frac{4}{5}}$
C. $7^{\frac{4}{5}} < 3^{\frac{1}{5}} < 5^{\frac{3}{5}}$ D. $3^{\frac{1}{5}} < 7^{\frac{4}{5}} < 5^{\frac{3}{5}}$

13. यदि $12 \times 4^{\frac{1}{3}}$ को $3\sqrt{2}$ से भाग दिया जाये तब भागफल का मान होगा—

A. 2 B. $\sqrt{15}$
C. 3 D. $2^{13/6}$

14. यदि $4^{\frac{1}{3}}, 6^{\frac{1}{6}}$ तथा $\sqrt{5}$ का गुणा किया जाये तो गुणनफल का मान होगा—

A. $(12000)^{\frac{1}{6}}$ B. $(12009)^{\frac{1}{6}}$
C. $(14000)^{\frac{1}{6}}$ D. $(15000)^{\frac{1}{4}}$

15. व्यंजक $\left(2+\sqrt{2}+\frac{1}{2+\sqrt{2}}+\frac{1}{\sqrt{2}-2}\right)$ का मान होगा—

A. 5 B. 2
C. 3 D. 8

16. व्यंजक $\left(\frac{\sqrt{7}+\sqrt{5}}{\sqrt{7}-\sqrt{5}}\right)$ का मान होगा।

A. $6-\sqrt{35}$ B. $2+\sqrt{35}$
C. $4-\sqrt{35}$ D. $6+\sqrt{35}$

17. निम्न में से किसका मान सबसे अधिक होगा—

$6 \times (5)^{\frac{1}{5}}, 8 \times 2^{\frac{1}{3}}, 2 \times (130)^{\frac{1}{3}}, (900)^{\frac{1}{3}}$

A. $8 \times (2)^{\frac{1}{3}}$ B. $6 \times (5)^{\frac{1}{3}}$
C. $2 \times (130)^{\frac{1}{3}}$ D. $(900)^{\frac{1}{3}}$

18. व्यंजक $\left(2+\sqrt{2}\right)+\left(\frac{1}{2+\sqrt{2}}\right)$ का मान क्या होगा?

A. $\frac{6+\sqrt{2}}{2}$ B. $\frac{3+\sqrt{2}}{2}$
C. $\frac{6-\sqrt{2}}{2}$ D. $\frac{6+\sqrt{2}}{4}$

19. $3\sqrt{15}\sqrt{5} - 4\sqrt{27}$ किसके बराबर होगा?

A. $\sqrt{24}$ B. $\sqrt{27}$
C. $\sqrt{25}$ D. $3\sqrt{5}$

20. $\left(\frac{\sqrt{9}+\sqrt{4}}{\sqrt{8}-\sqrt{4}}\right)$ व्यंजक में हर का परिमेयीकरण करने पर मान होगा—

A. $4+\sqrt{8}$ B. $3+\sqrt{8}$
C. $2-\sqrt{8}$ D. $3-\sqrt{8}$

उत्तरमाला

1	2	3	4	5	6	7	8	9	10
A	C	B	D	A	C	B	B	A	B
11	**12**	**13**	**14**	**15**	**16**	**17**	**18**	**19**	**20**
A	B	D	A	B	D	B	A	B	B

व्याख्यात्मक उत्तर

1. $\because \frac{1}{\sqrt{3}} = \frac{1}{\sqrt{3}} \times \frac{\sqrt{3}}{\sqrt{3}} = \frac{\sqrt{3}}{3} = \frac{1.732}{3} = 0.577.$

2. $\because \frac{1}{2}\left(\frac{\sqrt{2}-1}{\sqrt{2}+1}\right) = \frac{1}{2} \times \frac{\sqrt{2}-1}{\sqrt{2}+1} \times \frac{\sqrt{2}-1}{\sqrt{2}-1}$

$= \frac{1}{2} \times \frac{\left(\sqrt{2}-1\right)^2}{\left(\sqrt{2}\right)^2 - 1^2} = \frac{1}{2} \times \frac{2+1-2\sqrt{2}}{2-1}$

$= \frac{1}{2} \times \frac{3-2\sqrt{2}}{1} = \frac{1}{2} \times (3 - 2 \times 1.4142)$

$= \frac{1}{2} \times 0.1716 = 0.0858.$

3. $\because \sqrt{1936} = 44 \Rightarrow \sqrt{19.36} = 4.4$

$\Rightarrow \sqrt{0.1936} = 0.44 \Rightarrow \sqrt{.001936} = .044$

$\therefore \sqrt{19.36} + \sqrt{0.1936} + \sqrt{.001936}$

$= 4.4 + 0.44 + 0.044 = 4.884.$

4. $\because \sqrt{5+\frac{4}{9}} = \sqrt{\frac{45+4}{9}} = \sqrt{\frac{49}{9}} = \frac{7}{3} = 2\frac{1}{3}.$

5. $\because \frac{\sqrt{2}-1}{\sqrt{2}+1} = \frac{\sqrt{2}-1}{\sqrt{2}+1} \times \frac{\sqrt{2}-1}{\sqrt{2}-1}$

$= \frac{\left(\sqrt{2}-1\right)^2}{\left(\sqrt{2}\right)^2 - (1)^2} = \frac{2+1-2\sqrt{2}}{2-1}$

$= \frac{3-2\sqrt{2}}{1} = 3 - 2 \times 1.414 = 0.172.$

6. $\because \sqrt[3]{8^4} = (8)^{\frac{4}{3}} = \left(2^3\right)^{\frac{4}{3}}$

$= 2^{3\times\frac{4}{3}} = 2^4 = 16.$

7. $\because \sqrt{\frac{2}{3}} + 3\sqrt{\frac{3}{2}} = \frac{\sqrt{2}}{\sqrt{3}} \times \frac{\sqrt{3}}{\sqrt{3}} + 3 \times \frac{\sqrt{3}}{\sqrt{2}} \times \frac{\sqrt{2}}{\sqrt{2}}$

$= \frac{\sqrt{6}}{3} + \frac{3\sqrt{6}}{2} = \sqrt{6}\left[\frac{1}{3} + \frac{3}{2}\right]$

$= \sqrt{6} \times \frac{11}{6} = \frac{11}{6} \times 2.45 = 4.492.$

8. $\because \sqrt{72} = \sqrt{6 \times 6 \times 2} = \sqrt{6^2 \times 2} = 6\sqrt{2}.$

9. $\frac{\sqrt{2}}{\sqrt{2}+\sqrt{3}-\sqrt{5}}$

$= \frac{\sqrt{2}}{\sqrt{2}+\sqrt{3}-\sqrt{5}} \times \frac{\sqrt{2}+\sqrt{3}+\sqrt{5}}{\sqrt{2}+\sqrt{3}+\sqrt{5}}$

$= \frac{\sqrt{2}\left(\sqrt{2}+\sqrt{3}+\sqrt{5}\right)}{\left(\sqrt{2}+\sqrt{3}\right)^2 - \left(\sqrt{5}\right)^2}$

$= \frac{2+\sqrt{6}+\sqrt{10}}{2\sqrt{6}} = \frac{2+\sqrt{6}+\sqrt{10}}{2\sqrt{6}} \times \frac{\sqrt{6}}{\sqrt{6}}$

$= \frac{2\sqrt{6}+6+\sqrt{60}}{12} = \frac{3+\sqrt{6}+\sqrt{15}}{6}.$

10. $\because \sqrt{80} + 3 \times \sqrt{245} - \sqrt{125}$

$= \sqrt{16 \times 5} + 3 \times \sqrt{49 \times 5} - \sqrt{25 \times 5}$

$= 4\sqrt{5} + 21\sqrt{5} - 5\sqrt{5} = 20\sqrt{5}.$

11. $\because \dfrac{\sqrt{5}+\sqrt{3}}{\sqrt{5}-\sqrt{3}} = \dfrac{\sqrt{5}+\sqrt{3}}{\sqrt{5}-\sqrt{3}} \times \dfrac{\sqrt{5}+\sqrt{3}}{\sqrt{5}+\sqrt{3}}$

$= \dfrac{\left(\sqrt{5}+\sqrt{3}\right)^2}{\left(\sqrt{5}\right)^2-\left(\sqrt{3}\right)^2} = \dfrac{5+3+2\sqrt{15}}{5-3}$

$= \dfrac{8+2\sqrt{15}}{2} = 4+\sqrt{15}\cdot$

12. $\because 3^{\frac{1}{5}} = (3)^{\frac{1}{5}}$

$5^{\frac{3}{5}} = \left(5^3\right)^{\frac{1}{5}} = (125)^{\frac{1}{5}}$

तथा $7^{\frac{4}{5}} = \left(7^4\right)^{\frac{1}{5}} = (2401)^{\frac{1}{5}}$

अत: स्पष्ट है कि $(3)^{\frac{1}{5}} < (125)^{\frac{1}{5}} < (2401)^{\frac{1}{5}}$

अत: $3^{\frac{1}{5}} < 5^{\frac{3}{5}} < 7^{\frac{4}{5}}$ आरोही क्रम में होगी।

13. प्रश्नानुसार, $\dfrac{12\times 4^{\frac{1}{3}}}{3\sqrt{2}} = \dfrac{12\times 2^{\frac{2}{3}}}{3\times 2^{\frac{1}{2}}} \times \dfrac{2^{\frac{1}{2}}}{2^{\frac{1}{2}}}$

$= \dfrac{12\times 2^{\frac{7}{6}}}{3\times 2} = \dfrac{12\times 2^{\frac{7}{6}}}{6} = 2^{\frac{13}{6}}.$

14. $\because 4^{\frac{1}{3}} = 4^{\frac{2}{6}} = \left(4^2\right)^{\frac{1}{6}} = (16)^{\frac{1}{6}}$

$\because 6^{\frac{1}{6}} = (6)^{\frac{1}{6}}$

तथा $\sqrt{5} = 5^{\frac{1}{2}} = 5^{\frac{3}{6}} = \left(5^3\right)^{\frac{1}{6}} = (125)^{\frac{1}{6}}$

$4^{\frac{1}{3}} \times 6^{\frac{1}{6}} \times \sqrt{5} = (16)^{\frac{1}{6}} \times (6)^{\frac{1}{6}} \times (125)^{\frac{1}{6}}$

$= (16\times 6\times 125)^{\frac{1}{6}} = (12000)^{\frac{1}{6}}.$

15. $\because\ 2+\sqrt{2}+\dfrac{1}{2+\sqrt{2}}+\dfrac{1}{\sqrt{2}-2}$

$= 2+\sqrt{2}+\left(\dfrac{2-\sqrt{2}}{\left(2+\sqrt{2}\right)\left(2-\sqrt{2}\right)} + \dfrac{2+\sqrt{2}}{\left(\sqrt{2}-2\right)\left(2+\sqrt{2}\right)}\right)$

$= 2+\sqrt{2}+\left[\dfrac{2-\sqrt{2}}{4-2}+\dfrac{\sqrt{2}+2}{2-4}\right]$

$= 2+\sqrt{2}+\left[\dfrac{\left(2-\sqrt{2}\right)}{2}-\dfrac{\left(\sqrt{2}+2\right)}{2}\right]$

$= 2+\sqrt{2}+\left[\dfrac{2-\sqrt{2}-\sqrt{2}-2}{2}\right]$

$= 2+\sqrt{2}+\dfrac{\left(-2\sqrt{2}\right)}{2} = 2+\sqrt{2}-\sqrt{2} = 2.$

16. $\because \dfrac{\sqrt{7}+\sqrt{5}}{\sqrt{7}-\sqrt{5}} = \dfrac{\sqrt{7}+\sqrt{5}}{\sqrt{7}-\sqrt{5}} \times \dfrac{\sqrt{7}+\sqrt{5}}{\sqrt{7}+\sqrt{5}}$

$= \dfrac{\left(\sqrt{7}+\sqrt{5}\right)^2}{\left(\sqrt{7}\right)^2-\left(\sqrt{5}\right)^2} = \dfrac{7+5+2\sqrt{35}}{7-5}$

$= \dfrac{12+2\sqrt{35}}{2} = 6+\sqrt{35}\,.$

17. $\because 6\times 5^{\frac{1}{3}} = \left(6^3\right)^{\frac{1}{3}}.5^{\frac{1}{3}} = (216)^{\frac{1}{3}}.5^{\frac{1}{3}}$

$= (1080)^{\frac{1}{3}}$

$\because 8\times 2^{\frac{1}{3}} = \left(8^3\right)^{\frac{1}{3}}.2^{\frac{1}{3}} = (512)^{\frac{1}{3}}.2^{\frac{1}{3}}$

$= (1024)^{\frac{1}{3}}$

$\because 2\times(130)^{\frac{1}{3}} = \left(2^3\right)^{\frac{1}{3}}.(130)^{\frac{1}{3}}$

$= (8)^{\frac{1}{3}}.(130)^{\frac{1}{3}} = (1040)^{\frac{1}{3}}$

तथा $(900)^{\frac{1}{3}} = (900)^{\frac{1}{3}}$

अतः स्पष्ट है कि उपरोक्त में सबसे अधिक मान $(1080)^{\frac{1}{3}}$ का होगा

$\therefore\ 6 \times 5^{\frac{1}{5}}$ का मान सबसे अधिक होगा।

18. $\because 2 + \sqrt{2} + \dfrac{1}{2 + \sqrt{2}}$

$= 2 + \sqrt{2} + \dfrac{1}{2 + \sqrt{2}} \times \dfrac{2 - \sqrt{2}}{2 - \sqrt{2}}$

$= 2 + \sqrt{2} + \dfrac{2 - \sqrt{2}}{4 - 2} = 2 + \sqrt{2} + \dfrac{2 - \sqrt{2}}{2}$

$= \dfrac{4 + 2\sqrt{2} + 2 - \sqrt{2}}{2} = \dfrac{6 + \sqrt{2}}{2}$.

19. $\because 3 \times \sqrt{15}\sqrt{5} - 4 \times \sqrt{27}$

$= 3 \times \sqrt{3 \times 5} \times \sqrt{5} - 4 \times \sqrt{9 \times 3}$

$= 3 \times \left(\sqrt{5}\right)^2 \times \sqrt{3} - 4 \times \sqrt{9} \times \sqrt{3}$

$= 3 \times 5 \times \sqrt{3} - 4 \times 3 \times \sqrt{3}$

$= 15\sqrt{3} - 12\sqrt{3} = 3\sqrt{3} = \sqrt{27}$.

20. $\because \dfrac{\sqrt{8} + \sqrt{4}}{\sqrt{8} - \sqrt{4}} = \dfrac{\sqrt{8} + \sqrt{4}}{\sqrt{8} - \sqrt{4}} \times \dfrac{\sqrt{8} + \sqrt{4}}{\sqrt{8} + \sqrt{4}}$

$= \dfrac{\left(\sqrt{8} + \sqrt{4}\right)^2}{\left(\sqrt{8}\right)^2 - \left(\sqrt{4}\right)^2} = \dfrac{8 + 4 + 2\sqrt{32}}{8 - 4}$

$= \dfrac{12 + 4\sqrt{8}}{4} = 3 + \sqrt{8}$.

☆☆☆☆☆☆

7 औसत (Averages)

औसत निकालने के लिए पहले उन सब राशियों को जोड़ लें जिनका औसत निकालना हो; उसके बाद उस योगफल में उन राशियों की कुल संख्या से भाग दे दें। उदाहरण के लिए यदि आपको 8, 10, 12, और 14 का औसत निकालना है, तो पहले इन्हें जोड़ दें। 8 + 10 + 12 + 14 = 44 जिनका औसत निकालना है, वे संख्याएं 4 हैं। अतः 44 में 4 से भाग दे दें। $44 \div 4 = \frac{44}{4} = 11$ औसत आया। इसके लिए सूत्र हैंः

(i) $\frac{\text{राशियों का योगफल}}{\text{राशियों की संख्या}} = \text{औसत}$

(ii) औसत × राशियों की संख्या = राशियों का योगफल।

(iii) $\frac{\text{राशियों का जोड़}}{\text{औसत}} = \text{राशियों की संख्या}$

उदाहरण 1 : किसी कक्षा में 5 दिनों की दैनिक उपस्थिति 26, 23, 30, 29 और 17 थी। बताओ दैनिक औसत उपस्थिति क्या थी?

हल : ∵ 5 दिनों की कुल उपस्थिति = 26 + 23 + 30 + 29 + 17 = 125 थी।

$\therefore$ 1 दिन की औसत उपस्थिति $= \frac{\text{राशियों का योगफल}}{\text{राशियों की संख्या}}$

$= \frac{125}{5} = 25$

उदाहरण 2: एक दुकानदार 6 दिनों में 1950 रु. की बिक्री करता है। उसकी दैनिक औसत बिक्री कितनी है?

हलः कुल बिक्री = 1950 रु.

कुल दिन = 6

$\therefore$ दैनिक औसत बिक्री $= \frac{1950}{6} = 325$ रु.

उदाहरण 3: 4 पार्सलों का औसत वजन 12.5 कि.ग्रा. है। उनमें से 3 पार्सलों का औसत वजन 12.6 कि.ग्रा. है तो चौथे पार्सल का वजन कितना है?

हल : 4 पार्सलों का औसत वजन = 12.5 कि.ग्रा.

$\therefore$ चारों पार्सलों का कुल वजन = 12.5 × 4 = 50 कि.ग्रा.

$\therefore$ तीनों पार्सलों का औसत वजन = 12.6 कि.ग्रा.

$\therefore$ तीन पार्सलों का कुल वजन = 12.6 × 3 = 37.8 कि.ग्रा.

$\therefore$ चौथे पार्सल का वजन = 50 कि.ग्रा. – 37.8 कि.ग्रा.

= 12.2 कि.ग्रा.

उदाहरण 4 : 7 के प्रथम 20 गुणकों का औसत कितना होगा?

हल : 7 के प्रथम 20 गुणक क्रमशः 7, 14, 21, 28 .... 133, 140 होंगे।

∵ 7 के प्रथम 20 गुणकों का योग

$7 + 14 + 21 + ... 133 + 140$

$= 7(1+2+3+...+20) = 7 \times \frac{20(20+1)}{2}$

$= 70 \times 21 = 1470$

तथा 7 के प्रथम 20 गुणकों की संख्या = 20

$\therefore$ औसत $= \frac{1470}{20} = 73.5$

उदाहरण 5 : 20 से बड़ी पहली 5 अभाज्य संख्याओं का औसत कितना होगा?

हल : चूंकि 20 से बड़ी पहली 5 अभाज्य संख्यायें क्रमशः 23, 29, 31, 37, 41 होंगी।

$\therefore$ अभाज्य संख्याओं का योग = 23 + 29 + 31 + 37 + 41 = 161

तथा अभाज्य संख्याओं की गिनती = 5

$\therefore$ औसत मान $= \frac{161}{5} = 32.2$

उदाहरण 6 : किसी विद्यालय के विद्यार्थियों की औसत आयु 15 वर्ष है। विद्यालय में 10 नए विद्यार्थी आ गए जिनकी औसत आयु 12 वर्ष है। इसके कारण विद्यालय में विद्यार्थियों की औसत आयु घटकर 14.8 वर्ष रह गई। तो बताइये प्रारम्भ में विद्यार्थियों की संख्या कितनी थी?

हल : माना कि विद्यालय में प्रारम्भ में विद्यार्थियों की संख्या x थी।

$\therefore$ x विद्यार्थियों की औसत आयु = 15 वर्ष

$\therefore$ x विद्यार्थियों की आयु = $15x$ वर्ष

तथा 10 नए विद्यार्थियों की आयु का योग = 120 वर्ष

प्रश्नानुसार, $(x + 10)$ विद्यार्थियों की औसत आयु = 14.8 वर्ष

$\therefore$ $(x + 10)$ विद्यार्थियों की आयु का योग

= $(x + 10) \times 14.8$ वर्ष

$\therefore$ $(x + 10) \times 14.8 = 15x + 120$

$\Rightarrow$ $14.8x + 148 = 15x + 120$

$\Rightarrow$ $.2x = 148 - 120 = 28$

$\Rightarrow$ $x = \frac{28}{.2} = \frac{280}{2} = 140$

अतः विद्यालय में प्रारम्भ में विद्यार्थियों की संख्या = 140 थी।

उदाहरण 7: माना n संख्याएं $(n > 1)$ दी हुई हैं। जिनमें से एक $1 - \frac{1}{n}$ है तथा शेष प्रत्येक 1 है, तो n संख्याओं का औसत मान कितना होगा?

हल : प्रश्नानुसार, n संख्याओं का योग

$= \left(1 - \frac{1}{n}\right) + \left(1 + 1 + 1 + \ldots + (n-1)\text{तक}\right)$

$= 1 - \frac{1}{n} + (n-1) = n - \frac{1}{n}$

तथा संख्याओं की कुल गिनती = n

$\therefore$ औसत मान = $\frac{n - \frac{1}{n}}{n} = 1 - \frac{1}{n^2}.$

उदाहरण 8: एक कक्षा में 24 लड़कियों की औसत आयु 14 वर्ष 7 माह है। कक्षा में एक नई लड़की का प्रवेश होने के कारण उनकी औसत आयु 14 वर्ष 6 माह रह गई है। तो बताइये नई लड़की की आयु कितनी होगी?

हल : $\because$ 24 लड़कियों की औसत आयु = 14 वर्ष 7 माह

$= 14\frac{7}{12}$ वर्ष

$\therefore$ 24 लड़कियों की आयु का योग = 24×14 वर्ष 7 माह

$= 24 \times 14\frac{7}{12} = 24 \times \frac{175}{12} = 350$ वर्ष

चूंकि एक और लड़की का प्रवेश होने पर कक्षा में लड़कियों की संख्या = 25 होगी

$\therefore$ 25 लड़कियों की औसत आयु = 14 वर्ष 6 माह $14\frac{1}{2}$ वर्ष

$\therefore$ 25 लड़कियों की आयु का योग = $25 \times 14\frac{1}{2}$

$= 25 \times \frac{29}{2} = 362\frac{1}{2}$ वर्ष

$\therefore$ नई लड़की की आयु $362\frac{1}{2} - 350 = 12\frac{1}{2}$ वर्ष या 12 वर्ष 6 माह होगी।

उदाहरण 9 : क्रिकेट के एक खिलाड़ी का 16 पारियों में रन औसत कुछ था। 17वीं पारी में उसने 85 रन बनाए। इससे उसका रन औसत 3 बढ़ गया तो बताइये 17वीं पारी से पहले उसके रनों का औसत क्या था?

हल : चूंकि 17वीं पारी के औसत में वृद्धि = 3

$\therefore$ 17वीं पारियों के कुल रनों में वृद्धि = $17 \times 3 = 51$

परन्तु खिलाड़ी ने 17वीं पारी में 85 रन बनाए

$\therefore$ उसकी 16 पारियों का औसत रन = $85 - 51 = 34$ होगा।

उदाहरण 10 : आठ परिणामों का औसत 25 है। पहले दो का औसत 20, अगले तीन का औसत 26, छठा परिणाम सातवें से 4 कम तथा आठवें से 6 कम है तो अन्तिम परिणाम कितना होगा?

हल : माना कि अन्तिम परिणाम अर्थात् आठवाँ परिणाम x है।

$\therefore$ छठा परिणाम = $(x - 6)$ तथा सातवां परिणाम = $(x - 2)$ होगा।

चूंकि आठ परिणामों का औसत = 25

$\therefore$ आठ परिणामों का योग = $8 \times 25 = 200$

$\therefore$ पहले दो परिणामों का औसत = 20

$\therefore$ पहले दो परिणामें का योग = $2 \times 20 = 40$

अगले तीन परिणामों का औसत = 26

$\therefore$ अगले तीन परिणामों का योग = $3 \times 26 = 78$

$40 + 78 + (x - 6) + (x - 2) + x = 200$

$\Rightarrow$ $118 + 3x - 8 = 200$

$\Rightarrow$ $3x = 200 - 110$

$\Rightarrow$ $3x = 90$

$\Rightarrow$ $x = \frac{90}{3} = 30$

अतः अन्तिम परिणाम का मान = 30 होगा।

उदाहरण 11 : एक मोटरगाड़ी अपने शुरू के पाँच मिनट में क्रमशः 68 मी॰, 127 मी॰, 208 मी॰, 312 मी॰ तथा 535 मी॰ चलती है। इसके बाद पाँच मिनट में औसत चाल 33 किमी॰/घण्टा की गति से चलती है, तो गाड़ी की सम्पूर्ण यात्रा के दौरान औसत गति कितनी होगी?

हल : चूँकि पहले पाँच मिनट में चली गई दूरी = 68 + 127 + 208 + 312 + 535

$$= 1250 \text{ मी॰} = \frac{1250}{1000} = \frac{5}{4} \text{ किमी॰}$$

अगले पाँच मिनट में औसत चाल = 33 किमी॰/घण्टा

∴ अगले पाँच मिनट में चली गई दूरी

$$= \frac{33 \times 5}{60} = \frac{11}{4} \text{ किमी॰}$$

∴ मोटरगाड़ी द्वारा 10 मिनट में तय की गई कुल दूरी

$$= \frac{5}{4} + \frac{11}{4} = \frac{16}{4} = 4 \text{ किमी॰}$$

∴ औसत गति $= \dfrac{4}{10/60} = 4 \times 6 = 24$ किमी॰/घं॰।

उदाहरण 12: 9 जनवरी से 16 जनवरी तक का औसत तापक्रम 38.6° है, तथा 10 जनवरी से 17 जनवरी तक का औसत तापक्रम 39.2° है। यदि 9 जनवरी का तापक्रम 34.6° था तो बताइये 17 जनवरी का तापक्रम कितना होगा?

हलः चूंकि 9 जनवरी से 16 जनवरी तक दिनों की संख्या = 8

∴ 9 जनवरी से 16 जनवरी तक का कुल तापक्रम

$= 8 \times 38.6 = 308.8^\circ$

चूंकि 9 जनवरी का तापक्रम = 34.6° है।

∴ 10 जनवरी से 16 जनवरी तक का कुल तापक्रम

$= 308.8^\circ - 34.6^\circ$

$= 274.2^\circ$

परन्तु 10 जनवरी से 17 जनवरी तक का कुल तापक्रम

$= 8 \times 39.2 = 313.6^\circ$

∴ 17 जनवरी का तापक्रम $= 313.6^\circ - 274.2^\circ$

$= 39.4^\circ$ होगा।

प्रश्नमाला

1. 5 विद्यार्थियों की ऊँचाइयां (सेंमी में) 140, 135, 142, 138 व 140 है। उनकी औसत ऊँचाई हैः
A. 136 B. 138 C. 139 D. 140

2. 10 विद्यार्थियों द्वारा प्राप्तांक 22, 35, 37, 38, 29, 27, 34, 36, 28 और 34 हैं। उनके औसत अंक हैं:
A. 30 B. 31 C. 32 D. 34

3. एक लड़का जिसकी ऊँचाई 165 सेंमी है, के स्थान पर नया लड़का आ जाने से 34 लड़कों के एक समूह की औसत ऊँचाई 1 सेंमी कम हो जाती है। नये लड़के की ऊँचाई हैः
A. 132 सेंमी B. 129 सेंमी
C. 130 सेंमी D. 131 सेंमी

4. 2 से प्रारम्भ करके पांच लगातार सम संख्याओं का औसत हैः
A. 4 B. 6 C. 7 D. 5

5. 5 गेंदों का भार (ग्राम में) क्रमशः 50, 54, 53, 56 और 52 है। उनका औसत भार हैः
A. 53 B. 54 C. 52 D. 51

6. एक रस्सी के 5 टुकड़ों की लम्बाइयां (सेंमी में) 5, 5.2, 6.3, 7.2 और 6.3 हैं। टुकड़े की औसत लम्बाई हैः
A. 5.8 B. 6.0 C. 6.1 D. 6.2

7. 7 के प्रथम पांच गुणजों (Multiples) का औसत क्या होगा?
A. 21 B. 23 C. 24 D. 28

8. चार संख्याओं का औसत 18 है। यदि उनमें से पहली तीन संख्याएं क्रमशः 16, 22 व 28 हों तो बताइये अन्तिम संख्या क्या होगी?
A. 5 B. 8 C. 6 D. 9

9. 12 संख्याओं का औसत मान 30 है। यदि प्रत्येक संख्या में 3 से गुणा कर दिया जाये, तो बताइये नई संख्याओं का औसत मान कितना होगा?
A. 70 B. 80 C. 90 D. 100

10. एक व्यक्ति 50 रु॰ प्रति पुस्तक के हिसाब से 4 पुस्तकें, 60 रु॰ प्रति पुस्तक के हिसाब से 5 पुस्तकें, तथा 70 रु॰ प्रति पुस्तक के हिसाब से 6 पुस्तकें खरीदता है। बताइये पुस्तक का औसत मूल्य कितना होगा?

A. 62.33 रु॰ B. 41.50 रु॰
C. 61.33 रु॰ D. 61.75 रु॰

11. 25 राशियों का औसत 15 है, उनमें से 15 राशियों का औसत 17 है, तो शेष राशियों का औसत ज्ञात करो।
A. 10 B. 13 C. 11 D. 12

12. एक कक्षा में 23 छात्रों की औसत आयु 16 वर्ष है। यदि अध्यापक की आयु भी सम्मिलित कर ली जाए तो औसत आयु एक वर्ष बढ़ जाती है। अध्यापक की आयु क्या है?
A. 35 वर्ष B. 40 वर्ष C. 50 वर्ष D. 30 वर्ष

13. दी गई सात संख्याओं में से प्रथम चार संख्याओं का औसत 4 तथा अन्तिम चार संख्याओं का औसत भी 4 है। यदि इन सात संख्याओं का औसत 3 है, तो चौथी संख्या क्या है?
A. 11 B. 10 C. 12 D. 9

14. राजू, शशि और महेश के वेतनों का औसत 800 रुपये है और शशि, महेश और प्रभा के वेतनों का औसत 900 रुपये है। यदि प्रभा का वेतन 900 रुपये हो तो राजू का वेतन होगा।
A. 700 रु॰ B. 600 रु॰
C. 400 रु॰ D. 500 रु॰

15. एक बालक को 5 संख्याओं का औसत निकालने को कहा गया। परन्तु लिखते समय उसने 73 के स्थान पर 37 और 54 के स्थान पर 45 लिख दिया। इस प्रकार उसका औसत 59 प्राप्त हुआ तो वास्तविक संख्याओं का औसत ज्ञात करो।
A. 68 B. 86 C. 70 D. 67

16. 8 संख्याओं का औसत 12 है। यदि प्रत्येक संख्या में 2 की वृद्धि की जाए तो नयी प्राप्त संख्याओं का औसत होगा।
A. 12 B. 14 C. 13 D. 15

17. 5 वर्ष पहले A, B, C, D की औसत आयु 45 वर्ष थी। E को शामिल करने पर पांचों की वर्तमान आयु की औसत 49 है। E की वर्तमान आयु है।
A. 46 वर्ष B. 48 वर्ष
C. 45 वर्ष D. 50 वर्ष

18. तीन वर्ष पूर्व 5 सदस्यों के एक परिवार की औसत आयु 17 वर्ष थी। एक शिशु के जन्म लेने पर भी परिवार की औसत आयु आज भी 17 वर्ष ही है। शिशु की वर्तमान आयु है।
A. 1 वर्ष B. 3 वर्ष
C. 2 वर्ष D. 4 वर्ष

19. किसी कक्षा में 30 छात्रों की औसत आयु 12 वर्ष है। 5 छात्रों के एक समूह की औसत आयु 10 वर्ष है तथा 5 छात्रों के दूसरे समूह की औसत आयु 14 वर्ष है। बचे हुए छात्रों की औसत आयु है।
A. 13 वर्ष B. 10 वर्ष
C. 11 वर्ष D. 12 वर्ष

20. प्रथम पांच अभाज्य संख्याओं का औसत होगा।
A. 6.5 B. 5.6 C. 5.5 D. 6.6

उत्तरमाला

1	2	3	4	5	6	7	8	9	10
C	C	D	A	A	B	A	C	C	C
11	**12**	**13**	**14**	**15**	**16**	**17**	**18**	**19**	**20**
D	B	A	B	A	B	C	C	D	B

व्याख्यात्मक उत्तर

1. औसत ऊँचाई

$$= \frac{140+135+142+138+140}{5} = \frac{695}{5} = 139.$$

2. औसत अंक

$$= \frac{22+35+37+38+29+27+34+36+28+34}{10}$$

$$= \frac{320}{10} = 32.$$

3. 34 लड़कों की ऊँचाई में औसत कमी = 1 सेंमी
34 लड़कों की ऊँचाई में कुल कमी = 34 सेंमी
∴ नये लड़के की ऊँचाई = 165 − 34 = 131 सेंमी

4. 2 से प्रारम्भ करके 5 लगातार सम संख्याओं का औसत

$$= \frac{2+4+6+8+10}{5} = \frac{30}{5} = 6.$$

5. औसत भार

$$= \frac{50+54+53+56+52}{5} = \frac{265}{5} = 53.$$

6. औसत लम्बाई

$$= \frac{5+5.2+6.3+7.2+6.3}{5} = \frac{30.0}{5} = 6.0$$

7. $\because$ 7 के प्रथम 5 गुणज : 7, 14, 21, 28 व 35

$\therefore$ इनका औसत

$$= \frac{7+14+21+28+35}{5} = \frac{105}{5} = 21.$$

8. $\because$ चार संख्याओं का औसत = 18

$\therefore$ चारों संख्याओं का योग = 18 × 4 = 72

प्रश्नानुसार, उनमें से पहली तीन संख्याएं क्रमशः 16, 22 व 28 हैं।

$\therefore$ अन्तिम संख्या

= चारों संख्याओं का योग – (16 + 22 + 28)

= 72 – 66 = 6.

9. $\because$ 12 संख्याओं का औसत मान = 30

$\therefore$ 12 संख्याओं का कुल योग = 30 × 12 = 360

प्रश्नानुसार, प्रत्येक संख्या में 3 से गुणा करने पर 12 संख्याओं का कुल योग = 360 × 3 = 1080

12 नई संख्याओं का औसत मान = $\frac{1080}{12} = 90.$

10. $\because$ 50 रु॰ प्रति पुस्तक के हिसाब से 4 पुस्तकों का क्रय मूल्य = 200 रु॰

60 रु॰ प्रति पुस्तक के हिसाब से 5 पुस्तकों का क्रय मूल्य = 300 रु॰

तथा 70 रु॰ प्रति पुस्तक के हिसाब से 6 पुस्तकों का क्रय मूल्य = 420 रु॰

$\therefore$ 15 पुस्तकों का कुल क्रय मूल्य

= 200 + 300 + 420 = 920 रु॰

$\therefore$ औसत मूल्य = $\frac{920}{15} = 61.33$ रु॰।

11. $\because$ 25 राशियों का औसत = 15

$\therefore$ 25 राशियों योग = 25 × 15 = 375

इनमें से 15 राशियों का औसत = 17

$\therefore$ इन 15 राशियों का योग = 15 × 17 = 255

$\therefore$ शेष 25 –15 = 10 राशियों का योग

= 375 – 255 = 120

$\therefore$ शेष राशियों का औसत = $\frac{120}{10} = 12$

सूत्र द्वारा—

शेष 10 राशियों का औसत = $\frac{25 \times 15 - 15 \times 17}{25 - 15}$

$$= \frac{375 - 255}{10} = \frac{120}{10} = 12.$$

12. $\therefore$ 23 छात्रों की आयु का औसत = 16 वर्ष

$\therefore$ 23 छात्रों की आयु का योग = 23 × 16 = 368 वर्ष

$\therefore$ 23 + 1 = 24 जनों की आयु का औसत = 16 + 1 = 17 वर्ष

$\therefore$ इनकी आयु का योग = 24 × 17 = 408 वर्ष

$\therefore$ अध्यापक की आयु = 408 – 368 = 40 वर्ष।

13. $\therefore$ 7 संख्याओं का औसत = 3

$\therefore$ 7 संख्याओं का योगफल = 7 × 3 = 21

$\therefore$ प्रथम 4 संख्याओं का औसत = 4

$\therefore$ प्रथम चार संख्याओं का योग = 4 × 4 = 16

अन्तिम 4 संख्याओं का औसत = 4

$\therefore$ अन्तिम चार संख्याओं का योग = 4 × 4 = 16

$\therefore$ चौथी संख्या होगी = 16 + 16 – 21 = 11.

14. $\because$ राजू, शशि और महेश का औसत वेतन = 800 रुपये

$\therefore$ इनका कुल वेतन = 3 × 800 = 2400 रुपये

$\therefore$ शशि, महेश और प्रभा का औसत वेतन = 900 रुपये

$\therefore$ इन तीनों का कुल वेतन = 3 × 900 = 2700 रुपये

$\therefore$ प्रभा का वेतन = 900 रुपये

$\therefore$ राजू, शशि, महेश व प्रभा का कुल वेतन

= 2400 + 900 = 3300 रुपये

$\therefore$ राजू का वेतन = 3300 – 2700 = 600 रुपये।

15. $\because$ 73 – 37 = 36 तथा 54 – 45 = 9

$\therefore$ 5 संख्याओं के योग में कमी = 36 + 9 = 45

$\therefore$ 5 संख्याओं के ***औसत*** में कमी = $\frac{45}{5} = 9$

∴ वास्तविक संख्याओं का औसत = 59 + 9 = 68.

16. ∵ 8 संख्याओं का औसत = 12

∴ 8 संख्याओं का योग = 12 × 8 = 96

प्रत्येक संख्या में 2 की वृद्धि करने पर,

8 संख्याओं के योग में वृद्धि = 2 × 8 = 16

∴ नयी प्राप्त 8 संख्याओं का योग = 96 + 16 = 112

∴ नयी प्राप्त 8 संख्याओं का औसत $= \frac{112}{8} = 14$

नोट—यदि प्रत्येक संख्या में 2 की वृद्धि की जाए तो औसत भी 2 बढ़ जाएगा।

अतः नयी प्राप्त 8 संख्याओं का औसत = 12 + 2 = 14

इसी प्रकार, प्रत्येक संख्या में से 2 की कमी कर दी जाए, तो औसत 2 कम हो जाएगा।

17. A, B, C, D की 5 वर्ष पूर्व की औसत आयु = 45 वर्ष

∴ इन चारों की वर्तमान में औसत आयु

= 45 + 5 = 50 वर्ष

∴ इन चारों की वर्तमान आयु का योग

= 50 × 4 = 200 वर्ष

∴ A, B, C, D तथा E की वर्तमान औसत आयु = 49 वर्ष

∴ इनकी कुल आयु = 49 × 5 = 245 वर्ष

∴ E की वर्तमान आयु = 245 – 200 = 45 वर्ष।

18. 3 वर्ष पूर्व 5 सदस्यों की औसत आयु = 17 वर्ष

∴ वर्तमान में 5 सदस्यों की औसत आयु = 20 वर्ष

और वर्तमान में 6 सदस्यों की औसत आयु = 17 वर्ष

∴ शिशु की वर्तमान आयु = 17 × 6 – 20 × 5

= 102 – 100 = 2 वर्ष।

19. 30 छात्रों की कुल आयु = 30 × 12 = 360 वर्ष

5 छात्रों के पहले समूह की कुल आयु

= 5 × 10 = 50 वर्ष

और दूसरे समूह की कुल आयु = 5 × 14 = 70 वर्ष

∴ शेष (30–55) = 20 छात्रों की कुल आयु

= 360 – (50 + 70) = 240 वर्ष

∴ उनकी औसत आयु $= \frac{240}{20} = 12$ वर्ष।

20. प्रथम पांच अभाज्य संख्याएं = 2, 3, 5, 7, 11 हैं।

∴ उनका औसत $= \frac{2+3+5+7+11}{5} = \frac{28}{5} = 5.6.$

☆☆☆☆☆☆

8 प्रतिशत (Percentage)

1. प्रतिशत का अर्थ है–प्रत्येक सौ पर 1–इसका चिन्ह् है– %. 5% का अर्थ है–प्रत्येक सौ पर 5.

2. प्रतिशत को भिन्न में बदलने के लिए उसे 100 से भाग देते हैं। जैसे–20% = $\frac{20}{100} = \frac{1}{5}$

3. साधारण भिन्न को प्रतिशत में बदलने के लिए उसे 100 से गुणा करते हैं। जैसे–$\frac{1}{10} \times 100 = 10\%$

प्रतिशत को दशमलव में बदलने की विधि

प्रतिशत का चिह्न हटाकर बाईं ओर दो अंकों के बाद दशमलव का चिन्ह् लगाते हैं।

उदाहरण :25% को दशमलव में बदलें।

25% = .25 (बाईं ओर दो अंकों के बाद दशमलव बिन्दु लगा दिया।)

उदाहरण :1.5% को दशमलव में बदलिये।

1.5% = .015 (बाईं ओर दो अंकों के बाद दशमलव बिन्दु लगा दिया, यहां एक शून्य लगाकर दो अंक पूरे करने पड़े।)

दशमलव को प्रतिशत में बदलने की विधि

दशमलव बिन्दु के दाहिनी ओर दो अंक बढ़ा देते हैं और उसके बाद % का निशान लगाते हैं।

उदाहरण : .24 को प्रतिशत में बदलें।

हल : .24 = 24% (दशमलव बिन्दु के दाहिनी ओर दो अंक आगे बढ़ाने पर 24 बनेगा, अतः दशमलव बिन्दु (.) लगाने की जरूरत नहीं हैं।)

उदाहरण : .0043 को प्रतिशत में बदलें।

हल : .0043 = .43% (दशमलव बिन्दु को दाहिनी ओर दो अंक आगे बढ़ाने पर .43 बनेगा। उस पर % का निशान लगाते हैं।)

प्रश्नमाला

1. निम्नलिखित में से 20% का मान किसके बराबर होगा?

A. $\frac{1}{4}$ B. $\frac{1}{2}$

C. $\frac{1}{5}$ D. $\frac{1}{8}$

2. 36% का मान दशमलव भिन्न में होगा–

A. .36 B. .036

C. 3.6 D. .0036

3. $\frac{4}{5}$ को प्रतिशत भिन्न में बदलने पर मान होगा–

A. 80% B. 70%

C. 60% D. 40%

4. 36 का कितने %, 24 के बराबर होगा?

A. $16\frac{2}{3}\%$ B. $66\frac{2}{3}\%$

C. $11\frac{1}{9}\%$ D. $31\frac{1}{9}\%$

5. 3 मीटर का 15%, किसके बराबर होगा?

A. 44 सेंमी B. 45 सेंमी

C. 40 सेंमी D. 38 सेंमी

6. 26 का 18% = ?

A. 4.88 B. 4.65

C. 3.68 D. 4.68

7. 10% का 10% कितने % होगा?

A. 7 B. 6 C. 1 D. 5

8. किसी शहर की जनसंख्या 50,000 से बढ़कर 52,000 हो जाती हो, तो बताइये कितने प्रतिशत की वृद्धि होगी?

A. 3% B. 6%
C. 4% D. 5%

9. एक आदमी अपने वेतन का 75% खर्च करता है और 150 रु. मासिक बचाता है तो उसका मासिक वेतन है:

A. 750 रु. B. 600 रु.
C. 400 रु. D. 300 रु.

10. किसी विद्यालय में 97% विद्यार्थी उपस्थित थे और 18 विद्यार्थी अनुपस्थित थे। विद्यालय में कुल विद्यार्थियों की संख्या है:

A. 400 B. 450
C. 500 D. 600

11. किसी राशि का 7%, 35 रुपये है तो वह राशि ज्ञात कीजिए।

A. 550 रु. B. 700 रु.
C. 600 रु. D. 500 रु.

12. 3 किग्रा. कितने किग्रा. का 5% है:

A. 60 किग्रा. B. 50 किग्रा.
C. 65 किग्रा. D. 70 किग्रा.

13. किसी राशि का 5%, 500 रुपए के 12% के बराबर है तो राशि ज्ञात कीजिए।

A. 1100 रु. B. 1200 रु.
C. 1150 रु. D. 1250 रु.

14. अनिल ने अपनी पूंजी का 65% मशीनरी में तथा 20% कच्चा माल खरीदने में खर्च कर दिया। यदि उसके पास अब 1305 रुपये बचे हों तो उसने कितना खर्च कर दिया?

A. 7395 रु. B. 7350 रु.
C. 7390 रु. D. 7380 रु.

15. किसी पुस्तकालय में 20% पुस्तकें अंग्रेजी भाषा में हैं तथा शेष **की** 50% पुस्तकें हिन्दी भाषा में हैं। यदि शेष 900 पुस्तकें अन्य क्षेत्रीय भाषा में हैं तो पुस्तकालय में कुल कितनी पुस्तकें हैं?

A. 2300 B. 2250
C. 2290 D. 2280

16. 200 का 40% + 150 का 30% कितने के बराबर है?

A. 175 B. 200
C. 150 D. 125

17. 38 लड़कियों की एक कक्षा में तीन लड़कियां गैर हाजिर थीं। बाकि 20% गृह कार्य नहीं कर पाईं तो जिन लड़कियों ने गृह कार्य किया उनकी संख्या है:

A. 26 B. 27
C. 28 D. 29

18. विद्यालय में 800 छात्रों में से एक दिन $12\frac{1}{2}\%$ छात्र अनुपस्थित रहे। उपस्थित छात्रों की संख्या ज्ञात करो।

A. 700 B. 600 C. 650 D. 625

19. एक नगर में 35,600 हिन्दू, 12,240 मुसलमान और अन्य जाति के 2,160 लोग हैं। बताइए, हिन्दू कुल जनसंख्या के कितने प्रतिशत हैं?

A. 71.3% B. 71.2%
C. 71% D. 71.5%

20. जोसफ ने अपने धन का 40% बड़े पुत्र को और शेष का 70% छोटे पुत्र को दिया यदि अब उसके पास 5490 रुपये बच रहे, तो जोसफ का धन ज्ञात करो।

A. 32,000 रु.
B. 33,500 रु.
C. 32,500 रु.
D. 33,000 रु.

उत्तरमाला

1	2	3	4	5	6	7	8	9	10
C	A	A	B	B	D	C	C	B	C
11	**12**	**13**	**14**	**15**	**16**	**17**	**18**	**19**	**20**
D	A	B	A	B	D	C	A	B	D

व्याख्यात्मक उत्तर

1. $\because$ 20% = $\frac{20}{100} = \frac{1}{5}$

$\therefore$ 20% का मान, $\frac{1}{5}$ के बराबर होगा।

2. $\because$ 36% = $\frac{36}{100}$ = .36

$\therefore$ 36% का मान दशमलव भिन्न में .36 होगा।

3. चूंकि किसी भी साधारण या दशमलव भिन्न को प्रतिशत भिन्न में बदलने के लिए उसमें 100% से गुणा करना होता है अर्थात् $\frac{4}{5} = \frac{4}{5} \times 100\% = 80\%$

अतः $\frac{4}{5}$ का प्रतिशत भिन्न में मान = 80% होगा।

4. माना कि 36 का x% = 24

$\therefore 36 \times \frac{x}{100} = 24 \Rightarrow x = \frac{24 \times 100}{36} = 66\frac{2}{3}$

अतः 36 का $66\frac{2}{3}\%$, 24 के बराबर होगा।

5. $\because$ 3 मीटर का 15% = 300 सेंमी. $\times \frac{15}{100}$ = 45 सेंमी.

[$\because$ 3 मी. = 300 सेंमी.]

अतः 3 मीटर का 15%, 45 सेंमी. के बराबर होगा।

6. $\because$ 26 का 18% = $26 \times \frac{18}{100} = 4.68$

$\therefore$ (?) चिन्ह् के स्थान पर 4.68 होना चाहिए।

7. $\because$ 10% का 10% = $\frac{10}{100} \times \frac{10}{100} = \frac{1}{100} = 1\%$

अतः 10% का 10%, 1% के बराबर होगा।

8. प्रश्नानुसार, शहर की प्रारम्भिक जनसंख्या = 50,000

तथा शहर की वर्तमान जनसंख्या = 52,000

$\therefore$ जनसंख्या में वृद्धि = 52,000 – 50,000 = 2,000

$\therefore$ प्रतिशत वृद्धि = $\frac{2000}{50000} \times 100 = 4\%$

अतः शहर की जनसंख्या में 4% वृद्धि होगी।

9. बचत = 100% – 75% = 25% = 150 रु.

कुल वेतन = $\frac{100}{25} \times 150$ = 600 रु.।

10. अनुपस्थित विद्यार्थी = 100% – 97% = 3% = 18

माना कि कुल विद्यार्थियों की संख्या = x

तो, $x \times \frac{3}{100} = 18$ $\quad \therefore x = \frac{1800}{3} = 600.$

11. राशि का 7% = 35 रुपये

राशि = $\frac{35}{7\%} = \frac{35}{\frac{7}{100}} = \frac{35}{7} \times 100$

= 500 रुपये।

12. भार का 5% = 3 किग्रा.

भार = $\frac{3}{5\%} = \frac{3}{\frac{5}{100}} = \frac{3}{5} \times 100$

= 60 किग्रा. होगा।

13. 500 रुपये का 12% = $\frac{12}{100} \times 500$ रु. = 60 रुपये

$\because$ अभीष्ट राशि = 5% = 60 रुपये

$\therefore$ राशि = $\frac{60}{5\%} = \frac{60}{\frac{5}{100}} = \frac{60 \times 100}{5}$

= 1200 रुपये।

14. बची राशि की प्रतिशत संख्या = 100 – (65 + 20) = 15

$\because$ 15 रुपये बचते हैं तो खर्च की हुई राशि = 85 रुपये

$\therefore$ 1305 रुपये बचते हैं तो खर्च की हुई राशि

= $\frac{85 \times 1305}{15}$ = 7395 रुपये।

15. माना कुल पुस्तकें = 100

अत: अग्रेंजी भाषा की पुस्तकें = 20 पुस्तकें

शेष पुस्तकें = 100 – 20 = 80

हिन्दी भाषा की पुस्तकें = 80 का 50%

$$= 80 \times \frac{50}{100} = 40$$

शेष पुस्तकें = 100 – (20 + 40) = 40 पुस्तकें।

∵ 40 पुस्तकें अन्य क्षेत्रीय भाषाओं की है तो कुल पुस्तकें = 100

∴ 900 पुस्तकें अन्य क्षेत्रीय भाषाओं की है तो कुल पुस्तकें

$$= \frac{100}{40} \times 900 = 2250$$ पुस्तकें।

16. $\frac{40}{100} \times 200 + \frac{30}{100} \times 150 = 80 + 45 = 125.$

17. उपस्थित लड़कियों की संख्या = 38 – 3 = 35

लड़कियों की संख्या जिन्होंने गृह कार्य नहीं किया

= 20% × 35 = 7

∴ लड़कियों की संख्या जिन्होंने गृह कार्य किया

= 35 – 7 = 28.

18. छात्रों की कुल संख्या = 800

अनुपस्थित छात्रों का प्रतिशत = $12\frac{1}{2}\%$ या $\frac{25}{2}\%$

∵ अनुपस्थित छात्रों की संख्या

$$= 800 \times \frac{25}{2} \times \frac{1}{100} = 100$$

∴ उपस्थित छात्रों की संख्या = 800 – 100 = 700.

19. कुल जनसंख्या = 35600 + 12240 + 2160

= 50000

∵ 50000 में से हिन्दू = 35600

∴ 1 में से हिन्दू = $\frac{35600}{50000}$

∴ 100 में से हिन्दू = $\frac{35600}{50000} \times 100 = 71.2\%.$

20. माना जोसफ का धन = 100 रुपये है

∴ बड़े पुत्र को दिया = 40% = 40 रुपये

∴ शेष धन = 100 – 40 = 60 रुपये

∴ छोटे पुत्र को दिया = 60 का 70%

$$= 60 \times \frac{70}{100} = 42$$ रुपये

∴ उसके पास बचा = 60 – 42 = 18 रुपये

∵ 18 रुपये उसके पास बचे, तो कुल धन

= 100 रुपये

∴ 5940 रुपये उसके पास बचे तो कुल धन

$$= \frac{100}{18} \times 5940$$

= 33,000 रुपये।

☆☆☆☆☆☆

9

साधारण ब्याज
(Simple Interest)

ब्याज वह राशि है जो हमें दूसरों का धन प्रयोग करने के बदले में देनी पड़ती है। यदि यह वार्षिक देनी पड़े तो दर प्रतिशत वार्षिक कहते हैं। इस प्रकार 6% वार्षिक का अर्थ है कि 100 रु. पर 1 वर्ष में 6 रु. ब्याज है। जो धन उधार लिया जाता है उसे मूलधन कहते हैं। मूलधन और ब्याज के योग को समस्त धन (मिश्रधन) कहते हैं।

साधारण ब्याज के प्रश्नों के सूत्रः

$$\text{साधारण ब्याज} = \frac{\text{मूलधन} \times \text{दर\%} \times \text{समय (वर्षों में)}}{100}$$

समस्त धन = मूलधन + ब्याज

जब समय, दर % और ब्याज दिए गए हों तो,

$$\text{मूलधन} = \frac{\text{ब्याज} \times 100}{\text{दर} \times \text{समय}}$$

जब मूलधन, ब्याज और समय दिया गया हो तो,

$$\text{दर} = \frac{\text{ब्याज} \times 100}{\text{मूलधन} \times \text{समय}}$$

जब मूलधन, ब्याज और दर दी गई हो तो,

$$\text{समय} = \frac{\text{ब्याज} \times 100}{\text{मूलधन} \times \text{दर}}$$

प्रश्नमाला

1. किस धनराशि पर 4% वार्षिक ब्याज की दर से 5 वर्ष का साधारण ब्याज 64 रु. होगा?

A. 220 रु. B. 280 रु.
C. 320 रु. D. 300 रु.

2. 450 रु. पर 6% वार्षिक ब्याज दर से 4 मास का ब्याज कितना होगा?

A. 9 रु. B. 8 रु.
C. 6 रु. D. 5 रु.

3. कितने समय में 3600 रु. पर 6% वार्षिक दर से साधारण ब्याज 432 रु. होगा?

A. 1 वर्ष B. 2 वर्ष
C. $1\frac{1}{2}$ वर्ष D. $2\frac{1}{4}$ वर्ष

4. किस राशि पर 3% वार्षिक ब्याज की दर से 2 वर्ष का ब्याज 36 रु. होगा?

A. 500 रु. B. 575 रु.
C. 590 रु. D. 600 रु.

5. ब्याज की किस दर से कोई राशि 16 वर्षों में दोगुनी हो जाएगी?

A. $5\frac{1}{2}$ वर्ष B. $6\frac{1}{4}$ वर्ष
C. $4\frac{1}{3}$ वर्ष D. $2\frac{1}{2}$ वर्ष

6. 5000 रु. की राशि पर 10% वार्षिक दर से 5 वर्ष का साधारण ब्याज कितना होगा?

A. 2200 रु. B. 2500 रु.
C. 2300 रु. D. 2600 रु.

7. किस राशि का 6% वार्षिक ब्याज दर से 10 वर्ष का साधारण ब्याज 3 रु. होगा?

A. 4 रु. B. 8 रु.
C. 5 रु. D. 6 रु.

8. कितने वर्षों में कोई राशि 10% वार्षिक दर से अपने से दोगुनी हो जाएगी?

A. 10 वर्ष B. 8 वर्ष
C. 5 वर्ष D. 12 वर्ष

9. किस राशि का 5% दर से 5 वर्ष का साधारण ब्याज 80 रु. होगा?

A. 330 रु. B. 320 रु.

C. 340 रु. D. 380 रु.

10. यदि 5000 रु. पर 2 वर्ष का साधारण ब्याज 500 रु. हो, तो समस्त धन अर्थात् मिश्रधन कितना होगा?

A. 5600 रु. B. 5800 रु.

C. 5500 रु. D. 6000 रु.

11. 2000 रुपये पर $6\frac{1}{2}$ प्रतिशत वार्षिक ब्याज की दर से 8 महीने का साधारण ब्याज ज्ञात कीजिए।

A. $86\frac{2}{3}$ रु. B. $86\frac{3}{4}$ रु.

C. $86\frac{1}{3}$ रु. D. $86\frac{1}{2}$ रु.

12. कितने समय में 450 रुपये का 8% वार्षिक ब्याज की दर से साधारण ब्याज 90 रुपये हो जाएगा?

A. 2 वर्ष B. $2\frac{3}{4}$ वर्ष

C. $2\frac{1}{2}$ वर्ष D. 3 वर्ष

13. घनश्याम ने 2000 रुपये अपने मित्र से 5% सालाना ब्याज पर लिए और उसने पूरा पैसा 8 माह बाद चुका दिया। बताइये उसने कुल कितना धन चुकाया?

A. 2060.66 रु. B. 2066.66 रु.

C. 2066 रु. D. 2060 रु.

14. एक आदमी ने 600 रुपये 6 प्रतिशत वार्षिक ब्याज पर उधार लिए। 5 वर्ष बाद उसने 300 रुपये कीमत की एक घड़ी व कुछ धन उसको लौटाया तो बताओ उसने कितना धन लौटाया।

A. 480 रु. B. 485 रु.

C. 490 रु. D. 500 रु.

15. एक व्यक्ति अपने मित्र से 1000 रुपये 5% वार्षिक ब्याज की दर से उधार लेता है तीन वर्ष बाद वह उसे 500 रुपये नकद व एक रेडियो सैट लौटाता है तो रेडियो सेट की कीमत बताइये।

A. 675 रु. B. 600 रु.

C. 650 रु. D. 625 रु.

16. यदि 450 रुपये की एक राशि 3 वर्ष में साधारण ब्याज पर 504 रुपये हो जाती है तो ब्याज की दर ज्ञात कीजिए।

A. $4\frac{1}{2}\%$ B. $3\frac{1}{2}\%$

C. 5% D. 4%

17. संजय ने 800 रुपयों को 5% सालाना ब्याज पर मोहन से उधार लिया। यदि वह 9 माह पश्चात् 500 रुपये देता है तो उसको और कितनी धनराशि चुकानी बाकी है?

A. 300 रु. B. 330 रु.

C. 325 रु. D. 350 रु.

18. 2 पैसे प्रतिमाह की दर से 471 रुपए पर 7 माह का साधारण ब्याज क्या होगा?

A. 65.49 रु. B. 65.94 रु.

C. 65.84 रु. D. 55.94 रु.

19. $7\frac{1}{2}\%$ सरल ब्याज की दर से 2400 रुपये एक बैंक में जमा करवाये गए। कितने वर्ष बाद कुल राशि 2850 रुपये हो जाएगी?

A. 3 वर्ष B. 2 वर्ष

C. $2\frac{1}{2}$ वर्ष D. $3\frac{1}{2}$ वर्ष

20. 1800 रुपये का 2 वर्ष 4 मास 20 दिन का 9% की दर से साधारण ब्याज और मिश्रधन ज्ञात करो।

A. 2187 रु. B. 2178 रु.

C. 2190 रु. D. 2180 रु.

उत्तरमाला

1	2	3	4	5	6	7	8	9	10
C	A	B	D	B	B	C	A	B	C
11	**12**	**13**	**14**	**15**	**16**	**17**	**18**	**19**	**20**
A	C	B	A	C	D	B	B	C	A

व्याख्यात्मक उत्तर

1. $\because$ साधारण ब्याज = 64 रु॰, समय = 5 वर्ष तथा दर = 4%

$\therefore$ मूलधन (धनराशि) $= \dfrac{\text{साधारण ब्याज} \times 100}{\text{समय} \times \text{दर}}$

$= \dfrac{64 \times 100}{5 \times 4} = 320$ रु॰।

2. $\because$ मूलधन = 450 रु॰, दर = 6% वार्षिक, समय = 4 मास

$= \dfrac{1}{3}$ वर्ष

$\therefore$ साधारण ब्याज $= \dfrac{\text{मूलधन} \times \text{समय} \times \text{दर}}{100}$

$= \dfrac{450 \times \frac{1}{3} \times 6}{100} = 9$ रु॰।

3. $\because$ समय $= \dfrac{\text{साधारण ब्याज} \times 100}{\text{मूलधन} \times \text{दर}}$

$= \dfrac{432 \times 100}{6 \times 3600} = 2$ वर्ष।

4. $\because$ मूलधन $= \dfrac{\text{साधारण ब्याज} \times 100}{\text{समय} \times \text{दर}}$

$= \dfrac{36 \times 100}{2 \times 3} = 600$ रु॰।

5. $\because$ माना कि वह राशि = 100 रु॰

प्रश्नानुसार, 16 वर्षों बाद मिश्रधन = 200 रु॰

$\therefore$ साधारण ब्याज = मिश्रधन – मूलधन (राशि)

= 200 – 100 = 100 रु॰

$\therefore$ दर $= \dfrac{\text{साधारण ब्याज} \times 100}{\text{मूलधन} \times \text{समय}}$

$= \dfrac{100 \times 100}{100 \times 16} = 6\dfrac{1}{4}\%$।

6. $\because$ साधारण ब्याज $= \dfrac{\text{मूलधन} \times \text{समय} \times \text{दर}}{100}$

$= \dfrac{5000 \times 5 \times 10}{100} = 2500$ रु॰।

7. $\because$ मूलधन (राशि) $= \dfrac{\text{साधारण ब्याज} \times 100}{\text{समय} \times \text{दर}}$

$= \dfrac{3 \times 100}{10 \times 6} = 5$ रु॰।

8. $\because$ माना कि वह राशि = 100 रु॰ तथा मिश्रधन

= 2 × 100 = 200 रु॰

$\therefore$ साधारण ब्याज = 200 – 100 = 100 रु॰,

दर = 10%

$\therefore$ समय $= \dfrac{\text{साधारण ब्याज} \times 100}{\text{मूलधन (राशि)} \times \text{दर}}$

$= \dfrac{100 \times 100}{100 \times 10} = 10$ वर्ष।

9. $\because$ मूलधन (राशि) $= \dfrac{\text{साधारण ब्याज} \times 100}{\text{समय} \times \text{दर}}$

$= \dfrac{80 \times 100}{5 \times 5} = 320$ रु॰।

10. $\because$ समस्त धन अर्थात् मिश्रधन

= मूलधन + साधारण ब्याज

= 5000 + 500 = 5500 रु॰।

11. दर $6\dfrac{1}{2} = \dfrac{13}{2}\%$

समय = 8 महीने $= \dfrac{8}{12}$ वर्ष $= \dfrac{2}{3}$ वर्ष

साधारण ब्याज $= \dfrac{\text{मूलधन} \times \text{दर} \times \text{समय}}{100}$

$= \dfrac{2000 \times 13 \times 2}{100 \times 2 \times 3}$

$= \dfrac{260}{3} = 86\dfrac{2}{3}$ रुपये।

12. समय $= \dfrac{\text{साधारण ब्याज} \times 100}{\text{मूलधन} \times \text{दर}}$

$= \dfrac{90 \times 100}{450 \times 8} = \dfrac{5}{2}$ वर्ष

$= 2\dfrac{1}{2}$ वर्ष।

13. समय = 8 माह = $\frac{8}{12}$ वर्ष = $\frac{2}{3}$ वर्ष

साधारण ब्याज = $\frac{\text{मूलधन} \times \text{दर} \times \text{समय}}{100}$

$= \frac{2000 \times 2 \times 5}{3 \times 100} = \frac{200}{3}$ रुपये

मिश्रधन = मूलधन + साधारण ब्याज

$= \frac{2000}{1} + \frac{200}{3}$

$= \frac{6000 + 200}{3}$

$= \frac{6200}{3}$ रुपये

= 2066.66 रुपये।

14. 600 रुपये का 6% वार्षिक ब्याज से 5 वर्ष का ब्याज

$= \frac{600 \times 6 \times 5}{100} = 180$ रुपये

मिश्रधन = 600 + 180 = 780 रुपये

अत: उसको 780 रुपये लौटाने चाहिए थे, परन्तु 300 रु. की घड़ी उसने उसे दी तो उसका अतिरिक्त धन

= 780 – 300 = 480 रुपये।

15. 1000 रुपये का 5% दर से 3 वर्ष का ब्याज

$= \frac{1000 \times 5 \times 3}{100} = 150$ रुपये

मिश्रधन = मूलधन + ब्याज = 1000 + 150 = 1150 रुपये, अर्थात् उसको 1150 रुपये लौटाने चाहिए।

रेडियो सेट की कीमत = 1150 – 500 = 650 रुपये।

16. मिश्रधन = 504 रुपये

मूलधन = 450 रुपये

साधारण ब्याज = 504 – 450 = 54 रुपये

दर = $\frac{\text{साधारण ब्याज} \times 100}{\text{समय} \times \text{मूलधन}}$

$= \frac{54 \times 100}{3 \times 450} = 4\%$

दर = 4%.

17. समय = 9 माह = $\frac{9}{12}$ वर्ष = $\frac{3}{4}$ वर्ष

ब्याज = $\frac{800 \times 5 \times 3}{100 \times 4} = 30$ रुपये

मिश्रधन = 800 + 30 = 830 रुपये

शेष धनराशि = 830 – 500 = 330 रुपये

18. 1 रुपये पर 1 माह का ब्याज = 2 पैसे

$\therefore$ 1 रुपए का 7 माह का ब्याज = 14 पैसे

471 रुपए का 7 माह का ब्याज = 471 × 14

= 65.94 रुपए

अतः 7 माह का साधारण ब्याज 65 रुपये 94 पैसे होगा।

19. $\because$ मिश्रधन = 2850 रुपये तथा

मूलधन = 2400 रुपये

$\therefore$ ब्याज = 2850 – 2400 = 450 रुपये

दर = $7\frac{1}{2}\% = \frac{15}{2}\%$

समय = $\frac{100 \times \text{ब्याज}}{\text{मूलधन} \times \text{दर}}$

$= \frac{100 \times 450 \times 2}{2400 \times 15} = 2\frac{1}{2}$ वर्ष।

20. मूलधन = 1800 रुपये

समय = 2 वर्ष 4 मास 20 दिन

$= 2 \times 12 + 4 + \frac{20}{30}$

$= \frac{86}{3}$ मास $= \frac{86}{3 \times 12}$ वर्ष

$= \frac{43}{18}$ वर्ष, दर = 9%

$\therefore$ सरल ब्याज = $\frac{\text{मूलधन} \times \text{समय} \times \text{दर}}{100}$

$= \frac{1800 \times 43 \times 9}{100 \times 18} = 387$ रुपये

मिश्रधन = मूलधन + ब्याज

= 1800 + 387 = 2187 रुपये

☆☆☆☆☆☆

10 चक्रवृद्धि ब्याज (Compound Interest)

ब्याज की वह गणना, जिसमें ब्याज को मूलधन में जोड़कर प्राप्त मिश्रधन पर ब्याज लगाया जाए, **चक्रवृद्धि ब्याज** कहलाती है।

महत्वपूर्ण सूत्र :

1. चक्रवृद्धि मिश्रधन = मूलधन $\left(1+\frac{\text{दर}}{100}\right)^{\text{समय वर्ष में}}$
2. चक्रवृद्धि ब्याज = चक्रवृद्धि मिश्रधन – मूलधन

   $= \text{मूलधन}\left[\left(1+\frac{\text{दर}}{100}\right)^{\text{समय}}-1\right]$
3. यदि चक्रवृद्धि ब्याज की दर प्रत्येक वर्ष में बदल रही हो तो —

   मिश्रधन = मूलधन $\left(1+\frac{(\text{दर})\ 1}{100}\right)\left(1+\frac{(\text{दर})\ 2}{100}\right)\left(1+\frac{(\text{दर})\ 3}{100}\right)$

   [∴ समय, प्रत्येक दर के लिए 1 वर्ष है]
4. *(i)* यदि ब्याज की गणना **अर्द्धवार्षिक** है तो दर आधी तथा समय दुगुना कर दिया जाता हैं।

   (ii) यदि ब्याज की गणना त्रैमासिक है तो दर को 4 से भाग तथा समय को 4 से गुणा करते है।

नोट : एक वर्ष के लिए साधारण ब्याज तथा चक्रवृद्धि ब्याज बराबर होते हैं, जबकि ब्याज की दर वार्षिक हो।

प्रश्नमाला

1. 400 रु. की राशि पर 5% प्रतिवर्ष की दर से 2 वर्ष का चक्रवृद्धि ब्याज कितना होगा?

A. 40 रु. B. 41 रु.
C. 42 रु. D. 43 रु.

2. किसी राशि पर 6% चक्रवृद्धि ब्याज की दर से पहले वर्ष का ब्याज 60 रु. है, तो दूसरे वर्ष का ब्याज कितना होगा?

A. 120 रु. B. 66.60 रु.
C. 63.60 रु. D. 63 रु.

3. वह धनराशि ज्ञात करो, जिसका 5% ब्याज की दर से 2 वर्ष का चक्रवृद्धि ब्याज तथा साधारण ब्याज का अन्तर 3 रु. हो?

A. 1400 रु. B. 1500 रु.
C. 1350 रु. D. 1200 रु.

4. किस धन का 10% प्रतिवर्ष चक्रवृद्धि ब्याज की दर से 3 वर्ष में मिश्रधन 1331 रु. होगा?

A. 2000 रु. B. 1500 रु.
C. 1000 रु. D. 800 रु.

5. 2500 रु. का 6% ब्याज की दर से 2 वर्ष का चक्रवृद्धि ब्याज कितना होगा?

A. 306 रु. B. 150 रु.
C. 309 रु. D. 300 रु.

6. कोई राशि चक्रवृद्धि ब्याज की दर से 2 वर्ष में चार गुनी हो जाती है, तो कितने वर्ष में वह राशि 8 गुनी हो जायेगी?

A. 4 वर्ष B. $2\frac{1}{2}$ वर्ष
C. 3 वर्ष D. $3\frac{1}{2}$ वर्ष

7. 2400 रुपये पर 5% प्रतिवर्ष ब्याज की दर से 2 वर्ष में साधारण ब्याज तथा चक्रवृद्धि ब्याज का अन्तर होगा?

A. 8 रु. B. 10 रु.
C. 9 रु. D. 6 रु.

8. 8000 रु. **की राशि पर** 5% प्रतिवर्ष ब्याज की दर से 3 वर्ष का चक्रवृद्धि ब्याज कितना होगा?

A. 1361 B. 1261 रु.
C. 1141 रु. D. 1241 रु.

9. 2000 रु. का 2 वर्ष में किस चक्रवृद्धि ब्याज की दर से मिश्रधन 2205 रु. हो जायेगा?

A. 3% B. 4%
C. 5% D. 6%

10. 3200 रु. का 10% प्रतिवर्ष चक्रवृद्धि ब्याज की दर से कितने समय में चक्रवृद्धि ब्याज 672 रु. हो जायेगा?

A. $2\frac{1}{2}$ वर्ष B. $1\frac{1}{2}$ वर्ष

C. 2 वर्ष D. $3\frac{1}{2}$ वर्ष

11. किसी राशि का 6% वार्षिक ब्याज की दर से 2 वर्ष का साधारण ब्याज 300 रु. है, तो उसी राशि का उसी दर से उतने ही समय में चक्रवृद्धि ब्याज कितना होगा?

A. 306 रु. B. 309 रु.

C. 308 रु. D. 300 रु.

12. 3600 रु. का 2 वर्ष का साधारण ब्याज 216 रु. है। यदि ब्याज की दर 2% अधिक कर दी जाये तो इसी धनराशि पर इतने ही समय के लिए चक्रवृद्धि ब्याज क्या होगा?

A. 369 रु. B. 400 रु.

C. 380 रु. D. 375 रु.

13. किसी राशि पर 2 वर्ष का साधारण ब्याज 100 रु. तथा चक्रवृद्धि ब्याज 103 रु. है, तो उस राशि पर ब्याज की **वार्षिक** दर कितने प्रतिशत होगी?

A. 2% B. 8%

C. 6% D. 10%

14. यदि ब्याज छमाही देय हो तो 1500 रु. का 4% वार्षिक ब्याज की दर से एक वर्ष का चक्रवृद्धि ब्याज कितना होगा?

A. 60.60 रु. B. 62 रु.

C. 63 रु. D. 64 रु.

15. यदि किसी धनराशि का 5% चक्रवृद्धि ब्याज की दर से पहले वर्ष का ब्याज 400 रु. है, तो उस राशि का तीसरे वर्ष का ब्याज कितना होगा?

A. 1261 रु. B. 1461 रु.

C. 1562 रु. D. 1462 रु.

16. वह धन ज्ञात करो, जिसका 4% वार्षिक ब्याज की दर से 4 वर्ष का साधारण ब्याज और 400 रुपये का 10% की दर से 2 वर्ष का चक्रवृद्धि ब्याज बराबर हो?

A. 500 रु. B. 550 रु.

C. 525 रु. D. 450 रु.

17. किसी राशि का 2 वर्ष के चक्रवृद्धि ब्याज से मिश्रधन 5408 रु. तथा 3 वर्ष में 5624.32 रु. हो जाता है, तो ब्याज की दर क्या है?

A. 8% B. 9%

C. 4% D. 6%

18. 500 रु. **का** 10% ब्याज की दर से 2 वर्ष का साधारण ब्याज तथा चक्रवृद्धि ब्याज का अन्तर कितना होगा?

A. 10 रु. B. 5 रु.

C. 8 रु. D. 6 रु.

19. किसी धनराशि का 2 वर्ष के लिए 5% ब्याज की दर से साधारण ब्याज और चक्रवृद्धि ब्याज का अन्तर 15 रुपये हो तो वह धनराशि कितनी होगी?

A. 5000 रु. B. 5990 रु.

C. 6000 रु. D. 6100 रु.

20. 1600 रु. का 25% ब्याज की दर से 3 वर्ष का चक्रवृद्धि ब्याज कितना होगा?

A. 1200 रु. B. 1425 रु.

C. 1525 रु. D. 1575 रु.

उत्तरमाला

1	**2**	**3**	**4**	**5**	**6**	**7**	**8**	**9**	**10**
B	C	D	C	C	C	D	B	C	C
11	**12**	**13**	**14**	**15**	**16**	**17**	**18**	**19**	**20**
B	A	C	A	A	C	C	B	C	C

व्याख्यात्मक उत्तर

1. मूलधन = 400 रु., दर = 5%, समय = 2 वर्ष

$$\therefore \text{चक्रवृद्धि ब्याज} = \text{मूलधन}\left[\left(1+\frac{\text{दर}}{100}\right)^{\text{समय}}-1\right]$$

$$\therefore \text{चक्रवृद्धि ब्याज} = 400\left[\left(1+\frac{5}{100}\right)^{2}-1\right]$$

$$= 400\left[\left(\frac{21}{20}\right)^{2}-1\right] = 400\left[\frac{21}{20}\times\frac{21}{20}-1\right]$$

$$= 400\times\frac{41}{400} = 41 \text{ रु.}$$

2. पहले वर्ष का साधारण ब्याज तथा चक्रवृद्धि ब्याज बराबर होगा

$$\therefore 60 = \frac{\text{मूलधन}\times 6\times 1}{100}$$

$\therefore$ मूलधन = 1000 रु.

$\therefore$ दूसरे वर्ष के लिए मूलधन = 1000 + 60 = 1060 रु.

$$\therefore \text{ब्याज} = \frac{1060\times 6\times 1}{100} = 63.60 \text{ रु.}$$

3. माना कि धनराशि x रु. है।

$\therefore$ 5% वार्षिक ब्याज की दर से 2 वर्ष का साधारण ब्याज

$$= \frac{x\times 5\times 2}{100} = \frac{x}{10} \text{ रु.}$$

$$\text{तथा चक्रवृद्धि ब्याज} = x\left[\left(1+\frac{5}{100}\right)^{2}-1\right]$$

$$= x\left[\left(\frac{21}{20}\right)^{2}-1\right]$$

$$= x\left[\frac{21}{20}\times\frac{21}{20}-1\right] = \frac{x\times 41}{400} \text{ रु.}$$

प्रश्नानुसार—

$$\frac{41x}{400}-\frac{x}{10} = 3$$

$\therefore 41x - 40x = 400\times 3$ या $x = 1200$ रु.

अतः वह धनराशि 1200 रु. है।

4. माना वह धनराशि x रु. है

$$\therefore \text{मिश्रधन} = \text{मूलधन}\left(1+\frac{\text{दर}}{100}\right)^{\text{समय}}$$

$$\text{या } 1331 = x\left(1+\frac{10}{100}\right)^{3}$$

$$\therefore 1331 = x\times\frac{11}{10}\times\frac{11}{10}\times\frac{11}{10}$$

$$\therefore x = \frac{1331\times 10\times 10\times 10}{11\times 11\times 11} = 1000 \text{ रु.}$$

5. $$\text{चक्रवृद्धि ब्याज} = 2500\left[\left(1+\frac{6}{100}\right)^{2}-1\right]$$

$$= 2500\left[\left(\frac{53}{50}\right)^{2}-1\right]$$

$$= 2500\left[\frac{53}{50}\times\frac{53}{50}-1\right]$$

$$= 2500\left[\frac{2809-2500}{2500}\right]$$

$$= \frac{2500\times 309}{2500} = 309 \text{ रु.}$$

6. माना वह राशि x रु. है

$$\therefore \text{मिश्रधन} = \text{मूलधन}\left(1+\frac{\text{दर}}{100}\right)^{\text{समय}}$$

प्रश्नानुसार—

$$\therefore 4x = x\left(1+\frac{\text{दर}}{100}\right)^{2} \text{ या } 4 = \left(1+\frac{\text{दर}}{100}\right)^{2}$$

$$\text{या } (2)^2 = \left(1+\frac{\text{दर}}{100}\right)^{2} \text{ या } 2 = \left(1+\frac{\text{दर}}{100}\right)$$

$\therefore$ मिश्रधन को 8 गुना करने के लिए

$$\therefore (2)^3 = \left(1+\frac{\text{दर}}{100}\right)^{3}$$

$$\therefore 8 = \left(1+\frac{\text{दर}}{100}\right)^{3}$$

अत : स्पष्ट है कि मिश्रधन को 8 गुना होने में लगा समय = 3 वर्ष

7. साधारण ब्याज = $\dfrac{2400 \times 5 \times 2}{100} = 240$ रु.

चक्रवृद्धि ब्याज = = $2400 \left[\left(1+\dfrac{5}{100}\right)^2 - 1\right]$

$= 2400 \left[\dfrac{21}{20} \times \dfrac{21}{20} - 1\right] = \dfrac{2400 \times 41}{400} = 246$ रु.

∴ अन्तर = 246 – 240 = 6 रु.

8. चक्रवृद्धि ब्याज = $8000 \left[\left(1+\dfrac{5}{100}\right)^3 - 1\right]$

$= 8000 \left[\dfrac{21}{20} \times \dfrac{21}{20} \times \dfrac{21}{20} - 1\right]$

$= 8000 \left[\dfrac{9261 - 8000}{8000}\right] = \dfrac{8000 \times 1261}{8000.} = 1261$ रु.

9. $2205 = 2000 \left(1 + \dfrac{\text{दर}}{100}\right)^2$

या $\dfrac{2205}{2000} = \left(1 + \dfrac{\text{दर}}{100}\right)^2$ या $\dfrac{441}{400} = \left(1 + \dfrac{\text{दर}}{100}\right)^2$

या $\left(\dfrac{21}{20}\right)^2 = \left(1 + \dfrac{\text{दर}}{100}\right)^2$ या $\dfrac{21}{20} = 1 + \dfrac{\text{दर}}{100}$

$\dfrac{\text{दर}}{100} = \dfrac{21}{20} - 1 = \dfrac{1}{20}$ या दर $= \dfrac{100}{20} = 5\%$

10. मूलधन = 3200 रु., चक्रवृद्धि ब्याज = 672 रु.

∴ चक्रवृद्धि मिश्रधन = मूलधन + चक्रवृद्धि ब्याज

= 3200 + 672 = 3872 रु.

∴ चक्रवृद्धि मिश्रधन = मूलधन $\left(1 + \dfrac{\text{दर}}{100}\right)^{\text{समय}}$

∴ $3872 = 3200 \left(1 + \dfrac{10}{100}\right)^{\text{समय}}$

या $\dfrac{3872}{3200} = \left(\dfrac{11}{10}\right)^{\text{समय}}$ या $\dfrac{121}{100} = \left(\dfrac{11}{10}\right)^{\text{समय}}$

या $\left(\dfrac{11}{10}\right)^2 = \left(\dfrac{11}{10}\right)^{\text{समय}}$

∴ समय = 2 वर्ष

11. माना वह धनराशि x रु. है

∴ $300 = \dfrac{x \times 6 \times 2}{100}$ या $x = 2500$ रु.

∴ चक्रवृद्धि ब्याज = $2500 \left[\left(1+\dfrac{6}{100}\right)^2 - 1\right]$

$= 2500 \left[\dfrac{53}{50} \times \dfrac{53}{50} - 1\right]$

$= 2500 \left[\dfrac{2809 - 2500}{2500}\right]$

$= \dfrac{2500 \times 309}{2500} = 309$ रु.

12. ∴ साधारण ब्याज = $\dfrac{\text{मूलधन} \times \text{दर} \times \text{समय}}{100}$

∴ $216 = \dfrac{3600 \times \text{दर} \times 2}{100}$

∴ दर = $\dfrac{216 \times 100}{3600 \times 2} = 3\%$

प्रश्नानुसार—

नयी दर = (3 + 2)% = 5%

∴ चक्रवृद्धि ब्याज = $3600 \left[\left(1+\dfrac{5}{100}\right)^2 - 1\right]$

$= 3600 \left[\dfrac{21}{20} \times \dfrac{21}{20} - 1\right] = \dfrac{3600 \times 41}{400} = 369$ रु.

13. माना किसी राशि पर ब्याज की दर $x\%$ है

∴ 2 वर्ष का साधारण ब्याज = 100 रु.

∴ 1 वर्ष का साधारण ब्याज = 50 रु.

चूंकि पहले वर्ष का साधारण ब्याज तथा चक्रवृद्धि ब्याज बराबर होता है

∴ पहले वर्ष का चक्रवृद्धि ब्याज = 50 रु.

∴ दूसरे वर्ष का चक्रवृद्धि ब्याज = 103 – 50 = 53 रु.

∴ दूसरे वर्ष का चक्रवृद्धि ब्याज = पहले वर्ष का ब्याज + पहले वर्ष के ब्याज पर ब्याज

या 53 = 50 + 50 रु. का $x\%$

या $3 = \dfrac{50 \times x}{100}$ या $3 = \dfrac{x}{2}$

∴ $x = 6$

अतः ब्याज की दर = 6% होगी।

14. दर = $\frac{4}{2}\%$ = 2%, समय = 1 वर्ष = 2 छमाही

$\therefore$ चक्रवृद्धि ब्याज $= 1500\left[\left(1+\frac{2}{100}\right)^2-1\right]$

$= 1500\left[\frac{51}{50}\times\frac{51}{50}-1\right] = \frac{1500\times 101}{50\times 50} = 60.60$ रु.

15. $\therefore 400 = \frac{\text{मूलधन}\times 5\times 1}{100}$

$\therefore$ मूलधन = 8000 रु.

$\therefore$ चक्रवृद्धि ब्याज $= 8000\left[\left(1+\frac{5}{100}\right)^3-1\right]$

$= 8000\left[\frac{21}{20}\times\frac{21}{20}\times\frac{21}{20}-1\right]$

$= 8000\left[\frac{9261-8000}{8000}\right]$

$= \frac{8000\times 1261}{8000} = 1261$ रु.

16. माना वह धन x रु. है।

$\therefore$ 4% की दर से 4 वर्ष का साधारण ब्याज

$= \frac{x\times 4\times 4}{100} = \frac{16x}{100}$ रु.

तथा चक्रवृद्धि ब्याज $= 400\left[\left(1+\frac{10}{100}\right)^2-1\right]$

$= 400\left[\frac{11}{10}\times\frac{11}{10}-1\right] = \frac{400\times 21}{100} = 84$ रु.

प्रश्नानुसार—

$\frac{16x}{100} = 84$

$\therefore x = \frac{84\times 100}{16} = 525$ रु.

17. माना वह धनराशि x रु. है

$\therefore \quad 5408 = x\left(1+\frac{\text{दर}}{100}\right)^2 \quad ...(1)$

तथा $\quad 5624.32 = x\left(1+\frac{\text{दर}}{100}\right)^3 \quad ...(2)$

समीकरण (2) में (1) से भाग देने पर—

$$\frac{5642.32}{5408} = \frac{x\left(1+\frac{\text{दर}}{100}\right)^3}{x\left(1+\frac{\text{दर}}{100}\right)^2} = \left(1+\frac{\text{दर}}{100}\right)$$

या $\frac{\text{दर}}{100} = \frac{5624.32}{5408} - 1 = \frac{216.32}{5408}$

या दर $= \frac{216.32\times 100}{5408} = 4\%$

18. साधारण ब्याज $= \frac{500\times 10\times 2}{100} = 100$ रु.

तथा चक्रवृद्धि ब्याज $= 500\left[\left(1+\frac{10}{100}\right)^2-1\right]$

$= 500\left[\frac{11}{10}\times\frac{11}{10}-1\right] = \frac{500\times 21}{100} = 105$ रु.

$\therefore$ अन्तर = 105 –100 = 5 रु.

19. माना वह धनराशि x रु. है

$\therefore$ साधारण ब्याज $= \frac{x\times 5\times 2}{100} = \frac{x}{10}$ रु.

तथा चक्रवृद्धि ब्याज $= x\left[\left(1+\frac{5}{100}\right)^2-1\right]$

$= x\left[\frac{21}{20}\times\frac{21}{20}-1\right]$

$= \frac{x[441-400]}{400} = \frac{41x}{400}$ रु.

प्रश्नानुसार—

$\frac{41x}{400} - \frac{x}{10} = 15$ या $\frac{41x-40x}{400} = 15$

या x = 15 × 400 = 6000 रु.

अतः **वह** धनराशि = 6000 रु. **होगी।**

20. चक्रवृद्धि ब्याज $= 1600\left[\left(1+\frac{25}{100}\right)^3-1\right]$

$= 1600\left[\frac{5}{4}\times\frac{5}{4}\times\frac{5}{4}-1\right]$

$= 1600\ \frac{[125-64]}{64} = \frac{1600\times 61}{64} = 1525$ रु.

☆☆☆☆☆☆

11 लाभ तथा हानि (Profit and Loss)

लाभ और हानि शब्द साधारणतया व्यापार में इस्तेमाल किए जाते हैं। प्रत्येक व्यापार का उद्देश्य लाभ कमाना होता है। लाभ और हानि से संबंधित सभी तरह के प्रश्नों को हल करने से पहले निम्नलिखित बातों को जानना आवश्यक है।

1. कोई वस्तु जिस मूल्य पर खरीदी जाती है उसे उस वस्तु का **लागत मूल्य** या **क्रय मूल्य** (Cost Price) कहते हैं। इसे क्रय मूल्य (C.P.) द्वारा भी निर्दिष्ट किया जाता है।

2. कोई वस्तु जिस मूल्य पर बेची जाती है, उसे उस वस्तु का **विक्रय मूल्य** (Sale Price) कहते हैं। इसे विक्रय मूल्य (S.P.) द्वारा भी निर्दिष्ट किया जाता है।

3. यदि वस्तु का क्रय मूल्य (Cost Price), वस्तु के विक्रय मूल्य (Sale Price) से अधिक हो तो उस वस्तु पर हमेशा **हानि** होगी। अर्थात्

हानि = क्रय मूल्य − विक्रय मूल्य

4. यदि किसी वस्तु का विक्रय मूल्य (Sale Price) वस्तु के क्रय मूल्य (Cost Price) से अधिक हो तो उस वस्तु पर हमेशा **लाभ** होगा। अर्थात्

लाभ = विक्रय मूल्य − क्रय मूल्य

5. लाभ और हानि दो प्रकार से व्यक्त किए जाते हैं:

(i) रुपयों में; *(ii)* प्रतिशत में।

उदाहरण : यदि किसी वस्तु का क्रय मूल्य 100 रु. तथा उसका विक्रय मूल्य 95 रु. हो तो वस्तु पर लाभ या हानि कितनी होगी?

हल : चूंकि वस्तु का क्रय मूल्य और उसके विक्रय मूल्य से अधिक है, इसलिए वस्तु पर हानि होगी। अर्थात् हानि = क्रय मूल्य − विक्रय मूल्य = 100 − 95 = 5 रु. हानि।

उपरोक्त उदाहरण में हमने वस्तु पर लाभ और हानि को रुपयों में समझाया है। अब हम लाभ-हानि को प्रतिशत में व्यक्त करते हैं। लाभ-हानि को प्रतिशत लाभ और प्रतिशत हानि में बदलने के लिए निम्नलिखित सूत्रों को याद रखें।

1. $\text{लाभ\%} = \dfrac{\text{लाभ} \times 100}{\text{क्रय मूल्य}}$

2. $\text{हानि\%} = \dfrac{\text{हानि} \times 100}{\text{क्रय मूल्य}}$

लाभ-हानि को **प्रतिशत लाभ** और **हानि** में बदलने के लिए नीचे कुछ उदाहरणों द्वारा समझाया गया है।

उदाहरण 1. यदि किसी वस्तु को 20 रु. में खरीद कर उसे 25 रु. में बेच दिया हो तो उस वस्तु पर कितने प्रतिशत लाभ या हानि होगी?

हल : चूंकि वस्तु का क्रय मूल्य वस्तु के विक्रय मूल्य से कम है इसलिए वस्तु पर लाभ होगा।

अर्थात्, लाभ = विक्रय मूल्य − क्रय मूल्य = 25 − 20 = 5 रु.

$$\therefore \text{ प्रतिशत लाभ} = \frac{\text{लाभ} \times 100}{\text{क्रय मूल्य}} = \frac{5 \times 100}{20} = 25\%$$

उदाहरण 2. एक किताब का अंकित मूल्य 64 रु. है। यदि उसे 48 रु. में बेचा जाता है तो कितने प्रतिशत हानि होगी?

हल : किताब का क्रय मूल्य = 64 रु.

तथा किताब का विक्रय मूल्य = 48 रु.

हानि = क्रय मूल्य − विक्रय मूल्य = 64 − 48 = 16 रु.

$$\text{हानि\%} = \frac{\text{हानि} \times 100}{\text{क्रय मूल्य}} = \frac{16 \times 100}{64} = 25\%$$

प्रश्नमाला

1. एक आदमी कोई वस्तु 25 रु. में खरीदकर 30 रु. में बेचता है। तो बताइये उसका लाभ क्या होगा?

A. 6 रु. B. 7.50 रु.
C. 5 रु. D. 8.10 रु.

2. यदि 15 रु. वाली कोई वस्तु 12 रु. में बेच दी जाए, तो कितने प्रतिशत हानि होगी?

A. 20% B. 16%
C. 22% D. 25%

3. यदि किसी वस्तु को 21 रु. में बेचने पर 12% का लाभ होता हो तो बताइये उस वस्तु का क्रय मूल्य कितना होगा?

A. 15.50 रु. B. 20.15 रु.
C. 18.75 रु. D. 17.50 रु.

4. यदि किसी वस्तु को 2040 रु. में बेचने पर 15% की हानि होती हो तो बताइये उस वस्तु का क्रय मूल्य कितना होगा?

A. 2300 रु. B. 2400 रु.
C. 2475 रु. D. 2800 रु.

5. एक वस्तु का क्रय मूल्य 150 रु. है। यदि इसे 13% लाभ पर बेचा जाए तो बताइये वस्तु का विक्रय मूल्य कितना होगा?

A. 170.75 रु. B. 169.50 रु.
C. 160.50 रु. D. 174.75 रु.

6. किसी वस्तु को 250 रु. में खरीदकर 300 रु. में बेच दिया गया। बताइये उस पर कितने प्रतिशत लाभ हुआ?

A. 16% B. 20%
C. 18% D. 17%

7. एक वस्तु को 38 रु. में बेचने पर 5% हानि होती है। यदि इसे 42 रु. में बेचा जाए तो कितने प्रतिशत लाभ या हानि होगी?

A. 6% लाभ B. 5% लाभ
C. 8% हानि D. 4% हानि

8. यदि किसी वस्तु को 5% हानि पर बेचने पर 3990 रु. मिले हों, तो उस वस्तु का क्रय मूल्य कितना होगा?

A. 4100 रु. B. 4200 रु.
C. 3890 रु. D. 4400 रु.

9. यदि 10 पेनों का क्रय मूल्य, 8 पेनों के विक्रय मूल्य के बराबर हो तो प्रतिशत लाभ कितना होगा?

A. 20% B. 16%
C. 25% D. 30%

10. राम ने एक टी.वी. 2475 रु. में खरीद कर उसे 3090 रु. में बेच दिया हो तो उसे कितने प्रतिशत लाभ हुआ?

A. 23.8% B. 34.5%
C. 37.6% D. 24.8%

11. एक फल विक्रेता ने 20 दर्जन केले 100 रुपये में खरीदकर 6 रुपये प्रति दर्जन के भाव से बेच दिए। उसका लाभ अथवा हानि ज्ञात करो।

A. 20 रु. B. 30 रु.
C. 25 रु. D. 35 रु.

12. एक ठेकेदार ने 7500 रुपये में एक खाली जमीन खरीदी और उस पर 2,65,000 रुपये खर्च कर मकान तैयार किया। यदि अब उस मकान को 3,25,000 रु. में बेच दिया तो उसका लाभ अथवा हानि ज्ञात करो।

A. 15550 रु. हानि B. 15550 रु. लाभ
C. 15000 रु. हानि D. 15000 रु. लाभ

13. सलमा ने एक मोटर साइकिल 25,250 रुपये में खरीदी। उस पर 750 का सामान लगाया। बाद में रकम की आवश्यकता पड़ने पर उसे 500 रुपये की हानि से बेच दिया। बताइये मोटर साइकिल कितने में बेची गयी?

A. 22550 रु. B. 22225 रु.
C. 22000 रु. D. 22500 रु.

14. एक दुकानदार ने 50 पुस्तकें 70 रुपये के हिसाब से खरीदी। उसमें से 5 पुस्तकों में प्रकाशन की खामी के कारण बिक न सकी। शेष पुस्तकों को 80 रुपये के हिसाब से बेचने पर उसका लाभ या हानि ज्ञात करो।

A. 100 रु. हानि B. 100 रु. लाभ
C. 150 रु. लाभ D. 150 रु. हानि

15. सलमान ने एक पुरानी साइकिल 500 रुपये में खरीदी। उसे ठीक कराने में 20 रुपये खर्च किए तथा 50 रुपये का नया सामान डलवाया। सलमान ने वह साइकिल 600 रुपये में बेच दी तो उसे कितना लाभ अथवा हानि हुई?

A. 25 रु. B. 20 रु.

C. 30 रु. D. 35 रु.

16. एक आदमी ने एक फ्रिज 8000 रुपये में खरीदकर 450 रुपये लाभ पर बेच दिया यदि उसने वह फ्रिज 9000 रुपये में बेचा होता तो उसे और कितना लाभ होता?

A. 550 रु. B. 525 रु.

C. 500 रु. D. 575 रु.

17. राधेश्याम ने 8 क्विंटल मक्का 165 रुपये प्रति क्विंटल के भाव से खरीदकर उसमें से 4 क्विंटल मक्का को 170 रुपये प्रति क्विंटल के भाव से और बाकी बची हुई को 172 रुपये प्रति क्विंटल के भाव से बेच दिया। बताओ, उसे कुल कितना लाभ हुआ।

A. 40 रु. B. 45 रु.

C. 48 रु. D. 50 रु.

18. रामा ने 50 प्लेटें 250 रुपये में खरीदी। उसमें से 8 प्लेटें टूट गयी। शेष प्लेटों को वह किस मूल्य से बेचे कि उसे 2 रुपये का लाभ हो। एक प्लेट का विक्रय मूल्य ज्ञात कीजिए।

A. 6 रु. B. 5.50 रु.

C. 6.25 रु. D. 5 रु.

19. एक आदमी ने दो वस्तुएं, प्रत्येक 120 रुपये में खरीदी। उसने उसमें से एक को 10% हानि पर तथा दूसरे को 10% लाभ पर बेचा। बताओ उसने दोनों कितने रुपये में बेची?

A. 250 रु. B. 200 रु.

C. 240 रु. D. 225 रु.

20. 40 वस्तुओं का क्रय मूल्य 35 वस्तुओं के विक्रय मूल्य के समान है। लाभ प्रतिशत ज्ञात करो।

A. $14\frac{2}{7}\%$ B. 14%

C. $15\frac{2}{7}\%$ D. 15%

उत्तरमाला

1	2	3	4	5	6	7	8	9	10
C	A	C	B	B	B	B	B	C	D
11	**12**	**13**	**14**	**15**	**16**	**17**	**18**	**19**	**20**
A	C	D	B	C	A	C	A	C	A

व्याख्यात्मक उत्तर

1. ∵ वस्तु का विक्रय मूल्य, उसके क्रय मूल्य से अधिक है।

∴ लाभ = विक्रय मूल्य – क्रय मूल्य

= 30 – 25 = 5 रु.।

2. ∵ वस्तु का क्रय मूल्य, उसके विक्रय मूल्य से अधिक है।

∴ हानि = क्रय मूल्य – विक्रय मूल्य

= 15 – 12 = 3 रु.

$$\therefore \text{ प्रतिशत हानि} = \frac{\text{हानि} \times 100}{\text{क्रय मूल्य}}$$

$$= \frac{3 \times 100}{15} = 20\%.$$

3. ∵ वस्तु का विक्रय मूल्य = 21 रु. तथा लाभ % = 12%

$$\therefore \text{ क्रय मूल्य} = \text{विक्रय मूल्य} \left(\frac{100}{100 + \text{लाभ}\%}\right)$$

$$= 21\left(\frac{100}{100+12}\right) = \frac{21 \times 100}{112} = 18.75 \text{ रु.।}$$

4. ∵ वस्तु का विक्रय मूल्य = 2040 रु.

तथा हानि % = 15%

$$\therefore \text{ क्रय मूल्य} = \text{विक्रय मूल्य} \left(\frac{100}{100 - \%\text{हानि}}\right)$$

$= 2040 \left(\frac{100}{100-15}\right) = \frac{2040 \times 100}{85} = 2400$ रु.।

5. $\because$ वस्तु का क्रय मूल्य = 150 रु. तथा
लाभ % = 13%

$\therefore$ वस्तु का विक्रय मूल्य

$$= \text{क्रय मूल्य} \left(\frac{100 + \text{लाभ\%}}{100}\right)$$

$$= 150 \times \left(\frac{100+13}{100}\right)$$

$$= \frac{150 \times 113}{100} = 169.50 \text{ रु.।}$$

6. $\because$ वस्तु का क्रय मूल्य = 250 रु.
तथा वस्तु का विक्रय मूल्य = 300 रु.

$\therefore$ लाभ = 300 – 250 = 50 रु.

$\therefore$ प्रतिशत लाभ $= \frac{\text{लाभ} \times 100}{\text{क्रय मूल्य}} = \frac{50 \times 100}{250} = 20\%.$

7. पहली स्थिति में, वस्तु का विक्रय मूल्य = 38 रु., हानि % = 5%

$\therefore$ वस्तु का क्रय मूल्य

$$= \text{विक्रय मूल्य} \left(\frac{100}{100 - \text{हानि\%}}\right)$$

$$= 38\left(\frac{100}{100-5}\right) = \frac{38 \times 100}{95} = 40 \text{ रु.}$$

दूसरी स्थिति में, क्रय मूल्य = 40 रु.,
विक्रय मूल्य = 42 रु.

$\therefore$ लाभ = विक्रय मूल्य – क्रय मूल्य

= 42 – 40 = 2 रु.

$\therefore$ प्रतिशत लाभ $= \frac{\text{लाभ} \times 100}{\text{क्रय मूल्य}} = \left(\frac{2 \times 100}{40}\right)$

= 5%.

8. $\therefore$ वस्तु का विक्रय मूल्य = 3990 रु., तथा
हानि % = 5%

$\therefore$ वस्तु का क्रय मूल्य

$$= \text{विक्रय मूल्य} \left(\frac{100}{100-5}\right)$$

$$= 3990 \times \frac{100}{95} = 4200 \text{ रु.।}$$

9. माना कि 10 पेनों का क्रय मूल्य = x रु.
प्रश्नानुसार, 8 पेनों का विक्रय मूल्य = x रु.

$\therefore$ 1 पेन का क्रय मूल्य $= \frac{x}{10}$ रु.

तथा 1 पेन का विक्रय मूल्य $= \frac{x}{8}$ रु.

$\therefore$ लाभ = विक्रय मूल्य – क्रय मूल्य

$$= \frac{x}{8} - \frac{x}{10} = \frac{x}{40} \text{ रु.}$$

$\therefore$ प्रतिशत लाभ $= \frac{\text{लाभ} \times 100}{\text{क्रय मूल्य}} = \frac{\frac{x}{40} \times 100}{\frac{x}{10}} = 25\%.$

10. $\because$ टी.वी. का खरीद मूल्य या क्रय मूल्य = 2475 रु.
तथा विक्रय मूल्य = 3090 रु.

लाभ = विक्रय मूल्य – क्रय मूल्य
= 3090 – 2475 = 615 रु.

प्रतिशत लाभ $= \frac{\text{हानि} \times 100}{\text{क्रय मूल्य}}$

$$= \frac{615 \times 100}{2475}$$

= 24.8%.

11. 20 दर्जन केलों का क्रय मूल्य = 100 रुपये
20 दर्जन केलों का विक्रय मूल्य

= 6 × 20 = 120 रुपये

लाभ = विक्रय मूल्य – क्रय मूल्य
= 120 – 100 = 20 रुपये लाभ।

12. ठेकेदार का वास्तविक क्रय मूल्य

= 75000 + 2,65,000
= 3,40,000 रुपये

$\because$ उसका विक्रय मूल्य उसके क्रय मूल्य से कम है अत: हानि होगी।

हानि = क्रय मूल्य – विक्रय मूल्य
= 3,40,000 – 3,25,000
= 15,000 रुपये हानि।

13. सलमा के लिए मोटर साईकिल का कुल क्रय मूल्य
$= 22{,}250 + 750 = 23{,}000$ रुपये

$\because$ 500 रुपये हानि पर मोटर साईकिल बेची जाती है अतः उसका विक्रय मूल्य क्रय मूल्य से 500 रुपये कम होगा।

विक्रय मूल्य $= 23000 - 500 = 22500$ रुपये।

14. दुकानदार का कुल क्रय मूल्य
$= 50 \times 70 = 3500$ रुपये

शेष पुस्तकें $= 50 - 5 = 45$ पुस्तकें

45 पुस्तकों का विक्रय मूल्य $= 45 \times 80$
$= 3600$ रुपये

लाभ = विक्रय मूल्य – क्रय मूल्य
$= 3600 - 3500$
$= 100$ रुपये लाभ।

15. साईकिल का वास्तविक क्रय मूल्य
$= (500 + 20 + 50)$ रुपये
$= 570$ रुपये

साईकिल का विक्रय मूल्य = 600 रुपये

अतः लाभ = विक्रय मूल्य – क्रय मूल्य
$= (600 - 570)$ रुपये = 30 रुपये।

16. 9000 रुपये में बेचने पर उसका लाभ
$= 9000 - 8000 = 1000$ रु.

इस सौदे में उसका अतिरिक्त लाभ
$= 1000 - 450 = 550$ रुपये।

17. 8 क्विंटल मक्का का कुल क्रय मूल्य
$= 8 \times 165 = 1320$ रुपये

8 क्विंटल मक्का का कुल विक्रय मूल्य
$= (4 \times 170) + (4 \times 172)$
$= 680 + 688 = 1368$ रुपये

$\because$ विक्रय मूल्य, क्रय मूल्य से अधिक है अतः लाभ होगा।

लाभ $= 1368 - 1320 = 48$ रुपये।

18. 50 प्लेटों का क्रय मूल्य = 250 रुपये

शेष प्लेटें $= 50 - 8 = 42$ प्लेटें

शेष प्लेटें क्रय मूल्य से 2 रुपये लाभ अर्थात् 2 रुपये अधिक में बेची गयी।

इसलिए 42 प्लेटों का विक्रय मूल्य
$= 250 + 2 = 252$ रुपये

इसलिए 1 प्लेट का विक्रय मूल्य
$= \frac{252}{42} = 6$ रुपये प्रति प्लेट।

19. प्रथम वस्तु का क्रय मूल्य = 120 रुपये

10% लाभ = 120 का 10%
$= \frac{120 \times 10}{100} = 12$ रुपये

अतः प्रथम वस्तु का विक्रय मूल्य
$= 120 + 12 = 132$ रुपये

द्वितीय वस्तु का क्रय मूल्य = 120 रुपये

द्वितीय वस्तु पर हानि = 120 रु. का 10%
$= \frac{120 \times 10}{100} = 12$ रुपये

अतः द्वितीय वस्तु का विक्रय मूल्य
$= 120 - 12 = 108$ रुपये

दोनों वस्तुओं का कुल विक्रय मूल्य
$= 132 + 108 = 240$ रुपये।

20. माना 40 वस्तुओं का क्रय मूल्य 100 रुपये है।

$\therefore$ 35 वस्तुओं का विक्रय मूल्य भी 100 रुपये होगा।

$\because$ 35 वस्तुओं का विक्रय मूल्य 100 रुपये है तो

40 वस्तु का विक्रय मूल्य $= \frac{100}{35} \times 40$
$= \frac{800}{7}$ रुपये

$\therefore$ लाभ = विक्रय मूल्य – क्रय मूल्य
$= \frac{800}{7} - 100 = \frac{100}{7}$ रुपये

$\because$ क्रय मूल्य 100 रुपये माना था।

अतः लाभ% $= \frac{100}{7} = 14\frac{2}{7}\%$.

☆☆☆☆☆☆

12 अनुपात एवं समानुपात (Ratio and Proportion)

अनुपात : अनुपात सदैव दो सजातीय राशियों में होता है। एक राशि का, दूसरी सजातीय राशि में भाग देने पर अनुपात ज्ञात होता है या जब हम एक ही प्रकार की दो वस्तुओं की तुलना करते हैं और यह देखते हैं कि एक वस्तु, दूसरी वस्तु का कौन-सा भाग है तो उन दोनों के बीच पारस्परिक सम्बन्ध को अनुपात कहते हैं।

उदाहरण : किसी कक्षा में 24 लड़के और 16 लड़कियां हैं तो बताइये लड़कों और लड़कियों का क्या अनुपात होगा?

हल : $\dfrac{\text{लड़कों की संख्या}}{\text{लड़कियों की संख्या}} = \dfrac{24}{16} = \dfrac{3}{2}$

$\therefore$ लड़कों और लड़कियों की संख्या का अनुपात = 3 : 2 होगा।

समानुपात : जब दो अनुपात बराबर होते हैं तो उनकी बराबरी को समानुपात कहते हैं। जैसे $a : b = c : d$ हो तो इसका अर्थ यह है कि $\dfrac{a}{b}$ समानुपात में है $\dfrac{c}{d}$ के और इसे हम निम्न प्रकार से लिख सकते हैं।

अतः $a : b : : c : d$ में a, b, c तथा d को क्रमशः प्रथम, द्वितीय, तृतीय और चतुर्थ अनुपाती कहते हैं। इस प्रकार समानुपात में चार पद होते हैं।

नियम : समानुपात $a : b : : c : d$ में सिरे वाले दोनों पदों के गुणनफल, मध्य वाले दोनों पदों के गुणनफल के बराबर होता है। अर्थात् $a \times d = b \times c$

साझा : साझा दो प्रकार का होता है:

1. **साधारण साझा :** वह साझा जिसमें दो या दो से अधिक व्यापारी अपनी-अपनी पूंजी का इस्तेमाल एक समान अवधि के लिए करते हैं, उसे **साधारण साझा** कहते हैं।
2. **मिश्रित साझा :** वह साझा जिसमें दो या दो से अधिक व्यापारी अपनी-अपनी पूंजी का इस्तेमाल अलग-अलग अवधि के लिए करते हैं उसे **मिश्रित साझा** कहते हैं।

महत्त्वपूर्ण नोट : 1. साधारण साझे से सम्बन्धित प्रश्नों में व्यापार में हुए लाभ अथवा हानि को उनकी पूंजियों के अनुपात में विभाजित करते हैं। 2. मिश्रित साझे से सम्बन्धित प्रश्नों में व्यापार में हुए लाभ अथवा हानि को उनकी पूंजियों तथा समय के गुणनफलों के अनुपात में बांटा जाता है।

उदाहरण 1. निम्नलिखित में से कौन-सा अनुपात बड़ा होगा?

7 : 3 या 19 : 9

हल : 7 : 3 या $\dfrac{7}{3}$ तथा 19 : 9 = $\dfrac{19}{9}$

$\therefore \dfrac{7}{3} = \dfrac{7 \times 3}{3 \times 3}$ तथा $\dfrac{19}{9}$ $\therefore \dfrac{21}{9} > \dfrac{19}{9}$

अतः 7 : 3, 19 : 9 से बड़ा है।

उदाहरण 2. यदि $5 : 3 : : 9 : x$ हो, तो x का मान क्या होगा?

हल : $\therefore$ समानुपात में दोनों बाहरी संख्याओं का गुणनफल मध्य की दोनों संख्याओं के गुणनफल के बराबर होता है।

$$5 \times x = 3 \times 9$$

$$x = \frac{3 \times 9}{5} = \frac{27}{5} = 5\frac{2}{5}$$

उदाहरण 3: यदि $15 : 18 : : 25 : x$ हो तो x का मान कितना होगा?

हल: चूँकि समानुपात में दोनों बाहरी संख्याओं का गुणनफल मध्य की दोनों संख्याओं के गुणनफल के बराबर होता है।

$$\therefore \quad 15 \times x = 18 \times 25$$

$$\Rightarrow \quad x = \frac{18 \times 25}{15} = 30$$

अतः x का मान 30 होगा।

प्रश्नमाला

1. यदि 3 : 8 = 9 : x, तो x का मान कितना होगा?
A. 20 B. 27 C. 24 D. 25

2. यदि A : B = 3 : 4 तथा B : C = 5 : 6, तो A : B : C में क्या अनुपात होगा?
A. 20 : 15 : 24 B. 15 : 20 : 24
C. 15 : 24 : 20 D. 20 : 24 : 15

3. यदि 18 : x = x : 8 हो, तो x किसके बराबर होगा?
A. 11 B. 10 C. 16 D. 12

4. 8 : 12 : 10 : : ? है तो प्रश्न चिन्ह् (?) के स्थान पर क्या मान होगा?
A. 14 B. 15 C. 16 D. 18

5. 5 और 125 का मध्य समानुपात कितना है?
A. 20 B. 25 C. 28 D. 27

6. 3, 4 और 15 का चौथा अनुपात होगा?
A. 16 B. 18 C. 20 D. 15

7. 12 और 30 का तृतीय समानुपात कितना होगा?
A. 75 B. 125 C. 60 D. 70

8. दो संख्याओं का अनुपात 3 : 4 है। यदि दोनों संख्याओं का योग 490 हो तो वे संख्याएं क्रमशः क्या होंगी?
A. 220, 270 B. 210, 280
C. 120, 160 D. 180, 290

9. यदि एक त्रिभुज के कोणों में 1 : 2 : 3 का अनुपात हो तो उस त्रिभुज के सबसे बड़े कोण का मान होगा।
A. 90° B. 70°
C. 105° D. 110°

10. यदि किसी अनुपात का दूसरा पद 15 तथा अनुपात का मान $\frac{3}{5}$ हो तो उस अनुपात का पहला पद क्या होगा?
A. 8 B. 14 C. 9 D. 12

11. 1100 रुपये को सुधा, कमला और सलमा में इस प्रकार बांटो कि उनके धन में $\frac{1}{3}:\frac{2}{5}:\frac{1}{2}$ का अनुपात हो तो सुधा को मिलने वाला धन क्या है?
A. 300 रु. B. 350 रु.
C. 250 रु. D. 200 रु.

12. एक मिश्रधातु में तांबा, जस्ता और लोहा 7 : 6 : 9 के अनुपात में हैं। यदि मिश्रण में तांबे की मात्रा 560 ग्राम हो तो मिश्रधातु का कुल भार ज्ञात करो।
A. 1 किग्रा. 600 ग्रा. B. 2 किग्रा. 760 ग्रा.
C. 1 किग्रा. 760 ग्रा. D. 1 किग्रा. 700 ग्रा.

13. तीन संख्याओं का योग 16 है। दूसरी और तीसरी संख्याओं का अनुपात 9 : 16 है तथा प्रथम और तीसरी संख्याओं का अनुपात 1 : 4 है। दूसरी संख्या ज्ञात करो।
A. 38 B. 36 C. 40 D. 34

14. 1530 रुपये A, B, C में इस प्रकार वितरित **किए गए** कि यदि तीनों के हिस्सों में से क्रमशः 5, 10 और 15 कम कर दिए जाएं तो शेष भागों में 3 : 4 : 5 का अनुपात होगा। B का हिस्सा ज्ञात करो।
A. 505 रु. B. 500 रु.
C. 515 रु. D. 510 रु.

15. यदि A के पास B से 20% कम रुपये और B के पास C से 25% अधिक रुपये हों तो तीनों के धन का अनुपात ज्ञात करो।
A. 4 : 5 : 5 B. 4 : 5 : 4
C. 5 : 4 : 4 D. 4 : 4 : 5

16. एक थैली में एक रुपये, पचास पैसे और पच्चीस पैसे के सिक्के 2 : 3 : 4 के अनुपात में हैं। यदि थैली में कुल 45 रुपये हैं तो सिक्कों की कुल संख्या ज्ञात करो।
A. 90 B. 80
C. 85 D. 100

17. दूध और पानी के 20 लीटर मिश्रण में दूध और पानी का अनुपात 3 : 1 है। इस मिश्रण में कितना दूध और मिलाया जाए कि दूध और पानी का अनुपात 4 : 1 हो जाए?
A. 6 लीटर B. 7 लीटर
C. 5 लीटर D. 4 लीटर

उत्तरमाला

1	2	3	4	5	6	7	8	9	10
C	B	D	B	B	C	A	B	A	C
11	**12**	**13**	**14**	**15**	**16**	**17**			
A	C	B	D	B	A	C			

व्याख्यात्मक उत्तर

1. $\because 3 : 8 = 9 : x \Rightarrow \frac{3}{8} = \frac{9}{x}$

$\Rightarrow \quad x = \frac{8 \times 9}{3} = 24$

अतः x का मान = 24 होगा।

2. $\because$ दिया हुआ है : A : B = 3 : 4 तथा B : C = 5 : 6 दोनों अनुपातों में B को बराबर करने के लिए पहले अनुपात में 5 से तथा दूसरे अनुपात में 4 से गुणा करने पर,

$\therefore \quad A : B = 3 : 4 = 3 \times 5 : 4 \times 5 = 15 : 20$

तथा $B : C = 5 : 6 = 5 \times 4 : 6 \times 4 = 20 : 24$

$\therefore \quad A : B : C = 15 : 20 : 24$

3. $\because 18 : x = x : 8 \Rightarrow \frac{18}{x} = \frac{x}{8}$

$\Rightarrow x \times x = 18 \times 8 \Rightarrow x^2 = 144$

$\Rightarrow x = \sqrt{144} = 12$

अतः x, 12 के बराबर होगा।

4. चूंकि समानुपात में दोनों बाहरी संख्याओं का गुणनफल, मध्य की दोनों संख्याओं के गुणनफल के बराबर होता है।

$\because \quad 8 : 12 : : 10 : ?$

$\therefore \quad 8 \times ? = 12 \times 10 \Rightarrow ? = \frac{12 \times 10}{8} = 15$

अतः प्रश्न चिन्ह् (?) के स्थान पर मान = 15 होगा।

5. माना कि 5 और 125 का मध्य समानुपात = x है

$\therefore \quad 5 : x : : x : 125$

$\therefore \quad x \times x = 5 \times 125 \Rightarrow x^2 = 625$

$\Rightarrow \quad x = \sqrt{625} = 25$

अतः 5 और 125 का मध्य समानुपात = 25 है।

6. माना कि 3, 4 और 15 का चौथा अनुपात = x

$\therefore \quad 3 : 4 = 15 : x$

$\therefore \quad x \times 3 = 4 \times 15$

$\therefore \quad x = \frac{4 \times 15}{3} = 20$

अतः 3, 4 और 15 का चौथा अनुपात = 20 होगा।

7. माना कि 12 और 30 का तृतीय अनुपात = x

$\therefore \quad 12 : 30 = 30 : x$

$\therefore \quad 12 \times x = 30 \times 30 \Rightarrow x = \frac{30 \times 30}{12} = 75$

अतः 12 और 30 का तृतीय अनुपात = 75 होगा।

8. माना कि वे संख्याएं क्रमशः $3x$ व $4x$ हैं।

प्रश्नानुसार, $3x + 4x = 490 \Rightarrow 7x = 490$

$\Rightarrow \quad x = \frac{490}{7} = 70$

अतः वे संख्याएं क्रमशः $(3 \times 70 = 210)$ व $(4 \times 70 = 280)$ होंगी।

9. चूंकि त्रिभुज के कोणों में अनुपात = 1 : 2 : 3

$\therefore$ अनुपात संख्याओं का योग = 1 + 2 + 3 = 6

परन्तु त्रिभुज के तीनों कोणों का योग = 180°

$\therefore$ सबसे बड़े कोण का मान = $\frac{3}{6} \times 180° = 90°$

अतः सबसे बड़े कोण का मान = 90° होगा।

10. माना कि अनुपात का पहला पद = x

प्रश्नानुसार, $x : 15 = \frac{3}{5} = 3 : 5$

या, $\frac{x}{15} = \frac{3}{5}$

$\therefore \quad x \times 5 = 15 \times 3 \Rightarrow x = \frac{15 \times 3}{5} = 9$

अतः अनुपात का पहला पद = 9 होगा।

11. सुधा : कमला : सलमा

$\frac{1}{3} : \frac{2}{5} : \frac{1}{2}$

सरल करने पर, अनुपात = 10 : 12 : 15

अनुपातों का योग = 10 + 12 + 15 = 37

∴ सुधा का भाग = $\frac{1110}{37} \times 10$ = 300 रुपये

कमला का भाग = $\frac{1110}{37} \times 12$ = 360 रुपये

सलमा का भाग = $\frac{1110}{37} \times 15$ = 450 रुपये।

12. तांबा : जस्ता : लोहा

अनुपातों का योग = 7 + 6 + 9 = 22

मिश्रधातु का कुल भार = $\frac{560}{7} \times 22$

= 1760 ग्राम

= 1 किलोग्राम 760 ग्राम।

13. ∵ दूसरी संख्या : तीसरी संख्या = 9 : 16 ....(1)

और प्रथम संख्या : तीसरी संख्या = 1 : 4 ....(2)

(1) तथा (2) में तीसरी संख्या उभयनिष्ठ है अत: उसके मान को समान करने के लिए अनुपात (2) को 4 से गुणा करने पर,

प्रथम संख्या : तीसरी संख्या = 4 : 16

अत: प्रथम संख्या : दूसरी संख्या : तीसरी संख्या

= 4 : 9 : 16

अनुपातों का योग = 4 + 9 + 16 = 29

∴ दूसरी संख्या = $\frac{116}{29} \times 9$ = 36.

14. कुल धन = 1530 रुपये

तीनों के भागों में से कुल कम की गई राशि 5 + 10 + 15 = 30 रुपये

∴ शेष राशि = 1530 – 30 = 1500 रुपये

दिया गया अनुपात = 3 : 4 : 5

अनुपातों का योग = 3 + 4 + 5 = 12

शेष राशि में B का हिस्सा = $\frac{1500}{12} \times 4$ = 500 रुपये

∴ 1530 रुपये में B का हिस्सा = 500 + 10 = 510 रुपये

15. ∵ A के पास B से 20% कम रुपये हैं

∴ A : B = 80 : 100 = 4 : 5 ....(1)

और B के पास C से 25% अधिक रुपये हैं,

∴ B : C = 125 : 100 = 5 : 4 ...(2)

∴ A : B : C = 4 : 5 : 4

नोट—यदि प्रश्न में कुल राशि दी गई होती तो उसे भी उक्त प्रक्रिया में बांटा जा सकता था।

16. ∵ सिक्कों की संख्या का अनुपात = 2 : 3 : 4

∴ सिक्कों **के** मूल्य **का** अनुपात

= 2 × 100 : 3 × 50 : 4 × 25

= 200 : 150 : 100 = 4 : 3 : 2

अनुपातों का योग = 4 + 3 + 2 = 9

∴ एक रुपये के सिक्कों का मूल्य

= $\frac{45}{9} \times 4$ = 20 रुपये

पचास पैसे के सिक्कों का मूल्य

= $\frac{45}{9} \times 3$ = 15 रुपये

पच्चीस पैसे के सिक्कों का मूल्य = $\frac{45}{9} \times 2$ =10 रुपये

∴ एक रुपये के सिक्कों की संख्या = 20 × 1 = 20

पचास पैसे के सिक्कों की संख्या = 15 × 2 = 30

पच्चीस पैसे के सिक्कों की संख्या = 10 × 4 = 40

∴ सिक्कों की कुल संख्या = 20 + 30 + 40 = 90

नोट—उपर्युक्त प्रश्न में सिक्कों की संख्या के अनुपात को मूल्य के अनुपात में बदलने के लिए, जितने पैसे का सिक्का हो उतने ही से गुणा किया गया है।

इसी प्रकार, मूल्य के अनुपात को संख्या के अनुपात में बदलने के लिए, एक रुपये में उस प्रकार के जितने सिक्के हों, उसका गुणा करते हैं। जैसे—25 पैसे, 10 पैसे तथा 5 पैसे के सिक्कों के मूल्य का अनुपात 3 : 4 : 7 हो तो उनकी संख्या का अनुपात

= 3 × 4 : 4 × 10 : 7 × 20

= 12 : 40 : 140 = 3 : 10 : 35

17. ∵ 20 लीटर मिश्रण में दूध = $\frac{3}{4} \times 20$ = 15 लीटर

और पानी = 20 – 15 = 5 लीटर

माना, x लीटर दूध और मिलाया जाए, तो प्रश्नानुसार,

$(15 + x) : 5 = 4 : 1$

या $\frac{15+x}{5} = \frac{4}{1}$ या $15 + x = 20$

या $x = 20 - 15 = 5$

अत: 5 लीटर दूध और मिलाया जाए।

☆☆☆☆☆☆

13 चाल, समय एवं दूरी (Speed, Time and Distance)

याद रखें :

(i) दूरी निकालने के लिए चाल में समय से गुणा करें, अर्थात् दूरी = चाल × समय

(ii) चाल निकालने के लिए दूरी में समय से भाग दें, अर्थात् चाल = $\frac{\text{दूरी}}{\text{समय}}$

(iii) समय निकालने के लिए दूरी में चाल से भाग दें, अर्थात् समय = $\frac{\text{दूरी}}{\text{चाल}}$

(iv) गाड़ी को खम्भा या वृक्ष पार करने में केवल अपनी लम्बाई पार करनी होती है।

(iv) गाड़ी को पुल या प्लेटफार्म पार करने में अपनी लम्बाई और पुल या प्लेटफार्म की लम्बाई दोनों पार करनी होती है।

(vi) जब दो गाड़ियां एक ही दिशा में जा रही हों, तो उनकी आपेक्षिक गति (एक दूसरे को पार करने की गति) निकालने के लिए दोनों गाड़ियों की गति का अंतर निकाला जाता है।

(vii) जब दो गाड़ियां विपरीत दिशा में जा रही हों, तो उनकी आपेक्षिक गति (एक दूसरे को पार करने की गति) निकालने के लिए दोनों गाड़ियों की गति को जोड़ दिया जाता है।

प्रश्नमाला

1. एक गतिमान कार की चाल 36 कि॰मी॰ प्रति घंटा है। इसकी चाल मी॰/से॰ में है:

A. 10 मी॰/से॰ B. 15 मी॰/से॰
C. 20 मी॰/से॰ D. 25 मी॰/से॰

2. दो रेलगाड़ियां एक ही समय दो स्टेशनों X तथा Y से, जिनके मध्य 900 कि॰मी॰ की दूरी है, एक-दूसरे की ओर चलना शुरू करती हैं। यदि उनकी औसत चाल क्रमशः 38 तथा 22 कि॰मी॰/घं॰ हो तो वे एक-दूसरे को कितने समय बाद मिलेंगी?

A. 12 घण्टे B. 13 घण्टे
C. 14 घण्टे D. 15 घण्टे

3. 100 मी॰ लम्बी रेलगाड़ी 60 कि॰मी॰ प्रति घंटा की चाल से जा रही है। इसे एक तार चौकी को पार करने में समय लगेगा:

A. 4 सेकेण्ड B. 5 सेकेण्ड
C. 6 सेकेण्ड D. 8 सेकेण्ड

4. 150 मी॰ लम्बी एक रेलगाड़ी 90 कि॰मी॰ प्रति घंटा की चाल से जा रही है। इसे एक पेड़ को पार करने में समय लगेगा:

A. 3 सेकेण्ड B. 4 सेकेण्ड
C. 6 सेकेण्ड D. 8 सेकेण्ड

5. 100 मी॰ लम्बी एक रेलगाड़ी 65 कि॰मी॰ प्रति घंटा की चाल से जा रही है। यह एक व्यक्ति को जो 5 कि॰मी॰/घंटा की चाल से रेलगाड़ी की दिशा में जा रहा है, कितने समय में पार करेगी?

A. 8 सेकेण्ड B. 6 सेकेण्ड
C. 4 सेकेण्ड D. 2 सेकेण्ड

6. एक व्यक्ति नदी के बहाव की दिशा में 6 कि॰मी॰ प्रति/घं॰ तथा विपरीत दिशा में 3 कि॰मी॰ प्रति/घं॰ की चाल से नाव चलाता है। स्थिर पानी में नाव की चाल है:

A. 9 कि॰मी॰/घं॰ B. 4.5 कि॰मी॰/घं॰
C. 1.5 कि॰मी॰/घं॰ D. 1.0 कि॰मी॰/घं॰

7. प्रश्न 6 में नदी के बहाव की चाल है

A. 1.5 कि॰मी॰/घं॰ B. 2.5 कि॰मी॰/घं॰
C. 4.5 कि॰मी॰/घं॰ D. 18.0 कि॰मी॰/घं॰

8. एक साइकिल सवार 3 मिनट में 1.2 किलोमीटर दूरी तय करता है, तो उसकी गति प्रति घंटा क्या होगी?

A. 24 कि॰मी॰/घंटा B. 24 मी॰/घंटा
C. 24 मी॰/से॰ D. 24 कि॰मी॰/मिनट

9. एक 100 मीटर लम्बी गाड़ी 90 कि॰मी॰/घ॰ की चाल से चल रही है। गाड़ी को पेड़ को पार करने में कितना समय लगेगा?

A. 4 से॰ B. 8 से॰
C. 11 से॰ D. 11 से॰

10. एक रेलगाड़ी जो 90 कि॰मी॰/घं॰ की गति से चली जा रही है। एक खम्भे को पार करने में 10 सेकेण्ड का समय लेती है। बताइये उस रेलगाड़ी की लम्बाई (मीटर में) कितनी होगी?

A. 250 B. 240
C. 280 D. 270

11. 18 किमी प्रति घंटा **की** चाल को मीटर प्रति **सेकेण्ड** में बदलिए।

A. 7 मी॰/से॰ B. 4 मी॰/से॰
C. 6 मी॰/से॰ D. 5 मी॰/से॰

12. 3 मीटर प्रति **सेकेण्ड** की चाल को किमी प्रति घण्टा में बदलिए।

A. 10 किमी॰/घंटा B. 10.8 किमी॰/घंटा
C. 8 किमी॰/घंटा D. 8.10 किमी॰/घंटा

13. 500 मीटर लम्बी रेलगाड़ी 220 मीटर लम्बे प्लेटफार्म को 36 **सेकेण्ड** में पार कर लेती है, तो गाड़ी की चाल किमी प्रति घण्टा ज्ञात करो

A. 60 किमी॰/घंटा B. 65 किमी॰/घंटा
C. 72 किमी॰/घंटा D. 70 किमी॰/घंटा

14. एक आदमी 5 किमी प्रति घण्टा की चाल से P से Q स्थान तक जाता है और 3 किमी प्रति घण्टा की चाल से Q से P स्थान पर वापस आ जाता है। उसकी सारी यात्रा में औसत चाल क्या रही?

A. $4\frac{3}{4}$ किमी॰/घंटा B. $3\frac{3}{4}$ किमी॰/घंटा
C. 4 किमी॰/घंटा D. 3 किमी॰/घंटा

15. एक रेलगाड़ी 60 किमी की दूरी 45 मिनट में तय करती है, यदि इसकी गति 5 किमी/घण्टा कम कर दी जाए तो उसी दूरी को वह कितने समय में तय करेगी?

A. 42 मिनट B. 40 मिनट
C. 45 मिनट D. 48 मिनट

16. एक कार तीन किमी॰ लम्बाई की चार लगातार दूरियों को क्रमशः 10 किमी॰/घण्टा 20 किमी/घण्टा, 30 किमी॰/घण्टा तथा 60 किमी॰/घण्टा की गति से पार करती है। कुल दूरी में उसकी औसत गति है।

A. 30 किमी॰/घंटा B. 35 किमी॰/घंटा
C. 20 किमी॰/घंटा D. 25 किमी॰/घंटा

17. एक **व्यक्ति** कुछ दूरी 5 किमी/घण्टा की चाल से 6 घण्टे में तय की और अगले 12 घण्टे वह 4 किमी/घण्टा की चाल से चला उसकी औसत चाल है।

A. $5\frac{1}{3}$ किमी॰/घंटा B. $5\frac{2}{3}$ किमी॰/घंटा
C. $4\frac{1}{3}$ किमी॰/घंटा D. $4\frac{2}{3}$ किमी॰/घंटा

18. राम एक घण्टे में 5 मील और मोहन 1 घण्टे में 3½ मील चलता है। यदि वे प्रातः काल 6 बजे तक एक साथ चल पड़े तो बताओ कि दोपहर के 11 बजे तक राम, मोहन से कितना आगे निकल जाएगा?

A. 7 मील B. 7½ मील
C. 8 मील D. 8½ मील

19. एक व्यक्ति किसी स्थान तक पैदल जाने और वहां से साईकिल पर आने में 6 घण्टा 15 मिनट लगाता है। अगर वह पैदल जाता और पैदल ही आता तो 7 घण्टा 45 मिनट लगाता। वह साईकिल से ही आता जाता तो कितना समय लगता?

A. 4 घंटा 45 मिनट B. 4 घंटा 50 मिनट
C. 4 घंटा 40 मिनट D. 4 घंटा 30 मिनट

20. एक ट्रेन ठहराव के साथ किसी दूरी तक 60 किमी प्रति घण्टे की रफ्तार से चली और बिना ठहराव के 90 किमी प्रति घंटे की रफ्तार से हर घण्टे के बाद ट्रेन कितने मिनट तक रुकती है?

A. 15 मिनट B. 30 मिनट
C. 20 मिनट D. 25 मिनट

उत्तरमाला

1	2	3	4	5	6	7	8	9	10
A	D	C	C	B	B	A	A	A	A
11	**12**	**13**	**14**	**15**	**16**	**17**	**18**	**19**	**20**
D	B	C	B	D	C	C	B	A	C

व्याख्यात्मक उत्तर

1. चाल $= \frac{36 \text{ कि॰मी॰}}{\text{घंटा}} = \frac{36000 \text{ मी॰}}{3600 \text{ से॰}} = 10$ मी॰/से॰

2. दो रेलगाड़ियों द्वारा 1 घंटे में तय की गई दूरी

$= 38 + 22 = 60$ कि॰मी॰

कुल दूरी = 900 कि॰मी॰

समय $= \frac{900}{60} = 15$ घंटे।

3. दूरी = 100 मी॰

चाल $= \frac{60 \text{ कि॰मी॰}}{\text{घंटा}}$

$= \frac{60000 \text{ मी॰}}{3600 \text{ से॰}} = \frac{50}{3}$ मी॰/से॰

समय $= \frac{\text{दूरी}}{\text{चाल}}$

$= \frac{100}{50/3} = \frac{100 \times 3}{50} = 6$ से॰

4. चाल $= \frac{90 \text{ कि॰मी॰}}{\text{घंटा}} = \frac{90000 \text{ मी॰}}{3600 \text{ से॰}}$

$= 25$ मी॰/से॰

दूरी = 150 मी॰

समय $= \frac{\text{दूरी}}{\text{चाल}} = \frac{150}{25} = 6$ से॰

5. वास्तविक चाल = रेलगाड़ी की चाल – व्यक्ति की चाल

$= 65 - 5 = 60$ कि॰मी॰/घं॰

चाल $= \frac{60 \text{ कि॰मी॰}}{\text{घंटा}} = \frac{60000 \text{ मी॰}}{3600 \text{ से॰}}$

$= \frac{50}{3}$ मी॰/से॰

समय $= \frac{\text{दूरी}}{\text{चाल}} = \frac{100}{50/3} = \frac{100 \times 3}{50}$

$= 6$ से॰

6. स्थिर पानी में नाव की चाल $= \frac{6+3}{2} = \frac{9}{2}$

$= 4.5$ कि॰मी॰/घं॰

7. नदी के बहाव की चाल $= \frac{6-3}{2} = \frac{3}{2}$

$= 1.5$ कि॰मी॰/घंटा

8. गति $= \frac{\text{दूरी}}{\text{समय}}$, दूरी = 1.2 कि॰मी॰

समय = 3 मिनट $= \frac{3}{60}$ घंटा

गति $= \frac{\text{दूरी}}{\text{समय}} = \frac{1.2}{\frac{3}{60}}$

$= \frac{1.2 \times 60}{3} = 24$ कि॰मी॰/घंटा

9. चूंकि रेलगाड़ी सिर्फ पेड़ को पार करती है।

∴ पेड़ को पार करने में लगा समय

$= \frac{100 \text{ मी॰}}{90 \text{ कि॰मी॰/ घं॰}}$

$= \frac{100 \text{ मी॰}}{90 \times \frac{5 \text{ मी॰}}{18 \text{ से॰}}} = 4$ सेकेण्ड

10. चूंकि रेलगाड़ी सिर्फ खम्भे को पार करती है।

∴ खम्भे को पार करने में लगा समय

$= \frac{\text{रेलगाड़ी की लम्बाई}}{\text{रेलगाड़ी की चाल}}$

$\therefore \quad 10 = \dfrac{\text{रेलगाड़ी की लम्बाई}}{90 \times \frac{5}{18} \text{ मी॰/से॰}}$

$\therefore$ रेलगाड़ी की लम्बाई $= 10 \times 90 \times \dfrac{5}{18} = 250$ मीटर।

11. $\because$ 1 किमी = 1000 मीटर और
1घण्टा = 3600 **सेकेण्ड**

$\therefore$ 18 किमी प्रतिघण्टा $= \dfrac{18 \times 1000}{3600} = 5$ मीटर/**सेकेण्ड**।

12. 3 मीटर/**सेकेण्ड** $= \dfrac{3 \times 3600}{1000} = 10.8$ किमी/घण्टा।

13. गाड़ी द्वारा प्लेटफार्म को पार करने में तय की गई दूरी = 500 + 220 = 720 मीटर, समय = 36 **सेकेण्ड**

$\therefore \quad \text{चाल} = \dfrac{\text{दूरी}}{\text{समय}}$

$\therefore$ गाड़ी की चाल $= \dfrac{720}{36}$ मीटर प्रति **सेकेण्ड**

$= \dfrac{720 \times 3600}{36 \times 1000} = 72$ किमी/घण्टा।

14. माना P से Q स्थान की दूरी 15 किमी
(3 और 5 का ल.स.प. 15 है, अत: गणना की सुविधा के लिए 15 किमी दूरी मानी है।)

$\therefore$ जाने में लगा समय $= \dfrac{15}{3} = 5$ घण्टे

और वापस आने में लगा समय $= \dfrac{15}{3} = 5$ घण्टे

कुल दूरी = 15 + 15 = 30 किमी
कुल समय = 3 + 5 = 8 घण्टे

औसत चाल $\dfrac{30}{8} = \dfrac{15}{4} = 3\dfrac{3}{4}$ किमी प्रति घण्टा।

15. $\therefore$ दूरी = 60 किमी, समय = 45 मिनट $= \dfrac{3}{4}$ घण्टा

$\therefore$ चाल $= \dfrac{60 \times 4}{3} =$ 80 किमी प्रति घण्टा
5 किमी/घण्टा, कम होने पर चाल = 75 किमी/घण्टा

$\therefore$ समय $= \dfrac{60}{75} = \dfrac{4}{5}$ घण्टा = 48 मिनट।

16. प्रत्येक तीन किमी की दूरी को तय करने में लगा समय क्रमश:,

$\dfrac{2}{10}, \dfrac{3}{20}, \dfrac{3}{30}, \dfrac{3}{60}$ घण्टा

$\therefore$ कुल समय

$= \left(\dfrac{3}{10} + \dfrac{3}{20} + \dfrac{3}{30} + \dfrac{3}{60}\right) = \dfrac{3}{5}$ घण्टा

दूरी = 3 × 4 = 12 किमी

$\therefore$ चाल $= \dfrac{12 \times 5}{3} = 20$ किमी/घण्टा।

17. कुल दूरी = 5 × 6 + 12 × 4 = 30 + 48
= 78 किमी/घण्टा
कुल समय = 12 + 6 = 18 घण्टे

$\therefore$ औसत चाल $= \dfrac{78}{18} = \dfrac{13}{3} = 4\dfrac{1}{3}$ किमी/घण्टा।

18. $\therefore$ एक घण्टे में राम मोहन से $\left(5 - \dfrac{7}{2}\right) = \dfrac{3}{2}$ मील अधिक चलता है।

$\therefore$ 5 घण्टे में राम मोहन से $\dfrac{3}{2} \times 5 = 7\dfrac{1}{2}$ मील अधिक।

19. एक तरफ पैदल जाना + एक तरफ साईकिल से आना
= 6 घंटा 15 मिनट
या दो तरफ पैदल जाना + दो तरफ साईकिल से आना
= 12 घण्टा 30 मिनट

$\therefore$ दो बार साईकिल से आना = 12 घण्टा 30 मिनट –2 तरफ पैदल जाना
= 12 घण्टा 30 मिनट – 7 घण्टा 45 मिनट
= 4 घण्टा 45 मिनट।

20. प्रति घण्टे रुकने में लगा समय 90 किमी प्रति घण्टे की रफ्तार से बाकी दूरी (90-60) किमी या 30 किमी की दूरी तय करने में लगे समय के बराबर होगा।

$\therefore$ ट्रेन प्रति घण्टे $\dfrac{30}{90} = \dfrac{1}{3}$ घंटा या मिनट 20 रुकती है।

☆☆☆☆☆☆

14 समय एवं कार्य (Time and Work)

ऐकिक नियम के प्रश्नों में पहले इकाई वस्तु का मूल्य ज्ञात करके प्रश्न में दी गई संख्या का मूल्य निकालते हैं। उदाहरण के लिए प्रश्न है–

7 बकरियों की कीमत 630 रु० है, तो 20 बकरियों की कीमत क्या होगी?

ऐकिक नियम विधि से इस प्रश्न को हल करने में पहले एक बकरी की कीमत निकालनी होगी। उसके बाद 20 बकरियों की कीमत निकाली जायेगी।

ऐसे प्रश्नों को हल करते समय जो भाषा लिखी जाती है, उसमें जिस राशि या मद का उत्तर निकालना हो, उसे सबसे बाद में लिखा जाता है। जैसे–

उदाहरण 1. 7 बकरियों की कीमत 630 रु० है, तो 20 बकरियों की कीमत क्या होगी? इस प्रश्न में हमें कीमत निकालनी है (रु० में), अतः प्रश्न की भाषा लिखते समय रु० दाँयी ओर लिखेंगे।

हलः $\because$ 7 बकरियों की कीमत = 630 रु०

$\therefore$ 1 बकरी (इकाई) की कीमत = $\frac{630}{7}$ रु०

$\therefore$ 20 बकरियों की कीमत = $\frac{630}{7} \times 20 = 1800$ रु०

उदाहरण 2. 10 आदमी 1 काम को 30 दिनों में पूरा करते हैं। उसी काम को 15 आदमी कितने दिनों में पूरा करेंगे?

हलः इस प्रश्न में हमें दिन निकालने हैं। इसलिए इसे निम्न प्रकार से हल करेंगे।

$\because$ 10 आदमी एक काम को करते हैं = 30 दिनों में

$\therefore$ 1 आदमी उस काम को करेगा = 10×30 दिनों में

$\therefore$ 15 आदमी उसी काम को करेंगे = $\frac{10 \times 30}{15}$

= 20 दिनों में

नोटः

(i) यदि एक आदमी एक काम को 10 दिनों में करता है, तो उसका एक दिन का काम होगा = $\frac{1}{10}$ भाग

(ii) यदि किसी आदमी का एक दिन का काम $\frac{1}{10}$ हो, तो वह पूरा काम 10 दिनों में करेगा।

(iii) ऐसे प्रश्नों में पहले एक दिन का काम निकाला जाता है।

(iv) यदि काम करने वाले आदमी बढ़ जायें, तो काम कम समय (कम दिनों) में पूरा होगा और यदि काम करने वाले आदमी कम हो जायें, तो काम अधिक समय (अधिक दिनों) में पूरा होगा।

उदाहरण 3. यदि 15 आदमी किसी काम को 24 दिनों में करते हैं, तो कितने आदमी उसी काम को 18 दिनों में पूरा करेंगे?

हलः इस प्रश्न में हमें आदमी निकालने हैं, अतः इसे निम्न प्रकार से हल करेंगेः

24 दिन में काम पूरा करते हैं = 15 आदमी

$\therefore$ 1 दिन में काम पूरा करेंगे = 15×24

$\therefore$ 18 दिन में काम पूरा करेंगे = $\frac{15 \times 24}{18}$ = 20 आदमी

उदाहरण 4. एक रेलगाड़ी 50 मिनट में 60 कि॰मी॰ की दूरी तय करती है 210 कि॰मी॰ की दूरी तय करने में उसे कितना समय लगेगा?

हलः इस प्रश्न में हमें समय निकालना है। अतः हल इस प्रकार निकाला जाएगा।

$\because$ 60 कि॰मी॰ की दूरी तय करती है = 50 मिनट में

$\therefore$ 1 कि॰मी॰ की दूरी तय करेगी = $\frac{50}{60}$ मिनट में

$\therefore$ 210 कि॰मी॰ की दूरी तय करेगी = $\frac{50}{60} \times 210$

= 175 मिनट में

प्रश्नमाला

1. A एक काम को 6 दिन में तथा B उसे 10 दिन में कर सकता है। A तथा B मिलकर उसे पूरा करेंगे।

A. 10 दिन से कम तथा 6 दिन से अधिक दिनों में

B. 10 दिन से अधिक दिनों में

C. 6 दिन से कम दिनों में

D. 2 दिन में

2. A एक मेज को 3 दिन में तथा उसका मित्र उसे 6 दिन में बना सकता है। A और उसका मित्र मिलकर उसे पूरा बनाएंगेः

A. 3 दिन में B. 2 दिन में

C. 1 दिन में D. $\frac{1}{2}$ दिन में

3. X और Y मिलकर किसी कार्य को 10 दिन में कर सकते हैं। X अकेला उसे 15 दिन में कर सकता है तो Y उसे कितने दिन में करेगा?

A. 15 दिन B. 20 दिन

C. 25 दिन D. 30 दिन

4. 24 आदमी एक मशीन को 12 दिन में तैयार करते हैं तो 36 आदमी उसे कितने दिनों में तैयार करेंगे?

A. 8 दिन B. 12 दिन

C. 16 दिन D. 20 दिन

5. X, Y और Z किसी काम को क्रमशः 8, 10 और 8 दिन में कर सकते हैं। तीनों मिलकर उस कार्य को कितने दिनों में कर सकेंगे?

A. $2\frac{1}{7}$ दिन B. $2\frac{3}{7}$ दिन

C. $2\frac{5}{7}$ दिन D. $2\frac{6}{7}$ दिन

6. A एक काम को 5 दिन में तथा B उसी काम को 10 दिन में पूरा करता है तो बताइये (A + B) उस काम को कितने दिनों में पूरा करेंगे?

A. $2\frac{3}{4}$ दिन B. $3\frac{3}{4}$ दिन

C. $3\frac{1}{3}$ दिन D. $2\frac{1}{4}$ दिन

7. 3 पेन और 5 पैन्सिलों का मूल्य 14 रु. है। 12 पेन और 20 पेन्सिलों का क्या मूल्य होगा?

A. 42 रु. B. 56 रु.

C. 20 रु. D. 112 रु.

8. x, y और z मिलकर एक कार्य को 8 दिन में पूरा कर सकते हैं। यदि x और z मिलकर उस कार्य को 12 दिन में पूरा कर सकते हों तो बताइये y अकेला उस कार्य को पूरा कितने दिन में करेगा?

A. 22 दिन B. 24 दिन

C. $17\frac{1}{4}$ दिन D. 23 दिन

9. यदि 75 संतरों की एक पेटी का मूल्य 60 रु. है तो 50 संतरों का मूल्य होगाः

A. 30 रु. B. 40 रु.

C. 50 रु. D. 60 रु.

10. एक नल एक हौज को 4 घण्टे में तथा दूसरा नल उस हौज को 5 घण्टे में भर सकता है। यदि दोनों नल एक साथ खोल दिए जाएं तो हौज को भरने में कितने घण्टे लगेंगे?

A. $3\frac{2}{9}$ घण्टे B. $2\frac{2}{9}$ घण्टे

C. $2\frac{1}{9}$ घण्टे D. $3\frac{5}{9}$ घण्टे

11. यदि 210 रुपए में 6 बाल्टियां खरीदी जा सकती है तो 140 रुपए में कितनी बाल्टियां खरीदी जा सकेंगी।

A. 4 B. 3

C. 5 D. 6

12. गणित की 14 पुस्तकों का मूल्य 105 रुपए है तो बताइए ऐसी ही 24 पुस्तकों के लिए क्या मूल्य देना होगा?

A. 170 रु. B. 175 रु.

C. 180 रु. D. 185 रु.

13. यदि 3000 रुपए में 12 रेडियो सैट खरीदे जा सकते हों, तो बताओ 3750 रुपए में कितने रेडियो सैट खरीदे जा सकेंगे।

A. 12 B. 15

C. 10 D. 17

14. किसी परिवार के 6 सदस्यों के लिए 20 दिन की भोजन सामग्री है, तो बताओ 4 सदस्यों वाले परिवार के लिए यही भोजन सामग्री कितने दिनों के लिए पर्याप्त होगी।

A. 25 दिन B. 35 दिन
C. 20 दिन D. 30 दिन

15. 15 मजदूर एक खेत की गुड़ाई 6 घण्टे में कर सकते हैं तो बताइये 2 घण्टे में उस खेत की गुड़ाई करने के लिए कितने मजदूर चाहिए?

A. 40 B. 45
C. 50 D. 55

16. यदि 20 पुरुष किसी काम को 3 दिन में पूरा कर सकते हैं तथा 12 महिलाएं उसी काम को 12 दिन में पूरा कर सकती हैं तो 20 पुरुष तथा 20 महिलाएं मिलकर उस काम को कितने दिन में पूरा कर लेंगे?

A. $3\frac{3}{17}$ दिन B. $2\frac{3}{17}$ दिन
C. $3\frac{2}{17}$ दिन D. $2\frac{2}{17}$ दिन

17. यदि 10 आदमी या 18 लड़के किसी काम को 15 दिन में कर सकते हैं तो 25 आदमी और 15 लड़के उससे दुगुने काम को कितने दिन में करेंगे?

A. 12 दिन B. 15 दिन
C. 10 दिन D. 17 दिन

उत्तरमाला

1	2	3	4	5	6	7	8	9	10
C	B	D	A	D	C	B	B	B	B
11	**12**	**13**	**14**	**15**	**16**	**17**			
A	C	B	D	B	D	B			

व्याख्यात्मक उत्तर

1. A का 1 दिन का काम $= \frac{1}{6}$

B का 1 दिन का काम $= \frac{1}{10}$

(A + B) का 1 दिन का काम $= \frac{1}{6}+\frac{1}{10}=\frac{8}{30}$

$\therefore$ A + B मिलकर उसे $\frac{30}{8}$ दिन में करेंगे

$= 3\frac{6}{8}$ दिन $= 3\frac{3}{4}$ दिन

जो 6 दिन से कम है।

2. A तथा उसके मित्र द्वारा 1 दिन में किया गया कार्य

$= \frac{1}{3}+\frac{1}{6}=\frac{3}{6}$

$\therefore$ दोनों मिलकर उसे पूरा करेंगे $= \frac{6}{3} = 2$ दिन में।

3. X और Y का दिन का काम $= \frac{1}{10}$

अकेले X का 1 दिन का काम $= \frac{1}{15}$

अकेले Y का 1 दिन का काम $= \frac{1}{10}-\frac{1}{15}=\frac{1}{30}$

$\therefore$ Y अकेला उस काम को 30 दिन में करेगा।

4. $\because$ 24 व्यक्ति एक मशीन को बनाते हैं = 12 दिन में

$\therefore$ 1 व्यक्ति एक मशीन को बनाता है $= 24 \times 12$ दिन में।

$\therefore$ 36 व्यक्ति एक मशीन को बनाते हैं

$= \frac{24 \times 12}{36} = 8$ दिन में।

5. X + Y + Z का 1 दिन का काम

$= \frac{1}{8}+\frac{1}{10}+\frac{1}{8}=\frac{7}{20}$

$\therefore$ X + Y + Z उसे पूरा करेंगे $= \frac{20}{7}$ दिन

$= 2\frac{6}{7}$ दिन में

6. $\because$ A का 1 दिन का काम $= \frac{1}{5}$

तथा B का 1 दिन का काम $= \frac{1}{10}$

$\therefore$ (A + B) का 1 दिन का काम

$= \frac{1}{5} + \frac{1}{10} = \frac{2+1}{10} = \frac{3}{10}$

चूंकि $\frac{3}{10}$ काम (A + B) करते हैं = 1 दिन में

$\therefore$ पूरा काम (A + B) करेंगे $= \frac{10}{3} = 3\frac{1}{3}$ दिन में

7. $\because$ 3 पेन तथा 5 पेन्सिलों का मूल्य = 14 रु॰

$\therefore$ 1 पेन तथा 1 पेन्सिल का मूल्य

$= \frac{14}{\text{3 पेन तथा 5 पेन्सिल}}$

$\therefore$ 4 × (3 पेन तथा 5 पेन्सिलों) का मूल्य

$= \frac{14 \times 4 \times (\text{3 पेन तथा 5 पेंसिल})}{\text{3 पेन तथा 5 पेंसिल}}$ = 56 रुपये।

8. $\because$ $z(x + y + z)$ का 1 दिन का काम $= \frac{1}{8}$

तथा $(x + z)$ का 1 दिन का काम $= \frac{1}{12}$

$\therefore$ y का 1 दिन का काम $= \frac{1}{8} - \frac{1}{12}$

$= \frac{3-2}{24} = \frac{1}{24}$

चूंकि $\frac{1}{24}$ काम y करता है = 1 दिन में

$\therefore$ पूरा काम y करेगा 24 दिन में।

9. $\because$ 75 संतरों का मूल्य = 60 रु॰

$\because$ 1 संतरे का मूल्य $= \frac{60}{75}$

$\therefore$ 50 संतरों का मूल्य $= \frac{60}{75} \times 50$ = 40 रु॰

10. पहले नल द्वारा 1 घण्टे में हौज का भरा भाग $= \frac{1}{4}$

तथा दूसरे नल द्वारा 1 घण्टे में हौज का भरा भाग $= \frac{1}{5}$

$\therefore$ (पहले + दूसरे) नल द्वारा 1 घण्टे में हौज का भरा भाग

$= \frac{1}{4} + \frac{1}{5} = \frac{5+4}{20} = \frac{9}{20}$

चूंकि हौज का $\frac{9}{20}$ भाग (पहले + दूसरे) नल भरते हैं = 1 घण्टे में

$\therefore$ पूरा भाग (पहले + दूसरे) नल भरेंगे $\frac{20}{9} = 2\frac{2}{9}$ घण्टे में।

11.

रुपए	बाल्टियां
210	6
140	?

$\because$ 210 रुपए में खरीदी जाने वाली बाल्टियों की संख्या = 6

$\therefore$ 1 रुपए में खरीदी जाने वाली बाल्टियां $= \frac{6}{210}$

$\therefore$ 140 रुपए में खरीदी जाने वाली बाल्टियां

$= \frac{6}{210} \times 140$ = 4 बाल्टियां

अत: 140 रुपए में 4 बाल्टियां खरीदी जा सकेंगी।

12.

पुस्तक	मूल्य
14	105 रुपए
24	?

$\because$ गणित की 14 पुस्तकों का मूल्य = 105 रुपए

$\therefore$ गणित की 1 पुस्तक का मूल्य $= \frac{105}{14}$ रुपए

$\therefore$ गणित की 24 पुस्तकों का मूल्य

$= \frac{105}{14} \times 24$ रुपए

= **180 रुपए**

अत: गणित की 24 पुस्तकों का मूल्य = 180 रुपए **होगा।**

13.

रुपए	रेडियो सैट
3000	12
3750	?

$\because$ 3000 रुपए में खरीदे जा सकते हैं = 12 रेडियो सैट

$\therefore$ 1 रुपए में खरीदे जा सकते हैं $= \frac{12}{3000}$ रेडियो सैट

$\therefore$ 3750 रुपए में खरीदे जा सकते हैं

$= \frac{12}{3000} \times 3750$ रेडियो सैट = 15 रेडियो सैट

अत: 3750 रुपए में 15 रेडियो सैट खरीदे जा सकेंगे।

14.

सदस्य	**दिन**
6	20
4	?

$\because$ 6 सदस्यों के लिए भोजन सामग्री है = 20 दिनों के लिए

$\therefore$ 1 सदस्य के लिए भोजन सामग्री है = 20 × 6 दिनों के लिए

$\therefore$ 4 सदस्यों के लिए भोजन सामग्री है = $\frac{20 \times 6}{4}$ दिनों के लिए = 30 दिन के लिए

अत: 4 सदस्यों वाले परिवार के लिए यही भोजन सामग्री 30 दिन के लिए पर्याप्त होगी।

15. *(i)*

घंटे	**मजदूर**
6	15
2	?

(ii)

मजदूर	**घंटे**
15	6
20	?

(i) $\because$ 6 घंटे में खेत की गुड़ाई करते है = 15 मजदूर

$\therefore$ 1 घंटे में खेत की गुड़ाई करेंगे = 15 × 6 मजदूर

$\therefore$ 2 घंटे में खेत की गुड़ाई करेंगे = $\frac{15 \times 6}{2}$ मजदूर

= 45 मजदूर

अत: 2 घंटे में उस खेत की गुड़ाई करने के लिए 45 मजदूर चाहिए।

16. $\because$ 3 दिन में पूरा काम करते हैं = 20 पुरुष

$\therefore$ 1 दिन में पूरा काम करते हैं = 20 × 3 = 60 पुरुष

$\because$ 12 दिन में पूरा करती हैं = 12 महिलाएं

$\therefore$ 1 दिन में पूरा करती है = 12 × 12

= 144 महिलाएं

$\therefore$ 60 पुरुषों का काम = 144 महिलाओं का काम

$\therefore$ 1 पुरुष का काम = $\frac{144}{60}$

$\therefore$ 20 पुरुषों का काम = $\frac{144 \times 20}{60}$

= 48 महिलाओं का काम

$\therefore$ 20 पुरुष + 20 महिलाओं का काम = 48 + 20

= 68 महिलाओं के काम के

$\because$ 48 महिलाएं 1 काम करती है = 3 दिन में

$\therefore$ 1 महिला 1 काम करती है = 3 × 48 दिन में

$\therefore$ 68 महिलाएं 1 काम करती है = $\frac{3 \times 48}{68}$

$= \frac{36}{17} = 2\frac{2}{17}$ दिन में।

17. $\because$ 10 आदमियों का काम = 18 लड़कों का काम

$\therefore$ 1 आदमी का काम = $\frac{18}{10}$ लड़कों का काम

$\therefore$ 25 आदमियों का काम = $\frac{18}{10} \times 25$

= 45 लड़कों का काम

$\therefore$ 25 आदमी + 15 लड़कों का काम = 45 + 15

= 60 लड़कों का काम

$\because$ 18 लड़के 1 काम को करते हैं = 15 दिन में

$\therefore$ 1 लड़का 1 काम को करता है = 15 × 18 दिन में

$\because$ 60 लड़के 2 काम को करते हैं = $\frac{15 \times 18}{60} \times 2$

= 9 दिन में।

☆☆☆☆☆☆

15 समय एवं दूरी (Time and Distance)

समय पर आधारित प्रश्नों के उत्तर देने के लिए निम्न बातें जानना आवश्यक है।

(i) 12 मध्यरात्रि से 12 मध्याह्न के समय पूर्वाह्न तथा 12 मध्याह्न से 12 मध्यरात्रि तक के समय को अपराह्न कहा जाता है।

(ii) 12 मध्यरात्रि को 24:00 बजे या 00:00 बजे लिखा जाता है।

(iii) 12 मध्यरात्रि को 12:00 बजे लिखा जाता है।

(iv) दाईं ओर के दो अंकों से बनने वाली संख्या मिनटों की संख्या दर्शाती है।
जैसे–10 : 15

(v) यदि बाईं ओर के दो अंकों से बनने वाली संख्या 12 से कम हो तो यह (मध्यरात्रि के बाद का समय) पूर्वाह्न कहलाती है। जैसे–
10:30 बजे = 10:30 पूर्वाह्न
11:45 बजे = 11:45 पूर्वाह्न

(vi) यदि बाईं ओर के दो अंकों से बनने वाली संख्या 12 से अधिक हो तो यह (दोपहर के बाद का समय) अपराह्न कहलाती है, जैसे–
18 : 15 बजे = 6 : 15 अपराह्न
20 : 30 बजे = 8 : 30 अपराह्न

उदाहरण 1. एक रेलगाड़ी सायं 5:40 बजे मुम्बई से चलती है और अगले दिन प्रातः 10:55 बजे नई दिल्ली पहुंचती है। रेलगाड़ी द्वारा तय यात्रा में लिया गया समय है।

हलः मुम्बई से प्रस्थान समय = 5:40
नई दिल्ली आगमन समय = 10:55 (अगले दिन)
कुल समय = 5:40 से 5:40 (अगले दिन) = 12 घंटा
तथा 5:40 से 10:55 तक = 5 घंटे 15 मिनट
= 17 घंटे 15 मिनट

प्रश्नमाला

1. वैशाली सुपर फास्ट गाड़ी दिल्ली से 19:45 बजे रवाना होती है और अगले दिन 15:20 बजे मुज़फ्फरपुर पहुंचती है। बताओ यह मुज़फ्फरपुर पहुंचने में कितना समय लेती है?
A. 19 घंटा 25 मिनट
B. 18 घंटा 35 मिनट
C. 19 घंटा 35 मिनट
D. 18 घंटा 20 मिनट

2. मनु किसी सोमवार को रात में 9:30 पर सोया और अगले दिन 5:50 पर जागा। उसके सोने की अवधि कितनी थी?
A. 8 घंटे 20 मिनट
B. 8 घंटे 10 मिनट
C. 7 घंटे 40 मिनट
D. 7 घंटे 20 मिनट

3. इन्टरसिटी रेलगाड़ी रक्सौल से सुबह 9:15 पर चलती है तथा उसी दिन 11 बजे पीपरा पहुंचती है। रेलगाड़ी द्वारा यात्रा में लिया गया कुल समय है?
A. 1 घंटा 15 मिनट
B. 10 घंटे 45 मिनट
C. 1 घंटा 45 मिनट
D. 10 घंटे 15 मिनट

4. यदि किसी दिन सूर्य 6:20 पूर्वाह्न पर उदय हो तथा 6:57 अपराह्न पर अस्त हो तो उस दिन की लम्बाई होगी।

A. 12 घंटे 27 मिनट
B. 12 घंटे 17 मिनट
C. 12 घंटे 37 मिनट
D. 12 घंटे

5. 9 घंटे 30 मिनट बराबर है।
A. 0.90 बजे
B. 9:30 पूर्व॰ के
C. 8 घंटे 90 मिनट के
D. 9:30 अप॰ के

6. एक बस शिमला से दिल्ली के लिए 7:20 बजे प्रातः प्रस्थान करती है और दिल्ली पहुंचने में 9 घंटे का समय लेती है। बस कितने बजे दिल्ली पहुंचती है?
A. 4:20 बजे अप॰
B. 3:30 बजे अप॰
C. 6:30 बजे अप॰
D. 7:30 बजे अप॰

7. एक वायुयान मुम्बई से 7:50 बजे उड़ान भरता है। यह चेन्नई 10:30 बजे हवाई हड्डे पर उतरता है। यह चेन्नई पहुंचने में कितना समय लेता है।
A. 2 घंटे 30 मिनट
B. 2 घंटे
C. 3 घंटे लगभग
D. 2 घंटे 40 मिनट

8. एक लड़का रात्रि 8:30 बजे सोने के लिए गया तथा प्रातः 6:15 पर जागा। वह लड़का कितनी देर तक सोया?
A. 9 घंटे 45 मिनट
B. 9 घंटे 15 मिनट
C. 2 घंटे 15 मिनट
D. 4 घंटे 45 मिनट

9. एक छात्र अपने घर से विद्यालय के लिए प्रातः 8:30 बजे साईकिल से चला। वह विद्यालय से पढ़ाई करने के बाद सांय 4:50 बजे घर वापस आया। वह कितने समय तक घर से बाहर रहा।
A. 7 घंटे 20 मिनट
B. 8 घंटे 20 मिनट
C. 9 घंटे 20 मिनट
D. 7 घंटे 90 मिनट

10. एक स्कूल की वार्षिक परीक्षा 18 मार्च, 2002 को आरम्भ हुई और 23 मार्च, 2002 को समाप्त हुई। परीक्षा कितने दिन तक चली?
A. एक सप्ताह B. 8 दिन
C. 6 दिन D. 1 महीना

उत्तरमाला

1	2	3	4	5	6	7	8	9	10
C	A	C	C	B	A	D	A	B	C

व्याख्यात्मक उत्तर

1. दिल्ली से प्रस्थान का समय = 19:45
मुज़फ्फरपुर में आगमन समय = 15:20
कुल समय = 19:45 से 24:00
= 4 घंटे 15 मिनट
= 00:00 से 15:20
= 15 घंटे 20 मिनट
= 19 घंटे 35 मिनट

2. सोने का समय = 9:30
जागने का समय = 5:30
कुल समय = 9:30 से 12:00 बजे मध्य रात्रि तक
= 2 घंटे 30 मिनट
= 12:00 से 5:50 बजे सुबह तक
= 5 घंटे 50 मिनट
अर्थात् 7 घंटे 80 मिनट
= 8 घंटे 20 मिनट

3. रक्सौल से प्रस्थान समय = 9:15
पीपरा में आगमन समय = 11:00
कुल समय = आगमन समय – प्रस्थान समय
= 11:00 – 9:15 = 1 घंटा 45 मिनट

4. सूर्योदय होने का समय = 6:20
अस्त होने का समय = 6:57
कुल समय = प्रातः 6:20 से 6:20 शाम तक
= 12 घंटे
= शेष 37 मिनट
कुल समय = 12 घंटे 37 मिनट

5. दो अंकों से बनने वाली संख्या 12 से कम हो, तो वह पूर्वाह्न कहलाती है।
इस प्रकार 9:30 दर्शाता है 9:30 पूर्वाह्न

6. शिमला से प्रस्थान का समय = 7:20 प्रातः
दिल्ली पहुंचने में लगा समय = 9 घंटे
= 7:20 से 7:20 तक = 12 घंटे
9 घंटे के लिए = 7:20 – 3 = 4 : 20 अप॰

7. मुम्बई से उड़ान भरने का समय = 7:50
चेन्नई पहुंचने का समय = 10:30
कुल समय = आगमन का समय – प्रस्थान का समय
= 10:30 – 7:50
= 2 घंटे 40 मिनट

8. सोने का समय = 8:30 शाम
जागने का समय = 6:15 सुबह
कुल समय = 8:30 से 12 बजे रात तक
= 3 घंटे 30 मिनट
= 12 बजे रात से 6:15 सुबह तक
= 6 घंटे 15 मिनट
कुल समय = 9 घंटे 45 मिनट

9. विद्यालय जाने का समय = 8:30 प्रातः
वापस आने का समय = 4:50 शाम
= 8:30 से 12 बजे दिन तक = 3:30
= 12 बजे दिन से 4:50 बजे शाम तक
= 4:50
अर्थात् 7:80
= 8 घंटे 20 मिनट

10. परीक्षा की शुरुआत = 18 मार्च, 2002
परीक्षा की समाप्ति = 23 मार्च, 2002
कुल समय = 23 मार्च, 2002 से — 18 मार्च, 2002 तक = 6 दिन

☆☆☆☆☆☆

16 क्षेत्रमिति : रेखीय आकृति एवं वृत्त (Mensuration: Plane Figures and Circles)

क्षेत्रमिति से सम्बंधित प्रश्नों को हल करने के लिए निम्नलिखित प्रमुख सूत्रों का जानना आवश्यक होता है :

1. आयत:

(*a*) आयत का क्षेत्रफल = लम्बाई × चौड़ाई

(*b*) आयत की परिमिति = 2 (लम्बाई + चौड़ाई)

(*c*) आयत का विकर्ण = $\sqrt{(\text{लं.})^2 + (\text{चौ.})^2}$

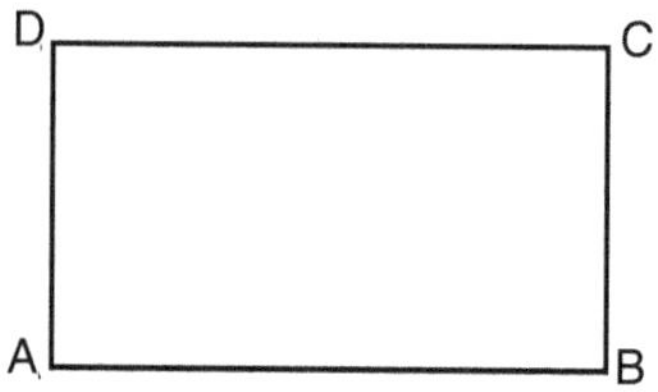

∴ AB = CD तथा BC = AD

2. वर्ग:

(*a*) वर्ग का क्षेत्रफल = (भुजा)^2

(*b*) वर्ग का परिमाप = 4 × भुजा

(*c*) वर्ग का विकर्ण = $\sqrt{2}$ × भुजा

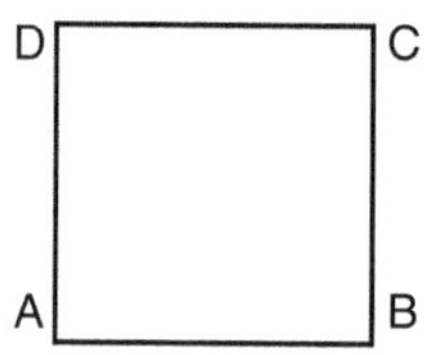

∴ AB = BC = CD = DA = भुजा

3. वृत्त:

(*a*) वृत्त का क्षेत्रफल = π × (त्रिज्या)^2

(*b*) वृत्त की परिधि = 2π × (त्रिज्या)

(*c*) त्रिज्या = $\frac{\text{व्यास}}{2}$ या व्यास = 2 × त्रिज्या

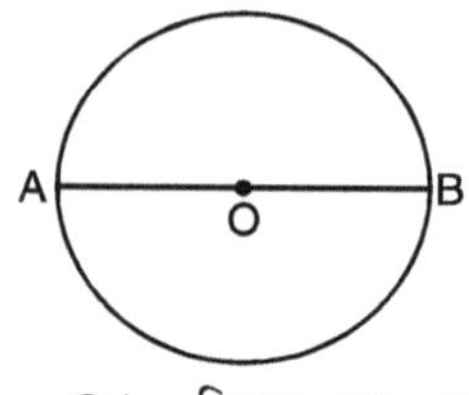

∴ OA = त्रिज्या, AB = व्यास

4. त्रिभुज :

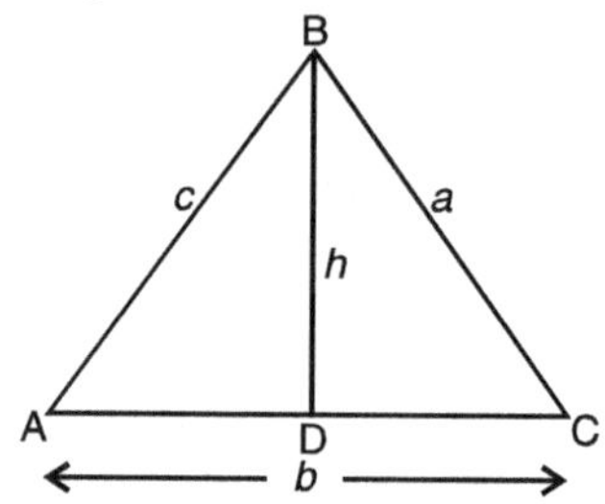

(*a*) त्रिभुज का क्षेत्रफल = $\sqrt{s(s-a)(s-b)(s-c)}$

जहां $s = \frac{a+b+c}{2}$

(*b*) यदि त्रिभुज समकोण हो तब

क्षेत्रफल = $\frac{1}{2}$ × आधार (*b*) × ऊंचाई (*h*)

(*c*) समबाहु त्रिभुज का क्षेत्रफल = $\frac{\sqrt{3}}{4}$ × (भुजा)^2

5. चतुर्भुज:

(*a*) चतुर्भुज का क्षेत्रफल = $\frac{1}{2}$ × विकर्ण × (शीर्ष लम्बों का योग)

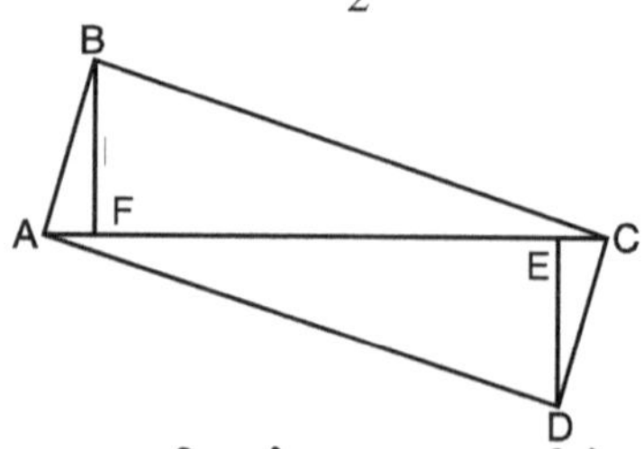

∴ AC = विकर्ण, BF व DE = शीर्ष लम्ब

(*b*) समान्तर चतुर्भुज का क्षेत्रफल = आधार × ऊंचाई

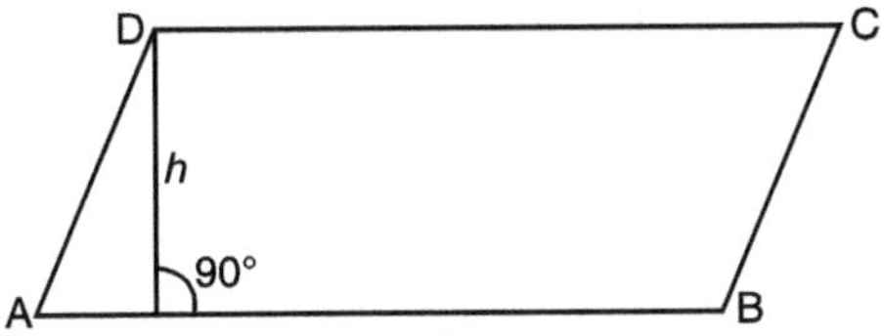

AB = आधार, ऊंचाई = *h*

(*c*) सम चतुर्भुज का क्षेत्रफल = $\frac{1}{2}$ × विकर्णों का गुणनफल

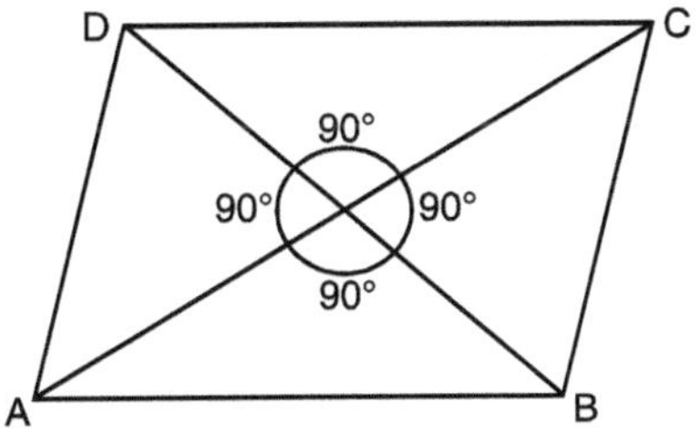

AC, BD = विकर्ण

AB = BC = CD = DA

(*d*) समलम्ब चतर्भुज का क्षेत्रफल = $\frac{1}{2}$ × ऊंचाई × समान्तर भुजाओं का योग

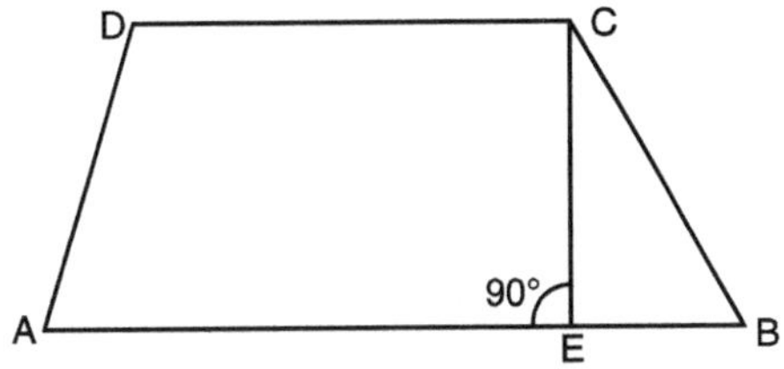

AB, CD = समान्तर भुजाएं, CE = ऊँचाई

6. चार दीवारों का:

(*a*) चार दीवारों का क्षेत्रफल = 2 × ऊंचाई (लम्बाई + चौड़ाई)

(*b*) ऊंचाई = $\dfrac{\text{क्षेत्रफल}}{2\ (\text{लम्बाई + चौड़ाई})}$

प्रश्नमाला

1. एक आयत की लम्बाई व चौड़ाई क्रमशः 50 **सेंमी.** व 25 **सेंमी.** है, तो उसका क्षेत्रफल कितना होगा?

A. 1150 वर्ग **सेंमी.** B. 1250 वर्ग **सेंमी.**
C. 1275 वर्ग **सेंमी.** D. 1280 वर्ग **सेंमी.**

2. एक वर्गाकार मैदान का परिमाप 580 मी. है, तो बताइये उस मैदान का क्षेत्रफल कितना होगा?

A. 21025 वर्ग मी. B. 20225 वर्ग मी.
C. 30025 वर्ग मी. D. 19975 वर्ग मी.

3. एक वर्ग की प्रत्येक भुजा 20 **सेंमी.** है, तो इसका क्षेत्रफल कितना होगा?

A. 300 वर्ग **सेंमी.** B. 380 वर्ग **सेंमी.**
C. 360 वर्ग **सेंमी.** D. 400 वर्ग **सेंमी.**

4. एक वृत्त का क्षेत्रफल 154 वर्ग **सेंमी.** है। वृत्त की परिधि कितनी होगी?

A. 44 **सेंमी.** B. 48 **सेंमी.**
C. 54 **सेंमी.** D. 68 **सेंमी.**

5. यदि किसी त्रिभुज का आधार 8 सेमी तथा ऊंचाई 10 **सेंमी.** हो तो उस त्रिभुज का क्षेत्रफल कितना होगा?

A. 40 वर्ग **सेंमी.** B. 20 वर्ग **सेंमी.**
C. 49 वर्ग **सेंमी.** D. 64 वर्ग **सेंमी.**

6. एक समलम्ब चतुर्भज की समान्तर भुजाएं क्रमशः 15 मी. तथा 25 मी. हैं तथा उनके बीच की दूरी 10 मी. है, तो इसका क्षेत्रफल क्या होगा?

A. 150 वर्ग मी. B. 225 वर्ग मी.
C. 200 वर्ग मी. D. 270 वर्ग मी.

7. एक आयताकार खेत का परिमाप 760 मी. है तथा उसकी लम्बाई व चौड़ाई में 11 : 8 का अनुपात है। तो बताइये आयताकार खेत का क्षेत्रफल क्या होगा?

A. 35200 वर्ग मी. B. 34700 वर्ग मी.
C. 35600 वर्ग मी. D. 45200 वर्ग मी.

8. यदि किसी वर्ग की भुजा में 50% की कमी कर दी जाये, तो उसका क्षेत्रफल कितने प्रतिशत घट जायेगा?

A. 50% B. 75%
C. 80% D. 60%

9. उस वर्ग की एक भुजा की लम्बाई क्या होगी जिसका क्षेत्रफल क्रमशः 6.4 मी. लम्बे तथा 2.5 मी. चौड़े आयत के क्षेत्रफल के बराबर हो?

A. 8 मी. B. 5.4 मी.

C. 3.8 मी. D. 4 मी.

10. यदि एक समकोण त्रिभुज का परिमाप उसकी सबसे छोटी भुजा का छः गुना हो तो उस त्रिभुज की तीनों भुजाओं के बीच क्या अनुपात होगा?

A. 13 : 5 : 12 B. 13 : 12 : 5

C. 12 : 5 : 13 D. 13 : 5 : 10

11. एक वर्ग का परिमाप 24 मी. तथा दूसरे वर्ग का परिमाप 32 मी. है। तो उस वर्ग का परिमाप क्या होगा जिसका क्षेत्रफल दोनों वर्गों के क्षेत्रफल के बराबर है?

A. 40 मी. B. 51 मी.

C. 37 मी. D. 42 मी.

12. यदि किसी वर्ग की भुजा को दुगुना कर दिया जाए तो उस वर्ग का क्षेत्रफल कितने गुना बढ़ जाएगा?

A. दो गुना B. चार गुना

C. तीन गुना D. आठ गुना

13. दो वर्गों के क्षेत्रफल में 225 वर्ग मी. अन्तर है। यदि बड़े वर्ग की भुजा 25 मी. हो तो छोटे वर्ग की भुजा कितनी होगी?

A. 18 मी. B. 21 मी.

C. 20 मी. D. 22 मी.

14. यदि एक समबाहु त्रिभुज का परिमाप 72 **सेंमी.** है तो उस समबाहु त्रिभुज का क्षेत्रफल क्या होगा?

A. $144\sqrt{3}$ वर्ग **सेंमी.** B. $142\sqrt{3}$ वर्ग **सेंमी.**

C. $154\sqrt{2}$ वर्ग **सेंमी.** D. $144\sqrt{2}$ वर्ग **सेंमी.**

15. दो वृत्तों की त्रिज्या क्रमशः 5 **सेंमी.** तथा 12 **सेंमी.** हो तो उस नए वृत्त की त्रिज्या क्या होगी जिसका क्षेत्रफल दोनों वृत्तों के क्षेत्रफल के बराबर हो?

A. 15 **सेंमी.** B. 13 **सेंमी.**

C. 10 **सेंमी.** D. 8 **सेंमी.**

16. एक वृत्त की परिधि तथा एक वर्ग का परिमाप बराबर है। तो बताइये उनके क्षेत्रफलों का अनुपात क्या होगा?

A. 14 : 11 B. 7 : 8

C. 14 : 13 D. 13 : 11

17. एक त्रिभुज की भुजाएं क्रमशः 17 : 15 : 8 के अनुपात में हैं। यदि उस त्रिभुज का परिमाप 40 मी. हो तो त्रिभुज का क्षेत्रफल कितना होगा?

A. 50 वर्ग मी. B. 49 वर्ग मी.

C. 60 वर्ग मी. D. 69 वर्ग मी.

18. यदि किसी आयत की लम्बाई में 20% वृद्धि तथा चौड़ाई में 15% कमी कर दी जाये तो उसके क्षेत्रफल में कितने प्रतिशत वृद्धि या कमी हो जाएगी?

A. 4% कमी B. 2% वृद्धि

C. 2% कमी D. 3% वृद्धि

19. यदि किसी समचतुर्भुज के दो विकर्णों की लम्बाई क्रमशः 16 **सेंमी.** व 12 **सेंमी.** हो तो समचतुर्भुज का परिमाप क्या होगा?

A. 38 **सेंमी.** B. 40 **सेंमी.**

C. 41 **सेंमी.** D. 46 **सेंमी.**

20. यदि किसी वृत्त की परिधि तथा उसके अर्द्धव्यास के बीच 37 **सेंमी.** का अन्तर हो, तो वृत्त का व्यास कितना होगा?

$\left(\pi = \frac{22}{7}\right)$

A. 11 **सेंमी.** B. 12 **सेंमी.**

C. 16 **सेंमी.** D. 14 **सेंमी.**

उत्तरमाला

1	**2**	**3**	**4**	**5**	**6**	**7**	**8**	**9**	**10**
B	A	D	A	A	C	A	B	D	B
11	**12**	**13**	**14**	**15**	**16**	**17**	**18**	**19**	**20**
A	B	C	A	B	A	C	B	B	D

व्याख्यात्मक उत्तर

1. आयत का क्षेत्रफल = लम्बाई × चौड़ाई = 50×25

$= 1250$ वर्ग **सेंमी.**।

2. $\therefore$ वर्गाकार मैदान का परिमाप = $4 \times$ भुजा

प्रश्नानुसार, $\therefore$ $4 \times$ भुजा $= 580 \Rightarrow$ भुजा $= \frac{580}{4}$

$= 145$ **सेंमी.**

$\therefore$ क्षेत्रफल = (भुजा)^2 $= (145)^2 = 21025$ वर्ग **सेंमी.**।

3. वर्ग का क्षेत्रफल = (भुजा)^2 = $(20)^2 = 400$ वर्ग **सेंमी.**

4. $\therefore$ वृत्त का क्षेत्रफल = $\pi \times$ (त्रिज्या)^2

$\therefore$ $\pi \times$ (त्रिज्या)^2 $= 154$

$\Rightarrow$ (त्रिज्या)$^2 = \frac{154}{\pi} = \frac{154}{\frac{22}{7}}$

$\Rightarrow$ (त्रिज्या)$^2 = \frac{154 \times 7}{22} = 7 \times 7 \Rightarrow$ त्रिज्या = 7 **सेंमी.**

$\therefore$ वृत्त की परिधि = $2\pi \times$ (त्रिज्या)

$= 2 \times \frac{22}{7} \times 7 = 44$ **सेंमी.**।

5. त्रिभुज का क्षेत्रफल = $\frac{1}{2} \times$ आधार × ऊंचाई

$= \frac{1}{2} \times 8 \times 10 = 40$ वर्ग **सेंमी.**।

6. चूंकि समलम्ब चतुर्भुज का क्षेत्रफल = $\frac{1}{2} \times$ ऊंचाई × समानान्तर भुजाओं का योग

$\therefore$ क्षेत्रफल $= \frac{1}{2} \times 10 \times (15 + 25)$

$= \frac{1}{2} \times 10 \times 40 = 200$ वर्ग मी।

7. माना कि आयताकार खेत की लम्बाई व चौड़ाई क्रमशः $11x$ मी. व $8x$ मी. है

$\therefore$ खेत का परिमाप $= 2(11x + 8x) = 2 \times 19x = 38x$ मी.

प्रश्नानुसार, आयताकार खेत का परिमाप = 760 है

$\therefore 38x = 760 \Rightarrow x = \frac{760}{38} = 20$

$\therefore$ खेत की लम्बाई व चौड़ाई क्रमशः $(11 \times 20 = 220$ मी.) व $(8 \times 20 = 160$ मी.) होगी।

$\therefore$ आयातकार खेत का क्षेत्रफल $= 220 \times 160$

$= 35200$ वर्ग मी.।

8. माना कि वर्ग की भुजा x मी. है

$\therefore$ **पहली स्थिति में,** वर्ग का क्षेत्रफल $= x^2$ वर्ग मी.

दूसरी स्थिति में, वर्ग की भुजा में 50% की कमी के कारण

नए वर्ग की भुजा $= x - x$ का $50\% = \frac{x}{2}$ मी.

$\therefore$ नए वर्ग का क्षेत्रफल $= \left(\frac{x}{2}\right)^2 = \frac{x^2}{4}$ वर्ग मी.

$\therefore$ वर्ग के क्षेत्रफल में कमी $= x^2 - \frac{x^2}{4} = \frac{3x^2}{4}$ वर्ग मी.

$\therefore$ प्रतिशत कमी $= \frac{\frac{3x^2}{4}}{x^2} \times 100 = 75\%$

अतः वर्ग का क्षेत्रफल 75% घट जायेगा।

9. $\therefore$ आयत का क्षेत्रफल $= 6.4 \times 2.5 = 16.00$ वर्ग मी.

प्रश्नानुसार, वर्ग का क्षेत्रफल = आयत का क्षेत्रफल

$\therefore$ वर्ग का क्षेत्रफल = 16 वर्ग मी.

$\therefore$ वर्ग की भुजा $= \sqrt{16} = \sqrt{4 \times 4} = 4$ मी.।

10. माना कि समकोण त्रिभुज की तीन भुजाओं a, b और c में से सबसे बड़ी व सबसे छोटी भुजा क्रमशः a व c हैं

$\therefore a^2 = b^2 + c^2$ ... (i)

तथा समकोण त्रिभुज का परिमाप $= a + b + c$

प्रश्नानुसार,

$(a + b + c) = c \times 6 \Rightarrow a + b = 5c$ ... (ii)

समीकरण (i) से,

$a^2 - b^2 = c^2 \Rightarrow (a + b)(a - b) = c^2$

$\Rightarrow 5c(a - b) = c^2 \Rightarrow a - b = \frac{c}{5}$ ... (iii)

$[\because a + b = 5c]$

समीकरण (ii) व (iii) से, $a + b = 5c$, $a - b = \frac{c}{5}$

$\Rightarrow \quad 2a = 5c + \frac{c}{5} = \frac{26c}{5}$

$\Rightarrow \quad a = \frac{13}{5}c \Rightarrow a : c = 13 : 5$

a का मान समीकरण (ii) में रखने पर,

$b = 5c - \frac{13c}{5} = \frac{12c}{5} \Rightarrow b : c = 12 : 5$

अतः समकोण त्रिभुज की तीनों भुजाओं में क्रमशः 13 : 12 : 5

11. $\because$ पहले वर्ग का परिमाप = 24 मी.

$\therefore$ पहले वर्ग की भुजा = $\frac{24}{4}$ = 6 मी.

तथा दूसरे वर्ग की परिमाप = 32 मी.

$\therefore$ दूसरे वर्ग की भुजा = $\frac{32}{4}$ = 8 मी.

प्रश्नानुसार, तीसरे वर्ग का क्षेत्रफल = दो वर्गों का क्षेत्रफल

$\therefore$ तीसरे वर्ग का क्षेत्रफल = पहले वर्ग का क्षेत्रफल + दूसरे वर्ग का क्षेत्रफल

= $(6)^2 + (8)^2 = 36 + 64 = 100$ वर्ग मी.

$\therefore$ तीसरे वर्ग की भुजा = $\sqrt{100}$ = 10 मी.।

12. पहली स्थिति मे, वर्ग की भुजा = x मी.

$\therefore$ वर्ग का क्षेत्रफल = x^2 वर्ग मी.

दूसरी स्थिति में, वर्ग की भुजा = $2x$ मी.

$\therefore$ वर्ग का क्षेत्रफल = $(2x)^2 = 4x^2$ वर्ग मी.

अतः स्पष्ट है कि वर्ग की भुजा को दो गुना कर देने से उसका क्षेत्रफल चार गुना बढ़ जाएगा।

13. माना कि छोटे वर्ग की भुजा x मी. है

चूंकि बड़े वर्ग का क्षेत्रफल = $(25)^2 = 625$ वर्ग मी.

तथा छोटे वर्ग का क्षेत्रफल = x^2 वर्ग मी.

प्रश्नानुसार, दोनों वर्गों के क्षेत्रफल में अन्तर = 225 वर्ग मी.

$\therefore 625 - x^2 = 225 \Rightarrow x^2 = 625 - 225 = 400$

$\Rightarrow x = \sqrt{20 \times 20}$ = 20 मी.

अतः छोटे वर्ग की भुजा 20 मी. होगी।

14. माना कि समबाहु त्रिभुज की भुजा = x **सेंमी.**

$\therefore$ समबाहु त्रिभुज का परिमाप = $3x$ **सेंमी.**

प्रश्नानुसार, $3x = 72 \Rightarrow x = \frac{72}{3}$ = 24 **सेंमी.**

$\therefore$ समबाहु त्रिभुज का क्षेत्रफल = $\frac{\sqrt{3}}{4} \times (x)^2$

= $\frac{\sqrt{3}}{4} \times (24)^2 = 144\sqrt{3}$ वर्ग **सेंमी.**।

15. पहले वृत्त की त्रिज्या = 5 **सेंमी.**

$\therefore$ पहले वृत्त का क्षेत्रफल = $\pi \times (5)^2 = 25\pi$ वर्ग **सेंमी.**

तथा दूसरे वृत्त की त्रिज्या = 12 **सेंमी.**

$\therefore$ दूसरे वृत्त का क्षेत्रफल = $\pi \times (12)^2 = 144\pi$ वर्ग **सेंमी.**

प्रश्नानुसार,

नए वृत्त का क्षेत्रफल = दोनों वृत्तों का क्षेत्रफल

$\therefore$ नए वृत्त का क्षेत्रफल = $25\pi + 144\pi = 169\pi$ वर्ग **सेंमी.**

$\therefore$ नए वृत्त का क्षेत्रफल = $\pi \times (13)^2$ वर्ग **सेंमी.**

अतः स्पष्ट है कि नए वृत्त की त्रिज्या 13 **सेंमी.** होगी।

16. माना कि वृत्त की त्रिज्या R **सेंमी.** तथा वर्ग की भुजा x **सेंमी.** है

$\therefore$ वृत्त की परिधि = $2\pi R$ **सेंमी.** वर्ग का परिमाप = $4x$ **सेंमी.**

प्रश्नानुसार, $2\pi R = 4x \Rightarrow R = \frac{2x}{\pi}$

$\therefore$ वृत्त तथा वर्ग के क्षेत्रफलों में अनुपात = $\pi R^2 : x^2$

$\Rightarrow \pi \times \left(\frac{2x}{\pi}\right)^2 : x^2 \Rightarrow \frac{4x^2}{\pi} : x^2$

$\Rightarrow 4 : \pi \Rightarrow 4 : \frac{22}{7} \Rightarrow 14 : 11.$

17. माना कि त्रिभुज की भुजाएं क्रमशः $17x$ मी., $15x$ मी. तथा $8x$ मी.

$\therefore$ त्रिभुज का परिमाप = $17x + 15x + 8x = 40x$ मी.

प्रश्नानुसार, त्रिभुज का परिमाप = 40 मी.

$\therefore 40x = 40 \Rightarrow x = \frac{40}{40}$ = 1 मी.

अतः त्रिभुज की भुजाएं क्रमशः (17 × 1 = 17 मी.)

(15 × 1 = 15 मी.)

तथा (8 × 1 = 8 मी.) होंगी

चूंकि $(17)^2 = (15)^2 + (8)^2$ अर्थात् त्रिभुज समकोण त्रिभुज होगा।

$\therefore$ समकोण त्रिभुज का क्षेत्रफल $= \frac{1}{2} \times$ आधार $\times$ ऊंचाई

$= \frac{1}{2} \times 8 \times 15 = 60$ वर्ग मी.।

18. माना कि आयत की लम्बाई व चौड़ाई क्रमशः x मी. व y मी. है।

$\therefore$ आयत का क्षेत्रफल $= xy$ वर्ग मी.

प्रश्नानुसार, आयत की लम्बाई में 20% वृद्धि तथा चौड़ाई में 15% कमी के कारण, उन आयत की लम्बाई

$= x + x$ का $20\% = 1.2x$ मी.

तथा नए आयत की चौड़ाई $= y - y$ का $15\% = .85y$ मी.

$\therefore$ नए आयत का क्षेत्रफल $= 1.2x \times .85y$

$= 1.020xy$ वर्ग मी.

$\therefore$ आयत के क्षेत्रफल में वृद्धि $= 1.02xy - xy$

$= .02xy$ वर्ग मी.

$\therefore$ प्रतिशत वृद्धि $= \frac{.02xy}{xy} \times 100 = 2\%$

अतः आयत के क्षेत्रफल में 2% की वृद्धि हो जाएगी।

19. चूंकि समचतुर्भुज की भुजा

$$= \sqrt{\left(\frac{\text{पहले विकर्ण की लं.}}{2}\right)^2 + \left(\frac{\text{दूसरे विकर्ण की लं.}}{2}\right)^2}$$

$$= \sqrt{\left(\frac{16}{2}\right)^2 + \left(\frac{12}{2}\right)^2} = \sqrt{(8)^2 + (6)^2}$$

$$= \sqrt{64 + 36} = \sqrt{100}$$

$\therefore$ समचतुर्भुज की भुजा $= \sqrt{100} = \sqrt{10 \times 10}$

$= 10$ **सेंमी.**

$\therefore$ समचतुर्भुज का परिमाप $= 4 \times$ भुजा $= 4 \times 10$

$= 40$ **सेंमी.**।

20. माना कि वृत्त का अर्द्धव्यास = R **सेंमी.**

$\therefore$ वृत्त की परिधि $= 2\pi R$ **सेंमी.**

प्रश्नानुसार,

$$2\pi R - R = 37 \Rightarrow R\left(2 \times \frac{22}{7} - 1\right) = 37$$

$$\Rightarrow R(44 - 7) = 37 \times 7 \Rightarrow R \times 37 = 37 \times 7$$

$$\Rightarrow R = \frac{37 \times 7}{37} = 7$$

अतः वृत्त का अर्द्धव्यास 7 **सेंमी.** होगा।

$\therefore$ वृत्त का व्यास $= 2R = 2 \times 7 = 14$ **सेंमी.**।

☆☆☆☆☆☆

17 क्षेत्रमिति : ठोस आकृतियाँ (Mensuration: Solid Figures)

ठोस : कोई वस्तु जो स्थान घेरती है, भार रखती है तथा जिसका आकार निश्चित होता है, ठोस कहलाती है। इस प्रकार ठोस में तीन मापें होती हैं—1. लम्बाई 2. चौड़ाई 3. ऊंचाई (मोटाई)।

आयतन : ठोस के तलों द्वारा घिरी हुई जगह ठोस का आयतन कहलाती है।

घनाभ : एक ठोस जो 6 आयताकार तलों द्वारा घिरा होता है, घनाभ कहलाता है।

घन : एक ठोस जो 6 वर्गाकार तलों द्वारा घिरा होता है, घन कहलाता है।

ठोस आकृतियों से संबंधित समस्याओं को हल करने के लिए निम्नलिखित सूत्रों का जानना आवश्यक है :

1. गोला :

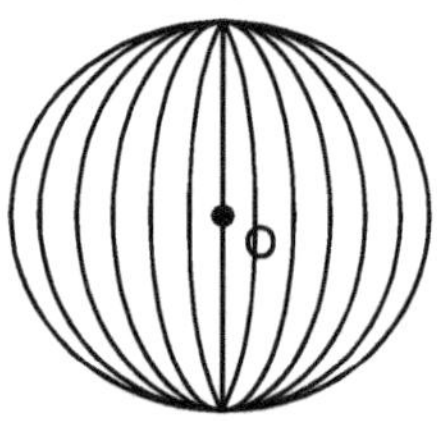

(*a*) गोले का आयतन = $\frac{4}{3}\pi r^3$ (जहां r गोले की त्रिज्या है)

(*b*) गोले के धरातल का क्षेत्रफल या वक्रपृष्ठ का क्षेत्रफल $= 4\pi r^2$

2. घनाभ :

(*a*) घनाभ का आयतन = लम्बाई × चौड़ाई × ऊंचाई

(*b*) घनाभ का पृष्ठ $= 2(l \times b + b \times h + h \times l)$ जहां l = लं., b = चौ., h = ऊं.

(*c*) किसी घनाभ का सबसे लम्बा विकर्ण $= \sqrt{l^2+b^2+h^2}$

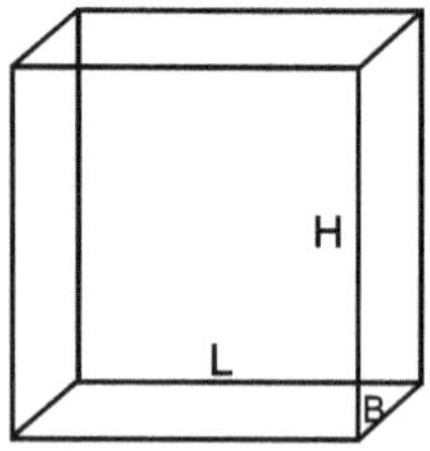

3. घन :

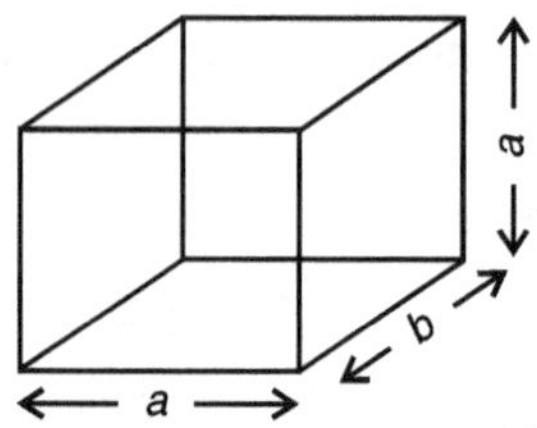

(*a*) घन का आयतन = (भुजा)^3 ∵ [भुजा = ल. = चौ = ऊं.]

(*b*) घन का पृष्ठ = 6 × (भुजा)^2

(*c*) किसी घन का सबसे लम्बा विकर्ण = $\sqrt{3}$ × भुजा

4. लम्ब वृत्तीय बेलन :

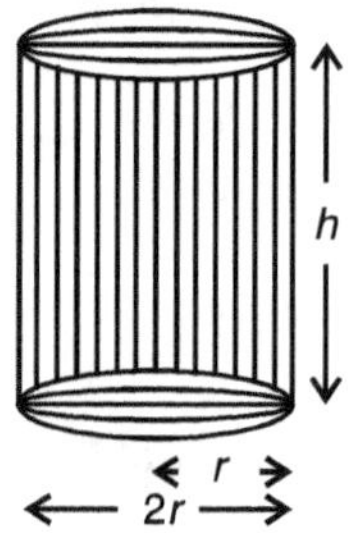

(*a*) बेलन का आयतन = आधार (वृत्त) का क्षेत्रफल × ऊँ. $= \pi r^2 \times h = \pi r^2 h$

(*b*) बेलन का वक्रपृष्ठ = आधार (वृत्त) की परिधि × ऊँचाई $= 2\pi r \times h = 2\pi rh$

(*c*) बेलन का सम्पूर्ण पृष्ठ = वक्र पृष्ठ + दोनों सिरों का क्षेत्रफल $= 2\pi rh + 2\pi r^2 = 2\pi r(h + r)$

5. शंकु :

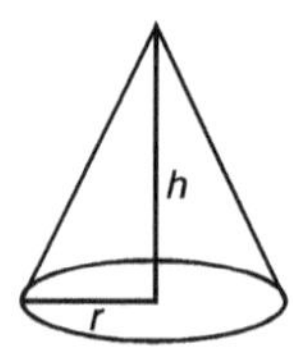

(*a*) शंकु का आयतन = $\frac{1}{3}\pi r^2 h$

(*b*) शंकु की तिर्यक ऊंचाई = $\sqrt{r^2+h^2}$

(*c*) शंकु के वक्र पृष्ठ का क्षेत्रफल = πr × तिर्यक ऊंचाई $= \pi r\sqrt{r^2+h^2}$

प्रश्नमाला

1. एक घनाभ की कोरें क्रमशः 4 **सेंमी.**, 3 **सेंमी.** तथा 2 **सेंमी.** हैं, तो उस घनाभ का आयतन कितना होगा?
A. 20 घन **सेंमी.** B. 22 घन **सेंमी.**
C. 28 घन **सेंमी.** D. 24 घन **सेंमी.**

2. एक टंकी 3 मी. लम्बी, 2 मी. चौड़ी तथा 1 मी. गहरी है। उसकी क्षमता (ली. में) क्या होगी?
A. 8000 ली. B. 10000 ली.
C. 6500 ली. D. 6000 ली.

3. एक घन का पृष्ठ क्षेत्रफल 1014 वर्ग **सेंमी.** है। इसका आयतन कितना होगा?
A. 2197 घन **सेंमी.** B. 2297 घन **सेंमी.**
C. 2179 घन **सेंमी.** D. 2117 घन **सेंमी.**

4. यदि दो घनाकृतियों के आयतन में 8 : 1 का अनुपात हो तो उनकी कोरों में क्या अनुपात होगा?
A. 1 : 2 B. 2 : 1
C. 4 : 1 D. 2 : 3

5. दो गोलों के पृष्ठ क्षेत्रफल में 9 : 16 का अनुपात है, तो बताइये उनके आयतनों में क्या अनुपात होगा?
A. 64 : 27 B. 27 : 64
C. 16 : 27 D. 11 : 27

6. एक कमरे की लं., चौ. व ऊँ. क्रमशः 12 मी., 9 मी. तथा 8 मी. है, तो बताइये उस छड़ की अधिक-से-अधिक लम्बाई क्या होगी जो कमरे में ठीक प्रकार रखी जो सके?
A. 17 मी. B. 18 मी.
C. 25 मी. D. 16 मी.

7. किसी लम्बवृत्तीय शंकु की त्रिज्या तथा ऊंचाई में 3 : 5 का अनुपात है। यदि शंकु का आयतन 120π घन मी. हो तो उसकी तिरछी ऊँचाई कितनी होगी?
A. $3\sqrt{34}$ मी. B. $2\sqrt{28}$ मी.
C. $2\sqrt{44}$ मी. D. $2\sqrt{34}$ मी.

8. यदि किसी बेलन के आधार की परिधि 88 **सेंमी.** तथा ऊंचाई 42 **सेंमी.** हो तो उस बेलन का आयतन कितना होगा?
A. 25872 घन **सेंमी.** B. 28572 घन **सेंमी.**
C. 25870 घन **सेंमी.** D. 22584 घन **सेंमी.**

9. 10 **सेंमी.** भुजा के दो घनों को आपस में सटाकर रखने से प्राप्त घनाभ का पृष्ठ क्या होगा?
A. 1200 वर्ग **सेंमी.** B. 5000 वर्ग **सेंमी.**
C. 1000 वर्ग **सेंमी.** D. 1250 वर्ग **सेंमी.**

10. एक आयताकार कागज के टुकडे की लम्बाई व चौड़ाई क्रमशः 30 **सेंमी.** तथा 20 **सेंमी.** है। यदि कागज को मोड़कर एक बेलन का वक्रपृष्ठ बनाया जाये तो बेलन कितने तरीके से बनाया जा सकता है?
A. तीन तरीके से B. दो तरीके से
C. एक तरीके से D. चार तरीके से

11. उपरोक्त प्रश्न में बने बेलनों के आयतनों में अनुपात क्या होगा।
A. 2 : 3 B. 3 : 1
C. 3 : 2 D. 2 : 1

12. यदि 3 **सेंमी.** त्रिज्या के एक ठोस गोले को पिघलाकर उसी त्रिज्या के आधार पर एक शंकु बनाया जाये तो शंकु की ऊंचाई कितनी होगी?
A. 8 **सेंमी.** B. 12 **सेंमी.**
C. 6 **सेंमी.** D. 5 **सेंमी.**

13. किसी रोलर का व्यास 2.4 मी. तथा लम्बाई 1.68 मी. है। यदि किसी मैदान को समतल करने में रोलर को 1000 पूर्ण चक्कर लगाने पड़े तो उस मैदान का क्षेत्रफल क्या होगा?
A. 12672 वर्ग मी. B. 12671 वर्ग मी.
C. 12762 वर्ग मी. D. 11768 वर्ग मी.

14. एक घन के किनारे की लम्बाई में 10% वृद्धि करने से घन के धरातल के क्षेत्रफल में कितने प्रतिशत वृद्धि हो जाएगी?
A. 21% B. 18%
C. 15% D. 20%

15. 14 मी. लम्बे तथा 4 मी. त्रिज्या वाले एक ठोस बेलन को पिघलाकर शंकु बनाया जाता है। यदि शंकु की त्रिज्या बेलन की त्रिज्या के बराबर हो तो शंकु की ऊंचाई कितनी होगी?
A. 21 मी. B. 42 मी.
C. 48 मी. D. 54 मी.

16. एक घनाकार कमरे की भुजा 10 मी है। यदि एक विद्यार्थी 5 घन मी. की जगह घेरता हो तो कमरे में कितने विद्यार्थी बैठ सकते हैं?

A. 100 B. 175
C. 200 D. 225

17. तीन घन, जिनके किनारे क्रमशः 2 **सेंमी.** 3 **सेंमी.** तथा 4 **सेंमी.** हैं, को पिघलाकर एक नया घन बनाया जाता है। उस नए घन का किनारा कितना होगा?

A. $\sqrt{99}$ **सेंमी.** B. $3\sqrt{99}$ **सेंमी.**
C. $\sqrt[3]{99}$ **सेंमी.** D. 99 **सेंमी.**

18. किसी घन के पृष्ठ भाग का क्षेत्रफल 600 वर्ग **सेंमी.** है, तो उसके विकर्ण की लम्बाई क्या होगी?

A. $10\sqrt{3}$ **सेंमी.** B. $5\sqrt{3}$ **सेंमी.**
C. $4\sqrt{2}$ **सेंमी.** D. $10\sqrt{2}$ **सेंमी.**

19. एक शंक्वाकार मकबरे का व्यास तथा उसकी ढलवां ऊँचाई क्रमशः 28 मी. तथा 50 मी. है, तो बताइये 80 पैसे प्रति वर्ग मी. की दर से उसकी गोलाकर सतह पर सफेदी कराने का खर्च क्या होगा?

A. 1860 रु. B. 1760 रु.
C. 1950 रु. D. 1875 रु.

20. किसी घनाभ (Cuboid) की लम्बाई व चौड़ाई में क्रमशः 8 : 7 का अनुपात है। यदि घनाभ का आयतन 1120 घन सेमी तथा ऊंचाई 5 **सेंमी.** हो तो घनाभ की चौड़ाई उसकी लम्बाई से कितनी कम होगी?

A. 4 **सेंमी.** B. 2 **सेंमी.**
C. 7 **सेंमी.** D. 5 **सेंमी.**

उत्तरमाला

1	2	3	4	5	6	7	8	9	10
D	D	A	B	B	A	D	A	C	B
11	**12**	**13**	**14**	**15**	**16**	**17**	**18**	**19**	**20**
C	B	A	A	B	C	C	A	B	B

व्याख्यात्मक उत्तर

1. ∵ घनाभ का आयतन = लं. × चौ. × ऊं.
= 4 × 3 ×2 = 24 घन **सेंमी.**

2. टंकी का आयतन = लं. × चौ. × ऊं. = 3 × 2 × 1
= 6 घन मी.
(∵ 1 घन मी. = 1000 ली.)
∴ टंकी की क्षमता = 6 × 1000 = 6000 ली.।

3. ∵ घन का पृष्ठ क्षेत्रफल = 6 × (भुजा)^2
∴ 6 × (भुजा)^2 = 1014
⇒ (भुजा)^2 = $\frac{1014}{6} = 169$
∴ घन की भुजा = $\sqrt{169}$ = 13 **सेंमी.**
∴ घन का आयतन = (भुजा)^3
= (13)^3 **सेंमी.**
= 2197 घन **सेंमी.**

4. माना दो घनों की भुजा क्रमशः a_1 व a_2 है।
∴ दोनों घनों का आयतन क्रमशः a_1^3 व a_2^3 होगा

प्रश्नानुसार, $a_1^3 : a_2^3 = 8 : 1$

$$\therefore \frac{a_1^3}{a_2^3} = \frac{8}{1}$$

$$\therefore \left(\frac{a_1}{a_2}\right)^3 = \left(\frac{2}{1}\right)^3 \Rightarrow a_1 : a_2 = 2 : 1$$

अतः उनकी कोरों में 2 : 1 का अनुपात होगा।

5. माना कि दो गोलों की त्रिज्या क्रमशः r_1 व r_2 है
दोनों गोलों का पृष्ठ क्षेत्रफल क्रमशः $4\pi r_1^2$ व $4\pi r_2^2$
प्रश्नानुसार, $4\pi r_1^2 : 4\pi r_2^2 = 9 : 16 \Rightarrow r_1^2 : r_2^2 = 9 : 16$

$$\Rightarrow \frac{r_1^2}{r_2^2} = \frac{9}{16} \Rightarrow \left(\frac{r_1}{r_2}\right)^2 = \left(\frac{3}{4}\right)^2 \Rightarrow r_1 : r_2 = 3 : 4$$

$$\Rightarrow \left(\frac{r_1}{r_2}\right)^3 = \left(\frac{3}{4}\right)^3 \Rightarrow \frac{r_1^3}{r_2^3} = \frac{27}{64}$$

$\Rightarrow r_1^3 : r_2^3 = 27 : 64$

$\because$ उनके आयतनों का अनुपात $= \frac{4}{3}\pi r_1^3 : \frac{4}{3}\pi r_2^3$

$\Rightarrow r_1^3 : r_2^3 = 27 : 64$

6. $\because$ अधिक-से-अधिक लम्बाई की छड़ = घनाभ के विकर्ण की लम्बाई

$= \sqrt{(\text{लं.})^2 + (\text{चौ.})^2 + (\text{ऊं.})^2}$

$= \sqrt{(12)^2 + (9)^2 + (8)^2}$

$= \sqrt{144 + 81 + 64} = \sqrt{289} = 17$ मी.

अतः उस छड़ की अधिक-से-अधिक लम्बाई जो ठीक प्रकार से कमरे में रखी जा सके 17 मी. होगी।

7. माना कि लम्बवृत्तीय शंकु की त्रिज्या व ऊंचाई क्रमशः $3x$ मी. व $5x$ मी. है

$\therefore$ शंकु का आयतन $= \frac{1}{3}\pi r^2 h = \frac{1}{3}\pi \times (3x)^2 \times 5x$ घन मी.

प्रश्नानुसार, शंकु का आयतन $= 120\pi$ घन मी. (दिया है)

$\therefore \quad \frac{1}{3}\pi \times 9x^2 \times 5x = 120\pi \Rightarrow x^3 = \frac{120 \times 3}{9 \times 5}$

$\Rightarrow x^3 = 8 \Rightarrow x^3 = (2)^3 \Rightarrow x = 2$ मी.

$\therefore$ लम्बवृत्तीय शंकु की त्रिज्या व ऊंचाई क्रमशः $3 \times 2 = 6$ मी. तथा $5 \times 2 = 10$ मी. होगी।

$\therefore$ तिर्यक ऊंचाई $= \sqrt{(\text{त्रिज्या})^2 + (\text{ऊंचाई})^2}$

$= \sqrt{(6)^2 + (10)^2}$

$= \sqrt{36 + 100} = \sqrt{136} = 2\sqrt{34}$ मी. ।

8. माना कि बेलन के आधार की त्रिज्या $= r$ **सेंमी.**

$\therefore$ बेलन के आधार की परिधि $= 2\pi r$ **सेंमी.**

प्रश्नानुसार, $2\pi r = 88$

$\Rightarrow r = \frac{88}{2\pi} = \frac{88}{2 \times \frac{22}{7}} = \frac{88 \times 7}{2 \times 22} = 14$ **सेंमी.**

$\therefore$ बेलन का आयतन $= \pi r^2 h = \frac{22}{7} \times (14)^2 \times 42$

$= 22 \times 2 \times 14 \times 42 = 25872$ घन **सेंमी.**।

9. विद्यार्थियों को इस प्रकार के प्रश्नों में हमेशा ध्यान रखना चाहिए कि दो घनों को आपस में सटाकर रखने पर प्राप्त घनाभ की भुजाओं में केवल लम्बाई में ही वृद्धि होगी। उसकी चौड़ाई तथा ऊंचाई घन की भुजा के ही बराबर होगी। $\therefore$ घनाभ की लम्बाई = पहले घन की भुजा की लम्बाई + दूसरे घन की भुजा की लम्बाई

अर्थात् घनाभ की लम्बाई $= 10 + 10 = 20$ **सेंमी.** होगी।

$\therefore$ घनाभ का पृष्ठ $= 2(20 \times 10 + 10 \times 10 + 10 \times 20)$

$= 2(200 + 100 + 200) = 2 \times 500 = 1000$ वर्ग **सेंमी.**।

10. कागज के टुकड़े को दो तरीके से मोड़ कर बेलन बनाया जा सकता है। **1.** आयताकार कागज को इस प्रकार मोड़ा जाए ताकि उसकी लम्बाई 30 **सेंमी.** तथा चौड़ाई 20 **सेंमी.** बेलन की क्रमशः वृत्तीय आधार की परिधि तथा ऊंचाई हो। **2.** पुनः आयताकार कागज को इस प्रकार से मोड़ा जाये ताकि उसकी लम्बाई 30 **सेंमी.** तथा चौड़ाई 20 **सेंमी.** बेलन की क्रमशः ऊंचाई व वृत्तीय आधार की परिधि हो।

11. **पहली स्थिति में,** $2\pi r = 30 \Rightarrow r = \frac{15}{\pi}$ **सेंमी.** तथा $h = 20$ **सेंमी.**

$\therefore \quad$ आयतन $(v_1) = \pi r^2 h = \frac{15 \times 15 \times 20}{\pi}$

$= \frac{4500}{\pi}$ घन **सेंमी.**

दूसरी स्थिति मे, $2\pi r = 20$

$\Rightarrow r = \frac{10}{\pi}$ **सेंमी.** तथा $h = 30$

$\therefore \quad$ आयतन $(v_2) = \pi r^2 h$

$= \frac{10 \times 10 \times 30}{\pi} = \frac{3000}{\pi}$ घन **सेंमी.**

$\because$ अनुपात $v_1 : v_2 = \frac{4500}{\pi} : \frac{3000}{\pi} = 3 : 2.$

12. $\because$ 3 **सेंमी.** त्रिज्या वाले गोले का आयतन

$= \frac{4}{3}\pi \times (3)^3 = \frac{4}{3}\pi \times 27$ घन **सेंमी.**

माना कि शंकु की ऊंचाई h **सेंमी.** है

$\therefore$ उसी त्रिज्या के आधार पर शंकु का आयतन

$= \frac{1}{3}\pi(3)^2 \times h$ घन **सेंमी.**

चूंकि शंकु का आयतन = गोले का आयतन

$\therefore \frac{1}{3}\pi \times (3)^2 \times h = \frac{4}{3}\pi \times 27 \Rightarrow h = 12$ **सेंमी.**

अत: शंकु की ऊंचाई 12 सेमी होगी।

13. $\because$ रोलर का व्यास = 2.4 मी. $\therefore$ रोलर की त्रिज्या = 1.2 **मी.** तथा रोलर की लम्बाई (ऊंचाई) = 1.68 मी.

$\therefore$ रोलर की वक्रपृष्ठ $= 2\pi rh = 2 \times \frac{22}{7} \times 1.2 \times 1.68$

= 12.672 वर्ग मी.

$\therefore$ 1 चक्कर में रोलर मैदान पर चला = 12.672 वर्ग मी.

$\therefore$ 1000 चक्कर में मैदान पर चलेगा $= 12.672 \times 1000$

= 12672 वर्ग मी.

अर्थात् मैदान का क्षेत्रफल = 12672 वर्ग मी. होगा।

14. $\because$ घन के धरातल के क्षेत्रफल दो कोरों में 10% की वृद्धि होती है। अर्थात् $x\% = y\% = 10\%$ तथा प्रतिशत वृद्धि की स्थिति में x, y के मान (+) धनात्मक होंगे।

$\therefore$ घन के धरातल के क्षेत्रफल में प्रतिशत वृद्धि

$$= \left(x + y + \frac{xy}{100}\right)\%$$

$$= \left(10 + 10 + \frac{10 \times 10}{100}\right)\% = 21\%$$

15. $\because$ ठोस बेलन का आयतन $= \pi r^2 h = \pi r^2 \times 14$ घन मी.

प्रश्नानुसार, शंकु की त्रिज्या = बेलन की त्रिज्या r मी = 4 मी.

चूंकि शंकु का आयतन = बेलन का आयतन

$\therefore \frac{1}{3}\pi r^2 \times$ ऊंचाई $= \pi r^2 \times 14$

$\therefore$ ऊंचाई = 14 × 3 = 42 मी.

अत: शंकु की ऊंचाई 42 मी. होगा।

16. $\because$ घनाकार कमरे का आयतन $= (10)^3 = 1000$ घन मी.

कमरे में बैठने वाले विद्यार्थियों की संख्या

$$= \frac{\text{कमरे का आयतन}}{\text{एक विद्यार्थी का आयतन}}$$

$$= \frac{1000}{5} = 200.$$

17. $\because$ तीन घन के किनारे क्रमश: 2 **सेंमी.**, 3 **सेंमी.** तथा 4 **सेंमी.** है।

$\therefore$ तीनों घनों के आयतन क्रमश: $(2)^3 = 8$ घन **सेंमी.**, $(3)^3 = 27$ घन **सेंमी.**

तथा $(4)^3 = 64$ घन **सेंमी.** होगी।

$\therefore$ नए घन का आयतन = तीनों घनों का आयतन

$\therefore$ नए घन का आयतन = 8 + 27 + 64 = 99 घन **सेंमी.**

$\therefore$ नए घन का किनारा $= \sqrt[3]{99}$ **सेंमी.**।

18. $\because$ घन के पृष्ठ भाग का क्षेत्रफल $= 6 \times (\text{भुजा})^2$

$\therefore 6 \times (\text{भुजा})^2 = 600 \Rightarrow (\text{भुजा})^2 = 100$

$\Rightarrow$ भुजा = 10 **सेंमी.**

$\therefore$ घन के विकर्ण की लम्बाई $= \sqrt{3} \times$ भुजा $= \sqrt{3} \times 10$

$= 10\sqrt{3}$ **सेंमी.**

19. $\because$ शंकु के वक्रतल का क्षेत्रफल $= \pi rl$

(जहां r = शंकु की त्रिज्या l = शंकु की ढलवां ऊंचाई)

$\therefore$ वक्रतल का क्षेत्रफल $= \frac{22}{7} \times \frac{28}{2} \times 50 = 2200$ वर्ग मी.

$\therefore$ 80 पैसे प्रति वर्ग मी. की दर से सफेदी कराने का खर्च

$= 2200 \times \frac{80}{100} = 1760$ रु. होगा।

20. माना कि घनाभ की लम्बाई व चौड़ाई क्रमश: $8x$ **सेंमी.** तथा $7x$ **सेंमी.** है।

$\therefore$ घनाभ का आयतन $= 8x \times 7x \times 5 = 280x^2$ घन **सेंमी.**

परन्तु घनाभ का आयतन = 1120 घन **सेंमी.**

(दिया हुआ है)

$\therefore 280x^2 = 1120 \Rightarrow x^2 = \frac{1120}{280} = 4 = (2)^2$

$\Rightarrow x = 2$

$\therefore$ घनाभ की लम्बाई = 8 × 2 = 16 **सेंमी.**

तथा घनाभ की चौड़ाई = 7 × 2 = 14 **सेंमी.**

अत: स्पष्ट है कि घनाभ की चौड़ाई उसकी लम्बाई से 2 सेमी कम होगी।

☆☆☆☆☆☆

18 सारणी एवं ग्राफ
(Tables and Graphs)

इस प्रकार के प्रश्नों में सारणी या ग्राफ दिया होता है, उससे सम्बन्धित प्रश्न पूछे जाते हैं। अतः अभ्यार्थियों को दिये गये प्रश्नों के सही उत्तर ज्ञात करने के लिए सारणी या ग्राफ का बहुत ही सावधानीपूर्वक अध्ययन करना चाहिए।

प्रश्नमाला

निर्देश (प्रश्न 1 से 4 तक) *निम्नांकित ग्राफ के अनुसार वर्ष 1998 में वर्षा ऋतु के दौरान हुई सड़क दुर्घटनाओं में मरने वालों की संख्या प्रदर्शित की गई है। ग्राफ पर आधारित ग्राफ के नीचे दिये गये प्रश्नों के उत्तर दीजिए।*

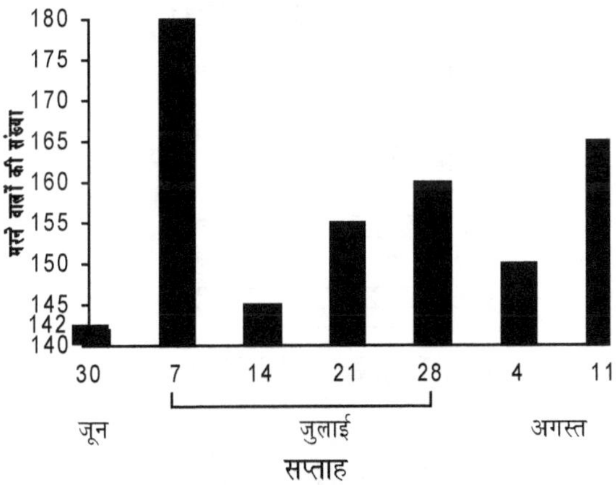

1. किन दो क्रमिक सप्ताहों के बीच मरने वालों की संख्या सबसे अधिक थी?

A. 4 अगस्त - 11 अगस्त
B. 14 जुलाई - 21 जुलाई
C. 30 जून - 7 जुलाई
D. 7 जुलाई - 28 जुलाई

2. कितने सप्ताहों में मरने वालों की संख्या 150 से अधिक थी?

A. 3 B. 2
C. 4 D. 1

3. कितने सप्ताहों में मरने वालों की संख्या 150 से कम थी?

A. 2 B. 0
C. 1 D. 3

4. किन दो क्रमिक सप्ताहों के बीच मरने वालों की संख्या में सबसे अधिक गिरावट थी?

A. 28 जुलाई – 4 अगस्त B. 7 जुलाई – 14 जुलाई
C. 30 जून – 7 जुलाई D. इनमें से कोई नहीं

निर्देश (प्रश्न 5 से 8 तक): *नीचे दी गई सारणी का सावधानी से अध्ययन कीजिए और उस पर आधारित नीचे दिये गये प्रश्नों के उत्तर दीजिए।*

किसी फैक्टरी के विविध विभागों में काम कर रहे कर्मचारियों की संख्या

विभाग / वर्ष	*उत्पादन*	*बिक्री*	*खरीद*	*प्रशासन एवं लेखा*	*अनुसंधान एवं विकास*
2001	150	25	50	45	75
2002	225	40	45	62	70
2003	450	65	30	90	73
2004	470	73	32	105	70
2005	500	80	35	132	74
2006	505	75	36	130	75

5. किस वर्ष उत्पादन में काम कर रहे कर्मचारियों की संख्या कुल कर्मचारियों के 50% से कम थी?

A. 2001 B. 2003
C. 2004 D. 2005

6. निम्न में से किस वर्ष प्रत्येक विभाग में काम कर रहे कर्मचारियों की संख्या प्रत्येक विभाग में उसके तुरन्त पिछले वर्ष के कर्मचारियों की संख्या से अधिक थी?

A. 2005 B. 2004
C. 2003 D. 2002

7. किस विभाग में वर्ष 2001 से 2006 तक कर्मचारियों की संख्या आसन्नतः समान रही है।

A. उत्पादन B. बिक्री
C. अनुसंधान एवं विकास D. प्रशासन एवं लेखा
E. खरीद

8. किस विभाग में वर्ष 2001 से 2006 तक लगातार कर्मचारियों की संख्या कुल कर्मचारियों की संख्या के 10% से कम रही है।

A. खरीद B. बिक्री
C. अनुसंधान एवं विकास D. प्रशासन एवं लेखा
E. बिक्री एवं खरीद

निर्देश (प्रश्न 9 से 12 तक): *नीचे दी गई पाई चार्ट किसी परिवार के विभिन्न मदों पर खर्च को दर्शाता है। इस पर आधारित नीचे दिये गये प्रश्नों के उत्तर दीजिए।*

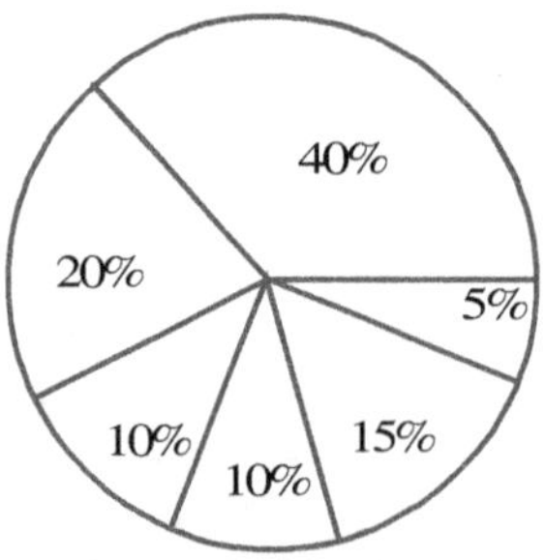

9. यदि शिक्षा पर 375 रु. खर्च होते हों, तो उतने ही रुपये निम्नलिखित में से किस पर खर्च होंगे?

A. दवा B. अन्य खर्च
C. किराया D. कपड़े

10. यदि भोजन पर खर्च 750 रु. प्रति माहवार हो, तो शिक्षा पर वार्षिक व्यय कितने रुपये होगा?

A. 2150 रु. B. 1022.50 रु.
C. 2250 रु. D. 1400 रु.

11. यदि परिवार का कुल खर्च 4500 रु. हो तो उस परिवार का कपड़े पर कितना खर्च होता है?

A. 800 रु. B. 900 रु.
C. 840 रु. D. 950 रु.

12. इस चार्ट में अन्य खर्च पर व्यय द्वारा केन्द्रीय कोण कितना होगा?

A. 40° B. 54°
C. 36° D. 15°

निर्देश (प्रश्न 13 से 16 तक): *निम्नलिखित आरेख का सावधानीपूर्वक अध्ययन करके उसे नीचे दिये गये प्रश्नों के उत्तर दीजिए।*

बिक्री तथा लाभ रिपोर्ट (1980-87)

बिक्री (लाख रुपयों में) आय रुपए दस हजार में

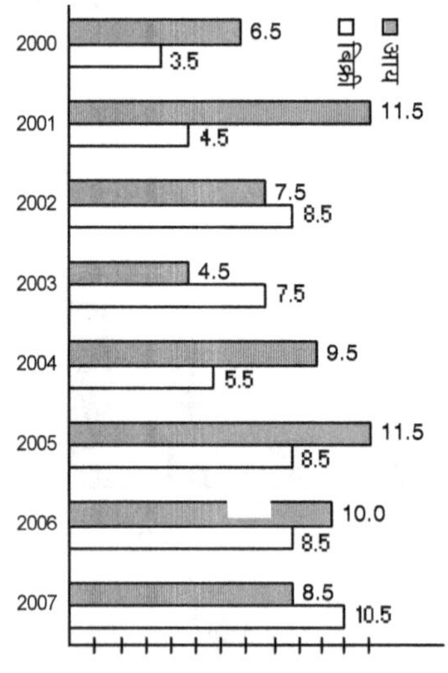

13. 2002 से 2007 तक बिक्री में वार्षिक बढ़ोत्तरी का माध्य (लाख रुपयों में) है–

A. 0.1 B. 0.2
C. 0.3 D. 0.4

14. स्टोर का वार्षिक माध्य लाभ (दस हजार रुपये में) निकटतम है–

A. 8.5 B. 8.6
C. 8.7 D. 9.0

15. किस वर्ष में लाभ का बिक्री से प्रतिशत अधिकतम था?

A. 2000 B. 2001
C. 2002 D. 2004

16. यदि 2000 के लाभ को आधार (100) माना जाए तो 2007 में कितना लाभ था?

A. 76 B. 105

C. 121 D. 131

निर्देश (प्रश्न 17 से 20 तक): *निम्नांकित तालिका किसी देश का विभिन्न वर्षों में बिस्कुटों का निर्यात प्रदर्शित करती है। तालिका का अध्ययन करके नीचे दिये गये प्रश्नों के उत्तर दीजिए।*

किसी देश का बिस्कुटों का कुछ वर्षों के लिए निर्यात

वर्ष	मात्रा (लाख टिनों में)	मूल्य (करोड़ रु. में)
2005	100	150
2006	75	150
2007	150	330
2008	160	400
2009	200	500

17. किस वर्ष प्रति टिन निर्यात मूल्य न्यूनतम था?

A. 2008 B. 2007

C. 2006 D. 2005

18. किन वर्षों में प्रति टिन मूल्य समान था?

A. 2006 और 2007 B. 2007 और 2008

C. 2008 और 2009 D. 2007 और 2009

19. 2005 से 2009 में निर्यात मूल्य में कितने प्रतिशत वृद्धि हुई?

A. 100 B. $116\frac{2}{3}$

C. $233\frac{1}{3}$ D. 350

20. 2008 से 2009 में निर्यात किये गये बिस्कुट टिनों की संख्या में कितना अन्तर था?

A. 40

B. 40,000

C. 4,00,000

D. 40,00,000

निर्देश (प्रश्न 21 से 25 तक): *निम्नलिखित आरेख का सावधानीपूर्वक अध्ययन करके उसे नीचे दिये गये प्रश्नों के उत्तर दीजिए।*

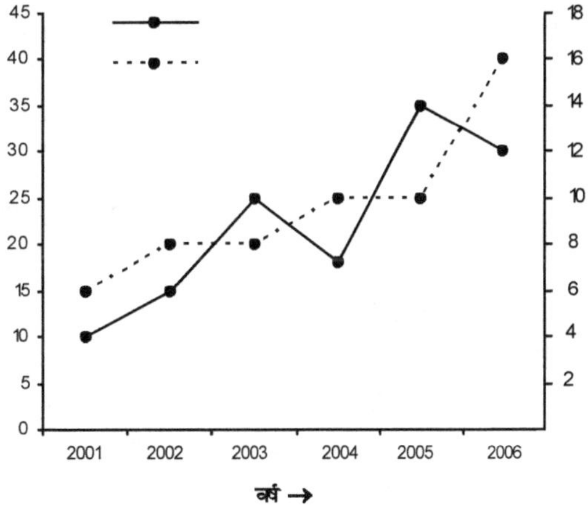

21. 2002 में प्रत्येक यंत्र की कीमत कितनी थी?

A. $5\frac{1}{3}$ हजार रु. B. 50 हजार रु.

C. 5103 रु. D. 3 हजार रु.

22. 2003 की अपेक्षा 2004 में यंत्रों के उत्पादन में कितने प्रतिशत कमी हुई?

A. 5 B. 20

C. 25 D. 30

23. 2004 तथा 2006 में यंत्रों की बिक्री से प्राप्त राजस्व में अन्तर कितना था?

A. 10 लाख रु. B. 1 करोड़ रु.

C. 4 करोड़ रु. D. 6 करोड़ रु.

24. यदि 2005 में प्रत्येक यंत्र की कीमत 25 प्रतिशत बढ़ाई जाती तो उस वर्ष उत्पादित यंत्रों की कुल कीमत क्या होती?

A. 32 करोड़ रु. B. 20 करोड़ रु.

C. 12.5 करोड़ रु. D. 15.5 करोड़ रु.

25. 2003 तथा 2004 में प्रत्येक यंत्र के मूल्य में कितना अन्तर था?

A. 1500 रु. B. 2500 रु.

C. 1800 रु. D. 3200 रु.

उत्तरमाला

1	2	3	4	5	6	7	8	9	10
A	C	D	B	A	A	C	B	C	C
11	**12**	**13**	**14**	**15**	**16**	**17**	**18**	**19**	**20**
B	B	D	C	B	D	D	C	C	D
21	**22**	**23**	**24**	**25**					
A	B	D	C	C					

व्याख्यात्मक उत्तर

1. ग्राफ के अनुसार दिये गये विकल्पों में 4 अगस्त – 11 अगस्त के दो क्रमिक सप्ताहों के बीच मरने वालों की संख्या में सबसे अधिक वृद्धि 165 – 150 = 15 थी।

2. चूँकि दिये गये ग्राफ में 7 जुलाई, 21 जुलाई, 28 जुलाई तथा 11 अगस्त के सप्ताहों में मरने वालों की संख्या 150 से अधिक थी अर्थात् सप्ताहों की गिनती = 4.

3. चूँकि ग्राफ से स्पष्ट है कि 30 जून, 14 जुलाई व 4 अगस्त के सप्ताहों में मरने वालों की संख्या 150 से कम थी। अर्थात् सप्ताहों की गिनती = 3.

4. ग्राफ के अनुसार 7 जुलाई से 14 जुलाई के दो क्रमिक सप्ताहों के बीच मरने वालों की संख्या में सबसे अधिक गिरावट आई थी।

5. 2001 में कुल कर्मचारियों की संख्या = 150 + 25 + 50 + 45 + 75 = 345

∴ उत्पादन में काम कर रहे कर्मचारियों की प्रतिशत संख्या

$$= \frac{150 \times 100}{345} = 43.48$$

2002 में कुल कर्मचारियों की संख्या = 225 + 40 + 45 + 62 + 70 = 442

∴ उत्पादन में काम कर रहे कर्मचारियों की प्रतिशत संख्या

$$= \frac{225 \times 100}{442} = 50.9$$

2003 में कुल कर्मचारियों की संख्या = 450 + 65 + 30 + 90 + 73 = 708

∴ उत्पादन में काम कर रहे कर्मचारियों की प्रतिशत संख्या

$$= \frac{450 \times 100}{708} = 63.56$$

2004 में कुल कर्मचारियों की संख्या = 470 + 73 + 32 + 105 + 70 = 750

∴ उत्पादन में काम कर रहे कर्मचारियों की प्रतिशत संख्या =

$$\frac{470 \times 100}{750} = 62.67$$

2005 में कुल कर्मचारियों की संख्या = 500 + 80 + 35 + 132 + 74 = 821

∴ उत्पादन में काम कर रहे कर्मचारियों की प्रतिशत संख्या =

$$\frac{500 \times 100}{821} = 60.9$$

2006 में कुल कर्मचारियों की संख्या = 505 + 75 + 36 + 130 + 75 = 821

∴ उत्पादन में काम कर रहे कर्मचारियों की प्रतिशत संख्या =

$$\frac{505 \times 100}{821} = 61.51$$

अतः 2001 में यह 50% से कम है।

6. सारणी से स्पष्ट है कि 2005 में प्रत्येक विभाग के कर्मचारियों की संख्या, पिछले वर्ष के प्रत्येक विभाग में कर्मचारियों की संख्या से अधिक थी।

7. सारणी के अनुसार अनुसंधान एवं विकास विभाग में वर्ष 2001 से 2006

9. ∵ केन्द्रीय कोण 36° शिक्षा तथा किराए के लिए एक ही है, अतः इन दोनों मदों पर खर्चा बराबर होगा। अर्थात् 375 रु. किराए पर खर्च होंगे।

10. ∵ भोजन पर खर्च = 750 रु.

∵ कुल खर्च $= \frac{100 \times 750}{40} = 1875$ रु.

∵ शिक्षा पर खर्च = 10%

∵ शिक्षा पर खर्च धनराशि $= 1875 \times \frac{10}{100}$

$= 187.50$ रु.

$\therefore$ शिक्षा पर वार्षिक खर्च = 187.50 × 12
= 2250.00 रु.

11. $\because$ कपड़े पर खर्च = 20%

$\therefore$ कपड़े पर कुल खर्च = $\frac{20}{100} \times 4500$ = 900 रु.।

12. 15% के लिए केन्द्रीय कोण $\frac{15}{100} \times 360^\circ = 54^\circ$.

13. 2002 से 2007 तक बिक्री में बढ़ोत्तरी का माध्य (लाख रुपये में) = $\frac{10.5 - 8.5}{5} = .4$.

14. स्टोर का वार्षिक माध्य लाभ (दस हजार रुपये में)

$$= \frac{(6.5 + 11.5 + 7.5 + 4.5 + 9.5 + 11.5 + 10.0 + 8.5)}{8}$$

$$= \frac{69.5}{8} = 8.7 \text{ (निकटतम)}$$

15. 2000 में लाभ का बिक्री से प्रतिशत

$$= \frac{6.5 \times 10000 \times 100}{3.5 \times 100000} = 1.86$$

2001 में लाभ का बिक्री से प्रतिशत

$$= \frac{11.5 \times 10000 \times 100}{4.5 \times 100000} = 25.56$$

2002 में लाभ का बिक्री से प्रतिशत

$$= \frac{7.5 \times 10000 \times 100}{8.5 \times 100000} = 8.82$$

तथा 2004 में लाभ का बिक्री से प्रतिशत

$$= \frac{9.5 \times 10000 \times 100}{5.5 \times 100000} = 17.27$$

$\therefore$ 2001 में लाभ का बिक्री से प्रतिशत अधिकतम था।

16. अभीष्ट लाभ = $\frac{100 \times 8.5}{6.5} = 131$.

17. 2005 में प्रति टिन निर्यात मूल्य = $\frac{150 \text{ करोड़}}{100 \text{ लाख}}$ = 150 रु.

2006 में प्रति टिन निर्यात मूल्य = $\frac{150 \text{ करोड़}}{75 \text{ लाख}}$ = 200 रु.

2007 में प्रति टिन निर्यात मूल्य = $\frac{330 \text{ करोड़}}{150 \text{ लाख}}$ = 220 रु.

2008 में प्रति टिन निर्यात मूल्य = $\frac{400 \text{ करोड़}}{160 \text{ लाख}}$ = 250 रु.

तथा 2009 में प्रति टिन निर्यात मूल्य

$$= \frac{500 \text{ करोड़}}{200 \text{ लाख}} = 250 \text{ रु.}$$

अतः स्पष्ट होता है कि 2005 में प्रति टिन निर्यात मूल्य न्यूनतम था।

18. उपरोक्त प्रश्न से स्पष्ट है कि 2008 तथा 2009 में प्रति टिन निर्यात मूल्य समान था।

19. 2005 व 2009 में निर्यात मूल्य में प्रतिशत वृद्धि

$$= \frac{(500 - 150)}{150} \times 100 = 233\frac{1}{3}.$$

20. अभीष्ट अन्तर = 200 – 160 = 40 लाख टिन या 40,00,000 टिन।

21. $\because$ 2002 में यंत्रों की संख्या = 15000
तथा यंत्रों का मूल्य = 80000000 रु.

$\therefore$ 2002 में 1 यंत्र का मूल्य = $\frac{80000000}{15000}$

$= 5\frac{1}{3}$ हजार रु.।

22. 2003 की अपेक्षा 2004 में यंत्रों के उत्पादन में प्रतिशत कमी = $\frac{(25 - 20) \times 100}{25}$ = 20%

23. 2004 में 2006 में यंत्रों की बिक्री से प्राप्त राजस्व में अन्तर = 16 – 10 = 6 करोड़ रु. था।

24. 2004 में 25% कीमत बढ़ने पर उत्पादित यंत्रों की कुल कीमत = $\frac{10 \times 125}{100}$ = 12.5 करोड़ रु.।

25. 2003 में प्रत्येक यंत्र का मूल्य = $\frac{80000000}{25000}$
= 3200 रु.

तथा 2004 में प्रत्येक यंत्र का मूल्य = $\frac{100000000}{20000}$
= 5000 रु.

$\therefore$ अभीष्ट अन्तर = 5000 – 3200 = 1800 रु.।

☆☆☆☆☆☆

19 प्रायिकता
(Probability)

प्रयोग

सुपरिभाषित परिणाम देने वाली क्रिया प्रयोग कहलाती है। प्रयोग दो प्रकार के होते हैं :

(*i*) यादृच्छिक प्रयोग

(*ii*) निर्धारणात्मक प्रयोग

(*i*) यादृच्छिक प्रयोग–वह प्रयोग जो समान परिस्थितियों में दुहराने पर असमान परिणाम देता है, यादृच्छिक प्रयोग कहलाता है।

जैसे–एक पासे को उछालने पर 1 से 6 तक के अंकों में से कोई भी परिणाम आ सकता है। परन्तु प्रत्येक बार समान परिणाम आए यह निश्चित नहीं है।

(*ii*) निर्धारणात्मक प्रयोग–वह प्रयोग जो समान परिस्थितियों के अन्तर्गत दुहराने पर समान परिणाम देता है।

जैसे–विज्ञान या अभियांत्रिकी में समान परिस्थितियों में प्रयोग को दुहराने पर हमेशा समान परिणाम आता है।

प्रतिदर्श समष्टि : किसी प्रयोग के सभी संभव परिणामों के समुच्चय प्रतिदर्श समष्टि कहलाता है।

जैसे– $S = \{1, 2, 3, 4, 5, 6\}$

किसी पासे को उछालने पर सभी संभव परिणाम हैं।

घटना : प्रतिदर्श समष्टि के सभी उप-समुच्चय एक घटना है। यह दो प्रकार के होते हैं–

(*i*) सरल घटना–वह घटना जिसमें केवल एक प्रतिदर्श बिन्दु होता है, सरल घटना कहलाती है।

जैसे–दो सिक्कों के उछालने पर प्रतिदर्श समष्टि $S = \{HH, HT, TH, TT\}$

यदि घटना, E = दो शीर्ष प्राप्त करने की घटना $= \{HH\}$

तब E सरल घटना है

(*ii*) संयुक्त घटना–वे घटनाएँ, जो सरल घटना नहीं है संयुक्त घटना कहलाती है।

जैसे–दो सिक्कों को उछालने पर प्रतिदर्श समष्टि

$$S = \{HH, HT, TH, TT\}$$

तो E = कम-से-कम एक पुच्छ (Tail) प्राप्त करने की घटना

$$E = \{TT, TH, HT\}$$

समसम्भावी घटनाएँ : किसी प्रयोग में यदि प्रत्येक घटना के घटित होने की संभावना समान हो तो वह घटनाएँ समसंभावी घटनाएँ कहलाती है।

जैसे–किसी सिक्का को उछालने पर शीर्ष एवं पुच्छ (Head and Tail) आने की संभावना समान है।

परस्पर अपवर्जी घटनाएँ : किसी प्रतिदर्श समष्टि S की दो घटनाएँ परस्पर अपवर्जी होगी यदि E_1 एवं E_2 साथ-साथ घटित ना हों अर्थात् $E_1 \cap E_2 = \phi$.

प्रायिकता : माना किसी यादृच्छिक प्रयोग में प्रतिदर्श समष्टि S तथा घटना $E \subseteq S$ है, तब घटना E के घटित होने की

प्रायिकता $P(E) = \dfrac{n(E)}{n(S)}$ होगी।

यदि $P(E) = 1$ तब E को निश्चित घटना तथा यदि $P(E) = 0$ तब E को असंभव घटना कहते हैं। अतः प्रायिकता हमेशा 0 से 1 के मध्य होता है अर्थात् $0 \le P(E) \le 1$

- यदि यादृच्छिक प्रयोग से संबंधित घटनाएँ E_1 एवं E_2 हो तब,

  $$P(E_1 \cup E_2) = P(E_1) + P(E_2) - P(E_1 \cap E_2)$$

- यदि E_1 एवं E_2 परस्पर अपवर्जी घटनाएँ हों तब

  $$P(E_1 \cup E_2) = P(E_1) + P(E_2)$$

- यदि $\bar{A}$, A नहीं है को सूचित करता है तब

$$P(\bar{A}) = 1 - P(A) \quad \text{या} \quad P(A') = 1 - P(A)$$

$$\Rightarrow \quad P(A) = 1 - P(\bar{A})$$

उदाहरण 1. दो सिक्कों को एक साथ उछाला जाता है तब (*i*) केवल एक शीर्ष (*ii*) कम-से-कम एक शीर्ष आने की प्रायिकता निकालें।

हल : दो सिक्कों को एक साथ उछालने पर प्रतिदर्श समष्टि की संख्या $= 2^2 = 4$

अतः $S = \{HH, HT, TH, TT\}$

माना E_1 केवल एक शीर्ष आने की घटना है तब

$$n(E_1) = \{HT, TH\} = 2$$

तथा E_2 = कम-से-कम एक शीर्ष आने की घटना

$$= \{HH, HT, TH\} = 3$$

अतः (*i*) $\quad P(E_1) = \dfrac{n(E_1)}{n(S)} = \dfrac{2}{4} = \dfrac{1}{2}$

(*ii*) $\quad P(E_2) = \dfrac{n(E_2)}{n(S)} = \dfrac{3}{4}$

उदाहरण 2. यदि दो पासे को एक साथ फेंका जाता है तो इसके पृष्ठ पर आने वाली अंकों का योग 7 से अधिक हो, की प्रायिकता ज्ञात करें।

हल : $n(3) = 6 \times 6 = 36$

माना E = पृष्ठ पर आने वाली अंकों का योग 7 से अधिक

$= \{(2, 6)(3, 5)(3, 6)(4, 4)(4, 5)(4, 6)(5, 3)(5, 4)(5, 5)(5, 6)(6, 2), (6, 3)(6, 4)(6, 5)(6, 6)\}$

$= 15$

$$\therefore \quad P(E) = \frac{n(E)}{n(S)} = \frac{15}{36} = \frac{5}{12}$$

उदाहरण 3. ताश की किसी गड्डी से 2 पत्ता यादृच्छया निकाला जाता है तो इसके बादशाह होने की प्रायिकता ज्ञात करें।

हलः $n(S) = 52\,C_2 = \dfrac{52 \times 51}{2 \times 1} = 26 \times 51 = 1326$

यदि E = दो बादशाह आने की घटना।

तब $\quad n(E) = 4C_2 = \dfrac{4 \times 3}{2} = 6$

अतः $\quad P(E) = \dfrac{n(E)}{n(S)} = \dfrac{6}{1326} = \dfrac{1}{221}$

उदाहरण 4. किसी थैला में 4 लाल, 6 काली, 8 हरी गेंद हैं। यादृच्छया 2 गेंद निकाला जाता है तब दोनों के काली होने की प्रायिकता ज्ञात करें।

हल : थैला में कुल गेंदों की संख्या $= 4 + 6 + 8 = 18$

$$\therefore \quad n(S) = 18C_2$$

माना E = दो काली गेंद आने की घटना

$$n(E) = 6C_2$$

अतः $\quad P(E) = \dfrac{n(E)}{n(S)} = \dfrac{6C_2}{18C_2}$

$$= \frac{\frac{6 \times 5}{2}}{\frac{18 \times 17}{2}} = \frac{6 \times 5}{18 \times 17} = \frac{5}{51}$$

$$\therefore \quad P(E) = \frac{5}{51}$$

उदाहरण 5. 1 से 20 तक की संख्याओं में से तीन संख्याओं को यादृच्छया चयन किया जाता है तो इसके लगातार (Consecutive) होने की प्रायिकता क्या होगी?

हल : 20 संख्याओं में से 3 संख्याओं को चयन करने के कुल तरीके $= 20C_3$

$$= \frac{20 \times 19 \times 18}{3 \times 2}$$

$$\therefore \quad n(S) = 20C3 = 1140$$

यदि E = तीन लगातार संख्याओं के चयन के तरीके

$= \{(1, 2, 3)(2, 3, 4)(3, 4, 5) \ldots. (18, 19, 20)\}$

$$n(E) = 18$$

अतः $\quad P(E) = \dfrac{n(E)}{n(S)} = \dfrac{18}{1140} = \dfrac{3}{190}$

उदाहरण 6. किसी थैला में 4 लाल, 5 हरी तथा 6 सफेद गेंद हैं। यदि यादृच्छया एक गेंद निकाली जाए तो इसके लाल या हरी होने की संभावना ज्ञात करें।

हल : कुल गेंदों की संख्या = 4 + 5 + 6 = 15

∴ $n(S) = 15$

माना E_1 = लाल गेंद होने की घटना = 4

E_2 = हरी गेंद होने की घटना = 5

तब $E_1 \cap E_2 = \phi$

अतः $P(E_1$ या $E_2) = P(E_1) + P(E_2)$

$$= \left(\frac{4}{15} + \frac{5}{15}\right) = \frac{9}{15} = \frac{3}{5}$$

उदाहरण 7. एक थैला में 2 लाल, 3 हरी तथा 2 सफेद गेंद हैं। यादृच्छया दो गेंद निकाली जाती हैं तो उसकी सफेद न होने की प्रायिकता ज्ञात करें।

हल : कुल गेंदों की संख्या = (2 + 3 + 2) = 7

$$\therefore \quad n(S) = 7C_2 = \frac{7 \times 6}{2} = 21$$

माना E = 2 गेंद निकलने की घटना जो सफेद न हो = (2 + 3) = 5

$$\therefore \quad n(E) = 5C_2 = 10$$

$$\therefore \quad P(E) = \frac{n(E)}{n(S)} = \frac{10}{21}$$

उदाहरण 8. किसी ताश की गड्डी से यादृच्छया दो पत्ता निकाला जाए तो इसकी क्या संभावना है कि दोनों या तो लाल हो या दोनों बादशाह?

हल : $n(S) = 52C_2 = \frac{52 \times 51}{2} = 1326$

माना E_1 = दोनों पत्ते को लाल होने की घटना

$$n(E_1) = 26C_2 = \frac{26 \times 25}{2} = 325$$

E_2 = दोनों पत्ते के बादशाह होने की घटना

$$n(E_2) = 4C_2 = \frac{4 \times 3}{2} = 6$$

तथा $(E_1 \cap E_2)$ = दोनों पत्ते लाल का बादशाह

$$\therefore \quad n(E_1 \cap E_2) = 2C_2 = 1$$

$$\therefore \quad P(E_1 \cup E_2) = P(E_1) + P(E_2) - P(E_1 \cap E_2)$$

$$= \frac{325}{1326} + \frac{6}{1326} - \frac{1}{1326}$$

$$= \frac{330}{1326} = \frac{55}{221}$$

उदाहरण 9. किसी कक्षा में 15 छात्र एवं 10 छात्राएँ हैं। यदि इसमें से 3 विद्यार्थी को चुनना हो तो इसकी क्या संभावना है कि उसमें 1 छात्रा एवं 2 छात्र होंगे।

हल : $n(S) = 25C_3 = \frac{25 \times 24 \times 23}{3 \times 2} = 2300$

यदि E = 1 छात्रा एवं 2 छात्र चुनने की घटना

$$\therefore \quad n(E) = 15\,C_2 \times 10\,C_1$$

$$= \frac{15 \times 14}{2} \times 10 = 1050$$

$$\therefore \quad P(E) = \frac{n(E)}{n(S)} = \frac{1050}{2300} = \frac{105}{230} = \frac{21}{46}$$

उदाहरण 10. यदि $P(A) = 0.25$, $P(B) = 0.50$ तथा $P(A \cap B) = 0.14$ तब $P(A \cap \overline{B})$ मान ज्ञात करें।

हल : दिया है, $P(A) = 0.25$, $P(B) = 0.50$

तथा $P(A \cap B) = 0.14$

अतः $P(A \cap \overline{B}) = P(A) - P(A \cap B)$

$= 0.25 - 0.14$

$= 0.11$

प्रश्नमाला

निर्देश : निम्नलिखित प्रश्नों को हल करें :

1. एक बर्तन में 2 लाल, 3 नीली तथा 4 काली गेंद हैं। यादृच्छया तीन गेंद निकाली जाती हैं, तो सभी के एक ही रंग के होने की प्रायिकता है–

A. $\frac{5}{84}$ B. $\frac{3}{9}$

C. $\frac{3}{7}$ D. $\frac{7}{17}$

2. तीन पासे एक साथ फेंके जाते हैं। उन पर आनेवाले अंकों का योग 17 या 18 होने की प्रायिकता है–

A. $\frac{1}{72}$ B. $\frac{1}{9}$

C. $\frac{1}{54}$ D. $\frac{4}{17}$

3. शब्द POSSESSIVE से एक अक्षर यादृच्छया चुना जाता है, तो इसके S होने की प्रायिकता है–

A. $\frac{3}{10}$ B. $\frac{4}{10}$

C. $\frac{3}{7}$ D. $\frac{4}{17}$

4. यदि A और B दो घटनाएँ हैं तथा $P(A') = 0.3$, $P(B) = 0.4$, $P(A \cap B') = 0.5$ तब $P(A \cap B')$ का मान–

A. 0.5 B. 0.8

C. 1 D. 0.1

5. किसी बक्से में 3 आम तथा 3 सेब हैं। यदि दो फल यादृच्छया चुने जाएँ तो एक आम तथा एक सेब होने की प्रायिकता–

A. $\frac{2}{3}$ B. $\frac{3}{5}$

C. $\frac{1}{3}$ D. $\frac{3}{4}$

6. छः (6) पुरस्कारों को तीन व्यक्ति में वितरण यादृच्छया किया जाता है, तो किसी एक व्यक्ति को सभी पुरस्कार नहीं मिलने की संभावना होगी।

A. $\frac{120}{216}$ B. $\frac{6}{216}$

C. $\frac{210}{216}$ D. $\frac{790}{216}$

7. 100 पत्तों की गड्डी जिन पर 1 से 100 तक संख्याएँ लिखी हैं, में से यादृच्छया एक पत्ता निकाला जाता है, तो पूर्ण वर्ग संख्या आने की प्रायिकता है–

A. $\frac{1}{5}$ B. $\frac{2}{5}$

C. $\frac{1}{10}$ D. $\frac{1}{15}$

8. तीन व्यक्ति एक समस्या पर स्वतंत्र रूप से कार्य करते हैं। उनके द्वारा समस्या का हल करने की प्रायिकताएँ क्रमशः $\frac{1}{3}, \frac{1}{4}$ एवं $\frac{1}{5}$ है तो किसी के द्वारा समस्या न हल होने की प्रायिकता है–

A. $\frac{1}{3}$ B. $\frac{3}{5}$

C. $\frac{2}{5}$ D. $\frac{1}{5}$

9. एक लॉटरी में 90 टिकट है, जिन पर 1 से 90 तक की संख्याएँ अंकित हैं। पाँच टिकट यादृच्छया चुने जाते हैं। इनमें से दो टिकटों पर 15 तथा 80 संख्या होने की प्रायिकता है–

A. $\frac{2}{801}$ B. $\frac{2}{623}$

C. $\frac{1}{267}$ D. $\frac{1}{623}$

10. A तथा B में से कम-से-कम एक के घटने की प्रायिकता 0.6 है। यदि A एवं B के साथ-साथ घटित होने की प्रायिकता 0.2 हो तब $P(A') + P(B')$ का मान–

A. 3.2 B. 1.5

C. 1.03 D. 1.2

11. किसी बक्से में 20 बल्ब हैं जिसमें से 4 खराब है। यादृच्छया दो बल्ब निकाला जाता है तो इसमें कम-से-कम 1 खराब होने की संभावना है–

A. $\frac{7}{19}$ B. $\frac{9}{19}$

C. $\frac{12}{19}$ D. $\frac{17}{19}$

12. दो पासे को फेंका जाता है तब इसके पृष्ठ पर आने वाले अंकों का योग अभाज्य संख्या होने की प्रायिकता–

A. $\frac{7}{9}$ B. $\frac{1}{12}$

C. $\frac{5}{12}$ D. $\frac{11}{12}$

13. किसी लॉटरी में 10 पुरस्कार एवं 25 खाली (पुरस्कार रहित) हैं। यदि एक टिकट यादृच्छया निकाला जाए तो पुरस्कार मिलने की प्रायिकता–

A. $\frac{1}{25}$ B. $\frac{1}{10}$

C. $\frac{1}{35}$ D. $\frac{2}{7}$

14. किसी बॉक्से में 5 हरी, 4 पीली एवं 3 सफेद शीशे की गोली है। तीन गोली यादृच्छया निकाला जाता है तब इसके एक ही रंग न होने की प्रायिकता–

A. $\frac{41}{44}$ B. $\frac{1}{44}$

C. $\frac{7}{55}$ D. $\frac{12}{55}$

15. यदि $N = \{1, 2, 3, ... 100\}$ से यादृच्छया 3 विभिन्न संख्या चुनी जाती है तो इन तीनों के 2 और 3 दोनों से विभाजित होने की प्रायिकता होगी–

A. $\frac{4}{25}$ B. $\frac{4}{35}$

C. $\frac{4}{33}$ D. $\frac{4}{1155}$

उत्तरमाला

1	2	3	4	5	6	7	8	9	10
A	C	B	B	B	C	C	C	A	D
11	**12**	**13**	**14**	**15**					
A	C	D	A	D					

व्याख्यात्मक उत्तर

1. कुल गेंद = 9

9 गेंद में से 3 गेंद निकालने के कुल तरीके = $9\,C_3$

$\therefore \quad n(S) = \frac{9 \times 8 \times 7}{3 \times 2} = 84$

E = सभी गेंद एक ही रंग के हो

$\therefore \quad n(E) = 3C_3 + 4C_3 = 1 + 4 = 5$

($\therefore$ लाल गेंद 2 ही है)

अतः अभीष्ट प्रायिकता $= \frac{n(E)}{n(S)} = \frac{5}{84}$.

2. तीन पासे फेंकने के कुल तरीके $= 6 \times 6 \times 6 = 216$

अतः $n(S) = 216$

माना E = योगफल 17 या 18 आने की घटना

$\therefore \quad = (6, 5, 6)\ (5, 6, 6)\ (6, 6, 5)\ (6, 6, 6)$

$n(E) = 4$

$\therefore \quad P(E) = \frac{n(E)}{n(S)} = \frac{4}{216} = \frac{1}{54}$.

3. कुल अक्षरों की संख्या = 10

$n(S) = 10$

E = S आने की घटना

$n(E) = 4$

$\therefore \quad P(E) = \frac{n(E)}{n(S)} = \frac{4}{10}$.

4. योग के प्रमेय से

$$P(A \cup B') = P(A) + P(B') - P(A \cap B')$$
$$= 1 - P(A') + 1 - P(B) - P(A \cap B')$$

$= 1 - 0.3 + 1 - 0.5 - 0.4$
$= 0.8.$

5. 6 में से दो फल चुनने के कुल तरीके $= 6\,C_2$

$\therefore \quad n(S) = 6\,C_2 = \frac{6 \times 5}{2} = 15$

E = 1आम तथा 1 सेब होने की घटना

$n(E) = 3\,C_1 \times 3\,C_1 = 3 \times 3$

$\therefore \quad P(E) = \frac{n(E)}{n(S)} = \frac{9}{15} = \frac{3}{5}.$

6. पुरस्कारों के वितरण करने के कुल तरीके $= 6 \times 6 \times 6$

अतः $n(S) = 216$

E = एक ही व्यक्ति को सभी पुरस्कार प्राप्त होने के तरीके

$n(E) = 6$

अतः किसी एक व्यक्ति को सभी पुरस्कार नहीं मिलने की प्रायिकता

= 1 – P (एक ही व्यक्ति को सभी पुरस्कार)

$= 1 - \frac{n(E)}{n(S)} = 1 - \frac{6}{216}$

$= \frac{210}{216}.$

7. एक पत्ता निकालने के कुल तरीके $= 100\,C_1 = 100$

अतः $n(S) = 100$

E = पूर्ण वर्ग संख्या आने की घटना

$= 1^2, 2^2, 3^2, 4^2, 5^2, 6^2, 7^2, 8^2, 9^2, 10^2$

$n(E) = 10$

$\therefore \quad P(E) = \frac{n(E)}{n(S)} = \frac{10}{100} = \frac{1}{10}.$

8. माना प्रत्येक व्यक्ति द्वारा समस्या का हल करने की प्रायिकता $P(A) = \frac{1}{3}, P(B) = \frac{1}{4}$ तथा $P(C) = \frac{1}{5}$ है तब प्रत्येक के द्वारा समस्या हल न होने की प्रायिकता

$P(\overline{A}) = 1 - \frac{1}{3} = \frac{2}{3}, \quad P(\overline{B}) = 1 - \frac{1}{4} = \frac{3}{4}$ तथा

$P(\overline{C}) = 1 - \frac{1}{5} = \frac{4}{5}.$

अतः तीनों में से किसी के द्वारा समस्या का हल न होने की प्रायिकता

$P(\overline{A} \cap \overline{B} \cap \overline{C}) = P(\overline{A}) \cdot P(\overline{B}) \cdot P(\overline{C})$

$= \frac{2}{3} \times \frac{3}{4} \times \frac{4}{5} = \frac{2}{5}.$

9. पाँच टिकटों में से दो टिकट (जिनकी संख्या 15 तथा 80 है) होने चाहिए अब शेष 88 में से तीन टिकट

$n(E)$ = चुनने के प्रकार $= 88\,C_3$

$n(S)$ = कुल चुनने के तरीके $= 90\,C_5$

अतः अभीष्ट प्रायिकता $= \frac{88\,C_3}{90\,C_5}$

$$= \frac{\dfrac{88 \times 87 \times 86}{3 \times 2}}{\dfrac{90 \times 89 \times 88 \times 87 \times 86}{5 \times 4 \times 3 \times 2}}$$

$= \frac{5 \times 4}{90 \times 89} = \frac{20}{8010} = \frac{2}{801}.$

10. दिया गया है $P(A \cup B) = 0.6$

तथा $P(A \cap B) = 0.2$

अब $P(A') + P(B') = 1 - P(A) + 1 - P(B)$

$= 2 - [P(A) + P(B)]$

$= 2 - [P(A) + P(B) - P(A \cap B) + P(A \cap B)]$

$= 2 - [P(A \cup B) + P(A \cap B)]$

$= 2 - (0.6 + 0.2)$

$= 2 - 0.8$

$= 1.2.$

11. 20 बल्ब में से 2 बल्ब चुनने के कुल तरीके

$En(S) = 20\,C_2$

माना E = कोई खराब बल्ब नहीं

$n(E) = 16\,C_2$

किसी बल्ब के खराब नहीं होने की प्रायिकता

$$P(E) = \frac{16\,C_2}{20\,C_2} = \frac{\dfrac{16 \times 15}{2}}{\dfrac{20 \times 19}{2}} = \frac{16 \times 15}{20 \times 19} = \frac{12}{19}$$

अतः कम-से-कम 1 बल्ब खराब होने की प्रायिकता

$$= 1-\frac{12}{19}=\frac{7}{19}.$$

12. $n(S) = 6 \times 6 = 36$

माना E = पासे पर आए अंकों का योग अभाज्य संख्या

E = {(1, 1) (1, 2) (1, 4) (1, 6) (2, 1) (2, 3) (2, 5) (3, 2) (3, 4) (4, 1) (4,3) (5, 2) (5, 6) (6, 1) (6, 5)}

$n(E) = 15$

$$P(E) = \frac{n(E)}{n(S)}=\frac{15}{36}=\frac{5}{12}.$$

13. कुल टिकट की संख्या = 25 + 10 = 35

$n(S) = 35$

E = पुरस्कार मिलने की घटना

$n(E) = 10$

$$\therefore \quad P(E) = \frac{n(E)}{n(S)}=\frac{10}{35}=\frac{2}{7}.$$

14. 12 गोली में से 3 गोली निकालने के कुल तरीके

$$n(S) = 12\,C_3 = \frac{12\times 11\times 10}{3\times 2} = 220$$

माना E = एक ही रंग के 3 गोली निकलने के तरीके

= (5 में से 3) या (4 में से 3) या (3 में से 3)

$n(E) = 5\,C_3 + 4\,C_3 + 3\,C_3$

$= 10 + 4 + 1 = 15$

$$P(E) = \frac{n(E)}{n(S)}=\frac{15}{220}=\frac{3}{44}$$

$\therefore$ अभीष्ट प्रायिकता $= 1-\frac{3}{44}=\frac{41}{44}.$

15. 1 से 100 के बीच 6 से विभाज्य संख्याएँ 6, 12, 18 .... 96. यदि ऐसी n संख्याएं हैं तब $96 = 6 + (n-1)\times 6$

$\Rightarrow n = 16$

अतः प्रायिकता $= \frac{16C_3}{100C_3}=\frac{4}{1155}.$

☆☆☆☆☆☆

सामान्य बुद्धिमत्ता एवं तर्कशक्ति
(General Intelligence and Reasoning)

भाषिक

श्रृंखला (SERIES)

भाग-I अक्षर श्रृंखला (Letter Series)

अक्षर श्रृंखला में निहित अक्षरों का एक निश्चित क्रम होता है। दी गई अक्षर श्रृंखला में अक्षर वर्णमाला के सीधे क्रम में भी हो सकते हैं और वर्णमाला के विपरीत क्रम में भी। यही नहीं, एक ही श्रृंखला में अक्षर वर्णमाला के सीधे क्रम में और वर्णमाला के विपरीत या उल्टे क्रम में अर्थात् दोनों ही अनुक्रमों में भी हो सकते हैं। श्रृंखला में दिए गए क्रम में कुछ अक्षर छोड़े भी गए हो सकते हैं या ऐसा भी हो सकता है कि श्रृंखला में कुछ अक्षरों को एकाधिक बार प्रयुक्त किया गया हो या फिर वे क्रमागत हों। श्रृंखला एकल भी हो सकती है और एक ही श्रृंखला में एकांतर क्रम में दो अलग-अलग श्रृंखलाएं भी निहित हो सकती हैं। अक्षर श्रृंखला पर आधारित प्रश्नों को हल करते समय श्रृंखला के पैटर्न पर ध्यान दिया जाना आवश्यक होता है।

वर्णमाला के सीधे क्रम में अक्षरों की श्रृंखला है :

A B C D E F G H I J K L M N O P Q R S T U V W X Y Z

A ↓ पहला, E ↓ 5वाँ, J ↓ 10वाँ, O ↓ 15वाँ, T ↓ 20वाँ, Y ↓ 25वाँ

वर्णमाला के विपरीत या उल्टे क्रम में अक्षरों की श्रृंखला है :

Z Y X W V U T S R Q P O N M L K J I H G F E D C B A

Z ↓ पहला, V ↓ 5वाँ, Q ↓ 10वाँ, L ↓ 15वाँ, G ↓ 20वाँ, B ↓ 25वाँ

टिप्पणी : Z पर पहुंच कर श्रृंखला A से पुनः शुरू होती है और A पर पहुंच कर श्रृंखला Z से पुनः शुरू होती है।

हल किए गए उदाहरण

निर्देश: *नीचे दी गई श्रृंखला में प्रश्न चिह्न को प्रतिस्थापित करने के लिए दिए गए विकल्पों में से सही अक्षर का चयन करें :*

1. B D F H J ?

(*a*) L (*b*) O (*c*) M (*d*) K

उत्तर (*a*) : श्रृंखला में प्रत्येक दो अक्षरों के बीच वर्णमाला के सीधे क्रम में एक अक्षर छूट गया है।

B →(+2) D →(+2) F →(+2) H →(+2) J →(+2) L

2. A Z B Y C ?
(*a*) D (*b*) X (*c*) U (*d*) E

उत्तर *(b)* : इस शृंखला में बारी-बारी से दो शृंखलाएं अंतर्निहित हैं :

शृंखला *I* : A B C (प्राकृतिक क्रम अर्थात् वर्णमाला के सीधे क्रम में क्रमागत अक्षर)

शृंखला *II* : Z Y X (वर्णमाला के विपरीत क्रम में क्रमागत अक्षर)

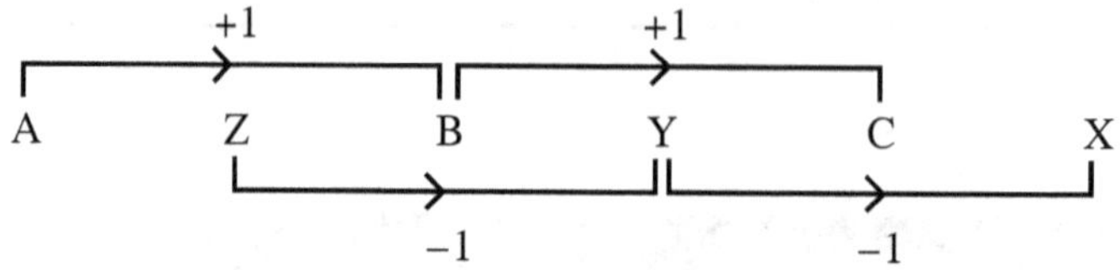

अभ्यास

निर्देश (प्र.सं. 1–10): *नीचे दी गई प्रत्येक शृंखला में अक्षरों का क्रम निर्धारित करें। तत्पश्चात् दिए गए विकल्पों में से उस विकल्प का चयन करें जिससे दी गई शृंखला में प्रश्न चिह्न प्रतिस्थापित होता हो।*

1. B Y C X D W E ?
(*a*) S (*b*) T
(*c*) U (*d*) V

2. A D C G E ?
(*a*) G (*b*) J
(*c*) I (*d*) L

3. L N P R T ?
(*a*) U (*b*) V
(*c*) W (*d*) Y

4. X O I F ?
(*a*) D (*b*) F
(*c*) B (*d*) E

5. B A F E J I P O ? U
(*a*) V (*b*) T
(*c*) S (*d*) Q

6. Z A A Y B B X C ?
(*a*) W (*b*) C
(*c*) V (*d*) D

7. A Z Y B X W C V U D T S E ?
(*a*) R S (*b*) S T
(*c*) R Q (*d*) Q R

8. C A B F D E I G H ?
(*a*) J L K (*b*) J K L
(*c*) L K J (*d*) L J K

9. B F K Q ?
(*a*) U (*b*) T
(*c*) X (*d*) Y

10. R K F ? B
(*a*) D (*b*) C
(*c*) E (*d*) B

व्याख्यात्मक उत्तर

1. *(d)* : दी गई शृंखला में बारी-बारी से दो अक्षर शृंखलाएं अंतर्निहित हैं।

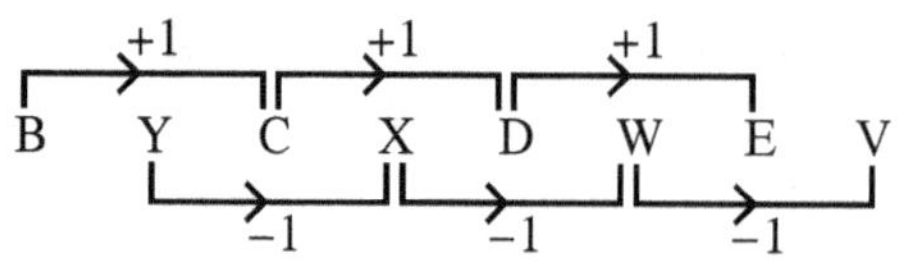

शृंखला I : BCDE (वर्णमला के सीधे क्रम में)

शृंखला II : YXWV (वर्णमाला के विपरीत क्रम में)

2. *(b)* : दी गई शृंखला में बारी-बारी से दो अक्षर शृंखलाएं अंतर्निहित हैं।

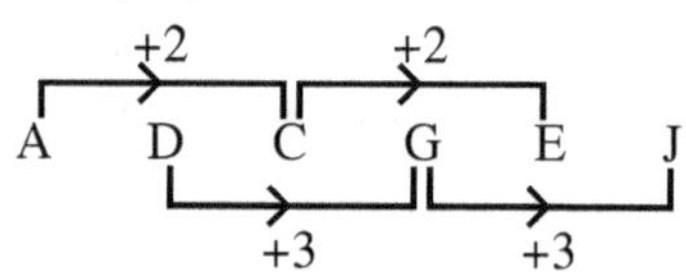

शृंखला I : ACE (शृंखला +2 पैटर्न का अनुपालन करती है)

शृंखला II : DGJ (शृंखला +3 पैटर्न का अनुपालन करती है)

3. (*b*) : शृंखला +2 पैटर्न का अनुपालन करती है, अर्थात्

L N P R T V

+2 +2 +2 +2 +2

4. (*b*) : शृंखला में दो सन्निकट अक्षरों के बीच वर्णमाला के विपरीत क्रम में क्रमश: 3 की कमी होती जाती है, अर्थात्

X O I F F

−9 −6 −3 −0

5. (*a*) : शृंखला में अंग्रेजी वर्णमाला के पांच स्वर (vowel) हैं अर्थात् (AEIOU) जिनमें से प्रत्येक के पहले वर्णमाला के सीधे क्रम में उसके ठीक बाद का क्रमागत अक्षर लिखा गया है।

B A F E J I P O V U

6. (*b*) : शृंखला में बारी-बारी से तीन शृंखलाएं अंतर्निहित हैं जिनमें से दूसरी और तीसरी शृंखलाएं एक जैसी हैं, अर्थात्

−1 −1

Z AA Y BB X CC

+1 +1

शृंखला I : ZYX (वर्णमाला के विपरीत क्रम में)

शृंखला II और III : ABC (वर्णमाला के सीधे क्रम में) अक्षर 'C' शृंखला II और III में उभयनिष्ठ है।

7. (*c*) : शृंखला में बारी-बारी से दो शृंखलाएं अंतर्निहित हैं।

+1 +1 +1 +1

A Z Y B X W C V U D T S E R Q

−1 −1 −1 −1 −1 −1 −1 −1 −1

शृंखला I : ABCDE (वर्णमाला के सीधे क्रम में)

शृंखला II : ZY XW VU TS RQ (वर्णमाला के विपरीत क्रम में एक साथ दो अक्षर)

8. (*d*) : वर्णमाला के सीधे क्रम में 3 अक्षरों के समूह से एक खंड निर्मित होता है। प्रत्येक खंड में 3 अक्षरों के समूह में पहला अक्षर बीच में है जिसकी दाहिनी ओर उसका क्रमागत अक्षर है तथा तीसरा क्रमागत अक्षर बीच के अक्षर की बायीं ओर अवस्थित है।

<u>CAB</u> <u>FDE</u> <u>IGH</u> <u>LJK</u>

9. (*c*) : शृंखला में दो सन्निकट अक्षरों के बीच अंतर में प्रत्येक चरण में एक की वृद्धि होती जाती है।

B F K Q X

+4 +5 +6 +7

10. (*b*) : शृंखला में दो क्रमागत अक्षरों के बीच वर्णमाला के विपरीत क्रम में अंतर में क्रमश: 2 की कमी होती जाती है।

R K F C B

−7 −5 −3 −1

भाग-II गलत या बेमेल अक्षर-शृंखला (Wrong Letter Series)

इस प्रकार के प्रश्नों में दी गई शृंखला में अभ्यर्थियों को ऐसे अक्षर या अक्षर-समूह ज्ञात करने की आवश्यकता नहीं होती जिनसे दी गई शृंखला पूर्ण होती है बल्कि उन्हें ऐसे अक्षर का पता लगाना होता है जो शृंखला में गलत या बेमेल हो।

हल किए गए उदाहरण

दी गई शृंखला में कौन-सा अक्षर गलत या बेमेल है?

J M P T V Y

(*a*) J (*b*) P (*c*) T (*d*) Y

उत्तर (*c*) : शृंखला में दो सन्निकट अक्षरों के बीच वर्णमाला के क्रम में +3 का अंतर है।

J M P S V Y

+3 +3 +3 +3 +3

अत: अक्षर T के स्थान पर S होना चाहिए।

अभ्यास

निर्देश (प्र.सं. 1–10): *नीचे के प्रत्येक प्रश्न में दी गई अक्षर-शृंखला में कौन-सा अक्षर या अक्षर-समूह गलत या बेमेल है?*

1. A E H O U
(*a*) U (*b*) O
(*c*) H (*d*) E

2. C H M S W B
(*a*) C (*b*) S
(*c*) B (*d*) W

3. X S N I C Y
(*a*) Y (*b*) C
(*c*) S (*d*) I

4. Z A W B X C
(*a*) D (*b*) C
(*c*) X (*d*) W

5. M L O N Q P R
(*a*) R (*b*) O
(*c*) Q (*d*) L

6. D K R Y F L
(*a*) L (*b*) D
(*c*) R (*d*) Y

7. L N Q T W Z C F
(*a*) C (*b*) Q
(*c*) L (*d*) F

8. XW, DC, CB, NM, PQ
(*a*) NM (*b*) CB
(*c*) PQ (*d*) XW

9. B E I N S A I
(*a*) A (*b*) E
(*c*) S (*d*) I

10. Z T P K H F
(*a*) Z (*b*) P
(*c*) T (*d*) F

व्याख्यात्मक उत्तर

1. (*c*) : शृंखला अंग्रेजी वर्णमाला के केवल स्वरों AEIOU से निर्मित है। अत: H के स्थान पर I होना चाहिए।

2. (*b*) : शृंखला में दो सन्निकट अक्षरों के बीच वर्णमाला के सीधे क्रम में +5 का अंतर है।

C H M R W B
+5 +5 +5 +5 +5

अत: शृंखला में S के स्थान पर R होना चाहिए।
(शृंखला Z पर पहुंचने के बाद A से पुन: शुरू होती है।)

3. (*b*) : शृंखला में दो सन्निकट अक्षरों के बीच वर्णमाला के उल्टे क्रम में –5 का अंतर है।

X S N I D Y
–5 –5 –5 –5 –5

अत: C के स्थान पर D होना चाहिए।

4. (*d*) : दी गई शृंखला में दो शृंखलाएं अंतर्निहित हैं :

A → Y (+1), B → C (+1)
Z A Y B X C
Z → Y (–1), Y → X (–1)

शृंखला I : ZYX (वर्णमाला के विपरीत क्रम में)

शृंखला II : ABC (वर्णमाला के सीधे क्रम में)
अत: शृंखला में W के स्थान पर Y होना चाहिए।

5. (*a*) : शृंखला में दो क्रमागत अक्षर विपरीत क्रम में लिखे गए हैं।

<u>ML</u> <u>ON</u> <u>QP</u> <u>SR</u>

अत: शृंखला में R के स्थान पर S होना चाहिए।

6. (*a*) : शृंखला में दो सन्निकट अक्षरों के बीच +7 का अंतर है।

D K R Y F M
+7 +7 +7 +7 +7

अत: शृंखला में L के स्थान पर M होना चाहिए।

7. (*c*) : शृंखला में दो सन्निकट अक्षरों के बीच +3 का अंतर है।

K N Q T W Z C F
+3 +3 +3 +3 +3 +3 +3

अत: L के स्थान पर K होना चाहिए।

8. (*c*) : शृंखला कोई भी दो क्रमागत अक्षरों को वर्णमाला के विपरीत क्रम में शामिल करके निर्मित की गई है।

XW ← DC ← CB ← NM ← QP ←

अत: शृंखला में P से पहले Q आना चाहिए।

9. (*c*) : शृंखला में प्रत्येक चरण में दो सन्निकट अक्षरों के बीच अंतर में एक की वृद्धि होती जाती है।

B E I N T A I

+3 +4 +5 +6 +7 +8

अत: शृंखला में S के स्थान पर T होना चाहिए।

10. (*b*) : वर्णमाला के विपरीत क्रम में लिखी गई इस शृंखला में प्रत्येक चरण में दो सन्निकट अक्षरों के बीच अंतर में एक की कमी होती जाती है।

Z T O K H F

−6 −5 −4 −3 −2

अत: P के स्थान पर O होना चाहिए।

भाग-III संख्या-शृंखला (Number Series)

इस प्रकार की शृंखला में दी गई संख्याओं के समुच्चय एक दूसरे से एक विशेष पैटर्न या रुप में संबंधित होते हैं। संख्याओं के बीच संबंध *(i)* क्रमागत विषम/सम संख्याओं; *(ii)* क्रमागत अविभाज्य संख्याओं; *(iii)* किसी संख्या (या संख्याओं) का वर्गफल/घनफल जिसमें किसी संख्या को जोड़ने या घटाने पर परिवर्तन होता है/नहीं होता; *(iv)* पूर्ववर्ती संख्याओं का योग/गुणनफल/अंतर; *(v)* किसी संख्या से योग/घटाव/गुणा/भाग; और *(vi)* उपर्युक्त संबंधों के अनेक और भी संयोजनों पर आधारित होता है।

हल किए गए उदाहरण

1. नीचे दी गई संख्या-शृंखला को पूरा करने के लिए कौन-सा विकल्प उपयुक्त है?

4, 8, 12, 16, ?

(*a*) 18 (*b*) 20 (*c*) 22 (*d*) 24

उत्तर (*b*): शृंखला में अंतर्निहित संख्याएं 4 की गुणज (multiples) हैं। शृंखला में अंतर्निहित अवयवों की एक अन्य व्याख्या यह है कि शृंखला की दो आनुक्रमिक संख्याओं के बीच 4 का अंतर है।

4 8 12 16 20

×2 ×3 ×4 ×5

या

4 8 12 16 20

+4 +4 +4 +4

2. दी गई शृंखला में प्रश्न चिह्न के स्थान पर क्या होगा?

2, 14, 98, 686, ?

(*a*) 1976 (*b*) 2548 (*c*) 980 (*d*) 4802

उत्तर (*d*) : शृंखला में अंतर्निहित संख्याएं 7 की गुणज हैं।

2 14 98 686 4802

×7 ×7 ×7 ×7

(किसी दी गई संख्या-शृंखला में बारी-बारी से एकाधिक शृंखलाएं भी अंतर्निहित हो सकती हैं।)

अभ्यास

निर्देश (प्र.सं. 1–10): *शृंखलाओं को पूरा करने के लिए दिए गए विकल्पों में से लुप्त पद/संख्या ज्ञात करें।*

1. 3, 9, 27, 81, 243, ?
(*a*) 486 (*b*) 729
(*c*) 972 (*d*) 359

2. 1, 6, 12, 19, 27, ?
(*a*) 38 (*b*) 35
(*c*) 36 (*d*) 54

3. 8, 48, 16, 96, 32, ?
(*a*) 192 (*b*) 150
(*c*) 64 (*d*) 288

4. 2, 3, 6, 18, 108, ?
(*a*) 1944 (*b*) 1658
(*c*) 648 (*d*) 1008

5. 1, 2, 3, 2, 3, 5, 4, 5, ?
(*a*) 9 (*b*) 6
(*c*) 10 (*d*) 7

6. 3, 8, 13, 24, 41, ?
(*a*) 65 (*b*) 75
(*c*) 70 (*d*) 80

7. 0, 8, 24, 48, 80, ?
(*a*) 110 (*b*) 96
(*c*) 120 (*d*) 140

8. 0, 5, 22, 57, ?, 205
(*a*) 198 (*b*) 116
(*c*) 172 (*d*) 92

9. 6, 9, 18, 45, 126, 369, ?
(*a*) 1059 (*b*) 1095
(*c*) 1098 (*d*) 1089

10. 1, 2, 5, 12, 27, 58, 121, ?
(*a*) 246 (*b*) 247
(*c*) 248 (*d*) 249

व्याख्यात्मक उत्तर

1. (*b*) : शृंखला में निहित संख्याओं को अगली संख्या प्राप्त करने के लिए 3 से गुणा किया गया है।

2. (*c*) : शृंखला के आरंभिक पदों अर्थात् 1 और 6 के बीच 5 का अंतर है और तत्पश्चात् शृंखला की आनुक्रमिक संख्याओं के बीच अंतर में क्रमशः 1 की वृद्धि होती जाती है।

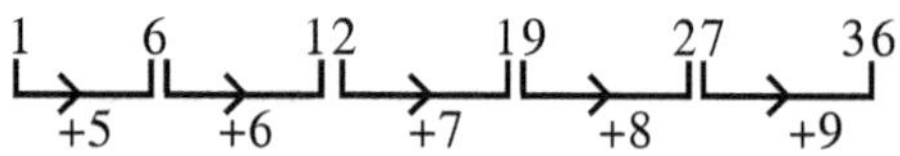

3. (*a*) : *व्याख्या I* : शृंखला में पहले 6 से गुणा करने और तत्पश्चात् 3 से भाग करने का पैटर्न अपनाया गया है जिसकी पुनरावृत्ति होती है।

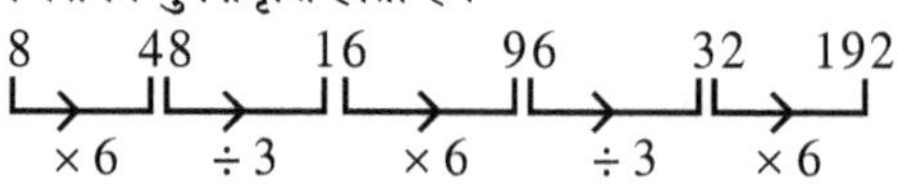

व्याख्या II : शृंखला में बारी-बारी से दो शृंखलाएं अंतर्निहित हैं और प्रत्येक शृंखला में पहले की संख्या को 2 से गुणा करने पर आनुक्रमिक संख्या प्राप्त होती है।

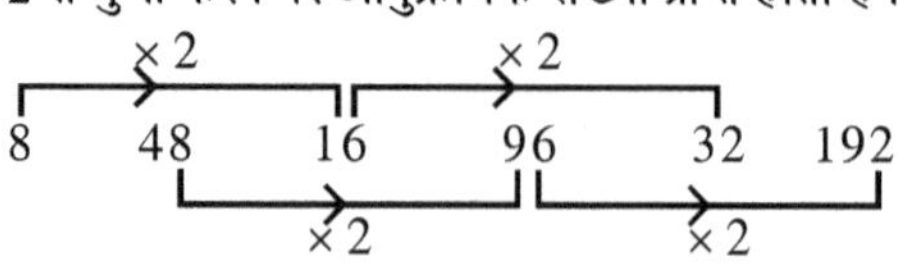

शृंखला I : 8, 16, 32
शृंखला II : 48, 96, 192

4. (*a*) : शृंखला में हर तीसरी संख्या पूर्ववर्ती दो संख्याओं का गुणनफल है।

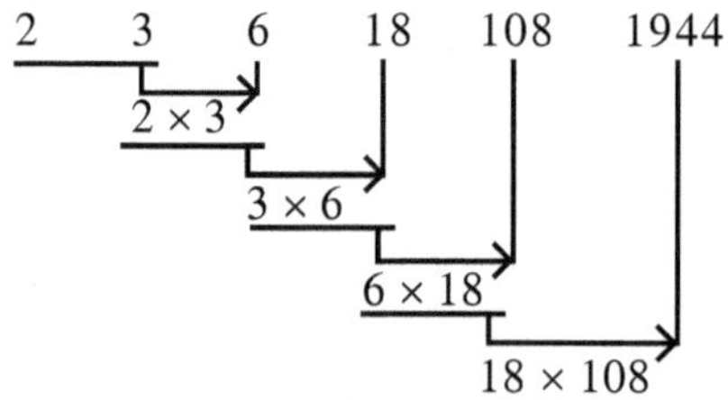

5. (*a*) : इस शृंखला में तीन संख्याओं से एक समुच्चय निर्मित होता है जिनमें से प्रत्येक समुच्चय में पहली दो संख्याएं सीधे क्रम में हैं तथा तीसरी संख्या पहली और दूसरी संख्याओं का योग है। अगले समुच्चय की पहली संख्या पूर्ववर्ती समुच्चय की पहली संख्या की दोगुनी है।

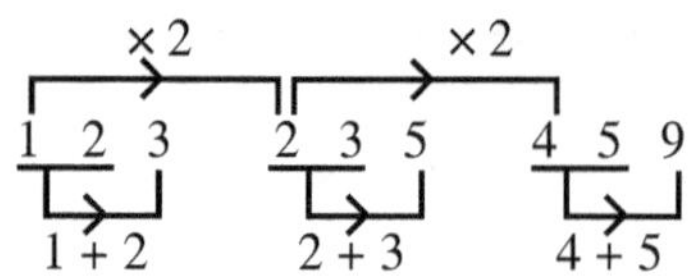

6. *(c)*: शृंखला में निम्नलिखित पैटर्न का अनुपालन किया जाता है :
(दी गई संख्या + अगली संख्या) +2 से आरंभ करके प्रत्येक चरण में 1 की वृद्धि करते हुए क्रमागत प्राकृतिक संख्या का योग :

3 8 13 24 41 70

(3+8) + 2, (8 + 13) + 3, (13 + 24) + 4, (24 + 41) + 5

7. *(c)*: शृंखला की संख्याएं प्राकृतिक क्रम में दो सम संख्याओं का गुणनफल हैं, अर्थात्

0	8	24	48	80	120
↓	↓	↓	↓	↓	↓
(0×2)	(2×4)	(4×6)	(6×8)	(8×10)	(10×12)

8. *(b)*: शृंखला निम्नलिखित पैटर्न का अनुपालन करती है : 1 से आरंभ करके प्राकृतिक संख्याओं का घनफल घटा 1 से आरंभ करके एकांतर विषम संख्याएं

0	5	22	57	116	205
↓	↓	↓	↓	↓	↓
1^3-1	2^3-3	3^3-5	4^3-7	5^3-9	6^3-11

9. *(c)*: शृंखला की आनुक्रमिक संख्याओं के बीच अंतर 3 की घात में वृद्धि के साथ बढ़ता है।

6 9 18 45 126 369 1098

$+3$, $+9 = 3^2$, $+27 = 3^3$, $+81 = 3^4$, $+243 = 3^5$, $+729 = 3^6$

10. *(c)*: शृंखला में निहित संख्या को 2 से गुणा करके 0 से आरंभ करके प्राकृतिक क्रम में संख्याओं को जोड़ने पर अगली संख्या प्राप्त होती है।

1 2 5 12 27 58 121 248

$(1 \times 2)+0$, $(2 \times 2)+1$, $(5 \times 2)+2$, $(12 \times 2)+3$, $(27 \times 2)+4$, $(58 \times 2)+5$, $(121 \times 2)+6$

भाग-IV मिश्रित-शृंखला (Mixed Series)

मिश्रित-शृंखला में अक्षरों और संख्याओं का संयोजन होता है। इस प्रकार की शृंखला में अक्षरों और संख्याओं का एक सर्वनिष्ठ पैटर्न या अलग-अलग अनुक्रम पैटर्न हो सकता है।

हल किए गए उदाहरण

1. निम्नलिखित अक्षर-संख्या संयोजन शृंखला में प्रश्न चिह्न के स्थान पर क्या आएगा?
F6, H8, J10, L12, ?
(*a*) N15 (*b*) O14 (*c*) N14 (*d*) O13

उत्तर *(c)*: शृंखला में अक्षर वर्णमाला के सीधे क्रम में दो स्थान आगे की ओर बढ़ते हैं तथा संख्या वर्णमाला में अक्षरों के स्थान को इंगित करती है।

F6 H8 J10 L12 N14

+2 +2 +2 +2

2. दिए गए विकल्पों में से कौन-सा विकल्प निम्नलिखित शृंखला को पूरा करता है?
R(2)S, T(4)U, V(6)W, ?
(*a*) X(8)Y (*b*) Y(10)Z (*c*) Z(8)A (*d*) Y(6)Z

उत्तर *(a)*: अक्षर वर्णमाला के सीधे क्रम में हैं जबकि संख्याएं 2 की आनुक्रमिक गुणज हैं।

अभ्यास

निर्देश (प्र.सं. 1–3): *नीचे की प्रत्येक शृंखला में प्रश्न चिह्न के स्थान पर क्या आएगा?*

1. 2B, 4C, 8E, 14H, ?
(*a*) 20L (*b*) 22L
(*c*) 21I (*d*) 16K

2. W(1)A, X(4)Z, Y(9)Y, ?, A(25)W
(*a*) X(11)Z (*b*) Z(21)A
(*c*) Z(16)X (*d*) Z(14)X

3. D2, I3, N6, S18, ?
(*a*) V72 (*b*) W36
(*c*) Y90 (*d*) X108

निर्देश (प्र.सं. 4 और 5): *नीचे की प्रत्येक अक्षर-संख्या शृंखला में कौन-सा पद बेमेल/शृंखला में उपयुक्त नहीं है?*

4. G4T, J10R, M20P, P43N, S90L
(*a*) J10R (*b*) S90L
(*c*) M20P (*d*) G4T

5. B0R, G3U, E3P, J7S, H9N
(*a*) E3P (*b*) J7S
(*c*) H9N (*d*) G3U

व्याख्यात्मक उत्तर

1. (*b*): शृंखला में संख्याओं का अनुक्रम +2, +4, +6 +8 का तथा अक्षरों का अनुक्रम +1, +2, +3, +4 का है।

2. (*c*): शृंखला में दिए गए समूहों में बायीं ओर के अक्षर वर्णमाला के विपरीत क्रम में हैं और दाहिनी ओर के अक्षर वर्णमाला के सीधे क्रम में हैं तथा संख्याएं 1 से आरंभ करके प्राकृतिक क्रम में क्रमागत संख्याओं के वर्ग हैं।

3. (*d*): अक्षर +5 पैटर्न का अनुपालन करते हैं और हर तीसरी संख्या अपनी पूर्ववर्ती दो संख्याओं का गुणनफल है।

4. (*a*): शृंखला में दिए गए समूहों में बायीं ओर के अक्षर +3 पैटर्न का, दायीं ओर के अक्षर –2 पैटर्न का अनुपालन करते हैं तथा संख्याओं द्वारा $(4 \times 2) + 1$, $(9 \times 2) + 2$, $(20 \times 2) + 3$, $(43 \times 2) + 4$ पैटर्न का अनुपालन किया जाता है। अतः J10R के स्थान पर शृंखला में J9R होना चाहिए।

5. (*b*): शृंखला के दिए गए समूहों में बायीं ओर के अक्षर +5, –2 (5 चरण आगे, 2 चरण पीछे) पैटर्न का अनुपालन करते हैं जिसकी आगे भी पुनरावृत्ति होती है। समूहों में दायीं ओर +3, –5 (3 चरण आगे, 5 चरण पीछे) पैटर्न का अनुपालन किया जाता है जिसकी पुनरावृत्ति होती है। शृंखला की संख्याएं शृंखला में अपने पूर्ववर्ती दो संख्याओं के योग के बराबर हैं। अतः J7S के स्थान पर J6S होना चाहिए।

सादृश्य या संबंध
(ANALOGIES OR RELATIONSHIPS)

भाग-I शब्द सादृश्य (Word Analogy)

संबंध या सादृश्य परीक्षा में दिए गए दो शब्दों के बीच संबंध स्थापित किया जाता है और उसी संबंध को दिए गए अन्य शब्दों पर अनुप्रयुक्त किया जाता है। दिए गए दो शब्दों के बीच विभिन्न प्रकार के संबंध हो सकते हैं, अत: इस प्रकार के प्रश्नों को हल करते समय सर्वप्रथम यह ज्ञात करना होता है कि दिए गए दो शब्दों के बीच किस प्रकार का संबंध है। शब्दों के बीच विभिन्न संबंधों पर नीचे चर्चा की गई है :

हल किए गए उदाहरण

1. क्रिया-साधन संबंध **(Action Object Relationship)**

उदाहरण : जैसे गोली चलाना और 'बंदूक' का संबंध है उसी प्रकार 'खाने' से किसका संबंध है?

(*a*) भूख (*b*) प्यास (*c*) रात्रि-भोज (*d*) फल

उत्तर (*d*) : दिए गए शब्दों के बीच संबंध यह है कि गोली चलाना एक क्रिया है और 'बंदूक' उस क्रिया को करने का एक विशिष्ट साधन या उपकरण है। इसी प्रकार 'खाना' एक क्रिया है और 'फल' इस क्रिया को करने अर्थात् खाने का साधन या उपकरण है।

2. साहचर्य संबंध (Association Relationship)

उदाहरण : जो संबंध 'ग्लैमर' और 'प्रसिद्धि' में है, ठीक वैसा ही संबंध 'रंग' का किससे है?

(*a*) इंद्रधनुष (*b*) छाया (*c*) कला (*d*) चित्रकारी

उत्तर (*d*) : जिस प्रकार ग्लैमर से प्रसिद्धि प्राप्त होती है उसी प्रकार 'रंग' से चित्रकारी की जाती है।

3. विपर्याय (विलोम) संबंध (Antonym Relationship)

उदाहरण : अंतर्मुखी : बहिर्मुखी

(*a*) कोण : स्पर्श रेखा (*b*) चरम : अंतरिम (*c*) प्रतिकूल : अनुकूल (*d*) क्रिया : नियम

उत्तर (*c*) : संबंधित शब्द विपरीतार्थक हैं।

4. कार्य-कारण संबंध (Cause and Effect Relationship)

उदाहरण : चोट : दर्द

(*a*) कोटि : योग्यता (*b*) बादल गरजना : बिजली चमकना

(*c*) घूमाना : बिलोना (*d*) धन : परिश्रम

उत्तर (*b*) : जिस प्रकार चोट के कारण दर्द होता है उसी प्रकार बादल गरजने के कारण बिजली चमकती है।

5. कोटि या अंश संबंध (Degree Relationship)

उदाहरण : गुनगुना का जो संबंध 'गरम' से वही संबंध बिलखना या विलाप करने का किससे है?

(*a*) सिसकना (*b*) चिल्लाना (*c*) मुस्कराना (*d*) शांत रहना

उत्तर (*a*) : 'गुनगुना' का अर्थ है 'थोड़ा गरम'। इसी प्रकार बिलखने या विलाप करने की निम्न कोटि है 'सिसकना'।

अभ्यास

निर्देश (प्र.सं. 1–5): *पूछे गए प्रत्येक प्रश्न में पहले दिए गए दो शब्दों के बीच संबंध स्थापित करें। तत्पश्चात् दिए गए विकल्पों में से उस विकल्प का चयन करें जिसके शब्द और प्रश्न में दिए गए तीसरे शब्द के बीच ठीक वैसा ही संबंध या सादृश्य हो जैसा कि पहले के दो शब्दों के बीच है।*

1. जो संबंध 'उन्माद' और 'सनक' में है वही संबंध 'भय' और निम्नलिखित में से किसमें है?

(*a*) इच्छा (*b*) शौक
(*c*) आवश्यकता (*d*) डर

2. 'हकलाना' जिस प्रकार 'वाणी' से संबंधित है उसी प्रकार 'बहरापन' का संबंध निम्नलिखित में से किससे है?

(*a*) कान (*b*) सुनना
(*c*) शोर (*d*) चुप्पी

3. जिस प्रकार 'नेता', 'अनुयायी' से संबंधित है, उसी प्रकार .... संबंधित है सिपाही से।

(*a*) कैप्टन (*b*) यूनिट
(*c*) सेना (*d*) बैरक

4. जिस प्रकार 'चिल्लाहट', 'फुसफुसाहट' से संबंधित है, उसी प्रकार 'मारना' निम्नलिखित में से किससे संबंधित है?

(*a*) थप्पड़ मारने (*b*) छूना
(*c*) क्रोध (*d*) शोरगुल

5. जिस प्रकार 'पंजा', 'बिल्ली' से संबंधित है उसी प्रकार 'खुर' निम्नलिखित में से किससे संबंधित है?

(*a*) घोड़ा (*b*) मेमना
(*c*) हाथी (*d*) शेर

निर्देश (प्र.सं. 6–10): *नीचे दिए गए प्रत्येक प्रश्न में :: चिह्न की बाईं ओर दो शब्द दिए गए हैं। इन दोनों शब्दों में कुछ संबंध है। वैसा ही संबंध :: चिह्न की दाईं ओर के दो शब्दों में है जिनमें से एक शब्द के स्थान पर प्रश्नवाचक चिह्न (?) है। प्रश्नवाचक चिह्न (?) के स्थान पर दिए गए विकल्पों में से एक उपयुक्त विकल्प का चयन करें।*

6. शिकारी : बंदूक :: लेखक : ?

(*a*) पुस्तक (*b*) कलम
(*c*) कविता (*d*) पृष्ठ

7. भोजन : आमाशय :: ईंधन : ?

(*a*) इंजन (*b*) ऑटोमोबाइल
(*c*) रेल (*d*) वायुयान

8. जल : रेत :: महासागर : ?

(*a*) द्वीप (*b*) नदी
(*c*) मरुभूमि (*d*) तरंगें

9. वयस्क : बच्चा :: फूल : ?

(*a*) बीज (*b*) कली
(*c*) फल (*d*) तितली

10. मोती : कंठहार :: फूल : ?

(*a*) पौधा (*b*) बगीचा
(*c*) पँखुड़ी (*d*) गुलदस्ता

व्याख्यात्मक उत्तर

1. (*d*) : संबंधित शब्द पर्यायवाची हैं।

2. (*b*) : 'वाणी' के दोष से 'हकलाने' की समस्या उत्पन्न होती है जबकि 'सुनने' में कठिनाई से 'बहरापन' उत्पन्न होता है।

3. (*a*) : जिस प्रकार 'अनुयायी' अपने 'नेता' से मार्गदर्शन प्राप्त करते हैं उसी प्रकार 'सिपाही' को अपने 'कैप्टन' से मार्गदर्शन प्राप्त होता है।

4. (*b*): 'चिल्लाहट' की तीव्रता में अत्यधिक कमी कर दी जाए तो वह 'फुसफुसाहट' का रूप ले लेती है और यदि 'मारने' की तीव्रता कम कर दी जाए तो वैसी क्रिया 'छूना' मात्र रह जाएगी।

5. (*a*): 'बिल्ली' के 'पैर में' 'पंजा' होता है जबकि 'घोड़ा' के पैर में 'खुर' होता है।

6. (*b*): 'शिकारी' का हथियार 'बंदूक' है और 'लेखक' का हथियार 'कलम' है।

7. (*a*): 'भोजन', 'आमाशय' में पचता है और 'ईंधन' की खपत 'इंजन' में होती है।

8. (*c*): संबंधित शब्द एक दूसरे के लगभग विपरीतार्थक शब्द हैं।

9. (*b*): 'बच्चा' विकसित होकर 'वयस्क' बनता है और 'कली' खिलकर 'फूल' बनती है।

10. (*d*): बहुत से मोतियों को मिला कर 'कंठहार' और बहुत से फूलों को मिलाकर 'गुलदस्ता' बनाया जाता है।

भाग-II अक्षर सादृश्य (Letter Analogy)

इस प्रकार के सादृश्य में अक्षरों के दो दिए गए समुच्चयों के बीच संबंध स्थापित किया जाता है और तत्पश्चात् अक्षरों के दिए गए तीसरे समुच्चय पर पहले दो अक्षर समुच्चयों के बीच के संबंध को अनुप्रयुक्त करके अक्षरों के चौथे अपेक्षित समुच्चय को ज्ञात किया जाता है। दिए गए दो अक्षर समुच्चयों में से पहले समुच्चय के अक्षरों को कुछ चरण आगे या पीछे करके, संपूर्ण समुच्चय के अक्षरों को या समुच्चय के कुछ अक्षरों को उलटे क्रम में लिखकर दूसरे समुच्चय के अक्षरों को प्राप्त किया जा सकता है।

हल किए गए उदाहरण

निर्देश: *दिए गए विकल्पों में से कौन-सा अक्षर-समूह प्रश्नचिह्न (?) के स्थान पर आएगा?*

1. JILK : KLIJ : : MNPQ : ?

(*a*) QNPM (*b*) MPQN (*c*) QPNM (*d*) PNMQ

उत्तर (*c*) : :: की बायीं ओर के अक्षर-समूहों में से पहले अक्षर-समूह के अक्षरों को विपरीत क्रम में लिखकर दूसरा अक्षर-समूह प्राप्त किया गया है। यही संबंध :: की दाहिनी ओर के दिए गए अक्षर समूह के अक्षरों पर अनुप्रयुक्त करने पर अपेक्षित अक्षर-समूह प्राप्त होता है।

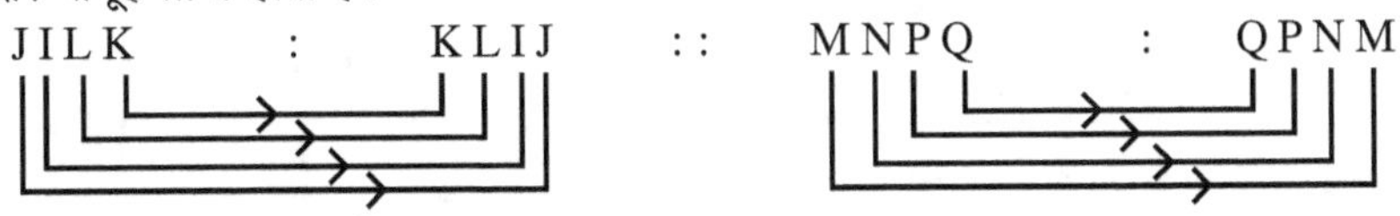

2. FLO : DOL : : RDP : ?

(*a*) PGM (*b*) MGP (*c*) GMP (*d*) MPG

उत्तर (*a*) : पहले और तीसरे अक्षरों को क्रमशः –2 और –3 चरण पीछे खिसका कर और दूसरे अक्षर को +3 चरण आगे बढ़ा कर :: चिह्न की बायीं ओर का दूसरा अक्षर समुच्चय प्राप्त होता है। यही संबंध :: चिह्न की दायीं ओर के पहले अक्षर समुच्चय पर लगाने पर प्रश्न चिह्न के स्थान पर अक्षर समुच्चय प्राप्त होता है।

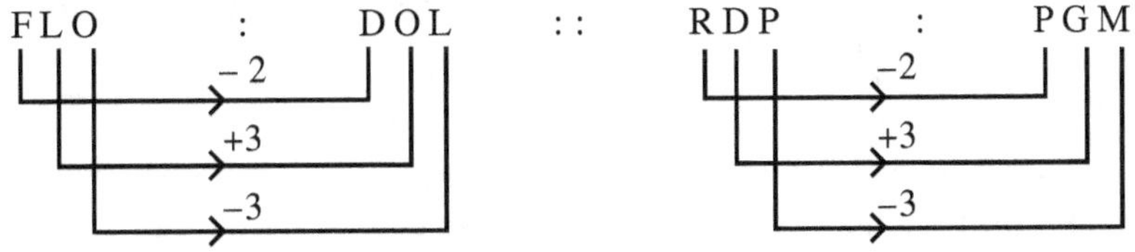

3. DumB : BonD : : RusT : ?

(*a*) MOst (*b*) TeNt (*c*) PaTH (*d*) WorK

उत्तर (*d*) : प्रत्येक समूह में सिरों पर स्थित दो अक्षर अंग्रेजी वर्णमाला के बड़े अक्षर हैं।

अभ्यास

निर्देश (प्र.सं. 1–10): *नीचे के प्रत्येक प्रश्न में एक लुप्त पद है। प्रश्न में :: चिह्न की बायीं ओर के दो अक्षर-समूहों में जो समानता या सादृश्य है वैसी ही समानता या सादृश्य :: चिह्न की दायीं ओर के दो अक्षर समूहों में है जिनमें से एक अक्षर समूह के स्थान पर प्रश्नवाचक चिह्न (?) लगा है। प्रश्नवाचक चिह्न (?) के स्थान पर लुप्त पद ज्ञात करें।*

1. GFC : CFG : : RPJ : ?
(*a*) JRP (*b*) JPR
(*c*) PJR (*d*) RJP

2. BCF : DEG : : MNQ : ?
(*a*) OPR (*b*) PQS
(*c*) OPP (*d*) QRT

3. NATION : ANITNO : : HUNGRY : ?
(*a*) HNUGRY (*b*) UNHGYR
(*c*) YRNGUH (*d*) UHGNYR

4. ACE : FGH : : LNP : ?
(*a*) QRS (*b*) PQR
(*c*) QST (*d*) MOQ

5. BOQD : ERTG : : ANPC : ?
(*a*) DQSF (*b*) FSHU
(*c*) SHFU (*d*) DSQF

6. BCDA : STUR : : KLMJ : ?
(*a*) VWXU (*b*) EFHG
(*c*) SRTU (*d*) QSRP

7. RUX : TRP : : BEH : ?
(*a*) SQN (*b*) QON
(*c*) QOM (*d*) QNL

8. BCDE : WVUT : : QRST : ?
(*a*) EFHG (*b*) JIHG
(*c*) POML (*d*) GEDC

9. AKU : AJS : : CRD : ?
(*a*) BQE (*b*) CQB
(*c*) DSB (*d*) APC

10. ODL : LOD : : PWN : ?
(*a*) WNP (*b*) NWP
(*c*) NPW (*d*) NMP

व्याख्यात्मक उत्तर

1. *(b)*: पहले समूह के अक्षरों को उलटे क्रम में लिखने पर दूसरा अक्षर-समूह प्राप्त होता है।

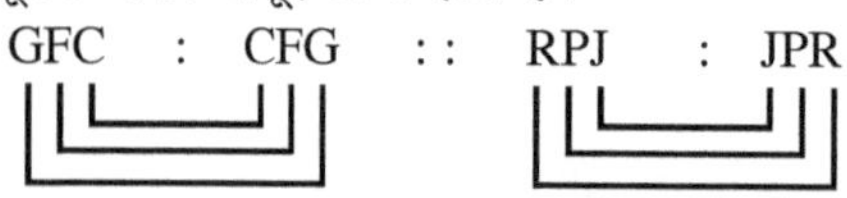

2. *(a)*: पहले और दूसरे समूह के तीनों अक्षरों के बीच वर्णमाला के सीधे क्रम में क्रमशः +2, +2 और +1 चरणों का अंतर है।

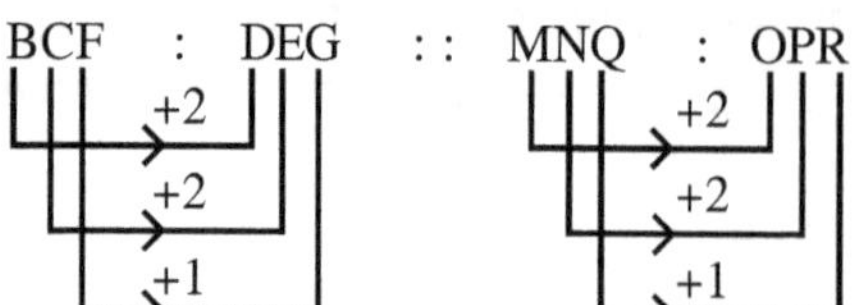

3. *(d)*: पहले समूह के अक्षरों को दो-दो अक्षरों के खंडों में विभाजित करके प्रत्येक खंड के अक्षरों को उल्टे क्रम में लिखने पर दूसरा अक्षर-समूह प्राप्त होता है।

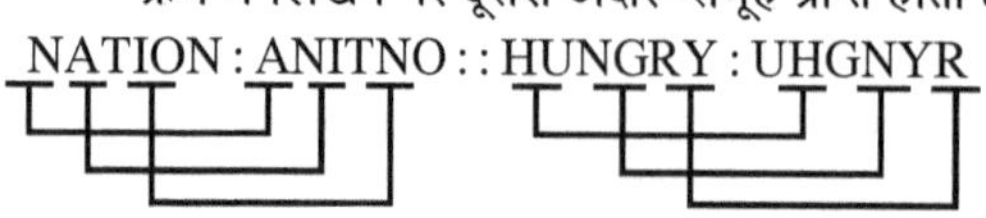

4. *(a)*: पहले और दूसरे समूह के तीनों अक्षरों के बीच वर्णमाला के सीधे क्रम में क्रमशः +5, +4, +3 चरणों का अंतर है।

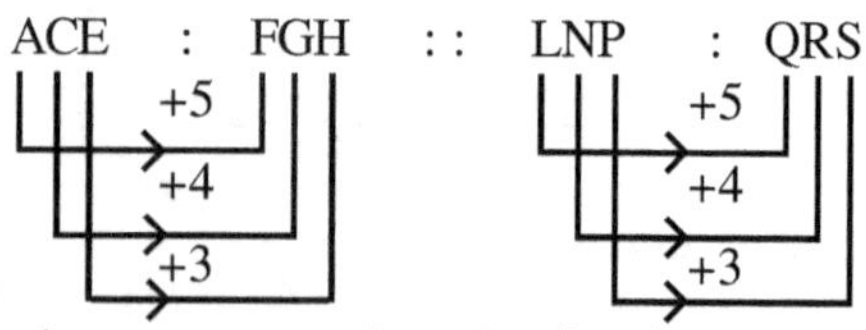

5. *(a)*: प्रत्येक अक्षर समूह में पहले और चौथे अक्षरों के बीच एक अक्षर छूटा हुआ है तथा दूसरे और तीसरे अक्षरों के बीच भी एक अक्षर छूटा हुआ है।

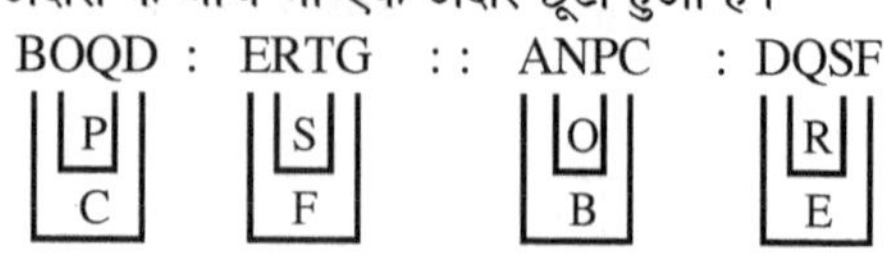

6. *(a)*: प्रत्येक अक्षर समूह में पहले तीन अक्षर क्रमागत हैं और उनके बाद अनुक्रम का आरंभिक चौथा अक्षर लिखा गया है।

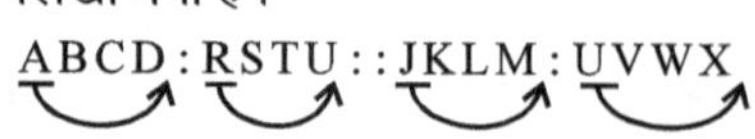

7. *(c)*: पहले समूह के अक्षरों में +3 का और दूसरे समूह के अक्षरों में –2 का अंतर है।

RUX : TRP :: BEH : QOM

(+3 +3) (–2 –2) (+3+3) (–2 –2)

8. *(b)*: पहले अक्षर-समूह के आनुक्रमिक अक्षर वर्णमाला के सीधे क्रम में हैं और दूसरे अक्षर समूह के आनुक्रमिक अक्षर वर्णमाला के उलटे क्रम में हैं।

BCDE → : WVUT ← :: QRST → : JIHG ←

9. *(b)*: पहले अक्षर समूह के तीन अक्षरों में से पहले अक्षर के स्थान को परिवर्तित किए बिना अन्य दो अक्षरों को वर्णमाला के विपरीत क्रम में क्रमशः –1 और –2 चरण पीछे खिसकाने पर दूसरा अक्षर-समूह प्राप्त होता है।

AKU : AJS :: CRD : CQB

(–1, –2) (–1, –2)

10. *(c)*: पहले अक्षर-समूह के पहले और दूसरे अक्षरों को तीसरे अक्षर के बाद रखने पर दूसरा अक्षर समूह प्राप्त होता है।

ODL : LOD :: PWN : NPW

भाग-III संख्या सादृश्य (Number Analogy)

संख्या सादृश्य में भी पहले दो दी गई संख्याओं के बीच संबंध स्थापित किया जाता है और तत्पश्चात् इस ज्ञात संबंध को संख्याओं के दूसरे जोड़े पर प्रयुक्त करके उसके लुप्त पद को ज्ञात किया जाता है। संख्याओं के बीच संबंध किसी भी एक पैटर्न पर आधारित हो सकता है, जैसे कि : *(i)* संख्याएं विषम/सम/अभाज्य संख्याएं हो सकती हैं; *(ii)* संख्याएं किसी एक संख्या का गुणज हो सकती हैं; *(iii)* संख्याएं भिन्न-भिन्न संख्याओं का वर्गफल/घनफल हो सकती हैं; *(iv)* दूसरी संख्या प्राप्त करने के लिए पहली संख्या में किसी संख्या को जोड़ा/घटाया/गुणा/ भाग किया जा सकता है; *(v)* दूसरी संख्या पहली संख्या के अंकों का योगफल/गुणनफल/अंतरफल हो सकती है, और *(vi)* दो दी गई संख्याओं के बीच संबंध उपर्युक्त किसी भी गणितीय परिकलनों के संयोजन द्वारा भी ज्ञात किया जा सकता है।

हल किए गए उदाहरण

निर्देश : *निम्नलिखित प्रश्नों में प्रश्न चिह्न (?) के स्थान पर लुप्त पद ज्ञात करें।*

1. 25 : 81 : : 36 : ?

(*a*) 121 (*b*) 93 (*c*) 65 (*d*) 103

उत्तर (*a*) : सभी संख्याएं भिन्न-भिन्न संख्याओं के वर्गफल को सूचित करती हैं।

25 : 81 :: 36 : 121

↓ ↓ ↓ ↓

5^2 9^2 6^2 11^2

2. 36 : 18 : : 72 : ?

(*a*) 164 (*b*) 134 (*c*) 94 (*d*) 14

उत्तर (*d*) : दूसरी संख्या पहली संख्या के अंकों का गुणनफल है।

36 : 18 :: 72 : 14

(3 × 6) (7 × 2)

अभ्यास

निर्देश (प्र.सं. 1–10): *नीचे के प्रत्येक प्रश्न में चिह्न '∷' के पहले दो संख्याएं दी गई हैं जिनमें आपस में एक संबंध है तथा '∷' चिह्न के बाद में एक तीसरी संख्या दी गई है। दिए गए विकल्पों में से उस संख्या का चयन करें जिसका तीसरी संख्या के साथ वैसा ही संबंध हो जैसा संबंध संख्याओं के पहले जोड़े के बीच है।*

1. 1 : 11 : : 2 : ?
(*a*) 20 (*b*) 22
(*c*) 24 (*d*) 44

2. 18 : 27 : : 22 : ?
(*a*) 42 (*b*) 39
(*c*) 33 (*d*) 54

3. 14 : 20 : : 16 : ?
(*a*) 23 (*b*) 10
(*c*) 48 (*d*) 32

4. 0.16 : 0.0016 : : 1.02 : ?
(*a*) 10.20 (*b*) 0.102
(*c*) 0.0102 (*d*) 1.020

5. 5 : 24 : : 8 : ?
(*a*) 65 (*b*) 63
(*c*) 62 (*d*) 64

6. 65 : 30 : : 44 : ?
(*a*) 79 (*b*) 62
(*c*) 28 (*d*) 16

7. 30 : 42 : : 56 : ?
(*a*) 92 (*b*) 21
(*c*) 38 (*d*) 72

8. 190 : 10 : : 102 : ?
(*a*) 4 (*b*) 7
(*c*) 3 (*d*) 5

9. 6 : 18 : : 4 : ?
(*a*) 2 (*b*) 6
(*c*) 8 (*d*) 16

10. 2 : 11 : : ?
(*a*) 6 : 17 (*b*) 8 : 43
(*c*) 5 : 41 (*d*) 7 : 35

व्याख्यात्मक उत्तर

1. *(b)*: पहली संख्या के अंक को दो बार लिखने पर दूसरी संख्या प्राप्त होती है।

2. *(c)*: पहले जोड़े की संख्याएं 9 का गुणज हैं और दूसरे जोड़े की संख्याएं 11 का गुणज हैं :

$$\underset{9\times 2}{18} : \underset{9\times 3}{27} :: \underset{11\times 2}{22} : \underset{11\times 3}{33}$$

3. *(a)*: संख्याओं के बीच संबंध निम्नवत् है :

$$\underset{7\times 2}{14} : \underset{(7\times 3)-1}{20} :: \underset{8\times 2}{16} : \underset{(8\times 3)-1}{23}$$

4. *(c)*: पहली दशमलव संख्या को 100 से भाग करने पर दूसरी दशमलव संख्या प्राप्त होती है :

$$0.16 \xrightarrow{\div 100} 0.0016 :: 1.02 \xrightarrow{\div 100} 0.0102$$

5. *(b)*: पहली संख्या के वर्ग से 1 घटाने पर दूसरी संख्या प्राप्त होती है :

$$5 \xrightarrow{(5^2)-1} 24 :: 8 \xrightarrow{(8^2)-1} 63$$

6. *(d)*: दूसरी संख्या पहली संख्या के अंकों का गुणनफल है :

$$\frac{65 : 30}{(6 \times 5)} :: \frac{44 : 16}{(4 \times 4)}$$

7. *(d)*: संख्याएं विभिन्न संख्याओं के वर्ग में उन्हीं संख्याओं को जोड़ने पर प्राप्त होती हैं :

$$\underset{5^2+5}{30} : \underset{6^2+6}{42} :: \underset{7^2+7}{56} : \underset{8^2+8}{72}$$

8. *(c)*: दूसरी संख्या पहली संख्या के अंकों का योगफल है :

$$\frac{190 : 10}{(1+9+0)} :: \frac{102 : 3}{(1+0+2)}$$

9. *(c)*: पहली संख्या के वर्ग को 2 से भाग करने पर दूसरी संख्या प्राप्त होती है :

$$6 \xrightarrow{6^2 \div 2} 18 :: 4 \xrightarrow{4^2 \div 2} 8$$

10. *(c)*: पहली संख्या दूसरी संख्या के अंकों का योगफल है :

$$2 : \underset{(1+1)}{11} :: 5 : \underset{(4+1)}{41}$$

वर्गीकरण या विजातीय छांटना
(CLASSIFICATION OR ODD ONE OUT)

भाग-I विजातीय छांटना – शब्दों पर आधारित समस्याएं

इस प्रकार के वर्गीकरण में **चार** शब्द दिए जाते हैं जिनमें से **तीन** शब्द तथ्य या अर्थ की दृष्टि से या अन्य किसी न किसी रूप में आपस में संबंधित होते हुए एक समूह बनाते हैं जबकि शेष केवल एक शब्द अन्य **तीनों** से भिन्न होता है। परीक्षार्थी को यह पता लगाना होता है कि वह एक कौन-सा शब्द है जो समूह से संबंधित नहीं है और इस कारण विजातीय है।

हल किए गए उदाहरण

निर्देश: *निम्नलिखित **चार** शब्दों में से उस एक शब्द का चयन करें जो अन्य **तीन** से भिन्न है :*

1. (*a*) पिता (*b*) माता (*c*) मित्र (*d*) भाई

उत्तर (*c*) : अन्य सभी के बीच रक्त-संबंध है।

2. (*a*) जल (*b*) जेली (*c*) नींबू शरबत (*d*) कॉफी

उत्तर (*b*) : अन्य सभी द्रव पदार्थ हैं।

अभ्यास

निर्देश (प्र.सं. 1–10): *यहां दिए गए प्रत्येक प्रश्न में **तीन** शब्द किसी न किसी प्रकार से समान हैं और इस कारण वे एक समूह बनाते हैं जबकि एक शब्द अन्य **तीनों** से भिन्न है। इस भिन्न या विजातीय शब्द को ज्ञात करें।*

1. (*a*) हरा (*b*) लाल
(*c*) रंग (*d*) नारंगी

2. (*a*) अस्तबल (*b*) बिल
(*c*) डोंगी (*d*) सुअर-बाड़ा

3. (*a*) बुध (*b*) चंद्रमा
(*c*) बृहस्पति (*d*) मंगल

4. (*a*) खुश (*b*) उदास
(*c*) प्रसन्नचित्त (*d*) प्रसन्न

5. (*a*) शंकु (*b*) वृत्त
(*c*) त्रिभुज (*d*) आयत

6. (*a*) सीसा (*b*) पारद
(*c*) तांबा (*d*) लोहा

7. (*a*) पतंग (*b*) चिड़िया
(*c*) रेडार (*d*) जेट

8. (*a*) अतिवृष्टि (*b*) अनावृष्टि
(*c*) भूस्खलन (*d*) युद्ध

9. (*a*) सिंहशावक (*b*) चूजा
(*c*) सूअर (*d*) पिल्ला

10. (*a*) खरगोश (*b*) मगरमच्छ
(*c*) केंचुआ (*d*) घोंघा

व्याख्यात्मक उत्तर

1. *(c)*: अन्य सभी विभिन्न प्रकार के रंग हैं।
2. *(c)*: डोंगी एक छोटी नाव होती है। अन्य सभी पशु–पक्षियों के निवासस्थलों के नाम हैं।
3. *(b)*: अन्य सभी ग्रहों के नाम हैं।
4. *(b)*: अन्य सभी आनन्द की अनुभूति को अभिव्यक्त करते हैं।
5. *(a)*: **अन्य सभी आकृतियाँ द्विविमीय आकृतियाँ हैं।**
6. *(b)*: अन्य सभी ठोस धातुएं हैं।
7. *(c)*: अन्य सभी हवा में उड़ने वाली वस्तुएं हैं। रेडार हवा में गमन करने वाली वस्तुओं की पहचान करता है।
8. *(d)*: अन्य सभी प्राकृतिक आपदाएं हैं। केवल युद्ध ही मानव द्वारा मानव समाज के समक्ष प्रस्तुत की जाने वाली एक कृत्रिम आपदा है।
9. *(c)*: अन्य सभी शब्द विभिन्न जंतुओं के शिशुओं के नाम हैं।
10. *(a)*: अन्य सभी रेंगने वाले जंतु हैं।

भाग-II विजातीय छांटना – अक्षरों पर आधारित समस्याएं

इस कोटि के अंतर्गत विकल्प के रूप में चार अक्षर-समूह या अक्षरों की एक शृंखला दी जाती है। परीक्षार्थी को इनमें से ऐसे विकल्प का चयन करना होता है जो अन्यों से भिन्न अर्थात् विजातीय हो।

हल किए गए उदाहरण

निर्देश: *निम्नलिखित अक्षर समूहों में से कौन-सा अक्षर समूह भिन्न या विजातीय स्वरूप का है?*

1. (*a*) NOP (*b*) RTU (*c*) JKL (*d*) EFG

उत्तर *(b)*: प्रत्येक समूह में अक्षर क्रमागत हैं, जबकि विकल्प (*b*) के अक्षर-समूह में पहले दो अक्षरों के बीच एक अक्षर 'S' छूटा हुआ है।

2. (*a*) RUX (*b*) CFI (*c*) BDG (*d*) FIL

उत्तर *(c)*: प्रत्येक समूह में अक्षरों के बीच समान संख्या में अक्षर छूटे हुए हैं जबकि विकल्प (*c*) में पहले दो अक्षरों B और D के बीच एक अक्षर और अंतिम दो अक्षरों D और G के बीच दो अक्षर छूटे हुए हैं।

अभ्यास

निर्देश (प्र.सं. 1–10): *नीचे के प्रत्येक प्रश्न में अक्षर समूहों के रूप में चार विकल्प दिए गए हैं जिनमें से तीन में किसी न किसी प्रकार की समानता है और इस कारण वे एक समूह बनाते हैं। उस अक्षर समूह का चयन करें जो समूह से संबंधित नहीं है।*

1. (*a*) ACE (*b*) LOR (*c*) GIK (*d*) VXZ

2. (*a*) TSR (*b*) LKJ (*c*) PQO (*d*) HGF

3. (*a*) EF LM (*b*) KJ SR (*c*) XW HG (*d*) ED YX

4. (*a*) JOPK (*b*) BOPC (*c*) QOPR (*d*) TOPS

5. (*a*) JKkL (*b*) OPpQ (*c*) DEEf (*d*) VWwX

6. (*a*) BdfH (*b*) FHJL (*c*) RTvX (*d*) uVwX

7. (*a*) DFHEG (*b*) TWXUV (*c*) OQSPR (*d*) JLNKM

8. (*a*) MKGA (*b*) PNID (*c*) RPLF (*d*) VTPJ

9. (*a*) ABJNM (*b*) QRTUZ (*c*) IXYOQ (*d*) WGFPO

10. (*a*) EFGH (*b*) IRST (*c*) ULMN (*d*) JKLO

व्याख्यात्मक उत्तर

1. *(b)*: शेष सभी अक्षर समूहों में अगला अक्षर अपने पूर्ववर्ती अक्षर से वर्णमाला के सीधे क्रम में 2 अक्षर आगे का है जबकि विकल्प (*b*) के अक्षर समूह में +3 अनुक्रम का पालन होता है।

A B C D E   L M N O P Q R
+2 +2   +3 +3

G H I J K   V W X Y Z
+2 +2   +2 +2

2. *(c)*: प्रत्येक समूह में अक्षर वर्णमाला के उलटे क्रम में हैं। केवल विकल्प *(c)* में अक्षरों का अनुक्रम बाधित हो रहा है।

3. *(a)*: शेष सभी समूहों में क्रमागत अक्षर वर्णमाला के उलटे क्रम में हैं।

KJ SR; XW HG; ED YX
−1 −1 −1 −1 −1 −1

केवल विकल्प (*a*) में ही क्रमागत अक्षर वर्णमाला के सीधे क्रम में है।

E F   L M
+1   +1

4. *(d)*: यहां दिए गए सभी अक्षर समूहों में बीच में 'OP' अक्षर हैं। विकल्प (*d*) में दोनों किनारों पर स्थित अक्षर वर्णमाला के उलटे क्रम में हैं, अर्थात्

TOPS
−1

जबकि शेष सभी अक्षर समूहों में दोनों किनारों पर स्थित अक्षर वर्णमाला के सीधे क्रम में हैं।

JOPK ; BOPC ; QOPR
+1 +1 +1

5. *(c)*: शेष समूहों में तीसरे अक्षर के रूप में दूसरे अक्षर की पुनरावृत्ति की गई है और उसे अंग्रेजी वर्णमाला के छोटे अक्षर के रूप में लिखा गया है जबकि विकल्प (*c*) के तीसरे अक्षर के रूप में दूसरे अक्षर की पुनरावृत्ति तो की जाती है किंतु उसे अंग्रेजी वर्णमाला के बड़े अक्षर के रूप में लिखा जाता है।

6. *(d)*: शेष समूहों में अंग्रेजी वर्णमाला के अक्षर चाहे छोटे हों या बड़े, किंतु दूसरे, तीसरे और चौथे स्थान पर स्थित अक्षर अपने पूर्ववर्ती अक्षरों से वर्णमाला के सीधे क्रम में 2 अक्षर आगे के हैं, अर्थात्

B D f H ; F H J L ; R T v X
+2 +2 +2   +2 +2 +2   +2 +2 +2

केवल विकल्प (*d*) में अक्षर वर्णमाला के सहज क्रम (+1) में हैं, अर्थात्

u V w X
+1 +1 +1

7. *(b)*: शेष समूहों में पहले, चौथे, दूसरे, पांचवें और तीसरे स्थानों पर स्थित अक्षरों से वर्णमाला का सीधा अनुक्रम बनता है। विकल्प (*b*), में पहले, चौथे, पांचवें, दूसरे और तीसरे स्थानों पर स्थित अक्षरों के मेल से वर्णमाला का सीधा अनुक्रम बनता है।

8. *(b)*: शेष समूहों में अक्षरों का अनुक्रम −2, −4, −6 के पैटर्न का पालन करता है, अर्थात्

M K G A ; R P L F
−2 −4 −6   −2 −4 −6

V T P J
−2 −4 −6

विकल्प (*b*) में अनुक्रम का निम्नलिखित पैटर्न है:

P N I D
−2 −5 −5

अत: सही पैटर्न होना चाहिए → P N J D
−2 −4 −6

9. *(c)*: शेष समूहों में कम से कम दो जोड़े अक्षर वर्णमाला के क्रम में हैं, अर्थात्

A B J N M ; Q R T U Z ; W G F P O

विकल्प (*c*) में केवल एक जोड़ा अक्षर-ही वर्णमाला के क्रम में है।

I X Y O Q

10. *(d)*: शेष समूहों में पहला अक्षर 'स्वर' है जिसके बाद तीन क्रमागत अक्षर लिखे गए हैं।

भाग-III विजातीय छांटना – संख्याओं पर आधारित समस्याएं

इस प्रकार के वर्गीकरण में विकल्पों के रूप में विभिन्न संख्याएं दी जाती हैं। इन संख्याओं में से एक को छोड़कर जो अन्य से भिन्न होती है, शेष किसी न किसी रूप में आपस में संबंधित होती हैं और इस प्रकार एक समूह बनाती हैं। परीक्षार्थी को दी गई संख्याओं में यह समानता ज्ञात करनी होती है और तत्पश्चात् समूह से भिन्न संख्या का चयन करना होता है। विकल्पों के रूप में दी गई संख्याएं विषम/सम/क्रमागत संख्याएं, अभाज्य संख्याएं, किसी संख्या का गुणज, एक अंकीय, विभिन्न संख्याओं का वर्ग या घन, किसी अन्य संख्या का जोड़/घटा या किसी भी गणितीय परिकलन का संयोजन हो सकती है।

हल किए गए उदाहरण

निर्देश: *दिए गए विकल्पों में विषम संख्या ज्ञात करें।*

1. (*a*) 62 (*b*) 121 (*c*) 36 (*d*) 256

उत्तर (*a*) : अन्य संख्याएं क्रमशः 11, 6 और 16 के वर्ग द्वारा सूचित होती हैं।

2. (*a*) 27 (*b*) 132 (*c*) 93 (*d*) 154

उत्तर (*d*) : शेष संख्याएं 3 से विभाज्य हैं।

अभ्यास

निर्देश (प्र.सं. 1–10): *यहां प्रत्येक प्रश्न में चार विकल्प दिए गए हैं जिनमें से तीन किसी न किसी रूप में आपस में संबंधित होते हुए एक समूह बनाते हैं, जबकि शेष एक संख्या अन्य से भिन्न है। उस भिन्न संख्या का चयन करें जो समूह से संबंधित नहीं है।*

1. (*a*) 1948 (*b*) 2401 (*c*) 966 (*d*) 1449

2. (*a*) 182 (*b*) 169 (*c*) 130 (*d*) 158

3. (*a*) 3215 (*b*) 9309 (*c*) 4721 (*d*) 2850

4. (*a*) 1776 (*b*) 2364 (*c*) 1976 (*d*) 3776

5. (*a*) 7658 (*b*) 1234 (*c*) 9876 (*d*) 6543

6. (*a*) 18 (*b*) 12 (*c*) 30 (*d*) 20

7. (*a*) 9875432 (*b*) 98765 (*c*) 98756 (*d*) 9876543

8. (*a*) 5243 (*b*) 9251 (*c*) 4256 (*d*) 3257

9. (*a*) 2553 (*b*) 1224 (*c*) 7992 (*d*) 3885

10. (*a*) 3223 (*b*) 4554 (*c*) 6116 (*d*) 9887

व्याख्यात्मक उत्तर

1. (*a*): शेष संख्याएं 7 से विभाज्य हैं।

2. (*d*): शेष संख्याएं 13 का गुणज हैं।

3. (*b*): शेष संख्याओं में किसी भी अंक का दो बार प्रयोग नहीं किया गया है।

4. (*b*): शेष संख्याओं में आखिरी दो अंक एक से हैं।

5. (*a*): शेष संख्याओं में उनके अंक गिनती के सीधे या उलटे क्रम में क्रमागत (निरंतर) हैं।

6. (*a*): शेष सभी संख्याएं $3^2 + 3 = 12$, $5^2 + 5 = 30$, $4^2 + 4 = 20$ हैं।

7. (*c*): शेष सभी संख्याओं में 987 के बाद अंक अवरोही या घटते हुए क्रम (decreasing order) में हैं।

8. (*a*): शेष सभी संख्याओं में 25 बीच में है और सिरे के दो अंकों का योग 10 के बराबर है।

9. (*b*): शेष सभी संख्याओं में दो सिरों पर स्थित अंकों का योग बीच में स्थित अंक के बराबर है जिसे दो बार लिखा गया है।

10. (*d*): शेष सभी संख्याओं में अंतिम दो अंक पहले दो अंकों को उलटे क्रम में लिखने पर प्राप्त होते हैं।

भाग-IV विजातीय छांटना – शब्द समूहों से संबंधित समस्याएं

शब्दों, अक्षरों या संख्याओं के समूह का वर्गीकरण एकल शब्द, अक्षर या संख्या के वर्गीकरण से अधिक भिन्न नहीं होता। इसमें परीक्षार्थी को दो परस्पर संबंधित शब्दों के बीच संबंध की विशिष्टता या प्रकृति ज्ञात करनी होती है और तत्पश्चात् दिए गए विकल्पों में से उस शब्द युग्म का पता लगाना होता है, जो अन्य शब्द-युग्मों के संबंध पैटर्न का अनुपालन नहीं करता हो। संबंधित शब्द विपरीत या सदृश अर्थ या स्वरूप के हो सकते हैं अथवा उनकी अर्थ छटा और अर्थ निरुपण में भिन्नता हो सकती है या फिर उनमें एक विशेष तुकबंदी हो सकती है।

हल किए गए उदाहरण

निर्देश: *निम्नलिखित में से कौन-सा शब्द-युग्म अन्यों से भिन्न है?*

1. (*a*) अच्छा-बेहतर (*b*) गुनगुना-गरम (*c*) नफा-लाभ (*d*) फुसफुसाना-चिल्लाना

उत्तर *(c)* : अन्य शब्द-युग्मों में युग्म के शब्द सदृश अर्थ वाले हैं किंतु उनमें सादृश्यता या साम्यता की अवस्था या कोटि भिन्न-भिन्न है।

2. (*a*) कैंची-कपड़ा (*b*) चाकू-सब्जी (*c*) कुल्हाड़ी-लकड़ी (*d*) हथौड़ा-कील

उत्तर *(d)* : हालांकि शब्दों के बीच संबंध ठीक है किंतु कील को काटने के लिए हथौड़े का प्रयोग नहीं किया जाता है। शेष तीन युग्मों में बायीं ओर उपकरण का नाम दिया गया है जिसकी सहायता से दायीं ओर लिखी गई वस्तु को काट सकते हैं।

अभ्यास

निर्देश (प्र.सं. 1–20): *नीचे के प्रत्येक प्रश्न में शब्दों के उस जोड़े का चयन करें जो शेष तीन जोड़ों से भिन्न हो।*

1. (*a*) कुर्सी-फर्नीचर (*b*) शर्ट-वस्त्र (*c*) कंठहार-आभूषण (*d*) बोगी-इंजन

2. (*a*) चित्रांकनी-कागज (*b*) पेंसिल-लेड (*c*) कलम-स्याही (*d*) बुरुश-रंग

3. (*a*) युद्ध-शांति (*b*) वास्तविक-सहज (*c*) अग्रगण्य-प्रथम (*d*) क्रोध-गुस्सा

4. (*a*) अंगूली-अंगूठी (*b*) सिर-टोपी (*c*) कमर-मुकुट (*d*) पांव-जूता

5. (*a*) दिन-रात (*b*) चालाक-मूर्ख (*c*) स्पष्ट-धुंधला (*d*) पहुंचना-आना

6. (*a*) क्विंटल-गैलन (*b*) गुलदस्ता-फूल (*c*) पुस्तक-पृष्ठ (*d*) संसद-सांसद

7. (*a*) चिड़िया-चहचहाना (*b*) घोड़ा-भिनभिनाना (*c*) शेर-गरजना (*d*) सांप-फुफकारना

8. (*a*) भतीजी-भतीजा (*b*) भाई-बहन (*c*) पति-पत्नी (*d*) पिता-माता

9. (*a*) पेट्रोल-कार (*b*) तेल-लैम्प (*c*) डीजल-लकड़ी (*d*) मोम-मोमबत्ती

10. (*a*) गंगा-नर्मदा (*b*) थार-गोबी (*c*) आमाशय-हाथ (*d*) एवरेस्ट-पर्वत

11. (*a*) औषधि-चिकित्सक (*b*) फूल-कलाकार (*c*) जूता-मोची (*d*) त्वचा-त्वचारोग विशेषज्ञ

12. (*a*) प्राधिकार-मंजूरी
(*b*) प्रतिकर्षण-आकर्षण
(*c*) तुनकमिजाज-दुस्तोषणीय
(*d*) श्वास-अस्तित्व

13. (*a*) पोलो-बर्फ का मैदान (रिंक)
(*b*) गोल्फ-लॉन
(*c*) टेनिस-कोर्ट
(*d*) शतरंज-बोर्ड

14. (*a*) उमंग-तरंग (*b*) नीड़-पीड़ (*c*) अपराध-रोकथाम (*d*) आन-बान

15. (*a*) सेना-सेनापति (*b*) कॉलेज-प्रिंसिपल (*c*) जहाज-कैप्टन (*d*) नौसेना-लेफ्टिनेंट

16. (*a*) रेलगाड़ी-पटरी
(*b*) पक्षी-उड़ना
(*c*) हवाई जहाज-आकाश
(*d*) पनडुब्बी-समुद्र

17. (*a*) जेली-सौम्य (*b*) पत्थर-कठोर
(*c*) रोवां-मुलायम (*d*) कांच-चिकना

18. (*a*) शाखा-पेड़ (*b*) मिनट-घंटा
(*c*) वाक्य-पैराग्राफ (*d*) विद्यार्थी-शिक्षक

19. (*a*) कुल-जोड़ (*b*) अभी-वर्तमान
(*c*) बड़ी-धारणा (*d*) हां-सहमत

20. (*a*) चार-चौगुना (*b*) तीन-तेरह
(*c*) दो-दोगुना (*d*) छह-छहगुना

व्याख्यात्मक उत्तर

1. *(d)*: बोगी रेलगाड़ी का एक हिस्सा होता है जो परिवहन का एक साधन है। कुर्सी, शर्ट और कंठहार क्रमशः फर्नीचर, वस्त्र और आभूषण हैं।

2. *(a)*: पेंसिल, कलम और ब्रुश से लिखने का माध्यम क्रमशः लेड, स्याही और रंग है। चित्रांकनी (क्रेयॉन) से लिखने या चित्र बनाने का माध्यम मोम होता है।

3. *(a)*: शेष सभी शब्द-युग्म समानार्थक शब्दों के युग्म हैं जबकि विकल्प (*a*) में दिया गया शब्द-युग्म विपरीतार्थक शब्दों का युग्म है।

4. *(c)*: मुकुट सिर पर पहना जाता है।

5. *(d)*: शेष शब्द-युग्म एक दूसरे के विपरीतार्थक हैं।

6. *(a)*: शेष सभी शब्द युग्मों में पहला दूसरे का समेकित रूप हैं।

7. *(b)*: शेष सभी में दूसरी पहले की बोली है। घोड़े हिनहिनाते हैं।

8. *(a)*: संबंधित शब्द-युग्मों में पहला पुल्लिंग और दूसरा स्त्रीलिंग है। विकल्प (*a*) में पहले स्त्रीलिंग और तत्पश्चात् पुल्लिग दिया गया है।

9. *(c)*: पेट्रोल का उपयोग कार चलाने में, तेल का उपयोग लैम्प जलाने में और मोम का उपयोग मोमबत्ती जलाने में किया जाता है। डीजल और लकड़ी का आपस में ऐसा कोई संबंध नहीं है।

10. *(d)*: संबंधित शब्दों की पहचान एक जैसी है। (*a*) नदियों को, (*b*) मरुभूमि को और, (*c*) शरीर के अंगों को सूचित करते हैं जबकि विकल्प (*d*) में एवरेस्ट एक पर्वत शृंखला का नाम है।

11. *(b)*: चिकित्सक का औषधि, मोची का जूता और त्वचारोग विशेषज्ञ का संबंध त्वचारोग से है। फूलों की देख-रेख करने वाले व्यक्ति को माली कहते हैं।

12. *(b)*: शेष शब्द युग्म समानार्थक हैं जबकि प्रतिकर्षण और आकर्षण शब्द एक दूसरे के विपरीत अर्थ वाले हैं।

13. *(a)*: शब्द युग्मों में खेलों और उन्हें खेले जाने वाले स्थानों के बीच संबंध दर्शाया गया है। पोलो मैदान में खेला जाता है।

14. *(c)*: शेष शब्द-युग्मों में शब्दों के बीच एक विशेष लय है।

15. *(d)*: नौसेना का प्रमुख कमांडर होता है।

16. *(b)*: रेलगाड़ी पटरी पर, हवाई जहाज आकाश में और पनडुब्बी समुद्र के जल में चलती है। इसी प्रकार पक्षी हवा में उड़ते हैं और साथ ही ये सजीव प्राणी भी हैं।

17. *(a)*: शब्द युग्मों का दूसरा शब्द पहले शब्द की विशेषता बताता है। जेली मुलायम या अस्थिर होती है।

18. *(d)*: शेष समूहों में पहला शब्द दूसरे का हिस्सा है।

19. *(c)*: शेष समूहों के शब्द परस्पर समानार्थक हैं।

20. *(b)*: तीन से तिगुना

सांकेतिक भाषा परीक्षण
(CODING AND DECODING)

भाग-I

कूटलेखन या 'कोडिंग' संवाद-संप्रेषण की एक प्रक्रिया है जिसमें एक गुप्त भाषा का प्रयोग वास्तविक तथ्यों शब्दों/मूल्यों की अभिव्यक्ति या प्रस्तुतिकरण को एक ऐसी भाषा में परिवर्तित करने के लिए किया जाता है जिसे संवाद के प्रेषक और प्राप्तकर्ता के अतिरिक्त कोई तीसरा व्यक्ति समझ न सके। कूटभाषा में लिखने के लिए *(i)* शब्दों के अक्षरों के स्थान पर वर्णमाला के सीधे उलटे क्रम में एक या एकाधिक स्थान आगे या पीछे के अक्षरों को लिखा जाता है; *(ii)* अक्षरों के स्थान पर संख्याओं को या संख्याओं के स्थान पर अक्षरों को लिखा जाता है; *(iii)* दिए गए शब्द के कुछ या सभी अक्षरों को उलटे क्रम में लिखा जाता है; और *(iv)* शब्द के अक्षरों के स्थान पर वर्णमाला के उलटे क्रम में समस्थानिक अक्षरों को लिखा जाता है।

वर्णमाला को सीधे क्रम में लिखने पर प्राप्त शृंखला :

A B C D E F G H I J K L M N O P Q R S T U V W X Y Z

A	E	J	O	T	Y
↓	↓	↓	↓	↓	↓
प्रथम अक्षर	पांचवां अक्षर	दसवां अक्षर	पंद्रहवां अक्षर	बीसवां अक्षर	पच्चीसवां अक्षर

वर्णमाला को उलटे क्रम में लिखने पर प्राप्त शृंखला :

Z Y X W V U T S R Q P O N M L K J I H G F E D C B A

Z	V	Q	L	G	B
↓	↓	↓	↓	↓	↓
प्रथम अक्षर	पांचवां अक्षर	दसवां अक्षर	पंद्रहवां अक्षर	बीसवां अक्षर	पच्चीसवां अक्षर

टिप्पणी: Z पर पहुंचने के पश्चात् शृंखला A से पुनः शुरू होती है और A पर पहुंचने के पश्चात् शृंखला Z से पुनः शुरू होती है।

हल किए गए उदाहरण

1. यदि एक विशेष प्रकार की कूट भाषा में शब्द FACE को GBDF की तरह लिखा जाता हो तो इसी कूट भाषा में BADE को कैसे लिखा जाएगा?

(*a*) CBEF (*b*) CEBF (*c*) CFBE (*d*) CBFE

उत्तर *(a)* : शब्द के अक्षरों को वर्णमाला के सीधे क्रम में एक चरण आगे का अक्षर लिखकर कूटबद्ध किया गया है।

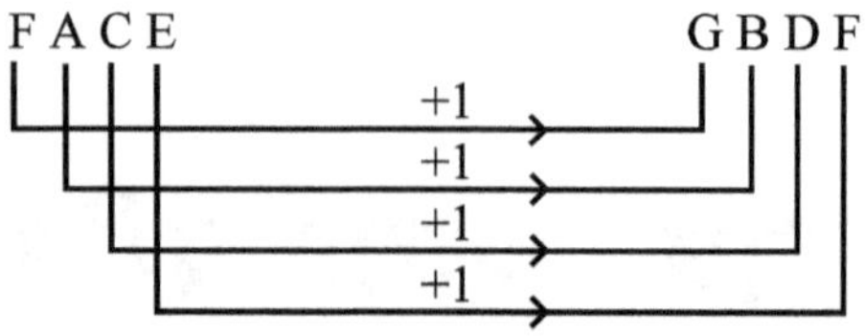

इसी प्रकार,

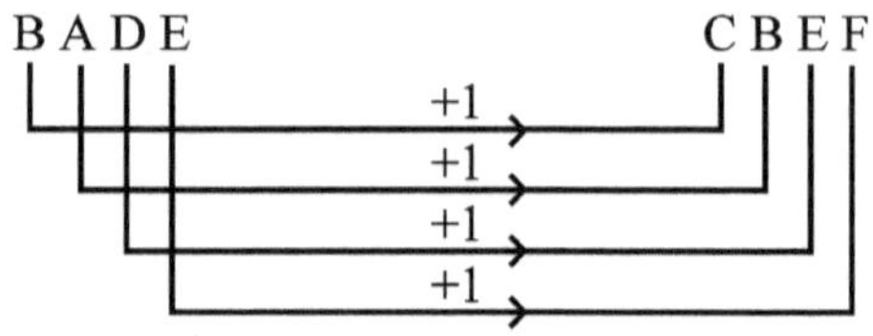

2. यदि किसी कूटभाषा में RESULT को 798206 लिखा गया हो तो उसी कूटभाषा में LET किस प्रकार लिखा जाएगा?
(*a*) 680 (*b*) 092 (*c*) 096 (*d*) 086

उत्तर *(c)* : अक्षरों को संख्याओं द्वारा कूटबद्ध किया गया है। दिए गए शब्द को कूटबद्ध करने के लिए संबंधित कूट संख्याएं ज्ञात करें।

R E S U L T → अक्षर
7 9 8 2 0 6 → कूट

अत: LET के लिए कूट संख्याएं निम्नवत् होगी :

L E T → अक्षर
0 9 6 → कूट

अभ्यास

निर्देश (प्र.सं. 1–10): *निम्नलिखित प्रश्नों में दिए गए शब्दों या अक्षरों के लिए इंगित कूटभाषा के शब्द या अक्षर ज्ञात करें।*

1. यदि किसी कूट भाषा में CHAIR को FKDLU के रूप में लिखा जाए तो उसी कूटभाषा में RAID शब्द को किस प्रकार लिखा जाएगा?
(*a*) ULGD (*b*) ULKG
(*c*) ULDG (*d*) UDLG

2. यदि किसी कूटभाषा में CONDEMN को CNODMEN लिखा जाता है तो उसी कूटभाषा में TEACHER को कैसे लिखा जाएगा?
(*a*) TEACHER (*b*) TAEECHR
(*c*) TCAEEHR (*d*) TAECEHR

3. किसी कूटभाषा में COME को XLNV और ABLE को ZYOV लिखा जाता है। इसी कूटभाषा में MOLLY किस प्रकार लिखा जाएगा?
(*a*) NLOBO (*b*) NLBOO
(*c*) LNOOB (*d*) NLOOB

4. यदि किसी कूटभाषा में ACTION को ZXGRLM लिखा जाता हो तो उसी कूटभाषा में HEALTH को कैसे लिखा जाएगा?
(*a*) SVZOGS (*b*) TVZOGT
(*c*) RUZPGR (*d*) QVGOZQ

5. यदि किसी विशेष कूटभाषा में EARTHQUAKE को MOGPENJOSM के रूप में लिखा जाता हो तो उसी कूटभाषा में EQUATE निम्नलिखित में से किस प्रकार लिखा जाएगा?
(*a*) MENOPM (*b*) MENOMP
(*c*) MJOGPM (*d*) MNJOPM

6. किसी विशेष सांकेतिक भाषा में COUNTRY शब्द को EMWLVPA के रूप में कूटबद्ध किया जाता है। इसी विशेष भाषा में ELECTORATE किस रूप में लिखा जाएगा?
(*a*) CJCEVQPYWC (*b*) GJGERQTYVG
(*c*) CNCERQPCRG (*d*) GJGAVMTYVC

7. यदि PHILOSOPHY को HPLISOPOYH लिखा जाता हो तो ORNAMENTAL कैसे लिखा जाएगा?
(*a*) ROANEMNTLA
(*b*) ONRAMNEALT
(*c*) ROANEMTNLA
(*d*) ROANEMNATL

8. यदि किसी कूटभाषा में लिखे गए शब्द OPFGBCST का अर्थवाचन NEAR के रूप में किया जाता हो तो उसी कूटभाषा में कूटबद्ध IJVWHI का अर्थ निम्नलिखित में से क्या होगा?
(*a*) HAG (*b*) HUG
(*c*) HUT (*d*) KEG

9. किसी विशेष कूटलिपि में PUNCTUAL को 16598623 के रूप में कूटबद्ध किया जाता है। इसी

कूटलिपि में ACTUPULN निम्नलिखित में से किस प्रकार लिखा जाएगा?

(*a*) 29861653 (*b*) 29861635
(*c*) 28916135 (*d*) 29851536

10. यदि OUT को 152120 के रूप में कूटबद्ध किया जाता हो तो इसी नियम का प्रयोग करके IN को निम्नलिखित में से कैसे लिखा जाएगा?

(*a*) 1015 (*b*) 819
(*c*) 1813 (*d*) 914

व्याख्यात्मक उत्तर

1. *(d)*: शब्द को कूटबद्ध करने के लिए उसके अक्षरों से वर्ण-माला के क्रम में +3 चरण आगे के अक्षर लिए गए हैं।

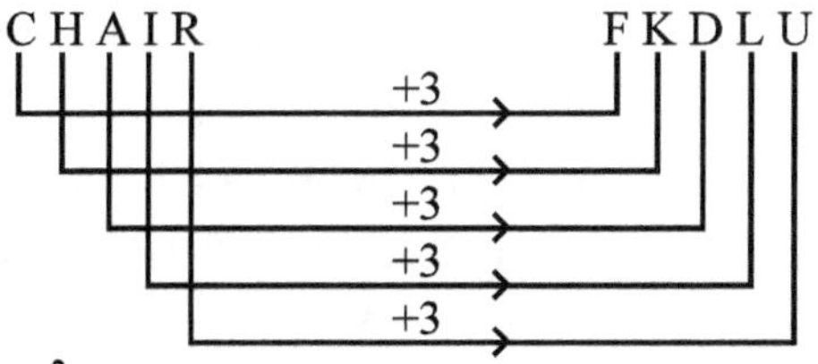

इसी प्रकार,

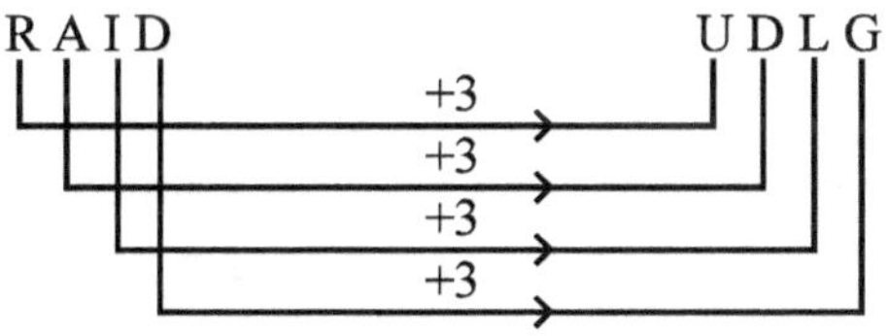

2. *(d)*: इस शब्द में दूसरे और तीसरे अक्षर एक दूसरे के स्थान पर आ जाते हैं और पांचवे और छठे अक्षरों द्वारा भी इसी नियम का पालन किया जाता है। शेष अक्षरों का स्थान अपरिवर्तित रहता है।

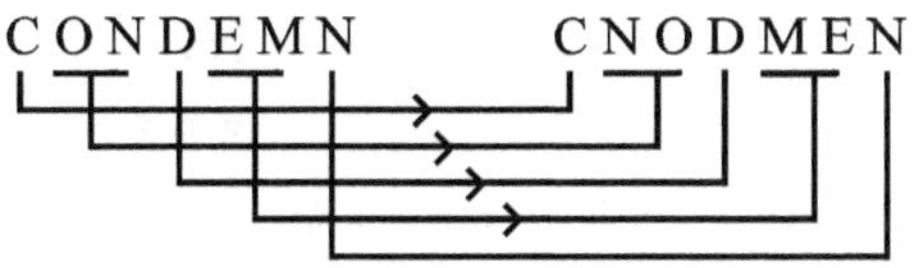

इसी प्रकार,

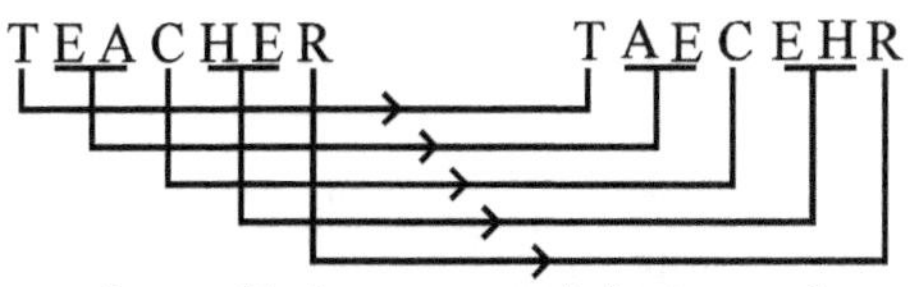

3. *(d)*: शब्द के अक्षरों को कूटबद्ध करने के लिए वर्णमाला के उलटे क्रम में समान स्थान वाले अक्षरों को लिया गया है।

C O M E → वर्णमाला के सीधे क्रम में अक्षर

X L N V → वर्णमाला के उलटे क्रम में समान स्थान वाले अक्षर

↓ ↓ ↓ ↓

3रा 15वां 13वां 5वां → वर्णमाला में अक्षरों का स्थान

A B L E → वर्णमाला के सीधे क्रम में अक्षर

Z Y O V → वर्णमाला के उलटे क्रम में समान स्थान वाले अक्षर

↓ ↓ ↓ ↓

1ला 2रा 12वां 5वां → वर्णमाला के अक्षरों का स्थान

इसी प्रकार,

M O L L Y → वर्णमाला के सीधे क्रम में अक्षर

N L O O B → वर्णमाला के उलटे क्रम में समान स्थान वाले अक्षर

↓ ↓ ↓ ↓ ↓

13वां 15वां 12वां 12वां 25वां → वर्णमाला में अक्षरों का स्थान

4. *(a)*: शब्द के अक्षरों को कूटबद्ध करने के लिए वर्णमाला के उलटे क्रम में समान स्थान वाले अक्षरों को लिया गया है।

A C T I O N → वर्णमाला के सीधे क्रम में अक्षर

Z X G R L M → वर्णमाला के उलटे क्रम में समान स्थान वाले अक्षर

↓ ↓ ↓ ↓ ↓ ↓

1ला 3रा 20वां 9वां 15वां 14वां → वर्णमाला में अक्षरों का स्थान

इसी प्रकार,

H E A L T H → वर्णमाला के क्रम में अक्षर

S V Z O G S → वर्णमाला के उलटे क्रम में समान स्थान वाले अक्षर

↓ ↓ ↓ ↓ ↓ ↓

8वां 5वां 1ला 12वां 20वां 8वां → वर्णमाला में अक्षरों का स्थान

5. *(d)*: EQUATE शब्द के अक्षर EARTHQUAKE शब्द से लिए गए हैं।
उत्तर कूट प्राप्त करने के लिए कूटबद्ध शब्द से अक्षरों का मिलान करें।

E A R T H Q U A K E → अक्षर

M O G P E N J O S M → कूट

E Q U A T E → कूटबद्ध किए जाने वाले अक्षर

M N J O P M → उत्तर कूट

6. *(d)*: शब्द को कूटबद्ध करने के लिए शब्द के अक्षरों से वर्णमाला के क्रम में क्रमशः 2 चरण आगे और दो चरण पीछे के अक्षर लिए गए हैं।

COUNTRY EMWLVPA

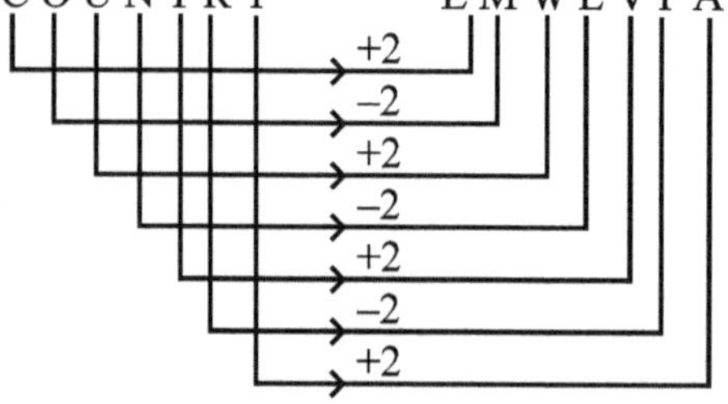

इसी प्रकार,

ELECTORATE GJGAVMTYVC

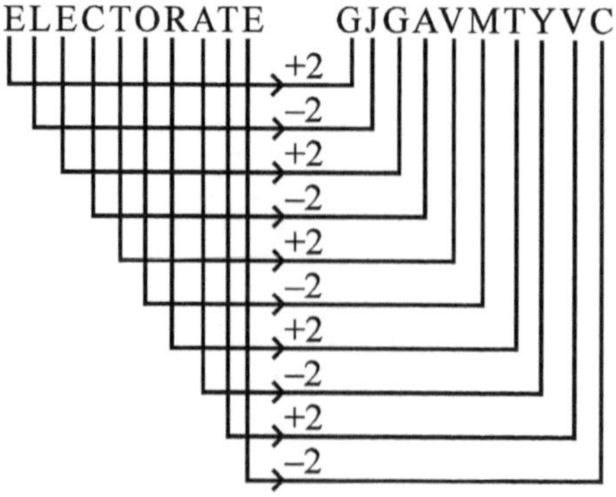

7. *(c)*: शब्द को कूटबद्ध करने के लिए उसके दो क्रमागत अक्षरों को एक दूसरे के स्थान पर लिखा जाता है।

PH IL OS OP HY HP LI SO PO YH

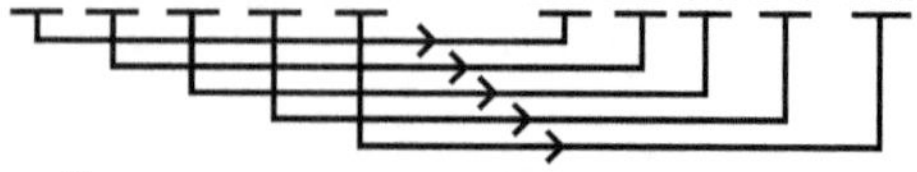

इसी प्रकार,

OR NA ME NT AL RO AN EM TN LA

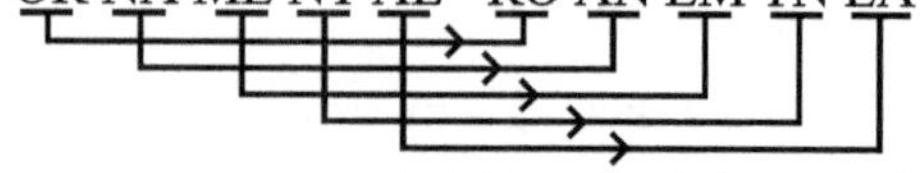

8. *(b)*: कूटबद्ध शब्द का अर्थ-निर्वचन निम्नलिखित रूप में किया गया है :

↓ OP ↓ FG ↓ BC ↓ ST → कूट

N E A R → दिया गया शब्द

अतः कूटबद्ध शब्द का अर्थ-निर्वचन करने के लिए वर्णमाला के अनुक्रम में दो क्रमागत अक्षरों से पहले के अक्षर लिए जाते हैं।

इसी प्रकार,

↓ IJ ↓ VW ↓ HI → दिया गया शब्द

H U G → उत्तर शब्द

9. *(b)*: शब्द PUNCTUAL के अक्षरों को यादृच्छिक क्रम में लेकर ACTUPULN शब्द लिखा गया है।
इसी प्रकार संख्या कूट भी लिखा जाएगा

P U N C T U A L → दिया गया शब्द

1 6 5 9 8 6 2 3 → कूट

इसी प्रकार,

A C T U P U L N → कूटबद्ध किया जाने वाला शब्द

2 9 8 6 1 6 3 5 → उत्तर कोड

10. *(d)*: कूट लेखन के लिए प्रयोग में लाई गई संख्याएं वर्णमाला के सीधे क्रम (ABCD...) में अक्षरों के स्थान को सूचित करती है।

O U T → OUT

↓ ↓ ↓

15वां 21वां 20वां → 152120

इसी प्रकार,

I N → IN

↓ ↓

9वां 14वां → 914

भाग-II

कूट लेखन विभिन्न प्रकार से किया जाता है। कूटभाषा का प्रयोग न केवल शब्दों और संख्याओं के लिए किया जाता है बल्कि किसी शब्द-समूह, विवरण या कभी-कभी वाक्यों को भी कूटभाषा द्वारा संप्रेषित किया जाता है। इस प्रकार की कूटभाषा से भ्रम की स्थिति उत्पन्न हो सकती है किंतु कुछ प्रश्नों को हल कर लेने के बाद ऐसी कूटभाषा को समझना और हल करना अत्यंत सरल हो जाता है। इस प्रकार की कूटभाषा पर आधारित प्रश्नों को हल करने के लिए अक्षरों को गिनने या छोड़ने अथवा गणितीय परिकलनों की श्रमसाध्य प्रक्रिया को अपनाने की आवश्यकता नहीं होती बल्कि इनके लिए तेजी से मिलान करने या सादृश्यता स्थापित करने की क्षमता ही अपेक्षित होती है। कूट के रूप में अक्षरों या संख्याओं का प्रयोग किया जा सकता है।

हल किए गए उदाहरण

1. यदि किसी कूटभाषा में 'ra mei ket' का अर्थ है 'he is rich'; 'rui pha jeu' का अर्थ है 'run for money'; और 'pha rui ket' का अर्थ है 'money for rich' उस **कूटभाषा** में 'rich' के लिए निम्नलिखित में से किस कूट का प्रयोग किया गया है?

(*a*) ra (*b*) pha (*c*) ket (*d*) jeu

उत्तर *(c)* : दी गई जानकारी है :

कूट	**वाक्य**
1. ra mei *ket*	he is *rich*
2. rui pha jeu	run for money
3. pha rui *ket*	money for *rich*

कूटों और वाक्यों की तुलना करने पर यह स्पष्ट होता है कि वाक्य 1 और 3 दोनों में 'rich' शब्द है और दोनों ही वाक्यों में इसके लिए 'ket' शब्द का प्रयोग किया गया है।

2. यदि किसी कूटभाषा में 'ni ra ge' का अर्थ है 'who are you'; 'boi wo dur' का अर्थ है 'going far away'; और 'wo ge chi' का अर्थ है 'you went away' तो उस कूटभाषा में 'went' के लिए निम्नलिखित में से किस कूट का प्रयोग किया गया है?

(*a*) ra (*b*) chi (*c*) wo (*d*) boi

उत्तर *(b)* : दी गई सूचना है :

कूट	**वाक्य**
1. ni ra *ge*	who are *you*
2. boi *wo* dur	going far *away*
3. *wo ge* **chi**	*you* **went** *away*

'went' शब्द केवल तीसरे वाक्य में है। 'you' शब्द पहले और तीसरे दोनों वाक्यों में है जिसके लिए इन वाक्यों में 'ge' कूट का प्रयोग किया गया है। शब्द 'away' दूसरे और तीसरे दोनों वाक्यों में है जिसके लिए 'wo' कूट का प्रयोग किया गया है। एकमात्र 'chi' कूट ही ऐसा बचता है जिसका अर्थ 'went' है।

अभ्यास

निर्देश (प्र.सं. 1–10): *नीचे के प्रत्येक प्रश्न में कूटलेखन के पैटर्न को ध्यान से देखें और दिए गए विकल्पों में से सही उत्तर का चयन करें।*

1. यदि किसी कूटभाषा में (a) 'go ju mi' का अर्थ है 'plenty of money'; (b) pao ju go nei vu' का अर्थ है 'money creates lots of problems'; (c) 'kol vu nei' का अर्थ है 'problems create tension'; और (d) 'sol tun ju haw' का अर्थ है 'still money is needed' तो उस कूट भाषा में निम्नलिखित में से किसका अर्थ 'money' है?

(*a*) nei (*b*) ju
(*c*) haw (*d*) go

2. किसी कूटभाषा में (a) 'FOR' का अर्थ है 'old is gold'; (b) 'ROT' का अर्थ है 'gold is pure'; (c) 'ROM' का अर्थ है 'gold is costly'। इसी कूटभाषा में 'pure old gold is costly' कैसे लिखा जाएगा?

(*a*) TFROM (*b*) FOTRM
(*c*) FTORM (*d*) TOMRF

3. यदि किसी कूटभाषा में '415' का अर्थ है 'milk is hot'; '18' का अर्थ है 'hot soup'; और '895' का अर्थ है 'soup is tasty' तो उसी कूटभाषा में 'tasty' शब्द किस संख्या द्वारा निरूपित होगा?

(*a*) 9 (*b*) 8
(*c*) 5 (*d*) 4

4. यदि किसी कूटभाषा में '643' का अर्थ है 'she is beautiful', '593' का अर्थ है 'he is handsome', और '567' का अर्थ है 'handsome meets beautiful' तो उसी कूटभाषा में 'meets' शब्द निम्नलिखित में से किस संख्या द्वारा सूचित होगा?

(*a*) 5 (*b*) 3
(*c*) 7 (*d*) 6

5. किसी कूटभाषा में (a) 'dugo hui mul zo' का अर्थ है 'work is very hard'; (b) 'hui dugo ba ki' का अर्थ है 'Bingo is very smart'; (c) 'nano mul dugo' का अर्थ है 'cake is hard', और (d) 'mul ki qu' का अर्थ है 'smart and hard' इस कूट भाषा में 'Bingo' के लिए किस कूटशब्द का प्रयोग किया गया है?

(*a*) jalu (*b*) dugo
(*c*) ki (*d*) ba

6. किसी कूटभाषा में (a) 'pic vic nic' का अर्थ है 'winter is cold'; (b) 'to nic re' का अर्थ है 'summer is hot'; (c) 're pic boo' का अर्थ है 'winter and summer' और (d) 'vic tho pa' का अर्थ है 'nights are cold' इस कूटभाषा में 'summer' के लिए किस कूटशब्द का प्रयोग किया जाता है?

(*a*) nic (*b*) boo
(*c*) to (*d*) re

7. किसी कूटभाषा में (a) 'mx das sci' का अर्थ है 'good little frock'; (b) 'jm coz sci' का अर्थ है 'girl behaves good'; (c) 'ngv drs coz' का अर्थ है 'girl makes mischief'; और (d) 'das gp coz' का अर्थ है 'little girl fell' इस कूटभाषा में 'frock' के लिए किस कूट शब्द का प्रयोग किया गया है?

(*a*) mx (*b*) das
(*c*) sci (*d*) gp

8. किसी कूटभाषा में 'mu mit es' का अर्थ है 'who is she' और 'elb mu es' का अर्थ है 'where is she' इस कूटभाषा में 'where' के लिए किस कूटशब्द का प्रयोग किया जाता है?

(*a*) es (*b*) elb
(*c*) mu (*d*) mit

9. किसी कूटभाषा में '069' का अर्थ है 'grapes are sweet', '476' का अर्थ है 'very sweet fruit' और '509' का अर्थ है 'grapes are ripe'। इस कूटभाषा में निम्नलिखित में से किस अंक से 'ripe' शब्द सूचित होता है?

(*a*) 0 (*b*) 5
(*c*) 9 (*d*) 7

10. किसी कूटभाषा में 'roi ja kyo twa' का अर्थ है 'Moody is writing letters', 'pok ju ja twa' का अर्थ है 'Woody is writing cards', 'trn kyo pos un' का अर्थ है 'they are writing letters', और 'koi rus pok' का अर्थ है 'gifts and cards'। इसी कूटभाषा में 'Moody' के लिए किस कूटशब्द का प्रयोग किया गया है?

(*a*) ja (*b*) twa
(*c*) roi (*d*) kyo

व्याख्यात्मक उत्तर

1. *(b)*:

	कूट	वाक्य
1.	go *ju* mi	plenty of *money*
2.	pao *ju* go nei vu	*money* creates lots of problems
3.	kol vu nei	problems create tension
4.	sol tun *ju* haw	still *money* is needed

ऊपर के पहले, दूसरे और चौथे कूटों और संबंधित वाक्यों में 'ju' शब्द और उसके लिए 'money' शब्द लिखा गया है।

2. *(a)*: **कूट** **वाक्य**

1. FOR old is gold

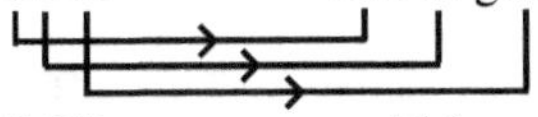

2. ROT gold is pure

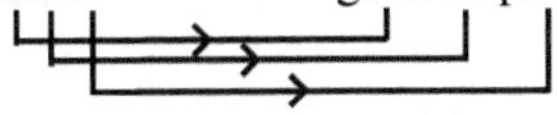

3. ROM gold is costly

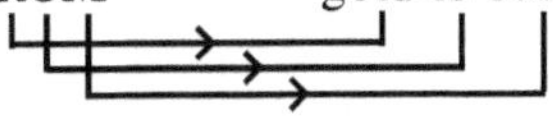

अतः,

F का अर्थ है old

O का अर्थ है is

R का अर्थ है gold

T का अर्थ है pure

M का अर्थ है costly

अत: 'pure old gold is costly' को 'TFROM' द्वारा व्यक्त किया जाएगा।

3. *(a)*: **कूट** **वाक्य**

1. 415 milk is hot
2. 18 hot soup
3. 895 soup is *tasty*

तीसरे कूट और उससे संबंधित वाक्य में दी गई न तो संख्या '9' और न ही शब्द 'tasty' को किसी अन्य कूट और वाक्य में दोहराया गया है।

4. *(c)*: **कूट** **वाक्य**

1. 643 she is beautiful
2. 593 he is handsome
3. 56*7* handsome *meets* beautiful

तीसरे कूट और उससे संबंधित वाक्य में दी गई न तो संख्या '7' और न ही शब्द 'meets' को किसी अन्य कूट और वाक्य में दोहराया गया है।

5. *(d)*: **कूट** **वाक्य**

1. *dugo hui* mul zo work *is very* hard
2. *hui dugo* **ba** *ki* **Bingo** *is very smart*
3. nano mul *dugo* cake is *hard*
4. mul *ki* qu *smart* and hard

दूसरे कूट और संबंधित वाक्य में निहित न तो 'ba' और न ही अर्थ शब्द 'Bingo' की पुनरावृत्ति होती है। (जिन शब्दों की पुनरावृत्ति होती है उन्हें तिरछे अक्षरों में लिखा गया है)

6. *(d)*: **कूट** **वाक्य**

1. pic vic nic winter is cold
2. to nic *re* *summer* is hot
3. *re* pic boo winter and *summer*
4. vic tho pa nights are cold

शब्द 'summer' और कूट 're' की दूसरे और तीसरे वाक्यों में पुनरावृत्ति होती है।

7. *(a)*: **कूट** **वाक्य**

1. **mx** *das sci* *good little* **frock**
2. jm coz *sci* girl behaves *good*
3. ngv drs coz girl makes mischief
4. *das* gp coz *little* girl fell

शब्द 'frock' केवल पहले वाक्य में है। कूट शब्द 'das' को चौथे वाक्य में और 'sci' को दूसरे वाक्य में दोहराया गया है। अत: स्पष्ट है कि 'frock' के लिए कूट शब्द 'mx' का प्रयोग किया गया है।

8. *(b)*: **कूट** **वाक्य**

1. *mu* mit *es* who *is she*
2. **elb** *mu* es **where** *is she*

कूट शब्दों 'mu' और 'es' को दोनों वाक्यों में दोहराया गया है। केवल कूट शब्द 'elb' ही बचता है जिसका अर्थ 'where' है।

9. *(b)*: **कूट** **वाक्य**

1. 069 *grapes are* sweet
2. 476 very sweet fruit
3. **5**09 *grapes are* **ripe**

पहले और तीसरे वाक्यों में कूट संख्याओं '0' और '9' की पुनरावृत्ति होती है। अत: स्पष्ट है कि शेष कूट संख्या '5' का ही 'ripe' के लिए प्रयोग किया गया है।

10. *(c)*: **कूट** **वाक्य**

1. **roi** *ja kyo twa* **Moody** *is writing letters*
2. pok ju *ja twa* Woody *is writing* cards
3. trn *kyo* pos un they are writing *letters*
4. koi rus pok gifts and cards

'Moody' शब्द केवल पहले वाक्य में है। पहले वाक्य के कूट शब्दों 'ja' और 'twa' की दूसरे वाक्य में पुनरावृत्ति होती है और 'kyo' की तीसरे वाक्य में पुनरावृत्ति होती है। केवल कूट शब्द 'roi' ही बचता है जिसका अर्थ 'Moody' है।

भाग-III

एक अन्य प्रकार के कूट लेखन में किसी शब्द को कूट नाम दिए जाते हैं जिन्हें आगे भी कूटबद्ध किया जाता है। इस पैटर्न पर आधारित प्रश्न अर्थहीन प्रतीत हो सकते हैं किंतु कूट यथार्थता की बुनियादी बातों से हट कर नहीं होने चाहिए।

हल किए गए उदाहरण

1. यदि किसी कूट भाषा में 'केला' को 'जेली' कहा जाए, 'जेली' को 'हरा' कहा जाए, 'हरा' को 'सेब' कहा जाए, 'सेब' को 'आम' कहा जाए तो उसी कूटभाषा में पत्ते के रंग को क्या कहेंगे?

(*a*) हरा (*b*) आम (*c*) सेब (*d*) केला

उत्तर *(c)* : पत्ता हरे रंग का होता है और प्रश्न में उल्लिखित कूटों के अनुसार 'हरा' को 'सेब' कहा जाता है।

2. यदि 'धूसर' को 'भूरा', 'सफेद' को 'गुलाबी', 'लाल' को 'धूसर', 'काला' को 'लाल' और 'भूरा' को 'सफेद' कहा जाए तो 'कोयला' किस रंग का है?

(*a*) भूरा (*b*) सफेद (*c*) काला (*d*) लाल

उत्तर *(d)* : 'कोयला' काले रंग का होता है और प्रश्न में दिए गए कूटों के अनुसार 'काला' को 'लाल' कहा जाता है।

अभ्यास

निर्देश (प्र.सं. 1–10): *प्रत्येक प्रश्न में दी गई कूटबद्ध सूचना को अच्छी तरह समझें और दिए गए विकल्पों में से सही उत्तर का चयन करें।*

1. यदि किसी कूटभाषा में 'पानी' को 'नीला', 'नीला' को 'लाल', 'लाल' को 'सफेद', 'सफेद' को 'आकाश', 'आकाश' को 'वर्षा', 'वर्षा' को 'हरा', 'हरा' को 'हवा' और 'हवा' को 'मेज' कहा जाए, तो इस कूटभाषा में दूध के रंग को क्या कहेंगे?

(*a*) सफेद (*b*) वर्षा
(*c*) आकाश (*d*) हरा

2. यदि किसी कूटभाषा में 'प्रकाश' को 'अंधकार', 'अंधकार' को 'हरा', 'हरा' को 'नीला', 'नीला' को 'लाल', 'लाल' को 'सफेद' और 'सफेद' को 'पीला' कहा जाता हो तो इस कूटभाषा में रक्त का रंग क्या कहलाएगा?

(*a*) लाल (*b*) अंधकार
(*c*) सफेद (*d*) पीला

3. यदि किसी कूटभाषा में 'आकाश' को 'समुद्र', 'समुद्र' को 'पानी', 'पानी' को 'हवा', 'हवा' को 'बादल' और 'बादल' को 'नदी' कहा जाता हो तो प्यास लगने पर इस कूटभाषा में पीने के लिए किस चीज की मांग करेंगे?

(*a*) आकाश (*b*) हवा
(*c*) पानी (*d*) समुद्र

4. यदि किसी कूटभाषा में 'पीला' का अर्थ 'लाल', 'सफेद' का अर्थ 'हरा', 'लाल' का अर्थ 'नारंगी', 'नीला' का अर्थ 'सफेद' और 'हरा' का अर्थ 'नीला' हो तो उस कूटभाषा में आकाश का रंग क्या है?

(*a*) सफेद (*b*) हरा
(*c*) नीला (*d*) पीला

5. यदि किसी कूटभाषा में 'घर' को 'झोपड़ी', 'झोपड़ी' को 'नहर', 'नहर' को 'स्कूल', 'स्कूल' को 'मैदान', 'मैदान' को 'सुराही' और 'सुराही' को 'तार' कहा जाए तो इस कूटभाषा में छात्रों के पढ़ने की जगह को क्या कहेंगे?

(*a*) मैदान (*b*) सुराही
(*c*) झोपड़ी (*d*) स्कूल

6. यदि किसी कूटभाषा में 'बिल्ली' को 'घोड़ा', 'घोड़ा' को 'चूहा', 'कुत्ता' को 'खरगोश', 'खरगोश' को 'बिल्ली', 'चूहा' को 'कुत्ता' और 'शेर' को 'चींटी' कहा जाए तो इस कूटभाषा मे प्रयुक्त कूटों के आधार पर भौंकने वाले पशु को क्या कहेंगे?

(*a*) कुत्ता (*b*) बिल्ली
(*c*) शेर (*d*) खरगोश

7. यदि 'भूमि' को 'झील', 'झील' को 'पत्थर', 'पत्थर' को 'भारी', 'भारी' को 'स्टेडियम', 'स्टेडियम' को 'महासागर', 'महासागर' को 'वर्षा' और 'वर्षा' को 'आग' कहा जाए तो क्रिकेट के टेस्ट मैच खेले जाने वाले स्थान क्या कहलाते हैं?
(*a*) भारी (*b*) महासागर
(*c*) पत्थर (*d*) भूमि

8. यदि किसी कूटभाषा में 'चिड़िया' को 'राजा', 'राजा' को 'फूल', 'फूल' को 'घन', 'घन' को 'मेज', 'मेज' को 'मनुष्य' और 'मनुष्य' को 'चिड़िया' कहा जाए तो इस कूटभाषा में 'गुलाब' क्या है?
(*a*) मेज (*b*) फूल
(*c*) घन (*d*) मनुष्य

9. यदि किसी कूटभाषा में 'पानी' को 'पत्थर', 'पत्थर' को 'तेल', 'तेल' को 'हवा', 'हवा' को 'लकड़ी', 'लकड़ी' को 'गैस' और 'गैस' को 'द्रव' कहा जाए तो इस कूटभाषा में फर्नीचर किस चीज से बनता है?
(*a*) गैस (*b*) हवा
(*c*) तेल (*d*) द्रव

10. यदि किसी कूटभाषा में 'पिंजड़ा' को 'रॉकेट', 'रॉकेट' को 'फंदा', 'फंदा' को 'ग्रह', 'ग्रह' को 'हवाई जहाज', 'हवाई जहाज' को 'साइकिल' और 'साइकिल' को 'कार' कहा जाए तो इस कूटभाषा में पृथ्वी को क्या कहेंगे?
(*a*) साइकिल (*b*) रॉकेट
(*c*) ग्रह (*d*) हवाई जहाज

व्याख्यात्मक उत्तर

1. *(c)*: दूध का रंग 'सफेद' होता है और इस कूटभाषा में 'सफेद' को 'आकाश' कहते हैं।

2. *(c)*: रक्त का रंग 'लाल' होता है और इस कूटभाषा में 'लाल' को 'सफेद' कहते हैं।

3. *(b)*: प्यास लगने पर हम 'पानी' पीते हैं और इस कूटभाषा में 'पानी' को 'हवा' कहते हैं।

4. *(a)*: आकाश का रंग 'नीला' होता है और नीला का अर्थ 'सफेद' है।

5. *(a)*: छात्र 'स्कूल' में पढ़ते हैं और 'स्कूल' को इस कूटभाषा में 'मैदान' कहा जाता है।

6. *(d)*: भौंकने वाला पशु 'कुत्ता' है और 'कुत्ता' को इस कूटभाषा में 'खरगोश' कहते हैं।

7. *(b)*: टैस्ट मैच 'स्टेडियम' में खेले जाते हैं और 'स्टेडियम' को इस कूटभाषा में 'महासागर' कहा जाता है।

8. *(c)*: गुलाब एक 'फूल' है और 'फूल' को इस कूटभाषा में 'घन' कहा जाता है।

9. *(a)*: फर्नीचर 'लकड़ी' से बनता है और 'लकड़ी' को इस कूटभाषा में गैस कहते हैं।

10. *(d)*: पृथ्वी एक 'ग्रह' है 'ग्रह' को इस कूटभाषा में हवाई जहाज कहते हैं।

कथन विश्लेषण
(STATEMENT ANALYSIS)

तर्कबुद्धि परीक्षण से संबंधित इस प्रकार के प्रश्नों में कुछ कथन दिए जाते हैं। इन कथनों में कतिपय तथ्यों को अलग-अलग रूपों में तोड़-मरोड़ कर प्रस्तुत किया जाता है। ऐसे प्रश्नों को हल करने के लिए अभ्यर्थियों से यह अपेक्षा की जाती है कि वे दिए गए कथनों का विश्लेषण करें, दिए गए तथ्यों को सुव्यवस्थित और वर्गीकृत करें तथा तत्पश्चात् दिए गए कथनों से संबंधित प्रश्नों के उत्तर दें।

हल किए गए उदाहरण

1. आइसक्रीम बर्फ के समान ठंडा होता है। बर्फ ओले जितनी ठंडी नहीं होती। हिमकण बर्फ जितने ठंडे नहीं होते किंतु ये आइसक्रीम से अधिक ठंडे होते हैं। इनमें से सर्वाधिक ठंडा क्या है?

(*a*) ओला (*b*) आइसक्रीम (*c*) हिमकण (*d*) हिम

उत्तर *(a)* : ठंडक में वृद्धि को दर्शाने वाला क्रम है—आइसक्रीम, बर्फ, हिमकण, हिम, ओला।

2. नीचे दिए गए कथन को सावधानीपूर्वक पढ़ें और पूछे गए प्रश्नों *(i)* और *(ii)* के उत्तर दें :

पांच आदमी जिनमें से एक वजनी, दूसरा मोटा, तीसरा दुबला-पतला, चौथा नाटा और पांचवां लंबा है, एक दूसरे के पीछे दौड़ रहे हैं। वजनी और लंबे आदमियों में से एक तो कलाकार है और दूसरा बातुनी। दुबला-पतला आदमी जो बुद्धिमान भी है, बीच में दौड़ रहा है। नाटा आदमी काला नहीं है और गोरे रंग का आदमी दुबले-पतले आदमी से आगे दौड़ रहा है। वजनी आदमी जो कलाकार नहीं है, मोटे आदमी के सामने दौड़ रहा है।

(i) गोरा कौन है?

(*a*) लंबा आदमी (*b*) मोटा आदमी (*c*) नाटा आदमी (*d*) वजनी आदमी

उत्तर : *(b)*

(ii) लंबा आदमी क्या है?

(*a*) बुद्धिमान (*b*) बातुनी (*c*) कलाकार (*d*) काला

उत्तर : *(c)*

पांचों आदमियों के गुणों का चार्ट इस प्रकार है :

वजनी आदमी बातुनी है।
मोटा आदमी गोरा है।
दुबला-पतला आदमी बुद्धिमान है।
नाटा आदमी काला नहीं है।
लंबा आदमी कलाकार है।

अभ्यास

1. A, B, C, D और E पांच मित्र हैं जिनमें से A का वजन B से अधिक है, C का वजन D से कम है, B का वजन D से कम है किंतु E से अधिक है। इनमें से किसका वजन सबसे अधिक है?

(*a*) B (*b*) C
(*c*) A (*d*) **कहा नहीं जा सकता**

2. झांसी की तुलना में पुणे एक बड़ा शहर है, तथा चित्तौड़ की तुलना में सीतापुर एक बड़ा शहर है। रायगढ़ झांसी जितना बड़ा शहर नहीं है किंतु यह सीतापुर की तुलना में बड़ा शहर है। चित्तौड़ सीतापुर जितना बड़ा शहर नहीं है। इनमें से सबसे छोटा शहर कौन है?

(*a*) झांसी (*b*) पुणे
(*c*) चित्तौड़ (*d*) सीतापुर

3. राम के मुकाबले अजय अधिक काम करता है। आलोक और राजू दोनों एक जितना काम करते हैं। पंकज आलोक के मुकाबले कम काम करता है। राम आलोक के मुकाबले अधिक काम करता है। इनमें से सबसे अधिक काम कौन करता है?

(*a*) अजय (*b*) राम
(*c*) आलोक (*d*) राजू

4. विपुल, हंस से लंबा है। हंस, आनंद से लंबा है। आलोक, अशोक से लंबा है। अशोक, हंस से लंबा है। इन पांचों मित्रों से कौन सबसे अधिक लंबा है?

(*a*) विपुल (*b*) आलोक
(*c*) अशोक (*d*) कहा नहीं जा सकता

5. प्रमोद, गोपाल से लंबा है। गोपाल, मधु से कम लंबा है। यह जानने के लिए कि इनमें सबसे अधिक लंबा कौन है, निम्नलिखित में से कौन-सी अतिरिक्त जानकारी आवश्यक है?

(*a*) मधु, गोपाल से लंबी है
(*b*) मधु, प्रमोद के भाई से कम लंबी है
(*c*) प्रमोद, मधु से लंबा है
(*d*) प्रमोद, मधु के भाई से लंबा है

6. A की आयु B से अधिक है जबकि C और D की आयु E से अधिक है तथा E की आयु A और B की आयुओं के बीच है। यदि C की आयु B की तुलना में अधिक हो तो बताएं कि निम्नलिखित में से कौन-सा कथन अनिवार्यत: सत्य है?

(*a*) E की आयु B से अधिक है
(*b*) A की आयु C से अधिक है
(*c*) C की आयु D से अधिक है
(*d*) D की आयु C से अधिक है

7. विक्रम की लंबाई राजन से अधिक किंतु ऐनी से कम है। जमाल, ऐनी से अधिक लंबा है। सीता, विक्रम से अधिक लंबी है। राजन, सीता से कम लंबा है। इस समूह में सबसे कम लंबाई किसकी है?

(*a*) सीता (*b*) राजन
(*c*) विक्रम (*d*) कहा नहीं जा सकता

8. सुरेश की आयु कमल से उतनी ही अधिक है जितनी कि उसकी आयु प्रबोध से कम है। नवीन और कमल की आयु एक जैसी है। निम्नलिखित में से कौन-सा कथन असत्य है?

(*a*) सुरेश की आयु नवीन से अधिक है
(*b*) कमल की आयु सुरेश से कम है
(*c*) प्रबोध सबसे अधिक आयु का नहीं है
(*d*) नवीन की आयु प्रबोध से कम है

9. प्रमोद आयु में जयेश और सुधीर से बड़ा है। विकास, अनिल से छोटा है। इनमें किसकी आयु सब से अधिक है, यह जानने के लिए निम्नलिखित में से कौन-सी अतिरिक्त जानकारी अपेक्षित है?

(*a*) सुधीर, जयेश से बड़ा है
(*b*) अनिल, जयेश से बड़ा है
(*c*) विकास, प्रमोद से बड़ा है
(*d*) विकास, प्रमोद से छोटा है

10. पांच लड़कों में बसंत, मनोहर से लंबा है किंतु वह राजू जितना लंबा नहीं है। जयंत, दत्ता से लंबा है किंतु मनोहर से उसकी लंबाई कम है। इनमें सबसे अधिक लंबा लड़का कौन है?

(*a*) राजू (*b*) मनोहर
(*c*) बसंत (*d*) कहा नहीं जा सकता

11. A और D एक ही कक्षा में पढ़ते हैं। K और L एक ही कक्षा में पढ़ते हैं। D किस कक्षा में पढ़ता है? इस प्रश्न का उत्तर ज्ञात करने के लिए निम्नलिखित A और B कथनों में से किसमें दी गई सूचना आवश्यक है?

A. D, L से एक कक्षा कम में पढ़ता है
B. A का बड़ा भाई K के साथ पढ़ता है

(*a*) उपर्युक्त A और B दोनों में दी गई सूचनाएं पर्याप्त नहीं हैं
(*b*) उपर्युक्त A और B दोनों में दी गई सूचनाएं अपेक्षित हैं

(*c*) केवल A में दी गई सूचना पर्याप्त है

(*d*) केवल B में दी गई सूचना आवश्यक है

निर्देश (प्र.सं. 12 और 13): (A) गोपाल की लंबाई अशोक से कम किंतु केशव से अधिक है; (B) नवीन की लंबाई केशव से कम है; (C) जयेश की लंबाई नवीन से अधिक है; (D) अशोक की लंबाई जयेश से अधिक है।

12. इनमें सबसे अधिक लंबा कौन है ?

(*a*) गोपाल (*b*) अशोक

(*c*) जयेश (*d*) नवीन

13. उपर्युक्त प्रश्न का उत्तर देने के लिए निम्नलिखित में से कौन-सी सूचना आवश्यक नहीं है ?

(*a*) A (*b*) B

(*c*) C (*d*) D

निर्देश (प्र.सं. 14–16): *नीचे दिए गए कथन को ध्यानपूर्वक पढ़ें और इसमें दी गई सूचना के आधार पर पूछे गए प्रश्नों के उत्तर दें:*

रवि, हरी, मनु और जतिन चार मित्र हैं। इनमें से एक कानपुर में रहता है और उसे लिखने-पढ़ने का शौक है। हरी और जतिन लखनऊ में रहते हैं। हरी को डाक टिकटें एकत्रित करने का शौक है। लखनऊ में रहने वाले दोनों मित्रों में से प्रत्येक को सिक्के एकत्रित करने का शौक है। रवि इलाहाबाद में रहता है। लखनऊ में रहने वाला एक लड़का संगीत सुनना भी पंसद करता है। इलाहाबाद में रहने वाले लड़के को यात्रा करने और कॉमिक्स पढ़ने का शौक है। यदि सभी लड़कों में से प्रत्येक को दो शौक हों तो निम्नलिखित प्रश्नों के उत्तर दें :

14. कानपुर में कौन रहता है ?

(*a*) जतिन (*b*) मनु

(*c*) रवि (*d*) हरी

15. सिक्के एकत्रित करने और संगीत सुनने का शौक निम्नलिखित में से किसे है ?

(*a*) मनु (*b*) रवि

(*c*) हरी (*d*) जतिन

16. निम्नलिखित में से कौन-सा शौक रवि को नहीं है ?

(*a*) कॉमिक्स पढ़ना (*b*) पढ़ना

(*c*) यात्रा करना (*d*) कहा नहीं जा सकता

व्याख्यात्मक उत्तर

1. *(d)*: वजन के घटते क्रम में इन मित्रों को निम्नवत् श्रेणीबद्ध किया जा सकता है : A/D, B/C, E या A/D, B, C/E अत: इन मित्रों में से A या D का वजन सबसे अधिक है।

2. *(c)*: आकार के घटते क्रम में शहरों के नाम हैं: पुणे, झांसी, रायगढ़, सीतापुर, चित्तौड़।

3. *(a)*: इन व्यक्तियों के नामों का इनके द्वारा किए जाने वाले काम की मात्रा के घटते क्रम में निम्नलिखित अनुक्रम होगा :

अजय, राम, आलोक/राजू, पंकज।

4. *(d)*: लंबाई के घटते क्रम में इन व्यक्तियों के नाम हैं : विपुल/आलोक, अशोक, हंस, आनंद। अत: विपुल या आलोक में से कोई एक सबसे अधिक लंबा है।

5. *(c)*: दी गई सूचना के अनुसार प्रमोद और मधु दोनों ही गोपाल से अधिक लंबे हैं। विकल्प *(c)* में दी गई जानकारी से ही यह पता चलता है कि सबसे अधिक लंबा कौन है।

6. *(a)*: आयु के घटते क्रम में इन व्यक्तियों को निम्नवत् विन्यस्त किया जा सकता है :

A/C/D, E, B.

7. *(b)*: लंबाई के घटते क्रम में इन व्यक्तियों को निम्नवत् विन्यस्त किया जा सकता है:

जमाल/सीमा, ऐनी, विक्रम, राजन

या

जमाल, सीता/ऐनी, विक्रम, राजन

8. *(c)*: आयु के घटते क्रम में इन व्यक्तियों को निम्नवत् विन्यस्त किया जा सकता है :

प्रबोध, सुरेश, कमल/नवीन

9. *(c)*: आयु के घटते क्रम में इन व्यक्तियों को निम्नवत् विन्यस्त किया जा सकता है:

1. प्रमोद, जयेश/सुधीर और 2. अनिल, विकास

विकल्प (c) इन दोनों कथनों के बीच संबंध स्थापित करता है।

10. *(a)*: लंबाई के घटते क्रम में इन लड़कों को निम्नवत् विन्यस्त किया जा सकता है:

राजू, बसंत, मनोहर, जयंत, दत्ता

11. *(a)*: दोनों में से किसी भी कथन में उपयोगी सूचना नहीं दी गई है।

12. *(b)*: लंबाई के घटते क्रम में इन व्यक्तियों को निम्नवत् विन्यस्त किया जा सकता है:

अशोक, गोपाल/जयेश, केशव, नवीन

या

अशोक, गोपाल, केशव/जयेश, नवीन

13. *(c)* **14. *(b)*** **15. *(d)*** **16. *(b)***

स्थान व्यवस्थीकरण
(PLACE ARRANGEMENT)

स्थान व्यवस्थीकरण का सामान्य अर्थ है दी गई सूचनाओं के आधार पर व्यक्तियों या वस्तुओं का स्थान-क्रम निर्धारित करना। इसके लिए आवश्यक है कि स्थान-क्रम को अच्छी तरह समझा जाए और तत्पश्चात् दिए गए प्रश्नों को उपलब्ध कराई गई सूचना के आधार पर हल करने का प्रयास किया जाए।

हल किए गए उदाहरण

1. पांच लड़के एक सीढ़ी पर चढ़ रहे हैं। सीढ़ी पर डेविड लड़कों के बीच में है। कार्तिक सबसे पीछे है। अनमोल नीतिन से आगे है जो अनमोल और डैनी दोनों के पीछे है। सीढ़ी पर सबसे आगे कौन है?

(*a*) डैनी (*b*) अनमोल

(*c*) डैनी या अनमोल (*d*) कहा नहीं जा सकता

उत्तर *(c)* : लड़कों के सीढ़ी पर चढ़ने का निम्नलिखित क्रम है :

डैनी		अनमोल
अनमोल		डैनी
डेविड	या	डेविड
नीतिन		नीतिन
कार्तिक		कार्तिक

अतः इस बात की पूर्ण संभावना है कि सीढ़ी पर सबसे आगे डैनी या अनमोल है।

2. पांच व्यक्ति किसी पंक्ति में एक दूसरे के पीछे चल रहे हैं। पंक्ति में सबसे आगे और सबसे पीछे चल रहे व्यक्तियों में एक व्यक्ति बुद्धिमान और दूसरा मूर्ख है। एक नाटे व्यक्ति के पीछे एक मजबूत कद काठी का व्यक्ति चल रहा है। मूर्ख व्यक्ति के सामने एक दुबला व्यक्ति चल रहा है। नाटा व्यक्ति बुद्धिमान व्यक्ति और मजबूत कद काठी के व्यक्ति के बीच में है। पंक्ति में बीचों-बीच कौन चल रहा है?

(*a*) नाटा व्यक्ति (*b*) मजबूत कद-काठी का व्यक्ति

(*c*) दुबला व्यक्ति (*d*) बुद्धिमान व्यक्ति

उत्तर *(b)* : पांचों व्यक्तियों का पंक्ति में स्थान-क्रम निम्नवत् है :

मूर्ख, दुबला व्यक्ति, मजबूत कद-काठी का व्यक्ति, नाटा व्यक्ति, बुद्धिमान व्यक्ति।

अभ्यास

निर्देश (प्र.सं. 1–10): *निम्नलिखित प्रश्नों में व्यवस्थीकरण के पैटर्न को समझें और तत्पश्चात् दिए गए विकल्पों में से सही उत्तर का चयन करें:*

1. पांच लड़के एक पंक्ति में बैठे हैं। रघु, श्याम या अमित की बगल में नहीं बैठा है। अजय, श्याम की बगल में नहीं बैठा है। रघु, मयंक की बगल में बैठा है। यदि मयंक पंक्ति में बीच में बैठा हो तो अजय निम्नलिखित में से किसकी बगल में बैठा है?

(*a*) अमित (*b*) रघु
(*c*) मयंक (*d*) श्याम

2. मिनी, रजनी के दाएं और अनंता के बाएं बैठी है। सत्या, मिनी के दाएं बैठी है किंतु वह जया के बाएं है। यदि सभी लड़कियां उत्तर दिशा की ओर मुंह किए बैठी हों तो इनमें से सबसे बाएं छोर पर कौन बैठी है?

(*a*) जया (*b*) मिनी
(*c*) रजनी (*d*) सत्या

3. किट्टू, मोहन और सोहन के बीच बैठा है। राजू, सोहन की बायीं ओर और श्याम, मोहन की दाहिनी ओर बैठा है। यदि ये सभी मित्र दक्षिण दिशा की ओर मुंह करके बैठे हों, तो सबसे दाहिने छोर पर कौन बैठा है?

(*a*) मोहन (*b*) सोहन
(*c*) किट्टू (*d*) श्याम

4. A, B, C, D और E एक दूसरे के पीछे दौड़ रहे हैं। C, E के निकट नहीं है और A, D के निकट नहीं है। B, A के पीछे है और E, D के निकट नहीं है। इनके बीच में कौन व्यक्ति है?

(*a*) B (*b*) E
(*c*) A (*d*) कहा नहीं जा सकता

5. O, P, Q, R, S और T एक बेंच पर अपनी लंबाई के घटते क्रम में खड़े हैं। P, O से अधिक लंबा है किंतु S से उसकी लंबाई कम है। केवल S ही T से अधिक लंबा है। R, P से कम लंबा है किंतु वह Q से अधिक लंबा है। इनमें किसकी लंबाई सबसे कम है?

(*a*) O (*b*) Q
(*c*) P (*d*) कहा नहीं जा सकता

6. छह मित्र एक गोल घेरे में बैठ कर ताश खेल रहे हैं। केनी, डैनी की बायीं ओर बैठा है। माइकल, बॉब और जॉन के बीच बैठा है। रॉजर, केनी और बॉब के बीच बैठा है। माइकल की दाहिनी ओर कौन बैठा है?

(*a*) डैनी (*b*) जॉन
(*c*) केनी (*d*) बॉब

7. चार लड़कियां A, B, C और D एक गोल घेरे में बैठी हैं। B और C का मुंह एक दूसरे की ओर है। निम्नलिखित कथनों में से कौन-सा निश्चित रूप से सत्य है?

(*a*) A, C की बायीं ओर बैठी है
(*b*) D, C की बायीं ओर बैठी है
(*c*) A और D एक दूसरे के आमने-सामने बैठी हैं
(*d*) A, B और C के बीच नहीं बैठी है

8. 10 पुस्तकों के एक ढेर में 3 पुस्तकें इतिहास की, 3 हिंदी की, 2 गणित की और 2 अंग्रेजी की पुस्तकें हैं। यदि ऊपर से देखा जाए तो इतिहास और गणित की एक-एक पुस्तकों के बीच अंग्रेजी की एक पुस्तक है, गणित और अंग्रेजी की एक-एक पुस्तकों के बीच इतिहास की एक पुस्तक है, अंग्रेजी और गणित की एक-एक पुस्तकों के बीच एक हिंदी की पुस्तक है, हिंदी की दो पुस्तकों के बीच गणित की एक पुस्तक है तथा गणित और इतिहास की एक-एक पुस्तकों के बीच हिंदी की दो पुस्तकें हैं। इस ढेर में किस विषय की पुस्तक ऊपर से छठे स्थान पर है?

(*a*) अंग्रेजी (*b*) हिंदी
(*c*) इतिहास (*d*) गणित

9. पांच व्यक्ति A, B, C, D और E एक पंक्ति में आपकी ओर मुंह करके इस प्रकार बैठे हैं कि D, C की बायीं ओर बैठा है और B, E की दाहिनी ओर बैठा है। A, C की दाहिनी ओर बैठा है और B, D की बायीं ओर बैठा है। यदि E कोने में बैठा हो तो बीच में कौन बैठा है?

(*a*) A (*b*) B
(*c*) C (*d*) D

10. छह मित्र A, B, C, D, E और F एक गोल घेरे में खड़े हैं। B, F और C के बीच में है, A, E और D के बीच में है, F, D की बायीं ओर है। A और F के बीच कौन है?

(*a*) C (*b*) B
(*c*) D (*d*) E

निर्देश (प्र.सं. 11–13): *नीचे दिए गए कथन को ध्यानपूर्वक पढ़ें और पूछे गए प्रश्नों के उत्तर दें :*

A, B, C, D और E एक पंक्ति में खड़े हैं। पंक्ति के एक छोर पर D और दूसरे छोर पर C है। B, E की दाहिनी ओर खड़ा है। A, C की बायीं ओर खड़ा है तथा E, D और B के बीच खड़ा है।

11. पंक्ति के बीच में कौन खड़ा है ?
(*a*) E (*b*) D
(*c*) B (*d*) A

12. A निम्नलिखित में से किसके बीच खड़ा है ?
(*a*) B और D (*b*) E और B
(*c*) C और E (*d*) B और C

13. B की दाहिनी ओर कौन खड़ा है ?
(*a*) C (*b*) E
(*c*) A (*d*) D

निर्देश (प्र.सं. 14 और 15): *निम्नलिखित कथनों को सावधानी पूर्वक पढ़ें और पूछे गए प्रश्नों के उत्तर दें :*

एक शेल्फ में पांच कमीजें एक ढेर में एक के ऊपर एक रखी हुई हैं। इस ढेर में लाल कमीज नीली कमीज के ऊपर रखी गई है और हरे रंग की कमीज नारंगी रंग की कमीज के नीचे रखी गई है। नीली कमीज नारंगी रंग की कमीज के ऊपर तथा सफेद कमीज हरी कमीज के नीचे रखी गई है।

14. लाल और नारंगी रंग की कमीजों के बीच रखी कमीज किस रंग की है ?
(*a*) सफेद रंग की (*b*) हरे रंग की
(*c*) नीले रंग की (*d*) आंकड़े अपर्याप्त हैं

15. सबसे नीचे किस रंग की कमीज है ?
(*a*) लाल (*b*) सफेद
(*c*) नारंगी (*d*) कहा नहीं जा सकता

निर्देश (प्र.सं. 16–18): *निम्नलिखित प्रश्नों को ध्यानपूर्वक पढ़ें और पूछे गए प्रश्नों के उत्तर दें :*

(*i*) A, B, C, D और E एक पांच मंजिली इमारत में रहते हैं।
(*ii*) B और E भूतल पर नहीं रहते।
(*iii*) D, A से एक मंजिल ऊपर और C से एक मंजिल नीचे के तल पर रहता है
(*iv*) E सबसे ऊपर वाली मंजिल पर नहीं रहता।

16. D किस मंजिल पर रहता है ?
(*a*) दूसरी (*b*) चौथी
(*c*) पांचवीं (*d*) पहली

17. इनमें से कितने व्यक्ति C से ऊपर वाली मंजिल पर रहते हैं ?
(*a*) 3 (*b*) 2
(*c*) 4 (*d*) 1

18. उपर्युक्त दोनों प्रश्नों का उत्तर ज्ञात करने के लिए दिए गए चार कथनों में से किसे छोड़ा जा सकता है ?
(*a*) केवल (*iv*) (*b*) केवल (*ii*) और (*iii*)
(*c*) कोई नहीं (*d*) केवल (*i*)

निर्देश (प्र.सं. 19 और 20): *निम्नलिखित सूचना को ध्यान से पढ़ें और नीचे पूछे गए प्रश्नों के उत्तर दें :*

(*i*) एक मेज पर एक के ऊपर एक मनोविज्ञान, हिंदी, अंग्रेजी, समाज विज्ञान, अर्थशास्त्र, शिक्षाशास्त्र और लेखाशास्त्र विषयों की सात पुस्तकें रखी हैं।
(*ii*) इनमें समाज विज्ञान की पुस्तक सभी पुस्तकों के ऊपर है।
(*iii*) लेखाशास्त्र की पुस्तक शिक्षाशास्त्र की पुस्तक के ठीक नीचे है जो समाज विज्ञान की पुस्तक के ठीक नीचे रखी गई है।
(*iv*) अर्थशास्त्र की पुस्तक मनोविज्ञान की पुस्तक के ठीक ऊपर किंतु सभी पुस्तकों के बीच में नहीं रखी गई है।
(*v*) हिंदी की पुस्तक मनोविज्ञान की पुस्तक के ठीक नीचे रखी गई है।

19. लेखाशास्त्र और हिंदी की पुस्तकों के बीच किन विषयों की तीन पुस्तकें रखी गई हैं ?
(*a*) अर्थशास्त्र, मनोविज्ञान और हिंदी
(*b*) अर्थशास्त्र, मनोविज्ञान और शिक्षाशास्त्र
(*c*) अंग्रेजी, अर्थशास्त्र और मनोविज्ञान
(*d*) कहा नहीं जा सकता

20. अर्थशास्त्र की पुस्तक निम्नलिखित में से किन पुस्तकों के बीच रखी गई है ?
(*a*) लेखाशास्त्र और शिक्षाशास्त्र
(*b*) मनोविज्ञान और हिंदी
(*c*) अंग्रेजी और मनोविज्ञान
(*d*) कहा नहीं जा सकता

व्याख्यात्मक उत्तर

1. *(b)*: पांचों लड़कों के पंक्ति में बैठने का निम्नलिखित क्रम है:
अमित, श्याम, मयंक, अजय, रघु
या
अजय, रघु, मयंक, अमित, श्याम

2. *(c)*: इन सभी लड़कियों के बैठने का निम्नलिखित क्रम है:
रजनी, मिनी, अनंता, सत्या, जया
या
सत्या, जया, अनंता
या
सत्या, अनंता, जया

3. *(d)*: दक्षिण दिशा की ओर मुंह करके बैठने पर इन मित्रों के बैठने का निम्नलिखित क्रम होगा:
श्याम, मोहन, किट्टू, सोहन, राजू

4. (a): दौड़ते समय ये व्यक्ति निम्नलिखित क्रम में एक दूसरे के पीछे होंगे:

E		E
A		A
B	या	B
C		D
D		C

5. (d): लंबाई के घटते क्रम में ये व्यक्ति बेंच पर निम्नलिखित विन्यास में खड़े होंगे:

S		S
T		T
P	या	P
R		R
O		Q
Q		O

इनमें या तो O या फिर Q सबसे छोटा है। दी गई सूचना उत्तर ज्ञात करने के लिए पर्याप्त नहीं है।

6. (d): इन छह मित्रों के बैठने का निम्नलिखित क्रम है:

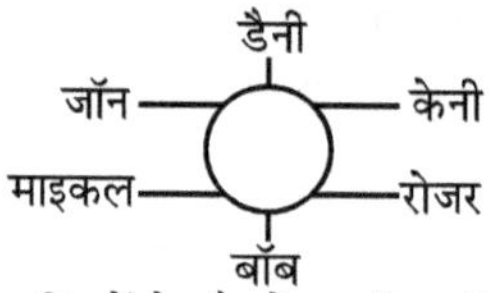

7. (c): इन लड़कियों के बैठने का निम्नलिखित क्रम होगा:

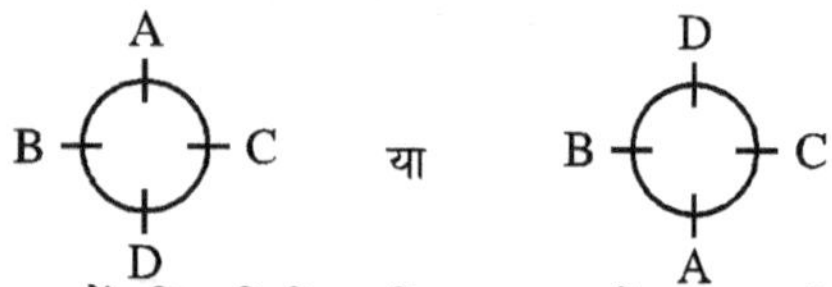

8. (b): पुस्तकें निम्नलिखित विषय-क्रम में एक दूसरे के ऊपर रखी गई हैं:

पहला — इतिहास
अंग्रेजी
गणित
इतिहास
अंग्रेजी
छठा — हिंदी
गणित
हिंदी
हिंदी
दसवां — इतिहास

9. (d): हमारी ओर मुंह किए बैठे इन व्यक्तियों का निम्नलिखित क्रम होगा:
A, C, D, B, E

10. (c): ये मित्र निम्नलिखित क्रम में एक दूसरे की बगल में खड़े हैं

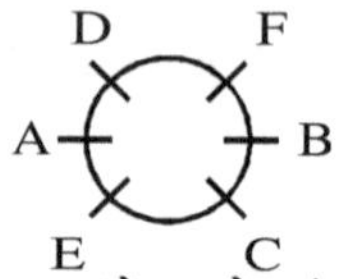

11. (c): प्रश्न संख्या 16 से 18 के संदर्भ में बताए गए पांच व्यक्ति पंक्ति में निम्नलिखित क्रम में खड़े हैं:
D, E, B, A, C.

12. (d) **13. (c)**

14. (c): प्रश्न संख्या 14 और 15 के संदर्भ में शेल्फ में कमीजों को निम्नलिखित क्रम में रखा गया है:

लाल कमीज
नीली कमीज
नारंगी रंग की कमीज
हरे रंग की कमीज
सफेद कमीज

15. (b)

प्रश्न संख्या 16 से 18 के संदर्भ में दी गई सूचना के अनुसार पांच मंजिली इमारत में A, B, C, D और E निम्नलिखित क्रम में रहते हैं:

B
E
C
D
A – भूतल

16. (d) **17. (b)** **18. (c)**

19. (c): पुस्तकें निम्नलिखित क्रम में एक दूसरे के ऊपर रखी गई हैं:

समाज विज्ञान
शिक्षाशास्त्र
लेखाशास्त्र
अंग्रेजी
अर्थशास्त्र
मनोविज्ञान
हिंदी

20. (c)

प्रश्न संख्या 21 से 25 के संदर्भ में दिए गए कथनों के अनुसार आवंटित किए गए फ्लैटों की अवस्थिति निम्नवत् है:

Q	T	S	↑N	इनका मुख्य दरवाजा उत्तर दिशा में खुलता है
U	R	P	↓S	इनका मुख्य दरवाजा दक्षिण दिशा में खुलता है

दिशा ज्ञान परीक्षण
(DIRECTION SENSE)

इस प्रकार के प्रश्न अभ्यर्थियों की सही दिशा-निर्देशों को समझने की योग्यता की जांच करने हेतु पूछे जाते हैं। ऐसे प्रश्न दिशा-चार्ट पर आधारित होते हैं:

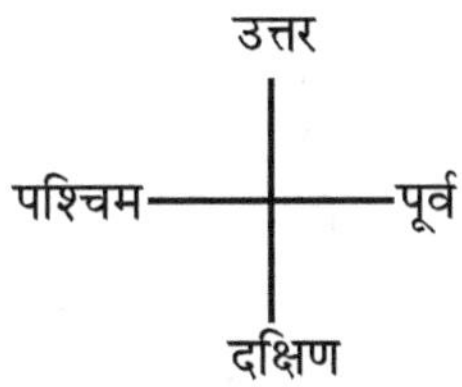

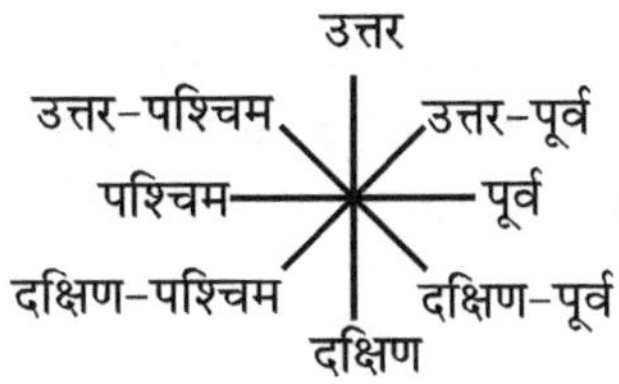

विभिन्न दिशाओं का बोध बाएं या दाएं मोड़ या कोणीय मोड़ों द्वारा निर्देशित होता है।

हल किए गए उदाहरण

1. एक व्यक्ति उत्तर दिशा में चल रहा है। वह दो बार दाहिने मुड़ता है और फिर चलने लगता है अब वह किस दिशा में चल रहा है?

(*a*) उत्तर (*b*) दक्षिण (*c*) पूर्व (*d*) पश्चिम

उत्तर *(b)*:

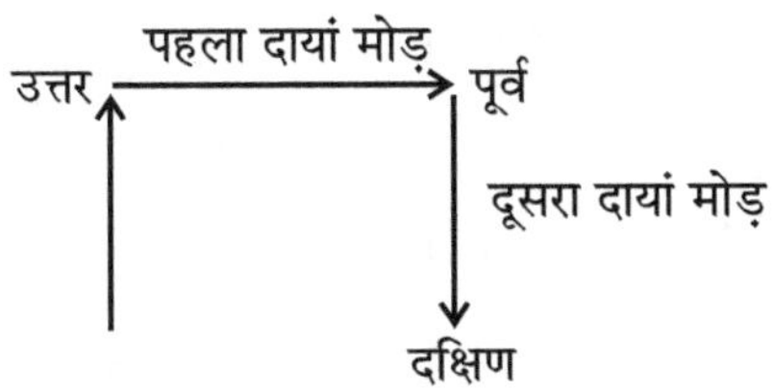

दिशा चार्ट का अनुसरण करने पर यह स्पष्ट होता है कि वह व्यक्ति अब दक्षिण दिशा में चल रहा है।

2. एक व्यक्ति पूर्व दिशा में चल रहा है। वह पहले 45° बाएं और तब 90° दाएं मुड़ता है। अब वह किस दिशा में चल रहा है?

(*a*) उत्तर (*b*) उत्तर-पश्चिम (*c*) ***दक्षिण***-पूर्व (*d*) पश्चिम

उत्तर *(c)* : 45° मोड़ का अर्थ है, सीधी दिशा न होकर दो दिशाओं के बीच में जाना। 90° मोड़ में भी दो दिशाएं शामिल हैं और व्यक्ति उत्तर-पूर्व में न जाकर **दक्षिण**-पूर्व दिशा में जाने लगता है।

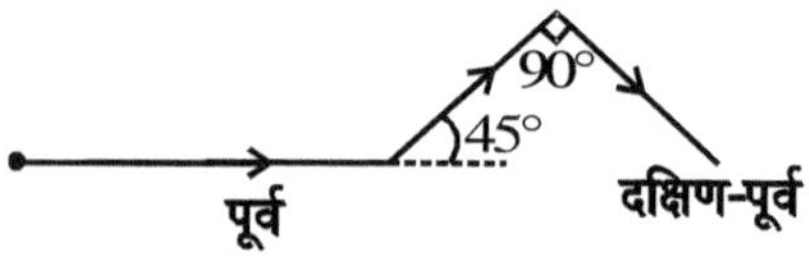

एक दिशा को छोड़कर दूसरी दिशा में जाने पर व्यक्ति किस दिशा में गति कर रहा है, इसे जानने के लिए सही दिशा-निर्देशों को समझने की आवश्यकता है। साथ ही अभ्यर्थियों को कागज पर दिशा की जानकारी होना भी आवश्यक है। दिशा चार्ट की सहायता से दूरियों को भी सरलतापूर्वक मापा जा सकता है।

अभ्यास

निर्देश (प्र.सं. 1–12): *नीचे के प्रत्येक प्रश्न में सही दिशा/दूरी दर्शाने के लिए दिए गए विकल्पों से सही उत्तर का चयन करें।*

1. किट्टू पहले पूर्व दिशा में चलता है और तब दक्षिण दिशा में चलता है। दक्षिण दिशा में कुछ दूरी तय करने के बाद वह पश्चिम दिशा में मुड़ जाता है और तब अपने बाएं मुड़ जाता है। अब वह किस दिशा में चल रहा है?

(*a*) उत्तर (*b*) दक्षिण
(*c*) पूर्व (*d*) पश्चिम

2. एक व्यक्ति पश्चिम दिशा में अपनी गाड़ी चला रहा है। वह दक्षिण दिशा में चले इसके लिए उसे निम्नलिखित में से कौन से मोड़ मुड़ने चाहिए?

(*a*) बायीं ओर, दायीं ओर, दायीं ओर
(*b*) दायीं ओर, दायीं ओर, बायीं ओर
(*c*) बायीं ओर, बायीं ओर, बायीं ओर
(*d*) दायीं ओर, दायीं ओर, दायीं ओर

3. ऋचा अपनी गाड़ी से दक्षिण दिशा में 8 किमी आगे चलकर बायीं ओर मुड़ जाती है और 5 किमी. आगे चलती है। वहां वह एक बार फिर से बायीं ओर मुड़कर 8 किमी. आगे चलती है। अब वह अपने शुरु के स्थान से कितनी दूरी पर है?

(*a*) 3 किमी.
(*b*) 5 किमी.
(*c*) 8 किमी.
(*d*) 13 किमी.

4. डिंगी अपनी गाड़ी से उत्तर की ओर 40 किमी. की दूरी तय करती है, वहां वह दायीं ओर मुड़कर 50 किमी आगे जाती है जहां वह एक बार फिर से दायीं ओर मुड़कर 30 किमी. आगे जाती है, और तब फिर से दायीं ओर मुड़कर 50 किमी. और आगे जाती है। यहां वह अपने आरंभिक बिंदु से कितनी दूरी पर है?

(*a*) 90 किमी.
(*b*) 50 किमी.
(*c*) 10 किमी.
(*d*) 5 किमी.

5. देबू पहले पूर्व की ओर और तब उत्तर की ओर चलता है तथा वहां वह 45° दायें मुड़कर कुछ देर आगे चलता है और अंततः बायीं ओर मुड़ जाता है। अब वह किस दिशा में चल रहा है?

(*a*) उत्तर
(*b*) पूर्व
(*c*) दक्षिण-पूर्व
(*d*) उत्तर-पश्चिम

6. यदि उत्तर का उत्तर-पश्चिम, उत्तर-पश्चिम का पश्चिम, पश्चिम का दक्षिण-पश्चिम और इसी प्रकार अन्य दिशाओं का भी नामकरण किया जाए तो दक्षिण पूर्व को क्या कहा जाएगा?

(*a*) पूर्व (*b*) पश्चिम
(*c*) उत्तर-पूर्व (*d*) दक्षिण-पूर्व

7. मैं अपने घर से उत्तर दिशा में 15 मीटर चला, तब पश्चिम दिशा में मुड़कर 10 मीटर और आगे चला, यहां दक्षिण दिशा में मुड़कर मैंने 5 मीटर की एक अन्य दूरी तय की और तब पूर्व की ओर मुड़कर 10 मीटर की दूरी तय की। बताइए कि मैं अपने आरंभिक स्थान से किस दिशा में हूँ?

(*a*) पूर्व (*b*) पश्चिम
(*c*) उत्तर (*d*) दक्षिण

8. मैं अपने घर से उत्तर दिशा में चला और तब बायीं ओर मुड़ गया। अब कुछ देर तक आगे चलने के बाद मैं फिर से बायीं ओर मुड़ा और तब दायीं ओर मुड़ गया। बाद में आगे चलते हुए मैं बायीं ओर और एक बार फिर से बायीं ओर मुड़ा। बताइए कि अब मैं किस दिशा में चल रहा हूँ?

(*a*) उत्तर (*b*) दक्षिण
(*c*) पूर्व (*d*) पश्चिम

9. राज पश्चिम दिशा में चल रहा है। वह आगे चलते हुए अपने दाएं, फिर दाएं और तब बाएं, हर बार 135° के कोण पर मुड़ा। बताइए कि अब वह किस दिशा में चल रहा है?

(*a*) उत्तर-पूर्व (*b*) दक्षिण-पूर्व
(*c*) पूर्व (*d*) पश्चिम

10. जतिन अपने घर से उत्तर दिशा में 12 किमी. चलता है। तब वह अपनी दायीं ओर मुड़कर 12 किमी. की एक अन्य दूरी तय करता है। वह एक बार फिर से दायीं ओर मुड़ता है और 12 किमी. की एक अन्य दूरी तय करके बायीं ओर मुड़ता है ओर तब 5 किमी. आगे चलता है। बताइए कि इस समय वह अपने घर से कितनी दूरी पर है और किस दिशा में है?

(*a*) 7 किमी., पूर्व दिशा
(*b*) 10 किमी., पूर्व दिशा
(*c*) 17 किमी., पूर्व दिशा
(*d*) 24 किमी., पूर्व दिशा

11. एक महिला उत्तर दिशा में 12 किमी. चलती है, तब वह दक्षिण दिशा में 6 किमी. चलती है और तत्पश्चात् पूर्व दिशा में 8 किमी चलती है। इस समय वह अपने आरंभिक बिंदु से कितनी दूरी पर है और किस दिशा में चल रही है?

(*a*) 5 किमी., उत्तर-पूर्व (*b*) 5 किमी., पूर्व
(*c*) 10 किमी., उत्तर-पूर्व (*d*) 10 किमी., पश्चिम

12. दिव्या पूर्व दिशा में 10 किमी. की यात्रा करती है, और तब दक्षिण-पश्चिम दिशा में 10 किमी. की यात्रा करती है। वह एक बार फिर से मुड़कर उत्तर-पश्चिम दिशा में 10 किमी. चलती है। बताइए कि अब वह अपने आरंभिक बिंदु से किस दिशा में चल रही है?

(*a*) दक्षिण (*b*) उत्तर
(*c*) पश्चिम (*d*) पूर्व

व्याख्यात्मक उत्तर

1. (*b*)

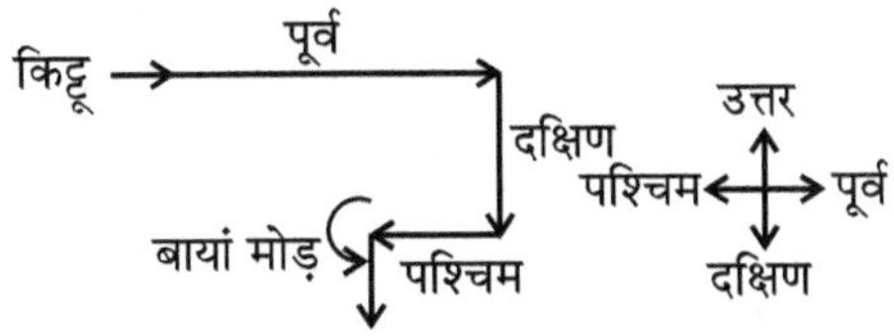

2. (*d*):

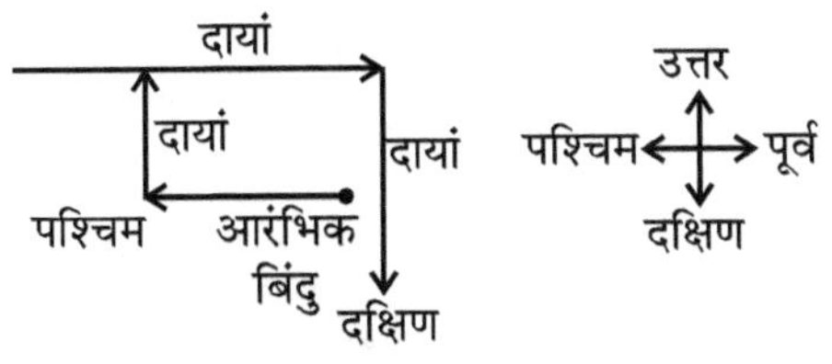

3. (*b*):

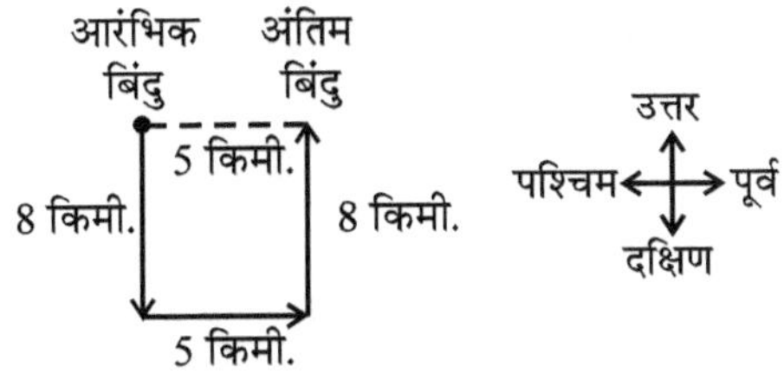

4. (*c*):

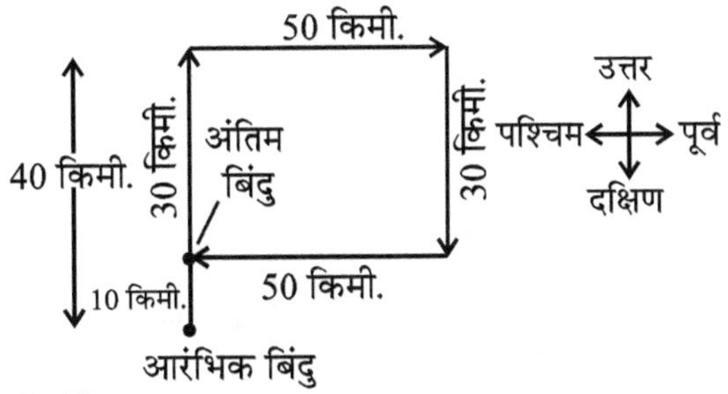

5. (*d*):

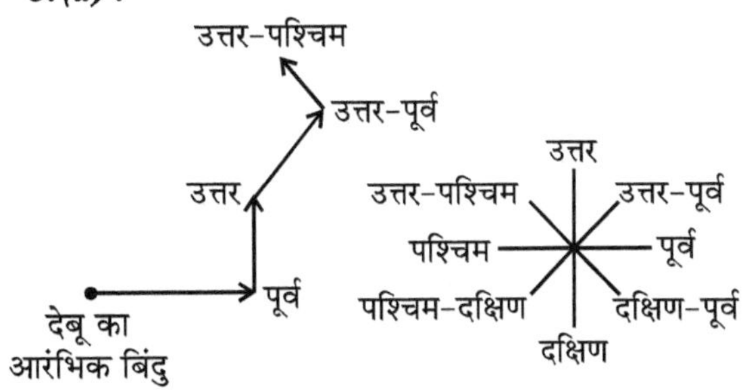

6. *(a)*:

मूल दिशाएं

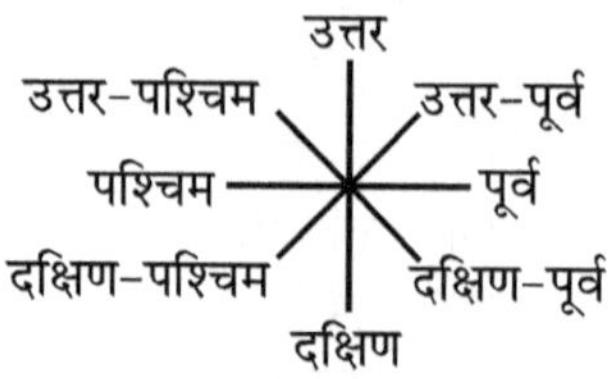

बदली हुई दिशाएं

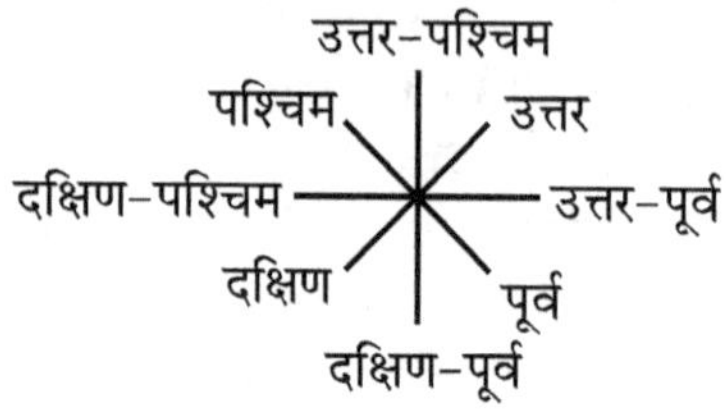

7. *(c)*:

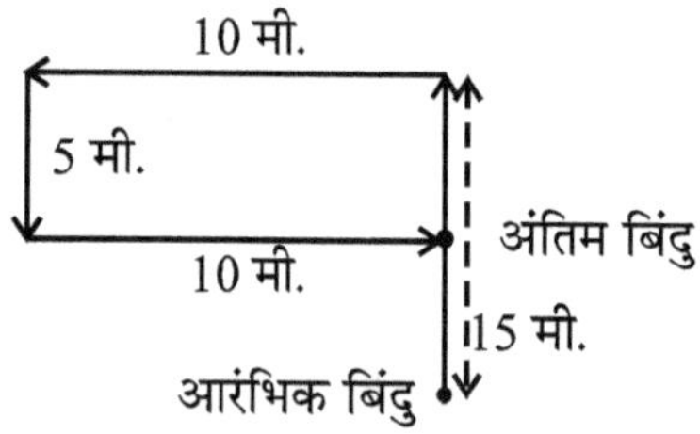

अंतिम बिंदु आरंभिक बिंदु से 10 मीटर उत्तर की ओर है।

8. *(c)*:

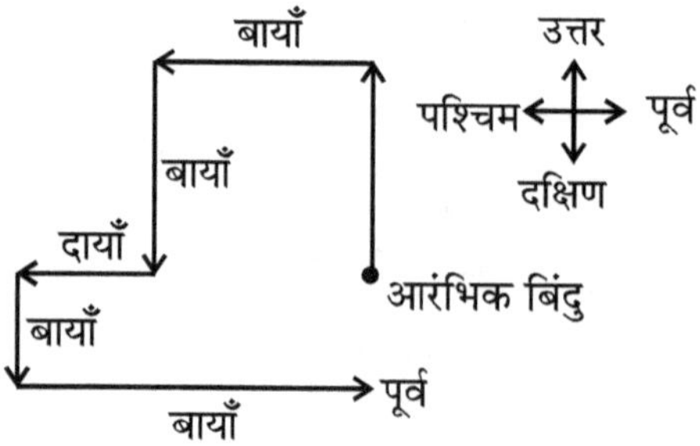

9. *(a)*:

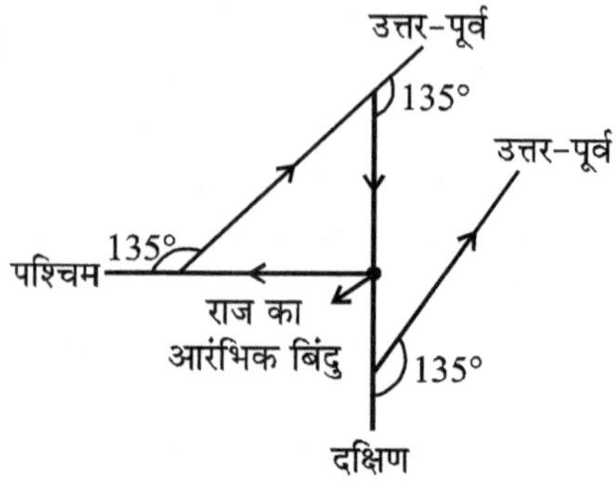

10. *(c)*: (12 किमी. + 5 किमी. = 17 किमी.)

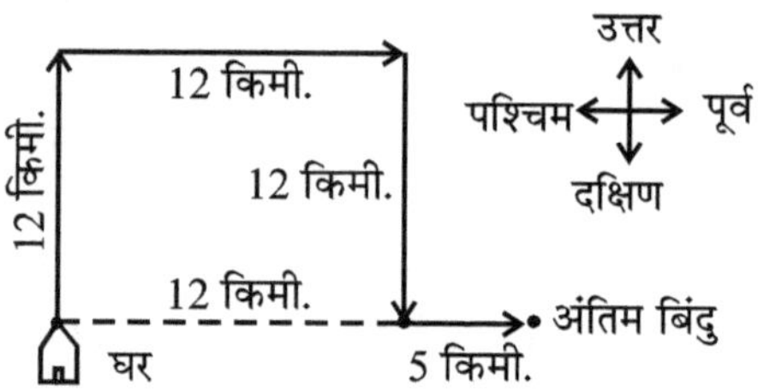

11. *(c)*: $ab = \sqrt{ac^2 + bc^2}$

$ab = \sqrt{8^2 + 6^2} = \sqrt{64 + 36} = \sqrt{100} = 10$

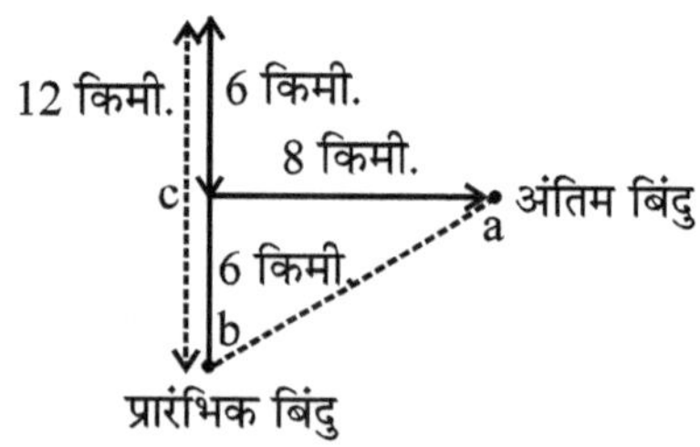

12. *(c)*:

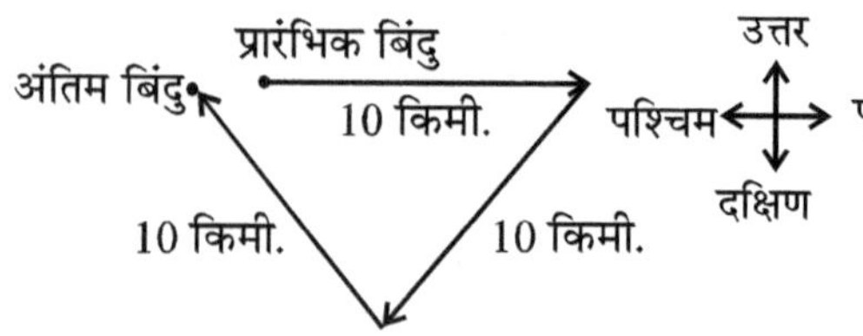

रक्त संबंधी परीक्षण
(BLOOD RELATIONSHIPS)

रक्त संबंधों पर आधारित प्रश्नों को हल करने के लिए यह आवश्यक है कि परीक्षार्थी रिश्तों की जटिलता को तत्काल समझ सकें और किन्हीं दो व्यक्तियों के बीच किस प्रकार के संबंध हो सकते हैं, इस बारे में उन्हें स्पष्ट जानकारी हो। इस प्रकार के प्रश्नों को पूछने का अभिप्राय मुख्यत: यह सुनिश्चित करना है कि परीक्षार्थी कतिपय जटिल भाषा में व्यक्त रिश्तों को कितनी तत्परता से समझ सकते हैं और उत्तर के रूप में सही विकल्प का चयन कर सकते हैं।

इन प्रश्नों को हल करने में सहायक कुछ संबंधों के पैटर्न नीचे दर्शाए गए हैं :

पिता का पिता	—	दादा
मां का पिता	—	नाना
पिता की मां	—	दादी
मां की मां	—	नानी
पिता या मां का पुत्र	—	भाई
पिता या मां की पुत्री	—	बहन
पिता का भाई	—	चाचा
पिता की बहन	—	बुआ
मां का भाई	—	मामा
मां की बहन	—	मौसी
चाचा या चाची का पुत्र या पुत्री	—	चचेरा भाई, चचेरी बहन
पुत्र की पत्नी	—	पुत्रवधु
पुत्री का पति	—	दामाद
पति का भाई	—	देवर
पत्नी का भाई	—	साला
पति की बहन	—	ननद
पत्नी की बहन	—	साली
भाई की पत्नी	—	भाभी
बहन का पति	—	बहनोई
भाई का पुत्र	—	भतीजा
भाई की पुत्री	—	भतीजी

हल किए गए उदाहरण

1. एक फोटो की ओर संकेत करते हुए एक महिला ने कहा ''इस व्यक्ति के पुत्र की बहन मेरी सास है''। उस महिला के पति का उस व्यक्ति से क्या संबंध है जिसका वह फोटो है?

(*a*) पुत्र (*b*) नाती (*c*) भतीजा (*d*) दामाद

उत्तर (*b*) : दिए गए प्रश्न के अनुसार संबंध चार्ट निम्नवत् दर्शाया जा सकता है :

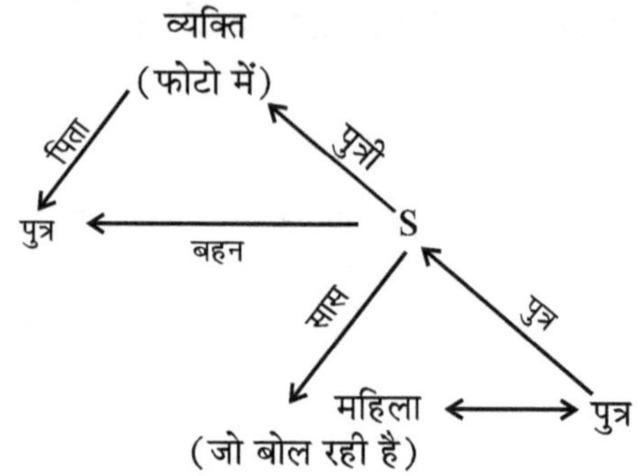

उस व्यक्ति के पुत्र की बहन (मान लें S) उस व्यक्ति की पुत्री है। यदि यह महिला 'S' उस महिला (जो बोल रही है) की सास है तो उसका विवाह 'S' के पुत्र से हुआ है। उस महिला के पति की मां S है और S फोटो वाले व्यक्ति की पुत्री है। अत: उस बोल रही महिला का पति फोटो वाले व्यक्ति का नाती है।

2. 'X', 'Y' की पत्नी है और 'Y', 'Z' का भाई है। 'Z', 'P' का पुत्र है। 'P' का 'X' से क्या संबंध है?

(*a*) बहन (*b*) चाची (*c*) भाई (*d*) श्वसुर

उत्तर (*d*) : दिए गए प्रश्न के अनुसार संबंध चार्ट निम्नवत् दर्शाया जा सकता है :

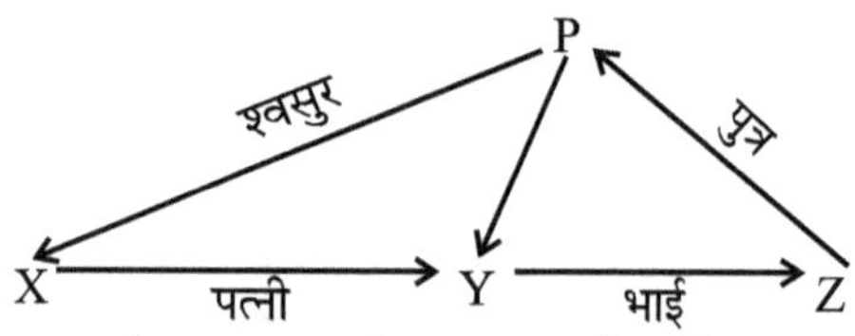

'Y', 'Z' का भाई है जो 'P' का पुत्र है। अत: 'Z' भी 'P' का पुत्र है। चूंकि 'P', 'Y' का पिता है और 'X', 'Y' की पत्नी है अत: 'P', 'X' का श्वसुर है।

अभ्यास

निर्देश (प्र.सं. 1–10): *नीचे के प्रत्येक प्रश्न में व्यक्तियों के बीच उल्लिखित संबंधों को सावधानीपूर्वक समझें और तब दिए गए विकल्पों में से सही उत्तर का चयन करें :*

1. A, B और C का पिता है। B, A का पुत्र है किंतु C, A का पुत्र नहीं है। C का A से क्या संबंध है?

(*a*) पुत्री (*b*) पुत्र

(*c*) भतीजी (*d*) भतीजा

2. एक महिला ने कहा, ''वहां खड़ी लड़की मेरे दादा जी के एकमात्र पुत्र की पुत्री है''। उस महिला का उस लड़की से क्या संबंध है?

(*a*) बहन (*b*) मां

(*c*) चाची (*d*) भतीजा

3. रवि अमित के पुत्र के पुत्र का भाई है। अमित, रवि का क्या है?

(*a*) चचेरा भाई (*b*) पिता

(*c*) दादा (*d*) पुत्र

4. मयंक ने कहा, ''मेरी मां रजत के भाई की बहन है''। रजत का मयंक से क्या संबंध है?

(*a*) चचेरा भाई (*b*) मामा

(*c*) चाचा (*d*) साला

5. लिली से परिचय कराते हुए राघव ने कहा, ''इसके पिता मेरी मां के एकमात्र पुत्र हैं''। लिली का राघव से क्या संबंध है?

(*a*) चाची (*b*) पुत्री

(*c*) मां (*d*) बहन

6. अजय, विजय का भाई है। शुभा, अजय की बहन है। संजय, राहुल का भाई है और मेहुल विजय की पुत्री है। संजय का चाचा कौन है?

(*a*) राहुल

(*b*) अजय

(*c*) मेहुल

(*d*) दी गई सूचना अपर्याप्त है

7. आदित्य, रवि का भाई है। भरत, जयंत के पिता हैं। ईला, रवि की मां है। आदित्य और जयंत आपस में भाई हैं। ईला का भरत से क्या संबंध है?

(*a*) बहन (*b*) मां

(*c*) पुत्री (*d*) पत्नी

8. एक व्यक्ति ने अपने साथ आ रहे लड़के का परिचय देते हुए कहा, ''यह मेरी पत्नी की पुत्री के पिता का पुत्र है।'' वह लड़का उस व्यक्ति का क्या है?

(*a*) दामाद (*b*) पुत्र

(*c*) भाई (*d*) पिता

9. A और B दो भाई हैं। C, B की बहन है। D, E की बहन है। E, A का पुत्र है। D का चाचा कौन है?

(*a*) D (*b*) E

(*c*) B (*d*) C

10. वरुण ने अरुण की ओर संकेत करते हुए कहा, ''वह मेरी बहन के एकमात्र भाई का पुत्र है।'' अरुण का वरूण से क्या संबंध है?

(*a*) पुत्र

(*b*) भाई

(*c*) भतीजा

(*d*) दी गई सूचना अपर्याप्त है

व्याख्यात्मक उत्तर

1. (*a*) :

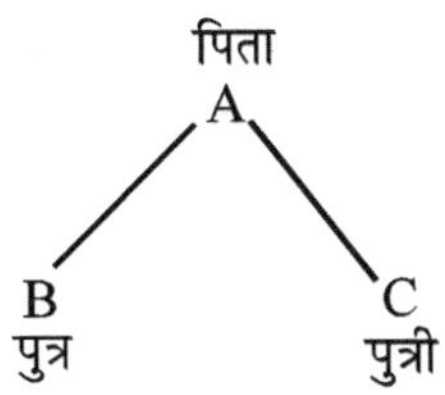

C, A का पुत्र नहीं है किंतु A, C का पिता है। अत: C, A की पुत्री है।

2. (*a*) :

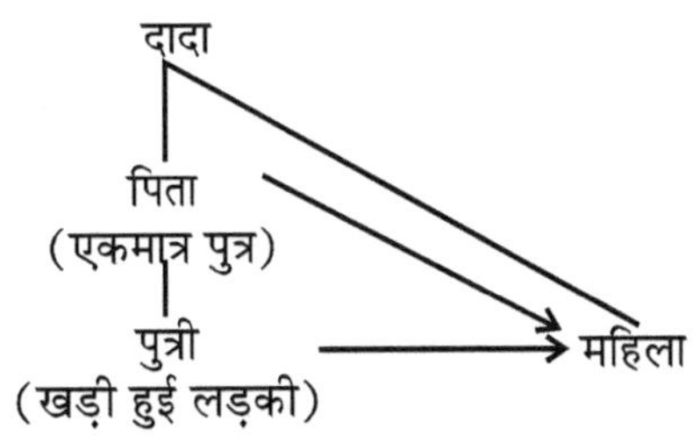

उस महिला के दादा का पुत्र उसके पिता हैं तथा पिता की पुत्री निश्चित ही उस महिला की बहन होगी।

3. (*c*) :

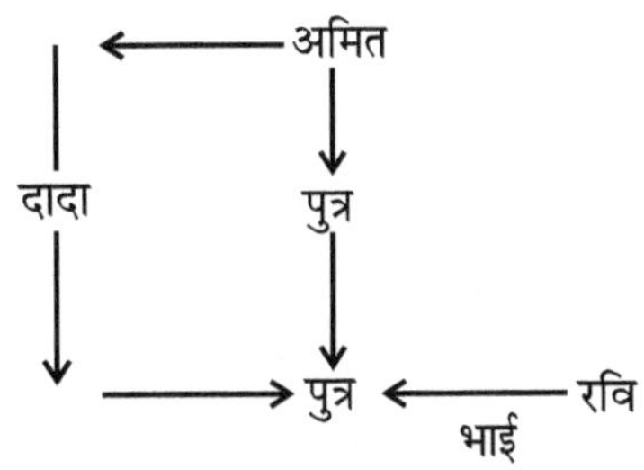

अमित के पुत्र का पुत्र अमित का पोता होगा। रवि अमित के पुत्र के पुत्र का भाई है, अत: अमित रवि के भी दादाजी हैं।

4. (*b*) :

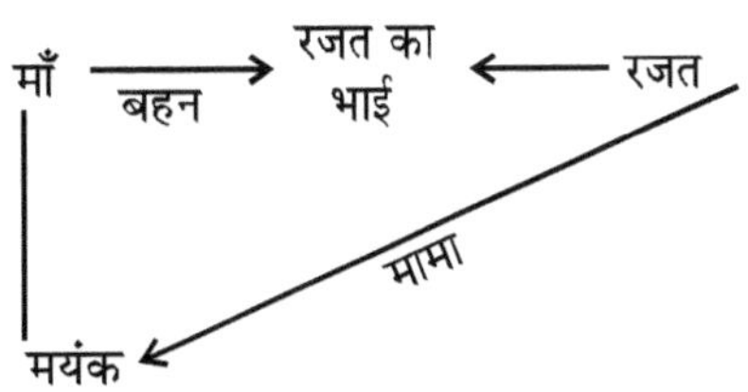

मयंक की मां रजत के भाई की बहन है। अतः रजत भी मयंक की मां का भाई है। इस प्रकार रजत, मयंक का मामा हुआ।

5. (*b*) : संबंध चार्ट निम्नवत् है : माँ

↑ पुत्र

राघव

↓ पिता

लिली (पुत्री)

राघव जब कहता है, ''मेरी मां का एकमात्र पुत्र'' तो वह स्वयं अपने बारे में ही कह रहा होता है। इसके पिता का आशय है, 'लिली के पिता' अर्थात् स्वयं राघव। अतः लिली, राघव की पुत्री है।

6. (*d*) : 1. शुभा ⟶ अजय ⟶ विजय ↓ मेहुल (पुत्री)

2. संजय ⟶ राहुल (भाई)

यहां दो संबंध-समुच्चयों का उल्लेख किया गया है। दी गई सूचना अपर्याप्त है और इन दो भिन्न संबंध-समुच्चयों के बीच कोई संबंध स्थापित नहीं किया जा सकता।

7. (*d*) : प्रश्न पर आधारित संबंध चार्ट है :

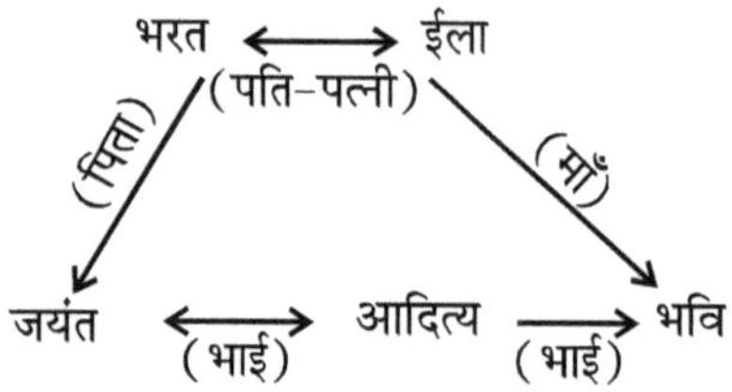

जयंत और आदित्य भाई हैं। यदि आदित्य, रवि का भाई है तो जयंत भी रवि का भाई है। यदि भरत, जयंत का पिता है तो वह आदित्य और रवि का भी पिता है। यदि ईला, रवि की मां है तो वह आदित्य और जयंत की भी मां है। इसका अर्थ है कि भरत और ईला पति-पत्नी हैं और तीनों बच्चों के माता-पिता हैं।

8. (*b*) : प्रश्न पर आधारित संबंध-चार्ट है :

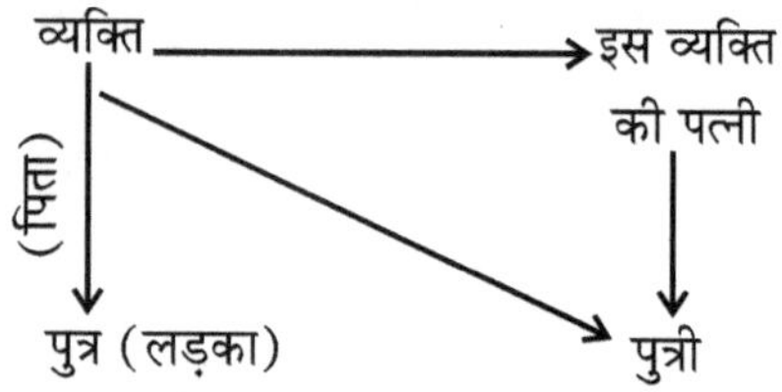

'उस व्यक्ति की पत्नी की पुत्री के पिता' का आशय है कि वह व्यक्ति स्वयं अपने बारे में बात कर रहा है, अतः वह लड़का उस व्यक्ति का पुत्र है।

9. (*c*) : प्रश्न पर आधारित संबंध-चार्ट है :

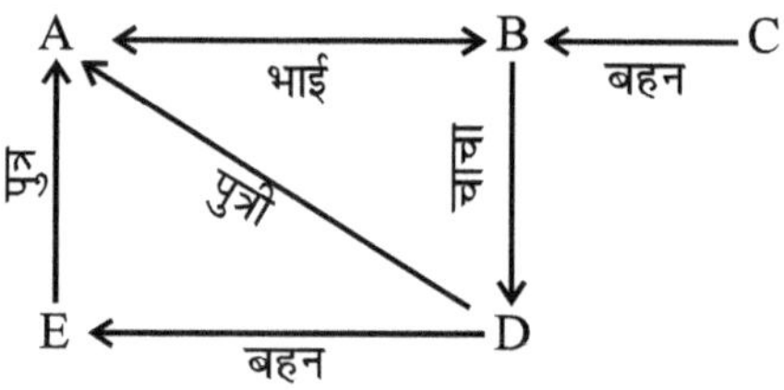

D, E की बहन है और E, A का पुत्र है। अतः D, A की पुत्री है। चूंकि A का भाई B है, अतः B, D का चाचा है।

10. (*a*) :

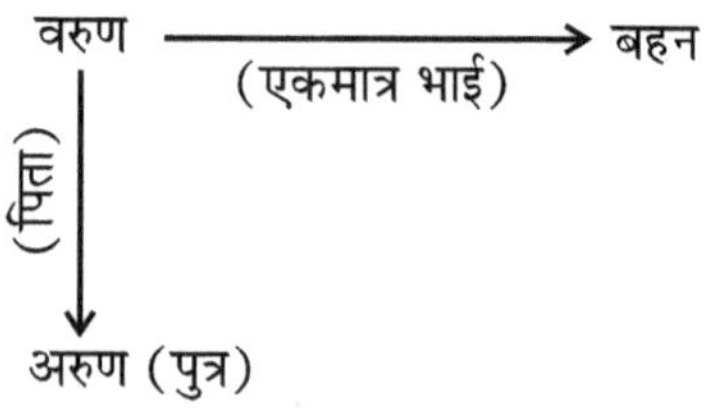

वरुण की बहन का एकमात्र भाई स्वयं वरुण है और उसका पुत्र अरुण है।

क्रम व्यवस्था और काल परीक्षण

(ROWS AND RANKS)

इस प्रकार के प्रश्न किसी पंक्ति या लाइन में व्यवस्थित वस्तुओं की संख्या या कुछ छात्रों की एक कक्षा में किसी छात्र के क्रम-स्थान (कोटि) या कक्षा में छात्रों की कुल संख्या ज्ञात करने के लिए कतिपय सरल गणितीय परिकलनों पर आधारित होते हैं।

हल किए गए उदाहरण

1. पेड़ों की किसी पंक्ति में कोई एक पेड़ किसी एक सिरे से आठवें और दूसरे सिरे से तीसरे स्थान पर है। बताइए कि इस पंक्ति में कुल कितने पेड़ हैं?

(*a*) 11 (*b*) 9 (*c*) 10 (*d*) 12

उत्तर (*c*) : इस पंक्ति में पेड़ों की संख्या

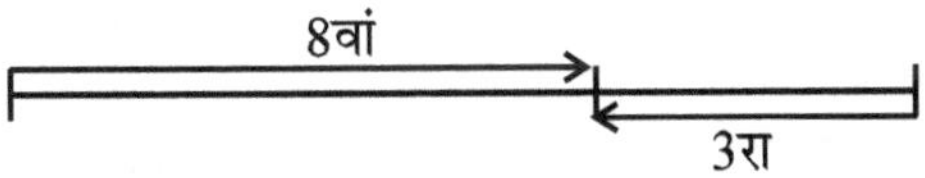

$(8 + 3) - 1 = 10$

2. यदि किसी कक्षा में योग्यता-क्रम में जानकी, पल्लवी से 12 स्थान आगे है और पल्लवी का कक्षा में 15वां स्थान है तथा जानकी का कक्षा में योग्यता-क्रम में चौथा स्थान है तो बताइए कि इस कक्षा में कुल कितने छात्र हैं?

(*a*) 23 (*b*) 27 (*c*) 31 (*d*) 33

उत्तर (*c*) : परिकलन करने पर निम्नलिखित उत्तर प्राप्त होता है :

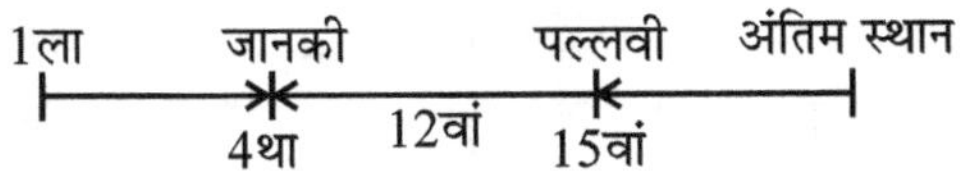

कक्षा में छात्रों की कुल संख्या $= 4 + 12 + 15 = 31$

अभ्यास

1. पेड़ों की एक पंक्ति में कोई एक पेड़ पंक्ति के दोनों छोरों से पांचवें स्थान पर है। इस पंक्ति में कुल कितने पेड़ हैं?

(*a*) 11 (*b*) 8
(*c*) 10 (*d*) 9

2. 53 छात्रों की एक कक्षा में जया का योग्यता-क्रम में 5 वां स्थान है। कक्षा में योग्यता-क्रम में नीचे से उसका क्रम-स्थान क्या है?

(*a*) 49 वां (*b*) 48 वां
(*c*) 47 वां (*d*) 50 वां

3. पैंसठ छात्रों की एक कक्षा में योग्यता-क्रम में मोहन का क्रम स्थान इक्कीसवां है। यदि योग्यता-क्रम में सबसे नीचे के छात्र का क्रम-स्थान 1 माना जाए तो योग्यता-क्रम में नीचे से मोहन का क्रम-स्थान क्या होगा?

(*a*) 44 वां
(*b*) 45 वां
(*c*) 46 वां
(*d*) दी गई सूचना अपर्याप्त है

4. लड़कों की एक पंक्ति में राहुल दाहिने से 12 वें स्थान पर और बाएं से चौथे स्थान पर खड़ा है। इस पंक्ति में और कितने लड़कों को शामिल करने पर पंक्ति में लड़कों की कुल संख्या 28 हो जाएगी?

(*a*) 12 (*b*) 14
(*c*) 20 (*d*) 13

5. लड़कों की एक पंक्ति में राजन दाहिने से दसवें स्थान पर है और सूरज बाएं से दसवें स्थान पर है। यदि राजन और सूरज आपस में अपना स्थान बदल लें तो सूरज बाएं से सताइसवें स्थान पर आ जाएगा। राजन अब पंक्ति में दाहिने से कितने स्थान पर खड़ा है?

(*a*) दसवें (*b*) छब्बीसवें
(*c*) उन्तीसवें (*d*) **सताइसवें**

6. 41 छात्रों की एक कक्षा में महेश और सुरेश योग्यता-क्रम में ऊपर से क्रमशः 11 वें और 12 वें स्थान पर हैं। योग्यता-क्रम में नीचे से इनका क्रम-स्थान क्या है?

(*a*) 32 वां और 33 वां (*b*) 29 वां और 30 वां
(*c*) 30 वां और 31 वां (*d*) 31 वां और 30 वां

7. किसी कक्षा में उमा योग्यता-क्रम में ऊपर से 8 वें और नीचे से 37 वें स्थान पर है। इस कक्षा में कुल कितने छात्र हैं?

(*a*) 47 (*b*) 46
(*c*) 45 (*d*) 44

8. एक पंक्ति में सादिक सामने से 14 वें स्थान पर और जोसफ अंत से 17 वें स्थान पर खड़ा है जबकि जेन, सादिक और जोसफ के बीच खड़ा है। यदि सादिक, जोसफ से आगे खड़ा है और पंक्ति में कुल 48 व्यक्ति खड़ें हो, तो सादिक और जेन के बीच पंक्ति में कितने व्यक्ति खड़े हैं?

(*a*) 5 (*b*) 6
(*c*) 7 (*d*) 8

9. किसी कक्षा में वार्षिक परीक्षा में उत्तीर्ण हुए छात्रों में योग्यता-क्रम में रोहन नीचे से सताइसवें स्थान पर और ऊपर से ग्यारहवें स्थान पर आया। यदि वार्षिक परीक्षा में इस कक्षा के 12 छात्र अनुत्तीर्ण घोषित किए गए हों तो परीक्षा में इस कक्षा के कितने छात्र शामिल हुए थे?

(*a*) 48 (*b*) 49
(*c*) 50 (*d*) कहा नहीं जा सकता

10. कुछ लड़के एक पंक्ति में बैठे हैं। P पंक्ति में बाएं से चौदहवें स्थान पर और Q दाहिने से सातवें स्थान पर बैठा है। यदि P और Q के बीच चार लड़के बैठे हों, तो इस पंक्ति में कुल कितने लड़के हैं?

(*a*) 19 (*b*) 21
(*c*) 25 (*d*) 23

11. एक पंक्ति में A, B, C, D और E कुल पांच मकान बने हैं। A, B की दाहिनी ओर, E, C की बायीं ओर और A की दाहिनी ओर अवस्थित है तथा B, D की दाहिनी ओर अवस्थित है। इनमें से कौन-सा मकान बीच में है?

(*a*) B (*b*) A
(*c*) D (*d*) E

12. इकतीस छात्रों की एक कक्षा में योग्यता-क्रम में माधव का स्थान सतरहवां है। योग्यता-क्रम में नीचे से उसका स्थान कितना है?

(*a*) 13 (*b*) 14
(*c*) 15 (*d*) 16

व्याख्यात्मक उत्तर

1. (*d*):

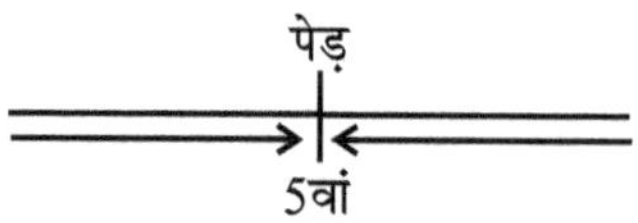

पंक्ति में पेड़ों की कुल संख्या
= (5 + 5) −1 = 9

2. (*a*) :

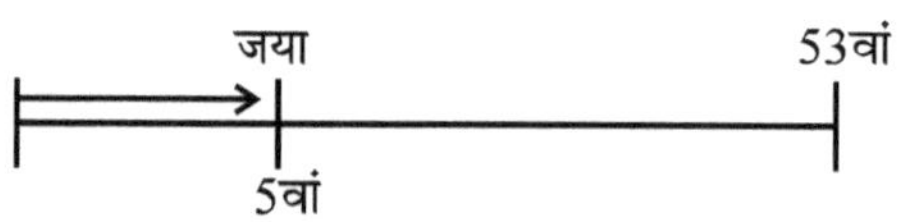

योग्यता-क्रम में नीचे से जया का स्थान
= (53 − 5) +1 = 49 वां

3. (*b*) : 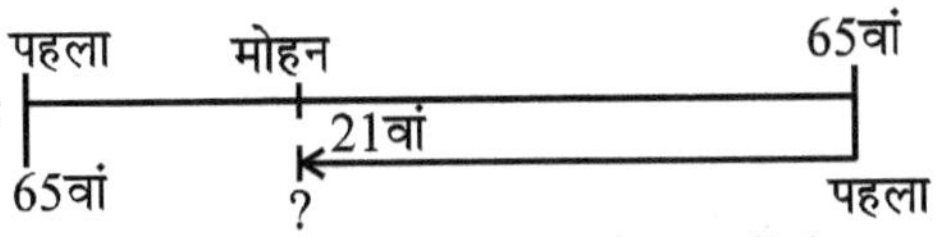

टिप्पणी : प्रश्न पूछने का अभिप्राय है कक्षा में योग्यता-क्रम में नीचे से मोहन का स्थान जानना।

मोहन का स्थान है = (65 – 21) +1 = 45 वां

4. (*d*) : 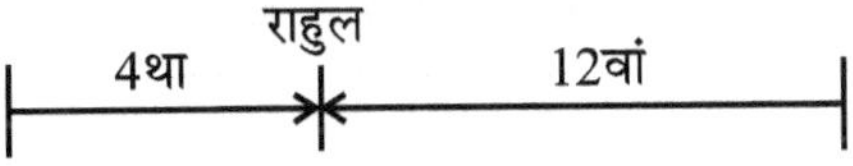

पंक्ति में लड़कों की कुल संख्या :
(4 + 12) – 1 = 15
पंक्ति में लड़कों की कुल संख्या 28 करने के लिए इसमें (28 –15) अर्थात् 13 लड़कों को शामिल करने की आवश्यकता है।

5. (*d*) : 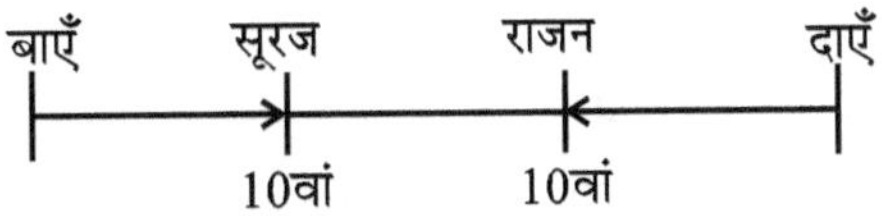

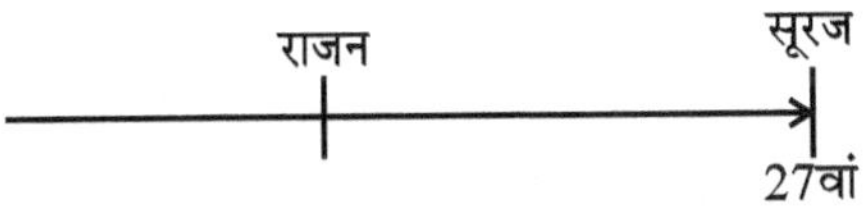

चूंकि लड़कों का क्रम-स्थान दोनों छोरों से समान है, अत: स्थान बदलने के बाद राजन का क्रम स्थान दाहिने से 27 वां होगा।

6. (*d*) : 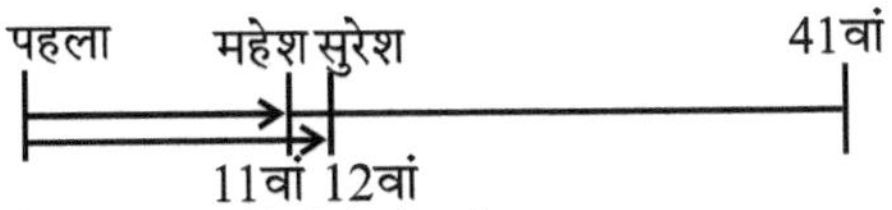

योग्यता-क्रम में नीचे से महेश का स्थान
= (41 – 11) + 1 = 31 वां
योग्यता-क्रम में नीचे से सुरेश का स्थान
= (41 – 12) +1 = 30 वां

7. (*d*) : 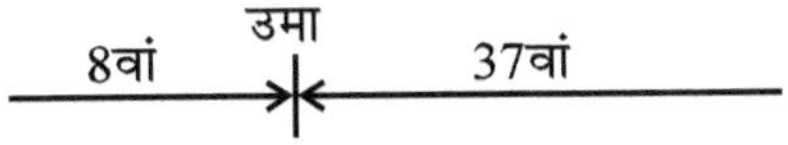

कक्षा में छात्रों की कुल संख्या
= (8 + 37) – 1 = 44

8. (*d*) : 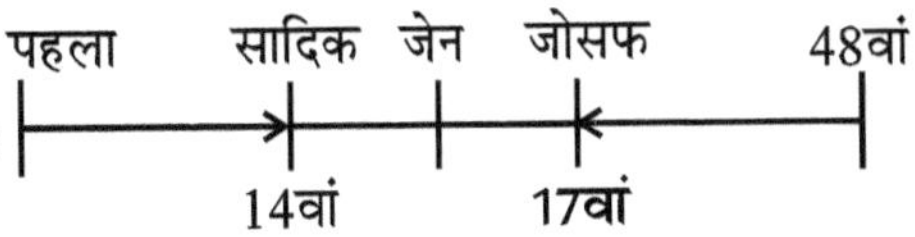

अंत से सादिक का क्रम स्थान:
(48 – 14) + 1 = 35 वां
सादिक और जोसफ के बीच व्यक्तियों की संख्या
= (35 – 17) – 1 = 17
जेन, सादिक और जोसफ के बीच में है, अर्थात् वह दोनों लड़कों से नौवें स्थान पर है।
∴ सादिक और जेन के बीच 8 व्यक्ति हैं।

टिप्पणी : (8 + 8) – 1 = 17

9. (*b*) : 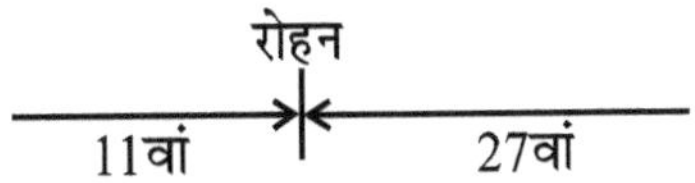

परीक्षा में उत्तीर्ण होने वाले छात्रों की संख्या
= (11+ 27) – 1 = 37
परीक्षा में अनुत्तीर्ण हुए छात्रों की संख्या = 12
परीक्षा में भाग लेने वाले छात्रों की कुल संख्या
= 37 + 12 = 49.

10. (*c*) : 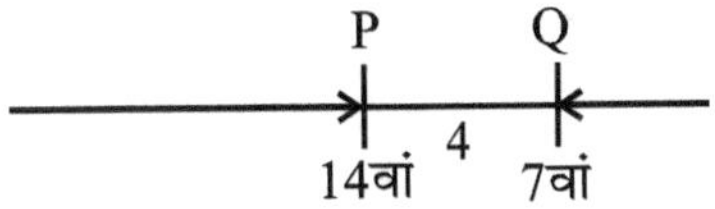

पंक्ति में लड़कों की संख्या
= (14 + 4 + 7) = 25

11. (*b*) : पंक्ति में अवस्थित मकान निम्नलिखित क्रम में हैं:
D B A E C

12. (*c*) : 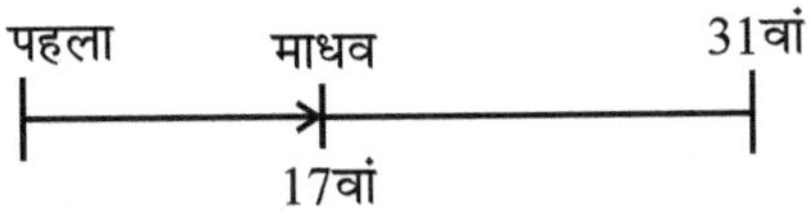

योग्यता-क्रम में नीचे से माधव का स्थान है:
(31 – 17) + 1 = 15 वां

प्रतीक (चिह्न) प्रतिस्थापन
(SYMBOL SUBSTITUTION)

इस प्रकार के प्रश्नों को हल करना अत्यधिक सरल है। ऐसे प्रश्नों को हल करने की एकमात्र अपेक्षा यह है कि उम्मीदवार दिए गए प्रतीकों या चिह्नों को प्रतिस्थापित करने और परिकलन की विद्या में पारंगत हों और अत्यधिक त्वरित गति से दिए गए प्रश्नों का हल ज्ञात कर सके। इस श्रेणी में पूछे गए कुछ सामान्य प्रकार के प्रश्न नीचे हल किए गए हैं।

हल किए गए उदाहरण

1. यदि '+' का अर्थ '×' हो, '×' का अर्थ '÷' हो, '÷' का अर्थ '–' हो और '–' का अर्थ '+' हो, तो $2 - 8 \times 2 + 6 \div 7$ का मान क्या होगा?

(*a*) 32 (*b*) 19 (*c*) 23 (*d*) 9

उत्तर (*b*) : दिए गए व्यंजक में गणितीय चिह्नों को प्रतिस्थापित करने पर नया व्यंजक होगा :

$2 + 8 \div 2 \times 6 - 7$

इस व्यंजक को हल करने के निम्नलिखित चरण होंगे :

$2 + 4 \times 6 - 7$

$2 + 24 - 7$

$26 - 7 = 19$

2. यदि '▲' का अर्थ '+' हो,

'■' का अर्थ '–' हो,

'●' का अर्थ '÷' हो,

'∗' का अर्थ '×' हो, तो

13 ▲ 5 ∗ 20 ● 10 ■ 9 = ?

(*a*) 26 (*b*) 37 (*c*) 14 (*d*) 55

उत्तर (*c*) : चिह्नों को प्रतिस्थापित करने पर प्राप्त हुआ नया व्यंजक है :

$13 + 5 \times 20 \div 10 - 9$

इस व्यंजक को हल करने के चरण होंगे :

$13 + 5 \times 2 - 9$

$13 + 10 - 9$

$23 - 9 = 14$

अभ्यास

1. यदि "+" का अर्थ "–" **हो**; "–" का अर्थ "×" हो; "×" का अर्थ "÷" हो और "÷" का अर्थ "+" हो, तो
$15 \times 5 \div 10 + 5 - 3 = ?$
(*a*) 9.5 (*b*) 0
(*c*) – 2 (*d*) 24

2. यदि "+" का अर्थ "–" हो; "–" का अर्थ "×" हो; "×" का अर्थ "÷" हो; और "÷" का अर्थ "+" हो, तो
$15 \times 3 \div 15 + 5 - 2 = ?$
(*a*) 0 (*b*) 10
(*c*) 20 (*d*) 6

3. यदि "+" का अर्थ "÷" हो; "×" का अर्थ "–" हो; "÷" का अर्थ "+" हो और "–" का अर्थ "×" हो, तो
$16 \div 8 \times 6 - 2 + 12 = ?$
(*a*) 22 (*b*) 24
(*c*) 23 (*d*) 20

4. यदि "+" का अर्थ "×" हो; "–" का अर्थ "÷" हो; "×" का अर्थ "–" हो और "÷" का अर्थ "+" हो, तो
$5 + 8 - 4 \times 2 \div 9 = ?$
(*a*) 15 (*b*) 13
(*c*) 17 (*d*) 11

5. यदि × का आशय जोड़ की संक्रिया से हो, ÷ का आशय घटाव की संक्रिया से हो, + का आशय गुणा की संक्रिया से हो और – का आशय भाग की संक्रिया से हो तो $(20 \times 6 \div 6 \times 4)$ निम्नलिखित में से किसके बराबर है?
(*a*) 5 (*b*) 24
(*c*) 25 (*d*) 80

6. यदि A + B > C + D, B + E = 2 C और C + D > B + E **हो**, तो इसका निश्चित अर्थ यह है कि :
(*a*) A > C (*b*) A + B > 2D
(*c*) A + B > 2C (*d*) A + B > 2E

7. यदि A + D > C + E, C + D = 2B और B + E > C + D हो, तो इसका निश्चित अर्थ यह है कि :
(*a*) A + D > B + E (*b*) A + D > B + C
(*c*) A + B > 2D (*d*) B + D > C + E

8. यदि "+" का अर्थ "÷" हो; "÷" का अर्थ "–" हो; "–" का अर्थ "×" हो और "×" का अर्थ "+" हो, तो
$10 \div 2 - 15 + 3 \times 5 = ?$
(*a*) 10 (*b*) 15
(*c*) 25 (*d*) 5

9. यदि "+" का अर्थ "÷" हो; "×" का अर्थ "–" हो; "÷" का अर्थ "×" हो और "–" का अर्थ "+" हो, तो निम्नलिखित व्यंजक का मान क्या होगा?
$9 + 3 \div 4 - 8 \times 2 = ?$
(*a*) $6\frac{3}{4}$ (*b*) $-1\frac{3}{4}$
(*c*) $-6\frac{1}{4}$ (*d*) 18

10. यदि 'a' का आशय '÷' **हो**, 'b' का आशय '×' हो, 'c' का आशय '+' है और 'd' का आशय '–', **हो**, तो
5 c 20 a 4 b 2 d 10 = ?
(*a*) 5 (*b*) 10
(*c*) 15 (*d*) 20

व्याख्यात्मक उत्तर

1. (*c*) : $15 \div 5 + 10 - 5 \times 3$
$3 + 10 - 15 = -2$

2. (*b*) : $15 \div 3 + 15 - 5 \times 2$
$5 + 15 - 10 = 10$

3. (*c*) : $16 + 8 - 6 \times 2 \div 12$
$16 + 8 - 1 = 23$

4. (*c*) : $5 \times 8 \div 4 - 2 + 9$
$10 - 2 + 9 = 17$

5. (*b*) : $20 + 6 - 6 + 4 = 24$

6. (*c*) : A + B > C + D > B + E or 2 C
$\therefore$ A + B > 2C

7. (*b*) : 1. A + D > C + E
2. B + E > C + D or 2 B
चूँकि 1 और 2 के बीच संबंध स्पष्ट नहीं है, तथापि यह निश्चित है कि A + D > B + C.

8. (*d*) : $10 - 2 \times 15 \div 3 + 5$
$10 - 10 + 5 = 5$

9. (*d*) : $9 \div 3 \times 4 + 8 - 2$
$12 + 8 - 2 = 18$

10. (*a*) : $5 + 20 \div 4 \times 2 - 10$
$5 + 10 - 10 = 5$

कृत्रिम मान और लुप्त संख्याएँ

(ARTIFICIAL VALUES AND MISSING NUMBERS)

इस प्रकार के प्रश्नों को हल करने के लिए संख्या संबंधी प्रश्नों को हल करने में निपुणता और गणितीय कौशल का होना अपेक्षित है। उत्तर प्राप्त करने के लिए अभ्यर्थियों के लिए यह अपेक्षित है कि वे अंकगणितीय चिह्नों या प्रतीकों के सही संयोजन का चयन करें जिसे दिए गए प्रश्नों में प्रश्न चिह्न के स्थान पर प्रतिस्थापित किया जा सके।

हल किए गए उदाहरण

1. यहाँ प्रश्न में दिए गए प्रश्न चिह्न (?) के स्थान पर प्रतिस्थापित करने के लिए सही विकल्प का चयन करें :

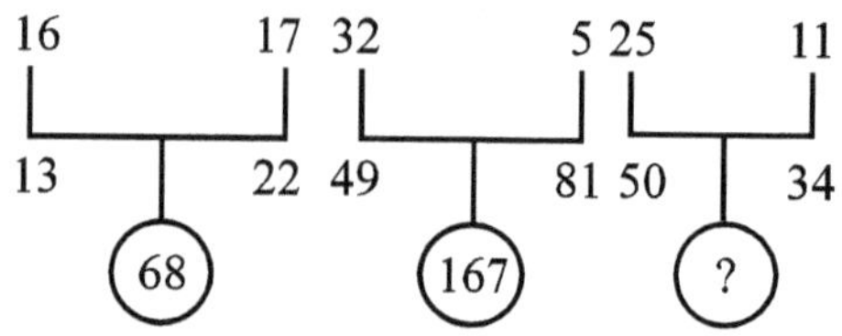

(*a*) 65 (*b*) 120 (*c*) 116 (*d*) 192

उत्तर (*b*) : गोल घेरे के भीतर दी गई संख्या शेष चार संख्याओं का योग है, अर्थात्

16 + 17 + 13 + 22 = 68

32 + 5 + 49 + 81 = 167, इसी प्रकार

25 + 11 + 50 + 34 = 120

2. यहाँ प्रश्न चिह्न के स्थान पर विकल्पों में दी गई कौन-सी संख्या आएगी ?

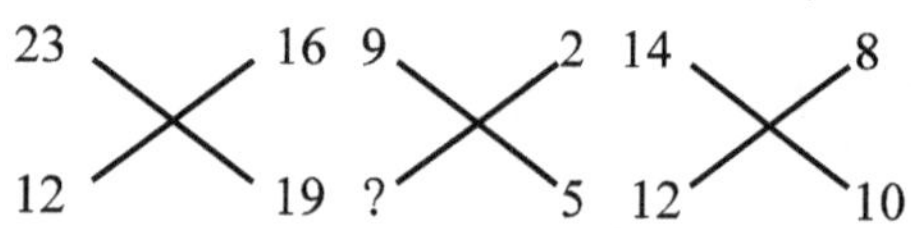

(*a*) 6 (*b*) 8 (*c*) 7 (*d*) 3

उत्तर (*a*) : दो सम्मुख संख्याओं का अंतर 4 है, अर्थात्

23 – 19 = 4 और 16 – 12 = 4

14 – 10 = 4 और 12 – 8 = 4, इसी प्रकार

9 – 5 = 4 और 6 – 2 = 4.

इस प्रकार के प्रश्नों में सही उत्तर ज्ञात करने का कोई निश्चित नियम नहीं है। सही उत्तर प्राप्त करने के विभिन्न तरीकों के बारे में जानने के लिए नीचे दिए गए अभ्यास में निहित प्रश्नों का हल ज्ञात करने का प्रयास करें।

अभ्यास

निर्देश (प्र.सं. 1–10): *नीचे दिए गए प्रत्येक प्रश्न में बताएँ कि प्रश्न चिह्न (?) के स्थान पर कौन-सी संख्या रखी जा सकती है?*

1.

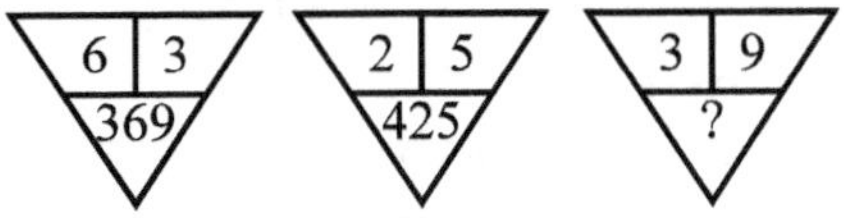

(*a*) 693 (*b*) 939
(*c*) 981 (*d*) 993

2.

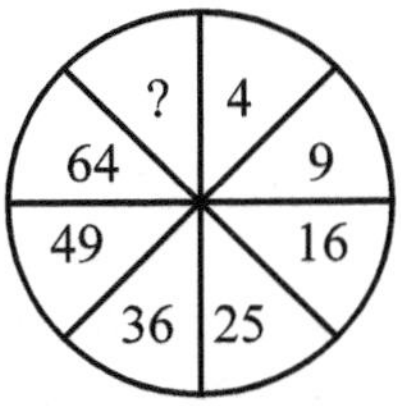

(*a*) 68 (*b*) 100
(*c*) 72 (*d*) 81

3.

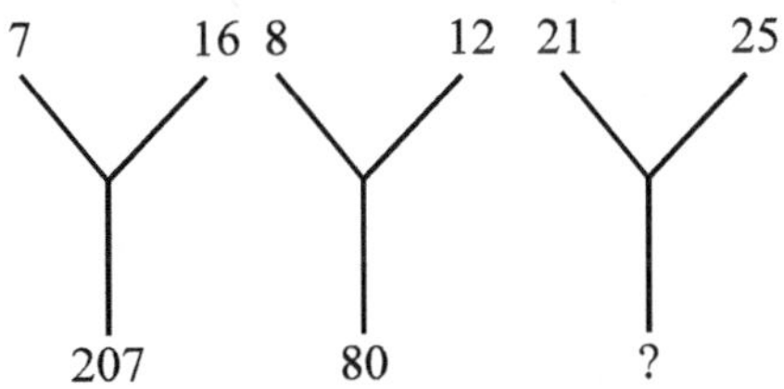

(*a*) 425 (*b*) 184
(*c*) 241 (*d*) 210

4.

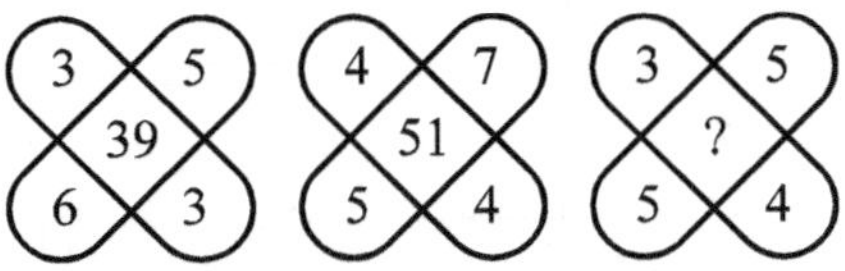

(*a*) 35 (*b*) 37
(*c*) 45 (*d*) 48

5.

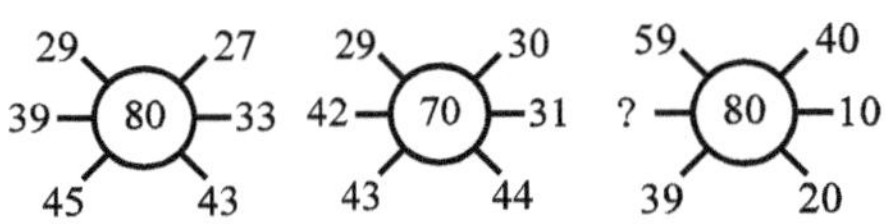

(*a*) 69 (*b*) 49
(*c*) 50 (*d*) 60

6.

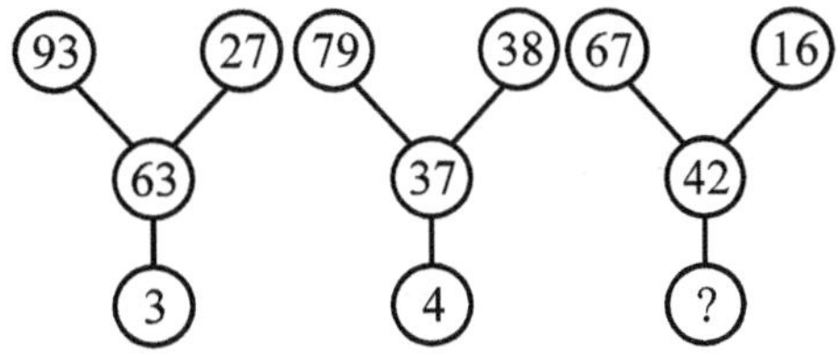

(*a*) 5 (*b*) 6
(*c*) 8 (*d*) 9

7.

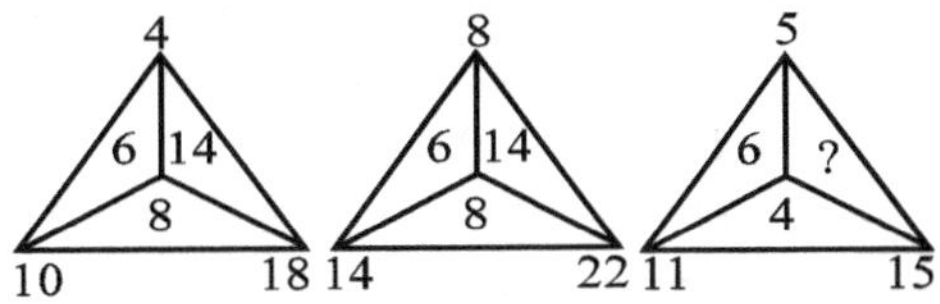

(*a*) 8 (*b*) 14
(*c*) 10 (*d*) 6

8.

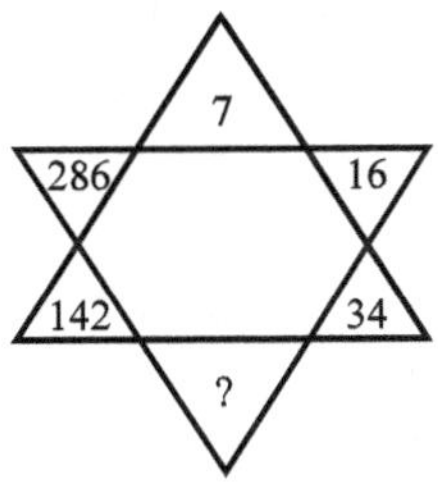

(*a*) 70 (*b*) 68
(*c*) 56 (*d*) 92

9.

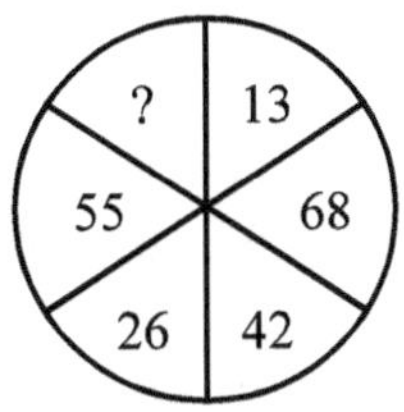

(*a*) 41 (*b*) 37
(*c*) 29 (*d*) 25

10.

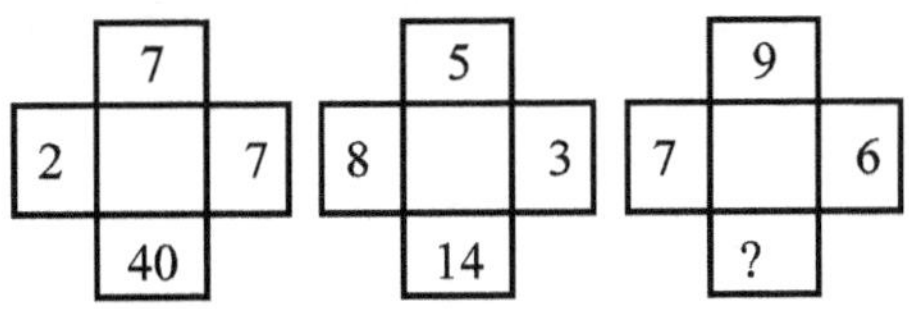

(*a*) 72 (*b*) 68
(*c*) 82 (*d*) 96

व्याख्यात्मक उत्तर

1. (***c***) **:** उलटे बने त्रिभुज के ऊपरी भाग के दोनों खानों में दी गई संख्याओं के वर्ग को एक दूसरे की बगल में रखने पर त्रिभुज के निचले शीर्ष की संख्या प्राप्त होती है, अर्थात्

6^2 और $3^2 = 369$

2^2 और $5^2 = 425$, इसी प्रकार

3^2 और $9^2 = 981$.

2. (***d***) **:** 4 से आरंभ करके प्रत्येक अनुवर्ती संख्या क्रमागत **प्राकृतिक** संख्या का वर्ग है। अर्थात् $2^2 = 4, 3^2 = 9, 4^2 = 16, \ldots 9^2 = 81$

3. (***b***) **:** नीचे की संख्या ऊपर की दोनों संख्याओं के वर्गों का अंतर है, अर्थात्

$16^2 - 7^2 = 256 - 49 = 207$

$12^2 - 8^2 = 144 - 64 = 80$, इसी प्रकार

$25^2 - 21^2 = 625 - 441 = 184$

4. (***b***) **:** बीच की संख्या विकर्णतः सम्मुख संख्याओं के गुणनफलों का योग है, अर्थात्

$(3 \times 3) + (5 \times 6) = 39$

$(4 \times 4) + (7 \times 5) = 51$, इसी प्रकार

$(3 \times 4) + (5 \times 5) = 37$

5. (***a***) **:** किसी भी एक आकृति में सरेखीय तीनों संख्याओं का योगफल समान है, अर्थात्

$29 + 80 + 43$ या $39 + 80 + 33$

या $45 + 80 + 27 = 152$

$29 + 70 + 44$ या $42 + 70 + 31$

या $43 + 70 + 30 = 143$, इसी प्रकार

$59 + 80 + 20$ या $39 + 80 + 40 = 159$.

अतः लुप्त संख्या है :

$$159 - (80 + 10) = 69$$

6. (***d***) **:** प्रत्येक आकृति में दाहिने और बीच के घेरों की संख्याओं के योगफल को बायीं ओर के घेरे की संख्या से घटाने पर आकृति में सबसे नीचे के घेरे की संख्या प्राप्त होती है, अर्थात्

$93 - (27 + 63) = 3$

$79 - (38 + 37) = 4$, इसी प्रकार

$67 - (16 + 42) = 9$

7. (***c***) **:** प्रत्येक त्रिभुजाकार आकृति के भीतर बने प्रत्येक त्रिभुज में आधार पर स्थित संख्याओं का अंतर त्रिभुज के भीतर स्थित संख्या के बराबर है, अर्थात्

$10 - 4 = 6, 18 - 4 = 14$ और $18 - 10 = 8$

$14 - 8 = 6, 22 - 8 = 14$ और $22 - 14 = 8$,

इसी प्रकार

$11 - 5 = 6, 15 - 5 = 10$ और $15 - 11 = 4$.

8. (***a***) **:** दी गई आकृति में 7 की संख्या से आरंभ करके दक्षिणावर्त अगली संख्या पहली संख्या के दोगुने से 2 अधिक है, अर्थात्

$(7 \times 2) + 2 = 16$

$(16 \times 2) + 2 = 34 \ldots$, इसी प्रकार

$(34 \times 2) + 2 = 70$

$(70 \times 2) + 2 = 142$

$(142 \times 2) + 2 = 286$

9. (***c***) **:** दी गई आकृति में सम्मुख त्रिज्यखंडों में दी गई संख्याओं का अंतर 13 है, अर्थात्

$26 - 13 = 13$

$68 - 55 = 13$, इसी प्रकार

अतः लुप्त संख्या है : $42 - 13 = 29$

($42 + 13 = 55$ विकल्पों में नहीं दिया गया है)

10. (***b***) **:** प्रत्येक आकृति में मध्यस्थ ग्रिड रेखा में दी गई संख्याओं के योगफल को ऊपर स्थित संख्या के वर्ग से घटाने पर आकृति में नीचे की संख्या प्राप्त होती है, अर्थात्

$7^2 - (2 + 7) = 40$

$5^2 - (8 + 3) = 14$, इसी प्रकार

$9^2 - (7 + 6) = 68$

अक्षर–अंक व्यवस्थापक मशीन संबंधी प्रश्न

(PROBLEMS BASED ON ENGLISH ALPHABET)

अंग्रेजी वर्णमाला पर आधारित प्रश्नों को हल करना अत्यधिक सरल है। इस प्रकार के प्रश्न वर्णमाला के सीधे क्रम में और साथ ही उलटे क्रम में भी दी गई शृंखलाओं पर आधारित होते हैं।

अंग्रेजी वर्णमाला का सीधा क्रम (Natural Order)

A B C D E F G H I J K L M N O P Q R S T U V W X Y Z

अंग्रेजी वर्णमाला का उलटा क्रम (Reverse Order)

Z Y X W V U T S R Q P O N M L K J I H G F E D C B A

शृंखला Z पर पहुँचने के बाद A से पुनः आरंभ होती है और उलटे क्रम में A पर पहुँचने के बाद Z से पुनः आरंभ होती है। इस शृंखला में A E I O U स्वर और शेष अक्षर व्यंजन कहलाते हैं।

हल किए गए उदाहरण

1. यदि वर्णमाला के पहले दस अक्षरों को उलटे क्रम में लिखा जाए तो निम्नलिखित में से कौन-सा अक्षर उस शृंखला के दाहिने छोर से बारहवें अक्षर की बायीं ओर का सातवाँ अक्षर होगा?

A B C D E F G H I J K L M N O P Q R S T U V W X Y Z

(*a*) H (*b*) C (*c*) I (*d*) B

उत्तर (*b*) : वर्णमाला के सीधे क्रम में दी गई शृंखला में पहले दस अक्षरों को उलटे क्रम में लिखने पर निम्नलिखित शृंखला प्राप्त होगी :

JIHGFEDCBAKLMNOPQRSTUVWXYZ

← 7th ← 12th

'Z' से गिनना आरंभ करने पर दाहिने छोर से बारहवाँ अक्षर 'O' है और 'O' की बायीं ओर का 7वाँ अक्षर 'C' है।

अभ्यास

निर्देश (प्र.सं. 1–10): *निम्नलिखित प्रश्न वर्णमाला के सीधे या उलटे क्रम में लिखी गई शृंखला पर तथा दिए गए शब्द में अक्षरों के स्थान परिवर्तन पर आधारित हैं।*

1. वर्णमाला के सीधे क्रम में लिखी गई शृंखला में बाएँ छोर से छठे अक्षर के ठीक पहले कौन-सा अक्षर होता है?

(*a*) U (*b*) E
(*c*) F (*d*) V

2. वर्णमाला में G और S के ठीक बीच में कौन-सा अक्षर है?

(*a*) L (*b*) N
(*c*) M (*d*) कोई अक्षर नहीं

3. यदि अंग्रेजी वर्णमाला में प्रथम अर्द्धांश के अक्षरों को उलटे क्रम में लिखा जाए तो दायीं ओर से नौंवें अक्षर की बायीं ओर का नौंवाँ अक्षर कौन-सा होगा?

(*a*) I (*b*) D
(*c*) F (*d*) E

4. यदि अंग्रेजी वर्णमाला को उलटे क्रम में लिखा जाए, तो दायीं और से सातवें अक्षर की बायीं ओर का आठवाँ अक्षर कौन-सा होगा?

(*a*) O (*b*) P
(*c*) N (*d*) Q

5. वर्णमाला में दाहिने छोर से तेरहवें अक्षर की दायीं ओर का पाँचवाँ अक्षर क्या होगा?

(*a*) R (*b*) S
(*c*) I (*d*) O

6. यदि अंग्रेजी वर्णमाला को उलटे क्रम में लिखा जाए तो P के दाएँ से छठा अक्षर कौन-सा होगा?

(*a*) J (*b*) W
(*c*) K (*d*) V

7. यदि अंग्रेजी वर्णमाला को दो बराबर हिस्सों में बाँट दिया जाए जिनमें पहले अर्द्धांश में A से M तक के और दूसरे अर्द्धांश में N से Z तक के अक्षर निहित हों, तो बाद वाले अर्द्धांश का कौन-सा अक्षर पहले वाले अर्द्धांश के J अक्षर के संगत होगा?

(*a*) W (*b*) Q
(*c*) V (*d*) R

8. यदि अंग्रेजी वर्णमाला को उलटे क्रम में लिखा जाए तो प्राप्त शृंखला में आपके बाएँ से सोलहवें अक्षर की बायीं ओर का बारहवाँ अक्षर कौन-सा होगा?

(*a*) X (*b*) W
(*c*) D (*d*) V

9. अंग्रेजी वर्णमाला में बाएँ से पाँचवें अक्षर से आंरभ करके यदि बारह अक्षरों को उलटे (विपरीत) क्रम में लिखा जाए तो प्राप्त शृंखला में दाएँ से चौदहवें अक्षर की बायीं ओर का सातवाँ अक्षर कौन-सा होगा?

(*a*) N (*b*) H
(*c*) L (*d*) O

10. यदि वर्णमाला में B से आरंभ करके सभी एकांतर स्थानों पर आने वाले अक्षरों को छोटे अक्षरों में और शेष अक्षरों को बड़े अक्षरों में लिखा जाए तो प्राप्त शृंखला के अक्षरों का प्रयोग करके 'September' माह को किस प्रकार लिखा जाएगा?

(*a*) SEptEMbEr (*b*) sePTemBeR
(*c*) SEptembER (*d*) SEpteMbeR

व्याख्यात्मक उत्तर

1. (*b*):

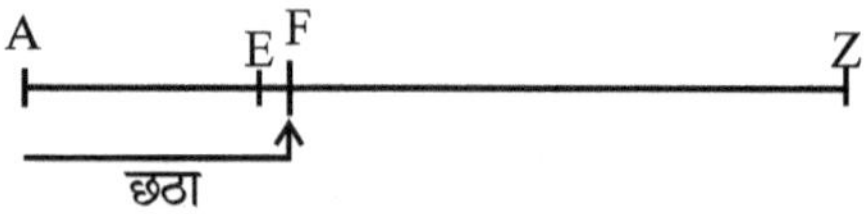

बाएँ से छठा अक्षर 'F' है और 'F' से ठीक पहले का अक्षर 'E' है।

2. (*c*):

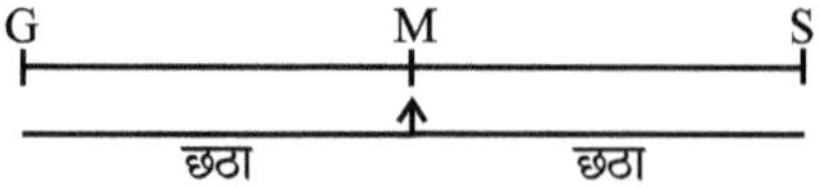

G और S के बीच का अक्षर M है।

3. (*d*): MLKJIGHFEDCBANOPQRSTUVWXYZ

नौंवाँ नौंवाँ

4. (*a*): ZYXWVUTSRQPONMLKJIHGFEDCBA

आठवाँ सातवाँ

5. (*b*):

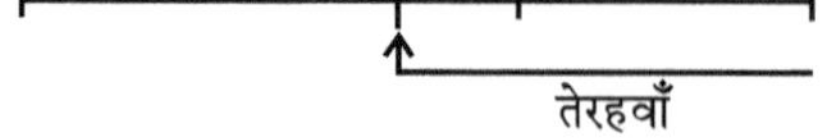

दाहिने छोर से तेरहवाँ अक्षर 'N' है और 'N' की दायीं ओर का पाँचवाँ अक्षर 'S' है।

6. (*a*):

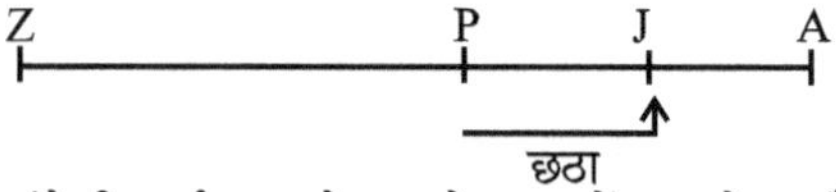

अंग्रेजी वर्णमाला के उलटे क्रम में 'P' के दाएँ से छठा अक्षर 'J' है।

7. (*a*): A B C D E F G H I J K L M
N O P Q R S T U V W X Y Z

8. (*b*):

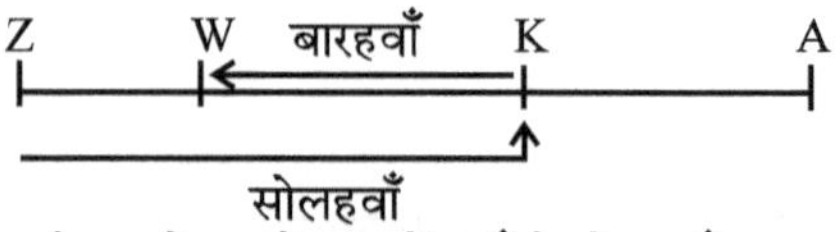

वर्णमाला के उलटे क्रम में बाएँ से सोलहवाँ अक्षर 'K' है और 'K' की बायीं ओर का बारहवाँ अक्षर 'W' है।

9. (*d*): ABCDPONMLKJIHGFEQRSTUVWXYZ

सातवाँ चौदहवाँ

10. (*a*): A b C d E f G h I j K l M n O p Q r S t U v W x Y z

कथन एवं वेन आरेख
(LOGICAL DIAGRAMS)

इस प्रकार के प्रश्नों में विकल्प के रूप में पाँच भिन्न-भिन्न आकृतियों का समुच्चय दिया जाता है। प्रत्येक आकृति संबंधित शब्दों के कुछ समूहों का एक तार्किक पैटर्न निरूपित करती है जिनमें प्रत्येक शब्द एक वर्ग को निरूपित करता है। अभ्यर्थी को दिए गए शब्दों के समुच्चय के लिए सर्वाधिक उपयुक्त तार्किक आकृति की पहचान करनी है। नीचे इन आरेखों द्वारा निरूपित कुछ संबंध दर्शाए गए हैं। संबंधित पैटर्नों को समझें और तत्पश्चात् दिए गए प्रश्नों के उत्तर दें।

हल किए गए उदाहरण

1. 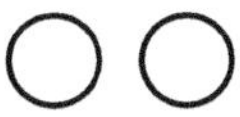

दिए गए वर्गों में कोई सदस्य समान (common) नहीं है।

उदाहरण : दूध, अंडे

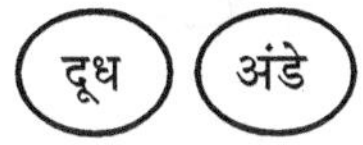

2. 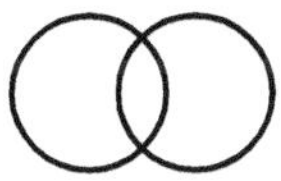

दिया गया आरेख यह दर्शाता है कि दोनों वर्गों में कुछ समान सदस्य हैं किंतु कोई भी वर्ग एक-दूसरे में पूर्णतः समाहित नहीं है।

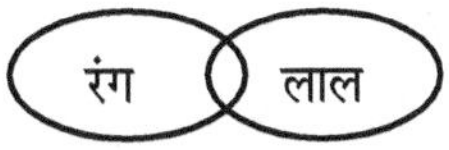

उदाहरण : रंग, लाल

3. 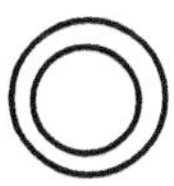

दिया गया आरेख यह दर्शाता है कि एक वर्ग दूसरे में पूर्णतः समाहित है किंतु दूसरा वर्ग पहले वर्ग में समाहित नहीं है अर्थात् ये दोनों वर्ग आपस में मिले-जुले नहीं हैं।

उदाहरण : फल, सेब

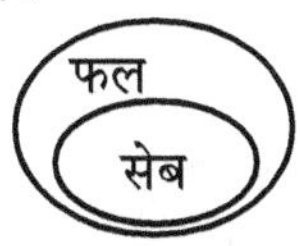

4. 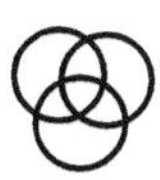

आकृति 2 के समान ही यह आकृति भी दर्शाती है कि तीनों वर्गों में कुछ समान (common) सदस्य हैं किंतु इनमें से कोई भी वर्ग एक-दूसरे में पूर्णतः समाहित नहीं है।

उदाहरण : लंबा, आदमी, शिक्षित

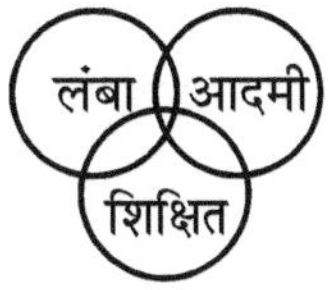

अभ्यास

निर्देश (प्र.सं. 1–5): *नीचे दिए गए पाँच तर्क आरेखों में से उस आरेख (आकृति) का चयन करें जो प्रश्न में दिए गए तीनों वर्गों के बीच संबंध को सर्वाधिक सुस्पष्ट रूप में प्रदर्शित करता है।*

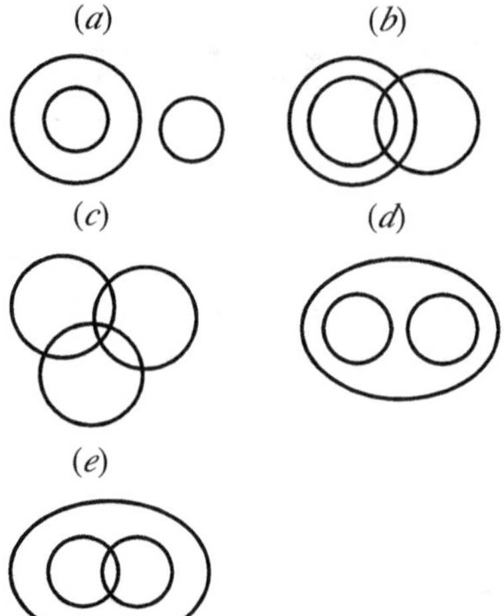

1. पक्षी, फल, आम
2. अपराधी, वकील, डकैत
3. तैराक, कुँआरा, पुरुष
4. स्मार्ट, इंजीनियर, महिला
5. सब्जियाँ, आलू, बैंगन

निर्देश (प्र.सं. 6–10): *नीचे दिए गए पाँच तर्क आरेखों में से उस आरेख (आकृति) का चयन करें जो प्रश्न में दिए गए तीनों वर्गों के बीच संबंध को सर्वाधिक सुस्पष्ट रूप में व्यक्त करता है।*

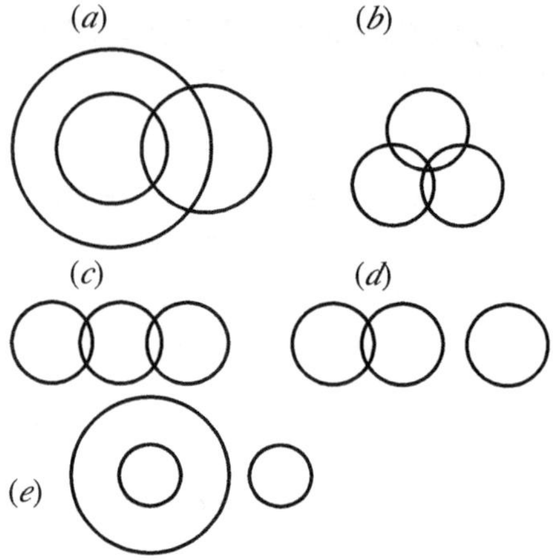

6. बहन, चचेरी-ममेरी-फुफेरी बहन, महिलाएँ
7. तारा, ग्रह, शनि
8. लोग, बुद्धिमान, धनी
9. पालतू पशु, बिल्लियाँ, कुत्ते
10. अभिनेता, मंच, फिल्म

व्याख्यात्मक उत्तर

1. (*a*) :

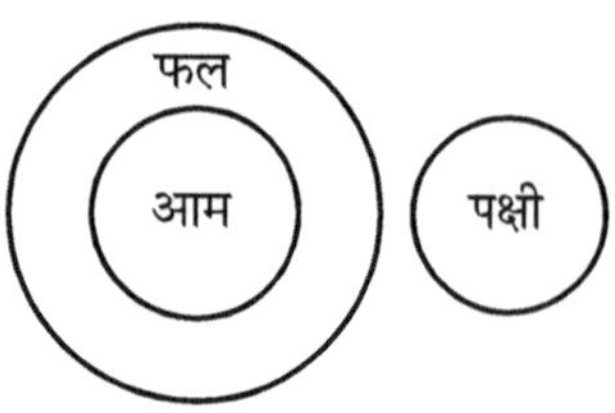

सभी आम फल हैं किंतु फल और आम में से कोई भी पक्षी नहीं है।

2. (*a*) :

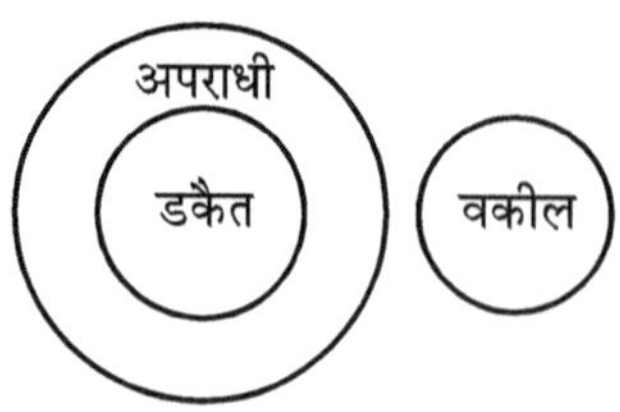

सभी डकैत अपराधी हैं किंतु अपराधी और डकैत में से कोई भी वकील नहीं हो सकता।

3. (*b*) :

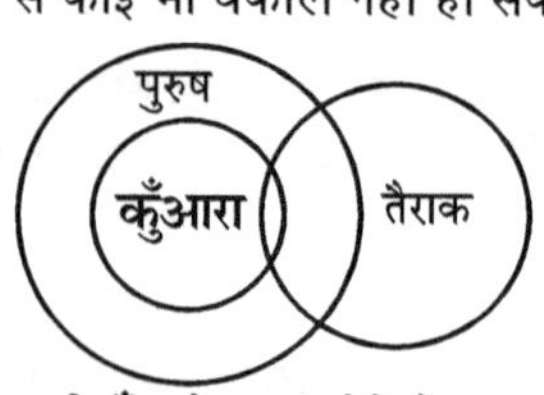

सभी कुँआरे पुरुष होते हैं तथा कुछ पुरुष और कुँआरे तैराक हो सकते हैं।

4. (*c*) :

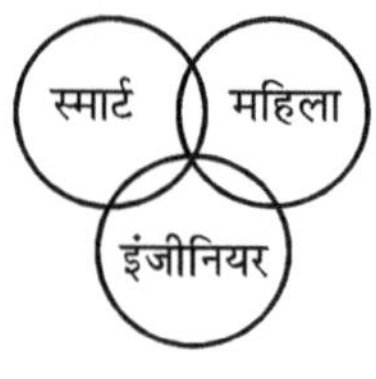

कुछ महिलाएँ स्मार्ट हो सकती हैं और कुछ महिलाएँ इंजीनियर हो सकती हैं तथा कुछ इंजीनियर स्मार्ट भी हो सकते हैं और महिला भी।

5. (*d*) :

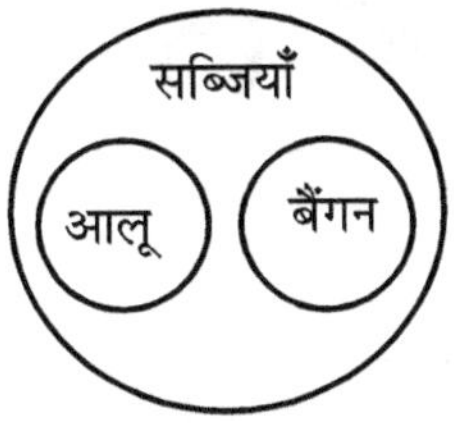

आलू और बैंगन दोनों सब्जियाँ हैं किंतु उनमें कोई समान गुण नहीं है। कुछ सब्जियाँ आलू हैं और कुछ बैंगन।

6. (*a*) :

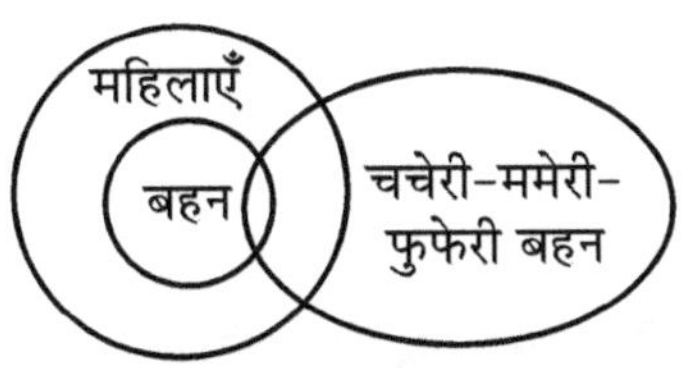

सभी बहनें महिलाएँ होती हैं। कुछ महिलाएँ जो बहनें हैं, चचेरी-ममेरी-फुफेरी बहनें हो सकती हैं या सभी चचेरी-ममेरी-फुफेरी बहनें कुछ महिलाएँ हैं।

7. (*e*) :

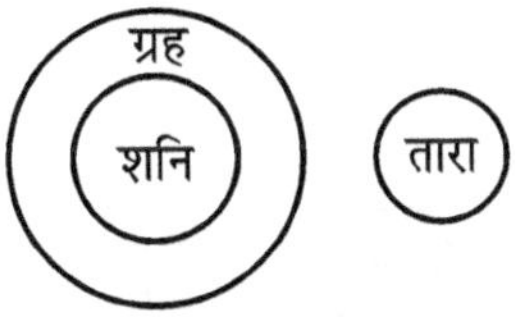

शनि एक ग्रह है। सौरमंडल के ग्रहों में एक ग्रह शनि है। तारा एक भिन्न वर्ग है।

8. (*b*) :

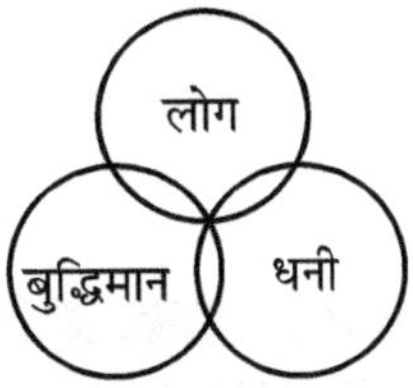

कुछ लोग बुद्धिमान हो सकते हैं और कुछ धनी हो सकते हैं तथा कुछ बुद्धिमान और धनी व्यक्ति लोगों की श्रेणी में शामिल हैं। कुछ बुद्धिमान धनी हो सकते हैं और कुछ बुद्धिमान व्यक्ति लोगों की श्रेणी में शामिल है या कुछ धनी बुद्धिमान हो सकते हैं और कुछ लोगों को बुद्धिमान कहा जा सकता है।

9. (*c*) :

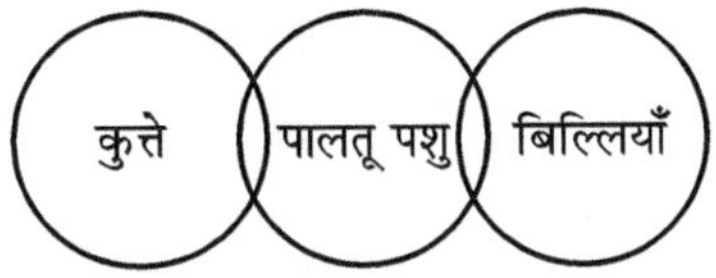

पालतू पशुओं में कुछ कुत्ते और कुछ बिल्लियाँ हो सकती हैं। कुछ कुत्ते और बिल्लियों को पालतू बनाया जा सकता है। किंतु कुत्ते और बिल्लियों का अलग-अलग वर्ग है।

10. (*b*) :

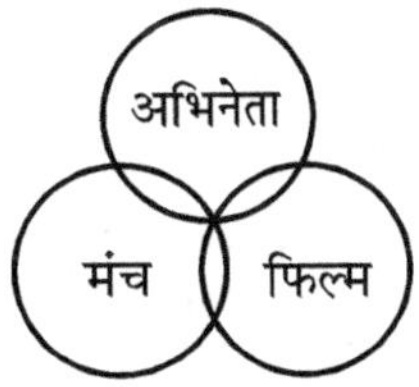

कुछ अभिनेता मंच से जुड़े होते हैं और कुछ फिल्मों से तथा मंच से जुड़े कुछ कलाकार और फिल्म से जुड़े कुछ कलाकार अभिनेता की श्रेणी में आते हैं।

अभाषिक

श्रृंखला (SERIES)

इस प्रकार की अभाषिक श्रृंखला (Non-Verbal Series) में, जो सर्वाधिक सामान्य प्रकार की श्रृंखला होती है, चार या पांच आनुक्रमिक प्रश्न आकृतियां एक निश्चित अनुक्रम निर्मित करते हैं और अभ्यर्थियों को दी गई उत्तर आकृतियों के सेट से उस एक आकृति का चयन करना होता है जिससे प्रश्न आकृतियों के समुच्चय की श्रृंखला सतत् हो जाए।

अभ्यर्थियों को प्रश्न आकृतियों के समुच्चय की श्रृंखला सतत् बनाने के लिए विभिन्न क्रियाएं, परिवर्तन, विस्थापन, क्रमावर्तन, पुनरावर्तन और बहुत से अन्य परिवर्तन करने की आवश्यकता होती है। निरंतर अभ्यास द्वारा श्रृंखला विषयक समस्याओं को हल करने में निपुणता प्राप्त की जा सकती है।

हल किए गए उदाहरण

नीचे पूछे गए प्रत्येक प्रश्न में उत्तर आकृतियों के समुच्चय से उस एक आकृति का चयन करें जिसे प्रश्न आकृतियों के बाद में रखने पर प्रश्न आकृतियों के समुच्चय की श्रृंखला सतत् हो जाए।

1. प्रश्न आकृतियां

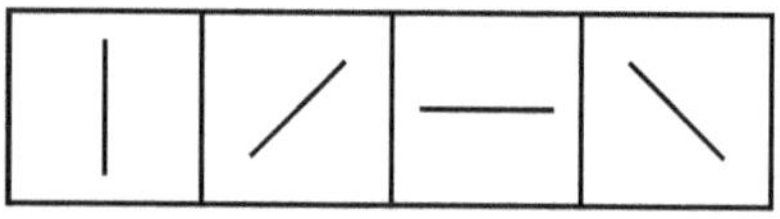

उत्तर आकृतियां

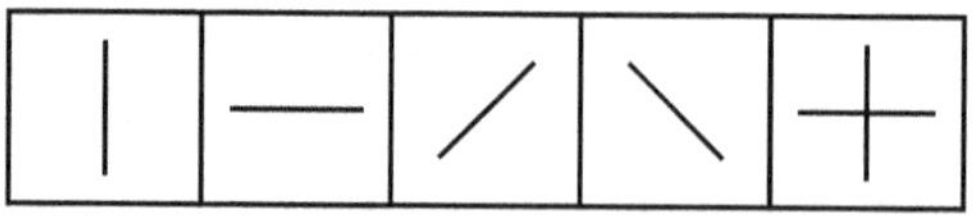

(*a*) (*b*) (*c*) (*d*) (*e*)

उत्तर (*a*): सभी आकृतियों में समान आकार की सीधी सरल रेखाएं दी गई हैं। उनकी दिशाएं और स्थिति परिवर्तित होती हैं। पहली आकृति में रेखा ऊर्ध्वाधर स्थिति में है। दूसरी आकृति में रेखा दक्षिणावर्त 45° के कोण से मुड़ जाती है और तीसरी आकृति में रेखा दक्षिणावर्त और 45° के कोण से मुड़ जाती है तथा चौथी आकृति में रेखा दक्षिणावर्त और 45° के कोण से मुड़ जाती है। अतः दो बातें स्पष्ट होती हैं: (i) रेखा दक्षिणावर्त घूमती है, और (ii) रेखा प्रत्येक चरण पर 45° के कोण से मुड़ती है।

अब चौथी आकृति (प्रश्न आकृति) भी दक्षिणावर्त 45° के कोण से मुड़नी चाहिए। अतः पांचवीं आकृति एक ऊर्ध्वाधर (उदग्र) रेखा होगी। इस प्रकार हमें ज्ञात होता है कि श्रृंखला को सतत् बनाने के लिए अगली आकृति एक ऊर्ध्वाधर या उदग्र सरल रेखा होगी।

2. प्रश्न आकृतियां

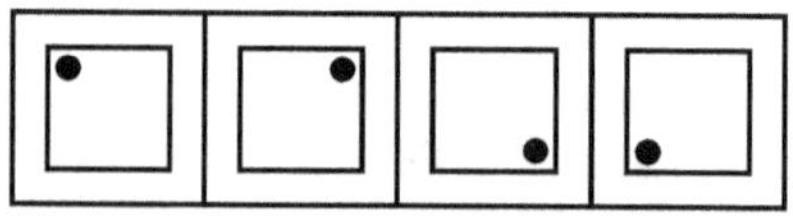

उत्तर आकृतियां

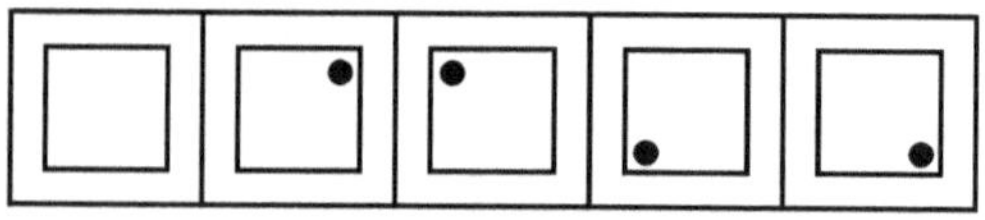

(*a*) (*b*) (*c*) (*d*) (*e*)

उत्तर (*c*): सभी चारों आकृतियां वर्ग हैं। जिनमें से प्रत्येक के भीतर एक काला बिंदु है। आकृतियों में वर्ग की अवस्थिति में परिवर्तन नहीं होता है बल्कि बिंदु की स्थिति परिवर्तित होती है। पहली आकृति में बिन्दु वर्ग के भीतर ऊपरी बाएं कोने पर अवस्थित है और दूसरी आकृति में बिन्दु वर्ग के भीतर ऊपरी दाएं

कोने पर पहुंच जाती है। तीसरी आकृति में बिन्दु निचले दाहिने कोने पर और चौथी आकृति में निचले बाएं कोने पर पहुंच जाती है। अतः दो तथ्यों का पता चलता है: (i) बिन्दु की अवस्थिति बाएं से दाएं अर्थात् दक्षिणावर्त परिवर्तित होती है, और (ii) यह प्रत्येक चरण पर वर्ग के एक कोने से दूसरे कोने पर पहुंच जाती है।

चौथी आकृति (प्रश्न आकृति) में बिन्दु निचले बाएं कोने पर अवस्थित है। अगले चरण में यह दक्षिणावर्त अगले कोने पर अर्थात् ऊपरी बाएं कोने पर पहुंच जाएगी। अतः प्रश्न आकृति में दी गई शृंखला को सतत् बनाने के लिए शृंखला की अगली अर्थात् पांचवीं आकृति में एक वर्ग होगा जिसके ऊपरी बाएं कोने पर एक बिन्दु अवस्थित होगा।

अभ्यास

निर्देश (प्र.सं. 1–30): *नीचे के प्रत्येक प्रश्न में आकृतियों के दो समुच्चय दिए गए हैं जिनमें से एक समुच्चय को* **प्रश्न आकृतियों** *का समुच्चय और दूसरे समुच्चय को* **उत्तर आकृतियों** *का समुच्चय कहा गया है। प्रश्न आकृतियों के समुच्चय से किसी न किसी प्रकार से एक शृंखला बनती है। उत्तर आकृतियों के समुच्चय से उस एक आकृति का चयन करें जिससे प्रश्न आकृतियों के समुच्चय की शृंखला संतत हो जाए।*

1. प्रश्न आकृतियां

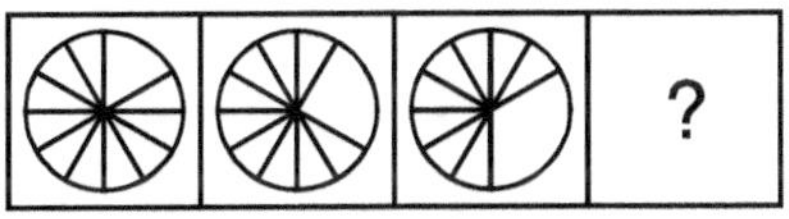

उत्तर आकृतियां

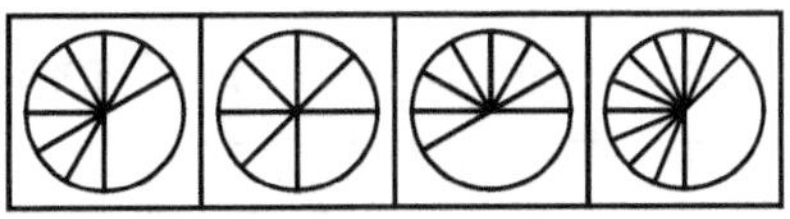

(*a*) (*b*) (*c*) (*d*)

2. प्रश्न आकृतियां

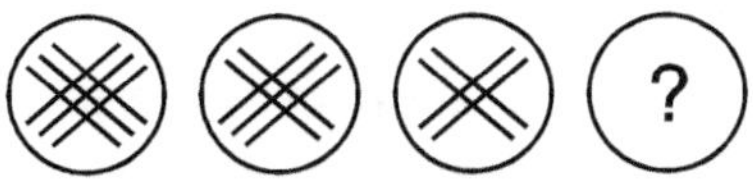

उत्तर आकृतियां

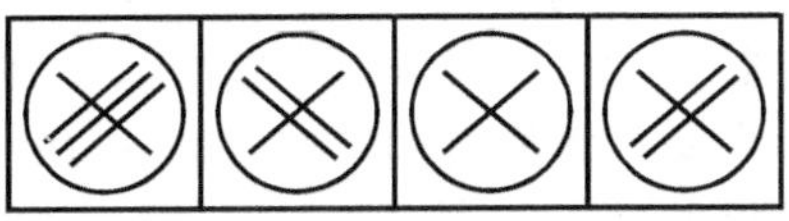

(*a*) (*b*) (*c*) (*d*)

3. प्रश्न आकृतियां

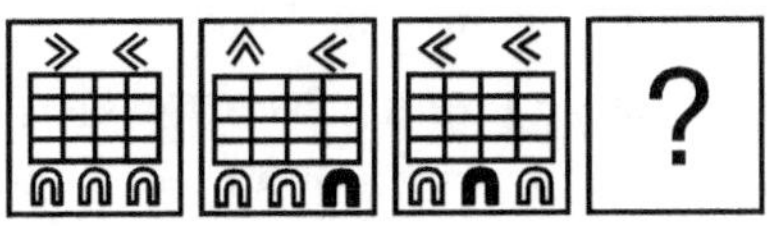

उत्तर आकृतियां

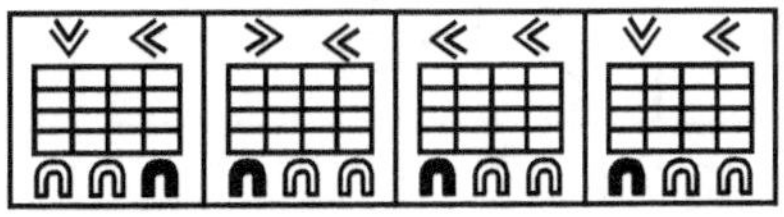

(*a*) (*b*) (*c*) (*d*)

4. प्रश्न आकृतियां

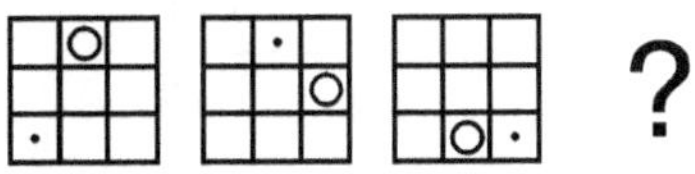

उत्तर आकृतियां

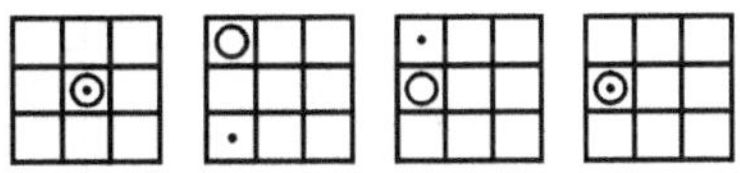

(*a*) (*b*) (*c*) (*d*)

5. प्रश्न आकृतियां

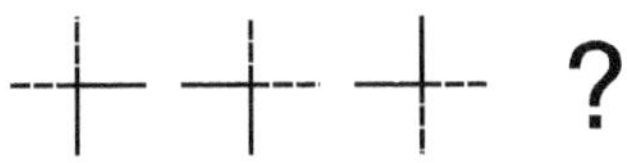

उत्तर आकृतियां

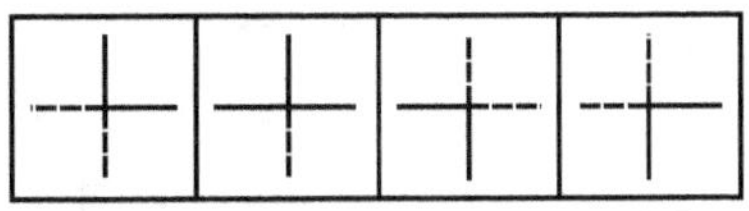

(*a*) (*b*) (*c*) (*d*)

6. प्रश्न आकृतियां

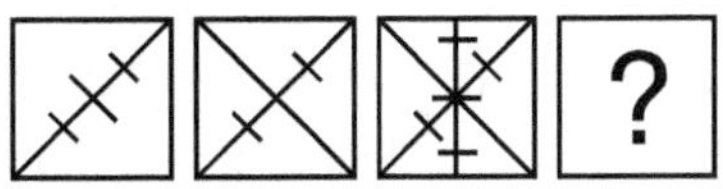

उत्तर आकृतियां

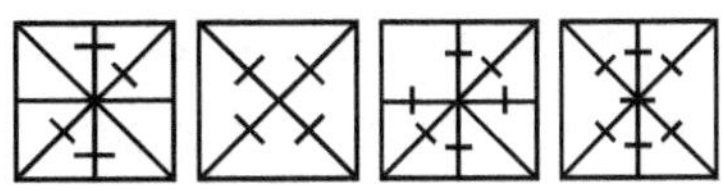

(*a*) (*b*) (*c*) (*d*)

7. प्रश्न आकृतियां

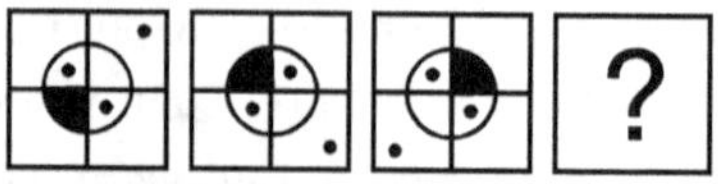

उत्तर आकृतियां

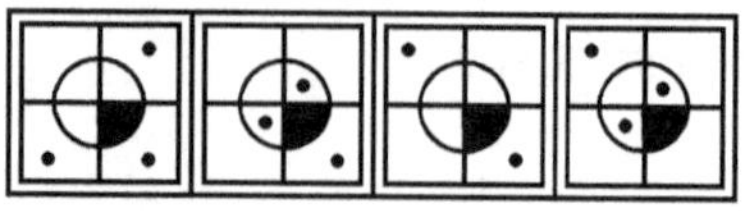

(*a*) (*b*) (*c*) (*d*)

8. प्रश्न आकृतियां

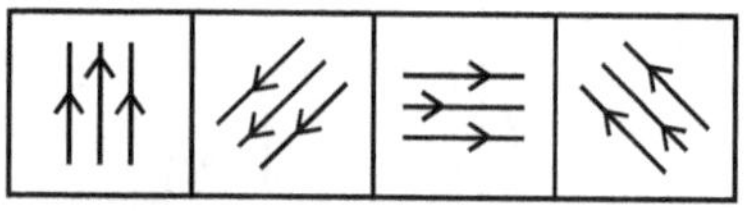

उत्तर आकृतियां

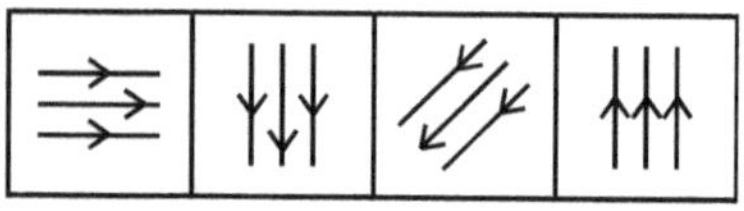

(*a*) (*b*) (*c*) (*d*)

9. प्रश्न आकृतियां

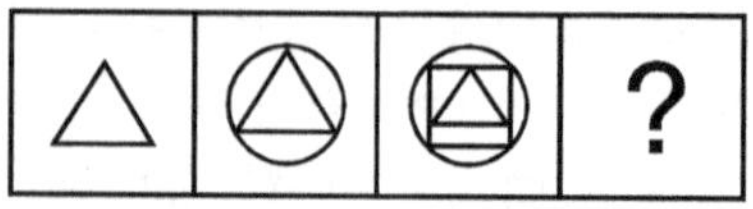

उत्तर आकृतियां

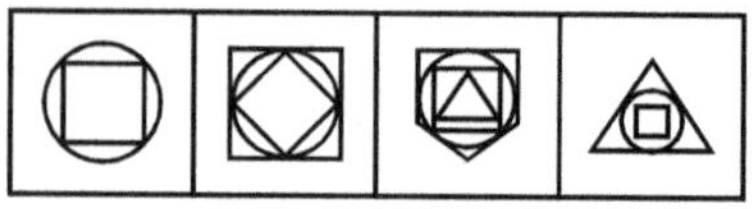

(*a*) (*b*) (*c*) (*d*)

10. प्रश्न आकृतियां

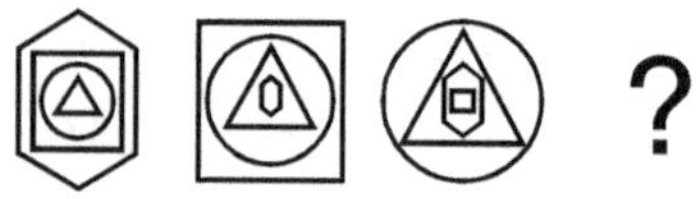

उत्तर आकृतियां

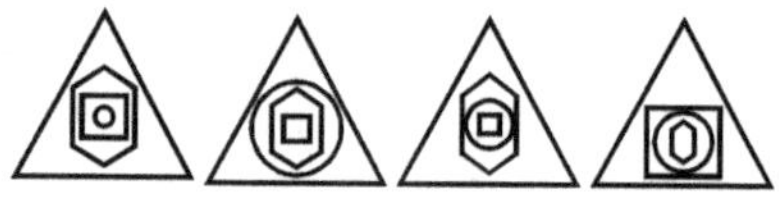

(*a*) (*b*) (*c*) (*d*)

व्याख्यात्मक उत्तर

1. (*c*) : एक आकृति से दूसरी आकृति में वृत्त क्रमशः दक्षिणावर्त 30° के कोण से घूम जाता है और प्रत्येक चरण में वृत्त के भीतर स्थित एक त्रिज्यीय रेखाखण्ड लुप्त होता जाता है।

2. (*d*) : तिरछे या विकर्णी रेखाखण्ड एक-एक करके एक निश्चित क्रम में लुप्त होते जाते हैं।

3. (*d*) : पहली आकृति में ऊपर बाएं स्थित >> अवयव क्रमशः अगली आकृति में वामावर्त 90° के कोण से घूम जाता है। आकृति में नीचे स्थित तीन अवयवों में से दाहिने ओर का एक अवयव दूसरी आकृति में छायांकित हो जाता है तथा उसके बाद की आकृति में इन तीनों में से दाहिने से बाएं के क्रम में केवल एक अवयव ही छायांकित होता जाता है।

4. (*d*) : वृत्त (गोल घेरा) और बिंदु अगली आकृति में दक्षिणावर्त क्रमशः दो और तीन खंड आगे खिसक जाते हैं।

5. (*a*) : प्रत्येक चरण में क्रॉस का चिह्न दक्षिणावर्त 90° के कोण से घूम जाता है।

6. (*a*) : पहली आकृति में विकर्ण पर बीच में स्थित रेखाखण्ड दूसरी आकृति में आगे बढ़कर वर्ग के सम्मुख कोनों को स्पर्श करता है। अगली आकृति में तीन रेखाखण्डों से युक्त एक नई रेखा जुड़ जाती है। शृंखला में निंरतरता स्थापित करने के लिए मध्यस्थ रेखाखण्ड को आगे बढ़ाकर वर्ग की भुजाओं से स्पर्श कराया जाना चाहिए।

7. (*d*) : प्रत्येक चरण पर संपूर्ण आकृति दक्षिणावर्त 90° के कोण से घूम जाती है।

8. (*b*) : एकांतर आकृतियों में तीर दक्षिणावर्त 90° के कोण से घूम जाते हैं और तीर के चिह्नों (वाणमुखों) की संस्थिति सामने से पीछे और पीछे से सामने होती जाती है।

9. (*c*) : प्रत्येक चरण पर पूर्ववर्ती आकृति-समुच्चय में एक नई आकृति जुड़ती जाती है।

10. (*a*) : पहली आकृति में सबसे बाहरी संरचना अगली आकृति में सबसे भीतर चली जाती है।

सादृश्य या संबंध

(ANALOGIES OR RELATIONSHIPS)

अभाषिक सादृश्य के प्रश्नों में दो प्रकार की आकृतियां दी जाती हैं जो (i) प्रश्न आकृतियां और (ii) उत्तर आकृतियां कहलाती हैं। प्रश्न आकृतियां दो भागों में विभाजित होती हैं। प्रश्न आकृतियों के नीचे उत्तर आकृतियां दी जाती है।

हल किए गए उदाहरण

1. प्रश्न आकृतियां

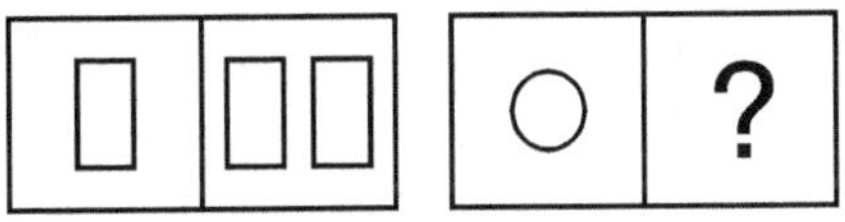

उत्तर आकृतियां

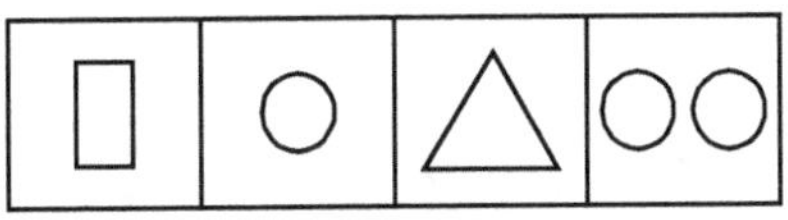

(*a*) (*b*) (*c*) (*d*)

उत्तर (*d*)**:** ऊपर दी गई प्रश्न आकृतियों के दो भाग हैं। पहले भाग में दो आकृतियां हैं जबकि दूसरे भाग में एक आकृति दी गई है जिसके बाद एक प्रश्न चिह्न (?) है। पहले भाग की आकृतियों के बीच एक विशेष संबंध है जिसके आधार पर दूसरे भाग की आकृतियों के बीच संबंध स्थापित किया जाना है।

प्रश्न आकृतियों के पहले भाग की दो आकृतियों में क्रमशः एक और दो आयत निहित हैं। पहली आकृति में एक आयत है जबकि दूसरी आकृति में दो आयत हैं। इसका अर्थ है कि उनके बीच संबंध यह है कि दूसरी आकृति में पहली आकृति में निहित आयत की संख्या की दोगुनी संख्या में आयत हैं।

दूसरे भाग की दोनों प्रश्न आकृतियों के बीच भी ठीक उसी प्रकार का संबंध होना आवश्यक है जैसा संबंध पहले भाग की दो प्रश्न आकृतियों के बीच है अर्थात् इस सादृश्य के आधार पर जबकि दूसरे भाग में पहली प्रश्न आकृति एक वृत्त है तो दूसरी प्रश्न आकृति में वृत्तों की संख्या दोगुनी अर्थात् 2 होगी।

2. प्रश्न आकृतियां

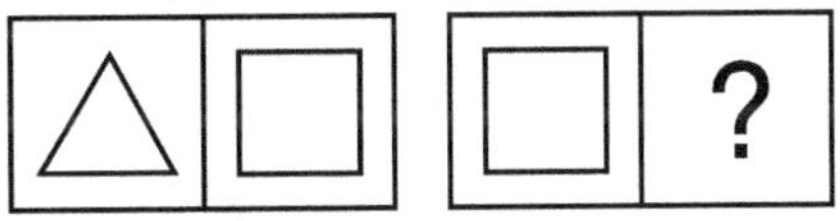

उत्तर आकृतियां

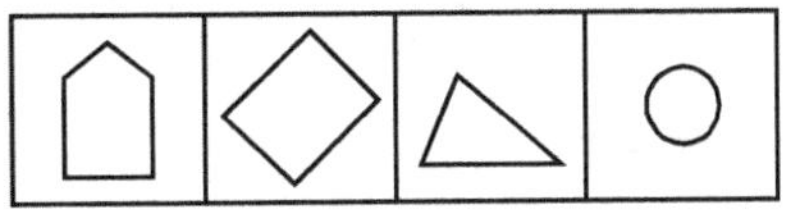

(*a*) (*b*) (*c*) (*d*)

उत्तर (*a*)**:** प्रश्न आकृतियों के पहले भाग में दी गई दोनों आकृतियों को देखें। पहली आकृति में एक त्रिभुज और दूसरी आकृति में एक वर्ग है। पहली आकृति (त्रिभुज) में तीन भुजाएं और तीन कोण हैं जबकि दूसरी आकृति (वर्ग) में चार भुजाएं और चार कोण हैं। इन दोनों आकृतियों के बीच संबंध यह है कि दूसरी आकृति में पहली आकृति की तुलना में एक भुजा और एक कोण अधिक है।

इस सादृश्य संबंध के आधार पर प्रश्न चिह्न (?) के स्थान पर रखी जाने वाली आकृति पाँच भुजाओं और पाँच कोणों वाली आकृति होनी चाहिए (जिसमें प्रश्न आकृतियों के दूसरे भाग की पहली आकृति से एक भुजा और एक कोण अधिक हो)।

अभ्यास

निर्देश (प्र.सं. 1–20): *प्रश्न आकृतियों में :: चिह्न के बाएं दी गई दो आकृतियों में से दूसरी आकृति का पहली आकृति के साथ एक विशेष संबंध है। :: चिह्न की दाईं ओर की दो आकृतियों के बीच भी ऐसा ही संबंध है। दिए गए विकल्पों से उस आकृति का चयन करें जिसे प्रश्न आकृतियों में प्रश्न चिह्न के स्थान पर रखा जा सकता है और जिसका :: चिह्न की दाईं ओर की पहली आकृति के साथ ठीक वैसा ही संबंध है जैसा कि :: चिह्न की बाईं ओर की दो आकृतियों के बीच है।*

1. प्रश्न आकृतियां

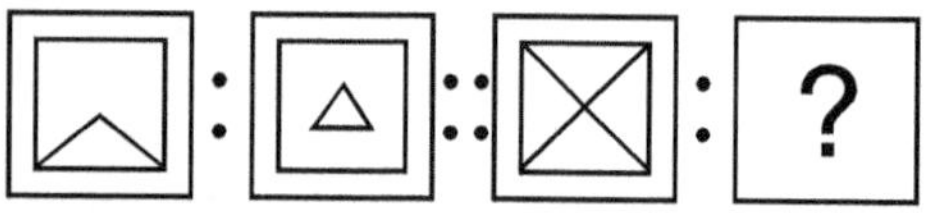

उत्तर आकृतियां

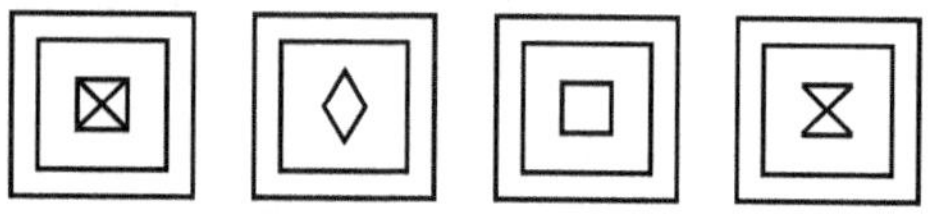

(*a*) (*b*) (*c*) (*d*)

2. प्रश्न आकृतियां

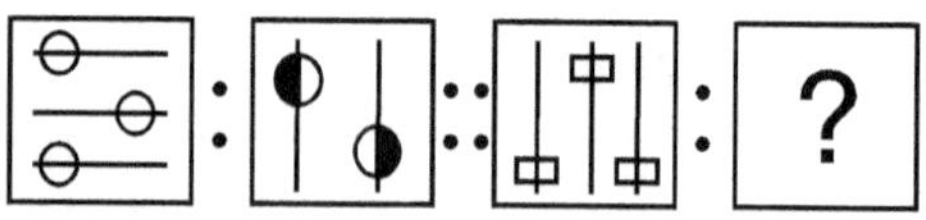

उत्तर आकृतियां

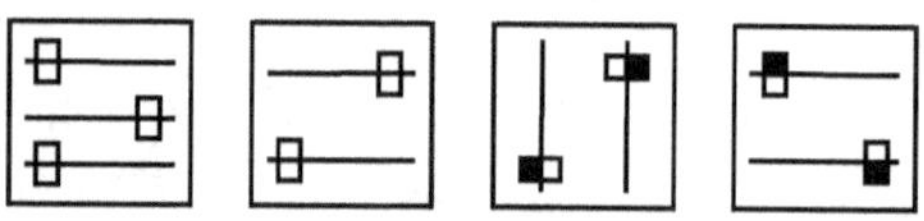

(*a*) (*b*) (*c*) (*d*)

3. प्रश्न आकृतियां

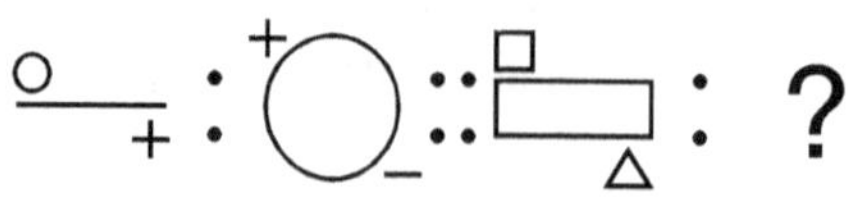

उत्तर आकृतियां

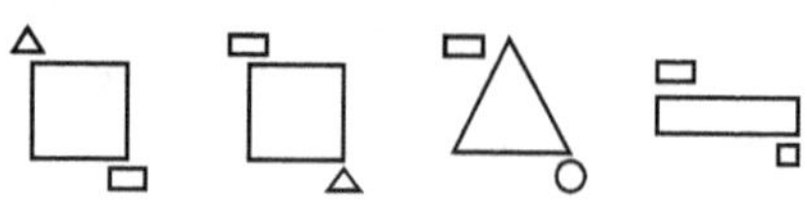

(*a*) (*b*) (*c*) (*d*)

4. प्रश्न आकृतियां

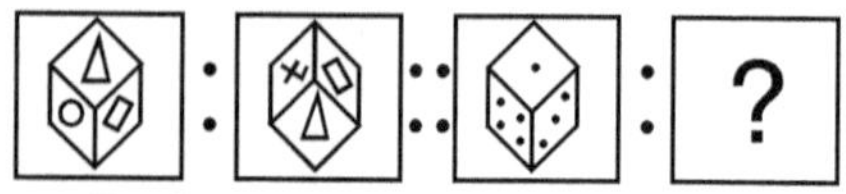

उत्तर आकृतियां

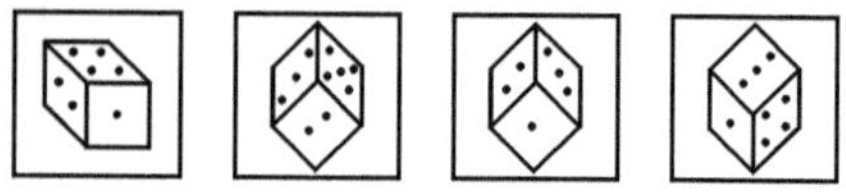

(*a*) (*b*) (*c*) (*d*)

5. प्रश्न आकृतियां

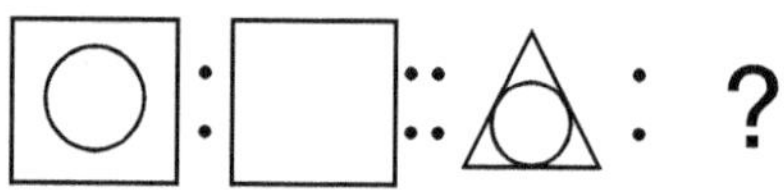

उत्तर आकृतियां

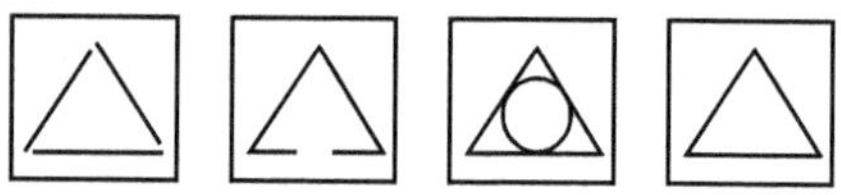

(*a*) (*b*) (*c*) (*d*)

6. प्रश्न आकृतियां

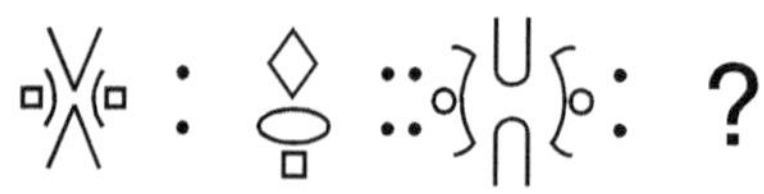

उत्तर आकृतियां

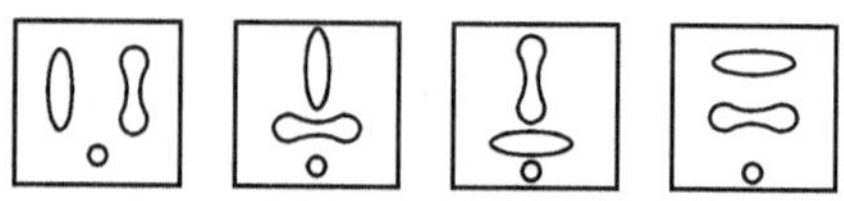

(*a*) (*b*) (*c*) (*d*)

7. प्रश्न आकृतियां

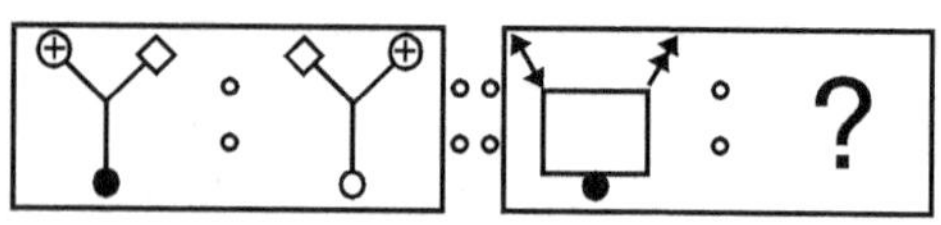

उत्तर आकृतियां

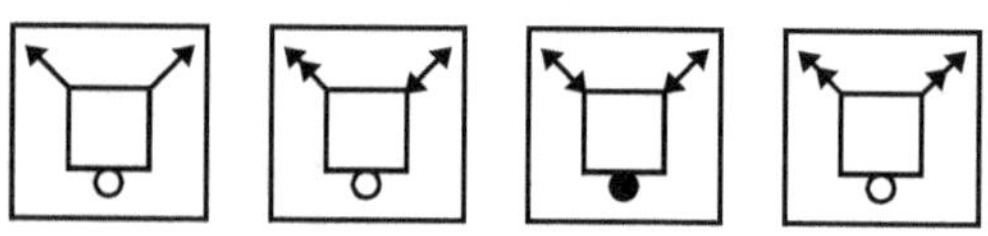

(*a*) (*b*) (*c*) (*d*)

8. प्रश्न आकृतियां

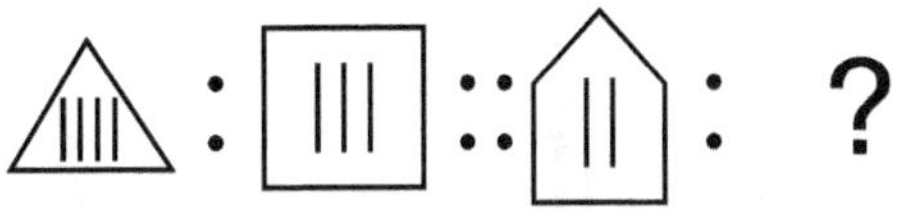

उत्तर आकृतियां

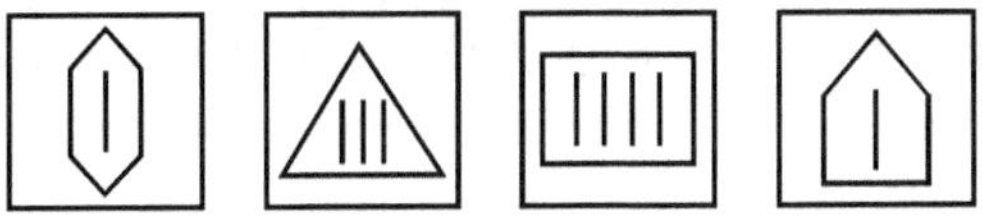

(*a*) (*b*) (*c*) (*d*)

9. प्रश्न आकृतियां

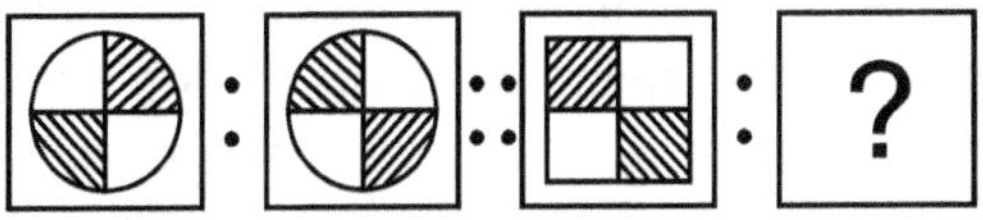

उत्तर आकृतियां

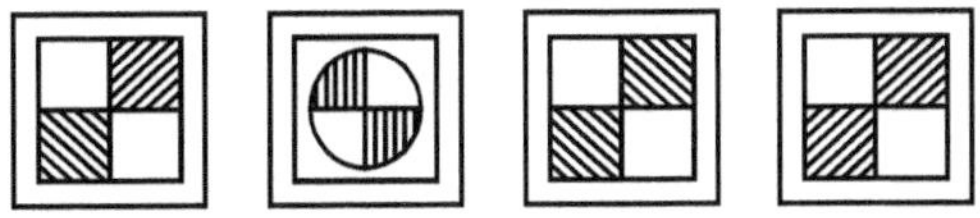

(*a*) (*b*) (*c*) (*d*)

10. प्रश्न आकृतियां

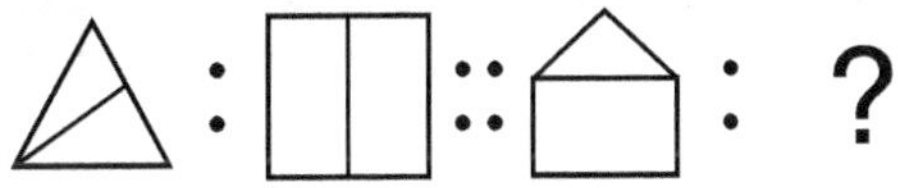

उत्तर आकृतियां

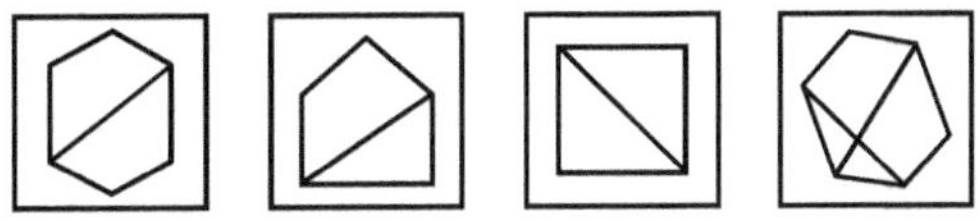

(*a*) (*b*) (*c*) (*d*)

व्याख्यात्मक उत्तर

1. (*d*) : पहली आकृति का त्रिभुज दूसरी आकृति में बीच में आ जाता है। इसी प्रकार शीर्ष पर जुड़े दो त्रिभुज भी उत्तर आकृति में बीच में आ जाते हैं।

2. (*d*) : पहली आकृति का संपूर्ण डिजाइन दूसरी आकृति में दक्षिणावर्त 90° के कोण से घूम जाता है और उसका एक अवयव लुप्त हो जाता है तथा रेखिका से जुड़े अवयव के परस्पर विपरीत दिशा वाले हिस्से छायांकित हो जाते हैं।

3. (*a*) : पहली आकृति से दूसरी आकृति में दाईं ओर नीचे का अवयव विकर्णतः सम्मुख कोने पर चला जाता है, बाईं ओर ऊपर का अवयव बड़ा हो जाता है और बीच में आ जाता है तथा बीच का अवयव छोटा होकर नीचे दाएँ कोने पर आ जाता है।

4. (*c*) : पहली आकृति से दूसरी आकृति में पाशे के फलक पर अंकित आकृति ऊपर से नीचे आ जाती है। दाहिनी ओर का डिजाइन अपरिवर्तित रहता है। जबकि बाईं ओर का डिजाइन बदल जाता है।

5. (*d*) : पहली आकृति में भीतर का अवयव दूसरी आकृति में लुप्त हो जाता है।

6. (*b*) : पहली आकृति के दो आधे अवयव दूसरी आकृति में ऊर्ध्वाधरतः पलट कर आपस में जुड जाते हैं और इस प्रकार निर्मित नया अवयव ऊपर शीर्ष पर पहुँच जाता है। पहली आकृति के दो क्षैतिजतः अवस्थित वक्र परस्पर जुड़कर एक नया अवयव निर्मित करते हैं और दूसरी आकृति में बीच में आ जाते हैं। पहली आकृति में दाएँ और बाएँ छोरों के दो सदृश अवयवों में से एक अवयव दूसरी आकृति में नीचे आ जाता है।

7. (*b*) : दूसरी आकृति में ऊपर के दो अवयव अपना स्थान बदल कर एक दूसरे के स्थान पर आ जाते हैं और वृत्त के भीतर का छायांकित भाग छायारहित हो जाता है।

8. (*a*) : पहली आकृति से दूसरी आकृति में एक ऊर्ध्वाधरतः रेखा कम हो जाती है और आकृति को निर्मित करने वाली रेखाओं की संख्या में एक की वृद्धि होती है।

9. (*a*) : पहली आकृति को वामावर्त 90° के कोण से घुमाने पर दूसरी आकृति प्राप्त होती है।

10. (*a*) : पहली आकृति से दूसरी आकृति में आकृति को निर्मित करने वाली रेखाओं की संख्या में एक की वृद्धि होती है।

विजातीय का चयन
(ODD-ONE OUT)

अभाषिक वर्गीकरण संबंधी तर्कबुद्धि परीक्षण विषयक प्रश्नों में आकृतियों का एक समूह दिया जाता है तथा अभ्यर्थियों से यह अपेक्षा की जाती है कि वे दी गई आकृतियों को उनके विशिष्ट गुणों या विशेषताओं के आधार पर अलग-अलग समूहों या वर्गों में वर्गीकृत करें। आकृतियों या मदों को उनकी बनावट, आकार, प्रतिरूप, संरचना, प्रकार, क्रम, रूप-रंग, कोटि, शैली, संघटक अवयवों और अन्य प्रकार की विशेषताओं में समानता के आधार पर समूहों या वर्गों में वर्गीकृत करना होता है और तत्पश्चात् उस समूह से भिन्न अर्थात् विजातीय आकृति की पहचान करनी होती है।

भाग–I

अभाषिक वर्गीकरण के इस प्रकार के प्रश्नों में प्रश्न आकृतियों और उत्तर आकृतियों के रूप में आकृतियों के दो समुच्चय नहीं दिए जाते बल्कि इनमें चार या पाँच आकृतियों का केवल एक ही समुच्चय दिया जाता है जिन्हें प्रश्न आकृतियाँ कहते हैं। इन प्रश्न आकृतियों में से एक आकृति शेष चार आकृतियों के समान या उनके सदृश नहीं होती। दूसरे शब्दों में तीन या चार आकृतियाँ किसी न किसी रूप में आपस में संबंधित होते हुए एक समूह बनाती हैं जबकि शेष केवल एक आकृति ही अन्यों से भिन्न अथवा विजातीय होता है जिसकी पहचान की जानी होती है।

हल किए गए उदाहरण

1.

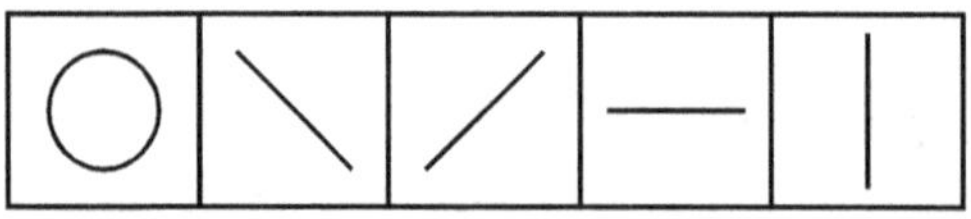

(*a*) (*b*) (*c*) (*d*) (*e*)

उत्तर (*a*)**:** दी गई आकृतियों में (*a*) एक वृत्त है जबकि (*b*), (*c*), (*d*) और (*e*) भिन्न-भिन्न दिशाओं को इंगित करने वाली सरल रेखाएं हैं। यहाँ ध्यान दें कि दी गई पाँच आकृतियों में से चार आकृतियों (*b*), (*c*), (*d*) और (*e*) में से प्रत्येक में एक सामान्य (सर्वनिष्ठ) विशेषता यह है कि ये सभी सरल रेखाएं हैं जो भिन्न-भिन्न दिशाओं को इंगित करती हैं, अतः ये चारों आकृतियां एक समूह या वर्ग निर्मित करती हैं। इन आकृतियों के विपरीत (*a*) एक वृत्त है जो अन्य आकृतियों से भिन्न अथवा विजातीय है।

अतः आकृति (*a*) समूह में शामिल न होने वाली आकृति अर्थात् एक विजातीय आकृति है।

2.

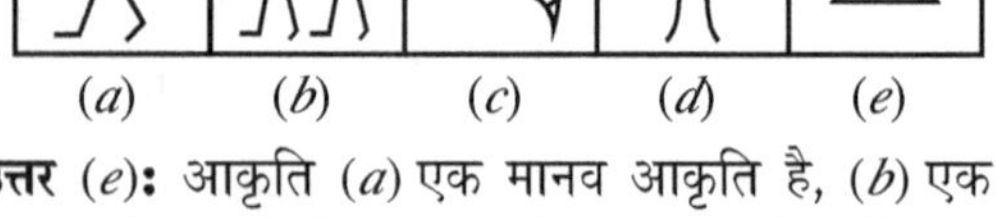

(*a*) (*b*) (*c*) (*d*) (*e*)

उत्तर (*e*)**:** आकृति (*a*) एक मानव आकृति है, (*b*) एक चौपाया पशु की आकृति है, (*c*) एक कीट, (*d*) एक पेड़ और (*e*) एक त्रिभुज है। इन पाँच अवयवों में से चार में एक सर्वनिष्ठ विशेषता है और वह यह है कि (*a*), (*b*), (*c*) और (*d*) (मानव, पशु, कीट और पेड़) सजीव जगत् से संबंधित हैं।

आकृति (*e*) एक त्रिभुज है और यह सजीव जगत् से संबंधित नहीं है। अतः आकृति (*e*) इस समूह में शामिल नहीं है।

अभ्यास

निर्देश (प्र.सं. 1–20): *नीचे के प्रत्येक प्रश्न में एक आकृति को छोड़कर अन्य सभी आकृतियाँ किसी-न-किसी रूप में आपस में संबंधित हैं और इस कारण वे एक समूह बनाती हैं। प्रत्येक प्रश्न में उस एक भिन्न आकृति का चयन करें जो अन्यों से संबंधित नहीं है अर्थात् जो भिन्न अथवा विजातीय है।*

1. 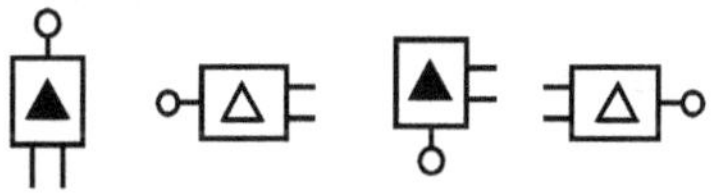

(*a*) (*b*) (*c*) (*d*)

2. 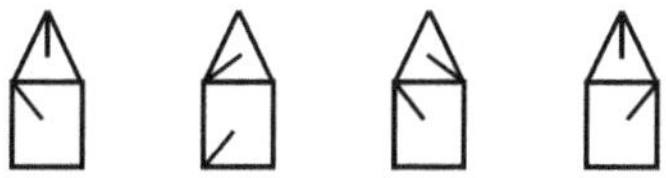

(*a*) (*b*) (*c*) (*d*)

3. 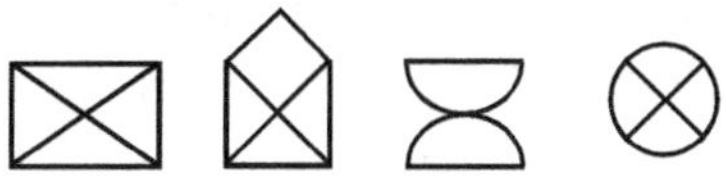

(*a*) (*b*) (*c*) (*d*)

4. 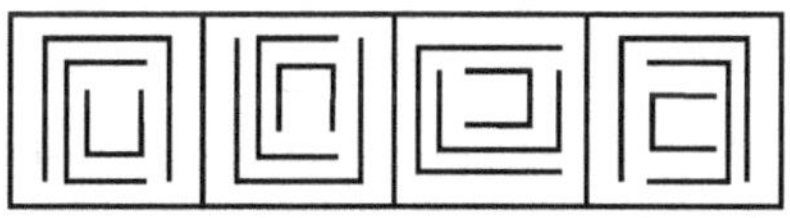

(*a*) (*b*) (*c*) (*d*)

5. 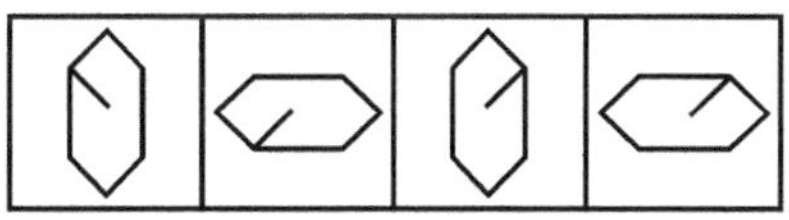

(*a*) (*b*) (*c*) (*d*)

6. 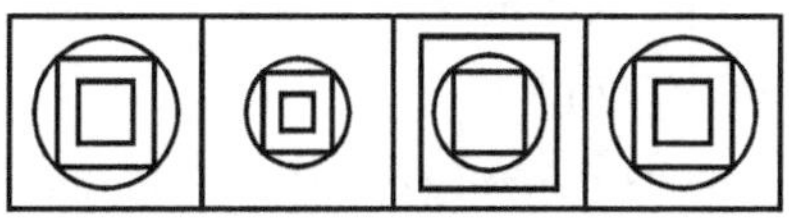

(*a*) (*b*) (*c*) (*d*)

7. 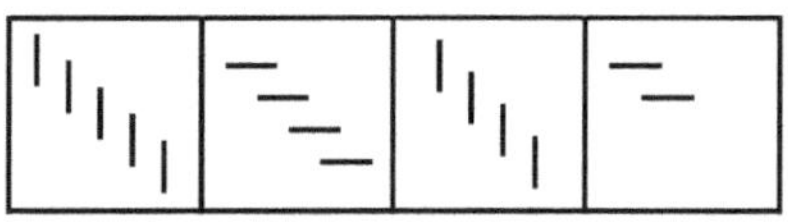

(*a*) (*b*) (*c*) (*d*)

8. 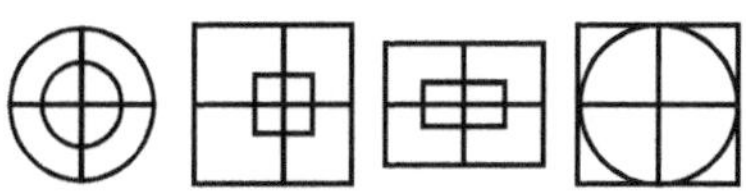

(*a*) (*b*) (*c*) (*d*)

9. 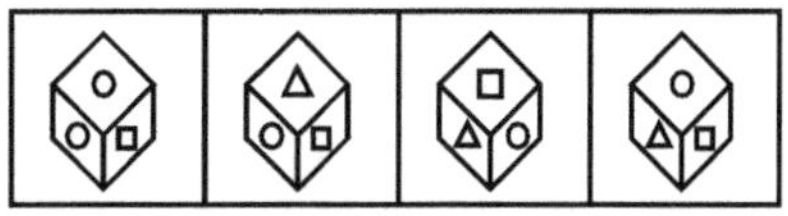

(*a*) (*b*) (*c*) (*d*)

10. 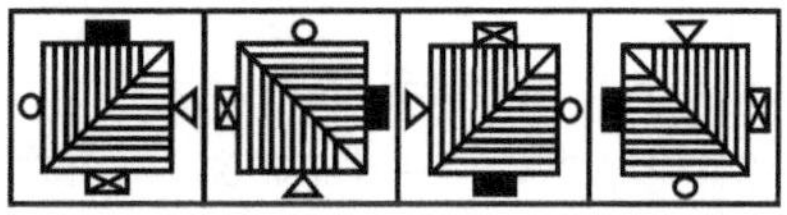

(*a*) (*b*) (*c*) (*d*)

11. 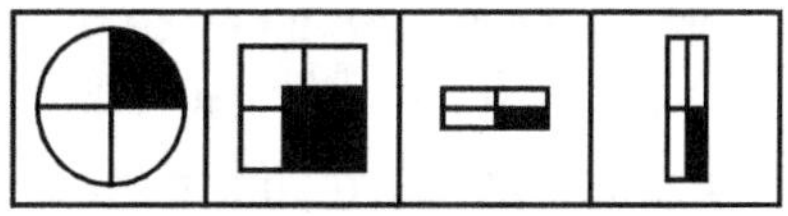

(*a*) (*b*) (*c*) (*d*)

12. 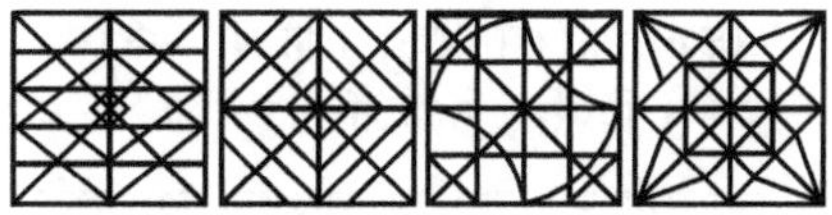

(*a*) (*b*) (*c*) (*d*)

13. 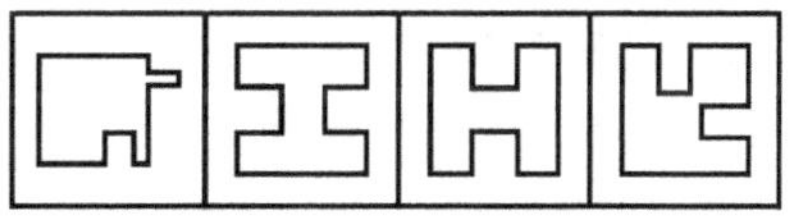

(*a*) (*b*) (*c*) (*d*)

14. 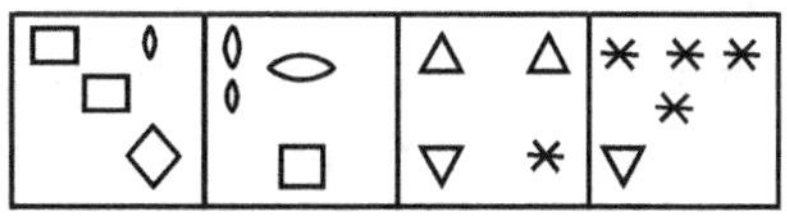

(*a*) (*b*) (*c*) (*d*)

15. 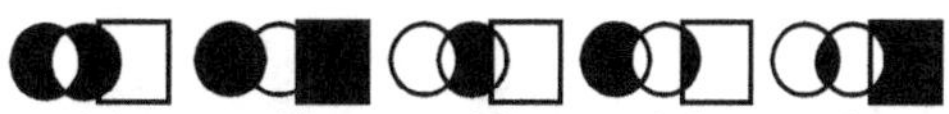

(*a*) (*b*) (*c*) (*d*) (*e*)

16. 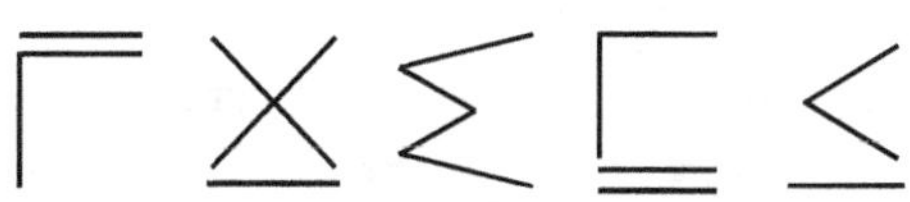

(*a*) (*b*) (*c*) (*d*) (*e*)

17. 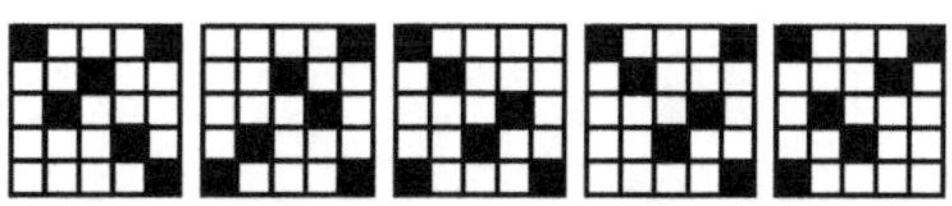

(*a*) (*b*) (*c*) (*d*) (*e*)

18. 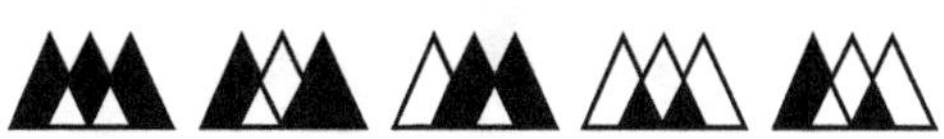

(*a*) (*b*) (*c*) (*d*) (*e*)

19. 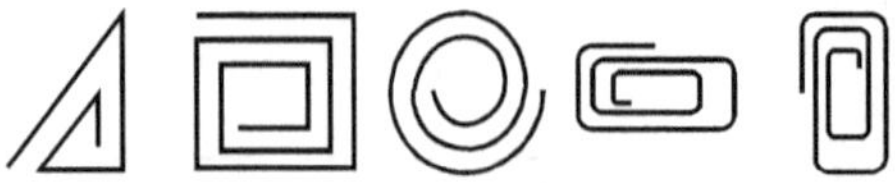

(a) (b) (c) (d) (e)

20. 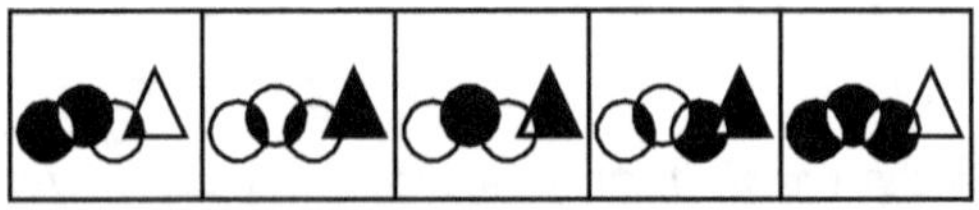

(a) (b) (c) (d) (e)

व्याख्यात्मक उत्तर

1. (*c*) : अन्य सभी आकृतियों में वृत्त युक्त रेखा और दो रेखाखंड वर्ग की सम्मुख भुजाओं पर अवस्थित हैं।

2. (*c*) : शेष सभी आकृतियों में एक रेखा के सिरों से एक ही दिशा में दो रेखाखंड खींचे जाते हैं। इस आकृति '(*c*)' में दो रेखाखंड दो विपरीत दिशाओं में खींचे जाते हैं।

3. (*c*) : शेष सभी आकृतियाँ चार भागों में विभक्त हैं।

4. (*d*) **:** केवल इसी आकृति में ही आकृति के मध्य में स्थित अवयव और दो अवयवों के बीच में स्थित अवयव परस्पर विपरीत दिशाओं में हैं।

5. (*c*) : शेष सभी आकृतियों को घुमा कर एक दूसरी आकृतियाँ प्राप्त की जा सकती हैं। इस आकृति में रेखाखंड गलत दिशा में है।

6. (*c*) : शेष सभी आकृतियों में बीच का और मध्यस्थ अवयव एक से हैं।

7. (*a*) : केवल इसी आकृति में रेखाखंडों की संख्या विषम है।

8. (*d*) : केवल इसी आकृति में दो अलग-अलग आकृतियाँ हैं जो दो समान भागों में विभाजित हैं।

9. (*a*) : केवल इसी आकृति में दो सदृश अवयव (वृत्त) निहित हैं।

10. (*c*) : शेष सभी आकृतियों को घुमाकर एक-दूसरी आकृतियाँ प्राप्त की जा सकती हैं।

11. (*b*) : शेष सभी आकृतियों में आकृति का केवल एक चौथाई भाग ही छायांकित है।

12. (*c*) : शेष सभी आकृतियों में वर्ग के सभी चारों खण्डों में एक जैसा पैटर्न है।

13. (*a*) : शेष सभी आकृतियों में वर्ग की दो भुजाओं पर कटान सदृश हैं।

14. (*d*) : केवल इसी आकृति में चार सदृश और एक भिन्न अवयव हैं। शेष सभी आकृतियों में तीन सदृश और एक भिन्न अवयव हैं।

15. (*d*) : आकृतियाँ (*a*) और (*e*) तथा आकृतियाँ (*b*) और (*c*) विपरीत युग्म निर्मित करती हैं। केवल आकृति (*d*) ही अकेला बचा रहता है।

16. (*c*) : अन्य सभी आकृतियाँ दक्षिणावर्त 90° के कोण से घूमी हुई रोमन संख्याएं हैं।

17. (*d*) : अन्य सभी आकृतियों में सदृश वर्ग ही छायांकित है। इस विकल्प में एक छायांकित वर्ग विकर्णतः सम्मुख कोने में है।

18. (*a*) : अन्य सभी आकृतियों में केवल दो रेखाखंड ही छायांकित हैं।

19. (*d*) : शेष सभी आकृतियों में पैटर्न (प्रतिरूप) को निर्मित करने वाली रेखाएं बाहर से भीतर की ओर दक्षिणावर्त खीची जाती हैं।

20. (*c*) : (*a*) और (*d*) तथा (*b*) और (*e*) आकृतियाँ सुमेलित विपरीत युग्म हैं। केवल आकृति (*c*) ही अकेली बच जाती है।

सामान्य सचेतता
(General Awareness)

हमारा भारत

भारत एक दृष्टि में

राजधानी-नई दिल्ली

क्षेत्रफल-32,87,263 वर्ग कि.मी.

क्षेत्रफल की दृष्टि से विश्व में स्थान-सातवां

स्थित-भूमध्य रेखा के उत्तर में 8°4′ और 37°6′ उत्तरी अक्षांश और 68°7′ तथा 97°25′ पूर्वी देशांतर के मध्य

विस्तार-उत्तर से दक्षिण तक 3,214 किमी., पूर्व से पश्चिम तक 2,933 किमी.

भूमि सीमा-15,200 किमी.

समुद्री तट-7,516.6 किमी.

सीमावर्ती देश-उत्तर-पश्चिम में पाकिस्तान और अफगानिस्तान, उत्तर में चीन, नेपाल और भूटान, पूर्व में म्यांमार और बंगलादेश, दक्षिण में मन्नार की खाड़ी और पाक-जलडमरूमध्य श्रीलंका से अलग करते हैं।

प्राकृतिक संरचना-मुख्य भूमि चार भागों में विभक्त–विस्तृत पर्वतीय क्षेत्र, सिंधु और गंगा के मैदान, रेगिस्तानी क्षेत्र, दक्षिणी प्रायद्वीप

प्रमुख नदियाँ-16–(क) हिमालय समूह : गंगा, यमुना, सिन्धु तथा ब्रह्मपुत्र; (ख) दक्षिणी नदियाँ : कृष्णा, कावेरी, गोदावरी, महानदी, दामोदर, भारत पुष्पा, नर्मदा, ताप्ती, पम्बा, पेरियार, पेण्णार, शरावती, नेत्रवती

जलवायु-ऊष्ण कटिबंधीय चार ऋतुएँ–शीत ऋतु, ग्रीष्म ऋतु, वर्षा ऋतु, शरद ऋतु

जीव-जंतु-लगभग 89,451 किस्म के

राष्ट्रीय उद्यान-103

वन्य जीव अभ्यारण्य-544

राजभाषा-हिन्दी, **मान्य भाषाएं-**22

उच्च न्यायालयों की संख्या-24

भारतीय संघ : राज्य व संघीय प्रदेश

संघ राज्य एवं संघीय प्रदेश	राजधानी	क्षेत्रफल (वर्ग कि॰मी॰)	भाषा
भारत	नई दिल्ली	32,87,263	हिन्दी-राजभाषा
		राज्य	
आंध्र प्रदेश	हैदराबाद	2,75,045	तेलुगू
असम	दिसपुर	78,438	असमिया
ओडिशा	भुवनेश्वर	1,55,707	ओडिया
उत्तर प्रदेश	लखनऊ	2,40,928	हिन्दी
केरल	तिरुवनन्तपुरम्	38,863	मलयालम
गुजरात	गांधीनगर	1,96,024	गुजराती
जम्मू-कश्मीर	श्रीनगर	2,22,236	कश्मीरी, उर्दू, डोगरी
तमिलनाडु	चेन्नई	1,30,058	तमिल
त्रिपुरा	अगरतला	10,492	त्रिपुरी, बंगला
नगालैण्ड	कोहिमा	16,579	अंग्रेजी, सेमा (सेमांग)
पंजाब	चण्डीगढ़	50,362	पंजाबी
प. बंगाल	कोलकाता	88,752	बांग्ला
बिहार	पटना	94,163	हिन्दी, मैथिली, भोजपुरी, मगही

मध्य प्रदेश	भोपाल	3,08,000	हिन्दी
महाराष्ट्र	मुम्बई	3,07,713	मराठी
मेघालय	शिलांग	22,429	खासा भारा
मणिपुर	इम्फाल	22,327	मणिपुरी, अंग्रेजी
राजस्थान	जयपुर	3,42,239	हिन्दी, मारवाड़ी
हरियाणा	चण्डीगढ़	44,212	हिन्दी
हिमाचल प्रदेश	शिमला	55,673	हिन्दी, पहाड़ी
कर्नाटक	बंगलुरू	1,91,791	कन्नड़
सिक्किम	गंगटोक	7,096	लेपचा, नेपाली, हिन्दी
मिजोरम	आइजल	20,987	मिजो, अंग्रेजी
अरुणाचल प्रदेश	ईटानगर	83,743	बिस्सी, वांची
गोवा	पणजी	3,702	कोंकणी, मराठी
छत्तीसगढ़	रायपुर	1,35,191	हिन्दी
झारखण्ड	रांची	79,714	हिन्दी, संथाली, बांग्ला तथा ओडिया
उत्तराखंड	देहरादून	53,483	हिन्दी, गढ़वाली, कुमायुँनी
तेलंगाना	हैदराबाद	1,14,840	तेलुगू
संघ शासित प्रदेश			
अण्डमान निकोबार द्वीप समूह	पोर्टब्लेयर	8,249	निकोबारी, हिन्दी
चण्डीगढ़	चण्डीगढ़	114	हिन्दी, पंजाबी
दिल्ली	दिल्ली	1,483	हिन्दी, पंजाबी
दमन-दीव	दमन	112	गुजराती
दादरा और नागर हवेली	सिलवासा	491	भीली, गुजराती
पुडुचेरी	पुडुचेरी	480	तमिल, हिन्दी
लक्षद्वीप	कावारत्ती	32	मलयालम

भारत की जनगणना 2011

भारत में जनगणना का विधिवत् कार्य 1881 में आरम्भ हुआ। 2011 की जनगणना (अंतिम) के अनुसार भारत की कुल जनसंख्या 121,08,54,977 थी। जबकि 10 वर्ष पूर्व 2001 में कुल जनसंख्या 102,70,15,247 थी। वर्ष 2011 की जनगणना के प्रमुख तथ्य निम्नलिखित हैं:

कुल जनसंख्या-121,08,54,977
पुरुष-62,32,70,258
महिला-58,75,84,719
कुल जनसंख्या में पुरुषों का प्रतिशत-51.53%
कुल जनसंख्या में महिलाओं का प्रतिशत-48.46%
भारत की जनसंख्या का विश्व जनसंख्या में भाग-17.5%
दशकीय वृद्धि दर (2001-2011)-17.7%
सर्वाधिक वृद्धि दर-मेघालय 27.9%
न्यूनतम वृद्धि दर-नगालैंड –0.6%
सर्वाधिक जनसंख्या वाला राज्य-उत्तर प्रदेश (19,98,12,341)
न्यूनतम जनसंख्या वाला राज्य-सिक्किम (6,10,577)
स्त्री-पुरुष अनुपात-943 : 1000
सर्वाधिक लिंगानुपात-केरल, 1084 : 1000
न्यूनतम लिंगानुपात-हरियाणा 879 : 1000
जनसंख्या घनत्व-382 व्यक्ति प्रति वर्ग किलोमीटर
सर्वाधिक घनत्व-बिहार (1,106)
न्यूनतम घनत्व-अरुणाचल प्रदेश (17)
केन्द्रशासित प्रदेशों में सर्वाधिक घनत्व-दिल्ली (11,320)
केन्द्रशासित प्रदेशों में न्यूनतम घनत्व-अण्डमान निकोबार द्वीप समूह (46)
साक्षरता प्रतिशत-73%
पुरुष साक्षरता-80.9%
महिला साक्षरता-64.6%
सर्वाधिक साक्षरता-केरल (94%)
न्यूनतम साक्षरता-बिहार (61.8%)

विभिन्न राज्यों में मिलने वाली जनजातियां

प्रदेश	जनजातियां
उत्तर प्रदेश, उत्तराखंड	बुक्सा, थारू, बिड़कोल, भोटिया, खरवार, जौनसारी, राजी
पश्चिम बंगाल, बिहार, झारखंड	संथाल, भुइया, कोरबा, उरांव, हो, विरहोर, असुर, मुंडा, कोल
राजस्थान	मीणा, भील, गरासिया, सहरिया, सांसी, दमोर, मेव, रावत, मेरात, कोली
अण्डमान-निकोबार द्वीप समूह	ओंग, सोपन, आरबा, अण्डमानी, निकोबारी
हिमाचल प्रदेश, जम्मू एवं कश्मीर	बकरवाल, गद्दी, गुर्जर, लाहौल लांबा, पंगवाला, किन्नर
असम, अरुणाचल प्रदेश, नगालैंड, मेघालय, मणिपुर	डफला, गुरूंग, रियांग, चकमा, मिनीपोंग, पासी, ग्लोंग, सिंगपो, रेंगमा, सेंगमा, यांग, नागा, गारो
मिजोरम	खासी
गुजरात	टोड़िया, भील, डाफर, रैवारी, पटेलिया, डूबला, कथोड़ी, सिद्दीस
केरल	कडर, इरुला, मुथुवन, कनिक्कर, मलनकुरावन, मलयारायन, मलावेतन, मलायन, मन्नान, उल्लातन, यूराली, पनियां, पुलायन, मल्लार, कुरुम्बा
तमिलनाडु, ओडिशा	जुवांग, खोंड, गोंड, बड़गा, बोंडो, जुआंग, परजा, भूमिज
महाराष्ट्र, आन्ध्र प्रदेश	भील, गोंड, अगरिया, असुरा, भारिया, कोया, वर्ली, कोली, डुका, बैगा, गडावास, कामर, खडिया, खोंडा, कोल, कोलम, कोरबा, मुन्डा
मध्य प्रदेश, छत्तीसगढ़	कोरकू, भील, बैगा, गोंड, अगरिया, भारिया, कोरबा, कोल, उरांव, प्रधान, नगेशिया, हल्वा, भतरा, माड़िया, सहरिया, कमार, कंवर
त्रिपुरा	लुभाई, माग, हलम, खशिया, भूटिया, मुन्डा, संथाल, भील, जमनिया, रियांग, उचाई
कर्नाटक	गौडालू, हक्की, पिक्की, इरुगा, जेनु, कुरुव, मलाईकुड, भील, गोंड, टोडा, वर्ली, चेन्चू, कोया, अर्नादन, चेरवा, होलेया, कोरमा
पंजाब	गद्दी, स्वांगला, भोट

विशेष दर्जा प्राप्त राज्य

राज्य	विशेष दर्जा प्राप्त करने का वर्ष	राज्य	विशेष दर्जा प्राप्त करने का वर्ष
असम	1969	त्रिपुरा	1972
नगालैंड	1969	सिक्किम	1975-76
जम्मू-कश्मीर	1969	मिजोरम	1986-87
हिमाचल प्रदेश	1971	अरुणाचल प्रदेश	1986-87
मणिपुर	1972	उत्तराखंड	2001-02
मेघालय	1972		

भारत में प्रथम

नोबेल पुरस्कार प्राप्तकर्ता

1. **साहित्यः** रवीन्द्रनाथ टैगोर (1913)
2. **भौतिकीः** सी॰वी॰ रमन (1929)
3. **शान्तिः** मदर टेरेसा (1979)
4. **अर्थशास्त्रः** अमर्त्य सेन (1998)

स्वतंत्र भारत के प्रथम एवं अंतिम भारतीय गवर्नर जनरल	चक्रवर्ती राजगोपालाचारी
महिला राष्ट्रपति	प्रतिभा पाटिल
महिला राज्यपाल	श्रीमती सरोजिनी नायडू
सुप्रीम कोर्ट की महिला न्यायाधीश	श्रीमती मीरा साहिब फातिमा बीबी
महिला प्रधानमंत्री	श्रीमती इंदिरा गांधी
भारतीय सेनापति	जनरल के॰ एम॰ करियप्पा
महिला मुख्यमंत्री	श्रीमती सुचेता कृपलानी
संयुक्त राष्ट्र महासभा की महिला अध्यक्ष	श्रीमती विजयालक्ष्मी पंडित (1954)
अंतर्राष्ट्रीय न्यायालय के भारतीय अध्यक्ष	डॉ॰ नगेन्द्र सिंह
इंगलिश चैनल तैरकर पार करने वाली भारतीय महिला	आरती गुप्ता
इंगलिश चैनल तैरकर पार करने वाला भारतीय पुरुष	मिहिर सेन
ब्रिटिश पार्लियामेंट के भारतीय सदस्य	दादा भाई नौरोजी
फील्ड मार्शल	एस॰एच॰एफ॰जे॰ मानेकशा
विक्टोरिया क्रॉस विजेता	खुदादाद खां
एवरेस्ट शिखर पर चढ़ने वाला भारतीय	शेरपा तेंजिंग (29 मई, 1953)
एवरेस्ट पर चढ़ने वाली भारतीय महिला	कु॰ बचेन्द्रीपाल (23 मई, 1984)
एवरेस्ट पर दो बार विजय प्राप्त करने वाली भारतीय महिला	संतोष यादव (10 मई, 1992; 10 मई, 1993)
भारतीय अंतरिक्ष यात्री (पुरुष)	राकेश शर्मा (3 अप्रैल, 1984)
भारतीय अंतरिक्ष यात्री (महिला)	कल्पना चावला (19 नवम्बर, 1997)
भारत रत्न से विभूषित महिला	श्रीमती इंदिरा गांधी
संयुक्त राष्ट्र संघ की महासभा में हिन्दी में भाषण देने वाला प्रथम भारतीय	अटल बिहारी वाजपेयी
भारतीय महिला मिस यूनिवर्स	कु॰ सुष्मिता सेन
भारतीय महिला मिस वर्ल्ड	रीता फारिया
समाचार-पत्र	बंगाल गजट (27 जनवरी, 1780)
डाक टिकट	1852
तार लाइन	1851 (कलकत्ता-डायमंड हार्बर)
रेल	16 अप्रैल, 1853 (बम्बई-थाणे)
विद्युत रेल	1925 (बम्बई-कुर्ला)
उपग्रह	आर्यभट्ट (1975)
रॉकेट	रोहिणी (1967)
आणविक रियेक्टर	अप्सरा (1956)
आणविक बिजलीघर	तारापुर आणविक बिजलीघर (1969)
भारतीय वायु सेना की महिला पायलट	हरित कौर देओल
फास्ट ब्रीडर आणविक रियेक्टर	कलपक्कम
बिना ऑक्सीजन एवरेस्ट की चोटी पर पहुंचने वाला भारतीय	फु दोरजी (1987)
मेट्रो रेलवे	कोलकाता (1984)

फिल्म (मूक)	राजा हरिश्चन्द्र (1913)
फीचर फिल्म (बोलती हुई)	आलम आरा (1931)
इंडियन नेशनल कांग्रेस की प्रथम महिला अध्यक्ष	श्रीमती एनी बेसेंट
इंडियन नेशनल कांग्रेस के प्रथम अध्यक्ष	व्योमेशचन्द्र बनर्जी (1888)
आई॰सी॰एस॰ में सफल होने वाला प्रथम भारतीय	सत्येन्द्र नाथ टैगोर

भारत में सबसे बड़ा/लम्बा/ऊँचा आदि

सबसे ऊंची चोटी*-के-2

सर्वाधिक आबादी वाला शहर-मुम्बई

सबसे लम्बी नदी-गंगा (2525 कि॰मी॰)

सबसे बड़ा राज्य (क्षेत्रफल में)-राजस्थान

सबसे बड़ा राज्य (आबादी में)-उत्तर प्रदेश

सबसे बड़ा पुल (सड़क)-असम में लोहित नदी पर भूपेन हजारिका सेतु (9.15 कि॰मी॰)

सर्वाधिक जनसंख्या घनत्व वाला राज्य-बिहार (1,106 प्रति वर्ग कि॰मी॰)

सर्वाधिक साक्षर राज्य-केरल (साक्षरता लगभग 94%)

सबसे बड़ा अजायबघर-इण्डिया म्यूजियम, कोलकाता

सबसे लम्बा बांध-हीराकुड (ओडिशा)

सबसे लम्बी सुरंग (रेलवे)-11.2 कि॰मी॰ (पीर पंजाल रेंज जम्मू-कश्मीर)

सबसे बड़ा चिड़ियाघर-जुलोजिकल गार्डन्स, कोलकाता

सबसे लम्बी सड़क-ग्राण्ड ट्रंक रोड (1500 मील)

सबसे ऊंची मीनार-कुतुबमीनार, दिल्ली (72.5 मी॰)

सबसे बड़ी मस्जिद-जामा मस्जिद, दिल्ली

बहादुरी के लिए सबसे बड़ा पुरस्कार-परमवीर चक्र

सबसे बड़ा रेगिस्तान-थार (राजस्थान)

सबसे बड़ा डेल्टा-सुन्दरवन डेल्टा, (75,000 वर्ग कि॰मी॰)

सबसे बड़ा गुम्बज-गोल गुम्बज (बीजापुर-42 मी॰ व्यास)

सबसे ऊँचा दरवाजा-बुलंद दरवाजा (फतेहपुर सीकरीः 176 फीट)

सबसे बड़ी मीठे पानी की झील-वुलर झील (कश्मीर)

सबसे बड़ा प्लेटफार्म-गोरखपुर (पूर्वोत्तर रेलवे)

सर्वाधिक वर्षा (वार्षिक औसत)-चेरापूंजी के निकट मासिनराम (12,000 मि॰मी॰)

झरना, सबसे ऊँचा-गरसोप्पा (कर्नाटक : 960 फीट)

सबसे बड़ा पशुओं का मेला-सोनपुर (बिहार)

सबसे बड़ा गुफा मंदिर-कैलाश मंदिर (एलोरा)

सबसे अधिक वन क्षेत्रफल वाला राज्य-मध्य प्रदेश

सबसे बड़ी कृत्रिम झील-गोविन्द सागर (भाखड़ा)

* विश्व की सबसे ऊंची चोटी मांउट एवरेस्ट है जो नेपाल में है। के-2 विश्व की दूसरी सबसे ऊँची और भारत की सबसे ऊँची (8611 मी॰) चोटी है।

✧✧✧✧✧

राष्ट्रीय प्रतीक

राष्ट्रीय ध्वज

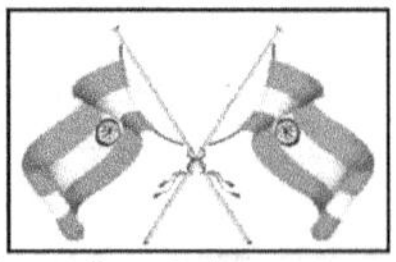

भारत का राष्ट्रीय ध्वज **तिरंगा** है। यह आयताकार तीन पट्टियों से बना है। इसमें सबसे ऊपर केसरिया, मध्य में श्वेत और नीचे हरा रंग है। केसरिया शक्ति, श्वेत शांति और हरा समृद्धि का प्रतीक माना जाता है। झण्डे की लम्बाई-चौड़ाई का अनुपात 3 : 2 है। श्वेत पट्टी के मध्य नीले रंग का एक चक्र है। चक्र में 24 तीलियाँ हैं। झण्डा फहराने के संबंध में भारत सरकार ने कुछ नियम बनाए हैं जिनका पालन करना अति आवश्यक है। संविधान सभा ने इसे 22 जुलाई 1947 को अंगीकार किया था।

राष्ट्रीय चिह्न

भारत का राष्ट्रीय चिह्न सारनाथ में अशोक निर्मित सिंह स्तम्भ की अनुकृति है। इस चिह्न में चार सिंह हैं, जो एक दूसरे के विपरीत दिशा में घूम कर बैठे हुए हैं। इन चार में से केवल तीन सिंह दिखाई देते हैं, चौथा पीछे की ओर छिपा हुआ है और दिखाई नहीं देता। नीचे चौरस पट्टी के मध्य में उभरी हुई नक्काशी में एक चक्र है, जिसके दाईं ओर एक सांड़ और बाईं ओर एक घोड़ा है। नीचे मुण्डकोपनिषद से लिया गया सूत्र 'सत्यमेव जयते' देवनागरी लिपि में लिखा गया है। इसका अर्थ है 'सत्य की ही विजय होती है'। सरकार ने राष्ट्रीय चिह्न को 26 जनवरी 1950 को स्वीकृत किया।

राष्ट्रीय गीत

श्री बंकिम चन्द्र चटर्जी द्वारा रचित गीत 'वन्दे मातरम्' को राष्ट्रीय गान के समकक्ष स्थान दिया गया है। उनके विख्यात उपन्यास 'आनन्द मठ' से उद्धृत यह गीत राष्ट्रीय आन्दोलन में एक महान प्रेरणा-स्रोत रहा है। इस गीत को सबसे पहले 1896 में भारतीय राष्ट्रीय कांग्रेस के अधिवेशन में गाया गया था।

राष्ट्रीय गान

रवीन्द्र नाथ टैगोर के गीत 'जन गण मन' को 24 जनवरी, 1950 को राष्ट्रीय गान के रूप में स्वीकार किया गया। यह गीत 'भारत-विधाता' शीर्षक से सर्वप्रथम 'तत्व-बोधिनी' पत्रिका के जनवरी 1912 के अंक में प्रकाशित हुआ था। यह गीत पहली बार 27 दिसम्बर 1911 को भारतीय कांग्रेस के कलकत्ता (कोलकाता) अधिवेशन में गाया गया था। पूरे गीत के 5 पद हैं। इसमें से प्रथम पद को राष्ट्रीय गान स्वीकार किया गया है। इसे गाने का निर्धारित समय लगभग 52 सेकण्ड है।

राष्ट्रीय पंचांग

सरकारी कार्यों में प्रयोग हेतु राष्ट्रीय पंचांग 22 मार्च, 1957 से अपनाया गया है। यह पंचांग शक संवत् पर आधारित है। 78 ई. में प्रारम्भ हुए शक संवत् का पहला महीना चैत्र है और वर्ष 365 दिन का है। इस पंचांग के दिन स्थायी रूप से ग्रेगेरियन कैलेंडर से सम्बद्ध दिनों के अनुरूप बैठते हैं। इस प्रकार सामान्य वर्षों में इस पंचांग का पहला दिन 22 मार्च के दिन आता है और लौंद (लीप) वर्ष में 21 मार्च के दिन।

राष्ट्रीय पंचांग के माह इस प्रकार हैं: 1. चैत्र, 2. बैशाख, 3.ज्येष्ठ, 4. आषाढ़, 5. श्रावण, 6. भाद्रपद, 7. आश्विन, 8. कार्तिक, 9. मार्गशीर्ष, 10. पौष, 11. माघ, 12. फाल्गुन।

राष्ट्रीय पशु : बाघ (पैंथरा टाइग्रिस-लिन्नायस)

राष्ट्रीय पक्षी : मोर (पावो क्रिस्टेटस)

राष्ट्रीय खेल : हॉकी

राष्ट्रीय पुष्प : कमल

✧✧✧✧✧

हमारी पृथ्वी

पृथ्वी सूर्य के अलावा आठ अन्य ग्रहों बुध, शुक्र, पृथ्वी, मंगल, बृहस्पति, शनि, यूरेनस और नेपच्यून वाले सौर मण्डल का एक सदस्य ग्रह है। ग्रहों के पास अपना स्वयं का प्रकाश नहीं होता और शुक्र और यूरेनस के अलावा सभी ग्रह अपनी धुरी पर पश्चिम से पूर्व की ओर परिक्रमा करते हैं। अनेक उपग्रह संबंधित ग्रह की परिक्रमा करते हैं। अंतरिक्ष में हजारों पुच्छल तारे और करोड़ों उल्काएं भी मौजूद हैं। पृथ्वी का एक ही उपग्रह है 'चन्द्रमा', शनि के पास 60 उपग्रह हैं जबकि बुध और शुक्र का कोई भी उपग्रह नहीं है। सूर्य से पृथ्वी की औसत दूरी 1,496 × 10^8 कि.मी. है। पृथ्वी सूर्य का तीसरा सबसे निकट और पांचवाँ सबसे बड़ा ग्रह है।

पृथ्वी : तथ्य और आँकड़े

पृथ्वी का द्रव्यमान	5.882 × 10^{21} टन
पृथ्वी का घनत्व	पानी की अपेक्षा 5.517 गुणा
पृथ्वी का आयतन	1.083 × 10^{11} घन किमी.
भूमध्यरेखीय परिधि	4.007 × 10^4 किमी.
ध्रुवीय व्यास	12,714 किमी.
विषुवतीय व्यास	12,756 किमी.
ध्रुवीय परिधि	4.0 × 10^4 किमी.
अनुमानित आयु	लगभग 4600 करोड़ वर्ष
भू-पृष्ठ	148,951,000 वर्ग किमी.
जलीय सतह	361,150,000 वर्ग किमी.
भू-सतह का सबसे उच्च बिन्दु	माउंट एवरेस्ट (8,848 मीटर)
भू-सतह का सबसे निम्न बिन्दु	मृत सागर का तट (समुद्र तल से 396 मीटर नीचे)
महासागर की सर्वाधिक गहराई	फिलीपींस के पूर्व में **प्रशान्त महासागर** में मेरियाना ट्रेंच (समुद्र तल से 11,033 मीटर नीचे)

सौरमण्डल

सबसे बड़ा ग्रह	बृहस्पति (Jupiter)
सबसे छोटा ग्रह	बुध (Mercury)
पृथ्वी का उपग्रह	चन्द्रमा (Moon)
सूर्य के सबसे निकट ग्रह	बुध (Mercury)
सूर्य से सबसे दूर स्थित ग्रह	वरुण (Neptune)
पृथ्वी के सबसे निकट स्थित ग्रह	शुक्र (Venus)
सबसे अधिक चमकीला ग्रह	शुक्र (Venus)
सबसे अधिक चमकीला तारा	साइरस (Dog Star)
सबसे अधिक उपग्रहों वाला ग्रह	बृहस्पति (Jupiter)
सबसे अधिक ठण्डा ग्रह	वरुण (Neptune)
सबसे अधिक गर्म ग्रह	शुक्र (Venus)
रात्रि में लाल दिखाई देने वाला ग्रह	मंगल (Mars)
सबसे बड़ा उपग्रह	गैनीमेड (Gannymede)
सबसे छोटा उपग्रह	डिमोस (Deimos)
नीला ग्रह	पृथ्वी (Earth)
भोर का तारा	शुक्र (Venus)
साँझ का तारा	शुक्र (Venus)
पृथ्वी की बहन	शुक्र (Venus)
हरा ग्रह	वरुण (Neptune)
विशाल लाल धब्बे वाला ग्रह	बृहस्पति (Jupiter)

पृथ्वी का आकार : पृथ्वी का आकार पूर्णरूप से वृत्तीय नहीं है बल्कि अंडाकार है। ऐसा इस वजह से है क्योंकि यह ध्रुवों पर चपटी और विषुवत पर उभरी हुई है। पृथ्वी का ध्रुवीय व्यास विषुवतीय व्यास से 42 किलोमीटर छोटा है। अत: पृथ्वी अंडाकार है।

पृथ्वी की गतियाँ : पृथ्वी अपनी धुरी पर किसी लट्टू की भांति घूमती है और 24 घंटे में एक चक्कर पूरा कर लेती है जबकि सूर्य की परिक्रमा करने में उसे 365 दिन, 5 घंटे, 45 मिनट और 46 सेकेंड लगते हैं। पृथ्वी की दैनिक गति के कारण रात और दिन होते हैं जबकि वार्षिक गति (परिक्रमा) के कारण ऋतु परिवर्तन होता है। पृथ्वी गैर-ज्योतिर्मय वृत्त है। पृथ्वी का जो भाग सूर्य के सामने आ जाता है वहाँ दिन होता है और जो भाग सूर्य के सामने नहीं होता वहाँ रात होती है। पृथ्वी का आवर्तन पश्चिम से पूर्व की तरफ होता है। इसी कारणवश हमें यह प्रतीत होता है कि सूर्य, चन्द्रमा और तारे विपरीत दिशा में घूम रहे हैं।

आवर्तन के प्रभाव : (क) दिन और रात होते हैं। (ख) देशांतर और समय में अंतर आ जाता है। (ग) वायु और तरंगों की दिशा में परिवर्तन होता है। (घ) दिन में दो बार समुद्र में लहरें उठती हैं।

परिक्रमा के प्रभाव : पृथ्वी दीर्घवृत्तीय कक्षा में सूर्य की परिक्रमा करती है। पृथ्वी को एक बार सूर्य का चक्कर लगाने में 365.25 दिन लग जाते हैं। एक सामान्य वर्ष 365 दिन का होता है जबकि चार वर्षों में 5 घंटे 45 मिनट और 46 सेकेंड एक दिन बना देते हैं और हर चौथा वर्ष अधि वर्ष (लीप ईयर) बन जाता है, जिसमें 366 दिन होते हैं। ऋतु में परिवर्तन मुख्यत: परिक्रमण की वजह से ही होता है।

21 जून : इस समय उत्तरी गोलार्द्ध में ग्रीष्मकाल होता है जबकि दक्षिणी गोलार्द्ध में शरदकाल होता है। दोपहर में सूर्य की सीधी किरणें कर्क रेखा पर पड़ती हैं।

22 दिसम्बर : इस समय उत्तरी गोलार्द्ध में शरदकाल और दक्षिणी गोलार्द्ध में ग्रीष्मकाल होता है। दोपहर में सूर्य की सीधी किरणें मकर रेखा पर पड़ती हैं।

सम्पात : 21 मार्च और 23 सितम्बर को पृथ्वी का प्रत्येक भाग सूर्य के सामने आ जाता है और सूर्य ठीक भूमध्य रेखा के ऊपर होता है। इन अवस्थाओं में पृथ्वी के प्रत्येक भाग में रात और दिन बराबर होते हैं। 21 मार्च को वसन्त सम्पात (Vernal equinox) और 23 सितम्बर को शरद सम्पात (Autumnal equinox) कहते हैं।

चट्टानों का रूपान्तरण

मूल चट्टान	रूपान्तरित चट्टान
शैल	स्लेट
चूना पत्थर	संगमरमर
चॉक तथा डोलोमाइट	संगमरमर
बलुआ पत्थर	क्वार्ट्जाइट
ग्रेनाइट	नीस
बेसाल्ट	सिस्ट
स्लेट	फाइलाइट
कांग्लोमरेट	क्वार्ट्जाइट

वायुमण्डल की संरचना

मण्डल	ऊँचाई (किमी)	विशेष तथ्य
क्षोभमण्डल	0-18	मौसमी घटनाएँ होती हैं।
समतापमण्डल	18-50	वायु परिवहन होता है तथा ओजोन परत पाई जाती है।
मध्यमण्डल	50-80	ऊँचाई के साथ तापमान में गिरावट होती है।
आयनमण्डल	80-640	विद्युत आवेशित कण पाए जाते हैं। रेडियो तरंगें इसी मण्डल से वापस पृथ्वी पर लौटती हैं।
बाह्यमण्डल	640 किमी से ऊपर	तापमान 5000ºC होता है।

✧✧✧✧✧

विश्व बोध

विभिन्न देशों के राष्ट्रीय प्रतीक

देश	प्रतीक
ऑस्ट्रेलिया	कंगारू
फ्रांस	लिली
ईरान	गुलाब
जापान	गुलदाउदी
यूनाइटेट किंगडम	गुलाब
कनाडा	सफेद लिली
जर्मनी	कार्न फ्लावर
आयरलैंड	तीन पत्ती वाली घास
पाकिस्तान	अर्द्धचंद्र
यू.एस.ए.	सुनहरी छड़ी
डेनमार्क	बुलिन
भारत	सिंह स्तम्भ
इटली	सफेद लिली
स्पेन	बाज

शहरों, राज्यों एवं देशों के परिवर्तित नाम

पुराना नाम	परिवर्तित नाम
एबिसीनिया	इथियोपिया
अंगोरा	अंकारा
औरंगाबाद	संभाजी नगर
बनारस	वाराणसी
बड़ौदा	बड़ोदरा
बताविया	जकार्ता
बसुतोलैण्ड	लिसोथो
बेचुआनालैण्ड	बोत्सवाना
बॉम्बे	मुम्बई
ब्रिटिश गुयाना	गुयाना
बर्मा	म्यांमार
कालीकट	कोझीकोड
कलकत्ता	कोलकाता
केप केनवरल	केप केनेडी
काउनपुर	कानपुर
सेंट्रल प्रोविंसेज	मध्य प्रदेश
अपर बोल्टा	बुर्कीना फासो
जुबुलपोर	जबलपुर
लियोपोलदविले	किन्हास
मेडागास्कर	मालागासी
मद्रास	चेन्नई
मलाया	मलेशिया
जुलन्धर	जालंधर
मंयुक्यिो	मंचूरिया
मैसोपोटामिया	इराक
सिलोन	श्रीलंका
क्रिस्टिना	ओस्लो
कांगो	जायरे
कांस्टेटिनपोल	इस्तान्बूल
डाका	ढाका
डहोमे	बेनिन
डच ईस्ट इंडीज	इंडोनेशिया
डच गुयाना	सूरीनाम
लोर सेई	पूर्वी तिमोर
एलिस आइसलैंड	तुवालू
फार्मोसा	ताइवान
गौहाटी	गुवाहाटी
गोल्ड कोस्ट	घाना
हालैण्ड	नीदरलैण्ड
रोडेशिया	जिम्बाब्वे
सैगोन	हो चिन मिन्ह सिटी
सेलिसबरी	हरारे
सैंडविच आइसलैंड	हवाईअन द्वीप
तंजानिका व जंजीबार	तंजानिया
सियाम	थाईलैंड
सिमला	शिमला
साउथ वेस्ट अफ्रीका	नामीबिया
स्पेनिस गुयाना	विषुवतीय गुयाना
न्यू हेब्रिडस	वनुआतु
उत्तरी रोडेशिया	जाम्बिया
न्यासालैण्ड	मालावी

पुराना नाम	परिवर्तित नाम
पंजिम	पणजी
पेट्रोगार्ड	लेनिनग्राड
पीकिंग	बीजिंग
पर्शिया	ईरान
पूना	पुणे
स्टालिनग्राड	वोल्गोगार्ड
सेंट पीट्सबर्ग	लेनिनग्राड
तंजौर	तंजावुर
यूनाइटेड प्रोविंसेज	उत्तर प्रदेश
यू.एस.एस.आर.	सीआईएस
विशाखापट्नम	विशाखापत्तनम
यूगोस्लाविया	सर्बिया
बंगलौर	बेंगलुरु
असम	असोम
उत्तरांचल	उत्तराखंड
पांडिचेरी	पुडुचेरी
पूर्वी पाकिस्तान	बांग्लादेश
रंगून	यांगून
मिस्त्र	संयुक्त अरब गणराज्य
उड़ीसा	ओडिशा

महत्त्वपूर्ण सीमा रेखाएं

- **डूरंड लाइन :** यह भारत और अफगानिस्तान के बीच सीमा के विभाजन को परिलक्षित करती थी। इसका सीमांकन सर मोर्टीमर डूरंड ने 1896 में किया था। **अब यह पाकिस्तान और अफगानिस्तान के बीच की सीमा रेखा है।**
- **हिंडेनवर्ग लाइन :** यह वह रेखा है जहां से विश्व युद्ध के दौरान जर्मनी की सेना वापस लौट गई थी। यह रेखा पोलैण्ड और जर्मनी के बीच की सीमा रेखा है।
- **मैकमोहन रेखा :** यह भारत और चीन के बीच सीमा रेखा है जिसका सीमांकन सर हेनरी मैकमोहन ने किया था।
- **मैगिनोट रेखा :** यह फ्रांस और जर्मनी के बीच सीमा रेखा है।
- **रेडक्लिफ रेखा :** यह भारत और पाकिस्तान के बीच सीमा रेखा है जिसका सीमांकन सर सिरिल रेडक्लिफ ने किया था।
- **17वां पैरेलल : यह उत्तरी एवं दक्षिणी वियतनाम के बीच की सीमा रेखा है।**
- **38वां पैरलल :** यह उत्तर और दक्षिण कोरिया के बीच सीमा रेखा है।
- **49वां पैरलल :** यह यू.एस. और कनाडा के बीच सीमा रेखा है।
- **अवूर निसे रेखा : यह रेखा पोलैण्ड और पूर्वी जर्मनी के बीच की सीमा रेखा है जो द्वितीय विश्व युद्ध में खींची गई थी।**
- **सिंगफ्रेड रेखा : प्रथम विश्व युद्ध में फ्रांस और जर्मनी के बीच की सीमा रेखा।**

विश्व के प्रमुख जल प्रपात

जल प्रपात	स्थान	ऊँचाई (मी॰)
एंजिल	वेनेजुएला	979 (यह कैरो नदी पर स्थित संसार का सबसे ऊँचा जल प्रपात है।)
योसेमाइट	कैलिफोर्निया	739
दक्षिण-मर्डाल्फोसेन	नार्वे	655
तुगेला	द॰ अफ्रीका	614
कुकवेनन	वेनेजुएला	610
सूथरलैंड	न्यूजीलैंड	580
रिब्बोन	कैलिफोर्निया	491
ग्रेट-कामारना	गुयाना	488
डेल्ला	कनाडा	440
गवार्नी	फ्रांस	422
जोग (गरसोप्पा)	भारत	255 (शरावती नदी पर स्थित इस जल प्रपात को महात्मा गाँधी जल प्रपात भी कहते हैं।)
नियाग्रा	कनाडा एवं अमेरिका की सीमा	120

विश्व की प्रमुख नहरें

नाम	स्थिति	स्थान
ईरी	ईरी झील और मिशीगन झील को जोड़ती है।	अमेरिका
सू नहर	सुपीरियर झील और ह्यूइन झील को जोड़ती है।	अमेरिका
कील नहर	उत्तरी सागर को बाल्टिक सागर से जोड़ती है।	जर्मनी
पनामा नहर	कैरीबियन सागर और प्रशांत महासागर	पनामा
स्वेज नहर	लाल सागर और भूमध्य सागर	मिस्र
मैनचेस्टर नहर	मैनचेस्टर एवं लिवरपूल के बीच	ग्रेट ब्रिटेन

विश्व की प्रमुख नदियाँ

नाम	उद्‌गम स्थल	गिरने का स्थान	लम्बाई (किमी)	प्रमुख स्थान
नील (विश्व की सबसे लम्बी नदी)	विक्टोरिया झील	भूमध्य सागर	6670	आस्वान बाँध व नासिर झील स्थित है।
अमेजन (आयतन की दृष्टि से विश्व की सबसे बड़ी नदी)	एण्डीज पर्वत	अटलांटिक महासागर	6448	
मिसीसिपी मिसौरी	अलास्का झील	मैक्सिको की खाड़ी	6300	पक्षीपाद डेल्टा बनाती है।
यांग्टिसीक्यांग	तिब्बत का पठार	चीन सागर	5494	
ह्वांग हो	कुललुन पर्वत	चीन की खाड़ी	4840	
कांगो / जायरे	लुआलिया और लुआपुआ का संगम	अटलाण्टिक महासागर	4800	विषुवत् रेखा को दो बार काटती है।
अमूर	शिल्का रूस, आरगून का संगम	टार्टइ स्ट्रेट	4510	चीन और रूस की सीमा बनाती है।
वोल्गा	बल्डाई पठार	कैस्पियन सागर	3700	यूरोप की सबसे लम्बी नदी
डेन्यूब	ब्लैक फॉरेस्ट	काला सागर	2820	बेलग्रेड, बुखारेस्ट, बुडापेस्ट और वियना शहर स्थित है।
सेंट लारेंस	आण्टेरियो झील	सेंट-लॉरेंस की खाड़ी	3058	नियाग्रा जल प्रपात स्थित है।
कोलोरेडो	ग्रैण्ड कंट्री	कैलीफोर्निया की खाड़ी	2333	ह्यूबर बाँध स्थित
नाइजर	गिनी	गिनी की खाड़ी	4800	तेल नदी कहलाती है।
मेकांग	तिब्बत का पठार	दक्षिण चीन सागर	4023	द.पू. एशिया की सबसे लम्बी नदी।
सिन्धु	मानसरोवर झील के पास	अरब सागर	3180	
ब्रह्मपुत्र	मानसरोवर झील	बंगाल की खाड़ी	2900	
डार्लिंग-मर्रे	ऑस्ट्रेलिया आल्पस	हिन्द महासागर	3720	ऑस्ट्रेलिया की सबसे बड़ी नदी।

विश्व की प्रमुख झीलें

झील का नाम	भौगोलिक क्षेत्र	क्षेत्रफल (वर्ग.किमी.)	विशेष तथ्य
कैस्पियन सागर	पूर्व सोवियत संघ तथा ईरान	3,94,299	खारे पानी की सबसे बड़ी झील
सुपीरियर झील	संयुक्त राज्य अमेरिका एवं कनाडा	82,414	ताजे पानी की सबसे बड़ी झील
विक्टोरिया झील	केन्या, युगाण्डा तथा तंजानिया	69,485	
अरल सागर झील	कजाकिस्तान एवं उज्बेकिस्तान	64,457	
ह्यूरन झील	संयुक्त राज्य अमेरिका तथा कनाडा	59,600	
मिशीगन झील	संयुक्त राज्य अमेरिका	57,800	
बैकाल झील	रूस	31,500	यह सबसे गहरी (1940 मी॰) झील है।

ग्रेट बेरियर झील	कनाडा	31,080	
ग्रेट स्लेव झील	कनाडा	28,438	
विनीपेग झील	कनाडा	24,341	
ओण्टेरियो झील	सं.रा. अमेरिका तथा कनाडा	19,529	
टिटिकाका	पेरू-बोलीविया	9,065	यह विश्व की सबसे ऊँची (3811 मी॰) झील है।
आयर झील	ऑस्ट्रेलिया	9,583	

विश्व की प्रमुख खाड़ियाँ

खाड़ी	क्षेत्रफल (वर्ग.किमी.)	खाड़ी	क्षेत्रफल (वर्ग.किमी.)
मैक्सिको की खाड़ी	15,44,000	हडसन की खाड़ी	12,33,000
अरब की खाड़ी	2,38,000	सेंट लॉरेन्स की खाड़ी	2,37,000
कैलिफोर्निया की खाड़ी	1,62,000		

महासागरों की प्रमुख जलधाराएं

जलधारा का नाम	प्रकृति	विशेष विवरण	महासागर का नाम
• उत्तरी विषुवतीय जलधारा	उष्ण अथवा गर्म		अटलांटिक महासागर
• गल्फस्ट्रीम धारा	उष्ण	हेटेरस अंतरीप तक इसे फ्लोरिडा धारा कहते हैं।	अटलांटिक महासागर
• कनारी धारा	ठंडी		अटलांटिक महासागर
• फ्लोरिडा की धारा	उष्ण		अटलांटिक महासागर
• लेब्राडोर की धारा	ठंडी		अटलांटिक महासागर
• बैंगुला की धारा	ठंडी		अटलांटिक महासागर
• फाकलैंड की धारा	ठंडी		अटलांटिक महासागर
• विपरीत भूमध्यरेखीय जलधारा	गर्म	इसे गिनी की धारा भी कहते हैं।	अटलांटिक महासागर
• उत्तरी भूमध्यरेखीय जलधारा	गर्म		प्रशांत महासागर
• क्यूरोसीवो जलधारा	गर्म	जापानी लोग इसे काली धारा भी कहते हैं।	प्रशांत महासागर
• कैलिफोर्निया जलधारा	ठंडी		प्रशांत महासागर
• पूर्वी ऑस्ट्रेलिया की जलधारा	गर्म	इसे न्यू साउथवेल्स की धारा के नाम से भी जाना जाता है।	प्रशांत महासागर
• अलास्का धारा	गर्म		प्रशांत महासागर
• दक्षिणी विषुवतीय जलधारा	गर्म		हिन्द महासागर
• मोजाम्बिक धारा	गर्म		हिन्द महासागर
• अगुलहास धारा	गर्म		हिन्द महासागर
• पश्चिमी ऑस्ट्रेलिया की धारा	ठंडी		हिन्द महासागर
• ग्रीष्मकाल मानसून प्रवाह	गर्म		हिन्द महासागर
• शीतकालीन मानसून प्रवाह	परिवर्तनशील		हिन्द महासागर

विश्व की प्रमुख जनजातियाँ

जनजाति	सम्बन्धित क्षेत्र/देश
माओरी	न्यूजीलैंड
बुशमैन	कालाहारी मरुस्थल (बोत्सवाना)
वेद्दा	श्रीलंका
बद्दू	अरब
आइनू	जापान
यूकाधिर	साइबेरिया
एस्कीमो	ग्रीनलैंड, कनाडा
मसाई	पूर्वी अफ्रीका
बोरो	ब्राजील
सेमांग	मलेशिया
जूलू	नेटाल (दक्षिण अफ्रीका)
खिरगीज	मध्य एशिया
रेड इंडियन	उ० अमेरिका
पिग्मीज	कांगो बेसिन
नीग्रो	मध्य एशिया
याइ	टुण्ड्रा प्रदेश

विश्व की प्रमुख भौगोलिक खोजें

1. **क्रिस्टोफर कोलम्बस**—प० द्वीप समूह (1492), द० अमेरिका (1498 ई०)
2. **जॉन कैवेट**—न्यूफाउण्डलैण्ड (1497 ई०)
3. **कोपरनिकस**—सौरमंडल (1540 ई०)
4. **केपलर**—ग्रहों की गति नियम (1600 ई०)
5. **मैगलन**—विश्व का भ्रमण, अटलांटिक के दक्षिण से प्रशांत महासागर की खोज (1519 ई०)
6. **वास्को-डि-गामा**—केप ऑफ गुड होप होकर भारत आगमन (1498 ई०)
7. **कैप्टन कुक**—हवाई द्वीप समूह (1770 ई०)
8. **फ्रिड्टजौफ नानसेन**—ग्रीनलैंड एवं उत्तरी ध्रुव का पहाड़ी भाग (1888 ई०)
9. **आर. एमण्डसन**—दक्षिणी ध्रुव पर पहुँचने वाला प्रथम व्यक्ति (1911 ई०)
10. **रॉबर्ट पियरे**—उत्तरी ध्रुव की खोज (1909 ई०)

विश्व के प्रसिद्ध स्थान

1. झुकी हुई मीनार : पीसा (इटली)
2. मर्डेका पैलेस : जकार्ता (इण्डोनेशिया)
3. रेड स्क्वायर, क्रेमलिन : मास्को
4. स्फिंक्स, पिरामिड : मिस्र
5. पोर्सलिन टावर : नानकिंग (चीन)
6. लोवर, एफिल टावर : पेरिस (फ्रांस)
7. पोटाला : ल्हासा (तिब्बत)
8. श्वेत डेगेन पैगोडा : रंगून
9. ओपेरा हाउस : सिडनी
10. ब्राडवे स्ट्रीट, स्टेच्यू ऑफ लिबर्टी, एंपायर स्टेट बिल्डिंग : न्यूयार्क (सं. रा. अमेरिका)
11. अल अक्सा, वेलिंग वाल, टेंपल माउंट : जेरूसलम (इजरायल)

विश्व के प्रमुख भौगोलिक उपनाम

उपनाम	देश
एण्टीलीज का मोती	क्यूबा
गगनचुम्बी इमारतों का नगर	न्यूयॉर्क (सं.रा.अमेरिका)
एटरनल सिटी (होली सिटी)	रोम
क्वेकर सिटी	फिलाडेल्फिया
चीन का शोक	ह्वांगहो नदी (पीली नदी)
निरंतर-बाही झरनों का शहर	क्विटो (इक्वेडोर)
शुगर बाऊल ऑफ द वर्ल्ड	क्यूबा
सात पहाड़ियों का नगर	रोम (इटली)
पर्ल ऑफ दी ऑरियण्ट	सिंगापुर
गार्डन सिटी	शिकागो
पूर्व का मोती	श्रीलंका
लैंड ऑफ मॉर्निंग काम	कोरिया
लैंड ऑफ थाउजेण्ड लेक्स	फिनलैंड
भूमध्यसागर का द्वार	जिब्राल्टर
लैंड ऑफ दी थाउजैंड एलीफैन्ट्स	लाओस
स्वर्णिम पैगोडा का देश	म्यांमार
सिटी ऑफ गोल्डन गेट	सैन फ्रांसिस्को
क्वीन ऑफ एड्रियाटिक	वेनिस (इटली)
पिलर्स ऑफ हरक्यूलिस	स्ट्रेट ऑफ जिब्राल्टर
श्वेत शहर	बेलग्रेड
पूर्व का मैनचेस्टर	ओसाका (जापान)
लिली का देश	कनाडा
होली लैंड	जेरूसलम (इजरायल)
सूर्योदय का देश	जापान
कॉकपिट ऑफ यूरोप	बेल्जियम

उपनाम	देश
आंसुओं का प्रवेश द्वार	बाब-अल-मंडब जलडमरूमध्य
लैंड ऑफ मिडनाइट सन	नार्वे
अरब सागर की रानी	कोच्चि (भारत)
लैंड ऑफ ह्वाइट एलीफैंट्स	थाइलैंड
दक्षिण का ब्रिटेन	न्यूजीलैंड
वेनिस ऑफ द वर्ल्ड	स्टॉकहोम (स्वीडन)
स्मारकों की नगरी	वियना (ऑस्ट्रिया)
पवनचक्कियों की भूमि	नीदरलैण्ड
आइलैंड ऑफ क्लोव्ज	जंजीवार (तंजानिया)
फॉरबिडन सिटी	ल्हासा (तिब्बत)
नील नदी का देश	मिस्र
एमराल्ड द्वीप	आयरलैंड
लैंड ऑफ थंडरवोल्ट	भूटान
मोतियों का द्वीप	बहरीन

नदियों के तट पर बसे विश्व के प्रमुख नगर

नगर	नदी
लन्दन (इंग्लैंड)	टेम्स
कैन्टन (चीन)	सीक्यांग
मास्को (रूस)	मस्कोवा
न्यूयार्क (सं.रा.अ.)	हडसन
बर्लिन (जर्मनी)	स्प्री
बेलग्रेड	डेन्यूब
पेरिस (फ्रांस)	सीन
बुडापेस्ट (हंगरी)	डेन्यूब
पर्थ (ऑस्ट्रेलिया)	स्वान
वाशिंगटन	पोटोमेक
बगदाद (इराक)	टाइग्रिस
वियाना (ऑस्ट्रिया)	डेन्यूब
आस्वान (मिस्र)	नील
टोकियो (जापान)	अराकावा
सेंट लुईस (अमेरिका)	मिसिसिपी
शंघाई (चीन)	यांग्टिसीक्यांग
रोम (इटली)	टाइबर
रंगून (म्यांमार)	इरावदी
प्राग	वितावा
ओटावा (कनाडा)	सेंट लारेंस
सिडनी (ऑस्ट्रेलिया)	डार्लिंग
मैड्रिड (स्पेन)	मैजेनसेस
लिस्बन	टेगस
लिस्बन (पुर्तगाल)	टंगस
अंकारा (तुर्की)	किजिल
लाहौर (पाकिस्तान)	रावी
मॉण्ट्रियल (कनाडा)	सेंट लारेंस
कराची (पाकिस्तान)	सिंधु
बोन (जर्मनी)	राइन
डबलिन (आयरलैंड)	लीफें
काहिरा (मिस्र)	नील
दिल्ली (भारत)	यमुना
ब्यूनस आयर्स (अर्जेंटीना)	लाप्लाटा
शिकागो (सं.रा.अ.)	शिकागो
लिवरपुल (इंग्लैंड)	मर्सी
ब्रिस्टल (इंग्लैंड)	एवन्
बसरा (इराक)	दजला एवं फरात
कीव (रूस)	नीपर

विश्व के प्रमुख घास के मैदान

घास के मैदान	सम्बन्धित देश
पम्पास	अर्जेन्टीना
प्रेयरी	अमेरिका
वेल्ड	दक्षिण अफ्रीका
डाउन्स	ऑस्ट्रेलिया
केन्टरबरी	न्यूजीलैण्ड
स्टेपी	यूरेशिया

प्रमुख देशों में स्थानान्तरित कृषि

कृषि	देश
चेन्ना	श्रीलंका
हुमा	जावा
कैंगिन	फिलीपीन्स
लैडान	इण्डोनेशिया एवं मलेशिया
रोका	ब्राजील
तमाराई	थाइलैण्ड
कोनुको	वेनेजुएला

✧✧✧✧✧

संयुक्त राष्ट्र संघ

स्थापना	:	24 अक्टूबर, 1945
संस्थापक सदस्य	:	50
मुख्यालय	:	न्यूयार्क
वर्तमान सदस्य संख्या	:	193 (इस संगठन का सदस्य बनने वाला अन्तिम देश दक्षिण सूडान है)।
ध्वज	:	ध्वज की पृष्ठभूमि हल्की नीली है और उस पर श्वेत रंग से राष्ट्र संघ का प्रतीक बना हुआ है।
कार्यकारी भाषाएँ	:	अंग्रेजी तथा फ्रेंच
अन्य मान्यता प्राप्त भाषाएँ	:	रशियन, अरबी, स्पेनिश तथा चीनी।

संयुक्त राष्ट्र संघ के लक्ष्य और उद्देश्य

संयुक्त राष्ट्र के कार्यों को तीन भागों में विभाजित किया जा सकता है, यथा–सुरक्षा, कल्याण और मानव अधिकार। संयुक्त राष्ट्र संघ के सदस्य-राष्ट्रों से चार कर्त्तव्यों के पालन की अपेक्षा की जाती है कि–(क) वे अपने विवादों को शांतिपूर्वक ढंग से निपटायेंगे, (ख) वे सैन्यबल का प्रयोग नहीं करेंगे, (ग) घोषणा-पत्र के पालन में सहायता करेंगे और (घ) आक्रामक की सहायता नहीं करेंगे। संयुक्त राष्ट्र संघ–जाति, भाषा, लिंग और धर्म का विचार किए बिना सब मनुष्यों के मानवीय अधिकारों को मान्यता देता है।

संयुक्त राष्ट्र संघ के प्रमुख अंग

प्रमुख अंग 6 हैं–**1.** साधारण महासभा, **2.** सुरक्षा परिषद्, **3.** आर्थिक व सामाजिक परिषद्, **4.** अंतर्राष्ट्रीय न्यायालय, **5.** प्रन्यास परिषद्, **6.** सचिवालय

प्रमुख अंतर्राष्ट्रीय संगठनों के मुख्यालय और स्थापना वर्ष

अंतर्राष्ट्रीय संगठन	मुख्यालय	स्थापना वर्ष
संयुक्त राष्ट्र संघ (UNO)	न्यूयार्क	1945
अंतर्राष्ट्रीय मुद्रा कोष (IMF)	वाशिंगटन	1945
विश्व स्वास्थ्य संगठन (WHO)	जेनेवा	1948
खाद्य एवं कृषि संगठन (FAO)	रोम	1943
अंतर्राष्ट्रीय श्रम संगठन (ILO)	जेनेवा	1919
यूनेस्को (UNESCO)	पेरिस	1946
अंतर्राष्ट्रीय न्यायालय	हेग	––
विश्व डाक संघ (UPU)	बर्न	1875
अंतर्राष्ट्रीय नागरिक उड्डयन संगठन (ICAO)	मांट्रियल	1944

अंतर्राष्ट्रीय संगठन	मुख्यालय	स्थापना वर्ष
सं॰ रा॰ औद्यो॰ विकास संगठन (UNIDO)	वियना	1967
अंतर्राष्ट्रीय परमाणु ऊर्जा अभिकरण (IAEA)	वियना	1957
अंतर्राष्ट्रीय वित्त निगम (IFC)	वाशिंगटन	1956
सं॰ रा॰ विकास कार्यक्रम (UNDP)	--	--
यूनिसेफ (UNICEF)	--	1946
अंतर्राष्ट्रीय समुद्री संगठन (IMO)	लंदन	1948
विश्व मौसम विज्ञान संगठन (WMO)	जेनेवा	1950
अंतर्राष्ट्रीय दूर संचार संघ (ITU)	जेनेवा	1932
अरब लीग	कैरो	1945
राष्ट्रमंडल (Commonwealth)	लंदन	1946
विश्व व्यापार संगठन (WTO)	जेनेवा	1995
अंतर्राष्ट्रीय विकास संघ (IDA)	--	1960
अंतर्राष्ट्रीय पुनर्निर्माण एवं विकास बैंक (विश्व बैंक) (IBRD)	वाशिंगटन	1945
विश्व बौद्धिक संपदा संगठन (WIPO)	जेनेवा	1967
मुस्लिम राष्ट्रों का संघ (OIC)	जेद्दा	1969
यूरोपीय आर्थिक समुदाय (EEC)	जेनेवा	1957
रेडक्रास	जेनेवा	1863
इंटरपोल (INTERPOL)	लियोन	1923
एशियाई विकास बैंक (ADB)	मनीला	1966
उत्तरी अटलांटिक संधि संगठन (NATO)	ब्रुसेल्स	1949
आसियान (ASEAN)	जकार्ता	1967
BRICS बैंक	शंघाई	2014

✧✧✧✧✧

भारत का भूगोल

प्रसिद्ध पर्वत शिखर

पर्वत शिखर	समुद्र तल से ऊंचाई (मीटर में)
1. K-2	8,611 पाकिस्तान के कब्जे में
2. कंचनजंगा	8,598
3. नंगा पर्वत	8,126
4. गशेर ब्रुम	8,068 पाकिस्तान के कब्जे में
5. ब्रॉड पीक	8,047 पाकिस्तान के कब्जे में
6. डिस्तगिल सर	7,885 पाकिस्तान के कब्जे में
7. माशेर ब्रुम (पूर्वी)	7,821
8. नंदा देवी	7,817
9. माशेर ब्रुम (पश्चिम)	7,806 पाकिस्तान के कब्जे में
10. राकापोशी	7,788 पाकिस्तान के कब्जे में

भारत के प्रमुख दर्रे

दर्रे	राज्य
काराकोरम	जम्मू-कश्मीर
माना	उत्तराखण्ड
जोजिला	जम्मू-कश्मीर
नीति	उत्तराखण्ड
पीरपंजाल	जम्मू-कश्मीर
नाथूला	सिक्किम
बनिहाल	जम्मू-कश्मीर
जैलेप्ला	सिक्किम
बुर्जिल	जम्मू-कश्मीर
बोम्डिला	अरुणाचल प्रदेश
शिपकी	हिमाचल प्रदेश
यांग्याप	अरुणाचल प्रदेश
रोहतांग	हिमाचल प्रदेश
दिफू	अरुणाचल प्रदेश
बड़ालाचा	हिमाचल प्रदेश
तुजु	मणिपुर
लिपुलेख	उत्तराखण्ड

पश्चिमी घाट के दर्रे

दर्रा	ऊं. (मी.)	स्थिति
थालघाट	580	नासिक एवं मुम्बई के बीच का संपर्क मार्ग
भोरघाट	520	मुम्बई एवं पुणे के बीच का संपर्क मार्ग
पालघाट	530	कोयंबटूर एवं कोचीन के बीच का संपर्क मार्ग
सिनकोट	280	त्रिवेन्द्रम एवं मदुरै के बीच का संपर्क मार्ग

प्रमुख जल–अन्तराल

नाम	अवस्थिति
8° चैनल	मालदीव व मिनीकॉय के मध्य
9° चैनल	लक्षद्वीप व मिनीकॉय के मध्य
10° चैनल	छोटा अंडमान व कारनिकोबार के मध्य
ग्रैण्ड चैनल	सुमात्रा (इंडोनेशिया) व निकोबार के मध्य
पाक स्ट्रेट	तमिलनाडु व श्रीलंका के मध्य
डुंकन पास	दक्षिण अंडमान व लघु अंडमान के मध्य
पाक खाड़ी	तमिलनाडु व श्रीलंका के मध्य
कोको स्ट्रेट	काको द्वीप (म्यांमार) व उ. अंडमान के मध्य
मन्नार खाड़ी	द.पू. तमिलनाडु व श्रीलंका के मध्य
लक्षद्वीप सागर	लक्षद्वीप व मालाबार तट के मध्य

भारत की महत्वपूर्ण झीलें

झीलें	राज्य
चिल्का	ओडिशा
कोलेरू, पुलीकट	आन्ध्र प्रदेश
लोकटक	मणिपुर
सुकना	चण्डीगढ़
लोनार	महाराष्ट्र
निजाम सागर	हैदराबाद
उमियम झील	मेघालय
नैनीताल, भीमताल	उत्तराखंड
वुलर, डल, पोगांग शो	जम्मू-कश्मीर
पुल्ह झील	उत्तर प्रदेश
अष्टमुदी	केरल
परशुराम कुण्ड	अरुणाचल प्रदेश

भारत की प्रमुख नदियाँ

नदी	उद्गम	मुहाना	लम्बाई (किमी.)	विशेष तथ्य
सिन्धु	मानसरोवर झील (तिब्बत)	अरब सागर	3100 (भारत में 1114)	सतलज, रावी, व्यास, झेलम इसकी सहायक नदियाँ हैं। लद्दाख में यह नदी गिलगित गॉर्ज का निर्माण करती है।
सतलज	राक्षसताल	चिनाब	1450 (भारत में 1050)	भाखड़ा, नांगल व नाथपा झांकरी बाँध।
गंगा	गंगोत्री के पास गोमुख से	बंगाल की खाड़ी	2525	देव प्रयाग में भागीरथी अलकनंदा से मिलती है और संयुक्त धारा का नाम गंगा हो जाता है। फरक्का बाँध एवं भागीरथी पर टिहरी बाँध।
यमुना	यमुनोत्री के पास बंदरपूंछ से	गंगा	1376	चम्बल, बेतवा, केन सहायक नदियाँ हैं।
चम्बल	महूँ (जानपाव पहाड़ी)	यमुना	1050	गाँधीनगर, राणासागर तथा जवाहर सागर बाँध स्थित है।
गण्डक	धौलाधार पर्वत	गंगा	300	त्रिवेणी के पास बाँध
सोन	अमरकंटक पहाड़ी	गंगा	784	बाणसागर व रिहन्द बाँध
ब्रह्मपुत्र	मानसरोवर झील (तिब्बत)	बंगाल की खाड़ी	2900 (भारत में 916)	ब्रह्मपुत्र नदी अरुणाचल प्रदेश में दिहांग, तिब्बत में शांग-पो और बांग्लादेश में 'जमुना' के नाम से प्रसिद्ध।
नर्मदा	अमरकंटक	अरब सागर	1290	इंदिरा सागर, महेश्वर, सरदार सरोवर बाँध। डेल्टा के बजाए एश्चुअरी बनाती है।
ताप्ती	मुलताई (बैतूल)	खम्भात की खाड़ी	720	काकरापार व ऊकाई बाँध/यह नदी डेल्टा के बजाए एश्चुअरी बनाती है।
महानदी	सिहावा के समीप	बंगाल की खाड़ी	890	हीराकुड, तिरकपाड़ा बाँध स्थित है, डेल्टा बनाती है।
कृष्णा	पश्चिमी घाट की पहाड़ी (महाबलेश्वर के पास)	बंगाल की खाड़ी	1290	शैलम तथा नागार्जुन सागर बाँध स्थित है। डेल्टा बनाती है।
गोदावरी	त्रयम्बक गाँव की पहाड़ी	बंगाल की खाड़ी	1450	दक्षिण की गंगा कहा जाता है। एनीकट बाँध स्थित है। डेल्टा बनाती है।
कावेरी	ब्रह्मगिरि की पहाड़ी	बंगाल की खाड़ी	760	शिवसमुद्रम जल प्रपात स्थित है। डेल्टा बनाती है।
तुंगभद्रा	कर्नाटक के पश्चिमी घाट	कृष्णा	331	कुमुदवती, वर्धा, मगारी आदि सहायक नदियाँ हैं।
माही	विन्ध्याचल पर्वत	खम्भात की खाड़ी	533	वनकवोरी बाँध।

भारत के महत्वपूर्ण जल प्रपात

जल प्रपात	ऊँचाई (मी.)	नदी	राज्य
शिवसमुद्रम	90	कावेरी	कर्नाटक
गरसोप्पा	260	शरावती	कर्नाटक
हुण्डरू	–	स्वर्णरेखा	झारखण्ड
केवटी	98	महाना	मध्य प्रदेश
रकीमकुण्ड	168	गायघाट	बिहार

नदियों के किनारे बसे प्रमुख नगर

नगर	नदी	नगर	नदी
दिल्ली	यमुना	गुवाहाटी	ब्रह्मपुत्र
आगरा	यमुना	जबलपुर	नर्मदा
बद्रीनाथ	अलकनंदा	कोटा	चम्बल
इलाहाबाद	गंगा, यमुना	कटक	महानदी
हरिद्वार	गंगा	नासिक	गोदावरी
कानपुर	गंगा	श्रीरंगपट्टनम	कावेरी
पटना	गंगा	जौनपुर	गोमती
श्रीनगर	झेलम	हैदराबाद	मूसी
अयोध्या	सरयु	मथुरा	यमुना
सूरत	ताप्ती	जमशेदपुर	स्वर्णरेखा
कोलकाता	हुगली	भागलपुर	गंगा
लखनऊ	गोमती	वाराणसी	गंगा
उज्जैन	क्षिप्रा		

प्रमुख बहुउद्देशीय नदी घाटी परियोजनाएँ

परियोजना का नाम	नदी	लाभान्वित राज्य
दामोदर घाटी परियोजना	दामोदर	झारखंड, पश्चिम बंगाल
टिहरी बाँध परियोजना	भागीरथी	उत्तराखंड
नागार्जुन सागर परियोजना	कृष्णा	आन्ध्र प्रदेश
कोसी परियोजना	कोसी	बिहार तथा नेपाल
हीराकुड बाँध परियोजना	महानदी	ओडिशा
व्यास परियोजना	व्यास	राजस्थान, पंजाब, हरियाणा, हिमाचल प्रदेश
चम्बल परियोजना	चम्बल	राजस्थान, मध्य प्रदेश
मयूराक्षी परियोजना	मयूराक्षी	पश्चिम बंगाल
तुंगभद्रा परियोजना	तुंगभद्रा	आन्ध्र प्रदेश, कर्नाटक
गण्डक परियोजना	गण्डक	बिहार, नेपाल
फरक्का परियोजना	गंगा, भागीरथी	पश्चिम बंगाल
काकरापारा परियोजना	ताप्ती	गुजरात
नागपुर शक्तिगृह परियोजना	कोराडी	महाराष्ट्र
इन्दिरा गाँधी नहर परियोजना	सतलज	राजस्थान, पंजाब तथा हरियाणा
रिहन्द परियोजना	रिहन्द	उत्तर प्रदेश
महानदी डेल्टा परियोजना	महानदी	ओडिशा
कुण्डा परियोजना	कुण्डा	तमिलनाडु
इडुक्की परियोजना	पेरियार	केरल
कोयना परियोजना	कोयना	महाराष्ट्र
सतलज परियोजना	चिनाब	जम्मू-कश्मीर
रंजीत सागर बाँध परियोजना	रावी	पंजाब
नाथपा-झाकरी परियोजना	सतलज	हिमाचल प्रदेश
शरावती परियोजना	शरावती	कर्नाटक
नर्मदा सागर परियोजना	नर्मदा	मध्य प्रदेश, गुजरात
जवाहर सागर परियोजना	चम्बल	राजस्थान
तुलबुल परियोजना	झेलम	जम्मू कश्मीर
सरदार सरोवर परियोजना	नर्मदा	गुजरात, मध्य प्रदेश, महाराष्ट्र एवं राजस्थान
दुलहस्ती परियोजना	चिनाब	जम्मू-कश्मीर
तिलैया परियोजना	बराकर	झारखंड

कृषि क्रांतियाँ

क्रांति	क्षेत्र
हरित क्रांति	*खाद्यान्न उत्पादन*
लाल क्रांति	*टमाटर उत्पादन*
श्वेत क्रांति	*दुग्ध उत्पादन*
गोल क्रांति	*आलू उत्पादन*
भूरी क्रांति	*उर्वरक उत्पादन*
रजत क्रांति	*अंडा उत्पादन*
नीली क्रांति	*मत्स्य उत्पादन*
सुनहरी क्रांति	*बागवानी उत्पादन*
पीली क्रांति	*तिलहन उत्पादन*
गुलाबी क्रांति	*झींगा उत्पादन*

राष्ट्रीय उद्यान और अभयारण्य

वर्तमान समय में हमारे देश में 103 राष्ट्रीय उद्यान और 544 वन्यजीव अभयारण्य हैं। कुछ महत्त्वपूर्ण अभयारण्यों और उद्यानों के नाम नीचे दिए गए हैं।

- कान्हा राष्ट्रीय उद्यान (म.प्र.)
- शिवपुरी राष्ट्रीय उद्यान (म.प्र.)
- जलदापाड़ा अभयारण्य (प. बंगाल)
- काजीरंगा अभयारण्य (असम)
- मानस अभयारण्य (असम)
- हजारीबाग राष्ट्रीय उद्यान (झारखंड)
- पलामू राष्ट्रीय उद्यान (झारखंड)
- डालमा वन्य जीव अभयारण्य (झारखंड)
- सेमलीपाल राष्ट्रीय पार्क (ओडिशा)
- वनकटना वन्य जीव अभयारण्य (उ.प्र.)
- भरतपुर वन्य जीव अभयारण्य (राजस्थान)
- डर्राह वन्य जीव अभयारण्य (राजस्थान)
- कॉर्बेट राष्ट्रीय उद्यान (उत्तराखंड)
- चन्द्रप्रभा अभयारण्य (उ.प्र.)
- डाचीगाम अभयारण्य (जम्मू-कश्मीर)
- दुधवा राष्ट्रीय उद्यान (उ.प्र.)
- नन्दा देवी कस्तूरी मृग वन (उत्तराखंड)
- माउंट आबू वन्य जीव अभयारण्य (राजस्थान)
- रणथम्भौर वन्य जीव अभयारण्य (राजस्थान)
- सरिस्का क्रीड़ा अभयारण्य (राजस्थान)
- रंगथिट्टू पक्षी अभयारण्य (कर्नाटक)
- बांदीपुर अभयारण्य (कर्नाटक)
- डंडेली अभयारण्य (कर्नाटक)
- महावीर अभयारण्य (गोवा-कर्नाटक सीमा)
- पेरियार अभयारण्य (केरल)
- वेदान्त-गाल पक्षी अभयारण्य (तमिलनाडु)
- गिरि वन (गुजरात)
- बोरीवल्ली राष्ट्रीय उद्यान (महाराष्ट्र)
- मोलेम क्रीड़ा अभयारण्य (गोवा)
- कोट्टीगांव क्रीड़ा अभयारण्य (गोवा)
- नागजीरा वन्य जीव अभयारण्य (महाराष्ट्र)
- वान्धवगढ़ राष्ट्रीय उद्यान (मध्य प्रदेश)
- घाट प्रभा पक्षी अभयारण्य (कर्नाटक)
- खगचन्दजेन्दा राष्ट्रीय उद्यान (सिक्किम)
- पेंच राष्ट्रीय उद्यान (महाराष्ट्र)
- रोहिया राष्ट्रीय उद्यान (हिमाचल प्रदेश)
- सुल्तानपुर सरोवर पक्षी अभयारण्य (हरियाणा)
- तोदोवा राष्ट्रीय उद्यान (महाराष्ट्र)
- मुदमलाई अभयारण्य (तमिलनाडु)
- नगर होल अभयारण्य (कर्नाटक)
- नाल सरोवर पक्षी अभयारण्य (गुजरात)
- बोंडला क्रीड़ा अभयारण्य (गोवा)
- तनसा झील वन्य जीव अभयारण्य (महाराष्ट्र)
- बनारघट्टा राष्ट्रीय उद्यान (कर्नाटक)
- ईराविकुलम राजमल्ली राष्ट्रीय उद्यान (केरल)

भारत के प्रसिद्ध पर्वतीय स्थल

स्थान	राज्य
अल्मोड़ा	उत्तराखंड
माउण्ट आबू	राजस्थान
चेरापूंजी	मेघालय
मसूरी	उत्तराखंड
कोडईकनाल	तमिलनाडु
नैनीताल	उत्तराखंड
डलहौजी	हिमाचल प्रदेश
ऊटकमंड	तमिलनाडु
दार्जिलिंग	पश्चिम बंगाल
पंचमढ़ी	मध्य प्रदेश
गुलमर्ग	कश्मीर
रानीखेत	उत्तराखंड
कसौली	हिमाचल प्रदेश
शिलांग	मेघालय
महाबलेश्वर	महाराष्ट्र
शिमला	हिमाचल प्रदेश

✧✧✧✧✧

रक्षा

भारत की रक्षा सेनाओं का सर्वोच्च कमाण्डर भारत का राष्ट्रपति होता है। भारत की सशस्त्र सेनाओं में तीन मुख्य सेवाएंहैं—थल सेना, नौ सेना और वायु सेना। तीनों सेनाओं के प्रमुख क्रमशः थल सेनाध्यक्ष, नौ सेनाध्यक्ष और वायु सेनाध्यक्ष होते हैं।

सेना में कमीशंड पद (Commissioned Ranks)

थल सेना

1. जनरल
2. लेफ्टिनेंट जनरल
3. मेजर जनरल
4. ब्रिगेडियर
5. कर्नल
6. लेफ्टिनेंट कर्नल
7. मेजर
8. कैप्टन
9. लेफ्टिनेंट

वायु सेना

1. एयर चीफ मार्शल
2. एयर मार्शल
3. एयर वाइस मार्शल
4. एयर कॉमोडोर
5. ग्रुप कैप्टन
6. विंग कमाण्डर
7. स्क्वाड्रन लीडर
8. फ्लाइट लेफ्टिनेंट
9. फ्लाइंग ऑफिसर

नौ सेना

1. एडमिरल
2. वाइस एडमिरल
3. रियर एडमिरल
4. कॉमोडोर
5. कैप्टन
6. कमाण्डर
7. लेफ्टिनेंट कमाण्डर
8. लेफ्टिनेंट
9. सब लेफ्टिनेंट

थल सेना कमाण्ड :

कमाण्ड	मुख्यालय
पश्चिमी कमाण्ड	चांडी मंदिर (चंडीगढ़)
पूर्वी कमाण्ड	कोलकाता
उत्तरी कमाण्ड	ऊधमपुर
दक्षिणी कमाण्ड	पुणे
मध्य कमाण्ड	लखनऊ
द.प. कमाण्ड	जयपुर
ट्रेनिंग कमाण्ड	शिमला

जल सेना कमाण्ड :

कमाण्ड	मुख्यालय
पूर्वी कमाण्ड	विशाखापट्टनम
दक्षिणी कमाण्ड	कोच्चि
पश्चिमी कमाण्ड	मुम्बई

वायु सेना कमाण्ड :

कमाण्ड	मुख्यालय
पूर्वी कमाण्ड	शिलांग
पश्चिमी कमाण्ड	नई दिल्ली
केन्द्रीय कमाण्ड	इलाहाबाद
दक्षिणी कमाण्ड	तिरुअनंतपुरम
द.-प. कमाण्ड	गांधीनगर
ट्रेनिंग कमाण्ड	बेंगलुरु
मेन्टेनेन्स कमाण्ड	नागपुर

थल सेना प्रशिक्षण संस्थान :

कमाण्ड	मुख्यालय
नेशनल डिफेन्स एकेडमी (NDA)	खड़कवासला
नेशनल डिफेन्स कॉलिज	नई दिल्ली
इंडियन मिलिट्री एकेडमी (IMA)	देहरादून
डिफेन्स सर्विस स्टाफ कॉलिज	विलिंग्टन
इन्फेनटरी स्कूल	महू
आर्म्ड सेण्टर	अहमदनगर
आर्टीलरी स्कूल	देवलाली

वायु सेना प्रशिक्षण संस्थान :

कमाण्ड	मुख्यालय
एयर फोर्स एडमिनिस्ट्रेटिव कॉलिज	कोयम्बटूर
एयर फोर्स एकेडमी	हैदराबाद
पैराटूपर ट्रेनिंग स्कूल	आगरा
एयर फोर्स टेक्निकल कॉलिज	जलाहली (बेंगलुरु)
एलीमेन्ट्री फ्लाइंग स्कूल	बिदर

नौ सेना प्रशिक्षण संस्थान :

कमाण्ड	मुख्यालय
आइ.एन.एस. चिल्का	भुवनेश्वर
आइ.एन., बेन्दुरथी	कोचीन
आइ.एन.एस. तसिरकार्स	विशाखापट्टनम
इण्डियन नेवल एकेडमी	कोचीन
आइ.एन.एस. शिवाजी	लोनावाला

आंतरिक सुरक्षा के संगठन

संगठन	स्थापना वर्ष	मुख्यालय
असम राइफल्स	1835	शिलांग
केन्द्रीय रिजर्व पुलिस बल	1939	नई दिल्ली
भारत-तिब्बत सीमा पुलिस	1962	नई दिल्ली
सीमा सुरक्षा बल (BSF)	1965	नई दिल्ली
केन्द्रीय औद्योगिक सुरक्षा बल	1969	नई दिल्ली
तट रक्षक बल	1978	नई दिल्ली
राष्ट्रीय सुरक्षा गार्ड	1984	नई दिल्ली

✧✧✧✧✧

कला एवं साहित्य

भारत के प्रमुख चित्रकार एवं उनकी कृतियां

अवनीन्द्र नाथ टैगोर	शाहजहाँ का ताज को देखना, बुद्ध और सुजाता, कमल के पत्ते पर अश्रुकण, वन साम्राज्ञी, औरंगजेब का बुढ़ापा, भारतमाता आदि।
गगनेन्द्र नाथ टैगोर	माँ से विदा लेते चैतन्य, कल्कि अवतार आदि।
राजा रवि वर्मा	दुष्यन्त को प्रेम-पत्र लिखती शकुन्तला, नायर लेडी, शकुन्तला वियोग आदि।
नन्द लाल बोस	उमा की तपस्या, घायल बकरी को ले जाते भगवान बुद्ध, कृष्णार्जुन, उड़ीसा की एक दुकान, प्रणाम, बसन्त, गोपिनी आदि।
के॰ वेंकटप्पा	हनुमान द्वारा लंका दहन, स्वर्ण मृग, राम और मृग तृष्णा आदि।
जॉर्ज कीट	कृष्ण जन्म, कर्ण जन्म, यम मार्कण्डेय, निराभरण गोपियाँ आदि।
भवेश चन्द्र सन्याल	आश्रयहीन लड़की, गोल मार्केट के भिखारी आदि।
मनीषी डे	नारी- शृंगार, पनघट की ओर, बंगाली शरणार्थी।
अमृता शेरगिल	एलिफेन्ट्स बाथिंग इन ग्रीन पुल, हिल साईड, भारतीय लड़कियाँ आदि।
नारायण श्रीधर बेन्द्रे	स्टेशन पर यात्री, बुद्ध पूजा आदि।
देवी प्रसाद राय चौधरी	लेपचा कुमारी, भौटिया आदि।
शोभा सिंह	हीर-रांझा
सतीश गुजराल	काला चांद

संगीत

भारत में चार प्रकार के संगीत-साज मिलते हैं—तंतु या तार वाले, समीर या वायु वाले, अवनाद अथवा थाप से संचालित होने वाले और घन जिसमें घंटियाँ, मंजीरे, घड़ियाल आदि शामिल हैं। तंतु या तार वाले सामान्य साज हैं जैसे—वीणा, सितार, सारंगी, सरोद, दिलरुबा, इसराज, एकतारा, तानपुरा और मयूरी। वायु संचालित साज हैं शहनाई, बाँसुरी, नादस्वरम, निनकिर्नस और पोंगी। थाप अथवा संघात से संचालित होने वाले साज हैं: तबला, मृदंग, ढोलक, पखावज, घटाम तथा कंजीरा-मंजीरा। करतल, जल तरंग आदि अन्य भारतीय साज हैं। गायन के क्षेत्र में **विष्णु नारायण भातखण्डे**, बेगम अख्तर, बड़े गुलाम अली, हीराबाई बरोडकर, भीमसेन जोशी, केसरभाई केलकर, ओंकारनाथ ठाकुर, सिद्धेश्वरी देवी, त्यागराज, विष्णु दिगंबर पलुसकर, पंकज मलिक, एम.एस. सुब्बालक्ष्मी, पंडित जसराज, गंगूभाई हंगल, मल्लिकार्जुन मंसूर, डागर बंधु, डी.के. जयरामन, के.जे. यशुदास, गुलाम मुस्तफा खान, कुमार गंधर्व, के.एल. वसंधा कुमारी, किशोरी अमोनकर, गिरिजा देवी, वी.के. नारायण स्वामी दीक्षित, तानसेन, श्यामा शास्त्री, स्वाति तिरूनल आदि साजपरक संगीत के कुछ दिग्गज कलाकार रहे हैं।

साजपरक संगीत के कुछ दिग्गज कलाकार निम्न हैं:-

बाँसुरी—हरि प्रसाद चौरसिया, पन्नालाल घोष, टी.आर. महालिंगम, एन. रमानी, विजय राघव राव, **रघुनाथ सेठ**, **राजेन्द्र कुलकर्णी**

जंजीरा—वी. नागराजन

घटाम—टी.एच. विनयाकरम

गिटार—पंडित विष्णु मोहन भट्ट, मोहन भट्ट, बृजभूषण कालरा, **श्रीकृष्ण नलिन**

हारमोनियम—पुरुषोत्तम वालावाकर, एम. धौलपुरी

मृदंग—पालघात आर. रघु, यू.एस. वर्मन

पखावज—गोविन्द राव, अनोखे लाल, कंठी महाराज

रूद्रवीणा—जिया मोहिउद्दीन डागर, **असद अली खान**

संतूर—शिव कुमार शर्मा, **तरुण भट्टाचार्य**

सितार—पंडित रविशंकर, बिलायत खान, देबू चौधरी, अब्दुल हलीम, जफर खान

सरोद—अली अकबर खान, अमजद अली खान, अलाउद्दीन खान, सरेन रानी, बज नारायण, **मुकेश शर्मा**, **चंदन राय**

शहनाई—बिस्मिल्ला खान, सुरबहार इमरत खान, **दयाशंकर जगन्नाथ**

वायलिन—लालगुडी जयारमण, एल. सुब्रह्मण्यम, एम.एस. गोपालकृष्णन, एस. सुब्रह्मण्यम, वी.जी. जोग, एन. राजन

तबला—अल्लारखा **खां**, गुदई महाराज, जाकिर हुसैन, लतीफ खाँ, **किशन महाराज** आदि।

नृत्य

- **भरतनाट्यम :** इस नृत्य शैली का ताल्लुक तमिलनाडु से है। यह कर्नाटक संगीत के साथ किया जाने वाला एकांतिक नृत्य है। अपने शुद्ध रूप में यह नृत्य शरीर की विभिन्न हलचलों, कोणों व घुमाव के जरिए लय-ताल का एक बेहतरीन नमूना पेश करता है।
- **ओडिसी :** इसकी उत्पत्ति **ओडिशा** में हुई है। यह नृत्य भरतनाट्यम के समानांतर है। 'गीत-गोविन्द' नामक काव्य की संरचना इस नृत्य शैली के काव्य तथा संगीत घटकों पर हावी रही है।
- **मणिपुरी :** यह मणिपुर का लयबद्ध नृत्य है। यह राधा-कृष्ण और गोपियों की अवधारणा के इर्द-गिर्द संकेद्रित रही है। नगाड़ों और मंजीरों पर बजने वाले कई प्रकार के ताल इस नृत्य के साथ-साथ चलते हैं।
- **कत्थक :** यह उत्तरी भारत का एक विशिष्ट शहरी नृत्य है। पूर्व में इसे दरबारों से जुड़ी नृत्य परंपरा के रूप में लिया जाता था। इस नृत्य के दौरान गायन चलता रहता है, मृदंग बजते रहते हैं तथा एक और कलाकार साज बजाता रहता है। कलाकारों का यह समूह सुर-ताल का आकर्षक नजारा पेश करता है।
- **कथकली :** यह केरल की शास्त्रीय नृत्य नाटिका है। अपने स्वरूप में यह नृत्य वर्णात्मक होने के बजाय नाट्यरूप में होता है। यह नृत्य महाकाव्यों के मिथकीय घटनाओं पर आधारित होता है जिसे अतिनाटकीय अंदाज में प्रस्तुत किया जाता है। नाटकीय कथा आँखों और भौहों के संचालन से, हाथों की भाव-भंगिमाओं से तथा शरीर के विशिष्ट संचालन से आगे बढ़ती है।
- **कुचिपुड़ी :** इस नृत्य का अभ्युदय आंध्र प्रदेश में हुआ माना जाता है। पारंपरिक रूप से यह नृत्य-नाटिका मंदिरों से संबद्ध रही है।

विभिन्न राज्यों के कुछ महत्वपूर्ण लोक-नृत्य :

- **महाराष्ट्र :** तमाशा, दही हण्डी, गोफ, दीपक, डिंडी
- **गुजरात :** गरबा, रासलीला, तिप्पनी, डांडिया
- **ओडिशा :** छऊ, माया शवरी, दलचाई
- **राजस्थान :** घूमर, कठपुतली, तेरा ताली
- **मध्य प्रदेश :** लोटा नृत्य, जवारा
- **हिमाचल प्रदेश :** दशहरा नृत्य, हिकत, नेतियो
- **पंजाब :** गिद्धा, भांगड़ा, पणिहारी
- **उत्तर प्रदेश :** रासलीला, नौटंकी, थाली, धुरंग, झुमेला, हुड़का बोल, **कजरी**
- **नगालैण्ड :** बांस नृत्य, केदोहोह
- **असोम :** बिहू, केली गोपाल, सतरिया
- **बंगाल :** कीर्तन, कालत्री, असुरबध, वृता, काली नाच
- **बिहार :** छऊ, मगही, दुर्गा नृत्य
- **तमिलनाडु :** तेरुकलथु, कबलतम, कर्गम, पुली वेशम
- **केरल :** मोहिनी अट्टम, पदायुनी
- **कर्नाटक :** यक्षगान, कुजीता, कोडवास
- **कश्मीर :** दुम्हल, हिकत, चाकरी
- **त्रिपुरा :** हजागिरि
- **आंध्र प्रदेश :** डंडारिया, बंजारा, घण्टा मरदाला
- **गोवा :** गोडे मोदनी, ढकनी
- **मेघालय :** नोंगकरेम, बांग्ला
- **मणिपुर :** ढोल चोलम, बसंत रस
- **हरियाणा :** धमचाल, लहूर, भांगड़ा, गिद्दा
- **झारखंड : सरहुल, सोहराई**

शास्त्रीय नृत्य के कुछ प्रख्यात कलाकार :

- **भरतनाट्यम** : यामिनी कृष्णमूर्ति, रुक्मिणी देवी अरुण्डेल, स्वप्न सुन्दरी, सोनल मानसिंह, वैजयंती माला, मृणालिनी साराभाई, चंद्रलेखा, इंद्राणी, राम गोपाल, बाल सरस्वती
- **कथकली** : गोपीनाथ, के.के. नायर, कुंजुकुरुप, टी.के. चंदू, **शांताराव, उदयशंकर**
- **कुचिपुड़ी** : स्वप्न सुंदरी, राजा रेड्डी, राधा रेड्डी, शोभा नायर, वेदांतम सत्यनारायण, विम्पत्ति चिन्ना सत्यम
- **कत्थक** : बिरजू महाराज, गोपीकृष्ण, शंभू महाराज, सितारा देवी, उमा शर्मा, दुर्गा लाल, शोभना नारायण
- **मणिपुरी** : उदय शंकर, दरोहरा झावेरी, चैतम्बि सिंह, बिपिन सिंह, सूर्यमुखी
- **ओडिसी** : केलुचरण महापात्र, इंद्राणी रहमान, माधवी मुद्गल, प्रोतिमा बेदी, संयुक्ता पाणिग्रही, सोनल मानसिंह, देवू दास, **प्रियवंदा मोहन्ती, मिनाती दास**

✧✧✧✧✧

महत्वपूर्ण दिवस

दिवस	महत्व
9 जनवरी	प्रवासी दिवस
15 जनवरी	थल सेना दिवस
25 जनवरी	भारतीय पर्यटन दिवस
26 जनवरी	भारतीय गणतंत्र दिवस
30 जनवरी	शहीद दिवस, विश्व कुष्ठ निवारण दिवस (महात्मा गाँधी की पुण्य तिथि)
1 फरवरी	तटरक्षक दिवस, डाक जीवन बीमा दिवस
4 फरवरी	विश्व कैंसर दिवस
20 फरवरी	विश्व सामाजिक न्याय दिवस
21 फरवरी	विश्व मातृभाषा दिवस
22 फरवरी	पल्स पोलियो दिवस
28 फरवरी	राष्ट्रीय विज्ञान दिवस (रमन प्रभाव की स्मृति में)
8 मार्च	अन्तर्राष्ट्रीय महिला दिवस
15 मार्च	विश्व उपभोक्ता अधिकार दिवस, विश्व विकलांगता दिवस
21 मार्च	विश्व वानिकी दिवस, विश्व रंगभेद उन्मूलन दिवस
22 मार्च	विश्व जल दिवस
23 मार्च	शहीद दिवस, विश्व मौसम विज्ञान दिवस
24 मार्च	विश्व तपेदिक दिवस
7 अप्रैल	विश्व स्वास्थ्य दिवस
18 अप्रैल	विश्व विरासत दिवस
22 अप्रैल	विश्व पृथ्वी दिवस
1 मई	मई दिवस (अन्तर्राष्ट्रीय श्रम दिवस)
8 मई	विश्व रेडक्रॉस दिवस
9 मई	अन्तर्राष्ट्रीय थैलीसीमिया दिवस
11 मई	राष्ट्रीय प्रौद्योगिकी दिवस
24 मई	कॉमनवेल्थ दिवस
31 मई	धूम्रपान विरोध दिवस

दिवस	महत्व
1 जून	अन्तर्राष्ट्रीय बाल दिवस
5 जून	विश्व पर्यावरण दिवस
14 जून	वर्ल्ड ब्लड डोनर डे
20 जून	शरणार्थी दिवस
21 जून	विश्व योग दिवस
11 जुलाई	विश्व जनसंख्या दिवस
6 अगस्त	विश्व शांति दिवस, हिरोशिमा दिवस
10 अगस्त	अंतर्राष्ट्रीय युवा दिवस
29 अगस्त	राष्ट्रीय खेल दिवस
5 सितम्बर	शिक्षक दिवस
8 सितम्बर	विश्व साक्षरता दिवस
14 सितम्बर	हिन्दी दिवस
16 सितम्बर	विश्व ओजोन दिवस
21 सितम्बर	अन्तर्राष्ट्रीय शांति दिवस
27 सितम्बर	विश्व पर्यटन दिवस
2 अक्टूबर	गाँधी जयन्ती / अन्तर्राष्ट्रीय अहिंसा दिवस
3 अक्टूबर	विश्व पर्यावास दिवस
5 अक्टूबर	विश्व आवास दिवस
9 अक्टूबर	विश्व डाक दिवस
16 अक्टूबर	विश्व खाद्य दिवस
17 अक्टूबर	विश्व गरीबी उन्मूलन दिवस
20 अक्टूबर	राष्ट्रीय एकता दिवस, विश्व सांख्यिकी दिवस
14 नवम्बर	विश्व मधुमेह दिवस
19 नवम्बर	अन्तर्राष्ट्रीय नागरिक दिवस
26 नवम्बर	विश्व पर्यावरण संरक्षण दिवस
1 दिसम्बर	विश्व एड्स दिवस
10 दिसम्बर	अन्तर्राष्ट्रीय मानवाधिकार दिवस
18 दिसम्बर	अन्तर्राष्ट्रीय प्रवास दिवस
29 दिसम्बर	विश्व जैव विविधता दिवस

✧✧✧✧✧

खेल जगत

खेलों से जुड़ी शब्दावली

- **एथलेटिक्सः** ऐली, स्प्रॉम, बैटन, बेंड, ब्लाइंड पास, बॉक्स, सर्किल, क्लियरेंस, क्रासबार, हीट्स, फाल्स स्टार्ट, फ्लॉप स्टाइल, फाउल, हर्डलेस, लेन, लैप, डेकाथलॉन, हैप्टेथलॉन, मैराथन, पेंटाथलोन, स्क्रैच, शॉट पुट, स्प्रिंट, स्टार्टिंग ब्लॉक स्टेपल चेज, स्ट्रैंडल, टाई, जोन।
- **बैडमिंटनः** एश, एली, बैक हैण्ड, ब्लाक, कैरी, चैकिंग द स्मैस, कोर्ट, क्रास कोर्ट, डबल हिट, ड्राप शाट, फाल्ट, फोरहैण्ड, फ्रेम, गेम प्वाइंट, किल, लोब, लव, नेट, रैकेट, रैली, सर्व, शार्ट सर्व, शटल (बर्ड भी कहते हैं) साइड आउट, अंडर हैंड।
- **बेसबॉलः** आर्म थ्रोअर, एराउंड द हार्न, बल्क, बाल, बाल हॉक, बेस ओपन बेस रनर, बैट, बैटर, कैचर, काक्ड आर्म, क्रास फायर, डाउनर, होम, हाट कार्नर, इनफील्ड फ्लाई, की स्टोन सैक, लेट अप, पेग, पिंच हिटर, पॉपी, पंच, रबर, इनअप, सिंकर, स्लाइडर, थ्री फुट लाइन।
- **बास्केट बॉलः** बैक डोर, बैंग बोर्ड, बैंक शाट, बाउंस पास, चार्ज, चेस्ट पास, कार्नर प्लेयर, कट, डेड बॉल, डबल फाउल, ड्रिबल, फेक, फील्ड गोल, फाउल, फ्री थ्रो, गोल, हेल्ड बॉल, जम्प बॉल, पायवोट, रिवाइंड, रिस्ट्रेनिंग सर्कल, टी, टैक्नीकल फाउल, थ्रो इन।
- **बिलियर्डस एंड स्नूकरः** एंगल, राउण्ड द टेबल, बल्क, बॉल, ब्रेक, ब्रिज, केनन, क्यू बॉल, कॉप, फॉलो, हजार्ड, पाकेट, पॉट, पिरामिड, रेडबॉल, रेस्ट्स, रन, सेट अप, शार्ट स्विंग, टेबल।
- **बॉक्सिंगः** स्प्रॉन, अटैक, ब्लैक पेडल, बैक हैंड पंच, ब्लाकिंग, बोली, बाउट, बट, चॉप, कम्बीनेशन, कट, डाइव, एलबोइंग, फर्स्ट ब्लड, फ्लोर, फुल काउंट, ग्लोब्स, हीलिंग, होल्डिंग, हुक, जब, माउथपीस, पंच, रिंग, स्कोरिंग, सेकेण्ड, स्पॉट, वार्निंग।
- **क्रिकेटः** ऑल राउण्डर, ऐशेज, बैकफुट, बेल्स, बॉल, बैट, बैटिंग, बैट्समैन, बीमर, बाउंसर, बाउण्ड्री, बॉलर, बॉलिंग क्रीज, बाई, कॉट एण्ड बोल्ड, कॉल, कैच, कॉट बिहाइंड, सेंचुरी, क्लीन बोल्ड, कवर प्वाइंट, क्रास बैट, कट, कटर, डेड बॉल, एक्स्ट्राज, फास्ट मीडियम, फॉलोआन, फ्रंट फुट, फुलटॉस, ग्लास, गुगली, गार्ड, गिल्ली, हाफ वॉली, हैट्रिक, हिट विकेट, हुक, इनस्वींगर, लेटकट, लेग ब्रेक, लेग साइड, मेडन, मिड ऑफ, मिड ऑन, मिड विकेट, नाइट वाचमैन, प्वांइट, ओपनर, ओवर, ओवर थ्रो, ओवर द विकेट, पिच, पुल-राउण्ड द विकेट, स्क्वायर कट, स्क्वायर लेग, स्वीप, टॉस, अम्पायर, विकेट कीपर, यार्कर।
- **गोल्फः** एश, एड्रेस, एयर शॉट, एप्रोन, अवे, बॉल मार्क, ब्रिडी, बोगी, बाई, चिप, क्लब, कप, ड्राइव, ईगल, फ्लफ्फ, हाल्वड्, हैण्डीकैप, हजार्ड, होल, ऑनर, हुक, जिग्गर, लाई, पार, पिन, पुट, रन, स्लाइस, स्टांस, स्विंग, टी, वेज।
- **हॉकीः** बैकपास, बुली, कैरिंग द बॉल, सेंटर फारवर्ड, चार्जिंग, कार्नर, डी, डिफेंडर, ड्रिवलिंग, फ्लिक, फारवर्ड, फाउल, फ्रीहिट, फुल बैक्स, गोल, हाब्स, हिट, हुकिंग, इंटरसेप्टिंग, लांग कार्नर, शार्ट पेनल्टी स्ट्रोक, पुश, रिवर्स स्टिक, स्कूप, सिक्सटीन यार्ड हिट, स्टिक, स्ट्राइकिंग सर्कल, टैकलिंग, थ्रू पास, ट्रैपिंग, ट्वेन्टी फाइव यार्ड लाइन, अंडरकटिंग।
- **सॉकरः** बाईसाईकिल किक, बाड़ी सर्व, बाक्स या पेनल्टी एरिया, कैरिंग, चेस्टिंग, क्लीयरिंग, कार्नर किक, कार्नर फ्लैग, क्रास, क्रास ओवर, डी, डायरेक्ट फ्री किक, डाइव, डबल फाउल, ड्रिवल, ड्राप वॉल, एक्स्ट्रा टाइम, फिनिशिंग, फ्लैंक, फाउल, गोल किक, गोल पोस्ट, गोल्स, हॉफ वॉली, हैट्रिक, हैडिंग, इनडायरेक्ट फ्री किक, इंटरसेप्सन, किक ऑफ, लाइंस मैन, लिंक मैन, लोब, मार्किंग, न्यूटमैग, ऑफ साइड, पास, पेनल्टी स्पॉट, रिवर्स पास, सीजर्स किक, शैडो मार्किंग, साइड लाइंस, स्ट्राइकर, स्वीपर, टेंकल, थ्रोइन, ड्रिपिंग, विंगर, येलो कार्ड।
- **स्क्वैशः** एंगल, बोर्ड कोर्ट, कट लाइन, ड्राइव, फुट फाउल्ट, हॉफ कोर्ट लाइन, हैमर, हैंड इन, किल, निक, पेनल्टी प्वाइंट, रैली, सर्विस बाक्स, सेट, शार्ट लाइन, वॉली, वेल्स।
- **स्वीमिंगः** बैकस्ट्रोक, बटरफ्लाई, ब्रेस्ट स्ट्रोक, कैसल, क्राउल, फाल्स स्टार्ट, फ्री स्टाइल, किकिंग, लेग, मेडले रिले, पुल, टच।

- **टेबल टेनिसः** एश, बैकहैण्ड, शॉट, ब्लेड, ब्लॉक शॉट, ड्यूस, ड्राप शॉट, गेम, ग्रिप, रैली, सर्विस, स्मैश, टॉप स्पिन, रिवर्स सेंटर लाइन।
- **टेनिसः** एश, एडवांटेज, बैक कोर्ट, बैक हैण्ड, बॉल ब्वाय या बॉल गर्ल, ब्रेक, बाई, सेंट्रल लाइन, चिप, चाप, कोर्ट, डेड, ड्यूस, डबल फाल्ट, डाउन द लाइन, ड्राप शॉट, ड्राप वॉली, इरर, फेस या रैकेट, फाउल्ट, फोर कोर्ट, फ्रेम, गेम, गेम प्वाइंट, ग्राउंड स्ट्रोक, लेट, लाइन बॉल, लोब, लव, मैच प्वाइंट, नेट, नेट बॉल, ओवर हैड, स्मैश, पासिंग शॉट, रैली रिटायर, रिटर्न, सर्व, सर्विस, सेट, सेटप्वाइंट, शार्ट बाल, स्मैश, स्ट्रोक, टॉस, अंडरहैंड, वॉली।
- **वॉलीबॉलः** एश, एड ऑन, बैकलाइन, ब्लॉक, बॉडी फाउल, कैरिंग द बॉल, चेस्टपास, कवर, क्रास कोर्ट शाट, ड्यूस, डिग, डबल हिट, फुट फाउल्ट, गेम प्वाइंट, किल, हेल्ड, बॉल, मल्टीपल टचेज, नेट, ओवर नेट, प्वाइंट, पावर सर्व, सर्व, सेट, साइड आउट, स्मैश, स्पाइकर टाइम आउट।

खेल के मैदान की माप

- **बैडमिंटन कोर्ट** : 20 फीट × 44 फीट (युगल); 17 फीट × 44 फीट (एकल)
- **बेसबॉल** : डायगोनल बेस में से निकटतम आधार के बीच की दूरी 90 फीट और 127 फीट 3⅜ इंच होती है। पिचर के सर्किल और बॉलर के बीच 60½ फीट की दूरी होती है।
- **बास्केटबॉल कोर्ट** : 85 फीट × 46 फीट।
- **बिलियर्ड्स टेबल** : 12 फीट × 6 *फीट* 1½ इंच।
- **बॉक्सिंग रिंग** : 20 फीट वर्ग।
- **क्रिकेट** : दोनों विकेट 22 गज की दूरी पर होते हैं। बॉल का व्यास लगभग 9 से.मी. और वजन 5½ से 5¾ ओंस होता है।
- **हैंडबॉल कोर्ट** : 126 से 147 फीट लम्बा और 60 से 73 फीट चौड़ा।
- **हॉकी का मैदान** : 100 गज × 55 गज।
- **रग्बी मैदान** : यह मैदान अंडाकार होता है जिसकी अधिकतम लम्बाई 150 से 200 गज और अधिकतम चौड़ाई 120 से 170 गज होती है।
- **रोविंग** : एकल नौका चालन हेतु नौका की लम्बाई 27 फीट और युगल के लिए 34 फीट होती है। कॉक्स्ड जोड़ा 35 फीट, काक्सलेस फोर 44 फीट, कॉक्स्ड फोर 45 फीट और कॉक्स्ड एट 62 फीट होता है।
- **फुटबॉल मैदान** : 100 से 130 गज लम्बा और 50 से 100 गज चौड़ा।
- **स्क्वैश कोर्ट** : 32 फीट × 21 फीट, कट लाइन 6 फीट का और टिन 19 इंच का होता है।
- **स्वीमिंग पुल** : 50 मीटर लम्बा।
- **टेबल टेनिस** : टेबल 9 फीट × 5 फीट का होता है तथा नेट की ऊंचाई 6 इंच होती है।
- **टेनिस कोर्ट** : एकल के लिए 78 फीट × 27 *फीट* और युगल के लिए 78 फीट × 36 फीट।
- **वालीबॉल कोर्ट** : 18 मीटर × 9 मीटर।
- **मैराथन दौड़** : 26 मील 385 गज।

ओलंपिक

प्राचीन काल में अपने नागरिकों को स्वस्थ एवं फिट बनाए रखने के लिए यूनानवासी प्रतियोगी खेल स्पर्द्धाओं का आयोजन करते थे। जौस देवता के सम्मान में प्रथम ओलम्पिक खेलों का आयोजन ओलम्पस माउंट में ईसा पूर्व 776 में किया गया था। इसके बाद 394 ईस्वी जबकि यूनानी सभ्यता का पतन हो गया, प्रत्येक 4 वर्षों के अंतराल के बाद ओलम्पिक खेलों का आयोजन किया जाता रहा। आधुनिक समय में फ्रांस के धनकुबेर पियरे डी कुबर्टिन ने आधुनिक खेलों को पुनर्जीवित किया। प्रथम आधुनिक ओलम्पिक खेल का आयोजन 1896 में एथेंस (यूनान) में किया गया। इसके बाद से विश्व युद्धों को छोड़कर प्रत्येक 4 वर्ष के अंतराल पर ओलम्पिक खेलों का आयोजन होता रहा है। ओलम्पिक खेलों का ध्वज श्वेत रंग का है जिस पर 5 रंगीन छल्ले बने हैं। प्रत्येक रिंग एक महादेश का प्रतिनिधित्व करता है। एक ही वर्ष में ग्रीष्मकालीन और शीतकालीन ओलंपिक खेलों का आयोजन किया जाता है।

वर्ष	ग्रीष्मकालीन ओलम्पिक (स्थल)
1896	एथेंस (यूनान)
1900	पेरिस (फ्रांस)
1904	सेंट लुईस (यूएसए)
1908	लंदन (ब्रिटेन)
1912	स्टॉकहोम (स्वीडन)
1920	एंटवर्प (बेल्जियम)
1924	पेरिस (फ्रांस)
1928	एम्सटर्डम (नीदरलैंड्स)
1932	लॉस एंजिल्स (यूएसए)
1936	बर्लिन (जर्मनी)
1948	लंदन (ब्रिटेन)
1952	हेलसिंकी (फिनलैण्ड)
1956	मेलबोर्न (ऑस्ट्रेलिया)
1960	रोम (इटली)
1964	टोकियो (जापान)
1968	मैक्सिको सिटी (मैक्सिको)
1972	म्यूनिख (जर्मनी)
1976	मांट्रियल (कनाडा)
1980	मास्को (यूएसएसआर)
1984	लॉस एंजिल्स (यूएसए)
1988	सियोल (दक्षिण कोरिया)
1992	बार्सिलोना (स्पेन)
1996	अटलांटा (अमेरिका)
2000	सिडनी (ऑस्ट्रेलिया)
2004	एथेंस (ग्रीस)
2008	बीजिंग (चीन)
2012	लंदन, (ब्रिटेन)
2016	रियो डि जनेरियो, ब्राजील
2020	टोक्यो, जापान (प्रस्तावित)

एशियाई खेल

द्वितीय विश्व युद्ध के पश्चात् अनेकों एशियाई देशों ने स्वतंत्रता प्राप्त की। ओलंपिक खेलों की तर्ज पर प्रत्येक चार वर्षों बाद एशियाई खेलों के आयोजन की योजना बनायी गई। भारत ने 1951 में नई दिल्ली में प्रथम एशियाई खेलों का आयोजन किया।

वर्ष	आयोजन स्थल
1951	नई दिल्ली (भारत)
1954	मनीला (फिलीपींस)
1958	टोकियो (जापान)
1962	जकार्ता (इंडोनेशिया)
1966	बैंकाक (थाईलैण्ड)
1970	बैंकाक (थाईलैण्ड)
1974	तेहरान (ईरान)
1978	बैंकाक (थाईलैण्ड)
1982	नई दिल्ली (भारत)
1986	सियोल (दक्षिण कोरिया)
1990	बीजिंग (चीन)
1994	हिरोशिमा (जापान)
1998	बैंकाक (थाईलैण्ड)
2002	बुसान (दक्षिण कोरिया)
2006	दोहा (कतर)
2010	ग्वांगझो (चीन)
2014	इंचियोन (द. कोरिया)
2018	जकार्ता (इंडोनेशिया)

राष्ट्रमंडल खेल

राष्ट्रमंडल खेल भी प्रत्येक चार वर्ष बाद आयोजित किए जाते हैं उसी वर्ष में जिसमें एशियाई खेल आयोजित होते हैं। सभी राष्ट्रमंडल देश (ब्रिटेन के पूर्व उपनिवेश) इसमें भाग ले सकते हैं। प्रथम राष्ट्रमंडल खेल 1930 में हैमिल्टन (कनाडा) में आयोजित हुआ। 2018 के राष्ट्रमंडल खेलों का आयोजन गोल्ड कोस्ट (ऑस्ट्रेलिया) में हुआ।

वर्ष	आयोजन-स्थल
1930	हेमिल्टन (कनाडा)
1934	लन्दन (ब्रिटेन)
1938	सिडनी (आस्ट्रेलिया)
1950	ऑकलैण्ड (न्यूजीलैण्ड)
1954	बैंकूवर (कनाडा)
1958	कारडिफ (ब्रिटेन)
1962	पर्थ (आस्ट्रेलिया)
1966	किंग्सटन (जमैका)
1970	एडिनबरा (स्कॉटलैण्ड)

वर्ष	आयोजन-स्थल
1974	क्राइस्ट चर्च (न्यूजीलैण्ड)
1978	एडमन्टन (कनाडा)
1982	ब्रिसबेन (आस्ट्रेलिया)
1986	एडिनबरा (स्कॉटलैण्ड)
1990	ऑकलैण्ड (न्यूजीलैण्ड)
1994	विक्टोरिया (कनाडा)
1998	क्वालालम्पुर (मलेशिया)
2002	मैनचेस्टर (ब्रिटेन)
2006	मेलबोर्न (आस्ट्रेलिया)
2010	नई दिल्ली (भारत)
2014	ग्लासगो (स्कॉटलैण्ड)
2018	गोल्ड कोस्ट (ऑस्ट्रेलिया)
2022	बर्मिंघम (ब्रिटेन) में प्रस्तावित

पहले राष्ट्रमंडल खेल, जो 1930 में कनाडा के हैमिल्टन में आयोजित किये गये थे, को ''ब्रिटिश अम्पायर गेम'' के नाम से जाना गया। 1954 में इनका नाम बदलकर ''ब्रिटिश अम्पायर एण्ड कॉमनवेल्थ गेम्स'' कर दिया गया। 1970 में एक बार फिर इनका नाम परिवर्तन कर 'ब्रिटिश कॉमनवेल्थ गेम्स' किया गया। वर्ष 1978 से इन्हें कामनवेल्थ गेम्स अथवा राष्ट्रमंडल खेलों के नाम से जाना जा रहा है।

विश्व कप फुटबॉल : एक दृष्टि में

वर्ष	आयोजक देश	विजेता	उप-विजेता
1930	उरुग्वे	उरुग्वे	अर्जेन्टीना
1934	इटली	इटली	चेकोस्लोवाकिया
1938	फ्रांस	इटली	हंगरी
1950	ब्राजील	उरुग्वे	ब्राजील
1954	स्विट्जरलैंड	प. जर्मनी	हंगरी
1958	स्वीडन	ब्राजील	स्वीडन
1962	चिली	ब्राजील	चेकोस्लोवाकिया
1966	इंग्लैंड	इंग्लैंड	प. जर्मनी
1970	मैक्सिको	ब्राजील	इटली
1974	प. जर्मनी	प. जर्मनी	हालैंड
1978	अर्जेन्टीना	अर्जेन्टीना	हालैंड
1982	स्पेन	इटली	प. जर्मनी
1986	मैक्सिको	अर्जेन्टीना	प. जर्मनी
1990	इटली	प. जर्मनी	अर्जेन्टीना
1994	अमेरिका	ब्राजील	इटली
1998	फ्रांस	फ्रांस	ब्राजील
2002	जापान और दक्षिण कोरिया	ब्राजील	जर्मनी
2006	जर्मनी	इटली	फ्रांस
2010	दक्षिण अफ्रीका	स्पेन	नीदरलैंड
2014	ब्राजील	जर्मनी	अर्जेन्टीना
2018	रूस	फ्रांस	क्रोएशिया
2022	कतर में प्रस्तावित		

विश्व कप क्रिकेट : एक दृष्टि में

वर्ष	आयोजक देश	विजेता	उप-विजेता
1975	इंग्लैंड	वेस्टइंडीज	ऑस्ट्रेलिया
1979	इंग्लैंड	वेस्टइंडीज	इंग्लैण्ड
1983	इंग्लैंड	भारत	वेस्टइण्डीज
1987	भारत-पाकिस्तान	आस्ट्रेलिया	इंग्लैंड
1992	आस्ट्रेलिया, न्यूजीलैंड	पाकिस्तान	इंग्लैंड
1996	भारत, पाकिस्तान, श्रीलंका	श्रीलंका	आस्ट्रेलिया
1999	इंग्लैंड	आस्ट्रेलिया	पाकिस्तान
2003	दक्षिण अफ्रीका	आस्ट्रेलिया	भारत
2007	वेस्टइण्डीज	आस्ट्रेलिया	श्रीलंका
2011	भारत, बांग्लादेश, श्रीलंका	भारत	श्रीलंका
2015	आस्ट्रेलिया, न्यूजीलैंड	आस्ट्रेलिया	न्यूजीलैंड
2019	इंग्लैंड में प्रस्तावित		

विश्व के प्रसिद्ध कप और ट्राफियाँ

- अमेरिकन कप — याच रेसिंग
- एशेज — क्रिकेट (इंग्लैंड बनाम आस्ट्रेलिया)
- कनाडा कप — गोल्फ (विश्व चैम्पियनशिप)
- कोलम्बो कप — सॉकर
- चैम्पियन ट्रॉफी — हॉकी (पुरुष) विश्व की 6 श्रेष्ठ टीमों के मध्य
- कोरबिलन कप — टेबल टेनिस (महिला) विश्व कप
- डेविस कप — लॉन टेनिस (पुरुष)
- डर्बी — घुड़ दौड़ (इंग्लैंड)

- जुल्स रिमेट कप — सॉकर—विश्व कप (पुरुष)
- किंग्स कप — एयर रेसेज (इंग्लैंड)
- मर्डेका कप — सॉकर (पुरुष) (मलेशिया)
- प्रिंस ऑफ वेल्स कप — गोल्फ (इंग्लैंड)
- रोथमेंस कप — क्रिकेट
- रायडर कप — गोल्फ (इंग्लैंड)
- स्वेथलिंग कप — विश्व टेबल टेनिस (पुरुष)
- थॉमस कप — विश्व बैडमिंटन (पुरुष)
- टुंकु अब्दुल रहमान कप — बैडमिंटन
- उबेर कप — विश्व बैडमिंटन (महिला)
- वाकर कप — गोल्फ (इंग्लैंड)
- विटमैन कप — लॉन टेनिस (महिला)
- विम्बलडन कप — लॉन टेनिस (इंग्लैंड)

प्रसिद्ध खेल मैदान एवं उनसे सम्बन्धित खेल

खेल-मैदान	खेल	स्थान
इन्द्रप्रस्थ स्टेडियम	इन्डोर गेम	दिल्ली
जवाहरलाल नेहरू स्टेडियम	एथलेटिक्स	दिल्ली
फिरोजशाह कोटला मैदान	क्रिकेट	दिल्ली
अम्बेडकर स्टेडियम	फुटबॉल	दिल्ली
शिवाजी स्टेडियम	हॉकी	दिल्ली
नेशनल स्टेडियम	हॉकी	दिल्ली
हेनले	रेगाटा	इंग्लैंड
नेशनल स्टेडियम	हॉकी	मुम्बई
वानखेडे स्टेडियम	क्रिकेट	मुम्बई
ब्रेबोर्न स्टेडियम	क्रिकेट	मुम्बई
ईडन गार्डन	क्रिकेट	कोलकाता
ग्रीन पार्क स्टेडियम	क्रिकेट	कानपुर
कीनन स्टेडियम	क्रिकेट	जमशेदपुर
नेहरू (चेपक) स्टेडियम	क्रिकेट	चेन्नई
वाराबती स्टेडियम	क्रिकेट	कटक
इप्सम	डर्बी घुड़दौड	ब्रिटेन
हेडिंग्ले मानचेस्टर	क्रिकेट	ब्रिटेन
लाईस, ओवल, लीड्स	क्रिकेट	ब्रिटेन
ब्लैक हीथ	रग्बी फुटबॉल	लन्दन
विम्बलडन	लॉन टेनिस	लन्दन
वेम्बले स्टेडियम	फुटबॉल	लन्दन
ब्रुकलैण्ड	फुटबॉल	इंग्लैंड
टिबंकहम	रग्बी फुटबॉल	इंग्लैंड
पटनी मार्टलेक	नौका दौड़	इंग्लैंड
टेंट ब्रिज	क्रिकेट	इंग्लैंड
एण्ट्री	घुड़दौड़	इंग्लैंड
व्हाइट सिटी	कुत्तों की दौड	इंग्लैंड
हरलिघम	पोलो	इंग्लैंड
पर्थ, ब्रिस्बेन, मेलबोर्न	क्रिकेट	आस्ट्रेलिया
यांकी स्टेडियम	बॉक्सिंग	न्यूयार्क
ब्रूकलिन	बेसबॉल	न्यूयार्क
फोरस्ट हिल	टेनिस	न्यूयार्क

✧✧✧✧✧

पुरस्कार एवं सम्मान

राष्ट्रीय पुरस्कार

भारत रत्न

यह भारत का सर्वोच्च असैनिक सम्मान है। यह कला, साहित्य, विज्ञान एवं खेलकूद के क्षेत्र में अतिविशिष्ट सेवाओं तथा सार्वजनिक क्षेत्र में उत्कृष्टतम योगदान के लिए प्रदान किया जाता है। सरकारी सेवाओं में लगे व्यक्तियों को यह पुरस्कार नहीं दिया जाता। निम्नलिखित व्यक्तियों को अब तक भारत रत्न से सम्मानित किया जा चुका हैः

भारत रत्न से अलंकृत व्यक्ति

1.	डा॰ एस॰ राधाकृष्णन	1954
2.	सी॰ राजगोपालाचारी	1954
3.	डा॰ सी॰वी॰ रमण	1954
4.	डा॰ भगवान दास	1955
5.	डा॰ एम॰ विश्वेश्वरैया	1955
6.	जवाहरलाल नेहरू	1955
7.	गोविन्द बल्लभ पन्त	1957
8.	डा॰ डी॰के॰ कर्वे	1958
9.	डा॰ विधानचंद्र राय	1961
10.	पुरुषोत्तम दास टंडन	1961
11.	डा॰ राजेन्द्र प्रसाद	1962
12.	डा॰ जाकिर हुसैन	1963
13.	डा॰ पाण्डुरंग वामन काणे	1963
14.	लालबहादुर शास्त्री*	1966
15.	इन्दिरा गांधी	1971
16.	वी॰वी॰ गिरि	1975
17.	के॰ कामराज*	1976
18.	मदर टेरेसा	1980
19.	आचार्य विनोबा भावे*	1983
20.	खान अब्दुल गफ्फार खां	1987
21.	एम॰जी॰ रामचन्द्रन*	1988
22.	डा॰ बी॰आर॰ अम्बेडकर*	1990
23.	डा॰ नेल्सन मण्डेला	1990
24.	मोरारजी देसाई	1991
25.	राजीव गांधी*	1991
26.	सरदार वल्लभभाई पटेल*	1991
27.	मौ॰ अबुल कलाम आजाद*	1992
28.	जे॰आर॰डी॰ टाटा	1992
29.	सत्यजीत रे	1992
30.	गुलजारी लाल नंदा	1997
31.	अरुणा आसफ अली*	1997
32.	डा॰ ए॰पी॰जे॰ अब्दुल कलाम	1998
33.	एम॰एस॰ सुब्बालक्ष्मी	1998
34.	सी॰ सुब्रह्मण्यम	1998
35.	जयप्रकाश नारायण*	1999
36.	अमर्त्य सेन	1999
37.	पंडित रविशंकर	1999
38.	गोपी नाथ बारदोलाई	1999
39.	लता मंगेशकर	2001
40.	बिस्मिल्ला खान	2001
41.	भीमसेन जोशी	2009
42.	सचिन तेंदुलकर	2014
43.	सीएनआर राव	2014
44.	पं. मदन मोहन मालवीय*	2015
45.	अटल बिहारी वाजपेयी	2015

* मरणोपरांत

पद्म विभूषण

यह अलंकरण सभी क्षेत्रों में उल्लेखनीय योगदान के लिए दिया जाता है। सरकारी सेवाओं में लगे व्यक्ति भी इसके पात्र माने जाते हैं।

पद्म भूषण

सभी क्षेत्रों में उल्लेखनीय योगदान के लिए यह उपाधि प्रदान की जाती है। सरकारी सेवाओं में रत व्यक्ति भी इसे पाने के हकदार हैं।

पद्म श्री

विविध क्षेत्रों में उत्तम कार्य करने के उपलक्ष्य में यह उपाधि प्रदान की जाती है। सरकारी सेवा में लगे लोगों को भी इस उपाधि से अलंकृत किया जा सकता है।

शौर्य पदक

परमवीर चक्र

शत्रु के समक्ष दृढ़ता से वीरता-प्रदर्शन के फलस्वरूप दिया जाने वाला यह सबसे बड़ा पुरस्कार है। यह अत्यन्त वीरतापूर्ण कार्य जल, थल तथा नभ में से किसी भी सेना के कर्मचारी द्वारा किये जाने पर दिया जाता है।

महावीर चक्र

यह दूसरा सर्वोच्च पदक है जो शत्रु के समक्ष अद्वितीय शौर्य प्रदर्शन के फलस्वरूप प्रदान किया जाता है। इस प्रकार का वीरतापूर्ण कार्य थल, जल एवं नभ सेनाओं में से किसी के भी द्वारा किया गया हो सकता है।

वीर चक्र

यह तीसरी श्रेणी का सेना पदक है जो शत्रु के समक्ष वीरता-प्रदर्शन करने के उपलक्ष्य में प्रदान किया जाता है। यह पदक जल, थल और नभ सेना के किसी भी वर्ग के कर्मचारी को वीरतापूर्ण कार्य के लिए प्राप्त हो सकता है।

अशोक चक्र

यह ऐसा पदक है जो जल, थल और नभ कहीं पर भी उत्कृष्ट वीरतापूर्ण कार्य करने अथवा आत्म-बलिदान होने के फलस्वरूप प्रदान किया जाता है। लेकिन इस प्रकार का काम शत्रु के समक्ष होना आवश्यक नहीं। गुणों के आधार पर इस पदक के तीन वर्ग हैं—प्रथम, द्वितीय तथा तृतीय। द्वितीय पदक का नाम कीर्ति चक्र तथा तृतीय पदक का नाम शौर्य चक्र है।

अन्य राष्ट्रीय पुरस्कार/सम्मान

ज्ञानपीठ पुरस्कार

यह पुरस्कार सांस्कृतिक एवं साहित्यिक संस्था 'भारतीय ज्ञानपीठ' द्वारा वर्ष 1965 से प्रदान किया जाता है। प्रत्येक वर्ष यह पुरस्कार संविधान की आठवीं अनुसूची में सम्मिलित 22 भारतीय भाषाओं में से चयनित भारतीय लेखकों को प्रदान किया जाता है। इस पुरस्कार से पुरस्कृत साहित्यकार को 11 लाख रुपए नकद, एक स्मृति चिह्न, एक प्रशस्ति-पत्र तथा वाग्देवी (सरस्वती) की प्रतिमा प्रदान की जाती है।

दादा साहब फाल्के पुरस्कार

इस पुरस्कार की स्थापना भारतीय फिल्म उद्योग के संस्थापक दादा साहब फाल्के की याद में भारत सरकार के सूचना एवं प्रसारण मंत्रालय द्वारा की गई है। इस पुरस्कार की धनराशि 10 लाख रुपए है। अब तक इस पुरस्कार से सम्मानित कलाकार निम्नलिखित हैं—

पुरस्कार प्राप्तकर्ता	वर्ष
श्रीमती देविका रानी	1969
बी॰एन॰ सरकार	1970
पृथ्वीराज कपूर	1971
पंकज मलिक	1972
सुलोचना रूबीमायर	1973
बी॰ एन॰ रेड्डी	1974
धीरेन गांगुली	1975
कानन देवी	1976
नितिन बोस	1977
आर॰सी॰ बोराल	1978
सोहराब मोदी	1979
पी॰ जयराज	1980
नौशाद अली	1981
एल॰वी॰ प्रसाद	1982
दुर्गा खोटे	1983
सत्यजीत रे	1984
व्ही॰ शांताराम	1985
बी॰ नागी रेड्डी	1986
राजकपूर	1987
अशोक कुमार	1988
लता मंगेशकर	1989
ए॰ नागेश्वर राव	1990
भालजी पेंढारकर	1991
भूपेन हजारिका	1992
मजरूह सुल्तानपुरी	1993
दिलीप कुमार	1994
डॉ॰ राजकुमार	1995

पुरस्कार प्राप्तकर्ता	वर्ष
शिवाजी गणेशन	1996
प्रदीप जी (कवि, गीतकार)	1997
बी॰आर॰ चोपड़ा	1998
ऋषिकेश मुखर्जी	1999
आशा भोंसले	2000
यश चोपड़ा	2001
देवानंद	2002
मृणाल सेन	2003
अडूर गोपालकृष्णन	2004
श्याम बेनेगल	2005
तपन सिन्हा	2006
मन्ना डे	2007
वी.के. मूर्ति	2008
डी. रामानायडू	2009
के. बालाचंदर	2010
सौमित्र चटर्जी	2011
प्राण	2012
गुलजार	2013
शशि कपूर	2014
मनोज कुमार	2015
के. विश्वनाथ	2016
विनोद खन्ना	2017

जमनालाल बजाज पुरस्कार

यह पुरस्कार रचनात्मक सामाजिक कार्य क्षेत्र में महत्त्वपूर्ण योगदान, ग्रामीण विकास हेतु विज्ञान एवं प्रौद्योगिकी के उपयोग तथा महिलाओं एवं बच्चों के उत्थान व कल्याण कार्यों हेतु प्रदान किया जाता है। इन पुरस्कारों के तहत 10-10 लाख की पुरस्कार राशि अब प्रदान की जाती है।

सरस्वती सम्मान

15 लाख रु॰ का यह पुरस्कार उत्कृष्ट साहित्यिक कृति पर दिया जाता है।

व्यास सम्मान

के॰ के॰ बिड़ला फाउंडेशन द्वारा स्थापित यह पुरस्कार किसी एक साहित्यिक कृति को प्रदान किया जाता है। इसके तहत एक प्रशस्ति पत्र तथा 3.5 लाख रुपये की धनराशि प्रदान की जाती है।

राजीव गांधी खेल रत्न पुरस्कार

1992 में स्थापित यह पुरस्कार भारत सरकार द्वारा खेलों में सराहनीय प्रदर्शन करने वाले खिलाड़ियों को प्रदान किया जाता है। इसमें 7.5 लाख रुपये की धनराशि, एक पदक और एक प्रशस्ति पत्र प्रदान किया जाता है।

अर्जुन पुरस्कार

1961 में स्थापित यह पुरस्कार भारत सरकार द्वारा विभिन्न खेलों में विशेष उपलब्धि प्राप्त करने वाले खिलड़ियों को प्रदान किया जाता है। इसमें अर्जुन की काँस्य प्रतिमा, प्रशस्ति पत्र तथा 5 लाख रुपये की धनराशि और समारोह परिधान प्रदान किया जाता है।

द्रोणाचार्य पुरस्कार

1985 में स्थापित यह पुरस्कार भारत सरकार द्वारा खेल प्रशिक्षकों द्वारा की गयी उत्कृष्ट सेवाओं के लिए प्रदान किया जाता है। इसमें गुरु द्रोणाचार्य की प्रतिमा, प्रशस्ति पत्र, 5 लाख रुपये तथा समारोह परिधान प्रदान किया जाता है।

अंतर्राष्ट्रीय पुरस्कार

नोबेल पुरस्कार

इस पुरस्कार का प्रवर्तन सन् 1901 में डाइनामाइट के आविष्कारक अल्फ्रेड बर्नहर्ड नोबेल (1833-1896 ई॰) द्वारा व्यक्त की गई इच्छा के परिणामस्वरूप किया गया था। नोबेल पुरस्कार प्रति वर्ष रसायन शास्त्र, भौतिकी, साहित्य, चिकित्सा, शान्ति-प्रोत्साहन और अर्थशास्त्र (अर्थशास्त्र के लिए यह पुरस्कार 1969 से दिया जाना शुरू किया गया) के क्षेत्र में दिये जाते हैं। निम्न भारतीय अब तक इस पुरस्कार से सम्मानित किए जा चुके हैं: (*i*) डॉ॰ रवीन्द्रनाथ टैगोर (1913) उनकी कृति 'गीतांजलि' के लिए, (*ii*) डा॰ सी॰ वी॰ रमन (1929) भौतिकी के लिए, (*iii*) मदर टेरेसा (1979) शान्ति के लिए, (*iv*) प्रो॰ अमर्त्य सेन (1998) अर्थशास्त्र के लिए और (*v*) कैलाश सत्यार्थी (2014) शान्ति के लिए।

रेमन मैग्सेसे पुरस्कार

एशिया महाद्वीप का सबसे बड़ा पुरस्कार फिलीपीन्स के भूतपूर्व राष्ट्रपति की स्मृति में वर्ष 1957 से प्रदान किया जाता है। इसमें एक स्वर्ण पदक तथा पचास हजार डॉलर

प्रदान किये जाते हैं। इसे एशिया का नोबेल पुरस्कार भी कहा जाता है।

शान्ति, निःशस्त्रीकरण व विकास के लिए इन्दिरा गांधी पुरस्कार

1986 में स्थापित यह पुरस्कार भारत सरकार द्वारा अन्तर्राष्ट्रीय शान्ति, निरस्त्रीकरण एवं विकास के क्षेत्र में उल्लेखनीय योगदान हेतु प्रदान किया जाता है। पुरस्कार राशि 25 लाख रुपये नगद व साथ में एक स्मृति-चिन्ह दिया जाता है।

महात्मा गांधी अन्तर्राष्ट्रीय पुरस्कार

एक करोड़ रु॰ की राशि का यह पुरस्कार भारत सरकार का सर्वोच्च असैनिक अन्तर्राष्ट्रीय पुरस्कार है जो 1995 में शुरू किया गया था। यह पुरस्कार अहिंसा के जरिए सामाजिक, आर्थिक और राजनीतिक परिवर्तन के लिए काम करने वाले व्यक्ति को दिया जाता है। वर्ष 2014 का यह पुरस्कार भारतीय अंतरिक्ष अनुसंधान संगठन (इसरो) को प्रदान किया गया है। (2015 से यह पुरस्कार किसी को नहीं दिया गया है)

मैन बुकर पुरस्कार

ब्रिटेन की संस्था बुकर मैकोनल कंपनी एंड पब्लिशर्स एसोसियेशन के द्वारा यह पुरस्कार 1969 में स्थापित हुआ। यह प्रतिवर्ष राष्ट्रमंडल देशों के किसी लेखक को अंग्रेजी भाषा की उत्कृष्ट रचना हेतु प्रदान किया जाता हैं। इसकी पुरस्कार राशि 50,000 पाउण्ड है।

ऑस्कर पुरस्कार

संयुक्त राज्य अमेरिका की 'नेशनल एकेडमी ऑफ मोशन पिक्चर आर्ट्स एण्ड साइंसेज' द्वारा फिल्म जगत का अत्यन्त प्रतिष्ठित यह पुरस्कार प्रतिवर्ष प्रदान किया जाता है।

अन्तर्राष्ट्रीय नेहरू पुरस्कार

भारत सरकार द्वारा 1964 में स्थापित यह पुरस्कार प्रत्येक वर्ष ऐसे व्यक्ति को प्रदान किया जाता है, जिसने विश्व में अन्तर्राष्ट्रीय सद्भावना और मित्रता का प्रसार करने में उल्लेखनीय भूमिका अदा की हो। वर्ष 1965 में पहला नेहरू सद्भावना पुरस्कार यू थांट (संयुक्त राष्ट्र संघ के तृतीय महासचिव) को प्रदान किया गया।

प्रमुख देशों के सर्वोच्च सम्मान

देश	सर्वोच्च सम्मान
भारत	भारत रत्न
पाकिस्तान	निशान-ए-पाकिस्तान
कुवैत	मुबारक अल कबीर पदक
सऊदी अरब	शाह अब्दुल अजीज पदक
अर्जेन्टीना	द ऑर्डर ऑफ सॉन मार्टिन
निकारागुआ	आगस्टोसीजर सैण्डिनो ऑर्डर
हंगरी	द ऑर्डर ऑफ वैनर
वियतनाम	द ऑर्डर ऑफ द गोल्डेन स्टार
ब्रिटेन	मेम्बर ऑफ ब्रिटिश एम्पायर, विक्टोरिया क्रॉस
जापान	ऑर्डर आफ मौलोवनिश सन
डेनमार्क	आर्डर ऑफ द डैने ब्रोग
फ्रांस	लेजेण्ड ऑफ ऑनर
अमेरिका	प्रेसिडेंशियल मेडल ऑफ फ्रीडम
जर्मनी	पोर ली मैरिट आयरन क्रॉस
नीदरलैण्ड्स	नीदरलैण्ड्स लॉयन

✧✧✧✧✧

सामान्य विज्ञान

विज्ञान की विविध शाखाएं

नाम	अध्ययन	नाम	अध्ययन
एरोनॉटिक्स	वैमानिकी का अध्ययन	फिलाटेली	टिकट संग्रह कला
एनाटोमी	मानव शरीर की रचना	हार्टीकल्चर	बागवानी
आर्कियोलॉजी	पुरातत्व अध्ययन	सीस्मोलॉजी	भूकंप का अध्ययन
एकॉस्टिक	ध्वनि से संबंधित अध्ययन	ऑस्टोलॉजी	हड्डियों का अध्ययन
एस्ट्रोनामी	खगोल अध्ययन	जेनेटिक्स	आनुवंशिकी का अध्ययन
एण्टोमोलॉजी	कीटाणुओं का अध्ययन	जूलॉजी	जन्तु विज्ञान
एस्ट्रोफिजिक्स	ग्रह-मंडल का अध्ययन	बायलॉजी	प्राणी विज्ञान
कैलिस्थेनिक्स	व्यायाम विद्या का अध्ययन	जिओलॉजी	भूगर्भ की बनावट का अध्ययन
क्रोनोलॉजी	ऐतिहासिक क्रम का अध्ययन	पैथॉलाजी	रोगों का अध्ययन
बॉटनी	वनस्पति का अध्ययन	फिजिक्स	भौतिक विज्ञान
केमिस्ट्री	रसायन का अध्ययन	बायोकेमिस्ट्री	प्राणी का रासायनिक अध्ययन
सेरामिक्स	चीनी के बर्तनों के निर्माण का अध्ययन	युजेनिक्स	नस्ल सुधार का अध्ययन
इकोलॉजी	जीव एवं पर्यावरण संबंधों का अध्ययन	एटिमोलॉजी	शब्द व्युत्पत्ति का अध्ययन
एन्टोमोलॉजी	कीट-पतंगों का अध्ययन		

आविष्कार और आविष्कारक

आविष्कार	आविष्कारक	देश	सन्
वायुयान	ओरविल और विलबर राइट	अमेरिका	1903
बॉल-पांइट	जॉन जे॰ लाउड	अमेरिका	1888
बैरोमीटर	इवेंजलिस्ता टौरीसेली	इटली	1644
बाईसिकिल	कर्कपैट्रिक मैकमिलन	इंग्लैंड	1839-40
बाईफोकल लेंस	बेन्जामिन फ्रैंकलिन	अमेरिका	1780
बनसेन बर्नर	आर॰ विल्हेम वोन बनसेन	जर्मनी	1855
कार (पेट्रोल)	कार्ल बेन्ज	जर्मनी	1888
सीमेंट (पोर्टलैंड)	जोसेफ एस्पडिन	इंग्लैंड	1824
सिनेमा	निकोलस और जीन लूमियर	फ्रांस	1895
क्लॉक (मैकेनिकल)	आई.सिंग और लियांग लिंग-तसान	चीन	1725
डीजल इंजन	रूडोल्फ डीजल	जर्मनी	1895
डायनेमो	हाइपोलाइट पिक्सी	फ्रांस	1832
इलैक्ट्रिक लैम्प	थॉमस अल्वा एडिसन	अमेरिका	1879
सेफ्टी पिन	वाल्टर हन्ट	अमेरिका	1849
सिलाई मशीन	बार्थलेमी थिम्मोनियर	फ्रांस	1829
जहाज (भाप)	जे॰सी॰ पेरियर	फ्रांस	1775

जहाज (टरबाइन)	होन॰ सर सी॰ पारसंस	इंग्लैंड	1894
स्लाइड रूल	विलियम ऑग्ट्रेड	इंग्लैंड	1621
भाप का इंजन	जेम्स वॉट	इंग्लैंड	1765
स्टेनलेस स्टील	हेरि ब्रियरले	इंग्लैंड	1913
समुद्री जहाज	डेविड बुशनेल	अमेरिका	1776
टैंक	सर अर्नस्ट स्विनटन	इंग्लैंड	1914
टेलीग्राफ	एम॰ लम्मोंड	फ्रांस	1787
टेलीग्राफ कोड	सैमुअल एफ॰ बी॰ मोर्स	अमेरिका	1837
टेलीफोन (परफैक्टेड)	अलेक्जैण्डर ग्राहम बेल	अमेरिका	1876
टेलीस्कोप	हेन्स लिप्परशे	नीदरलैंड्स	1608
टेलीविजन (मैकेनिकल)	जे॰एल॰ बेयर्ड	इंग्लैंड	1926
टेलीविजन (इलेक्ट्रॉनिक)	पी॰टी॰ फार्न्सवर्थ	अमेरिका	1927
थर्मामीटर	गैलिलियो गैलिली	इटली	1593
ट्रांसफार्मर	माइकल फैराडे	इंग्लैंड	1831
ट्रांजिस्टर	बरडीन, शोकले तथा ब्राट्टेन	अमेरिका	1948
टाइपराइटर	पेलेग्रिन टेर्री	इटली	1808
कपड़ा धोने की मशीन (विद्युत)	हर्ले मशीन कम्पनी	अमेरिका	1907
घड़ी	बारथोलोम्यू मैनफ्रेडी	इटली	1462

माप/तौल की इकाइयां

वॉट	बिजली की शक्ति की इकाई
ओम	विद्युत प्रतिरोध
हर्ट्ज	तरंगों की आवृत्ति
डाइन	बल की सापेक्ष इकाई
कैलोरी	ऊष्मा की इकाई
कूलम्ब	विद्युत की मात्रा
एम्पियर	विद्युत धारा
नॉट	समुद्र पोतों की गति
बार	वायुमंडलीय दाब की इकाई
डेसीबल	सापेक्ष ध्वनि की तीव्रता
एंगस्ट्रम	प्रकाश तरंगों की लम्बाई
कैरेट	बहुमूल्य पत्थर की तौल
फैदम	समुद्र की गहराई की इकाई
न्यूटन	बल
कैन्डला	ज्योति तीव्रता
प्रकाश वर्ष	आकाश के ग्रहों आदि की दूरी की इकाई

चिकित्सा विज्ञान संबंधी आविष्कार

रफ-बैटिन	इन्सुलिन (डायबिटीज के उपचार के लिए)
ब्रह्मचारी यू.एन.	काल-ज्वर बुखार की चिकित्सा
डॉ. क्रिश्चियन बर्नार्ड	हृदय प्रत्यारोपण
जी. डोमाग	सल्फा ड्रग्स
राबर्ट कोच	हैजे का टीका
डॉ. पाल मुलर	डी.डी.टी.
आइजकमेन	बेरी-बेरी की चिकित्सा
आर्थर बर्ग तथा जेम्स वाटसन	आर.एन.ए.
जेम्स वाटसन तथा क्रिक	डी.एन.ए.
ड्रेसर	एस्प्रिन
रेबी	क्लोरोक्वीन (कुनैन)
हरगोविन्द खुराना	कृत्रिम जीन
फिनले	टेरामाइसिन
ल्यूवेनहॉक	बैक्टीरिया
रोबर्थ	टायफायड के जीवाणु
रीड	पीले बुखार की चिकित्सा
फिन्सेन	अल्ट्रा वायलेट रेंज द्वारा चिकित्सा
पाल एरिक	सिफलिस की चिकित्सा
सर अलेक्जेंडर फ्लेमिंग और फ्लोरे	पेन्सिलिन
विलियम हार्वे	रक्त परिवहन (संचरण)
कार्ल लैंडस्टीनर	रक्त-आधान

हैनीमेन	होम्योपैथी की स्थापना
फंक	विटामिन
मैकुलन	विटामिन 'ए'
मैकुलन	विटामिन 'बी'
यूजोक्ट होल्कट	विटामिन 'सी'
एफ.जी. हॉपकिन्स	विटामिन 'डी'
एडवर्ड जेनर	चेचक का टीका
राबर्ट कोच	टी.बी. की चिकित्सा
लेनेक	स्टेथॉस्कोप
लार्डजोसेफ लिस्टर	एण्टीसेप्टिक द्वारा चिकित्सा
लुई पाश्चर	हाइड्रोफोबिया की चिकित्सा
डॉ. रोनेल्ड रॉस	मलेरिया की चिकित्सा
डॉ. जोन्स इ. साल्क	एण्टी पोलियो वैक्सीन
सर जेम्स हैरीसन	क्लोरोफार्म की खोज
वैक्समैन	स्ट्रेप्टोमाइसिन
हैनीमेन	होम्योपैथी

विटामिन की कमी से होने वाले रोग

विटामिन	रोग	स्रोत
विटामिन A	रतौंधी	गाजर, दूध, अंडा
विटामिन B_{12}	अरक्तता	कलेजी, अंडा
विटामिन B_1	बेरी-बेरी	दाल, अंडा, मूंगफली
विटामिन C	स्कर्वी	संतरा, टमाटर
विटामिन B_2	मुँह की त्वचा	कलेजी, दूध, मांस
विटामिन D	सूखा रोग	सूर्य का प्रकाश,
विटामिन B_6	एनीमिया और होंठ फटना	कलेजी, दूध, मांस मछली का तेल
विटामिन E	बांझपन	हरी सब्जियाँ, दूध, कलेजी
विटामिन B_7	पेलाग्रा	मछली, अंडा
विटामिन K	रक्त का थक्का जमने में कमी	हरी सब्जी

प्रमुख बीमारियों द्वारा प्रभावित अंग

बीमारी	प्रभावित अंग
निमोनिया	फेफड़े
टायफाइड	आँत
डिप्थीरिया	श्वसन नलिका
सिफलिस	जनन अंग
मेनिनजाइटिस	मस्तिष्क
आर्थ्राइटिस	जोड़ों की सूजन
एग्जीमा	चमड़ी
पीलिया	यकृत
अतिसार	आँत का अग्रभाग
सुजाक, श्वेत प्रदर	मूत्र मार्ग
प्लूरिसी	छाती
पायरिया	दाँत तथा मसूड़े
गठिया या ट्यूमैटिज्म	जोड़ों में
टिटनेस	तंत्रिका तंत्र, मांसपेशी
कुष्ठ	त्वचा, तंत्रिकाएं
हैजा	आँत, आहार नाल
रिकेट्स	हड्डियाँ
गोइटर (गण्डमाला)	थाइराइड ग्रंथि
काली खाँसी	श्वसन तंत्र
बॉट्यूलिज्म	तंत्रिका-तंत्र
एड्स	सम्पूर्ण शरीर
प्लेग	फेफड़े, लाल रक्त कणिकाएं
रेबीज या हाइड्रोफोबिया	तंत्रिका तंत्र
खसरा	सम्पूर्ण शरीर
कालाजार	रुधिर, प्लीहा व अस्थि मज्जा
हरपीस	त्वचा, श्लेष्मकला
क्षय रोग	शरीर का कोई भी अंग, विशेषकर फेफड़े
केटेरेक्ट, ग्लाइकोमा, ट्रेकोमा, मायोपिया	आँख
चेचक	सम्पूर्ण शरीर, विशेषकर चेहरा तथा हाथ-पैर

प्रमुख पाचक एन्जाइम एवं उनके कार्य

पाचक एन्जाइम	स्रोत	कार्य
टाइलिन	लार ग्रन्थि	स्टार्च का माल्टोस में परिवर्तन
एमाइलेज	लार ग्रन्थि, अग्न्याशय	पॉलीसैकेराइड का डाइसैकेराइड में परिवर्तन
पेप्सिन	आमाशय	प्रोटीन को पेप्टाइड खण्डों में तोड़ना
ट्रिप्सिन एवं काइमोट्रिप्सिन	अग्न्याशय	प्रोटीन एवं पॉलीपेप्टाइड को पेप्टाइड खण्डों में तोड़ना
लाइपेस	अग्न्याशय	ट्राइग्लिसराइड को वसीय अम्ल एवं मोनोग्लिसराइड में तोड़ना

मानव शरीर से सम्बन्धित महत्वपूर्ण तथ्य

तथ्य	स्थिति/मात्र
अस्थियों की कुल संख्या	206
सबसे छोटी अस्थि	स्टेपीज (मध्य कर्ण में)
सबसे लम्बी अस्थि	फीमर (जंघा में)
कशेरुकाओं की कुल संख्या	33
पेशियों की कुल संख्या	+639
सबसे लम्बी पेशी	सारटोरियस
बड़ी आँत की लम्बाई	1.5 मी (4.9 फीट)
छोटी आँत की लम्बाई	6.25 मी (20 फीट)
यकृत का भार (पुरुष में)	1.4-1.8 किग्रा
यकृत का भार (महिला में)	1.2-1.4 किग्रा
सबसे बड़ी ग्रन्थि	यकृत
सर्वाधिक पुनरुद्भवन की क्षमता	यकृत में
सबसे कम पुनरुद्भवन की क्षमता	मस्तिष्क में
शरीर का सबसे कठोर भाग	दाँत का इनेमल
सबसे बड़ी लार ग्रन्थि	पैरोटिड ग्रन्थि
शरीर का सामान्य तापमान	98.4°F (37°C)
शरीर में रुधिर की मात्रा	5.5 ली
हीमोग्लोबिन की औसत मात्रा (पुरुष में)	13.16 g/dl
हीमोग्लोबिन की औसत मात्रा (महिला में)	11.5-14 g/dl
श्वेत रुधिर कोशिकाओं (WBCs) की संख्या	5000-10000/cu mm
सबसे छोटी श्वेत रुधिर कोशिका	लिम्फोसाइट
सबसे बड़ी श्वेत रुधिर कोशिका	मोनोसाइट कोशिका
श्वेत रुधिर कोशिकाओं का जीवनकाल	120 दिन
लाल रुधिर कोशिकाओं (RBCs) का जीवनकाल	2-5 दिन
रुधिर का थक्का बनने का समय	3-6 मिनट
सर्वग्राही रुधिर वर्ग	AB
सर्वदाता रुधिर वर्ग	O
सामान्य रुधिर दाब	120/80 Hg
वयस्क में हृदय गति	72 बार प्रति मिनट

श्वसन अंग और उसके उदाहरण

श्वसन अंग	उदाहरण
फेफड़े	मनुष्य, मेंढक, पक्षी, छिपकली, पशु इत्यादि
त्वचा	मेंढक, केंचुआ
गिल्स	टैडपोल, मछली प्रॉन
श्वसन नाल	कीट
शरीर सतह	अमीबा, युग्लीना

जन्तु विज्ञान से सम्बन्धित महत्वपूर्ण तथ्य

विशेषता — नाम

- सबसे बड़ी स्तनी–**नीली व्हेल**
- सबसे विशाल स्थलीय स्तनी–**हाथी**
- सबसे बड़ी अस्थि–**फीमर (जंघा में)**
- सबसे बड़ा अण्डा–**शतुरमुर्ग**
- सबसे बड़ा शिरा–**इन्फीरियर वेना केवा**
- सबसे बड़ा स्थलीय पक्षी–**शतुरमुर्ग**
- विशालतम जीवित सरीसृप–**टर्टिल**
- विश्व में सबसे विषैला सर्प–**ऑस्ट्रेलिया का पेनिन्सुलर टाइगर सर्प**
- सबसे लम्बा स्तनी–**जिराफ**
- सबसे छोटी चिड़िया–**हमिंग बर्ड**
- दाँत रहित स्तनी–**चींटीखोर**
- शरीर का सबसे व्यस्त अंग–**यकृत**
- शरीर का सबसे भारी अंग–**यकृत**
- सबसे भारी कशेरुका–**लुम्बर**
- सबसे मजबूत पेशी–**जबड़े की पेशी**
- सबसे पुराना प्राइमेट–**लीमर**
- सबसे पुरानी स्तनी–***एकिडना***
- सबसे पुराना कपि–**गिब्बन**
- सबसे विषैला भारतीय सर्प–**किंग कोबरा**
- विषैली छिपकली–***हीलोडर्मा***
- विषैली मछली–**स्टोन मछली**
- अण्डा देने वाली स्तनी–***एकिडना,* डक बिल्ड प्लेटीपस**
- सबसे छोटा स्तनी–**छछुँदर**
- सबसे तेज दौड़ने वाला जन्तु–**चीता**
- सबसे बड़ा सर्प–**पाइथन**
- घोंसला बनाने वाला साँप–**किंग कोबरा**

✧✧✧✧✧

वस्तुनिष्ठ प्रश्नोत्तर

1. मोहनजोदड़ो और हड़प्पा के प्राचीन नगर अब कहाँस्थित हैं?
A. भारत में
B. पाकिस्तान में
C. बांग्लादेश में
D. तिब्बत में

2. सिन्धु सभ्यता से प्राप्त मुहरें निम्नलिखित में से किससे बनी थीं?
A. लाजवर्द
B. कांस्य
C. रजत
D. स्टेटाइट

3. निम्नलिखित में से कौन-सा वेद गद्य एवं पद्य में रचित है?
A. ऋग्वेद
B. यजुर्वेद
C. सामवेद
D. अथर्ववेद

4. ऋग्वैदिककालीन आर्यों के युद्ध के देवता कौन थे?
A. मंगल
B. इन्द्र
C. रुद्र
D. शिव

5. महावीर स्वामी को किस स्थान पर ज्ञान प्राप्त हुआ?
A. ऋजुपालिका नदी के तट पर
B. पुनपुन नदी के तट पर
C. गंगा नदी के तट पर
D. कोसी नदी के तट पर

6. अशोक के अभिलेखों को पढ़ने का प्रथम श्रेय प्राप्त है–
A. विल्किन्स को
B. विलियम जोन्स को
C. जेम्स विलियम को
D. जेम्स प्रिंसेप को

7. किसने भारत में सर्वप्रथम स्वर्ण सिक्के को चलाया था?
A. कुषाण
B. मौर्य
C. हिन्द यवन
D. गुप्त

8. गुप्तकाल में प्रमुख गणितज्ञ एवं खगोलशास्त्री था–
A. वराहमिहिर
B. आर्यभट्ट
C. रामानुजाचार्य
D. उपर्युक्त सभी

9. निम्नलिखित का काल क्रम है–
1. हल्दीघाटी युद्ध
2. बैरम खाँ का पतन
3. असीरगढ़ की विजय
4. अबुल फजल की हत्या

A. 1, 2, 3, 4
B. 3, 2, 4, 1
C. 1, 4, 2, 3
D. 2, 4, 3, 1

10. विदेशी आक्रमणकारियों को ऐतिहासिक क्रम में लिखिए–
1. मुहम्मद-बिन-कासिम
2. मुहम्मद गोरी
3. महमूद गजनवी
4. चंगेज खाँ

A. 1, 3, 4, 2
B. 4, 3, 2, 1
C. 1, 3, 2, 4
D. 4, 2, 3, 1

11. किस शासक के दरबार में सर्वाधिक हिन्दू पदाधिकारी थे?
A. अकबर
B. शाहजहाँ
C. जहाँगीर
D. औरंगजेब

12. किस शासक ने सिंचाई कर लगाया था?
A. मुहम्मद तुगलक
B. फिरोज तुगलक
C. अलाउद्दीन खिलजी
D. सिकन्दर लोदी

13. कबीर की मृत्यु किस स्थान पर हुई?
A. प्रयाग
B. काशी
C. मगहर
D. मथुरा

14. अंग्रेजों ने सर्वप्रथम अपना व्यापारिक कारखाना लगाया था–
A. मुम्बई में
B. हुगली में
C. सूरत में
D. बंगलौर में

15. भारतीय राष्ट्रीय कांग्रेस के प्रथम मुस्लिम अध्यक्ष थे–
A. बदरुद्दीन तैयबजी
B. मौलाना अबुल कलाम आजाद
C. सर सैयद अहमद खाँ
D. मो. जिन्ना

16. ऑल इण्डिया ट्रेड यूनियन के प्रथम अध्यक्ष थे–
A. लाला लाजपत राय
B. एम.एन. जोशी
C. स्वामी सदानन्द
D. बाल गंगाधर तिलक

17. भारत में सर्वप्रथम टेलीग्राफ व्यवस्था प्रारम्भ हुई थी–
A. 1850 में
B. 1853 में
C. 1854 में
D. 1856 में

18. असहयोग आन्दोलन वापस ले लिया गया था–
A. रौलट एक्ट के बाद
B. प्रथम विश्व युद्ध के बाद
C. जलियाँवाला बाग हत्याकाण्ड के बाद
D. चौरी-चौरा घटना के बाद

19. क्रिप्स मिशन को किसने 'उत्तर तिथिय चैक' की संज्ञा दी?
A. महात्मा गांधी B. पं. जवाहर लाल नेहरू
C. राजेन्द्र प्रसाद D. मोतीलाल नेहरू

20. थियोसोफिकल सोसाइटी का अन्तर्राष्ट्रीय मुख्यालय है–
A. अड्यार B. सैनफ्रांसिस्को
C. न्यूयार्क D. जेनेवा

21. सत्यशोधक समाज की स्थापना किसने की थी?
A. गोपाल कृष्ण गोखले B. महादेव गोविन्द रानाडे
C. ज्योतिबा फूले D. गोपाल हरि देशमुख

22. तैमूर ने किसके शासनकाल में भारत पर आक्रमण कियाथा?
A. बलबन
B. इल्तुतमिश
C. फिरोजशाह तुगलक
D. नासिरुद्दीन महमूदशाह तुगलक

23. समुद्रगुप्त ने अपने दक्षिण अभियान में किस वेंगी शासक को हराया था?
A. नंदी वर्मन B. हस्ती वर्मन
C. देव वर्मन D. नीरू वर्मन

24. मुहम्मद-बिन-तुगलक द्वारा अपनाया गया सांकेतिक मुद्रा किस धातु का बना हुआ था?
A. कांसा B. पीतल और तांबा
C. चाँदी D. लोहा

25. अकबर के शासन काल में मुगल सेना का सेनापति कौन था?
A. राजा मान सिंह B. टोडरमल
C. भगवंत दास D. फकीर अजीउद्दीन

26. इनमें से दिल्ली के सिंहासन पर बैठने वाला पहला अफगान शासक कौन था?
A. सिकन्दर लोदी B. शेरशाह
C. बहलोल लोदी D. इनमें से कोई नहीं

27. महमूद गवाँ का सम्बन्ध निम्नलिखित में किस दक्षिण राज्य से था?
A. बीजापुर B. वारंगल
C. काकतीय D. बहमनी

28. राष्ट्रीय कांग्रेस ने किस वर्ष ''पूर्ण स्वराज्य'' का प्रस्ताव पारित किया?
A. 1929 में B. 1916 में
C. 1924 में D. 1930 में

29. कांग्रेस तथा मुस्लिम लीग के बीच लखनऊ समझौता कब हुआ था?
A. 1906 में B. 1916 में
C. 1924 में D. 1929 में

30. सुभाष चन्द्र बोस के राजनीतिक गुरु कौन थे?
A. चित्तरंजन दास B. अरविन्द घोष
C. महात्मा गांधी D. बाल गंगाधर तिलक

31. पाकिस्तान के प्रथम प्रधानमंत्री कौन थे?
A. मुहम्मद अली जिन्ना
B. लियाकत अली खाँ
C. फीरोज खाँ नून
D. मौलाना मुहम्मद अली

32. भारतीय स्वतंत्रता के समय ब्रिटेन का प्रधानमंत्री कौन था?
A. लॉर्ड एटली B. विंस्टन चर्चिल
C. रैम्से मैक्डोनाल्ड D. रॉबर्ट वॉलपोल

33. 15 अगस्त, 1947 से 26 जनवरी, 1950 तक भारत का राजनीतिक दर्जा क्या था?
A. ब्रिटिश उपनिवेश
B. ब्रिटिश न्यास क्षेत्र
C. ब्रिटिश संरक्षण प्रदेश
D. ब्रिटिश राष्ट्रमंडल का एक अधिराज्य

34. किस वायसराय ने 1878 में भारतीय भाषाओं के समाचार-पत्रों पर अंकुश लगाया था?
A. लॉर्ड रिपन B. लॉर्ड नार्थबुक
C. लॉर्ड लिटन D. लॉर्ड एलगिन

35. निम्नलिखित में से किस अधिवेशन में राष्ट्रीय कांग्रेस के नरम एवं गरम दलों का पुनः विलय हो गया?
A. लाहौर (1929) B. पुणे (1917)
C. लखनऊ (1916) D. मद्रास (1915)

36. मुस्लिम लीग द्वारा ''प्रत्यक्ष कार्यवाही दिवस'' कब मनाया गया था?
A. 24 मार्च, 1946 B. 30 मार्च, 1946
C. 17 जून, 1946 D. 16 अगस्त, 1946

37. सिन्धु घाटी सभ्यता के लोग किस धातु से परिचित नहीं थे?
A. लोहा B. चाँदी
C. ताँबा D. सोना

38. सिन्धु घाटी सभ्यता का वह नगर कौन-सा है जहाँ बृहत् स्नानागार (Great Bath) के अवशेष मिले हैं?

A. लोथल B. मोहनजोदड़ो
C. कालीबंगा D. हड़प्पा

39. विक्रम संवत् कब-से प्रारम्भ हुआ?

A. 38 ई.पू. B. 58 ई.पू.
C. 78 ई.पू. D. 87 ई.पू.

40. पंचमार्क सिक्के सर्वाधिक रूप से किस धातु के बने थे?

A. सोना B. चाँदी
C. ताँबा D. काँच

41. निम्नलिखित में से कौन-सा ग्रह सबसे कम समय में सूर्य का चक्कर लगाता है?

A. शुक्र B. बुध
C. पृथ्वी D. शनि

42. पृथ्वी के अलावा किस आकाशीय पिंड पर जीवन की सम्भावना है, क्योंकि वहाँ का पर्यावरण जीवन के लिए अनुकूल है–

A. बृहस्पति
B. मंगल
C. यूरोपा-बृहस्पति का चन्द्रमा
D. चन्द्रमा-पृथ्वी का चन्द्रमा

43. दो ग्रह जिनके उपग्रह नहीं हैं, वे हैं–

A. पृथ्वी एवं बृहस्पति B. बुध एवं शुक्र
C. बुध एवं शनि D. शुक्र एवं मंगल

44. मानक समय क्या होता है?

A. किसी देशान्तर का सूर्य के अनुसार समय
B. ग्रीनविच औसत का समय
C. देश के लगभग बीच से गुजरने वाले देशान्तर का स्थानीय समय
D. उपर्युक्त में से कोई नहीं

45. रात और दिन होने की प्रक्रिया में कौन-सा तथ्य सही है?

A. पृथ्वी का अक्ष का 66½° अंश का झुका होना
B. पृथ्वी का सूर्य के चारों ओर परिक्रमण
C. पृथ्वी का अपनी (अक्ष) धुरी पर घूमना
D. उपर्युक्त में से कोई नहीं

46. ओजोन पर्त अवस्थित है–

A. क्षोभमंडल में B. क्षोभसीमा में
C. समतापमंडल में D. प्रकाशमंडल में

47. विली-विली है–

A. एक प्रकार का वृक्ष जो शीतोष्ण कटिबंध में उगता है
B. एक प्रकार की हवा जो मरुस्थल में चलती है
C. उत्तर-पश्चिम आस्ट्रेलिया का उष्णकटिबंधीय चक्रवात
D. लक्षद्वीप समूह के निकट सामान्यतः पाई जाने वाली मछली का एक प्रकार

48. चावल की खेती के लिए आदर्श जलवायु परिस्थितियाँ हैं–

A. 100 सेमी. से ऊपर वर्षा और 25°C से ऊपर ताप
B. फसल की पूरी अवधि के लिए ठण्डी और नम जलवायु
C. 100 सेमी. से कम वर्षा व 25°C से कम ताप
D. पूरी फसल अवधि में कुछ गरम और शुष्क जलवायु

49. सदाबहार वर्षा वन पाए जाते हैं–

A. आस्ट्रेलिया में B. ब्राजील में
C. कनाडा में D. फ्रांस में

50. सूची-I तथा सूची-II को सुमेलित कीजिए तथा सूचियों के नीचे दिए गए कूट का प्रयोग कर सही उत्तर चुनिए–

सूची-I (अग्रणी उत्पादक देश)	**सूची-II (पदार्थ)**
(*a*) चीन	1. प्राकृतिक रबड़
(*b*) भारत	2. दूध
(*c*) सउदी अरब	3. लौह-अयस्क
(*d*) थाइलैण्ड	4. पेट्रोलियम

कूट :

	(*a*)	(*b*)	(*c*)	(*d*)
A.	1	2	3	4
B.	4	3	2	1
C.	3	2	4	1
D.	2	3	1	4

51. किस घास के मैदान में वृक्ष नहीं पाए जाते हैं?

A. लैनॉस B. पम्पास
C. सवाना D. स्टेपी

52. माओरी जनजाति का निवास स्थान है–

A. इंग्लैण्ड B. न्यूजीलैण्ड
C. ग्रीनलैण्ड D. आयरलैण्ड

53. क्षेत्रफल की दृष्टि से भारत का सबसे बड़ा राज्य है–

A. बिहार B. पंजाब
C. राजस्थान D. उत्तर प्रदेश

54. पश्चिमी घाटों के मालाबार तट पर स्थित माहे निम्नलिखित में से किसका भाग है?
A. केरल B. महाराष्ट्र
C. पुदुचेरी D. तमिलनाडु

55. निम्नलिखित में से कहाँ प्राचीन चट्टानें पाई जाती हैं?
A. अरावली B. हिमालय
C. शिवालिक D. उपर्युक्त सभी

56. भारत में 'मरुस्थल की राजधानी' किसे कहते हैं?
A. उदयपुर B. जैसलमेर
C. जयपुर D. पालामऊ

57. 'मानसून प्रस्फोट' से क्या तात्पर्य है?
A. वर्षा की कृत्रिम वैज्ञानिक प्रक्रिया
B. आकाश में बादलों का गलत सघन रूप में आच्छादित होना
C. मेघाच्छन्न मौसम, जिसमें एक लम्बे समय तक वर्षा होती रहे
D. मानसून के समय विद्युत चमकने, बादल गरजने के साथ तीव्र मूसलाधार वर्षा

58. भारत में उगाई जाने वाली अधिकतर कॉफी की किस्म है–
A. ओल्ड चिक्स B. कुर्गुस
C. अरेबिका D. केन्ट्स

59. सूची-I को सूची-II से सुमेलित कीजिए तथा सूचियों के नीचे दिए गए कूट का प्रयोग कर सही उत्तर चुनिए–

सूची-I	**सूची-II**
(*a*) कोयम्बटूर	1. तेलशोधन
(*b*) राउरकेला	2. रेल डिब्बा
(*c*) कपूरथला	3. लौह-इस्पात
(*d*) बरौनी	4. सूती वस्त्र

कूट :

	(*a*)	(*b*)	(*c*)	(*d*)
A.	4	3	2	1
B.	1	2	3	4
C.	2	3	4	1
D.	4	2	3	1

60. 'दचिगाम अभयारण्य' भारत के किस राज्य में है?
A. जम्मू कश्मीर
B. महाराष्ट्र
C. हिमाचल प्रदेश
D. उत्तराखण्ड

61. सड़कों की कुल लम्बाई का सर्वाधिक हिस्सा निम्नलिखित में से किस प्रांत में है?
A. पंजाब B. महाराष्ट्र
C. उत्तर प्रदेश D. बिहार

62. भारत का सुदूर दक्षिण-बिन्दु कौन है?
A. कन्याकुमारी
B. लक्षद्वीप
C. रामेश्वरम्
D. ग्रेट निकोबार स्थित इंदिरा प्वाइंट

63. 'हजार झीलों की भूमि' किसे कहा जाता है?
A. स्वीडन B. फिनलैण्ड
C. डेनमार्क D. फ्रांस

64. नागार्जुन सागर बाँध किस नदी पर बनाया गया है?
A. कृष्णा (आन्ध्र प्रदेश) B. गोदावरी (महाराष्ट्र)
C. कृष्णा (कर्नाटक) D. गोदावरी (गुजरात)

65. निम्नलिखित में से किस प्रदेश में काली मिट्टी वाले क्षेत्र में सबसे अधिक खेती होती है?
A. बिहार B. उत्तर प्रदेश
C. महाराष्ट्र D. गुजरात

66. भू-वैज्ञानिकों की दृष्टि में भारत में सबसे पुरानी पर्वतमालाएँ कौन-सी हैं?
A. विन्ध्य B. सतपुड़ा
C. हिमालय D. अरावली

67. निम्नलिखित में से कौन-सी नदी समुद्र में नहीं मिलती है?
A. गंगा B. यमुना
C. नर्मदा D. गोदावरी

68. मानसून निवर्तन से अधिकतम वर्षा कहाँ पर होती है?
A. मुम्बई B. चेन्नई
C. दिल्ली D. कोलकाता

69. प्राचीन भारतीयों को वर्मा (म्यांमार) किस नाम से ज्ञात था?
A. सुवर्णभूमि B. सुवर्णद्वीप
C. यवद्वीप D. मलयमण्डलम्

70. विश्व का सबसे खारापन किस झील में है?
A. चाड झील (नाइजीरिया)
B. बैकाल झील (रूस)
C. वॉन झील (टर्की)
D. ग्रेट बियर झील (कनाडा)

71. चाय की खेती निम्नलिखित में से किसका उदाहरण है?
A. बृहत् (Extensive) कृषि
B. सघन (Intensive) कृषि
C. जीविकोपार्जन (Subsistence) कृषि
D. रोपण (Plantation) कृषि

72. मानचित्र में समुद्र तल से समान ऊँचाई वाले स्थानों को दर्शाने वाली रेखाओं को कहते हैं–
A. आइसोनेफ B. कंटूर रेखा
C. आइसोबार D. आइसोहेल

73. ब्राजील स्थित अमेजन बेसिन के वन कहलाते हैं–
A. पम्पास B. सेल्वास
C. कैम्पोस D. लानोस

74. किस महासागर में द्वीपों की संख्या सर्वाधिक है?
A. प्रशान्त महासागर में
B. हिन्द महासागर में
C. उत्तरी अटलाण्टिक महासागर में
D. दक्षिण अटलाण्टिक महासागर में

75. लूनी नदी किस राज्य में प्रवाहित होती है?
A. महाराष्ट्र B. बिहार
C. पंजाब D. राजस्थान

76. सम दिवारात्रि (Equinox) कब होता है?
A. 21 जून
B. 22 दिसम्बर
C. 21 मार्च एवं 22 सितम्बर
D. 21 जून एवं 22 दिसम्बर

77. दक्षिणी अमरीका के वृक्ष रहित घास के मैदान को क्या कहते हैं?
A. पम्पास B. डाउन्स
C. प्रेयरीज D. लानोस

78. मिट्‌टी का वैज्ञानिक एवं क्रमबद्ध अध्ययन कहलाता है–
A. विश्व रचना विज्ञान B. भौतिक भूगोल
C. मृत्तिका विज्ञान D. इनमें से कोई नहीं

79. गोबी रेगिस्तान कहाँ है?
A. पश्चिमी अफ्रीका में B. दक्षिणी अमरीका में
C. दक्षिणी आस्ट्रेलिया में D. मंगोलिया में

80. सौरमण्डल का सबसे बड़ा उपग्रह कौन-सा है?
A. टाइटन (बृहस्पति) B. गनिमेड (बृहस्पति)
C. मिरांडा (यूरेनस) D. ओबेरॉन (यूरेनस)

81. भारत की संविधान सभा का प्रथम अधिवेशन कब शुरूहुआ?
A. 10 जून, 1946 B. 9 दिसम्बर, 1946
C. 19 दिसम्बर, 1947 D. 30 जून, 1949

82. भारतीय संविधान सभा के किस अनुच्छेद में देवनागरी लिपि में हिन्दी को भारत की राजकीय भाषा के रूप में मान्यता दी गई है?
A. अनुच्छेद 343 B. अनुच्छेद 345
C. अनुच्छेद 348 D. अनुच्छेद 347

83. भारत के संविधान में अंतर्राष्ट्रीय शान्ति और सुरक्षा की अभिवृद्धि का उल्लेख है–
A. संविधान की उद्‌देशिका में
B. राज्य की नीति के निर्देशक तत्वों में
C. मूल कर्त्तव्यों में
D. नवीं अनुसूची में

84. सूची-I को सूची-II से सुमेलित कीजिए तथा सूचियों के नीचे दिए गए कूट का प्रयोग कर सही उत्तर चुनिए–

सूची-I	**सूची-II**
(*a*) अन्तर्राज्यीय परिषद्	1. अनुच्छेद 315
(*b*) वित्त आयोग	2. अनुच्छेद 280
(*c*) प्रशासनिक अधिकरण	3. अनुच्छेद 263
(*d*) संघ लोक सेवा आयोग	4. अनुच्छेद 323(ए)

कूट :

	(*a*)	(*b*)	(*c*)	(*d*)
A.	2	4	3	1
B.	3	2	1	4
C.	1	2	4	3
D.	3	2	4	1

85. राष्ट्रपति के उम्मीदवार के लिए क्या आवश्यक नहीं है?
A. आयु 35 वर्ष हो
B. पढ़ा-लिखा हो
C. सांसद चुने जाने की योग्यता रखता हो
D. देश का नागरिक हो

86. सर्वसम्मति से निर्वाचित भारत के राष्ट्रपति थे–
A. एस. राधाकृष्णन B. वी.वी. गिरि
C. एन. संजीवारेड्‌डी D. ज्ञानी जैल सिंह

87. संसद/विधान सभा के किसी सदस्य की सदस्यता तब समाप्त समझी जाती है, यदि वह बिना सदन को सूचित किए अनुपस्थित रहता है–
A. 60 दिन B. 90 दिन
C. 120 दिन D. 150 दिन

88. किस सभा का सभापति उसका सदस्य नहीं होता है?
A. राज्य सभा B. लोक सभा
C. विधान सभा D. विधान परिषद्

89. शिक्षा का विषय–
A. संघीय सूची में B. राज्य सूची में
C. समवर्ती सूची में है D. अवशिष्ट विषयों में है

90. सूची-I को सूची-II से सुमेलित कीजिए तथा सूचियों के नीचे दिए गए कूट का प्रयोग कर सही उत्तर चुनिए–

सूची-I (स्थापना वर्ष)	**सूची-II (राज्य)**
(*a*) 1960	1. सिक्किम
(*b*) 1962	2. गोआ
(*c*) 1975	3. महाराष्ट्र
(*d*) 1987	4. नागालैण्ड

कूट :

	(*a*)	(*b*)	(*c*)	(*d*)
A.	2	4	3	1
B.	3	4	1	2
C.	4	3	1	2
D.	3	4	2	1

91. प्रथम पंचायती राजव्यवस्था का उद्‌घाटन पं. जवाहर लाल नेहरू द्वारा 2 अक्टूबर, 1959 को किया गया था–
A. साबरमती में B. वर्धा में
C. नागौर में D. सीकर में

92. निम्नलिखित विधेयकों में से किसी एक का भारतीय संसद के दोनों सदनों द्वारा अलग-अलग विशेष बहुमत से पारित होना आवश्यक है?
A. साधारण विधेयक
B. धन विधेयक
C. वित्त विधेयक
D. संविधान संशोधन विधेयक

93. भाषा के आधार पर राज्यों के गठन हेतु राज्य पुनर्गठन आयोग की स्थापना कब की गई थी?
A. 1856 B. 1956
C. 1957 D. 1960

94. पंचायतों के निर्वाचन में चुनाव लड़ने के लिए उम्मीदवार की न्यूनतम आयु कितनी होनी चाहिए?
A. 21 वर्ष B. 18 वर्ष
C. 25 वर्ष D. 30 वर्ष

95. भारतीय संविधान के किस अनुच्छेद के तहत् जीवन रक्षा तथा व्यक्तिगत स्वतंत्रता का प्रावधान है?
A. अनुच्छेद 20 B. अनुच्छेद 21
C. अनुच्छेद 22 D. अनुच्छेद 23

96. संविधान निर्माण का कार्य पूरा करके संविधान सभा ने संविधान को कब स्वीकार किया?
A. 15 अगस्त, 1947 को B. 26 जनवरी, 1950 को
C. 26 नवम्बर, 1949 को D. 24 जनवरी, 1950 को

97. निम्नलिखित में से किस संविधान संशोधन के अनुसार राष्ट्रपति निर्वाचन के निर्वाचक मण्डल में पांडिचेरी तथा दिल्ली विधान सभा के निर्वाचित सदस्यों को भी रखागया है?
A. 71वाँ B. 42वाँ
C. 73वाँ D. इनमें से कोई नहीं

98. भारतीय संविधान के किस भाग को उसकी 'आत्मा' की संज्ञा दी जाती है?
A. मौलिक अधिकारों को
B. राज्य के नीति-निर्देशक सिद्धान्तों को
C. संविधान की प्रस्तावना को
D. अनुसूचियों को

99. भारत की संचित निधि से धन का व्यय निम्नलिखित में से किस माध्यम से किया जा सकता है?
A. संसद की अनुमति से
B. योजना आयोग की अनुमति से
C. भारत के नियंत्रक एवं महालेखा परीक्षक की अनुमति से
D. राष्ट्रपति की अनुमति से

100. योजना आयोग की स्थापना हुई थी–
A. 26 नवम्बर, 1950 B. 15 जून, 1950
C. 15 मार्च, 1950 D. 15 जनवरी, 1950

101. भारत में संविधान के किस अनुच्छेद में अस्पृश्यता समाप्त की गई है?
A. अनुच्छेद 42 B. अनुच्छेद 15
C. अनुच्छेद 14 D. अनुच्छेद 17

102. वह रिट, जो भारत में उच्च न्यायालय अथवा सर्वोच्च न्यायालय द्वारा किसी व्यक्ति अथवा व्यक्ति समुदाय को आदेश देती है कि वह अपना कर्त्तव्य पालन करे, है–
A. बन्दी प्रत्यक्षीकरण रिट
B. उत्प्रेक्षण रिट
C. परमादेश रिट
D. इनमें से कोई नहीं

103. संविधान में जोड़ी गई दसवीं अनुसूची किससे सम्बन्धित है?
A. मिजोरम राज्य के लिए विशेष प्रावधानों से
B. दल-बदल के आधार पर अयोग्यता सम्बन्धी प्रावधानोंसे
C. सिक्किम के स्तर से सम्बन्धित शर्तों से
D. उपर्युक्त में से किसी से नहीं

104. राज्यसभा के सदस्यों की कुल संख्या .... हो सकती है।
A. 240 B. 260
C. 241 D. 250

105. सर्वोच्च न्यायालय के न्यायाधीशों की नियुक्ति के पूर्व मुख्य न्यायाधीश से विचार-विमर्श करना राष्ट्रपति के लिए–
A. बाध्यकारी है
B. बाध्यकारी नहीं है
C. विवेक का प्रश्न है
D. संविधान इस विषय पर मौन है

106. निम्नलिखित में से कौन-सा पदाधिकारी संसद के किसी भी सदन की कार्यवाही में भाग ले सकता है?
A. भारत का मुख्य न्यायाधीश
B. भारत का महान्यायवादी (एटॉर्नी जनरल)
C. भारत का रक्षा सचिव
D. भारत का गृह सचिव

107. पंचवर्षीय योजना का अनुमोदन तथा पुनर्निरीक्षण निम्नलिखित में से किसके द्वारा किया जाता है?
A. नीति आयोग B. राष्ट्रीय विकास परिषद्
C. वित्त आयोग D. लोक सभा

108. भारतीय संविधान की कौन-सी विशेष व्यवस्था इंग्लैंड से ली गई है?
A. संसदीय प्रणाली B. संघीय प्रणाली
C. मूल अधिकार D. सर्वोच्च न्यायपालिका

109. संविधान के किस संशोधन द्वारा सम्पत्ति के अधिकार को मूल अधिकारों की श्रेणी से निकाल दिया गया है?
A. 42वें संशोधन B. 44वें संशोधन
C. 48वें संशोधन D. 24वें संशोधन

110. भारत के राष्ट्रपति की मर्जी तक निम्नलिखित में से कौन अपने पद पर रह सकता है?
A. सर्वोच्च न्यायालय के न्यायाधीश
B. चुनाव आयुक्त
C. राज्यपाल
D. लोकसभा अध्यक्ष

111. निम्न में से किसका उपयोग ऊँचाई नापने के लिए होता है?
A. बैरोमीटर B. प्लानोमीटर
C. अल्टीमीटर D. हाइड्रोमीटर

112. फ्लक्स घनता और चुम्बकीय क्षेत्र की क्षमता का अनुपात किसी माध्यम में होता है उसका–
A. चुम्बक की घनता B. ग्रहणशीलता
C. सम्बन्धित व्याकता D. पारगम्यता

113. ध्वनि तरंगें हैं–
A. अनुदैर्ध्य
B. अनुप्रस्थ
C. आंशिक लम्बवत्, आंशिक अनुदैर्ध्य
D. कभी-कभी अनुदैर्ध्य, कभी-कभी अनुप्रस्थ

114. कैमरे में किस प्रकार का लेन्स उपयोग में लाया जाता है?
A. उत्तल B. अवतल
C. वर्तुलाकार D. समान मोटाई का

115. एक स्वतंत्र रूप से लटका हुआ चुम्बक सदा ठहरता है (स्थिर होता है) वह दिशा है–
A. पूर्व-उत्तर B. उत्तर-पश्चिम
C. उत्तर-दक्षिण D. दक्षिण-पश्चिम

116. प्रकाश संश्लेषण में पौधे कौन-सी गैस का अवचूषण करते हैं?
A. CO_2 B. O_2
C. N_2 D. H_2

117. विद्युत मात्रा की इकाई है–
A. ऐम्पियर B. ओम
C. वोल्ट D. कूलॉम

118. 1 किग्रा. राशि का वजन है–
A. 1 न्यूटन B. 10 न्यूटन
C. 9.8 न्यूटन D. 9 न्यूटन

119. एक्स-रे के आविष्कारक थे–
A. आइन्स्टीन B. डब्ल्यू.एच. ब्रॅग
C. रॉन्जन D. हेनरी बेकरेल

120. नाड़ी गति द्वारा डॉक्टर ज्ञात करता है–
A. रक्तचाप B. साँस गति
C. हृदय की धड़कन D. उपर्युक्त में से कोई नहीं

121. निम्न में से कौन आवेश की इकाई नहीं है?
A. फैराडे B. फ्रैंकलीन
C. कुलम्ब D. एम्पीयर/सेकण्ड

122. मानव शरीर में क्रोमोसोम की संख्या होती है–
A. 46 B. 48
C. 49 D. 50

123. एक प्रकाशवर्ष इससे सर्वाधिक समीप है–
A. 10^8 मीटर B. 10^{12} मीटर
C. 10^{16} मीटर D. 10^{20} मीटर

124. हवाई जहाज के 'ब्लैक बॉक्स' का क्या रंग होता है?
A. काला B. लाल
C. बैंगनी D. नारंगी

125. निम्नांकित में से कौन एक कीट के शरीर से निकलास्राव है?
A. मोती B. मूँगा
C. लाख D. गोंद

126. निम्नांकित में से कौन-सी धातु किसी नगर की वायु को, जहाँ बहुत अधिक संख्या में मोटर कारें आदि हों, प्रदूषित करती है?
A. कैडमियम B. क्रोमियम
C. सीसा D. ताँबा

127. परमाणु के नाभिक में होते हैं–
A. इलेक्ट्रॉन तथा न्यूट्रॉन B. इलेक्ट्रॉन तथा प्रोट्रॉन
C. प्रोट्रॉन तथा न्यूट्रॉन D. प्रोट्रॉन तथा रेडान

128. निम्नांकित में कौन कठोरतम है?
A. सोना B. हीरा
C. लोहा D. टंगस्टन

129. शरीर के किस भाग में पित्त का निर्माण होता है?
A. यकृत B. तिल्ली
C. पित्ताशय की थैली D. पैन्क्रियाज

130. एन्जाइम मूलतः क्या है?
A. वसा B. शर्करा
C. प्रोटीन D. विटामिन

131. मानव शरीर में सबसे छोटी ग्रन्थि कौन है?
A. एड्रीनल B. थाइरॉइड
C. पैन्क्रियाज D. पिट्यूटरी

132. रेफ्रीजरेटर में थर्मोस्टेट का कार्य है–
A. तापमान को कम करना
B. हिमायन ताप को बढ़ाना
C. एक समान तापमान को बनाए रखना
D. गलनांक को घटाना

133. सूर्य की ऊर्जा उत्पन्न होती है–
A. आयनन द्वारा
B. नाभिकीय संलयन द्वारा
C. नाभिकीय विखण्डन द्वारा
D. ऑक्सीकरण द्वारा

134. द्रव क्रिस्टल प्रयुक्त होते हैं–
A. कलाई घड़ियों में B. प्रदर्शन युक्तियों में
C. पॉकेट कैलकुलेटरों में D. उपर्युक्त सभी में

135. निम्नांकित में से कौन-सा उर्वरक मृदा में सर्वाधिक अम्ल छोड़ता है?
A. यूरिया
B. अमोनियम सल्फेट
C. अमोनियम नाइट्रेट
D. कैल्सियम अमोनियम नाइट्रेट

136. खाद्य पदार्थों के संरक्षण हेतु निम्नांकित में से कौन-सा प्रयुक्त होता है?
A. सोडियम कार्बोनेट B. एसीटिलीन
C. बेंजोइक अम्ल D. सोडियम क्लोराइड

137. कृष्ण-छिद्र सिद्धान्त को प्रतिपादित किया था–
A. सी.वी. रमन ने B. एच.जे. भाभा ने
C. एस. चन्द्रशेखर ने D. हरगोविन्द खुराना ने

138. साइनोकोबालमिन है–
A. विटामिन सी B. विटामिन बी-2
C. विटामिन बी-6 D. विटामिन बी-12

139. निम्नांकित जोड़ों में किसका सुमेल है?
A. निमोनिया-फेफड़े
B. मोतिया बिन्द-थायराइड ग्रन्थि
C. पीलिया-आँख
D. मधुमेह-यकृत

140. दूध उदाहरण है–
A. एक श्लिषि का B. एक पायस का
C. एक निलम्बन का D. एक फेन का

141. भारत के राष्ट्रीय ध्वज में केसरिया, सफेद और हरे रंग की तीन–
A. आड़ी पट्टियाँ हैं
B. खड़ी पट्टियाँ हैं
C. एक दूसरे को काटती हुई पट्टियाँ हैं
D. तिरछी पट्टियाँ हैं

142. हमारे राष्ट्रीय ध्वज की लम्बाई और चौड़ाई का अनुपात–
A. 2 : 3 है
B. 3 : 4 है
C. 4 : 3 है
D. 3 : 2 है

143. भारत के राष्ट्रीय ध्वज के बीच में एक गोल चक्र है; यह चक्र–
A. तीनों रंग की पट्टियों पर है
B. केसरिया रंग की पट्टी पर है
C. सफेद रंग की पट्टी पर है
D. हरे रंग की पट्टी पर है

144. किसी भाषा को किसी राज्य की राजभाषा के रूप में अंगीकार करने का अधिकार किसे है?
A. राष्ट्रपति
B. संसद
C. राज्य विधान सभा
D. राजभाषा आयोग

145. हमारे राष्ट्रीय ध्वज में तीन पट्टियाँ हैं; उनमें सबसे नीचे वाली पट्टी किस रंग की है?
A. केसरिया
B. सफेद
C. हरे
D. इनमें से कोई नहीं

146. हमारे राष्ट्रगान 'जन-गण-मन' में कुल कितने पद हैं?
A. तीन
B. पाँच
C. चार
D. दो

147. राष्ट्रीय गीत 'वन्देमातरम्', 'आनन्दमठ' नामक ग्रंथ से लिया गया है, जिसके लेखक हैं–
A. बंकिम चन्द्र चटर्जी
B. रवीन्द्र नाथ टैगोर
C. व्योमेश चन्द्र बनर्जी
D. सुरेन्द्रनाथ बनर्जी

148. हमारे राष्ट्रीय चिन्ह में ऊपर तीन सिंह बने हैं और उनके नीचे देवनागरी लिपि में 'सत्यमेव जयते' लिखा है। यह 'सत्यमेव जयते' कहाँ से उद्धृत किया गया है?
A. भगवद्गीता से
B. मुण्डक उपनिषद से
C. ऋग्वेद से
D. स्कन्द पुराण से

149. भारत का राष्ट्रीय पंचांग–
A. शक् संवत् पर आधारित है
B. हिजरी संवत् पर आधारित है
C. विक्रमी संवत् पर आधारित है
D. विक्रमांक-चालुक्य संवत् पर आधारित है

150. भारत का राष्ट्रीय पशु है–
A. गाय
B. हाथी
C. अश्व
D. बाघ

151. होमगार्ड का गठन कब हुआ था?
A. 1972
B. 1962
C. 1968
D. 1965

152. स्थल सेना के निम्नलिखित पदों में सबसे छोटा कौन-सा है?
A. लेफ्टीनेंट
B. ब्रिगेडियर
C. कर्नल
D. कैप्टन

153. प्रादेशिक सेना का गठन कब हुआ था?
A. 1949
B. 1957
C. 1962
D. 1972

154. प्रादेशिक सेना में भर्ती होने के लिए क्या आयु होनी चाहिए?
A. 21 से 30 वर्ष
B. 21 से 35 वर्ष
C. 18 से 35 वर्ष
D. 20 से 35 वर्ष

155. एन.सी.सी. में कितने डिवीजन हैं?
A. चार
B. पांच
C. तीन
D. दो

156. एयरफोर्स अकादमी कहां है?
A. बेलगाम
B. कोयम्बटूर
C. हैदराबाद
D. सिकन्दराबाद

157. असम राइफल्स का मुख्यालय कहाँ है?
A. इंफाल
B. आइजोल
C. दिसपुर
D. शिलांग

158. हर साल 7 दिसम्बर को भारत में मनाया जाता है–
A. वायु सेना दिवस
B. झंडा दिवस
C. नौसेना दिवस
D. कोस्ट गार्ड दिवस

159. भारत में नौसेना दिवस किस दिन मनाया जाता है?
A. 8 अक्टूबर
B. 15 जनवरी
C. 21 दिसम्बर
D. 7 दिसम्बर

160. भारत की सेना के प्रथम भारतीय सेनापति थे–
A. जनरल के.एम. करियप्पा
B. फील्ड मार्शल मानेकशा
C. जनरल राजेन्द्र सिंह
D. उपरोक्त में से कोई भी नहीं

161. वीटो का अधिकार–
A. संयुक्त राष्ट्र के सभी सदस्यों को प्राप्त है
B. सुरक्षा परिषद् के सभी सदस्यों को प्राप्त है
C. सुरक्षा परिषद् के सभी स्थायी सदस्यों को प्राप्त है
D. सुरक्षा परिषद् के सभी अस्थायी सदस्यों को प्राप्त है

162. संयुक्त राष्ट्र संघ का मुख्यालय कहाँ है–
A. वाशिंगटन B. न्यूयार्क
C. बोस्टन D. शिकागो

163. संयुक्त राष्ट्र संघ का ध्वज किस रंग का है?
A. हल्के नीले रंग का
B. हल्के गुलाबी रंग का
C. गहरे केसरिया रंग का
D. आधा हल्के रंग का और आधा केसरिया रंग का

164. संयुक्त राष्ट्र संघ की बैठकों में आमतौर से काम-काज किस भाषा में होता है?
A. अंग्रेजी
B. रूसी
C. फ्रेंच
D. अंग्रेजी और फ्रेंच

165. अंतर्राष्ट्रीय न्यायालय का मुख्यालय कहाँ है?
A. हेग B. जेनेवा
C. रोम D. बर्न

166. राष्ट्रमंडल के सदस्य वे देश हैं, जो–
A. ब्रिटेन के अधीन हैं
B. ब्रिटेन से आर्थिक सहायता पाते हैं
C. पहले ब्रिटेन के अधीन थे किन्तु अब स्वाधीन हैं
D. ब्रिटेन से अस्त्र-शस्त्र प्राप्त करते हैं

167. सार्क (दक्षिण एशियाई सहयोग संगठन) में कितने देश सदस्य हैं?
A. पांच B. छः
C. आठ D. सात

168. निम्नलिखित देशों में से कौन-सा देश सार्क (SAARC) का सदस्य नहीं है?
A. भारत B. पाकिस्तान
C. बांग्लादेश D. म्यांमार

169. गुट निरपेक्ष आन्दोलन कब शुरू हुआ था?
A. 1955 में B. 1961 में
C. 1983 में D. 1976 में

170. गुट निरपेक्ष आन्दोलन के सदस्य देश–
A. शक्तिशाली देशों के गुटों से दूर रहते हैं
B. परस्पर एक-दूसरे की रक्षा के लिए वचनबद्ध हैं
C. एक दूसरे को सैनिक सहायता देते हैं
D. एक सैनिक संधि के सदस्य हैं

171. जमनालाल बजाज पुरस्कार किस क्षेत्र में सराहनीय योगदान के लिए प्रदान किया जाता है?
A. शांति व निःशस्त्रीकरण B. कृषि
C. रचनात्मक कार्य D. साहित्य

172. भारत वर्ष में प्रथम रमन मैग्सेसे पुरस्कार विजेता कौन था?
A. सी.डी. देशमुख B. जय प्रकाश नारायण
C. डॉ. वर्गीज कुरियन D. आचार्य विनोबा भावे

173. भारतीय ज्ञानपीठ पुरस्कार किसे प्रदान किया जाता है?
A. उत्कृष्ट हिन्दी कविता के लिए
B. भारतीय साहित्य में उत्कृष्ट योगदान के लिए
C. हिन्दी साहित्य में उत्कृष्ट योगदान के लिए
D. भारतीय दर्शन की उत्कृष्ट समीक्षा के लिए

174. अध्यापकों के लिए राष्ट्रीय पुरस्कारों की घोषणा कब की जाती है?
A. 14 नवम्बर B. 5 सितम्बर
C. 30 जनवरी D. 26 जनवरी

175. निम्नलिखित में से किस विषय पर नोबेल पुरस्कार नहीं दिया जाता है?
A. चिकित्सा B. गणित
C. अर्थशास्त्र D. रसायन शास्त्र

176. बुकर पुरस्कार किस क्षेत्र में प्रदान किया जाता है?
A. कल्पना साहित्य लेखन
B. औषधि
C. साहस के कार्य
D. विज्ञान

177. हर गोविन्द खुराना को नोबेल पुरस्कार किस क्षेत्र में योगदान के लिए मिला था?
A. चिकित्सा शास्त्र B. भौतिक शास्त्र
C. अर्थशास्त्र D. शांति

178. सर्वोच्च शौर्य पुरस्कार 'परमवीर चक्र' के प्रथम विजेता कौन थे?
A. मेजर ध्यान सिंह B. के. गुरुवचन सिंह
C. मेजर शैतान सिंह D. मेजर सोमनाथ शर्मा

179. धन्वन्तरि पुरस्कार किस क्षेत्र में विशिष्ट योगदान के लिए दिया जाता है?
A. संगीत B. नृत्य
C. दर्शन D. चिकित्सा

180. कलिंग पुरस्कार किस क्षेत्र में दिया जाता है?
A. साहित्य के क्षेत्र में
B. विज्ञान के क्षेत्र में
C. सामाजिक कल्याण के लिए किए गए कार्य के लिए
D. अन्तर्राष्ट्रीय शान्ति एवं सद्भावना के लिए

181. नोबेल पुरस्कार का आरम्भ कब से हुआ?
A. सन् 1901 से B. सन् 1905 से
C. सन् 1896 से D. सन् 1934 से

182. अर्थशास्त्र के लिए नोबेल पुरस्कार कब से आरम्भ हुआ?
A. सन् 1969 ई. से
B. सन् 1939 ई. से
C. सन् 1901 ई. से
D. सन् 1935 ई. से

183. निम्नलिखित किस अफ्रीकी नेता को भारत-रत्न से सम्मानित किया गया है?
A. होस्नी मुबारक B. जोमो केन्योटा
C. अनवर सादात D. नेल्सन मंडेला

184. विज्ञान को सर्वसुलभ व सर्वोपयोगी बनाने में सर्वाधिक योगदान देने वाले व्यक्ति को भारतीय नाम वाले किस अन्तर्राष्ट्रीय पुरस्कार से सम्मानित किया जाता है?
A. कालिंजर पुरस्कार
B. कलिंग पुरस्कार
C. मानवता पुरस्कार
D. ऐसा कोई पुरस्कार नहीं है

185. नेहरू पुरस्कार कौन-सी संस्था प्रदान करती है?
A. इंडियन कौंसिल ऑफ कल्चरल रिलेशन्स
B. इंडो-सोवियत कल्चरल सोसाइटी
C. भारतीय राष्ट्रीय कांग्रेस
D. भारतीय ज्ञानपीठ

186. वीरता का सर्वोच्च सम्मानसूचक पदक जो शत्रु के सामने असीम शौर्य और अदम्य साहस दिखाने या आत्म-बलिदान करने पर भेंट किया जाता है, उसका क्या नाम है?
A. चक्रव्यूह B. अशोक चक्र
C. महावीर चक्र D. परमवीर चक्र

187. प्रथम मरणोपरान्त 'भारत-रत्न' अलंकरण किसे प्रदान किया गया था?
A. के. कामराज नाडार B. आचार्य विनोबा भावे
C. लाल बहादुर शास्त्री D. एम.जी. रामचन्द्रन

188. निम्नलिखित में से कौन-सा पुरस्कार केवल एशियावासियों को दिया जाता है?
A. नेहरू सद्भावना पुरस्कार
B. पुलित्जर पुरस्कार
C. इन्दिरा गांधी शान्ति पुरस्कार
D. मैग्सेसे पुरस्कार

189. अर्जुन पुरस्कार कब से प्रारम्भ हुए?
A. 1961 ई. से B. 1962 ई. से
C. 1963 ई. से D. 1964 ई. से

190. ऑस्कर अवॉर्ड जीतने वाले पहले भारतीय थे–
A. नरगिस दत्त B. शशि कपूर
C. सत्यजीत रे D. भानु अथैया

191. अपर कट शब्द किस खेल में प्रयोग किया जाता है?
A. टेनिस B. वॉलीबॉल
C. क्रिकेट D. बॉक्सिंग

192. निम्नलिखित में से कौन-सा कप/ट्रॉफी फुटबॉल से सम्बन्धित नहीं है?
A. मर्डेका कप B. डूरण्ड कप
C. सन्तोष ट्रॉफी D. दिलीप ट्रॉफी

193. फिनिस शब्द का प्रयोग किस खेल में होता है?
A. शतरंज B. ब्रिज
C. बिलियर्ड्स D. रग्बी

194. एक दिवसीय क्रिकेट तथा टेस्ट मैंचों में सर्वाधिक रन बनाने का रिकॉर्ड किसके नाम है?
A. सौरभ गांगुली B. सचिन तेन्दुलकर
C. डॉन ब्रैडमैन D. ब्रायन लारा

195. निम्नलिखित में से कौन-सी अन्तर्राष्ट्रीय टेनिस खेल प्रतियोगिता घास के मैदान पर खेली जाती है?
A. यू.एस. ओपन B. फ्रेंच ओपन
C. विम्बलडन D. ऑस्ट्रेलियाई ओपन

196. 'विम्बलडन ट्रॉफी' का सम्बन्ध किस खेल से है?
A. पोलो (इंग्लैंड) से B. समुद्री दौड़ से
C. घुड़दौड़ से D. टेनिस से

197. निम्नलिखित में से किस पदक का सम्बन्ध हॉकी से नहीं है?
A. आगा खां कप B. वर्दवान ट्रॉफी
C. ध्यानचन्द ट्रॉफी D. बम्बई गोल्ड कप

198. 'रिवर्स स्विंग' एवं 'बीमर' नामक शब्दावलियां किस खेल से संबंधित हैं?
A. नौकायन B. क्रिकेट
C. फुटबॉल D. हॉकी

199. निम्नलिखित में से किस ट्रॉफी का सम्बन्ध हॉकी से है?
A. सिन्धिया गोल्ड कप B. संतोष ट्रॉफी
C. रोहिंगटन बेरिया ट्रॉफी D. सुब्रतो मुखर्जी ट्रॉफी

200. 'ज्यूल्स रिमेट ट्रॉफी का सम्बन्ध किस खेल से है?
A. फुटबॉल (विश्व) से B. गोल्फ से
C. हॉकी (भारत) से D. लॉन टेनिस (विश्व) से

201. 'मर्डेका' का सम्बन्ध किस खेल से है?
A. फुटबाल (विश्व) से
B. फुटबाल (भारत) से
C. फुटबाल (एशिया) से
D. क्रिकेट (आस्ट्रेलिया-इंग्लैंड) से

202. प्रथम ओलम्पिक खेल ओलम्पिया (ग्रीस) में कब खेले गए थे?
A. 233 ई.पू. में B. 1500 ई.पू. में
C. 500 ई.पू. में D. 776 ई.पू. में

203. 394 ई. में रोम के बाद एक सम्राट ने ओलम्पिक खेलों को बंद कर दिया था। इसको पुनः किसने शुरू किया?
A. मि. स्पोर्ट्समैन ने
B. बैरन पीयरे डी कोबर्टिन ने
C. जनरल फ्रेंको ने
D. अब्राहम लिंकन ने

204. सर्वप्रथम आधुनिक ओलिम्पिक ध्वज कब फहराया गया?
A. 1896 में B. 1908 में
C. 1920 में D. 1924 में

205. ग्रैंड स्लेम निम्नलिखित में से किस खेल से सम्बन्धित है?
A. फुटबॉल B. टेनिस
C. हॉकी D. पोलो

206. प्रथम आधुनिक ओलम्पिक खेल कब और कहां खेले गए?
A. रोम, 1894 ई. में B. मैड्रिड, 1840 ई. में
C. लिस्बन, 1800 ई. में D. एथेन्स, 1896 ई. में

207. जापान का राष्ट्रीय खेल क्या है?
A. हाराकीरी B. जूडो
C. निप्पोन D. टोजो

208. भारत में खेल सम्बन्धी दो राष्ट्रीय इंस्टीट्यूट हैं। एक नेताजी सुभाष बोस के नाम से पटियाला में है, दूसरा किसके नाम से ग्वालियर में है?
A. राणा प्रताप B. पृथ्वीराज चौहान
C. शिवाजी D. रानी लक्ष्मीबाई

209. सबसे बड़े मैदान में खेला जाने वाला खेल कौन-सा है?
A. हॉकी B. क्रिकेट
C. पोलो D. कबड्डी

210. लॉन टेनिस जाल की ऊँचाई कितनी होती है?
A. 2 फुट 6 इंच B. 3 फुट 6 इंच
C. 4 फुट D. 2 फुट 2 इंच

211. 'ए सूटेबल ब्वाय' पुस्तक का लेखक कौन है?
A. खुशवंत सिंह B. अरुण शोरी
C. विक्रम सेठ D. उपरोक्त में से कोई नहीं

212. 'कैन्टरबरी टेल्स' पुस्तक का लेखक कौन है?
A. ज्योफरी चासर B. लियो टॉलस्टाय
C. गुन्नार मिर्डल D. विलियम शेक्सपियर

213. निम्नलिखित में से कौन-सी पुस्तक प्रेमचन्द द्वारा रचित नहीं है?
A. गोदान B. गबन
C. प्रेम पचीसी D. आनंदमठ

214. बांग्लादेश की लेखिका तस्लीमा नसरीन को किस पुस्तक से ख्याति मिली?
A. शर्म B. लज्जा
C. नारी स्वातंत्र्य D. अबला

215. 'पावर्टी एण्ड अन-ब्रिटिश रूल इन इण्डिया' का लेखक कौन है?
A. लाला लाजपत राय
B. लाला हरदयाल
C. विनायक दामोदर सावरकर
D. दादाभाई नौरोजी

216. 'मुद्राराक्षस' ग्रंथ का लेखक कौन है?
A. विशाखदत्त B. कालिदास
C. भारवि D. माघ

217. 'माई प्रेसिडेंशल ईयर्स' पुस्तक का लेखक कौन है?
A. ज्ञानी जैल सिंह B. वी.वी. गिरि
C. आर. बेंकटरमन D. डॉ. शंकर दयाल शर्मा

218. 'जय सोमनाथ' किसकी कृति है?
A. के.एम. मुंशी B. वृन्दावन लाल वर्मा
C. अमृत लाल नागर D. मदन मोहन मालवीय

219. वर्शिपिंग फाल्स गॉड्स पुस्तक के लेखक हैं–
A. विक्रम सेठ B. अरुण शौरी
C. सलमान रुश्दी D. खुशवन्त सिंह

220. निम्नलिखित पुस्तकों में से कौन-सी पुस्तक सलमान रुश्दी की है?
A. दि वर्ल्ड ऑफ फतवाज
B. दि मूर्स लास्ट साई
C. दि अदर हॉफ
D. फूल्स पैराडाइज

221. मार्ग्रेट थैचर द्वारा रचित पुस्तक है–
A. लांग वॉक टु फ्रीडम B. दि पाथ टु पावर
C. इमेज एंड इमेजिनेशन D. 10 डाउनिंग स्ट्रीट

222. 'फ्रीडम एट मिडनाइट' के लेखक कौन हैं?
A. जवाहरलाल नेहरू तथा डॉ. राजेन्द्र प्रसाद
B. एम.ओ. मथाई तथा फ्रैंक मोरेस
C. मैक्सिम गोर्की तथा दोस्तोवस्की
D. लैरी कॉलिन्स और डोमिनिक लापियर

223. 'अंकल टॉम्स केबिन' के लेखक का क्या नाम है?
A. एच.बी. स्टोव B. एडम स्मिथ
C. टॉल्स्टॉय D. थामस मूर

224. 'वार एण्ड पीस' और 'अन्ना कैरेनिना' दोनों एक ही अन्तर्राष्ट्रीय ख्याति प्राप्त लेखक की कृतियाँ हैं; उस लेखक का क्या नाम है?
A. ओलीवर गोल्डस्मिथ B. श्वेतलाना
C. लुई ब्रोमफील्ड D. लियो टाल्स्टॉय

225. बोरिस पास्तरनाक ने एक बहुत ही विवादास्पद पुस्तक लिखी थी। उस पुस्तक का क्या नाम है?
A. डॉन क्विक्जोट B. फॉस्ट
C. डॉक्टर्स डिलेमा D. डॉ. जिवागो

226. 'दास कैपिटल' के लेखक कौन हैं?
A. शेक्सपियर B. कौटिल्य
C. कर्नल जॉन हण्ट D. कार्ल मार्क्स

227. 'मदर' के लेखक का क्या नाम है?
A. मैक्सिम गोर्की B. पर्ल एस. बक
C. कैथराइन मेयो D. टी.एस. इलियट

228. 'कलम का सिपाही' में किसकी जीवनी प्रस्तुत की गई है?
A. शरतचन्द्र B. प्रेमचन्द
C. राहुल सांकृत्यायन D. जोश मलीहाबादी

229. 'झण्डा ऊँचा रहे हमारा' गीत किस कवि की रचना है?
A. श्यामलाल गुप्त 'पार्षद' B. मैथिलीशरण गुप्त
C. सोहनलाल द्विवेदी D. रामधारी सिंह 'दिनकर'

230. 'आइने अकबरी' का लेखक कौन था?
A. इब्न बतूता B. अकबर
C. अबुल फजल D. अकबर मुरादाबादी

231. कम्प्यूटर–
A. एक उपकरण है जो गणितीय और तार्किक संक्रियायें सम्पन्न करता है
B. एक उपकरण है, जो केवल गणितीय संक्रियायें सम्पन्न करता है
C. एक स्मृति उपकरण है
D. एक गणना उपकरण है

232. 'PC' का अर्थ है–
A. प्राइवेट कम्प्यूटर B. पर्सनल कल्कुलेटर
C. पर्सनल कम्प्यूटर D. प्रोफेसनल कम्प्यूटर

233. 'बाइनरी अंक प्रणाली' में अधिकतम अंक (digit) कितने होते हैं?
A. 1 B. 10
C. 2 D. 4

234. निम्नलिखित में से कौन-सा 'इनपुट' उपकरण है?
A. मॉनीटर B. प्रिंटर
C. प्लॉटर D. माउस

235. CPU का पूरा नाम है–
A. सेन्ट्रल प्रोग्रामिंग यूनिट
B. सेन्ट्रल प्रोसेसिंग यूनिट
C. सेन्ट्रल प्रोग्रामिंग अण्डरस्टैंडिंग
D. सेन्ट्रल प्रोसेसिंग अण्डरस्टैंडिंग

236. गणना हेतु प्रयोग में लाया गया पहला उपकरण था
A. ENIAC B. ABACUS
C. एनालिटिकल इंजन D. EDSAC

237. ABACUS का प्रयोग कब शुरू हुआ था?
A. 250 ई. B. 450 ई.पू.
C. 1200 ई.पू. D. 1200 ई.

238. किस अंग्रेज को 'कम्प्यूटर का जनक' कहा जाता है?
A. ब्लेज पास्कल B. लेबनित्ज
C. चार्ल्स बैबेज D. जे.पी. एकर्ट

239. निम्नलिखित में से कौन-सी कम्प्यूटर की सेकेण्डरी मेमोरी है?
A. RAM B. ROM
C. रजिस्टर्स D. फ्लॉपी

240. निम्नलिखित में से कौन पैकेज नहीं है?
A. BASIC B. dBASE
C. वर्ड परफेक्ट D. पेज मेकर

241. कौन-सा बेमेल है?
A. वर्ड स्टार B. वर्ड परफेक्ट
C. DOS Editor D. विण्डो

242. डाटा के समुच्चय (Set) को क्या कहते हैं?
A. फील्ड B. रेकार्ड
C. फाइल D. इनमें से कोई नहीं

243. Keyboard है?
A. इनपुट यूनिट है
B. आउटपुट यूनिट है
C. इनपुट यूनिट और आउटपुट यूनिट दोनों हैं
D. उपरोक्त में से कोई भी नहीं है

244. प्रिंटर–
A. आउटपुट यूनिट है
B. इनपुट यूनिट है
C. उपरोक्त दोनों हैं
D. उपरोक्त में से कोई भी नहीं है

245. फ्लॉपी–
A. इनपुट यूनिट है
B. आउटपुट यूनिट है
C. इनपुट यूनिट और आउटपुट यूनिट दोनों हैं
D. उपरोक्त में से कोई भी नहीं है

246. कम्प्यूटर की विशेषताएं हैं–
1. तेज रफ्तार 2. स्वचालन
3. कार्यशीलता 4. परिवर्तनशीलता
निम्नलिखित में से कौन-सी विशेषता सही है?
A. 1 और 2 सही हैं B. 1, 2 और 4 सही हैं
C. 1, 2 और 3 सही हैं D. उपरोक्त सभी सही हैं

247. 1 बाइट बराबर है–
A. 8 बिट B. 16 बिट
C. 36 बिट D. 64 बिट

248. असंसाधित तथ्य को क्या कहा जाता है?
A. डाटम B. डाटा
C. फाइल D. फील्ड

249. कम्प्यूटर–
A. सूचना ग्रहण करता है
B. सूचना को निर्दिष्ट प्रयोजन के लिए अनुकूल बनाता है
C. परिणाम प्रदर्शित करता है
D. उपरोक्त सभी बातें सही हैं

250. डाटा क्या है–
A. संसाधित तथ्य
B. असंसाधित तथ्य
C. अंक और अक्षर
D. उपरोक्त में से कोई भी नहीं

251. 'जीने की कला' (आर्ट ऑफ लिविंग) के प्रतिपादक और प्रचारक कौन हैं?
A. महर्षि महेश योगी B. श्री श्री रवि शंकर
C. स्वामी चिन्मयानंद D. भगवान रजनीश

252. डंकन पैसेज निम्नलिखित में से किसके बीच स्थित है?
A. दक्षिणी और लिटिल अंडमान
B. उत्तरी और दक्षिणी अंडमान
C. उत्तरी और मध्य अंडमान
D. अंडमान और निकोबार

253. ₹ 2000 के नए नोट आरबीआई ने किस साल जारी किए हैं?
A. 2015 में B. 2014 में
C. 2016 में D. 2017 में

254. रासायनिक रूप से 'मिल्क ऑफ मैग्नेशिया' क्या होता है?
A. मैग्नीशियम कार्बोनेट
B. सोडियम बाइकार्बोनेट
C. कैल्सियम हाइड्रॉक्साइड
D. मैग्नीशियम हाइड्रॉक्साइड

255. वन अनुसंधान संस्थान कहाँ स्थित है?
A. देहरादून में
B. भोपाल में
C. लखनऊ में
D. दिल्ली में

256. निम्नलिखित कलाकारों और उनके कला-रूपों के मेल मिलाइए–

कलाकार	**कला-रूप**
(*a*) पन्नालाल घोष	1. चित्रकला
(*b*) पंडित भीमसेन जोशी	2. कर्नाटक संगीत (कंठ संगीत)
(*c*) अंजलि ईला मेनन	3. बाँसुरी
(*d*) मदुराई मणि अय्यर	4. हिन्दुस्तानी संगीत (कंठ संगीत)

कूट :

	(*a*)	(*b*)	(*c*)	(*d*)
A.	1	3	2	4
B.	2	1	4	3
C.	3	4	1	2
D.	4	2	3	1

257. त्वचा का रंग किसके कारण होता है?
A. एन्जाइम
B. एपीडरमिस
C. हारमोन्स
D. मेलानिन

258. किस क्षेत्र में अधिकांश मौसम सम्बन्धी गतिविधियाँ होती हैं?
A. आयनमंडल
B. क्षोभमंडल
C. समतापमंडल
D. क्षोभसीमा

259. निम्नलिखित में से वह पर्वत श्रेणी कौन-सी है जो भारत में सबसे पुरानी है?
A. हिमालय
B. विंध्याचल
C. अरावली
D. सहयाद्रि

260. निमज्जित वस्तु का पता लगाने के लिए किस उपकरण का प्रयोग किया जाता है?
A. राडार
B. सोनार
C. क्वासार
D. पल्सार

उत्तरमाला

1	**2**	**3**	**4**	**5**	**6**	**7**	**8**	**9**	**10**
B	D	B	B	A	D	C	B	A	C
11	**12**	**13**	**14**	**15**	**16**	**17**	**18**	**19**	**20**
D	B	C	C	A	A	B	D	A	A
21	**22**	**23**	**24**	**25**	**26**	**27**	**28**	**29**	**30**
C	D	B	B	C	C	D	A	B	A
31	**32**	**33**	**34**	**35**	**36**	**37**	**38**	**39**	**40**
B	A	D	C	C	D	A	B	B	B
41	**42**	**43**	**44**	**45**	**46**	**47**	**48**	**49**	**50**
B	B	B	C	C	C	C	A	B	C
51	**52**	**53**	**54**	**55**	**56**	**57**	**58**	**59**	**60**
D	B	C	C	A	B	D	C	A	A
61	**62**	**63**	**64**	**65**	**66**	**67**	**68**	**69**	**70**
B	D	B	A	C	D	B	B	A	C
71	**72**	**73**	**74**	**75**	**76**	**77**	**78**	**79**	**80**
D	B	B	A	D	C	A	C	D	B
81	**82**	**83**	**84**	**85**	**86**	**87**	**88**	**89**	**90**
B	A	B	D	B	C	A	A	C	B
91	**92**	**93**	**94**	**95**	**96**	**97**	**98**	**99**	**100**
C	D	B	A	B	C	D	C	A	C
101	**102**	**103**	**104**	**105**	**106**	**107**	**108**	**109**	**110**
D	C	B	D	A	B	B	A	B	C

111	**112**	**113**	**114**	**115**	**116**	**117**	**118**	**119**	**120**
C	B	A	A	C	A	D	C	C	C
121	**122**	**123**	**124**	**125**	**126**	**127**	**128**	**129**	**130**
D	A	C	D	C	C	C	B	A	C
131	**132**	**133**	**134**	**135**	**136**	**137**	**138**	**139**	**140**
D	C	B	D	B	C	C	D	A	B
141	**142**	**143**	**144**	**145**	**146**	**147**	**148**	**149**	**150**
A	D	C	C	C	B	A	B	A	D
151	**152**	**153**	**154**	**155**	**156**	**157**	**158**	**159**	**160**
B	A	A	C	C	C	D	B	C	A
161	**162**	**163**	**164**	**165**	**166**	**167**	**168**	**169**	**170**
C	B	A	D	A	C	C	D	B	A
171	**172**	**173**	**174**	**175**	**176**	**177**	**178**	**179**	**180**
C	D	B	B	B	A	A	D	D	B
181	**182**	**183**	**184**	**185**	**186**	**187**	**188**	**189**	**190**
A	A	D	B	A	D	C	D	A	D
191	**192**	**193**	**194**	**195**	**196**	**197**	**198**	**199**	**200**
D	D	B	B	C	D	B	B	A	A
201	**202**	**203**	**204**	**205**	**206**	**207**	**208**	**209**	**210**
C	D	B	B	B	D	B	D	C	B
211	**212**	**213**	**214**	**215**	**216**	**217**	**218**	**219**	**220**
C	A	D	B	D	A	C	A	B	B
221	**222**	**223**	**224**	**225**	**226**	**227**	**228**	**229**	**230**
B	D	A	D	D	D	A	B	A	C
231	**232**	**233**	**234**	**235**	**236**	**237**	**238**	**239**	**240**
A	C	C	D	B	B	A	C	D	A
241	**242**	**243**	**244**	**245**	**246**	**247**	**248**	**249**	**250**
D	A	A	A	C	D	A	B	D	B
251	**252**	**253**	**254**	**255**	**256**	**257**	**258**	**259**	**260**
B	A	C	D	A	C	D	B	C	B

✧✧✧✧✧

www.ingramcontent.com/pod-product-compliance
Lightning Source LLC
LaVergne TN
LVHW082027051026
849532LV00011B/3292
* 9 7 8 9 3 5 0 1 2 6 8 3 7 *